MAYO CLINIC
FAMILY HEALTH BOOK

MAYO CLINIC
FAMILY HEALTH BOOK

DAVID E. LARSON, M.D.
EDITOR-IN-CHIEF

WILLIAM MORROW AND COMPANY, INC.
NEW YORK

Mayo Clinic Family Health Book provides comprehensive health information in a single, authoritative source. *Mayo Clinic Health Letter,* our monthly, eight-page newsletter, offers the same kind of easy-to-understand, reliable information, with a special focus on timely topics. For information on how this award-winning newsletter can be delivered to your doorstep every month, call 1-800-333-9037.

Mayo Clinic Family Health Book provides reliable, practical, comprehensive, easy-to-understand information on issues relating to good health. Much of its information comes directly from the experience of Mayo's 1,100 physicians and research scientists.

The book supplements advice of your personal physician, whom you should consult for individual medical problems. *Mayo Clinic Family Health Book* does not endorse any company or product.

Library of Congress Cataloging-in-Publication Data

Mayo Clinic family health book
    p. cm.
  ISBN 0-688-07819-2
  1. Medicine Popular I. Mayo Clinic
  RC81. M473 1990
  613—dc20   90-6065
                                  CIP

Printed in the United States of America

BOOK DESIGN BY MARSHA COHEN/PARALLELOGRAM

FOREWORD

Since its beginning more than 100 years ago, Mayo Clinic has existed to offer, to both the sick and the well, comprehensive medical care of the highest standard through a coordinated and integrated group practice of medicine. Through the years, we have been privileged to serve more than 4 million individuals who have sought health care at Mayo facilities in Rochester, Minnesota; Jacksonville, Florida; and Scottsdale, Arizona. Annually, we welcome over 300,000 patients from around the world.

The goal of Mayo Clinic programs in medical education and medical research is to contribute to improved standards of medical care and a broader understanding of health and disease. Traditionally, such new knowledge has been shared with health care professionals through medical journals, textbooks, and seminars.

For Mayo, this book—a comprehensive medical guide for direct use by the public—marks a significant new step in an expanding health information program that began in 1983. All of us at Mayo hope that you will enjoy *Mayo Clinic Family Health Book* for years to come and will use it often as a source of authoritative health information.

Robert R. Waller, M.D.
Chairman of the Board
Mayo Foundation for Medical
Education and Research

EDITORIAL STAFF

PREFACE AND ACKNOWLEDGMENTS

Mayo Clinic Family Health Book is the result of the combined efforts of many members of Mayo Clinic's "extended family": the 17,000 physicians, scientists, paramedical personnel, and administrators who share a common goal. That goal is to offer each patient comprehensive medical care of the highest standard.

To achieve that goal, our founders, Dr. William J. Mayo and Dr. Charles H. Mayo, pioneered the concept of an integrated group practice. Our integrated group practice is composed of physicians who are recognized authorities in their specialty areas and who share their knowledge with each other for the benefit of our patients. This melding of medical knowledge is unified by extensive management systems and procedures.

Our medical team functions in a coordinated, noncompetitive atmosphere, supported by the most advanced equipment and by extensive programs in medical education and medical research. Together, our assembled personnel and systematic approach yield the high-quality patient care to which we are committed.

Mayo Clinic Family Health Book is an extension of our uniquely integrated medical practice. Each chapter has been carefully reviewed not only by specialists in the discipline but also by other physicians with interests and expertise in the area. In a sense, this book is a repository of the collective knowledge Mayo physicians have gained over the past century, during which we have earned an international reputation as a health care leader.

In addition to extensive review by Mayo Clinic physicians and scientists, further review and much of the actual production work was performed by members of various Mayo Clinic support sections. Medical illustrations were prepared by members of our Section of Medical Graphics. Virtually all of our medical illustrators played a role.

Research and sketches for the medical illustrations were submitted by medical illustrators Robert Benassi and Vincent Destro, who also served as consultants for all art in the book. Medical illustrator John Hagen prepared all of the finished medical illustrations, including those rendered in color in the Color Atlas of Human Anatomy, a section I am especially proud of.

All photographs included in our Photographic Guide to Common Skin Disorders came from Mayo Clinic's extensive collection of color photographs and were compiled by Dr. Sigfrid Muller and Donna Whipple, Department of Dermatology. (Patients who can be identified in these photographs gave us permission to publish their photographs.) All radiological illustrations (x-rays and imaging scans) were provided by the Mayo Clinic Department of Diagnostic Radiology and were compiled by Dr. J. William Charboneau.

Our Section of Publications provided complete manuscript preparation services, including editing, typing, cross-references (there are literally thousands of them), and proofreading. LeAnn Stee coordinated these efforts.

Joseph Kane, of our Photographic/Audiovisual Section, was principal photographer for the project. Mary Hedstrom coordinated this effort.

We did not, of course, prepare this book entirely by ourselves. The book was organized and initial drafts were prepared with the help of John Gallagher and Hugh Howard of Gallagher/Howard Associates, Inc. Our publisher is William Morrow and Company, Inc., where we were fortunate to work with Adrian Zackheim, the editor at Morrow in charge of this project. We also are grateful for the considerable help of Susan Halligan, Lisa Queen, Harvey Hoffman, Lori Ames, Nick Mazzella, Larry Norton, Deborah Weiss Geline, Karen Hansen, Pam Altschul, Will Schwalbe, Jim Landis, and Al Marchioni at Morrow. Marsha Cohen, Parallelogram Graphic Communications, prepared the design and layout. The index was done by Sydney Wolfe Cohen. The type was set by ComCom, Allentown, Pennsylvania, and the book was printed by R. R. Donnelley, Willard, Ohio.

This project was initiated after much discussion at Mayo under the direction of Dr. Glen Hartman and Rick Colvin, along with Paul Beyer and M. G. Brataas of Mayo Medical Ventures. Leadership also was provided by members of the Medical/Industry Relations Committee.

To help bring this enormous project to fruition required considerable help from my colleagues at Mayo Medical Ventures, including Lindsay Shorter, Mary Rysavy, Jo Ann Fox, and Bradley Schmidt, in addition to Nancy Skaran of our Section of Communications. Lillian Haapala provided not only superb secretarial and support skills but also the intangible assets of encouragement and attentiveness which sustained me throughout this project.

Special thanks also go to David Swanson, of Mayo Medical Ventures, for his patience, understanding, and ability to carefully craft words to make them active, understandable, and eminently useful to our readers.

Finally, a very special thanks to my wife, Julie, and children, Kirstin, Benjamin, and Jonathan. They wondered at times when this project would be completed but were always enthusiastic and supportive of the many extra hours during which much of the work for this book was done.

The following is a list of the more than 200 additional Mayo contributors to this project:

ADMINISTRATION

Jill A. Smith Beed, J.D.
Ann E. Decker, J.D.
Kathleen A. Meyerle, J.D.

Alan R. Schilmoeller
Richard C. Spavin
David J. Sperling

Stephen Q. Sponsel
Sharon A. Tennis, R.N.

ANESTHESIOLOGY
Glenn A. Fromme, M.D.

BIOCHEMISTRY AND MOLECULAR BIOLOGY

G. David Ball, Ph.D.	Paul J. Leibson, M.D.	Thomas C. Spelsberg, Ph.D.

CHAPLAIN SERVICE
Clyde J. Burmeister

DENTISTRY AND ORAL SURGERY

Ronald P. Desjardins, D.M.D.	Arnold J. Hill, Jr., D.D.S.	A. Howard Sather, D.D.S.
Joseph A. Gibilisco, D.D.S.	Bruce A. Lund, D.D.S.	Phillip J. Sheridan, D.D.S.

DERMATOLOGY

Charles H. Dicken, M.D.	Harold O. Perry, M.D.	Donna M. Whipple
Sigfrid A. Muller, M.D.	Henry W. Randle, M.D.	

FAMILY MEDICINE
John M. Wilkinson, M.D.

INTERNAL MEDICINE

Allergy

Lowell L. Henderson, M.D.	Harry A. Swedlund, M.D.	Richard G. Van Dellen, M.D.
James T. Li, M.D.		

Cardiovascular Diseases

William T. Bardsley, M.D.	David R. Holmes, Jr., M.D.	Richard J. Rodeheffer, M.D.
Robert O. Brandenburg, M.D.	Thomas E. Kottke, M.D.	Thom W. Rooke, M.D.
Gerald T. Gau, M.D.	Michael D. McGoon, M.D.	Clarence Shub, M.D.
Bernard J. Gersh, M.D.	Fletcher A. Miller, Jr., M.D.	Ray W. Squires, Ph.D.
Raymond J. Gibbons, M.D.	Jae K. Oh, M.D.	Douglas L. Wood, M.D.

Emergency Medicine
Larry F. Vukov, M.D.

Endocrinology/Metabolism

Paul C. Carpenter, M.D.	Roger L. Nelson, M.D.	Donald A. Scholz, M.D.
Clifford F. Gastineau, M.D.	P. J. Palumbo, M.D.	

Gastroenterology

William P. Baldus, M.D.	Christopher J. Gostout, M.D.	Alfred J. Schei
Alan J. Cameron, M.D.	Kenneth A. Huizenga, M.D.	Kenneth W. Schroeder, M.D.
Peter W. Carryer, M.D.	David E. Larson, M.D.	William J. Tremaine, M.D.
Albert J. Czaja, M.D.	Albert D. Newcomer, M.D.	Russell H. Wiesner, M.D.
Willard S. Gamble, M.D.		

General Internal Medicine

Darryl S. Chutka, M.D.	Frances L. McClain	Eric G. Tangalos, M.D.
Richard D. Hurt, M.D.		

Genetics

Hymie Gordon, M.D.	Virginia Michels, M.D.

Hematology

Edwin D. Bayrd, M.D.	Morie A. Gertz, M.D.	Mary Ann Morris
Dennis A. Gastineau, M.D.	Thomas M. Habermann, M.D.	William L. Nichols, M.D.

Hypertension
Gary L. Schwartz, M.D.

Infectious Diseases

Donald R. Nichols, M.D.	Alan J. Wright, M.D.

Nephrology
James T. McCarthy, M.D.

Preventive Medicine

Melvin A. Amundsen, M.D.	Michael A. Covalciuc, M.D.	Richard A. Owen, M.D.

Rheumatology

W. Leroy Griffing, M.D.	John G. Mayne, M.D.	Randall S. Vollertsen, M.D.

Thoracic Diseases

Howard A. Andersen, M.D.	James R. Jett, M.D.	Paul D. Scanlon, M.D.
W. Mark Brutinel, M.D.	Richard J. Pisani, M.D.	Bruce A. Staats, M.D.
Kathryn A. Cummings	Udaya B. S. Prakash, M.D.	Robert W. Viggiano, M.D.
Robert S. Fontana, M.D.	Jay H. Ryu, M.D.	

LABORATORY MEDICINE AND PATHOLOGY

Curtis L. Bakken, M.D.	Jurgen Ludwig, M.D.	S. Breanndan Moore, M.D.

MEDICAL GRAPHICS

Robert C. Benassi	Vincent P. Destro	John V. Hagen

MEDICAL LIBRARY
Dottie M. Hawthorne   Jean M. McDowall

NEUROLOGIC SURGERY
Chad D..Abernathey, M.D.   Dudley H. Davis, M.D.   Michael J. Ebersold, M.D.

NEUROLOGY
J. Eric Ahlskog, M.D.   Terrence L. Cascino, M.D.   Ronald C. Petersen, M.D.
J. Keith Campbell, M.D.   Bruce A. Evans, M.D.   Jerry W. Swanson, M.D.
Gregory D. Cascino, M.D.   Frank M. Howard, Jr., M.D.

NUTRITION/DIETETICS
Diane M. Huse, R.D.   Karen E. Moxness, R.D.   Jacalyn A. See, R.D.
Kathleen A. Lipari, R.D.   Jennifer K. Nelson, R.D.   N. Nicole Spelhaug, R.D.

OBSTETRICS AND GYNECOLOGY
Charles S. Field, M.D.   Edward O. Jorgensen, M.D.   Steven J. Ory, M.D.
Roger W. Harms, M.D.   George D. Malkasian, Jr., M.D. Richard E. Symmonds, M.D.

ONCOLOGY
David L. Ahmann, M.D.   John S. Kovach, M.D.   Michael J. O'Connell, M.D.
Harry F. Bisel, M.D.   Carole O. Lauger   Paula J. Schomberg, M.D.
M. Margaret Gillard   Harry J. Long, M.D.

OPHTHALMOLOGY
George B. Bartley, M.D.   George G. Hohberger, M.D.   Daniel T. Weaver, M.D.
Paul G. Belau, M.D.

ORTHOPEDICS
Peter C. Amadio, M.D.   Bernard F. Morrey, M.D.
James L. Graham, D.P.M.   Hamlet A. Peterson, M.D.   Thomas C. Shives, M.D.

OTORHINOLARYNGOLOGY
Christopher D. Bauch, Ph.D. Anna Mary Peterson   Martin S. Robinette, Ph.D.
Charles W. Beatty, M.D.

PEDIATRICS
Pediatric Allergy
Martin I. Sachs, D.O.

Pediatric Cardiology
William H. Weidman, M.D.

Community Pediatrics
Ann L. Beatty   Roy F. House, Jr., M.D.   Patricia S. Simmons, M.D.
Daniel D. Broughton, M.D.   Richard D. Olsen, M.D.
Edmund C. Burke, M.D.   Julia A. Rosekrans, M.D.

Pediatric Gastroenterology
Jean Perrault, M.D.

Pediatric Hematology/Oncology
Gerald S. Gilchrist, M.D.

Pediatric Neonatology
Fredric Kleinberg, M.D.   Robert V. Johnson, M.D.

Pediatric Nephrology
Dawn S. Milliner, M.D.

Pediatric Neurology
Sara E. Sacco, M.D.

Pediatric Rheumatology
Audrey M. Nelson, M.D.

PHOTOGRAPHY
James G. Bambenek   Mary E. Hedstrom   Carol J. Sparrow
Elman A. Hanken   Joseph M. Kane

PHYSICAL MEDICINE AND REHABILITATION
Tom R. Garrett   Steven G. Scott, D.O.   Lloyd T. Wood, M.D.
Timothy J. Madson   Gudni Thorsteinsson, M.D.

PSYCHIATRY AND PSYCHOLOGY
John E. Huxsahl, M.D.   Maurice J. Martin, M.D.   Lloyd A. Wells, M.D.
Alexander R. Lucas, M.D.   Robert M. Morse, M.D.   Donald E. Williams, Ph.D.
Lawrence M. Martin, M.D.   Wendell M. Swenson, Ph.D.

PUBLICATIONS
Virginia Dunt   Rose Ann Ptacek-Vitse   Roberta J. Schwartz
Jeanne Klein   Mary L. Schwager   LeAnn M. Stee

RADIATION SAFETY
Joel E. Gray, Ph.D.   Richard J. Vetter, Ph.D.

RADIOLOGY
Thomas H. Berquist, M.D.   Harley C. Carlson, M.D.   Glen W. Hartman, M.D.
Manuel L. Brown, M.D.   J. William Charboneau, M.D.   Michael J. Kiely, M.D.

SOCIAL SERVICE
Mary E. Ely   Ginny J. Rissmiller

SPEECH PATHOLOGY
Arnold E. Aronson, Ph.D.   Robert L. Keith   Jack E. Thomas

SURGERY
Philip E. Bernatz, M.D.   Bruce H. Kaufman, M.D.   Robert J. Spencer, M.D.
Richard M. Devine, M.D.   Peter Mucha, Jr., M.D.   John E. Woods, M.D.
John H. Donohue, M.D.   Thomas A. Orszulak, M.D.

UROLOGY
Stephen A. Kramer, M.D.   Ronald W. Lewis, M.D.   David E. Patterson, M.D.
Frank J. Leary, M.D.

To one and all, within and outside Mayo Medical Center, my sincere thanks.

David E. Larson, M.D.
Editor-in-Chief

CONTENTS

HOW TO USE THIS BOOK

Here you will find practical information about the book's organization, the content and purpose of each division, tips on how you can quickly and easily locate the information you need, and how to interpret your signs and symptoms.

PART I: LIFECYCLES

From entrance into the world to those "later years," our bodies and needs change. These introductory chapters review human growth and development and address some of the common ailments all of us may face during the course of our lives.

COLOR ATLAS OF HUMAN ANATOMY (Section A)

PART II: THE WORLD AROUND US

Look here for easy-to-understand, practical tips on first aid, preventing accidents, and treating injuries; dealing with the challenges of our environment; and staying healthy when traveling abroad.

PART III: KEEPING FIT

Maintaining or improving your health means eating right, exercising regularly, avoiding bad habits and substance abuse, and other preventive strategies.

PART IV: HUMAN DISEASE AND DISORDERS 445

If you are ill, look here to find detailed descriptions of signs and symptoms, causes, diagnosis, severity, and treatments for nearly 1,000 common and rare ailments.

PHOTOGRAPHIC GUIDE TO COMMON SKIN DISORDERS (Section B) 1154

PART V: MODERN MEDICAL CARE 1189

Here is your introduction to the complexities of modern medical practice. Also, there are chapters on understanding and coping with cancer, and on death and dying. Look for specific tips in understanding and using the numerous and sometimes perplexing health-care options available today.

APPENDICES 1279

INDEX 1331

"The object of all health education is to change the conduct of individual men, women and children by teaching them to care for their bodies well."

—C. H. Mayo, 1932

HOW TO USE THIS BOOK

This book is about answers: *Mayo Clinic Family Health Book* is designed to provide you with the kind of authoritative, comprehensive, and reliable information you need to live a healthier life.

THE ORGANIZATION

The book consists of five divisions. Parts I, II, and III address normal human growth and development, the changes to expect, and strategies for avoiding illness and dealing with habits or emergencies that can threaten your health. Parts IV and V mainly concern disease, its diagnosis, treatment, and modern medical care.

To use the book efficiently, you may find it helpful to understand in more detail how the divisions and chapters are arranged. The organization is as follows:

Part I: Lifecycles

If you are about to become a parent, or if you want to understand more about normal changes you might encounter in your children, your parents, or yourself, Part I, titled "Lifecycles," is the place to look.

Starting with the newborn, separate chapters address each stage of life, including infancy, the preschool years, school-age children, the teenage years, young adulthood, and the middle and later years.

Part II: The World Around Us

A lengthy chapter devoted to first aid anchors this section. In addition, there are chapters about safety and the environment. A closing chapter offers practical advice on special health concerns of the traveler.

Part III: Keeping Fit

Good habits are among the keys to good health. In Part III, separate chapters offer guidance on sound nutrition, exercise and fitness, care of your teeth, and controlling the stress all of us encounter in daily living. Chapters on tobacco, alcohol, medications, and drug abuse close the division.

Part IV: Human Disease and Disorders

For decades, Mayo Clinic has been a storehouse of the latest and best information on human disease and disorders. In this lengthy division we discuss individually most of the common, and many rare, health problems faced by humankind the world over. It is here that you can find detailed information about a specific ailment.

Each entry begins with a review of signs and symptoms. This is followed by a description of the disease and a discussion on how the diagnosis is made and the real or potential seriousness of the ailment. Then we provide complete information on prevention and the latest treatments—both those you can manage yourself and those for which you must secure professional help.

Part V: Modern Medical Care

The goal of Part V is to demystify the increasingly complex world of modern medicine, with chapters devoted to the organization and use of the health-care system and the modern pharmacy. There is a chapter that can help you avoid, understand, or cope with cancer, and one that addresses death and dying. We conclude with helpful advice about how you can secure home health care for yourself or for a loved one.

The Appendices

At the close of the book are appendices in which you can find explanations of many of the complex laboratory and other modern tests and procedures available; an index of commonly used generic and brand-name drugs; conversion charts for weights and measures; and a comprehensive glossary of medical, anatomical, and health-care terms.

Finding the Facts You Need

For speedy access to specific information, you will find, on the page that introduces each division, a complete listing of chapter titles included in that division. On the opening page of each chapter is a table of contents for that chapter. Throughout the book are numerous cross-references, and we end the book with a detailed index. But beyond these "tools" is an underlying rationale for the organization of this book.

Using Your Symptoms

You know when you are well: life's activities give you pleasure, whether in your work or play, the meal before you, or the joy of family and friends. There are no pains to distract you from life's satisfactions.

Equally, you know when you are ailing.

Yet, identifying the signs and symptoms of an illness, whether minor or major, is the very essence of caring for your health. For that matter, it is also at the heart of modern medical practice and of this book. A nagging ache, a regular cough, a minor or more significant change in your body's day-to-day messages to you—all are signs and symptoms, potentially meaningful pieces of information for you or your doctor.

This book is not intended to teach you to perform independent self-diagnosis. No book can be a substitute for your physician's years of medical school, clinical training, and practical experience. However, you can use this book to help you better understand your body and mind and to help you become a more active partner in your health care.

The fact is you know a great deal about your personal signs and symptoms. You live with them. If symptoms change, your doctor isn't the first to know—*you* are. Therefore, we organized *Mayo Clinic Family Health Book* to help you use signs and symptoms to recognize and better understand your health.

Because it deals with your personal health, this may be one of the most practical and valuable books in your home. We hope you will use it often and that the information in this book, complemented by the advice of your personal physician, will help you and your loved ones lead a healthier, more fulfilling life.

The Organization of an Entry

Most entries pertaining to human disease and disorders are organized in this format for quick, easy reference:

Name of disease

GINGIVITIS

Key indications

Signs and Symptoms
- Swollen, soft, red gums;
- Gums that bleed easily.

Basic description of the disease

The term "gingivitis" refers to inflammation of the gingiva or gums. It can be caused by deposits of plaque, the sticky film that forms on the exposed portion of teeth and irritates the gums.

Many people experience gingivitis first in their puberty and then at various degrees of severity throughout life. Mild forms of the disease are very common among adults. People with uncontrolled diabetes and pregnant women are particularly prone to the development of gum inflammation.

How the disorder is identified

The Diagnosis. Healthy gums are firm and pale pink. If you notice that your gums are swollen, very tender, and bleed easily, you may have gingivitis. Often, people first detect a change in their gums when they notice that the bristles of their toothbrushes are pink after brushing, a sign that their gums are bleeding even with the gentle pressure of brush bristles. Further examination usually reveals red, inflamed gums. Gingivitis often causes no direct pain or discomfort and thus is frequently overlooked.

If your gums seem swollen and red, consult your dentist. He or she will examine your gums carefully, looking for inflammation and excess deposits of plaque at the base of your teeth. As the gum margin swells, more plaque can be trapped, thus irritating the gum further.

Potential short- or long-term consequences

How Serious Is Gingivitis? Gingivitis often goes unnoticed because it usually is painless. If left unchecked, however, gingivitis can lead to periodontitis, a more serious disease that affects not only the gums but also the other supporting structures of the teeth, leading to tooth loss.

Latest information on treatment and prevention

Treatment. Your dentist will treat your gingivitis by using several techniques. The first step is a thorough cleaning of the teeth to remove the plaque and calculus (a chalky material composed of mineralized plaque, often called "tartar"). This cleaning can be uncomfortable, particularly if your gums are sensitive or if your teeth are encrusted with plaque and calculus. The removal procedure, known as "scaling," is designed to remove the deposits of bacteria, plaque, and calculus.

Sometimes the inflammation is enhanced by misaligned teeth, overhanging fillings, or poorly contoured restorations such as crowns and bridges that make plaque removal more difficult. Teeth can be straightened to minimize plaque accumulation, fillings can be replaced, and restorations can be recontoured.

PART I

LIFECYCLES

In the eight chapters that follow, you will find discussions, in chronological order, of human development. Each chapter is devoted to a specific time of life and reviews in detail the full range of concerns—medical, behavioral, developmental, and others, too—that constitute the common issues at each stage of life.

CONTENTS

COLOR ATLAS OF HUMAN ANATOMY

Your body never really sleeps. Day and night it is busy, constructing new cells, warding off illness, processing nutrients, and orchestrating a host of physical and biochemical actions, all of which contribute to your health and sense of well-being.

Within this COLOR ATLAS OF HUMAN ANATOMY you will find easy-to-understand drawings of the human body in all its wondrous grace and complexity. From your skin (your first line of defense against disease), to muscles, bones and organs (which control movement and bodily functions), to your immune system (where substances too small to be seen wage never-ending war against illness), the drawings in this atlas focus on normal human anatomy. Supporting the drawings are insets offering unique views of normal anatomy and a variety of common ailments as revealed by state-of-the-art imaging technology. In recent years, this remarkable equipment has significantly advanced the ability of physicians to diagnose illness at an early stage, when treatment often is most effective.

ATLAS CONTENTS

Epidermis

Dermis

Hypodermis
(subcutaneous
fatty tissue)

Hair Shaft

Sweat Pore

Arrector Pili
Muscle

Nerves

Hair Root

Oil (sebaceous)
Gland

Sweat Gland

YOUR SKIN

The two square yards of skin that cover your body constitutes your first line of defense against unwanted invaders, controls your body temperature, and protects vital internal organs. A single square inch of skin contains oil glands, hair roots (follicles), sweat glands, and millions of cells, as well as specialized nerve endings for sensing heat, cold, and pain.

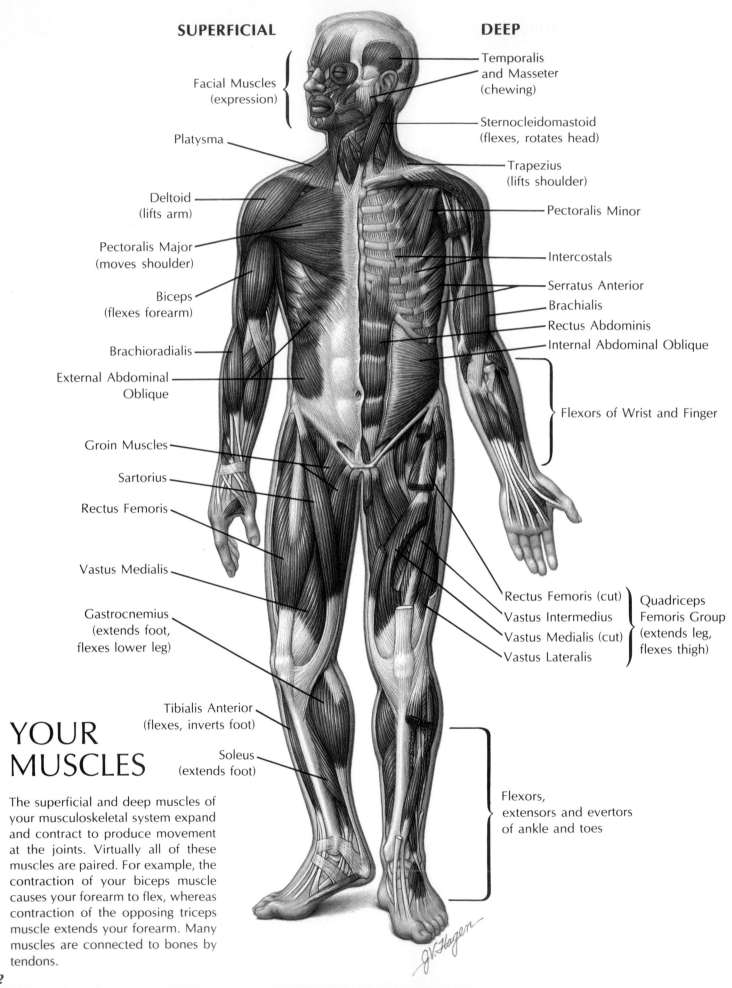

SUPERFICIAL   **DEEP**

Facial Muscles
(expression)

Temporalis
and Masseter
(chewing)

Platysma

Sternocleidomastoid
(flexes, rotates head)

Trapezius
(lifts shoulder)

Deltoid
(lifts arm)

Pectoralis Minor

Pectoralis Major
(moves shoulder)

Intercostals

Serratus Anterior

Biceps
(flexes forearm)

Brachialis

Rectus Abdominis

Brachioradialis

Internal Abdominal Oblique

External Abdominal
Oblique

Flexors of Wrist and Finger

Groin Muscles

Sartorius

Rectus Femoris

Vastus Medialis

Rectus Femoris (cut)

Quadriceps
Femoris Group
(extends leg,
flexes thigh)

Vastus Intermedius

Vastus Medialis (cut)

Vastus Lateralis

Gastrocnemius
(extends foot,
flexes lower leg)

Tibialis Anterior
(flexes, inverts foot)

YOUR
MUSCLES

Soleus
(extends foot)

Flexors,
extensors and evertors
of ankle and toes

The superficial and deep muscles of
your musculoskeletal system expand
and contract to produce movement
at the joints. Virtually all of these
muscles are paired. For example, the
contraction of your biceps muscle
causes your forearm to flex, whereas
contraction of the opposing triceps
muscle extends your forearm. Many
muscles are connected to bones by
tendons.

J.V. Hagen

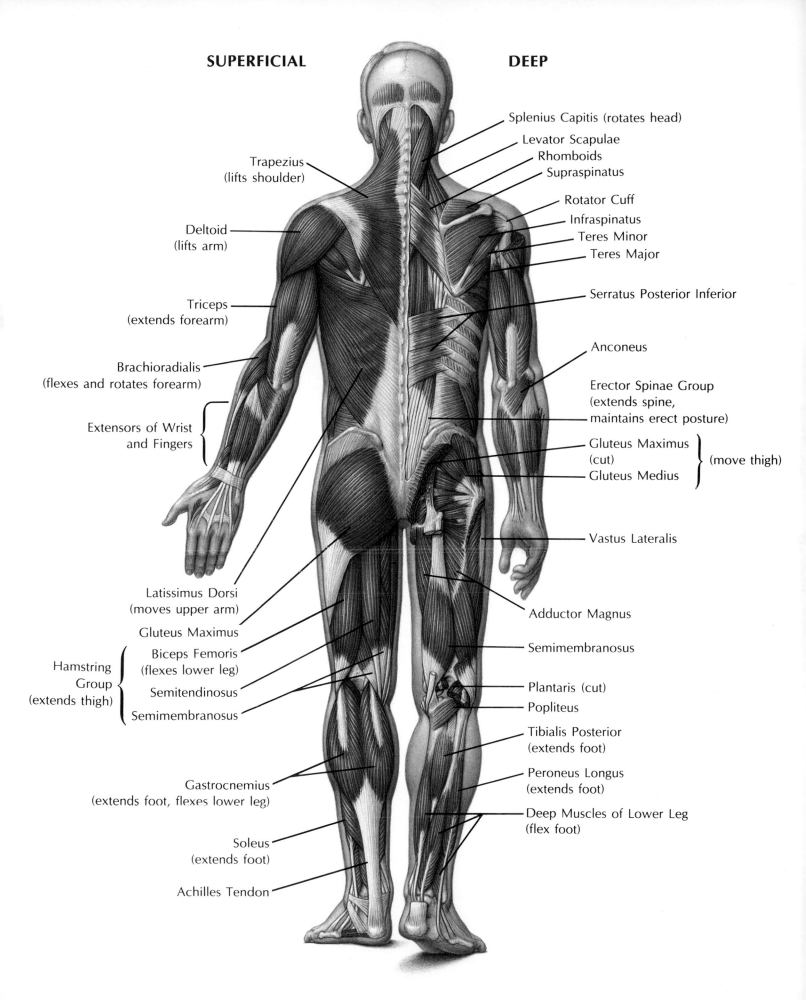

SUPERFICIAL

DEEP

Splenius Capitis (rotates head)

Levator Scapulae

Rhomboids

Supraspinatus

Trapezius
(lifts shoulder)

Rotator Cuff

Infraspinatus

Teres Minor

Teres Major

Deltoid
(lifts arm)

Serratus Posterior Inferior

Triceps
(extends forearm)

Anconeus

Brachioradialis
(flexes and rotates forearm)

Erector Spinae Group
(extends spine,
maintains erect posture)

Extensors of Wrist
and Fingers

Gluteus Maximus
(cut)

Gluteus Medius

(move thigh)

Vastus Lateralis

Latissimus Dorsi
(moves upper arm)

Adductor Magnus

Gluteus Maximus

Biceps Femoris
(flexes lower leg)

Semimembranosus

Hamstring
Group
(extends thigh)

Plantaris (cut)

Semitendinosus

Popliteus

Semimembranosus

Tibialis Posterior
(extends foot)

Peroneus Longus
(extends foot)

Gastrocnemius
(extends foot, flexes lower leg)

Deep Muscles of Lower Leg
(flex foot)

Soleus
(extends foot)

Achilles Tendon

A-3

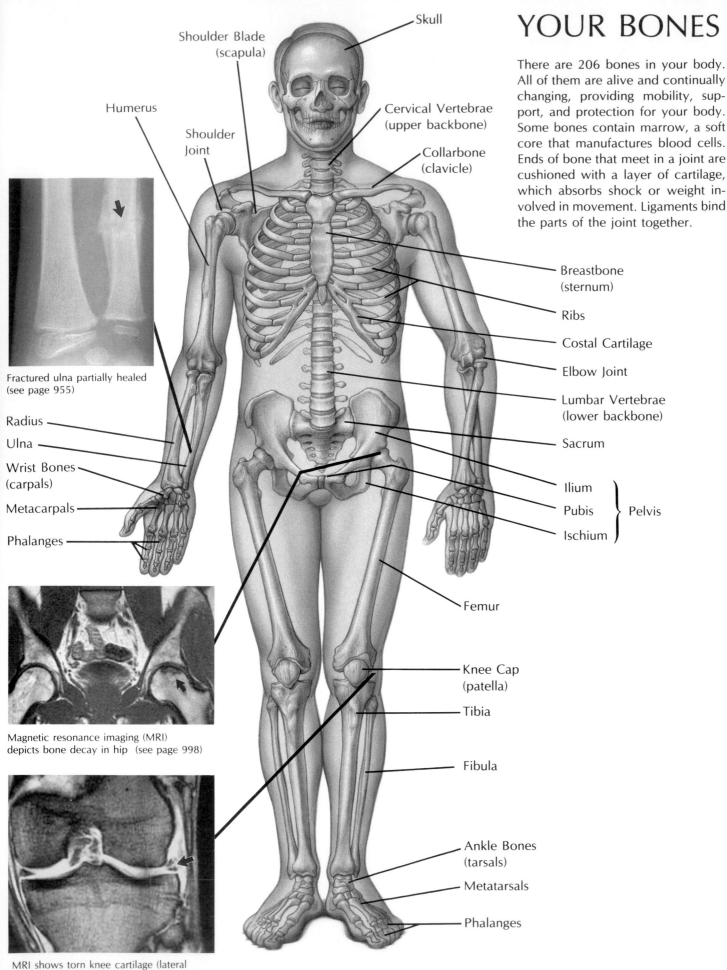

YOUR BONES

There are 206 bones in your body. All of them are alive and continually changing, providing mobility, support, and protection for your body. Some bones contain marrow, a soft core that manufactures blood cells. Ends of bone that meet in a joint are cushioned with a layer of cartilage, which absorbs shock or weight involved in movement. Ligaments bind the parts of the joint together.

Skull

Shoulder Blade (scapula)

Humerus

Shoulder Joint

Cervical Vertebrae (upper backbone)

Collarbone (clavicle)

Breastbone (sternum)

Ribs

Costal Cartilage

Elbow Joint

Lumbar Vertebrae (lower backbone)

Sacrum

Ilium

Pubis

Ischium

} Pelvis

Femur

Knee Cap (patella)

Tibia

Fibula

Ankle Bones (tarsals)

Metatarsals

Phalanges

Fractured ulna partially healed (see page 955)

Radius

Ulna

Wrist Bones (carpals)

Metacarpals

Phalanges

Magnetic resonance imaging (MRI) depicts bone decay in hip (see page 998)

MRI shows torn knee cartilage (lateral meniscus) (see page 966)

A-4

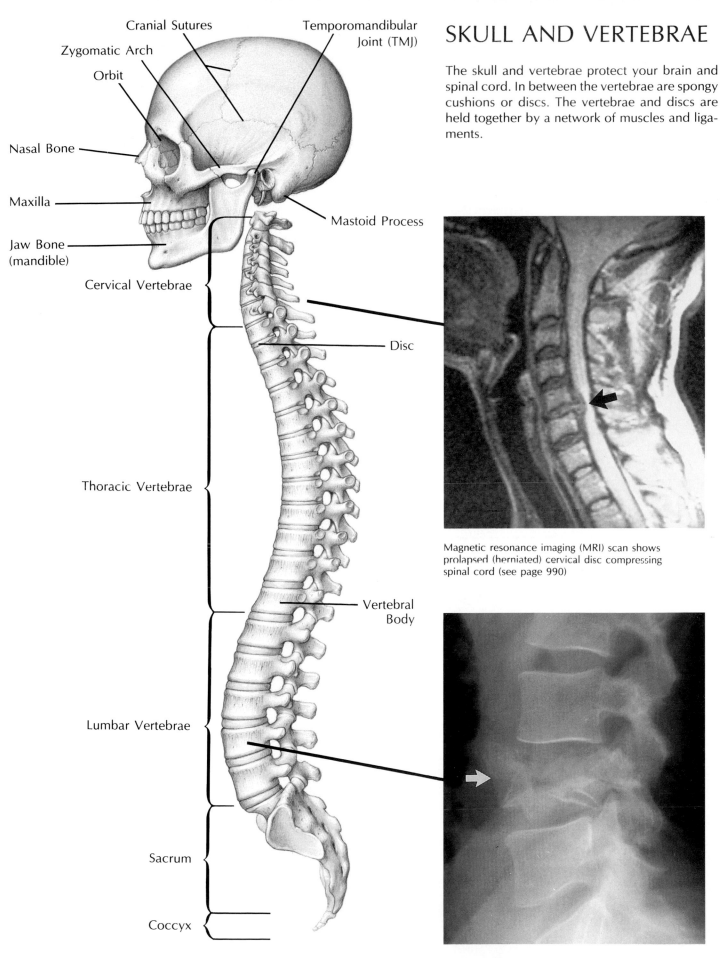

SKULL AND VERTEBRAE

The skull and vertebrae protect your brain and spinal cord. In between the vertebrae are spongy cushions or discs. The vertebrae and discs are held together by a network of muscles and ligaments.

Cranial Sutures

Temporomandibular Joint (TMJ)

Zygomatic Arch

Orbit

Nasal Bone

Maxilla

Jaw Bone (mandible)

Mastoid Process

Cervical Vertebrae

Disc

Thoracic Vertebrae

Vertebral Body

Lumbar Vertebrae

Sacrum

Coccyx

Magnetic resonance imaging (MRI) scan shows prolapsed (herniated) cervical disc compressing spinal cord (see page 990)

X-ray reveals severe fracture of low back (lumbar) vertebra

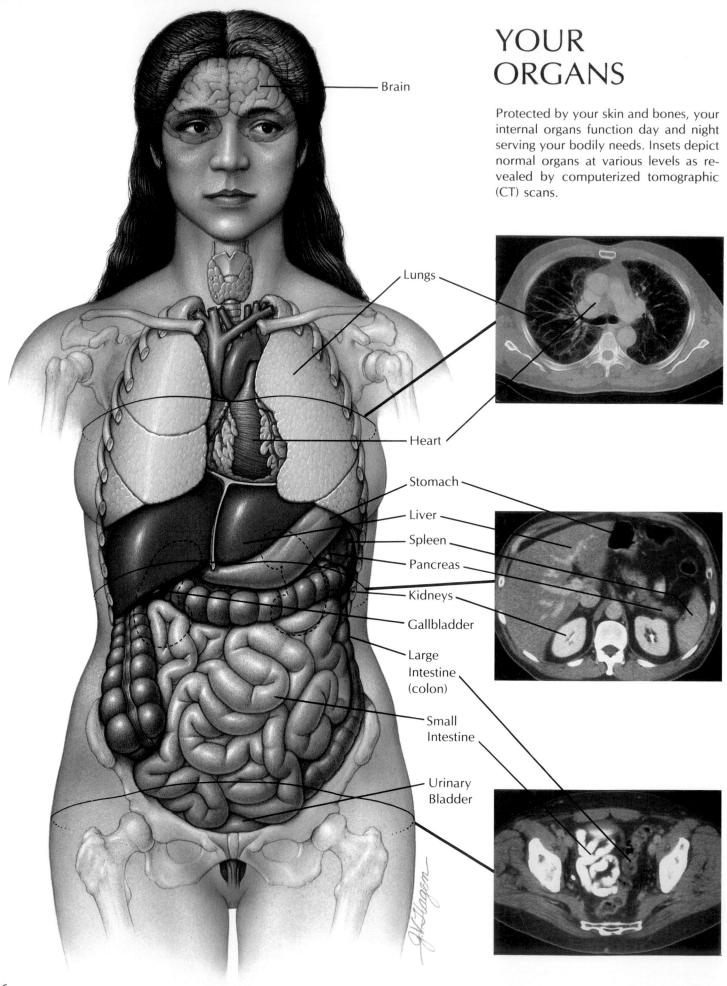

Brain

Protected by your skin and bones, your internal organs function day and night serving your bodily needs. Insets depict normal organs at various levels as revealed by computerized tomographic (CT) scans.

Lungs

Heart

Stomach

Liver

Spleen

Pancreas

Kidneys

Gallbladder

Large Intestine (colon)

Small Intestine

Urinary Bladder

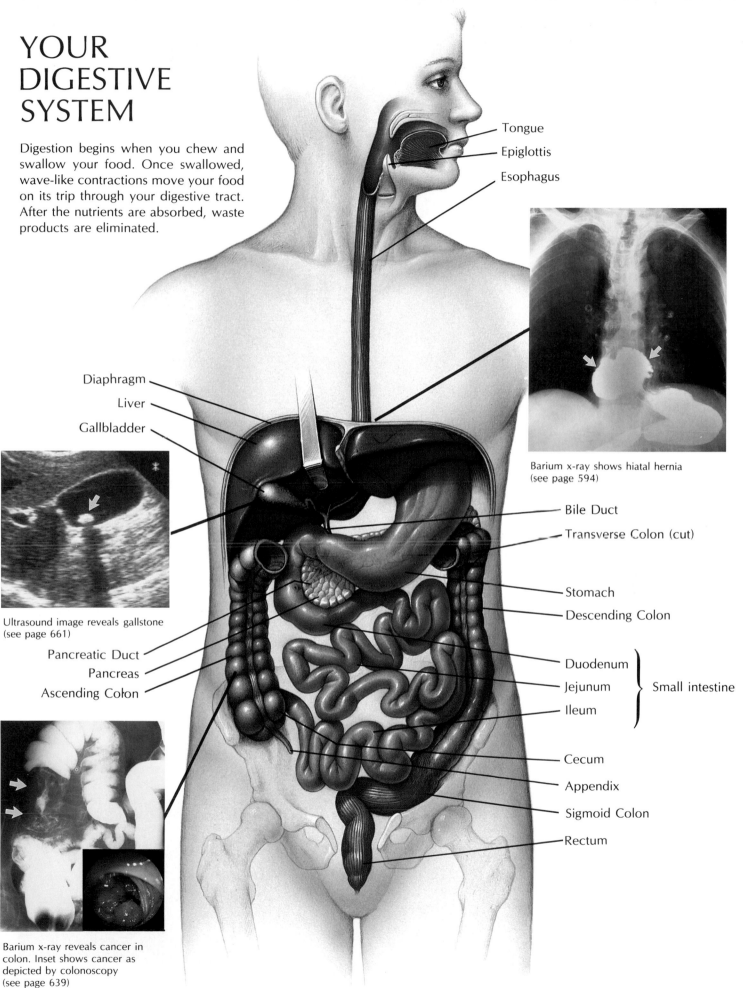

YOUR DIGESTIVE SYSTEM

Digestion begins when you chew and swallow your food. Once swallowed, wave-like contractions move your food on its trip through your digestive tract. After the nutrients are absorbed, waste products are eliminated.

Tongue

Epiglottis

Esophagus

Diaphragm

Liver

Gallbladder

Barium x-ray shows hiatal hernia (see page 594)

Ultrasound image reveals gallstone (see page 661)

Pancreatic Duct

Pancreas

Ascending Colon

Bile Duct

Transverse Colon (cut)

Stomach

Descending Colon

Duodenum

Jejunum

Small intestine

Ileum

Cecum

Appendix

Sigmoid Colon

Rectum

Barium x-ray reveals cancer in colon. Inset shows cancer as depicted by colonoscopy (see page 639)

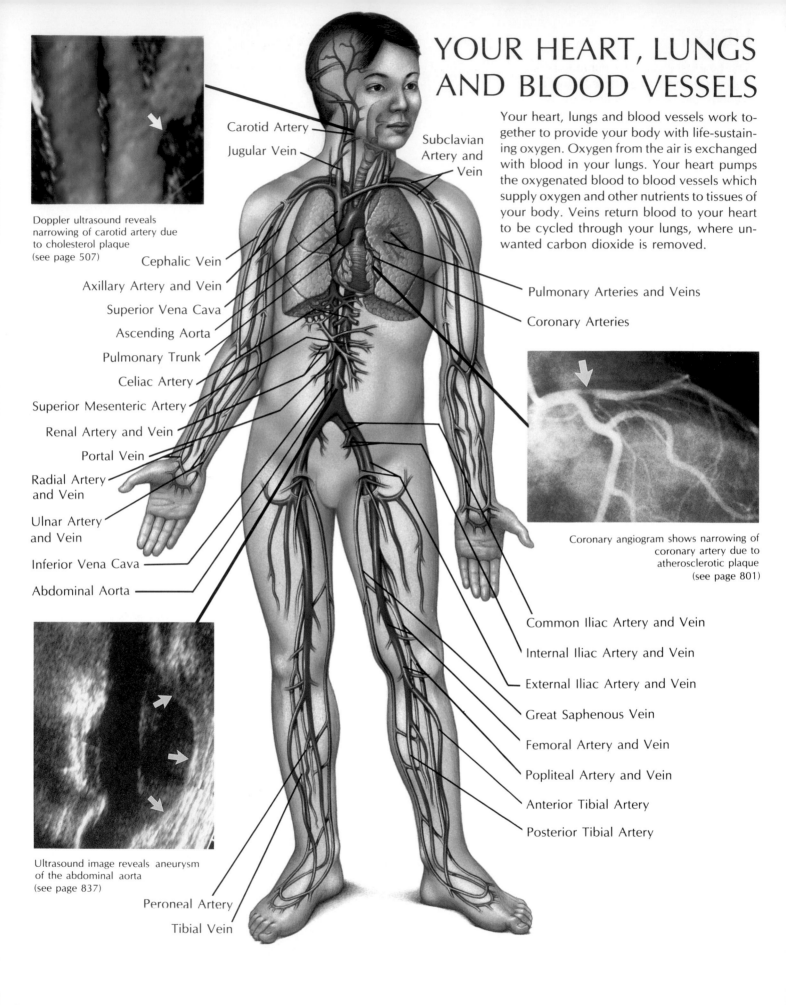

YOUR HEART, LUNGS AND BLOOD VESSELS

Your heart, lungs and blood vessels work together to provide your body with life-sustaining oxygen. Oxygen from the air is exchanged with blood in your lungs. Your heart pumps the oxygenated blood to blood vessels which supply oxygen and other nutrients to tissues of your body. Veins return blood to your heart to be cycled through your lungs, where unwanted carbon dioxide is removed.

Doppler ultrasound reveals narrowing of carotid artery due to cholesterol plaque (see page 507)

Coronary angiogram shows narrowing of coronary artery due to atherosclerotic plaque (see page 801)

Ultrasound image reveals aneurysm of the abdominal aorta (see page 837)

Carotid Artery
Jugular Vein
Subclavian Artery and Vein
Cephalic Vein
Axillary Artery and Vein
Superior Vena Cava
Ascending Aorta
Pulmonary Trunk
Celiac Artery
Superior Mesenteric Artery
Renal Artery and Vein
Portal Vein
Radial Artery and Vein
Ulnar Artery and Vein
Inferior Vena Cava
Abdominal Aorta
Pulmonary Arteries and Veins
Coronary Arteries
Common Iliac Artery and Vein
Internal Iliac Artery and Vein
External Iliac Artery and Vein
Great Saphenous Vein
Femoral Artery and Vein
Popliteal Artery and Vein
Anterior Tibial Artery
Posterior Tibial Artery
Peroneal Artery
Tibial Vein

HEART

The heart is a muscular pump containing four chambers connected by valves. Venous blood from your body flows through the superior and inferior vena cava into the right atrium, then through the tricuspid valve into your right ventricle. The right ventricle pumps blood through the pulmonary valve via pulmonary arteries into your lungs. From the lungs, blood enters the left atrium via the pulmonary veins and flows through the mitral valve into the left ventricle. The powerful left ventricle pumps oxygen-enriched blood through the aortic valve into the aorta for delivery to your body's tissues.

LUNGS

Your lungs supply oxygen to your blood and remove carbon dioxide from it. The exchange takes place in tiny air sacs called alveoli.

Superior Vena Cava
Ascending Aorta
Pulmonary Arteries
Pulmonary Veins
Right Atrium
Tricuspid Valve
Coronary Artery
Aortic Arch
Pulmonary Trunk
Pulmonary Arteries
Left Atrium
Pulmonary Veins
Pulmonary Valve
Aortic Valve
Mitral Valve
Left Ventricle
Inferior Vena Cava
Descending Aorta
Right Ventricle
Interventricular Septum

Nasal Cavity
Oral Cavity
Epiglottis
Thyroid Cartilage
Trachea
Lung
Bronchial Tree
Diaphragm

Normal lung tissue

Diseased lung tissue (emphysema) (see page 929)

Chest X-ray reveals cancer in left lung (see page 937)

YOUR BRAIN AND NERVES

Frontal Lobe

Parietal Lobe

Cerebrum

Temporal Lobe

Occipital Lobe

Cerebellum

Cervical Plexus

Brachial Plexus

Vertebra (cut)

Spinal Cord

Dura Mater

Spinal Nerves

Conus Medullaris

Cauda Equina

Lumbar Plexus

Sacral Plexus

Sciatic Nerve

Your brain and nerves are your means of receiving input from various body parts and from the outside world, and also your means of transmitting messages throughout your body. Your spinal cord transmits signals back and forth between your brain and the outermost regions of your peripheral nervous system.

Magnetic resonance image (MRI) scan depicts bleeding subdural hemorrhage (hematoma) (see page 511)

MRI scan reveals tumor in brain stem   (see page 537)

Parietal Lobe

Occipital Lobe

Corpus Callosum

Skull

Dura Mater

Frontal Lobe

Thalamus

Hypothalamus

Pituitary Gland

Pineal Body

Cerebellum

Spinal Cord

Pons

Midbrain

Medulla Oblongata

Brain Stem

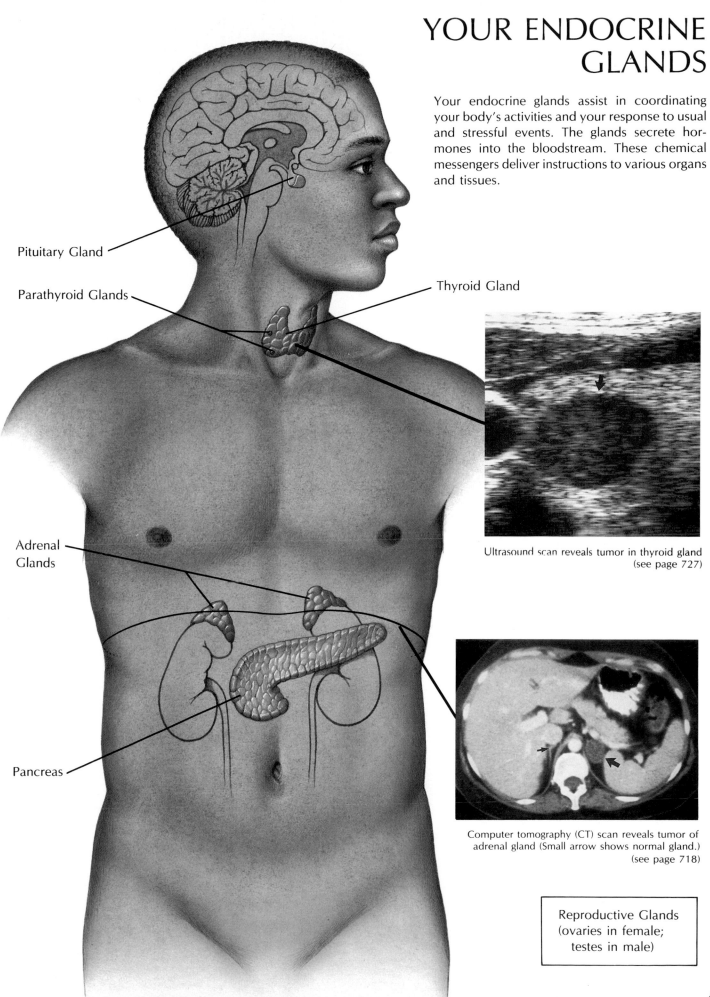

YOUR ENDOCRINE GLANDS

Your endocrine glands assist in coordinating your body's activities and your response to usual and stressful events. The glands secrete hormones into the bloodstream. These chemical messengers deliver instructions to various organs and tissues.

Pituitary Gland

Parathyroid Glands

Thyroid Gland

Adrenal Glands

Pancreas

Ultrasound scan reveals tumor in thyroid gland (see page 727)

Computer tomography (CT) scan reveals tumor of adrenal gland (Small arrow shows normal gland.) (see page 718)

Reproductive Glands
(ovaries in female;
testes in male)

YOUR REPRODUCTIVE ORGANS AND URINARY TRACT

Reproductive organs of the female include ovaries, which during menstruation release an egg; the fallopian tubes where the egg is fertilized; and the uterus where the egg implants itself and grows into a fetus. Reproductive organs of the male (opposite page) include testes, where sperm are produced, and the epididymis, which transports sperm for storage in the seminal vesicles. Fluids from the seminal vesicles and prostate are mixed with the sperm and ejaculated as semen through the urethra.

Your kidneys cleanse blood of excess fluid and waste products and pass the material through tube-like ureters to the bladder where it is stored and then expelled through the urethra.

Kidneys

Ureter

Fallopian Tube

Ovary

Uterus

Urinary Bladder

Vagina

Urethra

Contrast x-ray shows kidney stone at junction of kidney and ureter (see page 898)

Ultrasound scan reveals normal fetus in uterus   (see page 198)

Kidneys

CT scan reveals cancer
of the kidney
(see page 901)

Ureter

Urinary Bladder

Vas Deferens

Prostate
Gland

Seminal Vesicle

Urethra

Epididymis

Testes

Ultrasound scan reveals cancer within testes
(see page 1118)

A-13

YOUR SENSES

The five senses—sight, sound, smell, taste, and touch—allow you to perceive the world around you

Caruncle

Iris

Pupil

SIGHT

Images first pass through the opening at the front of your eye, the pupil, to the lens which inverts the image and projects it onto the retina. The retina processes the image and delivers it to your optic nerve which, in turn, transmits nerve impulses to your brain.

Canal of Schlemm

Eye Muscle

Sclera

Choroid

Retina

Fovea Centralis (focal point)

Optic Disc

Optic Nerve

Iris

Cornea

Lens

Anterior Chamber (aqueous humor)

U.S. MAIL

Suspensory Ligaments

Ciliary Body

Vitreous Chamber (vitreous humor)

Retinal Blood Vessels

Cataract (see page 768)

SOUND

Your eardrum transmits sound by means of tiny connective bones (hammer, anvil, stirrup) to the inner ear, where sound is transmitted as electrical impulses via the auditory nerve to the brain. The inner ear also contains the cochlea and semicircular canals, vestibular labyrinth, structures essential to balance.

Inner Ear

Middle Ear

Outer Ear

External Auditory Meatus

Stirrup (stapes)   Anvil (incus)   Hammer (malleus)

Skull

Semicircular Canals

Auditory Nerve   Vestibular Branch   Cochlear Branch

Cochlea

Eardrum (tympanic membrane)

Auditory (Eustachian) Tube

Sound Waves

Ruptured Eardrum (see page 678)

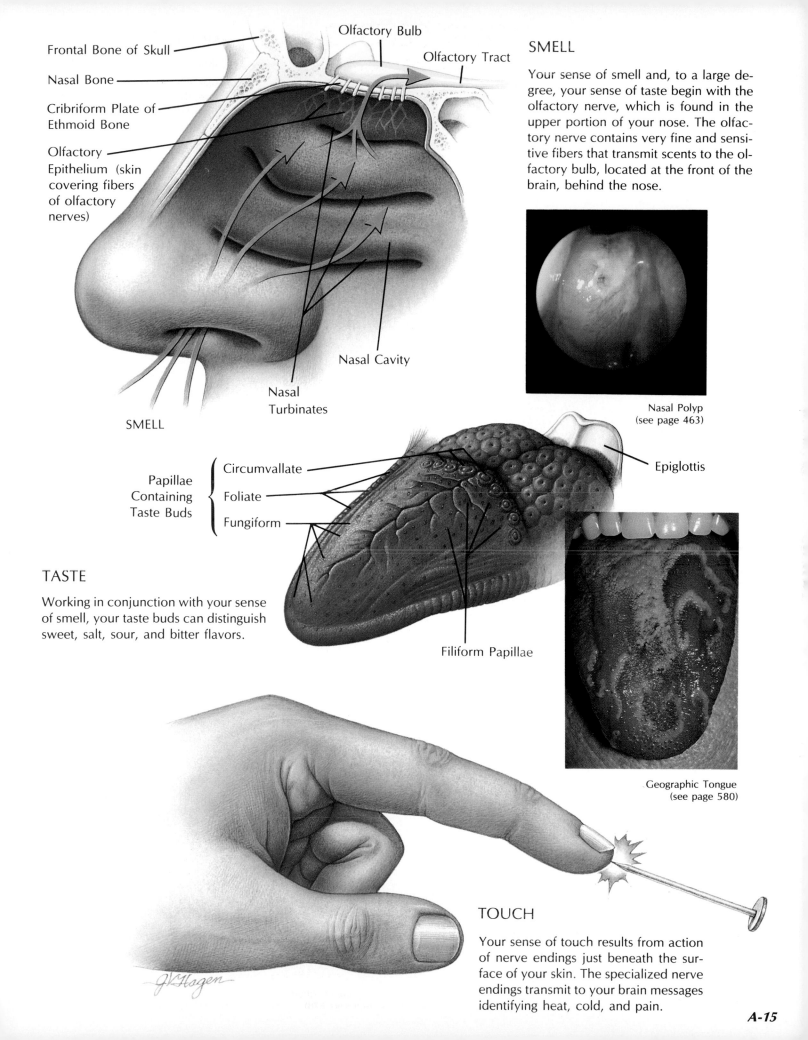

Frontal Bone of Skull

Nasal Bone

Cribriform Plate of
Ethmoid Bone

Olfactory
Epithelium (skin
covering fibers
of olfactory
nerves)

Olfactory Bulb

Olfactory Tract

Nasal Cavity

Nasal
Turbinates

SMELL

SMELL

Your sense of smell and, to a large degree, your sense of taste begin with the olfactory nerve, which is found in the upper portion of your nose. The olfactory nerve contains very fine and sensitive fibers that transmit scents to the olfactory bulb, located at the front of the brain, behind the nose.

Nasal Polyp
(see page 463)

Epiglottis

Papillae
Containing
Taste Buds

Circumvallate

Foliate

Fungiform

Filiform Papillae

TASTE

Working in conjunction with your sense of smell, your taste buds can distinguish sweet, salt, sour, and bitter flavors.

Geographic Tongue
(see page 580)

TOUCH

Your sense of touch results from action of nerve endings just beneath the surface of your skin. The specialized nerve endings transmit to your brain messages identifying heat, cold, and pain.

JVHagen

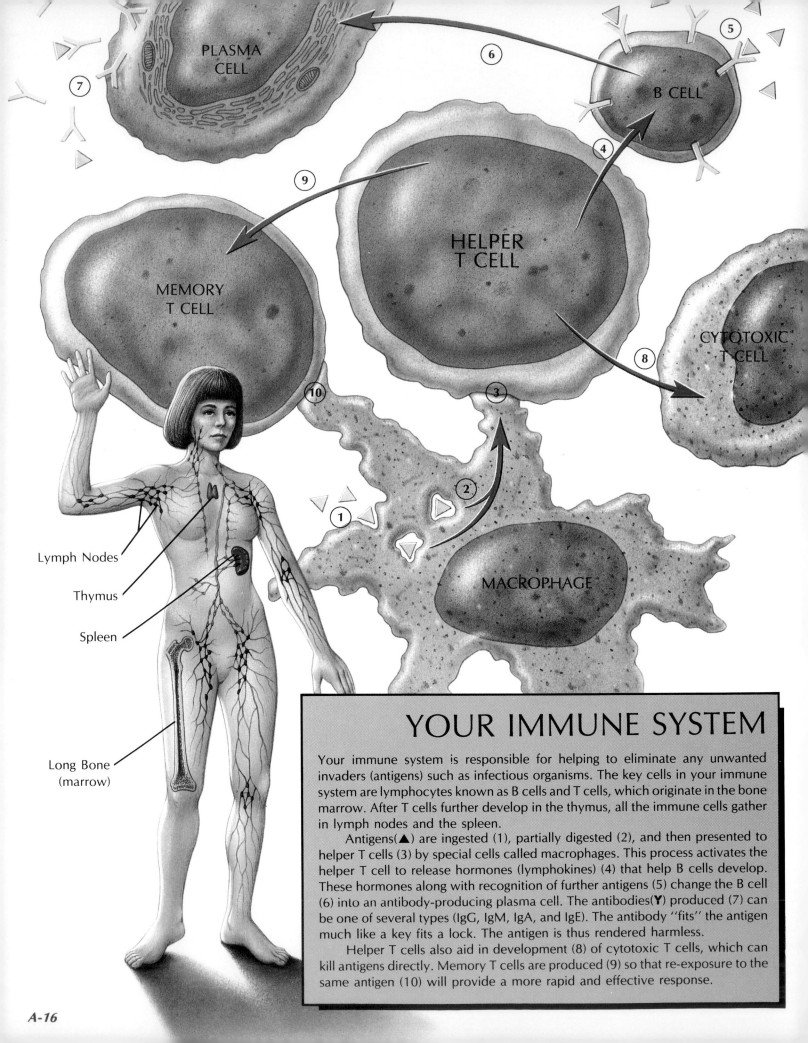

PLASMA CELL

B CELL

HELPER T CELL

MEMORY T CELL

CYTOTOXIC T CELL

Lymph Nodes

Thymus

Spleen

Long Bone (marrow)

MACROPHAGE

YOUR IMMUNE SYSTEM

Your immune system is responsible for helping to eliminate any unwanted invaders (antigens) such as infectious organisms. The key cells in your immune system are lymphocytes known as B cells and T cells, which originate in the bone marrow. After T cells further develop in the thymus, all the immune cells gather in lymph nodes and the spleen.

Antigens(▲) are ingested (1), partially digested (2), and then presented to helper T cells (3) by special cells called macrophages. This process activates the helper T cell to release hormones (lymphokines) (4) that help B cells develop. These hormones along with recognition of further antigens (5) change the B cell (6) into an antibody-producing plasma cell. The antibodies(Y) produced (7) can be one of several types (IgG, IgM, IgA, and IgE). The antibody "fits" the antigen much like a key fits a lock. The antigen is thus rendered harmless.

Helper T cells also aid in development (8) of cytotoxic T cells, which can kill antigens directly. Memory T cells are produced (9) so that re-exposure to the same antigen (10) will provide a more rapid and effective response.

CHAPTER 1

NEWBORN

THE FIRST MONTH OF LIFE

CHAPTER CONTENTS

THE FIRST MONTH OF LIFE

Few things are as exciting as the birth of a baby. After 9 months of wondering—Will my baby be a boy or girl? Who will he or she look like? Will he or she be normal? Will I automatically love my baby?—the questions suddenly have answers.

Despite the elation that comes with knowing they have a healthy newborn, first-time parents in particular may find themselves a bit overwhelmed—yesterday they were a couple, today they are a family.

The baby has needs that must take precedence over your own, and the baby depends on you for virtually everything. The responsibility may seem awesome at first, and you may feel as though you can do nothing right.

The newborn period—the first month of life—can be a trial for even the most experienced parents because every baby is different. Maybe you have given birth to three children, all of whom nursed well from the beginning, did not cry unless they were hungry, wet, or tired, and slept a good part of the day. Then comes the fourth child. This baby refuses to nurse half of the time, spends 3 hours crying every night for no apparent reason, and takes no more than two 1-hour catnaps during the day.

You are at the end of your rope. And you secretly wonder whether something is wrong with the child. Most likely, nothing is wrong. The first month of life is a period of adjustment for everyone closely involved in the baby's life.

For the parents, the adjustment can be equally difficult. The father may feel some jealousy toward the newborn, who is taking his wife's attention from him. Exhausted from lack of sleep and still recovering from the ordeal of giving birth, a new mother has many concerns. Can I take care of my child? Why am I not overwhelmed with love for the baby? Will I ever get rid of this fat? Will my husband still see me as an attractive woman and not just the mother of his child? It is little wonder that many a husband has come home to find both mother and child crying.

How then can you best get through your baby's first month? Physicians who specialize in the care of children offer this bit of advice: relax. If baby naps, a mother should too. Let a few dust balls accumulate. Forget about preparing gourmet meals. Do not feel duty bound to entertain all visitors who come for a peek at the baby.

As you and your baby begin to adjust to being home together, you may find that life gets easier.

Although most newborns (not all) spend a good part of the day sleeping and are alert only a small portion of the time they appear to be awake, you will discover how social the baby is during these brief but important moments. Holding and cuddling, cooing, establishing eye contact, and talking to your baby are all crucial to building a close relationship between the two of you.

Do not underestimate your newborn. Even at 1 month, the infant knows family and recognizes their voices, particularly his or her mother's.

A baby's abilities are limited, but not as much as you may think. Your baby was born with all the basic senses. He or she can see, hear, smell, and communicate by crying. The baby also is able to protect itself to some degree, thanks to some powerful reflexes.

For several days after birth, the gag reflex allows the infant to clear its airway of mucus in order to breathe. Its eyes are protected from bright light by a strong blink reflex. If one part of the infant's body becomes cold, the whole body changes color and temperature; the baby pulls its limbs toward the trunk to reduce the exposure and begins to shiver to generate heat.

Your newborn will try to avoid pain by drawing away from the source and batting with both arms or legs. Your baby also can avoid smothering if a blanket or something is placed over its head or face. First, the infant will mouth the object and then try to remove it by shaking its head violently from side to side. If that does not work, the baby will cross each arm over its face (see page 35).

Most new parents have many questions during their baby's first month. Your physician is an excellent source of information. Although you may be reluctant to "bother" the physician, most are accustomed to

fielding questions over the telephone. Many have pediatric nurse practitioners or other experienced nurses who can be of help. When in doubt, do not be afraid to ask.

If you suspect the infant may be ill, *call your baby's physician immediately.* Your baby is particularly vulnerable during the first month of life. A fever or cough that would be harmless for a 3-month-old may be serious enough to require hospitalization for a 3-week-old.

The purpose of this chapter is to provide a guide for parents with a newborn. Topics include normal growth and development, bonding between parents and child, signs of illness, nutrition, care of the newborn, and congenital abnormalities.

Since the beginning of time, when pain of delivery is past, the arrival of a new person is an especially joyous occasion for mother.

THE NORMAL BABY

For most expectant parents, the image of their baby begins to crystallize soon after

they learn that the results of a pregnancy test were positive. More often than not, the picture that emerges resembles the chubby, smiling 3- or 4-month-old that adorns disposable diaper boxes and baby food jars.

The reality is that the newborn your physician hands you in the delivery room is very different from that image. Wrinkled and often with a head that is molded from the trip down the birth canal, this baby is not exactly the beauty depicted in baby books.

The time from conception to birth may seem an eternity to prospective parents, although the process is completed in about 40 weeks. Babies born anywhere from 38 to 42 weeks after the last menstrual period are considered full-term.

Sometime within that 4-week period, most women go into labor, the climax of which is the delivery of an infant. The average full-term newborn weighs 5.5 to 10 pounds; boys weigh slightly more than girls. Most full-term babies are between 18 and 22 inches in length.

Immediately after delivery, suction is applied to your baby's mouth and nose to remove mucus and blood that could interfere with breathing. The umbilical cord, the former lifeline between mother and child, is cut. Your baby receives its first examination in the delivery room to ensure that there are no serious problems.

What does a normal baby look like? The infant may be quiet, or it may be screaming at the top of its lungs and flailing its arms and legs. Its skin may be discolored or mottled. Immediately after birth, the baby's color will be rather blue. This is the normal color for a baby before birth. During the first 5 to 10 minutes after birth, the baby becomes increasingly pink. Some infants have wrinkled and loose skin that gathers in body crevices. Others have pads of flesh that make them look fat. Many babies are born covered with vernix, a greasy white material that helps them slide through the birth canal.

Your baby may be totally bald or have a full head of hair, much of which will fall out by the fourth or fifth month. Fine, dark body hair (lanugo) may cover the infant's back, shoulders, and even parts of its face.

Most white babies are born with dark blue eyes. Black babies have eyes that appear dark brown. In white babies with dark complexions, the iris (the colored part of the eye) begins to darken within a few weeks. Brown eyes usually can be detected within the first 6 months.

You may notice that your baby's eyes are slightly swollen. This swelling is due to the erythromycin or silver nitrate ointment that, by law, is placed in the infant's eyes to protect them from possible infection from the birth canal. It is temporary and nothing to be concerned about.

The head looks large in relation to the body. When the infant is the mother's firstborn, the head is often pointed or swollen; this shape is caused by molding of the head to adjust to the size and shape of the birth canal. Although the sight of a misshapen head may be alarming to parents, the newborn's skull bones are pliable and made to overlap so the head can pass through the mother's narrow pelvis without injury. Molding does not result in any head or brain injury, and the infant's head returns to its normal shape in a few days. The top of the newborn's head contains a soft spot, which will remain until the bones close, usually between 9 and 18 months.

By the time your baby is 1 minute old, the infant will have been evaluated with the Apgar test, which is an assessment of the baby's apparent health. This test is repeated after 5 minutes. Babies with low Apgar scores require close observation (see The Apgar Test, page 7). An injection of vitamin K, which is a clotting agent, also is given shortly after birth to prevent internal bleeding.

If the baby is breathing well and appears healthy, he or she probably will be given to the mother wrapped in a warm blanket (to prevent heat loss). Many mothers opt to nurse their infants immediately. Even though the mother's body has not yet begun to produce milk, the breasts contain colostrum, a thin liquid that contains antibodies beneficial to the infant. The act of nursing itself helps develop a closeness or bond between mother and child.

Much has been written about bonding between parents and child. Simply put, bonding is the creation of emotional ties between the parents and their infant. By the time the infant is born, some bonding already has taken place. The parents, especially after going through childbirth, have an emotional attachment to their child. Beginning in the delivery room when the parents first hold the child, the infant begins to form a bond that will last the rest of his or her life (see Bonding, page 34).

For the first hour or two after birth, your baby is likely to be awake, alert, and quiet. This is a perfect time to begin to get to know your baby. Many parents like to unwrap the tight swaddling and examine the baby. All of us count fingers and toes to assure ourselves about our new child. Babies are born with hearing, and parents may observe the startle or jerk when the infant hears a loud noise in the delivery room. Newborns also can see and are able to focus on objects within 8 to 12 inches from them. Parents often are surprised to observe the infant staring intently at an object or face.

Birth is hard work, and the newborn's response to that stress is to sink into a deep sleep a couple of hours later. Usually this occurs after the infant has been taken to the hospital nursery. The newborn then is tightly swaddled and placed in a bassinet. During the first couple of days, most newborns rarely awaken fully. Occasionally, your baby may erupt into the crying fits that most people associate with newborns.

Newborns usually are brought to their mothers every 3 or 4 hours for bottle- or breast-feeding (some mothers elect to "room in" with the baby), but your newborn may not be interested in the breast or bottle for the first few days after birth. A newborn generally leaves the hospital weighing 6 to 10 percent less than at delivery. Usually by the third day—about the same time the mother's breasts fill with milk—the infant develops an appetite.

NORMAL GROWTH AND DEVELOPMENT

An amazing story is unfolding before your eyes. One day your infant is safe within the womb, and the next it has to breathe for itself, digest food, maintain its own body temperature, and stabilize a host of other functions that it must perform. Despite all of these requirements, your baby adapts and begins the long journey to independence.

Parents too must make many adjustments. Exhausted from giving birth, the mother's energies are taxed further by the demands of caring for this new person. Constant crying is a common complaint. Sometimes the baby will not eat; at other times a mother spends the better part of her day breast-feeding.

THE APGAR TEST

The Apgar test is used to evaluate the general health of the newborn at 1 minute and again at 5 minutes after birth. The Apgar score is an indication of whether any immediate measures must be taken to aid the baby in breathing.

The following areas are assessed: heart rate, respiratory effort, muscle tone, response to a tube (catheter) in the nostril, and color.

A score of 10 indicates that a baby is in the best possible condition. The heart rate is more than 100 per minute and the baby is breathing well and crying, is active, coughs or sneezes when the catheter is inserted in a nostril, and is completely pink, including the hands and feet.

If the score is 0 to 4, the baby has a slow or inaudible heart rate and is pale or even blue; the reflex response may be absent or depressed.

Most infants have a score of 7 to 9 and require nothing more than having the mucus suctioned from the airway.

Infants with a score of 4 or less at 1 minute after delivery require immediate assistance with their breathing. Further conclusions are not to be drawn from the test results: an Apgar score generally does not have long-term predictive value for a child's future development or intelligence.

Any parent with more than one child knows that there is no standard approach to caring for an infant. The following is a guide as to what to expect of your child during the first month of life; keep in mind that there are normal variations.

Weight. The average newborn weighs between 5.5 and 10 pounds and is between 18 and 22 inches in length. By the time the baby leaves the hospital, it probably will have lost anywhere from 6 to 10 percent of its birth weight because of fluid loss and initial lack of appetite. At the end of the first month, the average baby weighs 2 pounds more than it did at birth.

Posture and Motor Capabilities. The posture of the newborn simulates the fetal position. At birth, when placed on a firm surface, the baby can move its head from side to side. When held on an adult's shoulder, the infant can lift its head. When on its stomach, it lies in a frog-like position or rolled in a ball. When the baby is pulled to a sitting position, its head falls backward or forward. Fingers are balled into a fist.

At 1 month, the baby's unsupported head still flops but the infant may hold its head in

REQUIRED SCREENING FOR NEWBORNS

Some rare but serious defects in the metabolism of various substances can be treated effectively if they are diagnosed during an infant's first weeks after birth. If left untreated, however, these disorders can cause various devastating problems, including mental retardation, stunted physical growth, and cataracts.

Many states require that newborns be tested for these deficiencies to ensure that proper treatment is initiated immediately to enhance the chance of a normal life.

Your infant's physician or the nursing staff at the hospital where you give birth will inform you of any disorders for which testing is required in your particular state.

The following are three metabolic disorders for which your newborn may be tested.

Phenylketonuria

Phenylketonuria (PKU) is a congenital deficiency of a specific enzyme; it disrupts normal metabolism and causes brain damage. This inherited defect is rare in white infants and even rarer in black infants.

Infants born with PKU are normal at birth. These infants are often blonder than their siblings and have fair skin and blue eyes.

Those who are undiagnosed or who go untreated typically begin to deteriorate mentally. Generally, an infant with PKU whose IQ is normal at birth has lost 50 IQ points by the first birthday. The mental retardation in these children is so severe that institutional care is usually necessary.

Many states now require that all infants be tested for PKU to prevent this sequence of events. The test is a simple one, and only a few drops of the baby's blood are needed. Although PKU can be detected as early as 4 hours after birth, most testing for PKU is done after the baby's third day because the accuracy of the test depends on the baby having eaten an adequate amount of protein. Breast-fed babies, in particular, usually do not get much protein until the mother's milk comes in, usually on the third or fourth day after birth. Thus, if you are breast-feeding, you may have to bring the baby back to the hospital for the brief test a few days after you have been released.

If your baby has PKU, a special diet will be prescribed. If the abnormality is caught in time and corrected, your baby will be normal.

Galactosemia

This is also an enzyme deficiency; it affects the body's ability to metabolize galactose. One in 40,000 to 50,000 children is born with this inherited disorder.

This is a serious disease that, if left untreated, can cause brain damage, cataracts, and liver problems in an otherwise normal newborn.

A newborn who does not appear to be thriving or who has symptoms such as convulsions, marked lethargy, persistent jaundice, feeding difficulties, or hypoglycemia should have blood or urine tests to determine whether galactosemia is present.

Treatment involves a diet restricted in galactose content. When the diagnosis is made early, the infant's chance of a normal life is good.

Hypothyroidism

This is an inherited deficiency in the production of thyroid hormone.

Hypothyroidism is twice as common in females as in males. Neonatal screening programs that have tested 50 million infants worldwide have found that the disorder occurs in about 1 in every 4,000 births. Before massive screening, this defect often went unrecognized because there were few initial symptoms.

Symptoms might include sluggishness, constipation, and poor growth. Affected babies sleep more than normal infants and cry very little. Symptoms appear gradually over the first few months of life.

Because symptoms initially may be absent or mild and then progress slowly, it is very important that all newborns be screened with blood tests to rule out congenital hypothyroidism.

If left untreated, these children are usually mentally retarded and have short stature. Treatment with thyroid hormone is effective for preventing growth problems.

Experts agree that improved screening at birth has had a major impact on improving life for these children. Studies have shown that infants who begin treatment during the first month of life have normal IQs in the first grade. Further studies are needed to assess later school performance (see Hyperthyroidism, page 727).

---

line with its back when pulled to a sitting position. The baby can roll partway to its side from its back. When the baby's fingers are pried open, it can grasp a spoon but drops it right away.

Vision. Newborns can see. From the moment of birth, your newborn is capable of focusing and following objects within 8 to 12 inches of its face. Beyond that distance, the image is probably hazy.

At 1 month, your newborn continues to stare at objects but will not reach for them. The infant also is able to coordinate its eyes better. The baby makes eye-to-eye contact and is particularly interested in focusing on its mother's face.

Hearing. Babies are born with their sense of hearing and can distinguish volume. A sharp noise may startle the baby, whereas a soft voice may cause the baby to smile or to come close to smiling.

At 1 month, the infant distinguishes between the parents' voices.

Language. The language of the newborn is the cry. By 1 month, the infant's repertoire includes soft, throaty, and gurgling sounds.

Feeding. The newborn is hungry at irregular intervals. It is not uncommon for a baby to show little interest in feeding, particularly during the first couple of days after birth. By the end of the first week most infants eat every 2 to 5 hours.

Feeding is still somewhat disorganized at 1 month. Because breast milk is digested more quickly than formula, a breast-fed baby may eat as often as every 3 hours during the day and have two night feedings. Babies who are given formula may go longer between feedings. Gradually, over the course of the first month, the number of feedings may be reduced from seven or eight over a 24-hour period to five or six.

The length of feedings also is erratic. On one day a breast-fed infant might want to nurse for 40 minutes at each breast, and the next day it may nurse for only 10 minutes at each.

By 2 weeks of age, your newborn may drink 18 ounces of milk per day. At 1 month, the infant may increase the amount to 25 ounces each day.

Bowel Movements. The baby has the first bowel movement usually within 24 hours after birth. Called a meconium stool, it is composed of intestinal secretions and amniotic fluid and is dark green. After the baby begins to drink milk, the meconium stool is replaced by transitional stools, usually on the third or fourth day of life. These stools are usually greenish brown and may contain milk curds. After the passage of transitional stools, the stool resembles the bowel movement of an older infant.

By the end of the first week, most babies pass between three and five stools a day, although it is not uncommon for a baby, especially one that is breast-fed, to have more bowel movements each day. However, if your newborn goes for a day without having a bowel movement, do not worry. This does not mean that the baby is constipated.

The stool of the breast-fed baby is odorless and mushy and has been compared with the consistency of a thick soup. New parents initially may mistake it for diarrhea. It is not. The stool of a formula-fed baby has a characteristic fecal smell and is usually more formed.

By 1 month most babies have a bowel movement three or four times a day, often after a feeding. However, some infants, especially some nursing babies, occasionally may not have one for 1 to 3 days. This is normal and not a cause for concern.

Sleeping. The newborn often has an alert period immediately after birth. After this hour or two of alertness, the baby sinks into a deep sleep. During the next several days most newborns sleep anywhere from 14 to 18 hours a day and are alert for only 30 minutes out of every 4 hours.

A 1-month-old baby spends most of the time sleeping, usually at least 14 hours a day. Generally, as the baby moves toward the end of the first month, parents observe that the seven or eight daily sleep periods are reduced to three or four daily naps and a 5- or 6-hour block of sleep at night. Sleep patterns, however, are highly variable.

No matter how much or how little your infant sleeps, he or she is a light sleeper. Hence, even though the baby is asleep, you may see it grimace, cry out, startle, and move about—all without waking up.

Crying. Crying is your baby's first method of communication. Although not terribly sophisticated, it works in that it rarely fails to bring someone running. The amount a newborn cries, like many other facets of development, varies. Some babies cry only when hungry or wet; others cry more often.

One day your newborn may cry many times a day, for example, before a feeding, falling asleep, or having a bowel movement. On another day the crying may be infrequent.

Psychosocial Development and Personality.   These important areas of development are discussed on pages 33 through 41.

BIRTH INJURY

Between 2 and 7 of each 1,000 newborns have a birth injury. A birth injury is defined as trauma incurred by the infant during labor and delivery. Most often, the birth injury occurs despite excellent obstetric care.

Certain conditions make the possibility of a birth injury more likely. Prematurity, breech birth, prolonged pregnancy, an abnormally large fetus, an abnormal fetal position, and a small maternal pelvis are conditions that predispose infants to birth trauma.

Forceps sometimes are involved in birth injuries. Forceps are used to pull the baby from the birth canal when the mother is unable to push it out. Forceps injuries generally are minor, involving facial or scalp abrasions. Often, forceps delivery is the best way to end a labor that may threaten the life or health of mother or child.

In traveling down the vaginal canal, a newborn may sometimes sustain minor injury to the soft tissues of the scalp, causing a swelling of the head after birth. Called caput succedaneum, this swelling is not harmful and usually disappears in a few days when the baby's head assumes its normal shape.

Another useful technique is vacuum extraction. In this method, a metal or silicone cap is placed on the head of the fetus while it is in the birth canal. This creates suction, allowing for traction to be applied to enhance progress. Newer methods that prevent too much suction from being applied help protect the baby from injury.

The following are the most common birth injuries.

Caput succedaneum is swelling of the tissues of the scalp; it occurs because of pressure of the head against the rigid vaginal canal. The infant's face also may be swollen, discolored, or distorted. This swelling usually disappears after a few days and the baby's head assumes a normal shape.

Cephalhematoma is a collection of blood under the scalp. It is caused by slow bleeding, and the swelling usually is not visible until several hours after birth. A skull fracture occasionally is associated with this injury. Most cephalhematomas resolve within 2 weeks to 3 months. Treatment is rarely required.

A fractured collar bone (clavicle) is the most frequent bone injury during labor and delivery, particularly when there is difficulty in delivering the shoulder or during breech births.

An infant with this injury fails to move the arm on the affected side. The Moro reflex (the neck extends, and the arms and legs fling outward in response to sudden contact or a noise; see page 35) is abnormal on the affected side.

Infants with a fractured clavicle recover completely.

On occasion, a *nasal fracture* can occur. This is usually a dislocation of the cartilage in the septum. The infant may have difficulty nursing and some problems breathing through its nose. The nose appears asymmetric and flattened. A surgeon should be consulted to determine the specific treatment.

Facial nerve palsy usually results from pressure over the facial nerve in the uterus, a hard labor, or a forceps delivery. The paralysis may involve an entire side of the infant's face.

When the infant cries, the affected side of the face does not move and the mouth is drawn to one side. The eye on the paralyzed side cannot close and the corner of the mouth droops. The long-term outcome depends on whether the nerve was injured by pressure or whether nerve fibers were torn. If pressure is the cause, improvement is rapid and complete. Microsurgical repair of the nerve may be necessary if the paralysis continues.

COMMON CONCERNS DURING THE NEWBORN STAGE

The parent can be at a disadvantage when trying to determine whether a newborn is indeed sick or simply is having a bad day.

After living with a child, a parent becomes accustomed to the child's moods and patterns. Even before the child is old enough to communicate, you often can sense that something is not right by, for example, a change in your infant's eating or sleeping habits. In short, some behavior change triggers your suspicions. But the newborn and parents are just getting to know each other. What is "normal" behavior for this child has not yet been established. So how can a parent tell whether something is wrong?

SIGNS AND SYMPTOMS OF ILLNESS

Illness can be indicated in many ways. Some signs or symptoms always indicate that the baby is ill; others, such as excessive crying, may or may not be indicative of illness. For easy reference, the most common ones are discussed below in brief; in the pages that follow, most are discussed in detail.

Fever in the newborn is a rectal temperature of more than 100.5°F. Fever is the body's response to infection. Keep in mind, however, that in the first few months of life, particularly in premature infants, an infection may not cause a fever. The key is how your baby acts. If he or she is more listless than normal or if a fever is present, contact your physician.

Excessive crying also may indicate illness, especially if there are other symptoms. Some babies cry more than others—sometimes even for 2 or 3 hours—without being ill. Some babies have colic (severe gas attacks during which the baby may have episodes of crying, its legs are drawn up to its chest, and its abdomen is distended). Burping, rocking, or walking your baby often helps a colicky child (see Excessive Crying, page 12). If nothing seems to work and the crying continues for several hours, the baby may be crying because of illness.

Breathing difficulty is a sign of illness. If the baby is congested, wheezing, or having difficulty breathing, there may be a respiratory problem. Sneezing in an infant is common and normal.

Diarrhea is a serious condition; if untreated, it can lead to dehydration. Babies' stools are generally loose. As a rule, a baby with diarrhea has an increase in the number of stools and the consistency changes. A breast-fed baby's normal stool is the consistency of thick soup and contains curds. If the curds disappear and the stool becomes watery, the baby probably has diarrhea. A baby with diarrhea also looks sick (see page 14).

Vomiting is not the gentle spitting up after eating that occurs in most newborns. Rather, true vomiting is when the contents of the stomach are propelled forcefully from the baby's mouth. Although occasional vomiting usually is not cause for alarm, if it becomes frequent or contains green bile or blood, the baby could have a problem (see page 14).

Lethargy may be a bad sign. If your child is suddenly uninterested, limp, and sleeping more than usual, an infection or disease could be present.

Lack of appetite occurs in most sick newborns. A baby who has been eating well but suddenly refuses the bottle or breast may be sick.

Jaundice (yellowing of the skin) is common immediately after birth. If it persists for more than a few days after birth or if your newborn becomes jaundiced after you are released from the hospital, a serious infection or other disorder may be present.

Failure to move an extremity may be a sign of a fracture, dislocation, or nerve injury.

If your baby has any of the above symptoms or signs or is more irritable or lethargic than you think is warranted, or if you believe the baby just does not look right, call your baby's physician immediately.

FEVER

A fever is usually the body's response to infection. In the case of the newborn, it also may be the result of dehydration or overexposure in hot climates.

Regardless, a rectal temperature of more than 100.5°F warrants a call to your baby's physician. Any fever in a newborn is considered potentially serious and should be investigated.

When should you take your baby's temperature? Does the baby feel warm to the touch? Does the forehead feel warmer than your lips when you kiss it? Is the infant unusually fussy or unusually quiet? Have its sleep patterns abruptly changed? Is the baby vomiting or having diarrhea? Does its chest sound congested? Has the baby stopped wetting its diapers? If the answer to any of these questions is "yes" or if your instincts tell you that something is not right, take the infant's temperature.

The temperature of an infant is taken rectally, much to the dismay of many nervous parents. A special rectal thermometer—the

When taking a newborn's temperature with a rectal thermometer, insert the thermometer approximately one inch. Never let go of the thermometer while it is in your child.

bulb is rounded—is needed. You also will need some petroleum jelly or cold cream to lubricate the tip of the thermometer so that it will slide in easier.

Insert the thermometer into the rectum about an inch and hold it there for a couple of minutes. You should never let go of the thermometer while it is inside the baby because one squirm may push it deeper into the rectum and cause an injury.

An infant's temperature varies. It is often lower in the morning and increases in the afternoon or evening. As long as it is below 100.5°F, the baby does not have a fever.

If, however, it is above 100.5°F, call your pediatrician or family physician even if the child has no other symptoms. Your physician may want to examine the baby. It is not uncommon for a physician to hospitalize an infant who has a slight temperature with no other symptoms. It may be nothing more than a harmless virus, but because as many as 10 percent of infants develop infections during their first month, the physician may want to eliminate more serious possibilities such as meningitis (see page 527).

Many physicians recommend acetaminophen (never aspirin) for reducing fever. Do not, however, give your newborn any medicine unless instructed to do so by your physician.

EXCESSIVE CRYING

A baby cries for several reasons. The infant may cry when hungry, wet, or tired. The baby cries because of gas or just before a bowel movement. Sometimes the cry may be out of frustration or because the baby wants to be cuddled. The newborn cries because of illness or pain. And sometimes your baby will cry for no reason at all—at least none that you can determine.

Crying is your baby's first means of communication. Although the infant will develop more sophisticated methods, few will be any more effective for obtaining a response from the parent.

What is excessive crying during the first month of life? There is no easy answer to that question because every baby and every day are different. All babies cry, some more than others.

On some days your baby may cry for 20 or 30 minutes for four or five times—typically before eating, sleeping, and having a bowel movement. On another day, the infant may scream for hours.

Studies show that infants respond to the stresses of their environment by crying; the more stressful the situation, the longer and more intense the crying spell. Thus, if the parent has had a bad day, the baby may too. However, on days when the atmosphere at home is relaxed, the fussy periods decrease dramatically in proportion to how much attention the baby gets. First babies are more likely to have the long crying spells, presumably because parents become more relaxed with subsequent children.

The newborn's nervous and digestive systems are learning to adjust to the outside world. For some babies, this is a difficult task. If the bulk of your baby's crying occurs in the late afternoon or evening and its stomach is distended, the infant may have colic. Few common infant maladies make a parent feel as helpless as an attack of colic.

The following scenario may be familiar to countless parents. Your newborn is quiet in the hospital, but a few days after going home it begins to have crying spells that may last for several hours. You change the diapers, pick the newborn up, and even offer the breast or bottle. Nothing works. The infant cries so hard that its face becomes flushed. Its stomach is tense and distended and its legs are drawn up toward its abdomen. Its feet and hands may feel cold.

You wonder whether something is terribly wrong with your child and you call the baby's physician.

The infant with these symptoms is not seriously ill. The baby simply has colic, a common ailment that is more upsetting to the parents than it is harmful to the infant.

The term colic describes frequent attacks of abdominal pain, thought to originate in the infant's intestines. The infant hurts and responds by severe crying, often to the point of exhaustion. The severity and frequency of colic attacks vary. Some babies are predictable in that every evening they scream for hours; others spread their crying out in shorter intervals during the day. Some infants cry on and off during the day but sleep well at night, and others reserve their crying for the middle of the night.

A baby with colic generally begins to cry after a feeding, which is one sign that differentiates the cries of a colicky baby from those of a hungry one.

No one knows for certain what causes colic. Certain infants simply seem to be susceptible to abdominal upsets. Attacks may be associated with hunger and with swallowed air that has passed into the intestines. Foods that the breast-feeding mother has eaten, particularly those with a high carbohydrate content, may be responsible for excessive fermentation in the infant's intestines.

What should you do for excessive crying, colic-related or otherwise?

The first thing you should understand is that the end is in sight. The vast majority of babies—even those with severe colic—are over these crying episodes by the third month of life. Until that magic time, a parent can do several things (none is a panacea, unfortunately).

First, check for the obvious. Is the baby hungry? If the infant ate well and now is crying less than 2 hours later, it is unlikely to be hungry. However, you can try another feeding. Sometimes just the comfort of sucking will quiet a newborn.

Change the baby's diaper or try burping it. Some babies become quiet if you rock them; others like to be sung to. Some physicians contend that a baby held over the parent's heart cries less.

If the baby seems colicky, holding it upright sometimes helps. Most colicky babies are more comfortable lying on their abdomens. Try holding the baby, abdomen down, across your lap and massaging its back.

A hot water bottle placed against the abdomen helps relieve the symptoms of colic in some infants. If you decide to try this method, however, you must make sure the bottle is not so hot as to burn the infant. Test the temperature by holding your wrist against the bottle for a moment. If that is uncomfortable, the water is too hot.

Rocking or walking the baby sometimes helps. Do not be afraid of spoiling your newborn by excessive holding. That result is unlikely. Hold the baby if that seems to help.

Swaddling a colicky baby in a soft blanket sometimes helps. Other methods that may work include giving the baby a pacifier, putting the baby in a small space such as a bassinet or infant carrier (rather than the larger crib), or going for a short ride in the car.

Often a colic attack ends when the infant passes rectal gas or has a bowel movement. Sometimes the insertion of a thermometer into the baby's rectum will elicit gas or a bowel movement and the baby may feel better.

As a parent of a colicky baby, you also should pay particular attention to burping after every feeding. Even if it takes awhile, try to get the baby to burp.

If your baby's colic is persistent, your baby's physician may suggest you try another formula (if you are bottle-feeding) to see if there is an improvement.

And what about the baby who, despite your efforts, will not stop crying? If there are no signs of illness (see Signs and Symptoms of Illness, page 11), maybe the next step is to do nothing and see what happens. Some babies simply cannot fall asleep without crying for awhile. When all else fails, do not be afraid to let the baby cry for 20 minutes or so in its crib.

VOMITING AND SPITTING UP

It is not uncommon for a newborn or even an older infant to spit up after a feeding.

"Spitting up" (reflux) is the gentle spilling of what is typically a small amount of milk from the baby's mouth. This should not be confused with vomiting, during which the contents of the baby's stomach are ejected forcefully from its mouth.

One newborn may spit up after every feeding, and another may spit up only infrequently. Spitting up is messy for the parents (some have learned never to hold their baby unless a diaper is on their shoulder), but it rarely signifies a serious problem. Usually by the time the child is between 9 months and 1 year old—the age when the infant is sitting up and beginning to move about—the problem resolves itself.

The reason that a baby spits up is not completely understood, but it probably is related to its immature digestive system. Unlike the older child or adult, the young baby's muscle between the esophagus and the upper part of the stomach is not yet adept at holding the stomach's contents down. Thus, any movement, even something as gentle as laying the baby down or the act of digestion itself, can cause the milk to reflux.

Often the milk that spills from your baby's mouth smells slightly sour, and it also may be curdled. This is nothing to be concerned about; the milk was undergoing digestion when it was regurgitated.

What should you do if your baby spits up? Sometimes a baby spits up because of gas in its stomach. Thus, burping after each feeding is important. Even though it may take awhile, parents should try to get the baby to burp after every feeding. Some physicians also suggest keeping the baby upright in an infant seat for a half hour after feeding.

If your baby is a spitter, the problem probably will continue no matter what you do. As long as the baby seems healthy and is gaining weight, your physician will not be concerned and you should not be either.

Vomiting, however, can be a cause for concern.

A newborn may vomit mucus, often streaked with blood, a few hours after birth. This generally is not worrisome. It often is blood from the mother that the infant swallowed during delivery. Usually this vomiting subsides after a few feedings. If it continues, however, it can signify an obstruction in the esophagus or intestines that will need further evaluation.

Vomiting also can be the result of milk intolerance or an initial sign of another illness.

What should you do if your baby vomits?

Some spitty babies vomit large amounts as often as once a day. You should notify your baby's physician, but, again, as long as the baby seems healthy and is gaining weight, there is probably no reason to be alarmed.

If there is blood or green bile in the vomit, the baby should be examined immediately because this may suggest a serious illness.

When a baby who has never done much spitting up suddenly vomits, you should take the infant's temperature because vomiting is occasionally a symptom of infection. If the temperature is normal and the baby behaves normally, everything is probably all right. If the infant continues to vomit, call your pediatrician or family physician.

LOOSE STOOLS AND CONSTIPATION

The stool of a breast-fed newborn is naturally the consistency of thick soup. If your baby does have diarrhea during the first month, it may be caused by an infection. The stool is apt to be greenish, the frequency will increase, the stools will become watery, the curds contained in the normal stool of a breast-fed newborn will be absent, and there may be an unpleasant odor.

If you suspect your newborn has diarrhea, call your baby's physician. If the physician determines that the baby has only a mild case of diarrhea, you may be advised to change the frequency or amount of your baby's feedings. Let your nursing baby continue to nurse, but do not be surprised if the baby wants less than usual. If your physician thinks the diarrhea is more severe or thinks the baby is becoming dehydrated, your baby may need care in the hospital.

Constipation is rare in the newborn.

First, you should understand that constipation refers to the consistency of the stool and not to the frequency. Some breast-fed babies have a bowel movement after every feeding, and some newborns have only one a day or one every other day. The baby who has one only once a day or even less frequently is not necessarily constipated.

True constipation is the difficult passage of hard, dry stools. The breast-fed baby passes mushy stools that are the consistency of applesauce. Sometimes the baby may appear to be straining and yet the stool that passes is liquid. In such cases, some physicians believe that the stool is too soft to place pressure on the anus. Usually, no treatment is recommended.

The formula-fed newborn sometimes may have difficulty having a bowel movement. The stools may be hard.

Chronic constipation that develops after you have brought the newborn home also could indicate a congenital problem and should be discussed with your baby's physician.

NEONATAL JAUNDICE

Approximately 60 percent of all full-term newborns develop jaundice during their first week, and the proportion increases to 80 percent in premature infants.

Jaundice (yellowing of the skin) is not a disease itself but rather is the result of the inability of the immature liver of an infant to metabolize bilirubin. Thus, the bilirubin accumulates in the skin and gives it a yellowish tint.

Some babies are jaundiced at birth, and others develop jaundice later, depending on the condition responsible for the jaundice.

Jaundice that is present at birth or appears within the first 24 hours may be the result of several problems, including hemorrhage, sepsis (an infection in the blood), and a blood incompatibility between the baby and mother. If your physician is concerned about these possibilities, special blood tests will be done.

Typically, most jaundiced infants become so during the second or third day of life. This is called physiological jaundice and is due to the breakdown of fetal red blood cells in combination with the inability of the immature liver to excrete bilirubin.

Jaundice occurring after the third day but within the first week may be the result of an infection.

When an infant develops jaundice after the first week of life, the cause may be the mother's breast milk (this occurs in 1 in 200 breast-fed, full-term infants) or congenital blood or liver problems. If the jaundice persists during the first month, it may be due to a liver abnormality, severe infection, or enzyme deficiency.

Your physician will watch your newborn carefully for signs of jaundice. If your baby is getting progressively more jaundiced, your physician may order periodic blood tests to measure the bilirubin concentration.

Most infants with physiologic jaundice require little more than observation. Generally within a week to 10 days at the most, the condition is gone. However, the severity of physiological jaundice is influenced by race or ethnic background; Chinese, Japanese, Korean, and American Indian full-term newborns are affected more severely.

If your infant has a significantly increased amount of bilirubin, he or she may be placed under a high-intensity light (phototherapy). Bilirubin absorbs light and is then converted into a form that can be excreted in the bile and urine. This treatment is applied continuously until the amount of bilirubin has been reduced to a level considered safe for the infant.

Side effects of phototherapy can include loose stools, rash, and dehydration.

FAILURE TO GAIN WEIGHT

An infant who fails to gain weight may even lose weight.

Your physician may advise you to change formula, increase the number of feedings, or supplement your breast milk to correct the lack of weight gain.

Some babies do not gain weight because of physical abnormalities that interfere with the infant's ability to eat or to thrive. These include cleft palate, gastrointestinal diseases, chronic heart failure, lung and kidney diseases, malignancies, and endocrine disorders. Your physician may perform tests to rule out some of these conditions.

Treatment may involve hospitalization. In the hospital, the infant usually is given unlimited feedings to determine whether weight gain will result. Tests and x-rays also can be done if a physical abnormality is suspected.

The long-term outlook for babies who fail to gain weight varies, but most infants do well.

DIAPER RASH

Signs and Symptoms
• A rash in the region covered by the diaper.

Most infants develop a diaper rash; some even arrive home from the hospital with a slight rash. A diaper rash does not necessarily mean that an infant is receiving poor care (although an infant who is not cared for properly is more likely to get a diaper rash). It only means that the baby has sensitive skin.

Diaper rash can be the result of many different causes. The typical diaper rash is the reaction of the sensitive skin of a newborn to contact with urine and stool. This rash often goes away without treatment.

Babies can be plagued by a fungal infection. The infection may appear on the buttocks and genitals as bright red spots that come together to form a solid red area with a scalloped border. This common rash can be treated by the physician with a special ointment. It has a tendency to recur.

Treatment. If your baby has a diaper rash, the first step may be simply changing the diaper more often and a thorough washing of the skin every time the diaper is changed. If you have been using plastic pants to help keep the baby dry, stop using them until the rash has disappeared. Petroleum jelly or a zinc oxide paste can be applied to the rash several times a day. If the rash is particularly persistent and severe, a 0.5 to 1 percent hydrocortisone cream can be used for a limited time.

For persistent diaper rash, many physicians recommend taking the baby's diaper off and exposing the affected area to air. This can be messy, but it usually works. (See color photograph of diaper rash, page B-2.)

CRADLE CAP

Signs and Symptoms
• Dry, scaly skin on the scalp.

Cradle cap (seborrheic eczema) is a common problem that can occur at any age, but it is most common during infancy and adolescence. Cradle cap often begins during the infant's first month of life and may continue to be a problem throughout the first year. Its cause is unknown.

If your infant has cradle cap, you probably first will notice dry, scaly patches on the scalp that give it a dirty appearance. A thick, yellow crust may form over the scales. You may notice some scaly patches around the hairline, eyebrows, eyelids, nose, and ears. Sometimes the rash is so severe that the entire body is affected. (See color photograph of cradle cap, page B-2.)

Treatment. Cradle cap usually has a shorter course than many other rashes, and it responds to treatment. The best treatment for mild cradle cap is daily washing with soap and water. You may want to try oiling the affected areas, shampooing the baby's scalp with an antiseborrheic shampoo, and scraping off the scales with a soft toothbrush.

If the condition does not improve, your baby's physician may recommend a medication to apply to the affected area.

Cradle cap usually is not a problem after the first few months of life.

INFANTILE ECZEMA

Signs and Symptoms
• Rough, red patches of dry skin.

Infantile eczema (atopic dermatitis) is a rough, red, patchy rash that usually is associated with extremely dry skin.

The body's reaction to an irritant, such as food, clothing, baby powder, or urine, eczema is more likely to occur in infants whose relatives have allergies. These infants have a tendency to have asthma and hay fever later in their lives.

If your infant has eczema, you may first notice light red or tannish pink patches of rough, scaly skin. The patches later become red. Typically, the baby begins to try to rub the itchy patches against the crib to ease the tremendous itching. The result is trauma to the skin, which causes it to ooze and crust. Infection may follow. (See color photograph of infantile eczema, page B-2.)

The most common areas for eczema are the cheeks and forehead. The problem may spread to the ears and neck.

Treatment.   If you suspect your infant has eczema, see your baby's physician. In some infants, the rash can be traced to diet or a change in formula. Sometimes the offender may be a laundry detergent, a fabric such as wool, or excessive perspiration during hot weather. Rarely, eczema is a symptom of a serious disease. Often the cause is hard to identify.

The main complication of eczema is infection of the lesions with a virus or bacteria. Infants with eczema should not be exposed to persons with cold sores (herpes simplex). To decrease the chances of more bacteria being introduced into the open skin, keep your baby's nails clipped as short as possible. If your baby will tolerate them, a pair of cotton mittens, worn especially during sleep when most of the scratching is done, helps prevent further damage and infection.

Treatment is geared toward avoiding the source of irritation (if one has been determined). Avoid extremes of temperature. Most babies with eczema do better in a warm climate with moderate humidity because sweating seems to aggravate the rash. The baby's clothing should be cotton. Avoid wool; a baby with eczema should not even lie on wool carpeting.

Keep baths to a minimum, and use bath oil to lubricate the dry skin.

If the eczema is particularly severe, your baby's physician may recommend that you apply dressings soaked in a special solution to ease the redness and itching. Corticosteroid lotions and creams can be applied after the dressing is removed. Antihistamines such as diphenhydramine and hydroxyzine are often effective for controlling the problem. If your baby's lesions become infected, antibiotics will be necessary.

Particularly when severe and persistent, eczema can be a frustrating problem for a new parent. Infantile eczema disappears in most children between the ages of 3 and 5 years.

BIRTHMARKS

Birthmarks in the newborn are common. Generally, they are of no concern and no therapy is required.

The following are some of the more common birthmarks that occur in newborns.

Milia are small white bumps or cysts on the newborn's face that resemble whiteheads. They are harmless and disappear without treatment. (See color photograph of milia and salmon patches, page B-2.)

Salmon patches (often called stork bites) are small, light pink, flat spots that appear on 30 to 50 percent of normal newborns. They are collections of small blood vessels (capillaries). Occurring most frequently on the eyelids, upper lip, the area between the eyebrows, and the back of the neck, salmon patches become more noticeable during crying bouts or when the temperature changes. Facial salmon patches eventually fade, whereas those on the back of the neck often persist but are usually not noticeable once the infant's hair grows.

Hemangiomas are benign (noncancerous) tumors made of newly formed blood vessels. Characteristically, hemangiomas are bright red, protruding, sharply demarcated lesions that may appear anywhere on the body. A *strawberry hemangioma* usually appears on the face, scalp, back, or chest, but it may be anywhere on the body. More common in girls, it is seldom present at birth, more often appearing within the first 2 months of life.

Most strawberry hemangiomas grow rapidly, remain at a fixed size, and then begin to disappear. Usually no treatment is recommended. In 60 percent of cases these lesions disappear by the time the child is 5 years old, and 90 to 95 percent disappear by the time the child is 9. Approximately 10 percent of children with this birthmark have some discoloration or a slight puckering of the skin after the mark is gone.

A *cavernous hemangioma* is more deeply situated than a strawberry hemangioma. It is typically a red-blue spongy mass made up of tissue filled with blood.

The outcome of this lesion is hard to predict. Some lesions disappear on their own. Sometimes the corticosteroid medication prednisone is helpful for treating the lesion.

A *port-wine stain* is a flat hemangioma that consists of dilated blood capillaries; the face is the most common site. The size of the nevus varies; occasionally, half the body surface may be affected. This is a permanent defect. Laser therapy has become the treatment of choice, but it is most successful on adolescents and adults. (See color photograph of hemangiomas, page B-2.)

ERYTHEMA TOXICUM

Signs and Symptoms
• A rash characterized by white pimples or pustules on a red background.

An estimated 50 percent of full-term newborns (less in premature infants) develop erythema toxicum 1 to 3 days after birth. It generally appears on the face, trunk, and limbs and has the appearance of flea bites.

The cause is unknown. The rash is harmless and requires no treatment; it generally disappears in a few days.

THRUSH

Signs and Symptoms
• A thin layer of milky matter on, in, and around the baby's mouth.

An umbilical hernia is caused by a failure of the ring around the navel to close. This results in a soft swelling that may protrude further during coughing, straining, and crying.

Thrush is a mild fungal infection of the mouth that looks like whitish patches stuck to the inside of the cheeks and on the tongue and the roof of the mouth. If the white patch is scraped off, the skin beneath it looks inflamed and may bleed. Thrush occurs in healthy newborns. (See color photograph of thrush, page B-10.)

The Diagnosis.   A baby with thrush may have a sore mouth. The infant may show discomfort while nursing and even refuse to eat.

If you suspect your infant has thrush, consult the baby's physician. Often only a visual inspection is needed to make the diagnosis.

Treatment.   A healthy newborn generally can fight off the infection on its own, but treatment with an antifungal agent called nystatin four times a day will hasten the process, particularly if the thrush is extensive.

INNOCENT HEART MURMURS

At one time or another, most children have an innocent heart murmur. It is found frequently in newborns or after a child has had a fever, been anxious, or engaged in increased physical activity.

Most parents associate heart murmurs with serious heart problems. Although some heart murmurs are the result of congenital heart defects or infections such as rheumatic fever, an innocent heart murmur does not cause problems. Most children outgrow the murmur by the time they reach adolescence.

Innocent heart murmurs usually are discovered during routine examinations. Using a stethoscope, the infant's physician can hear the sounds made when the heart's ventricles contract and the heart valves open and close. If your child has a murmur, the physician hears an additional sound. There are several types of murmurs; each type creates its own sound, and the sounds vary in intensity.

If your baby's physician diagnoses an innocent murmur, do not be alarmed. Treatment is unnecessary. The tendency among some parents is to become overprotective of the child and, as he or she becomes older, forbid physical exertion. These precautions are not necessary.

UMBILICAL HERNIA

An infant with an umbilical hernia has a soft bulge of tissue around the naval that may protrude when the baby cries, coughs, or strains.

The problem is failure of the ring around the navel to close; as a result, a portion of the small intestine is allowed to slip through the umbilicus.

Umbilical hernia is more apt to occur in black infants and in those with a low birth weight.

Unlike other hernias, there is little danger associated with an umbilical hernia. Most that appear before the age of 6 months disappear by the time the baby is 1 year old. Operation is rarely necessary unless the hernia becomes progressively larger, fails to heal by the time the child is 5 years old, or causes an obstruction.

SPECIAL CONCERNS DURING THE NEWBORN STAGE

Most infants are born fully developed, healthy, and, after a few days, ready to be taken home.

Unfortunately, a few babies do not follow this pattern. For various reasons, some babies are born prematurely. Tiny and often with lungs and other organs that are not yet developed enough to function properly, these infants require special care, often for weeks or even months. Some babies are born with complications because of a disease that the mother has. And some babies do not survive for more than a few weeks or months.

The birth of a seriously ill or premature baby is heartbreaking. But today, the outlook is far from hopeless. The proliferation of specialized neonatal units for these ill newborns has been a dramatic force in improving their chances of survival.

The following section discusses infants who require specialized care.

PREMATURE BABIES

A premature baby is defined as one born before 35 weeks of gestation.

The word "premature" upsets many expectant parents, and it is true that not long ago the survival rates for premature infants were lower than those for full-term babies.

However, recent advances in the care of low-weight, premature infants have greatly improved the chances of survival. It is not an easy way to begin life, but more and more children are testimony to the fact that prematurity is a problem that can often be overcome successfully.

Many factors contribute to prematurity. Women who are undernourished, are anemic, or have little or no prenatal care are more likely to give birth prematurely. A history of infertility, stillbirths, abortions, and other premature births can increase the chance of premature birth, as can teenage pregnancy and smoking.

Often the stimulus for early labor comes from other factors. Premature separation of the placenta, uterine abnormalities, or a cervix that is too weak to bear the weight of the developing fetus are all associated with early delivery (see pages 209, 1092, and 205). In addition, urinary tract infections in the mother may predispose to a premature delivery.

To reduce the likelihood of premature delivery, seek early and regular prenatal care. If problems occur during pregnancy, contact your physician immediately.

A baby born too soon has not had time for adequate development of body systems that are essential to life. Thus, it is the role of the physician—often a neonatologist (a physician trained to care for sick newborns)—and the nursing staff of the neonatal intensive-care unit to allow the baby time to develop further in a protected environment.

As a rule, the longer the baby is in the womb, the better equipped it is to live outside, the fewer the complications, and the better the chances of not only surviving but also surviving with no long-term disabilities. Babies born after 26 weeks of gestation have a good chance of surviving.

Usually, although not always, the size of the baby is indicative of its age. For example, a baby born at 26 weeks of gestation is apt to be much smaller than one born at 32 weeks.

Although size is important, the older the gestational age of the infant at birth, the greater the chances of survival. Moreover, the younger the gestational age at birth and the lower the birth weight, the more likely the baby is to have a neurological or developmental handicap such as cerebral palsy, learning difficulties, or vision and hearing problems.

A host of problems seem to go hand in hand with premature birth. One of the biggest problems is underdeveloped lungs, a condition that results in hyaline membrane disease. This disease accounts for a significant percentage of all neonatal deaths.

An infant with hyaline membrane disease may have difficulty using its lungs properly to breathe. The result is severe respiratory distress. The smaller or more premature the baby, the more likely it is that hyaline membrane disease will be present. Boys have this disease more often than girls, and white babies are affected more often than black babies.

If your baby develops this disease, it usually becomes evident soon after birth. He or she will require constant monitoring and administration of oxygen through a tube placed down its windpipe (trachea). The goal is to maintain adequate oxygen exchange, blood circulation, and nutrition while allowing the baby's lungs to develop. In most cases, this occurs within 10 days to 2 weeks. (For a more detailed discussion, see Respiratory Distress Syndrome, this page.)

Other problems associated with premature birth include heart defects and other congenital abnormalities, pneumonia, low blood sugar concentration (hypoglycemia), anemia, and infection.

Babies born prematurely are taken to neonatal intensive-care units (see Respiratory and Intensive-Care Units, page 22), where they are placed in incubators to help conserve their body heat. The combination of very little body fat and underdeveloped mechanisms for regulating the heart prevents the premature infant from maintaining body heat.

Many premature infants have not yet developed the sucking reflex or are too weak to suck. These infants are fed through a tube inserted through their nostril or mouth into their stomach. Some premature infants have not developed digestive enzymes and must be fed intravenously.

After these beginning feedings are well established, these infants usually can be fed with a bottle containing either formula or milk pumped from the mother's breasts. When the sucking reflex is developed, nursing may begin.

The trend today in neonatal nurseries is toward greater parental involvement. Parents are encouraged to spend time with their infants and to stroke them even when tubes, wires, and other equipment make cuddling impossible. Whenever practical, parents are allowed to feed the child and to change a diaper. Some parents bring books and read to their babies, play music, or put pictures of themselves in the incubator.

Finally, one day your baby's physician will allow you to take the infant home. By now the baby may be weeks or even months old. This is an exciting moment but one that is often mixed with fear and anxiety.

Like countless other parents who have done it, you can too. You can be sure that your infant would not be dismissed from the hospital unless the physicians thought it was time. Moreover, you will be instructed fully on any special care the baby will require, and if you have any questions, help is only a telephone call away.

Try to relax. You have come through a difficult time. Now it is time to reap the rewards of parenthood.

RESPIRATORY DISTRESS SYNDROME

At birth, an infant must rapidly fill its lungs with air while at the same time clearing them of fluid. Simultaneously, the newborn must also increase the volume of blood in its lungs.

Somehow the newborn must breathe without the lungs collapsing every time they are expanded; most full-term infants are able to accomplish this because the lungs have had adequate time to develop fully. Many premature infants and even some full-term babies, however, have problems breathing.

Two types of respiratory distress occur in newborns: respiratory distress syndrome, which typically affects premature infants, and transient tachypnea (rapid, shallow breathing), which occurs in both premature and full-term babies.

Respiratory distress syndrome, also called hyaline membrane disease, is a major cause of death for newborns, accounting for a significant percentage of all neonatal deaths.

The severity of hyaline membrane disease correlates with the infant's gestational age and birth weight. Thus, the smaller and more premature the infant, the greater the chance the baby will have hyaline membrane disease. This disorder is rarely found in infants born at term.

The infant born with this disease has an inadequate amount of certain agents (called surfactants) in the lungs that help reduce surface tension and prevent collapse of the lungs' small air spaces every time a breath is drawn. Thus, greater pressure is needed to expand the lungs.

Respiratory distress syndrome generally is recognized within minutes after birth. In some babies the distress at birth is so severe that resuscitation is necessary. Symptoms include grunting, nasal flaring, and a dusky skin color. The baby's breathing is harsh and irregular. An x-ray of the lung and blood tests can establish the diagnosis.

If your child is born with respiratory distress syndrome, he or she will need to be in a neonatal intensive-care unit (see Respiratory and Intensive-Care Units, page 22), where vital signs will be monitored constantly. The baby will be placed in an incubator that is filled with warmed, humidified oxygen to aid breathing. Nutrition and fluids will be given intravenously.

Many infants with this disease require help in breathing. In such a case, a breathing tube may be inserted into the baby's trachea.

The goal in caring for infants with respiratory distress syndrome is to keep them complication-free until the lungs have had time to develop adequately. With the advent of special neonatal units and highly trained physicians and nurses, the mortality rate for these infants has declined steadily.

Transient tachypnea can occur after an uneventful vaginal delivery or cesarean section and in premature or full-term infants.

Infants born with this form of respiratory distress often have no symptoms other than rapid shallow breathing (tachypnea). In some babies the skin may have a bluish cast, which can be alleviated with small amounts of oxygen.

Unlike infants with hyaline membrane disease, these infants rarely appear severely ill. Moreover, most of them recover within 3 days.

Treatment often involves discontinuing feeding so as to avoid the aspiration of fluid into the lungs. Occasionally, intravenous feedings are necessary if the baby is breathing too fast to be fed orally. Usually no other treatment is necessary.

SUDDEN INFANT DEATH SYNDROME

Sudden infant death syndrome (SIDS) is the sudden and unexplained death of an apparently healthy infant.

Typically, the parents go to the baby's crib in the morning and find their baby dead. Sometimes the infant has had a slight cold but, more often than not, nothing seemed amiss when the parents put their baby to bed the night before. In most cases, an autopsy fails to establish the cause of death.

SIDS rarely occurs before 2 weeks or after 6 months of age, and the peak incidence is between the second and third months of life. The incidence in the United States is about 1 in 500 live births. Males are more likely to die of SIDS than females, and the syndrome strikes more often during cold weather.

The parents of a child who dies of SIDS are likely to be torn with grief and guilt. Common thoughts are, If only I had checked the baby during the night. . . . I should have known something was wrong. . . . I am responsible because the baby smothered under too many blankets.

The fact is that, although its cause remains unknown, experts do know what does not cause SIDS. A baby who dies under these mysterious circumstances did not choke, smother, or strangle. Nor was a slight cold the cause of death.

Researchers around the world are studying this perplexing syndrome and discovering that many of these children were not really as healthy as they appeared to be.

Some evidence now suggests that infants with SIDS may have had an abnormality of the central nervous system. Some also believe that infants who have prolonged breathing pauses during sleep (apnea) are more likely to die of the syndrome, although others have found no difference between the apnea of "normal" infants and the apnea of those who subsequently died of SIDS.

Although the cause remains elusive, physicians now know that certain infants

RESPIRATORY AND INTENSIVE-CARE UNITS

Babies born prematurely or who have a serious infection, a respiratory problem, or a major birth defect may require care in a neonatal intensive-care unit.

Any birthing place must be prepared to assist the newborn with problems at birth. For those hospitals or birthing places without a neonatal intensive-care unit, detailed arrangements should be made well in advance in case the need for transfer to such a unit arises.

Some hospitals have units equipped and staffed to handle all but the most serious cases; often one hospital in a particular area is designated as being the facility to which the sickest babies may be transported. The purpose of the intensive-care unit is to provide maximal care and monitoring of patients with life-threatening problems.

In the United States, the neonatal death rate has decreased substantially during the past 40 years, mainly as a result of vastly improved care for sick newborns.

The major elements of a neonatal intensive-care unit are the staff—neonatologists (physicians trained in caring for sick newborns), pediatric intensive-care nurses, and paramedical personnel; monitoring and alarm systems so that every vital sign of every baby can be watched; respiratory therapy and resuscitation equipment and drugs; access to physicians in every pediatric specialty, including surgery and anesthesiology; and 24-hour laboratory service.

If your newborn requires intensive care, the experience may seem overwhelming at first. Your infant will be placed in an incubator to conserve body heat and reduce the chance of infection from the environment. The baby will be connected to monitors that provide the nurses and physicians with information about heart rate, blood pressure, body temperature, and rate of respiration.

Depending on whether respiratory distress is present, the infant may be attached to a ventilator so that it can breathe through a tube inserted into its windpipe (trachea). The newborn may have a feeding tube through its nose or connected to a needle in a vein to provide liquid nutrition from a special container.

Important factors in the successful care of premature and ill infants are the skill and experience of the nurses and the number of nurses who care for these children. It is the nurse who provides most of the baby's care and informs the physician when something goes wrong. A typical neonatal intensive-care unit is crowded with nurses and it is not uncommon to see two nurses bent over one particularly sick baby.

Although an intensive-care unit is not the ideal place to begin your relationship with your newborn, parents are encouraged to spend as much time as possible in the unit. Even though you may not be able to hold your baby, eye contact, touch, and any other stimulation you can provide can be beneficial for both you and your newborn.

may be at greater risk than others, although infants who are not in this high-risk group also die of this syndrome. Premature or low-birth-weight babies, the babies of smokers or drug users, babies who have had a sibling die of SIDS, babies who have stopped breathing and then have been resuscitated, and babies with low Apgar scores (see The Apgar Test, page 7) are at higher risk.

In an effort to prevent SIDS, monitoring might be recommended for infants who are at especially high risk.

Little information is available, however, on which infants should be monitored and how useful monitoring is. Parents who opt for monitoring require special training in cardiopulmonary resuscitation and proper use of the monitoring equipment.

BRONCHOPULMONARY DYSPLASIA

Signs and Symptoms
- Rapid breathing;
- Wheezing;
- Coughing;
- Difficulty breathing;
- Bluish tinge to the lips and fingernail beds (cyanosis).

Bronchopulmonary dysplasia is a chronic lung disease that occurs in infants who have received high concentrations of oxygen and mechanical ventilator assistance during the newborn period. Often it is a complication of respiratory distress syndrome (see Respiratory Distress Syndrome, page 20).

Symptoms include wheezing, coughing, cyanosis (in which the lips and the fingernail beds turn blue), and difficulty breathing. Bronchopulmonary dysplasia often is suspected in infants with respiratory distress syndrome who do not recover quickly, and it is diagnosed from a chest x-ray.

If your infant has bronchopulmonary dysplasia, he or she will be hospitalized and monitored closely. Most infants recover slowly over several months. However, their lungs are somewhat fragile, and care should be taken to keep them warm and free of infection. These infants may require supplemental oxygen and medications such as theophylline to help breathing. Because their lungs tend to accumulate extra fluid easily, diuretics are used to help prevent water retention. These infants are at increased risk for infections (such as pneumonia) and must be followed closely. Therefore, your physician will want to examine your infant frequently.

CONGENITAL LOBAR EMPHYSEMA

Signs and Symptoms
* Persistent shortness of breath;
* Wheezing;
* Bluish tinge to the lips and fingernail beds (cyanosis).

Congenital lobar emphysema, also known as infantile lobar emphysema, occurs when air enters an infant's lungs but has trouble leaving. The lungs become overinflated, and air leaks out into the space around the lungs. In most cases, only one lobe is affected, usually an upper one.

Congenital lobar emphysema is almost always identified during the first 2 weeks of life. In most cases, no cause can be identified; the infant's lungs may not have developed completely or something may be obstructing the airway.

Symptoms include shortness of breath, wheezing, and sometimes cyanosis (the lips and fingernail beds turn bluish). A chest x-ray shows the overinflation of the lungs and may reveal a blockage of the air passage.

Treatment. In infants with no or only mild and intermittent symptoms, no specific treatment is necessary. However, surgical removal of the affected lobe may be necessary in some cases.

PNEUMOTHORAX IN INFANTS

Signs and Symptoms
* Increased activity;
* Shortness of breath;
* Rapid, grunting breathing;
* Bluish lips and fingernail beds (cyanosis).

Emergency Symptoms
* Sudden collapse.

Every infant is born with collapsed lungs. One of the miracles of birth is that, within a few breaths, the lungs inflate and the baby begins breathing. However, considerable pressure changes occur to inflate the lungs that first time. Occasionally the lungs do not immediately inflate all the way and the pressure changes cause small ruptures in the alveoli (air sacs) of the tiny lungs. These ruptures allow air to leak out into the spaces between the thin membranes (called pleura) lining the lung and the inner wall of the chest. If a large amount of air leaks into this area (called the pleural space), the lungs may collapse (pneumothorax) and breathing becomes difficult.

The Diagnosis. If a small amount of air leaks, the infant will have signs of increased activity, shortness of breath, and rapid, grunting breathing and may have cyanosis (bluish lips and fingernail beds). However, if a large amount of air leaks, the infant may collapse suddenly. Your physician may take a chest x-ray to try to identify where the leakage is occurring.

How Serious Is Pneumothorax?. Pneumothorax can be potentially serious if the lung collapses suddenly, but in most cases the leakage of air is small and the air is reabsorbed on its own.

Treatment. Sometimes no specific treatment is necessary. Occasionally, the pneumothorax can be corrected by giving the infant 100 percent oxygen to breathe for 1 to 2 hours. In the case of sudden collapse,

DRUG WITHDRAWAL IN INFANTS

The infant of a mother who took drugs frequently during her pregnancy may go through withdrawal at birth. Drugs that cause withdrawal in infants include narcotics (heroin, morphine, methadone), barbiturates (especially phenobarbital), analgesics (prescription pain medications), tranquilizers and sedatives, alcohol, amphetamines, and phencyclidine (PCP).

The infant whose mother was addicted to narcotics may show withdrawal symptoms within 72 hours after delivery. These symptoms include irritability, hyperactivity, sleep and feeding problems, diarrhea, vomiting, convulsions, a high-pitched cry, and increased depth and rate of respiration. If the mother was addicted to barbiturates, withdrawal symptoms in the infant may not appear until 7 to 10 days after birth. Symptoms include irritability, jitteriness, and fussing.

After birth, treatment may be required for the drug withdrawal syndrome. The infant is also at increased risk for problems resulting from retarded growth while within the uterus and from prematurity. The infant may need oxygen if it has difficulty breathing or if its respiration is depressed. If withdrawal symptoms are mild, they are treated simply by providing a quiet, comforting environment, with swaddling, gentle handling, and frequent feedings.

If symptoms are severe, drug therapy—usually consisting of phenobarbital, chlorpromazine, paregoric, or diazepam—may be required. The smallest dose possible to relieve the symptoms is given. After the newborn has no symptoms for several days, the physician will begin to decrease the dose until the child is no longer receiving any medication and the symptoms have disappeared.

Infants with drug withdrawal syndrome may be more susceptible to respiratory distress syndrome (see Respiratory Distress Syndrome, page 20) and to sudden infant death syndrome (see Sudden Infant Death Syndrome, page 21) and should be followed closely. Withdrawal syndrome is rarely fatal, but it may have long-term effects on the health and development of the child.

---

tube into the space between the ribs (chest wall) and the lung itself.

BABIES OF DIABETIC MOTHERS

Before the availability of insulin, many women with diabetes were too ill to conceive. Today, with improved maternal and prenatal care, more diabetic women than ever before are able to have babies.

Even so, if you are a diabetic, your child is at greater risk than one whose mother does not have diabetes. Children whose mothers have diabetes either before pregnancy or whose diabetes is a temporary result of pregnancy (gestational diabetes) have a higher mortality rate than do those whose mothers do not have diabetes. In addition, these babies are more apt to be born with problems such as respiratory distress and metabolic anomalies such as low blood sugar value (hypoglycemia).

If you have diabetes, seek the care of a specialist. Optimal care begins before conception. It is important for the diabetes to be well controlled, both before and during pregnancy, to minimize the risk of birth defects or other problems in the baby.

The degree to which the mother's diabetes is controlled correlates closely with the infant's outcome. With close monitoring of your diabetes by your physician, the large size and large head of infants born to diabetic mothers are less common than in the past.

Regardless of size, all babies of diabetic mothers should be initially monitored in an intensive-care unit. Blood sugar tests should be done within 1 hour after birth and then frequently thereafter.

In some infants, glucose will have to be given intravenously if the blood sugar value is too low after birth. These changes are temporary, and normal regulation is established within hours to several days (see Diabetes Mellitus, page 707).

---

the air that has leaked into the chest may need to be removed as an emergency procedure. This is accomplished by inserting a

---

GENERAL CARE

Many mothers discover that taking care of their healthy, happy newborn is quite natural: somehow, as if by instinct, you know what the proper approach should be for a given situation. Others are at a loss, afraid to make a mistake and afraid that they might endanger the well-being of the baby.

Regardless of how confident you are with your newborn, you should be aware of some everyday issues.

PROPER CLOTHING

Comfort and convenience should be the important features of any newborn's wardrobe. Keep in mind that it is not economical to buy too much of one item. You will be surprised at how quickly your newborn will grow. Thus, as a rule, try to stay away from newborn and layette sizes. There is no reason why a full-term newborn cannot wear clothing designated for babies 3 to 6 months old. Fit does not have to be perfect.

The following should give you an idea of the types of clothes you should have on hand when your newborn comes home. Of course, there are seasonal variations.

Knitted nightgowns are an essential part of the newborn's wardrobe. These usually have a drawstring at the bottom and mittens on the end of the sleeves that keep the baby from scratching himself or herself. Usually, three or four of these are adequate.

Stretch suits are comfortable for the newborn and can be worn day or night. Usually made of polyester, terry cloth, or cotton, they have snaps down one or both legs to make changing diapers easier.

Undershirts come in two styles: those that pull over the head and those that snap on. The latter often are preferred because they are easier to put on the newborn. Unless the weather is extremely cold, a short-sleeved, medium-weight undershirt usually is adequate.

Sweaters, usually made of acrylic, are useful in cool weather or to add extra warmth when the baby is out of bed. If you dress your baby in a sweater, make sure there is adequate room at the neck and that the buttons are sewn on securely.

A snowsuit, pram suit, or bunting is important if your infant will be taken out in cold weather. A bunting is a warm zippered bag in which baby is encased up to its shoulders. A pram suit or snowsuit is shaped like a pair of overalls and encloses the feet. These suits are usually made of warm, quilted, water-repellent material.

If the baby will be outside in cold weather, a cap is necessary. In the summer, a sun hat with a chin strap is needed if the baby will be in the sun any length of time.

Shoes are not recommended for newborns.

Booties and socks are useful for keeping the baby's feet warm in cold weather.

WHEN IS YOUR BABY WARM ENOUGH?

How can you tell whether your baby needs an extra sweater? The hands are not a good indicator of how warm a baby is because they tend to be cool even when the body is warm. The legs, arms, or neck are better indicators—but the baby's face is the best guide. If the infant is cold, the cheeks will lose all color. A cold baby also is very likely to be fussy.

Bedclothes should include fitted crib sheets (probably three to six), a mattress pad for protection, and two or three crib blankets, usually made of a combination of cotton and polyester. Cotton receiving blankets are not particularly warm as a covering but are good for swaddling the infant to keep the baby from kicking off the covers and for security.

Most parents are more likely to put too many clothes on their newborn rather than too few. Too many clothes can be detrimental because the baby's body loses its ability to adjust to climate changes and then becomes chilled more easily.

CAR SEATS

Not so long ago, parents thought that the safest place for their baby during a ride in the car was in someone's arms.

For all automobile rides, secure your newborn in an infant car seat that is fastened to the seat of your car.

Today, we know that a baby held in someone's arms is doomed should an accident occur. Even if the vehicle is traveling at only 30 miles per hour, a newborn will be ripped from your arms with a force comparable to that of falling from a three-story building. If you are not wearing a seat belt, the baby may be crushed between you and the windshield.

Many states have laws requiring that children be in a specially designed safety seat. Even if you live in a state that does not have such a law, a safety seat will be one of your most important purchases. Your baby should not leave the hospital without a car seat. In fact, some hospitals will not let a parent take an infant home unless they have a safety seat installed in the car. Many hospitals or civic groups either rent or lend safety seats for newborns.

A safety seat is designed to spread the forces of a crash over the child's entire body and to keep the child from being thrown out of the car or from striking anything inside the car. Although no one can predict the outcome of an accident, experts do know that an infant's chance of surviving even a serious accident is improved greatly when a safety seat is used properly.

Two types of safety seats are suitable for a newborn.

One is the infant safety seat designed for a baby weighing less than 20 pounds. It is installed so the baby faces the rear of the car when placed in the seat. This position is crucial because during a crash the back—the strongest part of the baby's body—absorbs the shock. The safety seat can be placed in the back or front seat of your car. Many parents, at least initially, like to put the seat in the front so that they can observe the baby while they are driving.

The other is a convertible seat that can be used from birth until the child weighs approximately 40 pounds. This seat can be converted from the reclining, back-facing position to an upright and forward-facing position when the child weighs about 20 pounds.

When you begin shopping for a safety seat, make sure you buy one that conforms to the Federal Motor Vehicle Safety Standard of 1981 or a later standard and that has been crash tested.

Whatever seat you choose, make sure you understand the instructions and then follow them. If the seat is not installed properly and used correctly, the baby does not have the benefit of its full protection.

INFANT CARRIERS

Infant carriers are inclined plastic seats and are useful for carrying the infant from place to place. The seat also is a good place to put your awake baby when your arms are full. If you decide to use an infant carrier, however, make sure you always strap the infant into it. Some parents put the seat on a kitchen counter or a high table so they can watch and talk to the baby; but the seat should never be placed on a high surface because of the danger of the baby falling. Instead, keep the seat on the floor or a low table. Make sure that any seat you buy has a large enough base so that it will not tip easily once your baby becomes more active. A car seat, not an infant carrier, should be used when the baby is riding in the car.

PACIFIERS

Should you give your infant a pacifier?

The answer to that question is somewhat controversial. Some physicians are adamantly against the use of pacifiers. Others believe that when used in moderation they can help quiet a baby; the key, they say, is to know when to throw the pacifier away.

There are several types of pacifiers. If you decide to use one, you will have to experiment to see which style your baby prefers.

Pacifiers generally are used to quiet a newborn. It is not known whether a pacifier quiets the baby because the sucking relieves some minor stomach discomfort or simply because it keeps the baby's mouth busy. Regardless, it works for many babies.

If you decide to try a pacifier, the most important thing is to use it properly. Do not pop it into your baby's mouth every time it opens. Do not let your baby or yourself become dependent on the pacifier. And take it away as soon as your baby's need for extra sucking is gone.

EXPOSURE TO SUN AND WIND

Parents often ask their baby's physician whether they can take their newborn outside. The answer is a qualified yes.

Babies love the motion of a ride in the stroller or carriage. You need not let winter keep you indoors as long as you bundle up the baby.

A baby can and should be exposed to some sunlight, but only in moderation. Direct sunlight contains ultraviolet rays, which create vitamin D in the skin, a vitamin necessary for growth of bones and teeth. Most babies also receive vitamin D supplements.

The main danger of sun exposure is sunburn. If a baby is left asleep in a carriage or stroller outside in the sun for an hour or two, the result may be a sunburn and overheating. The sunburn is not only extremely painful but also damaging to the baby's delicate skin.

Take into account the season and whether the area where the carriage is parked is partially shaded. An infant can take more sun on a cold winter day when the rays are not so strong than during the summer. Likewise, the closer you live to the equator, the stronger the sun's burning rays. Consider these factors before exposing your infant to the sun.

Most babies should not be out in the summer sun for more than 30 or 40 minutes. At the beach, where the sun is more intense, the infant should be in the shade whenever possible. Put a sun hat on your baby to protect its face. Although sunblock lotions are highly recommended for children and adults, they should be used with discretion for children younger than 6 months.

Do not allow your baby to become overheated. A flushed skin is a sign that your infant is too hot.

CARE OF THE EYES AND EARS

There is very little a parent has to do to care for the newborn's eyes and ears.

The newborn's eyes are bathed constantly by tears secreted by the tear ducts.

During the baby's bath, you can wash around your infant's eyes with a soft washcloth and plain water. Do not use soap or any other cleanser because it will irritate the delicate eyes. Never put anything in the baby's eyes.

Many newborns develop a slight inflammation of the eyes a few days after birth. This requires no treatment. If your baby's eyes are very red or pink, it is probably an infection and you should call the baby's

physician. Some parents may observe a white discharge from one eye. Typically, the infant awakens with the affected eye "glued" shut. The discharge may be due to a blocked tear duct. The lid is not being cleansed adequately by the ducts, and the result is a slight infection. A trip to the physician is warranted.

Your baby's ears also are easy to care for. The outer ear is the only part you need be concerned with during the baby's bath. Simply wash the ear with a soft cloth and mild soap. Do not be concerned about any wax in the ear canal. Wax is formed by the ears for protection. Parents should never attempt to remove the wax, nor should anything be inserted into the ear for cleaning purposes. If an excessive amount of ear wax makes it impossible for your physician to examine the child's ears, he or she will remove the wax with a special instrument.

Any blood or discharge from your infant's ears should be reported to the physician.

TRIMMING NAILS

Trimming an infant's nails—especially for the first time—can be intimidating. Thus, parents may put it off as long as possible. But infants whose nails are allowed to grow too long usually end up scratching themselves.

Select a good pair of scissors. Ideally, the scissors should have blunt ends to prevent injury to a squirming baby. Small manicure scissors work well. Some parents prefer nail clippers.

Trimming a baby's nails while it is asleep is probably the preferred way because the infant is still. However, access to the nails is difficult when the infant is lying down.

If you choose to perform the task while your infant is awake, do not expect cooperation. Babies usually start squirming the moment you bring the scissors toward them. That, of course, can produce a nervous parent who is understandably frightened of cutting the baby's finger instead of its nail. An effective method is to make this a two-person job. Have someone hold the baby's hand steady while you do the trimming.

FONTANELLE

Every baby is born with a soft spot (fontanelle) on the top of its head.

Your child's tiny skull consists of not one but several separate bones. Over the first year or two of life, these bones fuse to form a single protective bone mass. Until then, there will be a soft spot (fontanelle) at the main juncture of the bones.

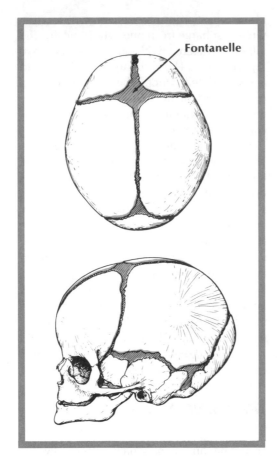

Fontanelle

During birth it is necessary for the baby's relatively large head to move down a narrower birth canal. To do so, the head must adapt itself to this smaller space. A completely formed skull could not do this. Thus, babies have a spot on the top part of the skull where four pieces of bone have not yet come together.

The size of the fontanelle varies. Generally, the larger the soft spot, the longer it takes to close. In some babies the bones come together by 9 months after birth; in others the process may take 2 years. The average is between 12 and 18 months.

New parents often are particularly concerned about this soft spot. Some mothers are afraid to shampoo the infant's hair for fear they will harm its brain. In fact, the baby's brain is well protected from normal handling by a membrane over the soft spot. This protective covering is as tough as canvas. Parents should not be afraid of inflicting damage by simply touching the top of the baby's head.

You may sometimes see the soft spot pulsing. This is nothing to be concerned about. However, if you ever observe marked bulging or if the spot appears to sink, especially if the baby is acting differently than usual, notify your pediatrician or family physician at once.

APPROPRIATE TOYS

A newborn infant does not need a room filled with toys. Does this mean then that your newborn does not need toys? No. A newborn placed in an empty crib with nothing to look at is going to be bored. The key is finding toys that are appropriate for the newborn's very limited physical abilities.

The word "toy" may not accurately describe what a newborn needs in that it implies a certain physical interaction that the newborn is not yet capable of. The baby cannot shake a rattle, cuddle a teddy bear, or spin the dials or pull the levers on a busy box attached to the crib. A cluttered crib may hinder baby's movements.

Although the newborn's physical abilities are limited, the baby has been born with the abilities to see, hear, touch, smell, and taste. In selecting toys, keep this in mind and find objects that will stimulate some of those senses. Even though the baby is not capable of shaking a colorful rattle, he or she can hear the interesting sound it makes when you shake it. It also can appreciate the color and pattern of a mobile hanging over the crib or the soft feel of a teddy bear's fur when you rub it against the baby's cheek.

What toys should a parent or prospective parent buy for the newborn?

Because your newborn spends a large portion of the day in bed, every effort should be made to make that environment as pleasant and as interesting as possible. Busy patterns rather than bright solid colors are more interesting to the young baby. Keeping that in mind, you can buy patterned sheets and bumper pad covers that give your baby something interesting to look at. Bedding with pictures of animals, colorful balloons, or geometric shapes is always preferable to plain-colored bedding.

Many parents buy a mobile to hang over the crib. Mobiles come in various styles. When choosing one, keep in mind the baby's perspective. Some mobiles may look great to parents who are seeing them at eye level, but there may not be much to see from baby's position in the crib. The most useful mobiles are designed so that the baby sees the mobile at its best. Some hang stationary, and others rotate and even play lullabies when you push a button. *Important:* Be sure to position the mobile out of the reach of your child; and it should be well secured.

A baby can appreciate music. Your newborn can enjoy a small music box in the nursery, a musical mobile, or even a radio playing soft music.

Some parents put small stuffed toys and animals in the crib, but do not expect the infant to pick them up and start playing. Again, any toy with an interesting pattern is going to capture baby's attention more readily than one without a pattern. If you do put stuffed toys in the crib, remember how soft they feel against skin and do not be afraid to let your baby feel them.

Several toys are designed to hang over infant seats or even car seats. Generally, these sets contain three or four colorful rattles or shapes. The newborn cannot reach up to grab these objects, but he or she can enjoy looking at them.

Walking into a toy store for the first time can be puzzling for the new parent. With thousands of toys to choose from, how does one make a decision? Most of the major toy companies indicate on the packages the age for which a particular toy was designed.

When you choose toys from a major company that are age-appropriate for your newborn, you can feel relatively confident that the toy is safe. However, you still should examine the toy to make sure there is nothing sharp or loose that could hurt the baby and nothing on which your child might choke.

BATHING

The first bath you give your baby probably will be the hardest. Many parents are terrified of bathing their baby, and babies rarely cooperate. Don't despair. Most hospitals give bath demonstrations in the newborn nursery. If not, ask your mother, another relative, or a friend for advice. After a time or two, giving a bath will be easy for you and enjoyable for your infant.

In the early months it may be more convenient to bathe the baby in the morning, usually before a feeding, because the baby is apt to be more alert then. Some mothers prefer the evenings, especially if the baby's father is on hand to help out.

How often you bathe the baby is up to you. Some physicians advocate daily baths, but others advise a bath every other day, particularly during the winter when a baby's skin is more prone to dryness. As long as the diaper area and the mouth are thoroughly cleansed daily, a baby can go several days without a bath.

The kitchen is an excellent place for bathing a newborn, especially in the winter, because in most houses it tends to be one of the warmer rooms.

Placing a tiny, slippery baby in an adult-sized bathtub can be difficult and uncomfortable for parents. Thus, many parents buy a baby bathtub that can be placed in the kitchen sink or in the tub. Large bowls or washbasins also can be used. If you do not feel comfortable with even the small tub, you can give the baby sponge baths initially. Many physicians recommend sponge baths until the baby's navel is healed (see page 32).

The trick to bathing a baby is to have everything ready ahead of time. Never leave the baby unattended in the tub for even a few seconds. The bathtub can be an extremely dangerous place if a baby is left alone, even if it contains only a small amount of water. A parent should *never* leave a baby alone in the bathtub. Let the telephone or doorbell ring. Do not let anything take your attention away from your infant. Hence, advance planning is important. Here are the items you will need: soap, washcloth, towel, cotton, lotion or powder (not necessary but it smells nice), clean diaper, undershirt, and sleeper or nightgown.

While bathing your newborn, support the baby's head with your wrist and place fingers of that hand in your baby's armpit. Never leave your child unattended in the bath, even for a moment.

After you have run the water in the tub (fill it to a depth of only an inch or two), touch the water with your elbow or wrist to make sure it is not hot. It should feel comfortably warm but not hot. Some parents prefer using a bath thermometer. If you have one, the temperature should be between 90°F and 100°F.

Undress the baby. Support its head with your wrist and place the fingers of that hand in its armpit; then place the baby in the tub. First, wash the face with a soft, wet cloth but no soap. Use a piece of cotton soaked in plain water to wipe around the baby's eyes. A shampoo is necessary only once or twice a week. For the scalp, use a mild soap or baby shampoo. Wipe the suds off the scalp with a damp rag. Do not pour water over the baby's face.

After the face is washed, soap the rest of the body. Most parents find it easier to soap the skin with their hand rather than a washcloth because the other hand is holding the baby. Wash the diaper area last.

When the soap has been rinsed away, hold your baby with both hands and move it to a soft bath towel. If the navel is still not healed, your baby's physician may want you to swab it with cotton soaked in alcohol.

After the baby is dried, you may want to use a lotion or powder. Lotion can help if the baby's skin is dry, and powder is good for a baby whose skin chafes easily. Neither is necessary most of the time. If you choose to use powder, never dust it directly on the baby because the particles can irritate the lungs. Instead, apply some to your hand (away from the baby) and gently pat it on thinly. Do not use baby oil. It can cause skin problems.

SELECTING A CRIB

The crib you choose should have slats that are less than 2⅜ inches apart, a mattress

that fits snugly, a locking mechanism that keeps the sides up, and no sharp edges. There should be at least 26 inches from the top of the rail to the mattress when the mattress is set at the lowest level. Most cribs on the market today meet these specifications. However, if someone has given you an older crib, measure the slats; if they are more than 2⅜ inches apart, the crib can be dangerous, especially if the mattress does not fit perfectly. Babies have been known to strangle as a result of getting their heads stuck between the slats. Another potential danger of an old crib is that it may have been painted with a lead-based paint. Make sure this is not the case. Infants sometimes chew the slats of their cribs, and lead-based paint, when consumed, can harm health (see Lead Poisoning, page 76).

Bumper pads should be used in the crib to prevent the baby from banging against the sides. A pillow is unnecessary and should not be used.

DIAPERS

The two basic types of diapers are disposable and cloth.

Disposable diapers are the choice of many parents because of their convenience; the diaper is worn and then thrown away. Disposable diapers come in various sizes and thicknesses. A disposable diaper is easy for even the most inexperienced parent to put on a baby because it is prefolded and secured around the baby with adhesive tape rather than pins. Parents who use these diapers do not have the age-old worry of sticking their newborn with a pin.

Despite their convenience, however, disposable diapers are not without their problems. One is cost. Babies diapered with disposables also have a higher incidence of diaper rash than those who wear cloth diapers. The final disadvantage is that they fill up your garbage can. Follow the disposal instructions.

If you choose to use cloth diapers, buy the largest size. Cloth diapers are made of several materials, including cotton, gauze, and flannel.

You can launder them or you can hire a diaper service. Those who choose to wash the diapers themselves—the most economical method—should buy at least 2 dozen, more if you do not want to be tied to the

---

DON'T LEAVE YOUR BABY ALONE

Leaving your baby alone, in the house or outside, is an invitation to trouble. An infant, or any young child, should never be left alone in the house. If you cannot find a trusted babysitter, take the baby with you. Some new parents take turns going out.

There is no mystery to changing a cloth diaper. First, fold the diaper approximately in half. Second, fold it again, this time on the diagonal, into a triangle. Third, position your baby on the diaper and pin the corners together carefully.

washing machine every day. You will need a covered diaper pail, partially filled with water, to put used diapers in. Empty bowel movements into the toilet and rinse the diaper before putting it into the pail. Diapers should be machine washed with a mild soap or detergent and rinsed two or three times. Rinsing is important. A diaper with soap residue on it may irritate your baby's skin.

If you hire a diaper service, the service will deliver sterilized diapers to your door and pick up the used ones (stored in a container) for about the same cost as disposable diapers.

When you put in the pin, slip two fingers between the baby and the diaper to avoid sticking the infant. Sometimes it helps to soap the pin so that it slides through the diaper more easily.

Some parents change their infants at least once and often twice during a feeding—usually at the beginning and at the end. This frequent changing is not really necessary unless the baby has had a bowel movement. Changing the infant after a feeding is usually adequate.

When changing a baby who has had a bowel movement, use a disposable wipe or a washcloth with soap and water to clean the area thoroughly. A girl should always be wiped from front to back to avoid getting stool bacteria into the urethra (a common cause of urinary infection).

PREVENTION OF DISEASE

Most of the medical care a newborn infant receives is geared toward the prevention of disease.

In most hospitals, newborns are kept in a nursery to limit the risk of infection that can come from exposure to people.

Occasionally, bacteria in the birth canal cause serious eye infections in a newborn. Therefore, immediately after birth, every newborn's eyes are protected with erythromycin ointment or silver nitrate drops.

An injection of vitamin K is given to prevent hemorrhage. In addition, tests for PKU (phenylketonuria), galactosemia, and a deficiency of thyroid hormone will be done (see Required Screening for Newborns, page 8).

Most hospitals prohibit anyone but the parents from unrestricted and unlimited contact with the infant, in part as a means of protecting the newborn from infection.

It may be wise to continue to limit your newborn's exposure to outsiders for awhile after you leave the hospital. In particular, avoid crowds. Remember, fever and other illnesses that may be considered minor in the older baby may be cause for alarm during the first month of life.

It is crucial that all infants be seen by a physician on a regular basis. Before your release from the hospital, your physician will discuss this schedule with you. Generally, the first follow-up visit occurs when the baby is about 2 weeks old. Some pediatricians or family physicians recommend monthly visits during the first year of life; others want to see the baby every 2 months, provided everything is going well.

CIRCUMCISION

Not long ago, male infants were circumcised routinely shortly after birth. It was believed that circumcision—the surgical removal of the foreskin of the penis—helped prevent problems such as penile infection and cancer because a circumcised penis could be kept cleaner than an uncircumcised one.

Today, however, physicians know that circumcision usually is not medically necessary. Good hygiene offers the advantages of circumcision without the potential risks. Thus, most circumcisions today are performed for cultural or religious reasons.

In considering whether to have your infant son circumcised, consider the pros and cons.

One of the advantages is that the glans (the end of the penis) is easier to keep clean. Also, a small percentage of males have to be circumcised because of problems that surface later in childhood or even adulthood.

The disadvantages include the possibility of complications, even though circumcision is a relatively easy procedure. Complications include bleeding that may require a dressing and occasionally stitches or an infection that may result in scarring and injury to the penis. Also, the procedure is painful.

If you choose not to have your son circumcised, be assured that the foreskin is easy to clean. Understand, however, that at birth the foreskin is firmly attached to the glans. Over time—an average of 3 years but often longer—the foreskin separates from the glans. Do not attempt to retract the foreskin during cleaning or you could cause an injury.

Clean the uncircumcised penis as you would any other part of your newborn's body. Simply wash the genitals thoroughly with a soft washcloth and soap and water. Rinse thoroughly.

As your child grows and the foreskin separates from the glans, you can teach him the importance of keeping clean. The foreskin should be retracted and the surface underneath cleaned during the daily bath or shower.

CARE OF THE UMBILICUS

The infant's lifeline to its mother is the umbilical cord. During its 9 months in the uterus, the baby receives its nourishment through the blood vessels of the cord. At birth, however, that connection is severed because it is no longer needed.

All that remains of the cord is a small stump, about an inch long, cut close to the infant's body. The cord begins to wither and separate, the raw area becomes covered by a thin layer of skin, scar tissue forms, and, in most babies, the cord drops off within 12 to 15 days after birth.

Most of the time the care of the umbilicus is relatively easy. Many physicians advise parents not to cover the area because this may impede healing. The cord should be kept dry. When diapering the newborn, fold over the top of the diaper so it does not cover the navel. This will allow it to stay dry.

Some physicians recommend sponge baths until the cord has dropped off. Others do not mind if you bathe your infant, provided you wipe the navel dry with sterile cotton.

In addition to these instructions, your baby's physician may advise you to clean the area several times a day with a piece of cotton dipped in alcohol. Do not simply swab delicately around the end of the stump. Gently pull on the stump and swab around the base of the navel. This procedure will help keep the area clean and will discourage infection.

Until the cord completely heals, infection is possible (although rare) because of the ease with which bacteria can enter the body through the opening. If your infant's navel area looks inflamed or there is any discharge, call your baby's physician. If the area is infected, medication and probably hospitalization will be needed.

Some babies develop small growths in this area, called umbilical granulomas. If your infant has a granuloma, the healing process is delayed. You will notice that the cord area looks dull red or pink and moist and there may be an unpleasant-smelling discharge.

Initially, the physician may recommend cleaning the area several times a day with alcohol. If the granuloma persists, your physician can cauterize or seal the cord with silver nitrate.

STERILIZATION

Remember the stories of your mother boiling all the utensils that a baby would use? Today, that is thought unnecessary.

The tap water in most communities is safe and bacteria-free. Bottles, nipples, caps, and baby's other feeding equipment can be washed with soap and hot tap water, rinsed in hot water, and allowed to air dry. They also can be run through a dishwasher.

Once it is in a nursing bottle, milk should not be stored for more than a few hours, and then only in the refrigerator. Discard milk in half-empty bottles.

Inform your physician of any bleeding from your baby's umbilicus.

PSYCHOSOCIAL DEVELOPMENT OF PERSONALITY AND BEHAVIOR

A newborn does not arrive as a "blank slate," as was once believed. Rather, from the moment of its birth, your newborn is unlike any other person ever born.

Some babies are quiet, some are noisy. Some stay awake for as long as 90 minutes after birth; others fall asleep within 15 minutes. Some suck better than others. One baby prefers visual stimulation; the newborn in the next bassinet may prefer sounds.

From one normal baby to the next, the variations are enormous. It is important, however, to be able to recognize the abnormal and to foster, reinforce, and recognize the changes, development, and various behaviors of your newborn.

NORMAL DEVELOPMENT

Your baby starts life with traits inherited from generations of your family. The events during pregnancy and birth are also important for shaping the infant. Did the mother eat well? Did she refrain from smoking, consuming alcohol, and taking drugs? Were labor and childbirth normal, or were there complications? These and other factors influence the person your baby is and will become.

A crucial factor in the development of your infant's personality is the relationship between parents and child. Love and affection are as critical to the infant's emotional survival as food is to the body's well-being. An infant deprived of human love and attention will wither emotionally and also often physically (see Bonding, page 34).

Your infant is a social creature from the beginning. Research has found that newborns prefer looking at figures that resemble human faces rather than at other pictures. Some scientists believe that a baby has an inborn tendency to perceive the human face as a source of potential reward. In addition, a newborn infant seems to prefer a female's voice.

During the first month your infant probably will show a preference for familiar persons. Babies also tend to form attachments based on the kind of stimulation they prefer. For instance, if your baby loves action, the aunt who rocks him or her may be preferred to the one who sings.

Do not be surprised to see your infant smile. Initially, the infant's smile is usually in response to something internal and is seen when the baby is sleeping or drowsy. Between the third and fifth weeks of life, however, most babies have their first social smile, typically in response to a face or voice. This is an exciting moment for most parents.

Your baby is born a mimic. Stick your tongue out and the newborn repeats the action. By the time most babies are 4 weeks old, they begin to make small throaty noises—their first attempt at conversation.

Your newborn responds positively to comfort. A crying baby often will quiet when picked up by familiar hands. The baby searches out its mother's face, makes eye contact, and then stops crying. The baby cries when wet or hungry and quiets when the diaper is changed or the bottle or breast is given.

Sometime during the newborn period you will notice that your baby is expressing a new emotion: enjoyment. For many babies, this is first seen in the bath. A crying infant may stop when put in the bath, relax, smile, and then begin crying (out of disappointment) when the bath is over.

Excitement is another emotion that emerges during the first month. Usually the source is a person or toy. Your baby may move its arms and legs, pant, coo, and even smile at you or at a particularly interesting object.

A newborn does not yet distinguish between actions and their results. Things seem to appear and reappear. By the time your baby is 1 month old, however, you will notice the infant begin to repeat actions for its own pleasure. Your baby may thrust out its legs, like the way that feels, and do it again to regain the good feeling.

A 1-month-old infant is beginning to take a little control over its environment. For example, your baby may discover that sucking its thumb or mouthing its fist is comforting. During a crying spell, you may see the baby pop its fist into its mouth. A moment later, things are quiet.

An infant's early weeks are consumed by adaptation. In the first few days of life, the infant begins to communicate and interact through signals. The baby is hungry, the baby cries, and then mother appears with food. The baby is wet, the baby cries, and the diaper is changed. It is through these and similar exchanges that the attachments between parent and child are formed. The infant learns that its needs will be met by someone who cares.

Thus, it is impossible to overemphasize the importance of security and consistency to the newborn. For normal emotional development, the infant must learn to trust, and trust can be learned only when a parent or parent-figure responds to the baby's needs in a prompt and loving manner. Infants who do not receive this responsive care learn that they have no influence over their environment. The results can be lifelong hostility, anxiety, the inability to develop close relationships, and other emotional problems.

BONDING

The bonding (nurturing) between parent and child begins long before the baby is born.

A couple discovers that the woman is pregnant. They begin to look through books for a name for their child. They furnish a nursery. They hear their baby's heartbeat on a visit to the obstetrician. They plan and dream, worry and hope. And finally the day arrives. After the effort of labor comes the greatest reward.

Bonding is the complex array of emotional ties and commitments that characterize the parent-child relationship. By the time a baby enters the world, there is already a strong emotional link on the parents' part, a link that is stronger for some than others. Over the course of the next few months, the infant begins to develop an attachment to the person or persons with whom it learns to associate protection, love, and guidance.

If your baby is healthy, bonding begins immediately. Most babies have an alert period for an hour or two after the delivery, making it a particularly good time for the parents and child to begin to know one another. It is not known whether the bonding between humans has a critical period. However, the key is not *when* it happens but that it *does:* it is most important that the bonding eventually take place.

How does a parent go about bonding with an infant? There is no easy recipe for bonding, just as there is no way to tell someone how to love. Bonding occurs during the day-to-day exchange of affectionate actions between parent and child.

A mother gently touches her infant, and that touch is pleasurable to the new baby. When the baby's cheek is touched, the infant turns toward the mother's face or toward the breast and begins to nuzzle and lick the nipple. This not only stimulates the production of milk but also is a powerful emotional stimulant. The baby gazes into the mother's eyes during breast- or bottle-feeding. The infant cries and the parent picks the baby up, strokes its cheek, and speaks in a soft and soothing voice.

The importance of bonding is well recognized by hospitals and health professionals. Thus, most hospitals give new parents almost unlimited opportunities to spend time with their newborn. If, however, your infant is born prematurely or is seriously ill, the situation is different. Your baby will probably be placed in an incubator and connected to machines that monitor its vital signs. Intravenous and feeding tubes may be present.

You may not be able to hold or even feed your infant. However, you will still be encouraged to spend as much time with your newborn as possible. You can stroke the baby's skin, hold its tiny fist, and soothe its cries with your voice. It is not the ideal bonding situation, but even this limited contact is important for both you and your baby and your ultimate relationship.

Once you bring your baby home from the hospital, the bonding process continues. In the hospital, a nurse often was the one to respond when the baby cried. Now, you are the one on duty. Whether breast- or bottle-feeding, you are feeding the infant every 2 to 4 hours, during which time you are cuddling, stroking, and providing comfort as well as nourishment. The infant may cry when picked up by someone other than you. You may notice after a few weeks that your infant recognizes your voice and quiets in response to it. The colicky baby cries, you spend hours walking the floor, and the baby learns that someone cares. These all are ways in which, over the course of the first few months, you and your baby form the life-long bonds that are the basis for the normal and loving parent-child relationship.

It is not uncommon for parents to wonder during pregnancy whether they will be able to love this new person who is about to enter and change their lives. Even after birth, many a parent has looked at the newborn expecting to feel a rush of love and, instead, felt nothing or, worse, disappointment or even dislike.

Do not be too hard on yourself if you do not immediately love your infant. Parenting is never easy, and at times it can be downright trying. Love for your baby comes gradually. Again, as you bond with the child, as the three of you get to know each other, as you see the baby's eyes light up when you come into the room, or when the infant smiles at you for the first time, you will find yourself loving your baby.

INFANT REFLEXES AND RESPONSES

Your newborn's movements are governed by reflexes. Stroke its cheek and the baby will root and try to suck. Prick the soles of its feet and the knees and feet flex. Make a sudden noise and your baby's head drops backward, its neck extends, and its arms and legs swing outward and sharply back.

All normal babies are born with predictable reflexes that disappear in a predictable order as the voluntary motor functions take control. However, the absence of reflex responses may indicate a possible neurological problem. Part of your newborn's first examination in the hospital includes attempts to elicit various reflexes and responses.

The reflexes and responses found in the newborn at birth are described below. All normal newborns should exhibit these responses, although they may be more subdued in a sleepy or recently fed baby.

The *Moro reflex* is one of the most frequent and dramatic newborn responses; it occurs when your infant hears a loud noise, has an abrupt change in position, or is handled roughly. The infant startles, arches its back, and throws its head back. At the same time, it throws out its arms and legs and then brings them abruptly back toward its body. The infant cries, then startles, and then cries because of the startle.

To calm your baby, apply steady but gentle pressure to any part of its body. In addition, if you hold its arm firmly flexed at its shoulder, the baby should calm down. The Moro reflex generally disappears by the third month of life.

Stroking your infant sets off several responses. The baby will grasp your finger when you stroke the palm of its hand *(palmar grasp)* or sole of its foot *(plantar grasp)*. The more premature the infant, the more reluctant it is to let go. Stroke the top of its foot or hand and the infant withdraws the limb, arches, and again grasps your finger. The palmar grasp disappears at age 6 months, and the plantar grasp continues until 10 months of age.

Rooting and sucking are two of your infant's important reflexes. Stroking the baby's cheek produces the rooting reflex. The baby turns toward the stroking object and begins to root for the nipple. The sucking reflex follows and can be initiated by stroking the baby's mouth, the inside of which is the area most sensitive to this reflex. Sucking and rooting reflexes usually stop by the time the infant is 4 months old. However, they can be produced in a sleeping infant until the seventh month.

The *tonic neck reflex* is seen when your baby is on its back and its head is turned to the side. The infant arches its body away from the face side, the arm on the face side extends while the other arm flexes, and the legs are drawn up.

Although present in newborns, this reflex is more prominent in the 2-month-old infant. It usually disappears by the sixth month.

The *orienting response* of your newborn is a response to a change in the environment. If, for example, the infant hears or sees something new, it becomes more alert and less active. Its head may turn toward the stimulus and its heartbeat changes. If the infant is adapting to a familiar stimulus the heartbeat slows; when the stimulus is unfamiliar the heartbeat accelerates.

An infant is able to protect itself because of several responses and reflexes. Because of a strong *gag reflex,* your newborn infant is able to spit up mucus to help clear its windpipe. If a part of the infant's body is exposed to cold air, its entire body changes color and temperature, its limbs are pulled in close to its body to reduce the exposed surface, and it begins to shiver and cry in an attempt to stay warm. In addition, a strong *blink reflex* protects the newborn's eyes from glaring light.

Your newborn does not like pain any more than you do and will do whatever possible to avoid it. If the baby's leg is hurt, for instance, it will pull the leg away. If that does not work, the other foot will attempt to push you away.

Even though your newborn's reflexes will disappear—most of them during the first year of life—their usefulness seems to be more than short-term. Studies indicate that your baby's brain stores information learned from these early reflexes. For example, when infants try to right themselves, this act,

even though unsuccessful, probably contributes to their development of the concept of space. Similarly, the strong tonic reflex helps a baby learn to use both sides of its body separately and to use its hands voluntarily rather than instinctively.

TWINS

"Twinship" is the closest of all human relationships. Twins need very little encouragement to remain close. As parents, the best gift you can give your twins is a sense of identity. Use their names frequently. Take pictures individually. Spend time alone with each child. These are just a few ways to strengthen their sense of uniqueness.

Caring for two or more babies can be physically and emotionally overwhelming for both new and experienced parents. Here are tips that will help ease your daily responsibilities and help preserve the quality of family life.

Attend to your own needs of adequate rest and good nutrition. Keep meals simple, and take naps often. This will help give you the energy you need to meet the high demands of caring for twins.

Share the workload. Cooperative parenting lightens the load for both parents. Working parents sometimes can shorten workdays during initial weeks to help out at home.

Give special attention to other siblings, and share general household duties.

If ever there was a time for a babysitter or parent's helper, this is it. Grandparents, neighbors, student nurses, and even school-aged helpers may enjoy the opportunity to share in this special experience. Call on them. Their help allows you some relief and personal time, and it is essential as routine activities such as grocery shopping and going to the post office become much more difficult tasks. These helpers also give your children opportunities to develop early social skills and foster outside relationships.

It is easy to be so involved in the daily demands of these two infants that you may overlook persons, organizations, or professionals that can offer assistance or advice. Other parents of twins are a natural source of practical advice. Some communities offer support groups for parents of twins. Pediatricians, psychologists, psychiatrists, and social workers often have special interests in, and valuable advice concerning, the more specific problems of nurturing twins.

SLEEPING PROBLEMS

The average newborn spends more time sleeping than on any other activity.

Your 1-week-old newborn spends about 80 percent of the day sleeping, in seven or eight daily naps. By the time your infant is 1 month old, sleeping time may be reduced to three or four daily naps and one 5- or 6-hour stretch of sleep at night.

The newborn not only sleeps more than you do but also sleeps differently. Newborns are light sleepers, and they catnap rather than sleep in long stretches. Studies of brain waves of infants during sleep have shown that a newborn spends at least half of its sleep time in restless sleep and 20 to 30 percent in deep sleep. Once the baby is 8 months old, it spends more time in deep sleep and less in restless sleep.

Most sleeping problems occur after the newborn period. However, the following are some that may develop during the first month of life.

Fussiness at bedtime may occur. Some babies sleep soundly during the day and then want to stay up all night. No one fully understands why some babies are more fussy at night, although colic may sometimes be the cause (see page 13).

You can try several things to get your baby to sleep at night. A pacifier may work. Try swaddling the baby in a receiving blanket. Some babies are happier in confined places, so try putting the infant to sleep in a bassinet or infant carrier rather than the crib. A ride in the baby carriage or the car settles some infants at bedtime (some infants, however, wake up the minute you lift them out of the car). A hot water bottle in the baby's bed also may help (make sure the bottle is not uncomfortably hot to the skin by touching it to your wrist first).

Difficulty in falling asleep may be the result of too much stimulation. When some babies have been awake longer than usual, are in a strange place, or are surrounded by strangers, they become tense and cranky. The result can be difficulty in falling asleep. Some babies simply need to cry in order to fall asleep. New parents often have a hard time understanding this. Instead of putting the baby to bed crying, they try walking, rocking, or feeding the infant, which usually serves to make the crying worse than ever.

If your crying baby has been awake for longer than usual, has been fed, and is dry, assume that he or she wants to go to sleep. It is not wrong to put a crying baby to bed. Initially, the infant's cries may intensify, but often after a few moments they slowly die down until they cease altogether. At any rate, give the infant a chance to go to sleep. If after 15 or 20 minutes the infant is still frantically screaming, pick it up.

Chronic resistance to sleep may have its origins during the newborn period, but it usually does not manifest itself until the infant is 2 or 3 months old.

Often babies who develop this problem have had problems with colic. Because of colic attacks they have spent more time awake than the average baby, usually being carried or rocked by the mother or father. One day the parents notice that the colic has subsided but the infant still expects the parents' attention at night. The result is a nightly struggle between parents and child.

Once parents realize what is happening, the only thing they can do is to put the child to bed at a reasonable time. Expect the infant to protest, loudly at first. After 20 or 30 minutes of crying, most babies give up the fight and fall asleep. Sometimes it takes several nights of crying before an infant will willingly accept sleep.

Some experts recommend you set a time limit—say 15 or 20 minutes—after which you enter the nursery, reassure the infant that everything is all right, and leave again without picking up the baby. The next night wait an additional 5 minutes before going to the infant.

HEARING

Babies are born with a sense of hearing. The normal newborn will blink and startle in response to sound and can distinguish differences in volume. Soft noises may produce something akin to a smile, whereas harsh or loud sounds may cause the infant to cry. Moreover, your newborn already has developed sound preferences, favoring a high-pitched voice such as mother's over lower pitches.

Hearing is essential in the acquisition of speech and language. Even a minor hearing loss can have a major impact on your infant's ability to understand and later to communicate with language.

Some newborns are in a high-risk group for hearing loss. They include infants who do not spontaneously begin breathing within 10 minutes after birth; those whose Apgar scores are between 0 and 3 (see pages 20 and 7); those born with infections such as rubella, syphilis, and herpes; those who have head or neck defects, severe jaundice, or a family history of hearing loss during childhood; and those who are born very prematurely.

The incidence of severe hearing loss in both ears among neonates with any of these conditions ranges between 2 and 5 percent.

Four types of hearing loss are found in infants and children.

Conductive hearing loss involves some type of interference with the external ear's ability to receive sound or with the transmission of sound from the external ear to the inner ear. The most common causes of this type of hearing loss are congenital abnormalities of the ear and ear infection. This type of hearing loss often can be treated with medication or operation.

Sensorineural hearing loss results from abnormalities of the cochlear hair cells within the ear or the auditory nerve. More than 50 percent of severe sensorineural hearing loss is hereditary, and other causes are severe jaundice, infection while in the uterus, and bacterial infections of the pharynx.

Sensorineural hearing loss is usually permanent.

Mixed hearing loss occurs when a child has both conductive and sensorineural hearing losses. This type of loss may be severe. Medication or operation or both may help restore a portion of the child's hearing loss.

Central auditory disorders result from a problem in the central auditory nervous system, the ear's nerve linkage with the brain. Children with these disorders can hear sound but only as a jumble of noise.

Before your baby is dismissed from the hospital, your physician routinely will test to detect abnormal responses. If a newborn's hearing loss is not detected during the first days of life in the hospital, it may not be discovered until the infant is 18 to 24 months old, when parents become concerned that the child's language is delayed. By this time, the child already has passed a critical period for language acquisition.

Thus, it is important that even a minor hearing loss be detected in infancy so that the proper steps can be initiated to avoid problems the loss can cause.

If your newborn is thought to be at high risk for hearing loss, hearing tests should be done while the baby is still in the hospital or arranged for in follow-up evaluations. Two tests currently are used: 1) observation of the infant's response to noise and 2) a special test (auditory brainstem-evoked responses), which can check for loss in one ear.

However, none of the current hearing tests used on newborns detects slight hearing loss or minimal loss that will progress as the child grows. Thus, if any hearing loss is suspected, your infant should have a follow-up hearing test between the ages of 3 and 6 months (see page 67).

Certain types of hearing loss can be corrected. When the loss is due to ear infection (see Acute Ear Infection, page 680), for example, antibiotics can eradicate the infection and the ear can function normally. Operation sometimes corrects congenital malformations of the ear.

Programs that help parents communicate with their deaf or hearing-impaired infants also are available in many communities. Parents are taught how to make the most of any hearing the child has and to acquaint the child with visual language through signing or lipreading.

VISION

At birth, your infant's eyes are about three-fourths the size of what they will be at adulthood. The white part of the eye (sclera) has a bluish tinge, and the colored part (iris) is usually a nondescript blue in whites and dark in other races. The pupils in the newborn are small and may not constrict readily in response to light. The eyes do not always appear to move together.

Your baby probably will keep its eyes shut much of the time. This does not mean the infant cannot see. In fact, physicians now know that babies see immediately after birth, although hazily. Your newborn will try to focus on objects held in front of its face. If the light is farther than 8 to 12 inches away, the image is hazy and the baby's eyes may wander, each in a different direction.

The newborn is attracted to patterns more

than to colors. Most interesting of all to the newborn is the human face, usually its mother's.

Your newborn's first eye examination occurs in the hospital, where the physician will examine its eyes closely and observe their response to light. Most infants are slightly farsighted, although some babies, particularly those born prematurely, are born nearsighted (unable to see objects far away). As the normal infant grows, its eyes change and become able to see both near and far objects more clearly.

Some infants are born with partial or total loss of vision. Common causes include developmental malformations, damage to the eyes due to infection, birth trauma, a significant loss of oxygen (hypoxia), and genetic diseases that affect the eye itself or the nerves to the brain's vision center.

Until the mid-1950s, the leading cause of blindness in infants was retrolental fibroplasia (now referred to as retinopathy of prematurity). This occurred when small or premature infants were given high concentrations of oxygen in incubators to help them survive. In some, this resulted in partial or total blindness.

Retinopathy of prematurity sometimes occurs today in very premature infants with low birth weight who survive because of advances in technology and neonatal care. Fortunately, blindness is less frequent as new understanding of this problem is gained and better treatments evolve.

The physician may notice immediately that the infant is partially or completely blind. There may be dense cataracts, the eyes may be abnormally small (microphthalmia), or the cornea may be opaque. Sometimes, however, the defect lies not in the eye or optic nerve but in the brain itself, requiring neurological evaluation and studies such as computed tomography or magnetic resonance imaging (see pages 1286 and 1287).

If a severe problem is not apparent in the infant's early days in the hospital, how does a parent know that something is wrong with the baby's vision? The first clue may be what is called nystagmus—the rapid movement of the baby's eyes. The baby's eyes suddenly may begin to move up and down, side to side, around and around, or a combination of all three movements. Another common sign is the baby's inability to develop skill in properly aligning both eyes on an object.

One eye fixes on an object, and the other deviates. The baby may squint and appear to be cross-eyed. As the baby grows, you may notice that he or she appears to be timid about crawling or seems unusually clumsy. Contrary to what many believe, an infant will not outgrow crossed eyes. Any baby with crossed or deviated eyes should be examined by an ophthalmologist (see page 750).

Treatment for congenital partial or complete blindness depends on the cause. Sometimes a defect can be corrected surgically. Cataracts, for example, can be removed. Whether or not vision is restored depends on whether the infant has other vision problems and whether they can be corrected.

Sometimes blindness is permanent. If your child is born blind, your pediatrician or family physician can direct you to social and community agencies that may be able to offer information and help in rearing a visually handicapped child.

BEHAVIOR MANAGEMENT

Many parents wonder whether you can spoil a newborn.

A century ago the prevailing wisdom was that a newborn could be spoiled and that it was easy to do so. Infants were put on strict schedules and handled only when absolutely necessary. If a newborn cried for any reason other than hunger or a diaper change, the wails often were ignored. No one wanted a spoiled child.

Today, physicians believe that it is unlikely that a newborn can be spoiled. The written-in-stone schedule has been cast aside in favor of a flexible schedule that takes into account the needs of each baby and the family into which it is born. Parents are encouraged to cuddle their child. Physicians advise parents to meet the immediate needs of the newborn, whether it be for food or comfort. In essence, enjoy your baby.

A baby's emotional needs are as important as its body's needs. Even a newborn needs affection. He or she needs comforting when in pain, needs to see a smile in order to return one, and needs to learn that someone cares about its wants and will fill them. A parent who does this will not spoil the newborn. One who does not may spoil the child's chances of emotional security.

Even though you should not worry about spoiling your newborn with too much attention, be aware that sometimes behavior patterns emerge during the newborn period that can backfire in the third or subsequent months of life, the result being a spoiled baby whose parents have become virtual slaves to their child's whims.

This sometimes occurs with infants who have been colicky. Night after night you walk the floor with your colicky newborn. For most infants, the colic passes by the third month. Your infant too seems to have weathered this uncomfortable period. The infant's abdomen is no longer distended and the child doesn't appear to be uncomfortable. Yet every evening when you put the baby in the crib, the screams start (see page 13).

The infant has learned how good it feels to be held and walked. Some would say this infant is slightly spoiled. To keep a slightly spoiled infant from becoming a very spoiled one, you might try being a little less eager to please. Put the infant to bed, say goodnight, and do not run immediately to the rescue when the baby begins to wail (see page 80).

Unlike the older infant, a newborn's environment and response to that environment are extremely limited. You are months away from having to worry about your child hitting a playmate, sticking its finger in an unprotected electrical socket, or telling you an emphatic "no."

Rather, the newborn's behavior is in response to its immediate physical needs. The typical newborn spends most of the day sleeping, interrupted by a need to eat every 2 to 4 hours. In between, it may spend a good part of the day crying.

Parents often worry that their child is not eating the correct amount, is not sleeping enough, or cries too much.

To some degree, a parent can manage the behavior of the newborn. However, you may first want to determine whether the infant's behavior is really upsetting or whether it is simply different from what you had expected. For example, most newborns sleep most of the day, but your infant is awake for several hours a day. Does this behavior in itself bother you or are you just concerned that it is not normal? When in doubt about so-called normal behavior, ask your physician.

Although the trend is toward letting the infant set the schedule, a parent can have some input. You are not the only one who has some adjustments to make; your newborn must adjust to being part of a family.

For example, you need not always let your baby dictate the feeding schedule. If your infant wakes at midnight for a feeding but you like to go to bed at 11 p.m., try waking the baby up before you go to bed. You can try to give the prior feeding a bit earlier so that the baby will be hungry when you wake him or her. Most babies do not mind being awakened for a feeding if it has been 3 or 4 hours since the last meal.

Parents can influence an infant's feeding schedule and help the baby learn to increase the time between feedings. If you automatically awaken the infant because a certain number of hours have elapsed since the last meal, the baby will learn to be hungry at that time. Similarly, if the infant wakes up between feedings and you rush in to feed him or her, you establish a pattern. Instead, wait a few moments and see whether the baby goes back to sleep. If not, try delaying the feeding with a pacifier or some water.

You also can help the infant establish sleep patterns. If it is best for you to put the infant to bed after a feeding, do it and be consistent. Moreover, do not make the common mistake of tiptoeing around the house whenever the infant is asleep. The baby will get used to this abnormal quiet and awaken at the slightest noise.

Often, especially for first-time parents, the worst thing about a baby's behavior is crying. Babies cry for various reasons. The infant may be hungry, wet, colicky, sick, tired, or simply unhappy. To some degree, you can help manage your infant's crying by responding to the baby's needs. Offer food when the infant is hungry or change a diaper when it is wet. Some babies need to cry in order to fall asleep. If nothing else works, try putting the infant to bed. Listening to a crying child, especially when it is your child, is difficult, but try to refrain from picking the baby up right away. Give it a few minutes to go to sleep.

Most important, realize that time does improve the situation. In a couple of months the crying spells should cease, and your infant will be much more responsive and generally much more pleasant to be around.

In the meantime, despite frayed nerves,

try to keep your cool. A crying baby can be unnerving, but you must *never* handle an infant roughly. Shaking or any other rough behavior can cause irreparable damage and even death. It might be best to ask for "time-out" and get out of the apartment or house for a short time while the baby is under the care of someone you trust.

NUTRITION IN THE NEWBORN

Your goal in feeding your newborn is to help the baby grow at an acceptable rate and to avoid any deficiencies that cause health problems.

Unlike the older baby, the newborn does not have a varied diet. If you are breast-feeding, your baby will be nourished by breast milk. If you are bottle-feeding, your infant will be given formula, usually a combination of specially processed cow's milk, vitamins, and minerals mixed with water. The formula closely approximates the natural composition of breast milk. Whichever method you choose, milk and water (if your baby wants water) are all that a healthy newborn needs to thrive.

Regardless of whether the source is mother's milk or formula, the following are the components of the basic diet of the newborn.

Water is absolutely essential for human life. Water accounts for 70 to 75 percent of your newborn's body weight, compared with only 60 to 65 percent of an adult's body weight. To remain healthy, an infant must take in larger amounts of water per unit of body weight than an adult. The daily amount of water required is between 10 and 15 percent of the infant's body weight, whereas in an adult the requirement is between 2 and 4 percent.

Fortunately, the water content of both breast milk and formula is very high. Some babies like to have water from a bottle between feedings, although water itself is seldom needed unless the baby has a fever or diarrhea or the environmental temperature is high. If the infant is feeding well, the amount of water being ingested is adequate.

A *calorie* is a measurement of the energy content of food. Everything we eat and much of what we drink contains calories. The distribution of calories in human milk and formula is similar: between 9 and 15 percent of the calories come from protein, 45 to 55 percent from carbohydrates, and 35 to 45 percent from fat.

Protein is essential for growth and for the repair of cells. Most of the major body organs are composed mainly of protein. If the body does not receive an adequate amount of protein, it begins to break down its muscles to supply protein to the brain and to make enzymes. An infant, or anyone else, deprived of protein for a long enough period will develop lethargy, a distended abdomen, and swelling. The result can be death.

Carbohydrates supply most of the body's energy needs. If the body has an inadequate carbohydrate intake, it improvises by using protein and fat for energy. Carbohydrates are stored in the liver and muscles. The infant's reserve is a fraction of that of the adult.

Fats are a concentrated source of energy. They help protect body organs, vessels, and nerves, provide insulation against changes in temperature, act as a vehicle for the absorption of some vitamins, and delay the time it takes for the stomach to empty, thus giving one a "full" sensation. Although it is important for adults to limit their fat intake, infants and young children should not be on a fat-restricted diet.

Minerals are important to the structure and workings of virtually every part of the body. For example, calcium and fluoride are necessary for the formation of strong bones and teeth, copper is required for the production of red blood cells, and sodium is needed to maintain the water balance in the body.

Vitamins are substances required by the body in minute amounts if every organ is to work properly. Some of the necessary vitamins include vitamin A, which is needed for the eyes and to keep the linings of the bronchial, urinary, and intestinal tracts healthy; vitamin C, which is needed for the development of bones, teeth, blood vessels, and other tissues; and vitamin D, which is also needed for the development of bones and teeth.

Although it is helpful for a parent to understand the rudiments of nutrition, the newborn's diet is simple. If you are breast-feeding your infant, the baby is getting the most complete food known. If you opt to feed your infant formula, your physician will recommend one that will provide the nutritional ingredients that satisfy its needs. (A supplemental vitamin may be prescribed, including fluoride to prevent the development of tooth decay.)

Parents often want to know how one can tell whether an infant is eating enough. The best rule is to trust your baby. He or she knows how much food is needed. When you offer the breast or bottle, your baby will eat as much as is needed, regardless of how much is left. When it is time to eat again, the baby cries.

If a baby does not get enough to eat, you will soon know it. He or she screams until you offer more food. An infant who needs more food than is being given will awaken more at night and will decrease rather than increase the time between feedings. Moreover, these infants finish their milk to the last drop and still do not seem satisfied. You may even observe the baby chewing his or her fist.

Some parents make the mistake of trying to overfeed the baby. Again, the infant will eat as much as is needed. When the baby stops feeding, do not push further feeding, even if you think it is not full.

The best indication that your baby is receiving the necessary nourishment is weight gain. Some babies gain weight slowly, and others gain it rapidly. Sometimes slow weight gain can be attributed to illness, but often nothing is wrong, although a slow gainer may require more visits to the pediatrician or family physician to make sure nothing is amiss. Sometimes these babies will gain weight if you offer more feedings.

As a rule, the average baby gains 2 pounds a month during the first 3 months of life. Most babies who weigh about 7 pounds at birth (the average weight of a newborn) have doubled their weight by the fifth month.

COMMON FEEDING PRACTICES

You have three options when it comes to feeding your newborn: breast, bottle, or a combination of the two.

A generation ago, breast-feeding was not the norm for many American women. Today, it has become a popular method, and it is believed by many to be the ideal feeding method because of its nutritional advantages and its enhancement of the mother-child bond (see page 43).

Even so, some women who decide to breast-feed need more flexibility than that method normally allows. Thus, they also introduce the infant to the bottle. If you want to supplement one or more breast-feedings a day with a bottle, you can pump your breasts and store the milk, which later can be given by someone else. Have your physician demonstrate the proper procedure for pumping your breasts. Or you can use formula, although this is not recommended for more than one or two daily feedings because your milk supply will be diminished.

Many parents prefer, and physicians recommend, that the newborn be allowed to set the schedule of feedings—at least to some degree. This method takes into account the differences in babies. Many newborns may be content to be fed every 4 hours, whereas other infants may demand a feeding every 2 or 3 hours.

Even if your infant has been on a 3-hour feeding schedule, the rules may suddenly change; he or she may shorten the time between feedings to every 2 hours. In short, a parent should be prepared for some ups and downs at feeding time during the first month of life.

Many breast-fed infants are allowed to nurse for the first time immediately after birth. Although a mother's milk does not fill the breasts until the third day after birth, bonding between mother and child is facilitated and the infant gets the health benefits of the mother's colostrum, a lemon-colored breast liquid believed to be beneficial in protecting the baby against some diseases.

If you choose to breast-feed your infant, you should know that breast milk is digested more easily than formula, the result being that you will be feeding more often than a mother who bottle-feeds. Do not be surprised if initially you are feeding the baby every 3 hours and sometimes every 2 hours.

It is important for a nursing mother to learn to relax. This enhances the ability of the "let down" reflex to fill your breasts with milk. Make sure you are comfortable, either lying down or sitting in a comfortable chair, preferably with an armrest. Support the baby comfortably with its face held close to your breast with one arm while the other hand supports the breast so the nipple is easily accessible to the infant's mouth. Make sure the nipple does not cover the baby's nose.

Nursing time per breast varies. Most physicians recommend that you start nursing gradually. Five minutes a side is generally a good start. Some babies can empty a breast in that time, but it may take more leisurely eaters 20 minutes a side. At any rate, half the milk is drained within the first 2 minutes and 80 to 90 percent within the first 4 minutes.

Be certain to empty at least one breast at each feeding, otherwise it will not be stimulated to refill.

Initially, a nursing mother may have sore nipples. Keep your nipples as dry as possible. Rubbing small quantities of lanolin on the nipples (after, not before, nursing) can help prevent cracking.

Your diet is important if you choose to nurse. Be wary of taking any medication unless approved by a physician. Avoid smoking and excessive alcohol intake. Lactation is

BOTTLE-FEEDING VERSUS BREAST-FEEDING

Which is better—bottle-feeding or breast-feeding?

Many pediatricians and family physicians recommend breast-feeding whenever possible. However, for various reasons, some mothers either cannot or do not want to breast-feed. If you opt to feed your newborn formula, do not feel guilty. Today's formulas are nutritionally sound. A bottle-fed baby is as well fed as a breast-fed infant.

Why, then, the preference for breast-feeding? Over the years the pendulum has swung back and forth on this issue. In the past, women often shunned breast-feeding in favor of the bottle. Today, many have embraced breast-feeding wholeheartedly.

With breast milk, the newborn gets a natural food. If the mother's diet is nutritionally sound, breast milk is all the baby needs for the first few months of life, with the exception of fluoride and vitamin D. These two items usually are given as supplements. The milk is fresh, free of contaminating bacteria, and readily available. Rather than preparing a bottle in the middle of the night, a nursing mother

The debate is forever: breast-feeding versus bottle-feeding, which is best? Your baby can thrive on either method.

only has to take the baby from the crib and put it to her breast.

A big advantage to breast-feeding is that breast milk contains antibodies. It is believed that a breast-fed infant receives some protection against viruses. A mother who breast-feeds does not have to worry about her infant being allergic to her milk.

Some believe that another advantage of breast-feeding is a psychological one. The mother is more personally involved because she is nourishing her child and gaining a feeling of accomplishment. Furthermore, the intimate contact between mother and child enhances the relationship. This is not to imply that a bottle-feeding mother and her child cannot establish the same closeness.

Nursing a baby has its disadvantages. In some ways, bottle-feeding is easier. The mother does not always have to be there for her baby. A babysitter can feed the baby, and the baby's father can help with feedings in the middle of the night so that the mother can rest.

Whatever method you choose—breast or bottle—you should know that studies have shown little difference in growth rate between infants fed breast milk and those given formula. Your baby can thrive no matter what method you choose.

not the time to begin a diet. If you are nursing you are expending hundreds of extra calories in the production of milk.

Most bottle-fed babies have their first feeding within 6 hours after delivery. A bottle-fed baby probably will want between six and nine feedings in a 24-hour period by the end of the first week of life.

The setting for bottle-feeding is similar to that for breast-feeding. A bottle should never be propped up against the infant. Rather, the parent should take the time to hold the child closely and give it the feeding.

The formula should be warmed to body temperature and the temperature tested by dropping a bit on your wrist. A word of caution: do not warm the bottle in a microwave oven. The formula can become very hot and severely burn your infant. A bottle-feeding may last from 5 to 25 minutes, depending on the eagerness and sucking ability of the infant.

Both bottle-fed and breast-fed babies should be burped after a feeding.

FEEDING PROBLEMS

The newborn period can be fraught with problems related to feeding the infant. Maybe your infant simply will not eat—or at least not as much as you want it to. Perhaps the baby falls asleep in the middle of a feeding and then wakes up an hour later screaming to be fed. Some babies do not gain weight.

An important step in dealing with an apparent feeding problem is for the new parent to relax. If your baby has had an off day or two, he or she is not going to starve. When you bring your infant home from the hospital, your pediatrician or family physician will prescribe a vitamin supplement, particularly if you plan to breast-feed, in the form of drops to be given daily. The drops contain fluoride and vitamins such as C and D that are in short supply in breast milk. So even when the infant eats poorly, some important nutrients are still being given.

Some common feeding problems are described below.

The infant who does not seem to eat enough may, in fact, be eating plenty. The average 2-week-old newborn takes between 2 and 3 ounces per feeding; by 3 or 4 weeks, the baby usually has increased the amount to between 4 and 5 ounces.

Do not expect your infant to eat the same amount every day at every feeding. Babies are like everyone else; they are hungrier on some days than on others. Trust your infant to know how much to eat. Do not force food on the infant or feeding problems may result later.

The infant who falls asleep during a feeding and wakes up crying before it is time for the next feeding may be hungry or simply need to be burped. If the baby's intake was just a little under the usual amount, the problem is probably not hunger but an abdominal upset. Many physicians advise trying to let the baby go back to sleep without an additional feeding. If that does not work, offer the breast or bottle again.

The infant who is underfed is an unhappy baby who is restless, cries a lot, may be constipated and unable to sleep, and fails to gain weight. This infant may be emptying the bottle or breast and still may not be getting enough.

The problem may be solved by simply increasing the number of feedings per day, enlarging the size of the nipple holes in the bottle so the infant gets more milk with every suck, or trying a different type of nipple. Deficiencies in vitamin and mineral intake may need correcting.

When an infant is overfed, it may regurgitate. Generally, most infants refuse to take more than they want. Sometimes, however, an infant will succumb to a well-intentioned parent's plea to eat more.

Many babies spit up or even vomit after a feeding. Spitting up is normal, but vomiting is not and may indicate a serious problem. Spitting up can be reduced by burping the infant after every feeding, handling the baby gently, placing the infant on its right side or abdomen after a feeding, and keeping the infant's head lower than the rest of the body immediately after a feeding (see Vomiting and Spitting Up, page 14).

Loose stools are the norm for breast-fed infants. If the mother uses laxatives or eats food with laxative properties, the baby's stools may become even looser. Although bottle-fed babies have firmer stools, even their stools may become loose, especially if they are overfed or if the sugar content of the formula is too high.

Mild diarrhea due to overfeeding usually can be treated by decreasing the amount of breast milk or formula and even eliminating one or more feedings altogether.

Constipation rarely occurs in breast-fed infants. Parents should not be concerned if their infant misses a bowel movement. This does not signify constipation because the consistency of the stool, and not the frequency of bowel movements, indicates constipation. A baby who passes hard, pellet-like stools is constipated.

If the constipation is present from birth, your baby's physician will want to examine the infant's rectum to make sure there is no obstruction or congenital abnormality. If your formula-fed infant becomes constipated, it may be due to an inadequate food or fluid intake. Increasing the amount of sugar or fluid in the formula should alleviate the problem (see page 70).

Failure of the infant to gain weight can be cause for alarm. The average baby gains 2 pounds a month; your infant may gain more or less. If your infant is not gaining weight at all or is losing weight, your pediatrician or family physician may want to try another formula if you are bottle-feeding. If you are breast-feeding, your pediatrician or family physician may want you to supplement your breast milk with one or two daily feedings of formula.

Your infant's rate of growth may simply be slower than average. However, if the baby seems hungry all the time, slow growth may be an indication that the infant is not getting enough to eat and some feeding modifications should be made.

GENETICS AND GENETIC DISORDERS

Will the child have blue or brown eyes, be short or tall, be chubby or thin? Will this new person's skin burn easily in the sun or take on a golden hue when exposed to sunlight? Will it be a boy or a girl? Will the child be healthy or have a birth defect or genetic disorder?

The answers to these questions are determined by the interaction of the genes (the biological units of heredity) with the social and physical environments in which the child develops.

Genetics is the study of heredity. It is concerned primarily with the study of the origin of the characteristics of the individual and their transmission to offspring. Medical genetics is the branch of human genetics concerned with the relationship between heredity and diseases.

At conception, the mother's egg (ovum) is penetrated by the father's sperm. The ovum and sperm, called germ cells, each contain 23 chromosomes. During the process of fertilization, the union of sperm and egg produces an individual with 46 chromosomes.

Each chromosome contains many genes. The genes determine many of your offspring's characteristics, which are passed from one generation to another. Usually this occurs uneventfully. Sometimes, however, unexpected changes or genetic defects occur. Although most causes of genetic defects in humans are largely unknown, various environmental agents, such as radiation,

viruses, and chemicals, are among the factors that have been identified.

The three basic categories of genetic defects are the single mutant gene, abnormalities of the chromosomes, and multifactorial disorders.

A *single mutant gene* is one discrete unit of genetic material that is defective. A disorder caused by the transmission of a single mutant gene shows one of three simple patterns of inheritance: 1) autosomal dominant, 2) autosomal recessive, or 3) X-linked.

The term autosomal is applied to a gene present in any chromosome other than a sex chromosome, and the term dominant applies to a gene that produces a recognizable defect if passed to the offspring from one parent. The risk of passing an autosomal dominant mutant gene to an offspring is 50 percent. The term recessive refers to a gene that does not produce a clinical effect unless both of the pair of genes are abnormal. Thus, a disease with autosomal recessive inheritance occurs only if an abnormal gene is received from both parents. The risk of passing an autosomal recessive mutant gene to an offspring is 25 percent. Diseases such as cystic fibrosis, sickle cell anemia, phenylketonuria, and color blindness are caused by mutations of single genes.

The genes responsible for X-linked disorders are located on the X chromosome. The female has two X chromosomes, and the male has only one X chromosome. An

TAKING THE FAMILY HISTORY

A genetic evaluation can be very helpful for family planning, especially for couples who already have had a child with a birth defect or who have a family history of a birth defect or a genetic disease. Such couples often are unsure whether they should have a baby. Sometimes the couple has no family history of birth defects but, because of the relatively advanced age of one or both of them, they might seek information about diagnostic tests that are available for the detection of possible defects in unborn babies. Detection of possible defects in unborn babies is important because some genetic disorders can be treated.

The first requirement in a genetic evaluation is an accurate diagnosis. A family history will be taken. The first step is to obtain information on the index patient—the person who has brought the family to the attention of the specialist in genetic or inherited disorders. This specialist is called a medical geneticist. In addition, information will be obtained on all first- and second-degree relatives of the index patient (that is, grandparents, aunts, uncles, cousins, parents, siblings, and offspring). This information includes the given name, surname, maiden name, birth date or current age, age at death, cause of death, and name or description of any disease or defect.

The second step is to ask questions designed to survey the family for the presence of a disease or a defect, such as the following.

1. Does any relative have an identical or similar trait?
2. Does any relative have a trait that is absent in the index patient but that is known to occur in some people with the same disease? The answers to this question give the medical geneticist knowledge about the manifestations of a given disease.
3. Does any relative have a trait that is recognized to be genetically determined? The purpose of this question is to determine the occurrence of an inherited disease in the family, even though the particular patient may not be known to be affected.
4. Does any relative have an unusual disease, or has any relative died of a rare condition? The purpose of these questions is to identify a condition that might be genetically determined although it is not recognized as such by the person giving the history.
5. Are any blood relatives married to each other?
6. What is the ethnic origin of the family? Persons of certain ethnic origins have increased chances of specific genetic diseases, such as sickle-cell disease in African-American blacks, cystic fibrosis in persons of northern European descent, and Tay-Sachs disease in Ashkenazi Jews.

important feature of all X-linked inheritance is the absence of transmission of the trait from male to male (that is, father to son). An X-linked trait cannot be transmitted from father to son because the father's Y chromosome, and never the X chromosome, is transmitted to his son. Alternatively, the male's X chromosome always is passed to a daughter.

Chromosome abnormalities result from the lack, excess, or abnormal arrangement of one or more chromosomes, which may produce either an excess or a deficiency in genetic material. Birth defects caused by abnormalities of the chromosomes occur in about 1 in 250 newborns. Moreover, in about 50 to 60 percent of early miscarriages, the fetus has a chromosome abnormality.

Down syndrome is an example of a chromosome abnormality. Chromosome abnormalities usually cause multiple defects, including various combinations of growth retardation, mental deficiency, skeletal disorders, and defects of vital organs.

Multifactorial inheritance is the process whereby abnormal genes interact with environmental factors to produce a congenital defect or disease. No one knows how many genes are involved. Some researchers believe that the genes are harmless under normal circumstances. However, in combination with certain environmental factors these genes can cause abnormalities in the developing baby. Some of these environmental factors include drugs ingested by the mother during pregnancy, alcohol, and maternal disease such as diabetes; in most cases, the external agents are not known.

Many of the common chronic diseases of adults, such as essential hypertension, coronary artery disease, diabetes mellitus, peptic ulcer disease, and schizophrenia, and also many of the common birth defects (such as cleft lip and palate, spina bifida, and congenital heart disease), long have been known to run in families. These fit best into the category of multifactorial diseases.

Most of the common birth defects, such as cleft lip or congenital heart defects, usually have a relatively small risk of recurrence—about 3 to 5 percent. However, in some families the risk could be much higher. Disorders caused by single mutant genes tend to have a much higher risk of recurrence—25 to 50 percent—but in some cases the risk could be almost 0. After carefully analyzing the family history and the nature of the birth defect or genetic disease, a geneticist usually can give the parents a fairly precise estimate of the risk of recurrence. Laboratory tests can determine whether a parent is a carrier of an abnormal chromosome. Similarly, they often can detect the carriers of single-gene disorders.

After a cause is established and you have more information about the defect and its chances of being transmitted to your child, you can decide whether to attempt pregnancy.

Sometimes parents blame themselves if their infant is born with a malformation or is mentally retarded. The mother may wonder, for example, whether the medication she took for an infection during pregnancy is responsible. Some medicines are known to cause defects; others are thought to be safe. In general, it is best to avoid any unnecessary drugs during pregnancy, particularly during the first 3 months. Sometimes, however, the medicine is necessary because, if untreated, the mother's illness would be more detrimental to the developing baby than is the medication.

The following pages discuss several birth defects.

ABNORMAL HANDS AND FEET

The Hands. *Congenital absence of a part or all of the upper extremities* is more common than absence of a part of the lower extremities. A child may be born with only part of one finger missing, or an entire arm may be absent.

A newborn with only one hand should be seen in a specialized facility as soon as possible. Once the baby is able to sit, a prosthesis, usually a paddle, can be fitted to allow the child to function as if it had two hands. If a prosthesis is not fitted early, the child develops one-handed patterns that are nearly impossible to break.

Polydactyly is the presence of an extra finger or fingers, most commonly a fifth finger or extra thumb. This defect is more common in black newborns. Frequently, the extra digit consists of skin and soft tissue and can be removed easily. However, if the extra finger contains bone or cartilage, removal may require operation on adjacent

structures, which can best be performed after the infant is a few months old.

Syndactyly (webbing) of the fingers, unlike syndactyly of the toes (see page 48), is best treated surgically. Because the bones in the fingers are of various lengths, the joints of the fused fingers do not line up and the fingers are difficult to use. If operation is not performed, the child will never acquire significant use of the fingers.

Camptodactyly is the permanent and irreducible flexion of one or more fingers. This is usually congenital and most often affects the little finger.

Clubhand is the rare absence of the radius (the bone on the thumb side of the forearm) or the ulna (the larger bone, on the opposite side of the forearm). Treatment involves stretching the soft tissues of the arm during infancy. Operation is then necessary to reposition the bone. However, retaining the new position is a problem. Several operations during childhood may be necessary.

This defect is associated with a higher incidence of cardiac disease and blood problems.

The Feet. The newborn's feet are proportionately longer and thinner than those of the older child, and the joints of the ankle and foot are extremely flexible. Although the feet often may appear to be in abnormal positions, there is rarely cause for concern because these minor problems resolve in time.

Both polydactyly (a congenital deformity of the hand in which the newborn has an extra finger) and syndactyly (webbing of the fingers) can be effectively treated surgically.

Your baby's feet may occasionally seem to be in an abnormal position, perhaps in-toeing as shown here. This common, minor problem rarely requires treatment.

In-toeing and *out-toeing* are common problems in which the foot or leg turns inward or outward. The condition is aggravated when the infant sleeps face down. They are usually positional or postural deformities that correct spontaneously with growth and development. They rarely require treatment.

Webbing (syndactyly) of the toes is rarely more than a cosmetic problem. The scars and contractures of operation may be more unsightly than the webbed toes. In contrast to webbed fingers, webbed toes usually function normally.

Clubfoot, which occurs in 1 of every 1,000 births, is the term used to describe several congenital foot abnormalities in which the foot is twisted out of shape or position. In about 95 percent of cases of clubfoot, the forefoot is twisted downward and inward, the arch is increased, and the heel is turned inward. This usually will not correct itself spontaneously or even with persistent stretching exercises.

Early treatment is essential and should be initiated soon after birth. The feet should be manipulated to the normal position and then held there by casts or adhesive tape. This process is repeated every few days during the first 2 weeks of treatment and then at 1- to 2-week intervals. If this method is successful, corrective shoes may then maintain this position. If this method does not correct the problem, an operation—usually when the infant is 2 or 3 months old—may be necessary.

Although the position of the corrected clubfoot may look relatively normal, the foot will never have completely normal contours, and the calf on the affected leg will be thinner than that on the normal leg. Orthopedic care throughout childhood is necessary for children born with clubfoot.

Extra toes can make it difficult to fit shoes and thus they often are surgically removed. However, operation should not be performed until the structures are large enough to be easily operated on, yet it should be done before the child begins to walk and wear shoes.

CONGENITAL DISORDERS OF THE SKELETON

Congenital dislocation of the hip is the result of abnormal development of one part or all parts of the hip joint. The problem may be detected during the initial examination at birth or later.

The newborn with a congenital dislocation of the hip is fitted with a brace or splint-like device to position the head of the thigh

Syndactyly (webbing of the toes) is rarely more than a cosmetic problem, requiring no treatment. In contrast, clubfoot (in which the foot is twisted out of shape or position) requires therapy soon after birth.

bone (femur) in the hip socket (acetabulum). This treatment is often successful within 6 to 8 weeks. Most dislocated hips that are diagnosed during the newborn period can be treated adequately in this manner.

Dwarfism (dysplasia) indicates several skeletal abnormalities, most of which have disproportionate lengths of limbs and trunk. Usually, the child's limbs are short initially. As the child grows, the trunk is also disproportionately short. Most dysplasias are not detected during the newborn period. These children may have other congenital problems such as hearing impairment, kidney problems, and immune deficiencies. There is no cure for the actual skeletal defect, but many of the accompanying problems can be treated.

Treatment involves a combination of orthopedic techniques to maximize the child's mobility and function and to correct deformities of the limbs and spine. Emotional support and psychological and genetic counseling are often beneficial.

PECTUS EXCAVATUM

Signs and Symptoms
- An indentation of the sternum (breastbone).

Pectus excavatum, also referred to as funnel chest, is a major indentation of the sternum; the lower part of the bone is depressed toward the spine, and the chest has a funnelled or hollow appearance.

This is usually a congenital defect, although rarely it is caused by rickets or a chronic airway obstruction. In the latter case, successful treatment of the obstruction sometimes results in the disappearance of the deformity.

Babies and children with pectus excavatum usually have normal respiratory function. Only rarely is heart function adversely affected. Some inherited muscle diseases also are associated with the malformation. This condition tends to run in families.

Treatment. Operation is usually not recommended for most children with pectus excavatum. However, in the case of a severe deformity, operation may be performed for cosmetic reasons.

DEFECTS OF THE SEXUAL ORGANS

Boys. The scrotum in the newborn boy is relatively large. The size can be increased by the trauma of a breech birth. In addition, a black newborn's scrotum usually is dark before the rest of the skin attains its dark color. It is not uncommon for a newborn's penis to be erect. If you cannot fully pull back the foreskin of your newborn's penis, do not be concerned. The skin is usually still attached to the end of the penis and should never be forced back.

None of these characteristics is cause for alarm. However, abnormalities of the male genitals are not uncommon, and some require treatment.

Phimosis is a tightness of the foreskin that results in the inability to pull back the fold of skin that covers the uncircumcised penis. It can be congenital or the result of inflamma-

Pectus excavatum, a congenital deformity of the chest, usually will not interfere with breathing. Surgery generally is not required for other than cosmetic reasons.

Phimosis is a tightness of the foreskin resulting in an inability to pull back the fold of skin that covers the uncircumcised penis. Sometimes this requires minor surgical treatment.

When one or both testes fail to travel from the abdomen to the scrotum, the condition is termed undescended testes and may require surgery.

The testis may be misplaced within the abdomen or be absent altogether. The latter condition is rare and usually occurs in a child born with ambiguous sex characteristics.

Two months before birth the testes normally descend from an area near the kidney through a small opening in the abdominal muscles into their normal position in the scrotum. In about 1 of 30 full-term newborns, they do not descend. The incidence of undescended testes is up to 17 percent in premature infants weighing less than 5 pounds, and it is up to 100 percent in infants weighing less than 2 pounds because the testicles do not descend until after the seventh month of gestation.

In up to 30 percent of cases, both testes are affected.

Sometimes hormones are given to bring the undescended testis into place. If it has not descended by the child's first birthday, however, it will not do so spontaneously and the condition should be treated surgically, at 12 to 15 months of age. Operation also is important because often the boy with an undescended testis also has a hernia due to the failure of the opening in the abdominal muscles to close properly. In such cases, the intestines or bladder may slip through the muscle opening and become trapped. The operation can be done on an outpatient basis. Occasionally a testis has shrunk or atrophied so severely that removal is indicated.

When left untreated, undescended testis may lead to infertility in adulthood, particularly if both testes are involved.

tion. Sometimes this requires minor surgical treatment.

Paraphimosis occurs when the foreskin of the uncircumcised penis is retracted too much and cannot be brought back over the end. This can cause severe and painful swelling. When discovered early, the condition can be treated by gentle but firm pressure applied to the end of the penis to reduce the swelling and to allow the foreskin to be brought back. Sometimes circumcision is required.

Undescended testes is the absence, at birth, of one or both testes from the scrotum.

A boy born with an undescended testis has a risk of testicular cancer, generally when he is in his 20s or 30s. Correction does not reduce the risk, but it does allow for better examination and earlier detection should a tumor develop. (See also Undescended Testicle, page 1118.)

Hypospadias occurs in approximately 1 of 500 newborns. In this congenital defect, the urethral opening is not in its normal position at the end of the penis. In its mildest form, the opening is just on the underside of the glans; in its most severe form, it may be as far away as the scrotum.

The more severe the degree of hypospadias, the more curved the penis. Ten percent of boys born with hypospadias also have undescended testes.

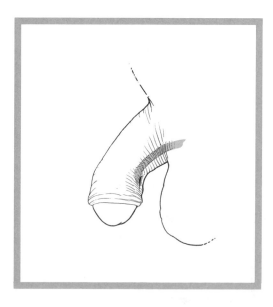

Hypospadias is a condition in which the urethral opening is not located at its normal position at the end of the penis. Surgery can correct this congenital defect.

Hypospadias is treated surgically. Circumcision should not be done because the foreskin is needed for the surgical repair. If the case is mild, the main reason for operation is cosmetic. The more severe the deformity, the greater the need for operation because of urination problems—the child will not be able to stand to urinate—and inability to function sexually later. The psychological consequences of having malformed genitals also are a factor in the consideration of operation.

When should the operation be performed? The current thinking is the earlier, the better. Many pediatric urologists believe the ideal age is during the first year, certainly before the child is toilet-trained.

A single surgical procedure is generally all that is necessary to bring the opening closer to the tip of the penis and also to straighten the penis.

A *hydrocele* is the accumulation of fluid in an area of the testis called the tunica vaginalis. This problem is not uncommon in newborn boys. If the testes can be examined easily and the amount of fluid remains constant, treatment is unnecessary. Small hydroceles usually disappear during the first year. However, if the sac changes size during the day, it may mean there is direct contact with the abdominal cavity. This is a hernia and requires operation.

Girls. Hormonal changes in the mother before birth often may cause changes in the breasts and genitals of her newborn daughter. Although they may be disturbing to the new parent, these changes are normal and temporary and require no treatment.

Enlarged breasts sometimes occur in both girls and boys during the first 2 weeks of life because of the large amounts of circulating hormones that reach the baby through the umbilical cord. This condition is temporary and no cause for alarm. Sometimes pressure on the breast can even elicit breast milk (known as witch's milk) from the infant's nipple. However, parents should not squeeze the infant's nipples because this can cause irritation or infection. Mastitis, an inflammation of the mammary gland, occasionally occurs as a result of a bacterial infection. Antibiotics and manual expression of the infant's breast milk under medical supervision then may be necessary.

A not uncommon problem in newborns is an accumulation of fluid near the testes called a hydrocele.

The *clitoris* of the newborn girl is often enlarged as a result of hormonal changes that affect the genital area. The size decreases shortly after birth. If the clitoris seems unusually large, tests may be indicated to affirm the child's sex (see Ambiguous Genitalia, below).

Vaginal discharge sometimes occurs in the newborn. During the first 3 weeks, many mothers notice a thick, white discharge from the baby's vagina. The discharge is the result of hormonal changes that took place in the mother before she gave birth. Treatment is unnecessary.

Vaginal withdrawal bleeding is sometimes the newborn girl's response to the absence of the maternal hormone estrogen after birth. This manifests as a few drops of blood shed from the vagina. Parents understandably are shocked to find blood in the diaper. Again, this is a temporary condition. The baby is not hemorrhaging or starting to menstruate, as some anxious parents at first suspect.

AMBIGUOUS GENITALIA

Ambiguous genitalia can manifest in several ways. Sometimes a female who has been exposed to an excess of male hormones in the womb is born with ovaries but male-like genitals (female pseudohermaphroditism). A male may be born with testes but with ambiguous or completely female genitals (male pseudohermaphroditism). Some newborns have both ovaries and testicles and ambiguous genitals (true hermaphroditism).

The numerous causes of ambiguous genitalia include tumors, chromosome abnormalities, and hormone excesses or deficiencies.

Treatment. When a newborn's sex is in question, a specialist in hormonal problems of infancy should be consulted promptly. Only after thorough testing and evaluation can a correct diagnosis be established and the correct assignment of sex be made. This is a serious problem with a significant impact on future life and emotional health. Hormones may be given to males to increase the size of the penis. Reconstructive procedures can be done.

SUPERNUMERARY NIPPLES

Rarely, an infant is born with one or more extra nipples.

The nipples may occur with or without breast tissue. Sometimes the nipple does not have an areola (the darker pigment that surrounds a nipple). Although supernumerary nipples usually are located around the breast area, they have been observed occasionally on the neck, back, thigh, and vulva.

An estimated 1 to 2 percent of North Americans have supernumerary nipples. The condition occurs equally in men and women, but it is more likely to occur in blacks, Japanese, and Jews.

The defect seems to be associated with urinary abnormalities.

Tears or a white or yellow discharge on the cheek of your infant may indicate an obstruction of the nasolacrimal duct. This can persist for several months. Your physician might prescribe an antibiotic to help prevent infection. Most often, cleansing your infant's eyelid with warm water and massaging the area will suffice.

If your newborn has supernumerary nipples, they can be removed for cosmetic purposes.

The nipples rarely present a medical problem, although they can respond to hormonal changes that occur during puberty, menstruation, and pregnancy. When this happens, the supernumerary nipple may enlarge and become painful. The presence of a third breast also can be emotionally traumatic. Moreover, a supernumerary nipple is at the same risk as a normal nipple of developing breast disorders such as mastitis, abscesses, and cancer.

An infant also can be born with absence of a breast or nipple. Sometimes the muscle underlying the breast also has failed to develop. When this occurs, nothing should be done during infancy or early childhood. However, operation can be performed for cosmetic reasons when the child reaches puberty.

EPSTEIN PEARLS

Eighty percent of newborns have Epstein pearls, which are small cysts on the palate. These cysts are cells that were trapped during the formation of the palate. Similar cysts also may form on the gums, leading parents to suspect the child has a tooth. Epstein pearls are painless, require no treatment, and disappear within a few weeks.

SUPERNUMERARY TEETH

Most infants are born toothless. Sometimes, however, a tooth can be observed in the newborn's mouth, usually in the lower front gum. It generally falls out before the infant starts teething.

An x-ray should be obtained to determine that the tooth is supernumerary and not a natal tooth, which is a prematurely erupted primary (baby) tooth.

Supernumerary teeth can interfere with the position and eruption of adjacent teeth.

CONGENITAL OBSTRUCTION OF THE NASOLACRIMAL DUCT

Congenital obstruction of the nasolacrimal duct results from incomplete development of the tear drainage system.

Normally, tears and secretions from the eye drain from the tear ducts, which lead from two small openings at the inner corner of the eyelids, first toward the nose and then down into the nasal cavity. If this drainage system is partially or completely obstructed, the tears are not drained from the eyes.

This problem is usually apparent within the first days or weeks after birth. A cold or exposure to wind or low temperature often aggravates the problem. The first sign a parent typically notices is the presence of tears in the baby's eyes. This can range from what appears to be a pool of tears to tears spilling onto the baby's cheeks. There also may be some white or yellow discharge in the corners of the eyes and some crusting that glues the eyes shut after the baby has been asleep for awhile.

Sometimes infants with nasolacrimal duct obstruction develop inflammation in the duct area. The area under the eye may become swollen, red, and tender. The baby also may have a fever and be irritable.

This is a fairly common condition and rarely injures the eye, even when it persists for several months. The main treatment involves cleansing the infant's lids with warm water and massaging the area two or three times a day. Antibacterial drops are used to prevent infection.

In most cases, this is the only treatment that is needed and the problem resolves within the first year. In persistent cases, the physician may need to dilate the duct. Occasionally, insertion of tubes or a reconstructive operation is necessary.

CLEFT LIP AND CLEFT PALATE

Cleft lip and cleft palate are separate birth defects that may or may not occur together.

The incidence of cleft lip with or without cleft palate is 1 per 1,000 births; the incidence of cleft palate alone is 1 in 2,500 births. Genetics seem to be more of a factor in cleft lip with or without cleft palate than in cleft palate alone.

An infant born with a cleft malformation, especially if it is a cleft palate alone, has a higher incidence of other defects including hearing impairment.

An infant born with a cleft lip has a fissure or elongated opening where the upper lip failed to fuse. This can vary from a small notch at the top of the lip to a complete separation extending to the nose. If the palate is also cleft, the roof of the baby's mouth has failed to close.

If your infant is born with either defect or both defects, the most immediate problem is feeding. Soon after birth, a specially designed obturator (prosthesis) can be fitted over the palate so that the baby can be fed. However, because the infant will be growing rapidly, this will have to be replaced every few weeks.

A baby with a cleft lip typically has an operation to close the lip at 1 or 2 months of age. Frequently, nasal widening is associated with cleft lip deformities. Closure of the cleft lip helps to narrow the nasal base. A definitive nasal operation, however, usually is deferred until the child has reached adolescence. The cosmetic results depend on the severity of the deformity, the absence of infection, and the surgeon's skill.

A cleft palate generally is closed within the first year of life to enhance normal speech development. The goals of operation are to make it possible for the child to speak in a normal voice and to reduce nasal regurgitation. If a child does not have the operation by age 3 years, a prosthesis may be used to help the child develop intelligible speech.

Complications of cleft lip or palate include recurring ear infections, hearing loss, an excessive amount of dental cavities, and dis-

Failure of the lip to fuse together results in a condition called cleft lip. When the roof of the mouth has also failed to close, this is termed a cleft palate. These conditions require surgical correction.

placement of the teeth, which requires orthodontic correction. Some children continue to have speech defects even after operation because of muscle problems in the palate. Speech therapy often is required (see page 135).

CONGENITAL HEART DISORDERS

Approximately 8 of every 1,000 newborns have a congenital heart disorder. These defects range from mild to severe. Two to three babies of every 1,000 show the first signs of a heart disorder during the first year of life.

The precise cause of a congenital heart disorder is rarely found, although, as a rule, multifactorial inheritance seems to be responsible (see page 46). Some chromosome abnormalities, such as the one that causes Down syndrome, also are associated with heart defects. Infections such as German measles, contracted by the mother during the first 2 months of pregnancy, also increase the risk of congenital heart defects.

With recent advances in heart surgery, children born with heart disorders often can lead normal lives. Some of the common congenital heart disorders are described.

VENTRICULAR SEPTAL DEFECT

Ventricular septal defect is the most common heart malformation, accounting for 25 percent of the cases of congenital heart disease. The infant born with this defect has an opening between the lower chambers (ventricles) of its heart so that there is an increased blood flow, under high pressure, to the lungs.

The symptoms vary depending on the size of the defect. Most children have a small opening that does not produce noticeable symptoms. The problem may be discovered during a routine stethoscopic examination when the physician may detect a slight murmur. Babies born with large defects develop hypertension, feeding difficulties, profuse perspiration, poor growth rates, recurrent pulmonary infections, and cardiac failure in early infancy.

Treatment depends on the size of the defect. Approximately 30 to 50 percent of small defects close spontaneously during the first year of life. Many children have no symptoms and no apparent heart damage.

Treatment for infants with symptoms is aimed at controlling the heart failure with drugs. If this is unsuccessful, an operation to close the defect should be done before the baby is 1 to 2 years old.

ATRIAL SEPTAL DEFECT

Atrial septal defect is an opening high in the heart between the upper chambers (atria); it produces abnormal blood flow. It is more common in female infants than in males, and it often occurs in children with Down syndrome.

The affected children frequently have no symptoms.

Surgical closure is the recommended treatment, usually between the ages of 3 and 6 years.

PATENT DUCTUS ARTERIOSUS

The ductus arteriosus is a vessel that leads from the pulmonary artery to the aorta. Normally, this closes immediately after birth. When it does not, blood flows between the pulmonary artery and the aorta; this condition is called patent ductus arteriosus.

An unwanted opening between two of the chambers of the heart—ventricular septal defect (see arrow)—allows blood to flow under high pressure to the lungs. In many cases, the defect resolves itself, but in some instances surgical correction is required.

In babies who are born prematurely, the ductus has not had time to close. In a full-term infant, failure to close is a congenital malformation.

Patent ductus arteriosus occurs more often in female infants, in children born at high altitude, and in the offspring of women who had German measles (rubella) during the first 3 months of pregnancy.

If the ductus is small, there are often no symptoms. A large ductus will produce a heart murmur, hypertension, and growth retardation.

In the premature infant, the ductus often closes spontaneously within weeks or months. In the full-term infant or the premature infant whose ductus fails to close, operation is necessary, usually between the first and second years of life.

COARCTATION OF THE AORTA

Coarctation (constriction) of the aorta results in increased blood pressure above the obstruction. There are usually no symptoms. However, heart failure may develop because of other associated heart abnormalities.

In the absence of symptoms, the obstruction should be surgically relieved between the ages of 2 and 5 years if it is determined to be significant; this will help prevent future complications.

TETRALOGY OF FALLOT

Tetralogy of Fallot consists of a large ventricular septal defect (see page 54), obstruction of blood flow from the heart's right ventricle to the lung (pulmonary) arteries, and a shift of the aorta to the right side of the heart. The right ventricle also is enlarged. The result is decreased blood flow to the lungs.

The main symptom of this disorder is a bluish cast to the skin (cyanosis), although this may not always be present at birth.

The symptoms of tetralogy of Fallot often begin slowly during the first year of life. Sometimes, however, the problem is apparent at birth. Treatment is geared toward providing an immediate increase in pulmonary blood flow. Infants with this disorder should be in specially equipped neonatal centers.

Corrective open heart operation is the usual treatment once your child is past infancy. However, occasionally an operation is performed during infancy to improve blood flow to the lung and to decrease cyanosis.

PULMONARY STENOSIS

Pulmonary stenosis is an obstruction of blood flow from the heart to the pulmonary artery.

With mild or moderate obstruction, there are often no symptoms. The newborn with a severe obstruction has a bluish cast to the skin and shows signs of heart failure.

Congestive heart failure (see page 807) occurs in the worst cases during the first month of life.

Children with mild to moderate stenosis can lead a normal life but they should be under the regular care of a physician. Those with more severe stenosis require operation.

AORTIC STENOSIS

Aortic stenosis—a narrowing of the valve through which blood leaves the heart to enter the aorta—is more common in male infants and accounts for 5 percent of cardiac malformations.

Severe stenosis generally is detected in early infancy. However, most children have no symptoms and the problem is found during a routine examination when the physician hears a heart murmur.

Operation is needed for severe stenosis. Children with mild or moderate obstruction should remain under medical care because of the possibility of the obstruction increasing in severity.

TRANSPOSITION OF THE GREAT VESSELS

Transposition of the great vessels is a complex defect in which the two arteries arising from the heart are reversed. Blood returning to the heart from the body is pumped back to the body without passage through the lungs. Infants with transposition are blue (severely cyanotic) and must have immediate medical care.

Several surgical procedures are available to relieve the problem.

CENTRAL NERVOUS SYSTEM DISORDERS

The central nervous system is the portion of the nervous system consisting of the brain and spinal cord. A neurological problem in infancy is most likely due to a congenital malformation.

The most common congenital abnormalities of the central nervous system are described below.

SPINA BIFIDA

Spina bifida is a defect in the arch of vertebrae that results in a failure to fuse. This can occur in any vertebra but is most common at the base of the back or lower spine. The clue to the presence of this condition is an abnormal tuft of hair, a collection of fat, or tiny vessels on the skin overlying the defect. Generally, this condition is an insignificant finding on an x-ray and is not associated with any underlying neurological defect because there is no involvement of the spinal nerves.

Babies born with spina bifida should receive a thorough neurological examination because a small percentage of them have neurological disturbances of the lower legs, bladder, or bowel.

HYDROCEPHALUS

A child born with hydrocephalus has an imbalance between the brain's ability to produce cerebrospinal fluid and its ability to absorb it. An infant with hydrocephalus has an accumulation of cerebrospinal fluid in its skull, which produces an extremely large head.

The incidence of this birth defect varies in different populations, but on the average it is 1 per 1,000 births.

The most obvious symptom of congenital hydrocephalus is an abnormally large head. Occasionally, the head of the fetus grows so large that a normal delivery is impossible. In less extreme cases, the head may seem normal at birth but immediately begins to grow.

A CT scan and an MRI scan (see pages 539, 1286, and 1287) are useful for differentiating hydrocephalus from other disorders and for looking for the cause of the hydrocephalus.

The goal of treatment is to establish equilibrium between the production and absorption of cerebrospinal fluid. Sometimes medication is effective, but generally the best treatment is the surgical insertion of a shunt in the skull to drain the fluid. The shunt is a permanent fixture in the child's skull and should be removed only in the event of infection or malfunction of the device itself.

The long-term outlook for children born with hydrocephalus has improved greatly as a result of shunt placement. If left untreated, more than half of infants born with this disorder die. With proper medical management, an estimated 70 percent of infants with hydrocephalus live beyond infancy. Of this group, 40 percent will have normal intelligence, and 60 percent (mainly those with other central nervous system disorders) will have severe intellectual and motor impairment.

An outpouching of membranes covering the spinal cord (meningomyelocele) occurs in some infants with spina bifida. This may result in neurological disturbances of the lower legs, bladder, or bowel.

CEREBRAL PALSY

Cerebral palsy is one of the most common crippling disorders of childhood. It is a result of damage to the motor function areas of the central nervous system before, during, or after birth.

There are many causes of cerebral palsy. One common cause is the absence of adequate oxygen in the brain tissue (anoxia). Studies also have shown that one-third of infants born with cerebral palsy weigh less than 5 pounds. Damage to the brain during labor and delivery also is a cause, as are infection, such as bacterial meningitis, and hemorrhage. Often, however, there is no obvious explanation.

There are four types of cerebral palsy: spastic cerebral palsy, extrapyramidal cerebral palsy, atonic cerebral palsy, and mixed types.

Spastic cerebral palsy is the most common type. An infant with spastic cerebral palsy has an abnormal persistence of some newborn reflexes. A hyperactive grasp reflex leaves the infant's hands in a tight fist. As the infant grows, the limbs become more spastic and rigid.

All four limbs may be involved (spastic quadriplegia). When this occurs, there is often some degree of mental retardation as well. Convulsions are common.

If all four limbs are affected but the arms are affected to a lesser degree, the condition is called diplegia. Children with diplegia may have good use of their hands. Their intelligence is often normal or near normal but they may have some difficulties learning to draw and write letters.

One-third of all children with cerebral palsy have spastic hemiplegia (paralysis on one side of the body only). Children with spastic hemiplegia tend to have intelligence in the low-normal range, although some have average or even above-average intelligence.

Extrapyramidal cerebral palsy manifests initially as weakness and floppiness of a baby's muscles. This form of cerebral palsy generally is not diagnosed until the infant is 6 months old. An early sign is abnormal positioning of the hands when the baby attempts to reach for something.

Atonic cerebral palsy has two forms: atonic diplegia and congenital cerebellar ataxia. The former is associated with severe mental retardation. Spasticity often develops later in childhood. Congenital cerebellar ataxia is a rare form of cerebral palsy that may be accompanied by mild mental retardation.

The outlook for a child with cerebral palsy depends largely on whether the child also has intellectual handicaps. Even when a child has severe motor problems that necessitate use of a wheelchair, adjustments are easier if the child is capable of going to school. The family's attitude toward the child's handicap has an impact on whether the child develops a positive self-image.

There is no cure for cerebral palsy. Treatment involves early stretching exercises to help the muscles stay loose and to prevent contractures, the use of aids such as wheelchairs and walkers to improve the child's mobility, and special educational methods to help compensate for the child's motor deficit and any learning disabilities.

DOWN SYNDROME

An estimated 1 in 600 to 800 infants is born with Down syndrome, a birth abnormality caused by the presence of an extra chromosome.

A woman's chances of giving birth to a child with Down syndrome increase with age. For example, the chance of having a baby with this syndrome is 1 in 1,205 for a 25-year-old woman but 1 in 365 for a 35-year-old woman.

An infant born with Down syndrome has a small, undersized, round head. The ears are set low and are oval. The eyes slant slightly upward. The mouth angles downward at the corners and tends to hang open. The tongue usually is enlarged and protruding. Gray-white specks are often seen on the iris of the eyes.

Infants born with Down syndrome may be average size, but typically they grow slowly and remain small. They have mental retardation that ranges from mild to severe. Congenital heart defects and gastrointestinal malformations are common.

The mortality rate during the first year is high. Many of these children succumb to respiratory infections, cardiac problems, or leukemia.

There is no treatment for Down syndrome. Heart or other associated defects often can be repaired successfully with operation. The severity of retardation plays a major role in determining the quality of the child's life. Many children with Down syndrome live with loving families, go to school, learn, and even enter the work force in sheltered workshops or other low-level jobs. Other children are profoundly retarded and spend their lives cared for by others.

CONGENITAL GASTROINTESTINAL TRACT DISORDERS

There are many congenital abnormalities of the gastrointestinal tract, some of which are responsible for partial or complete obstruction of the passage of food or fecal material. The most common obstructions involve the duodenum (the first section of the small intestine) or the rectum and anus at the lower end of the gastrointestinal tract.

The most frequent gastrointestinal abnormalities in the newborn are described.

PYLORIC STENOSIS

Pyloric stenosis is a narrowing of the pylorus, the part of the stomach through which food and other stomach contents pass to enter the small intestine.

Pyloric stenosis affects approximately 1 out of every 150 male newborns and 1 out of every 750 female infants. About 15 percent of those born with this condition have a family history of the malformation, but the precise cause is not known.

If your infant is born with pyloric stenosis, the symptoms usually begin during its second or third week of life. The initial symptom may be regurgitation and possibly vomiting, although not necessarily forceful or projectile vomiting. After the symptoms have been apparent for a week or so, the infant generally begins to vomit more violently (projectile vomiting). Rarely, the vomit will contain blood. The vomiting typically occurs during or shortly after a feeding, but it may be delayed for hours. After vomiting, the baby is hungry and wants another feeding.

The infant with pyloric stenosis has very small stools because little food is reaching the intestines. Soon the baby begins to lose weight and may become dehydrated. The infant's eyes may appear sunken and the cheeks wrinkled, giving the baby the appearance of an old person. The newborn with pyloric stenosis may appear uncomfortable but does not seem to be in great pain.

Pyloric stenosis usually can be diagnosed from a physical examination, the child's feeding history, and the identification of a pyloric mass during the abdominal part of the examination. If the mass cannot be felt, an ultrasonographic examination (see page 1287) can be done.

An infant born with pyloric stenosis requires operation as soon as possible after appropriate replacement of fluids through a vein.

Within 6 hours after the operation your baby will begin to receive oral feedings; the amount of the feeding is increased gradually. Most infants can go home 2 days after the operation.

The prognosis for an infant with pyloric stenosis is very good, depending on how early the diagnosis is made and on the overall condition of the infant. The incidence of death due to operation is less than 1 percent.

A narrowing of the opening of the stomach (pylorus) through which stomach contents pass into the small intestine is called pyloric stenosis. This condition requires prompt surgical treatment.

ESOPHAGEAL ATRESIA

An infant born with esophageal atresia has an esophagus (the tube leading from the throat to the stomach) that has not fully developed.

An estimated 1 in 3,000 to 4,500 infants is born with this malformation. One-third of babies with esophageal atresia are premature. This defect often is accompanied by other abnormalities, usually of the trachea (the tube from the larynx into the lungs). Moreover, at least 30 percent of infants with esophageal atresia have other life-threatening birth defects such as heart, urinary tract, and central nervous system problems.

The symptoms of this birth defect often are detected in the delivery room. The infant may have an abnormally large amount of secretions coming from its mouth or may choke, cough, or turn blue when the mother attempts a feeding. If the physician cannot pass a tube through the baby's mouth into the stomach, the infant has esophageal atresia.

If your baby has esophageal atresia, operation is needed immediately. If the underdeveloped esophageal segment is short, repair can be attempted immediately. If the segment is long, the surgeon might decide to permit growth of the esophagus before attempting repair; in this event, a tube is placed through the abdominal wall into the stomach to permit feeding.

BILE DUCT ATRESIA

Bile duct atresia (obstruction of the bile ducts) is an uncommon congenital defect, affecting an estimated 1 in 50,000 to 75,000 newborns.

It is often difficult to differentiate hepatitis from bile duct atresia in an infant. If the results of hepatitis tests are normal, a liver biopsy can be done to confirm the diagnosis.

Infants with bile duct atresia have an increased incidence of other abdominal abnormalities. The stools are free of bile, and the liver may be of abnormal size.

If your infant has bile duct atresia, your physician will probably perform an exploratory operation to determine the precise site. Rarely, the obstruction can be corrected surgically. However, drainage of bile can be achieved with a special connection to the intestine called hepatoportoenterostomy of Kasai. It is very important that the operation be performed during the first 3 months of life to ensure success.

Children with bile duct atresia often have persistent inflammation of the liver even after operation. Some may ultimately require liver transplantation.

INTESTINAL ATRESIA

Obstruction of the intestine occurs in about 1 out of 1,500 births. The obstruction can occur anywhere in the intestines.

If the obstruction is high, the infant's predominant symptom is vomiting, which tends to be persistent even when feedings have been discontinued. An infant with a low obstruction usually has a distended abdomen initially, although vomiting occurs later. Vomiting of bile should always be investigated by your physician. An infant with an intestinal obstruction generally does not have a bowel movement, although meconium stools (see page 9) may be passed during the first days of life if the obstruction is high in the small intestine.

The obstruction may be complete or partial. When the child has a partial obstruction, the symptoms may not be apparent immediately.

If your physician suspects that your infant has an intestinal obstruction, an x-ray of the abdomen will be taken.

Treatment depends on the obstruction. A complete obstruction requires prompt operation to prevent severe complications. An operation often is needed for partial obstruction, although a child with a partial obstruction may survive for weeks. Some minor obstructions may not require operation.

When the diagnosis is made promptly and the proper treatment is initiated, most infants tolerate the operation well and recover completely.

HIRSCHSPRUNG'S DISEASE

An infant born with Hirschsprung's disease (also called congenital megacolon) gradually develops an abnormally large or dilated colon. This condition is due to a failure of the lower rectum to propel stool through the anus. Rare in premature infants, Hirschsprung's disease accounts for about 33 percent of all neonatal obstructions in the colon.

Early signs in the newborn may include the failure to pass meconium stool, vomiting, abdominal distention, and the failure to have a bowel movement. After a rectal examination, the baby often has an explosive bowel movement. Sometimes a newborn even vomits fecal material. Dehydration and weight loss are common. Many infants have alternating constipation and diarrhea.

The best method of diagnosing megacolon in the newborn is by rectal biopsy.

The treatment for Hirschsprung's disease is an operation during which an opening on the outside of the abdomen is created so that the stool can pass into a disposable pouch. This is a temporary measure. The opening is closed during another operation when the child is between 12 and 18 months old.

The treatment is highly successful, although continued bouts of diarrhea are sometimes a problem.

IMPERFORATE ANUS

If your newborn is born with an imperforate anus, the anal opening is obstructed. Consequently, there is no passage of stool.

Congenital anomalies of the anus and rectum are fairly common, with minor abnormalities occurring in 1 out of 500 births and major ones in 1 out of 5,000 births.

Children born with anal and rectal abnormalities have a higher incidence of other birth defects such as urinary anomalies.

Imperforate anus is suspected when a baby fails to pass a meconium stool. X-ray and ultrasound studies can be done to establish whether the obstruction is high or low in the rectum.

Treatment depends on the location of the obstruction. If the anal opening is simply narrowed, an instrument can be used to dilate the opening. In other types of imperforate anus, operation is required; the higher the obstruction, the more major the surgical procedure. Some children require complete reconstruction of the anus; others need a temporary colostomy for the first 6 to 12 months of life (see also Hirschsprung's Disease, page 59).

Children with low anal obstruction generally do well after operation and develop bowel control. When the obstruction is higher, there may be some incontinence.

DIAPHRAGMATIC HERNIA

A diaphragmatic hernia occurs when an abnormal opening in the diaphragm enables part of the abdominal contents to poke through into the chest cavity. In severe cases, the stomach and a large part of the intestines displace the heart and lungs.

This abnormality may be detected shortly after birth if the child is in respiratory distress as a result of the hernia. It is then a life-threatening situation and requires emergency operation. Often, however, the hernia is not detected until months later.

Later-appearing symptoms of diaphragmatic hernia include vomiting, severe colicky pain, discomfort after eating, and constipation. Occasionally there are no symptoms and the problem is discovered on routine x-rays.

If your physician suspects that your infant has diaphragmatic hernia, x-rays will be taken to confirm the diagnosis.

Operation is the necessary treatment. In severely affected infants who are diagnosed during the first 3 days of life, the mortality rate is 50 percent. However, most of the infants who do not have respiratory distress survive.

CHAPTER 2
INFANCY
AGES 1 MONTH TO 1 YEAR

CHAPTER CONTENTS

THE FIRST YEAR

The second month of life is the point at which you and your baby have begun to adjust to one another. Mothers usually begin to recover some of their strength by the second month, and the relationship between parents and infant grows.

If you have found yourself adjusting to caring for your baby, think of the phenomenal transformation he or she has experienced in just a few short weeks. The physical changes in appearance from birth to 1 month are dramatic. Your 1-month-old baby also is beginning to fall into a somewhat predictable schedule of eating, sleeping, and eliminating. This is not to say that the schedule will not change. It will—frequently—during the first year of life. But between the changes there is a new-found sense of predictability in what to expect from your baby during a given day.

The first year of life is a time of continuous and rapid change. During this first year your baby will go from a diet of mother's milk or formula to feeding himself or herself table food and even drinking from a cup. The young baby who spends a good part of each day sleeping becomes the 11-month-old who is active the whole day except for an afternoon nap. The baby will progress from being able to sit up on his or her own, to creeping and then to walking, which generally occurs between ages 9 and 16 months.

You will watch your infant evolve from a being who communicates only by crying to one who coos and squeals with pleasure when you walk into the room and then to one who can say mama and dada and wave bye-bye.

This chapter is devoted to the infant ages 1 through 12 months. Within its pages we explore the developmental—both physical and psychological—milestones that you can expect during these important months. Common concerns such as diarrhea, rashes, and vomiting will be covered. We will emphasize general care, nutrition, feeding problems, and ways in which you can help keep your curious infant safe in your home.

NORMAL GROWTH AND DEVELOPMENT

How much weight gain is normal? How does a breast-feeding mother know whether her baby is getting enough to eat? How many hours a day should my infant be sleeping?

These are all common questions asked by parents, particularly those with a first child.

It is natural to worry whether your baby is developing normally, even though serious abnormalities are uncommon.

From the standpoint of reducing parental anxiety, it would be easier if your physician could tell you with absolute confidence that your baby will gain a specified amount of weight each month, turn over by itself at a definite time, and begin to walk at some exact age. Easier, perhaps, but not realistic.

What this chapter and your physician can offer you, however, are guidelines. There is a range within which development occurs in most infants. For example, a child may walk as early as 9 months or as late as 16 months and still fall within the normal range. Just because your baby walks at 15 months does not mean he or she is slow. On the contrary, your infant may have been directing energies toward language and as a result may be more verbally advanced than his or her peers.

What should you do if your baby fails to reach a developmental milestone within the normal time frame? This does not necessarily mean something is wrong, but you should take your concerns to your physician.

THE MILESTONES

The precise timetable is not fixed, yet human development does occur in a predictable sequence of events. An infant simply does not suddenly begin to walk; instead, he or she begins in the first weeks of life to lift his or her head and later to roll over, sit alone, crawl, stand, and then finally walk.

Although the steps involved in the mastery of a skill such as walking are the same for all children, the rate at which the steps occur varies considerably. This variation often leads to concern. Parents remember that their first child walked at 9 months and then become anxious when the second still is not walking at 14 months.

In this section we give you some guidelines for growth and development. Keep in mind, however, that these are only averages.

Growth. By the time your infant is 1 month old, he or she probably has gained 1 to 3 pounds over his or her birth weight and has grown 1 or 2 inches in length. The baby will probably double his or her birth weight by the age of 4 to 5 months and triple it by the first birthday. Your infant's height will increase about 10 to 12 inches over the course of the year. The circumference of the baby's head will increase about 4 or 5 inches during the first year of life.

Your baby will likely develop a first tooth between 5 and 9 months. Most children have between six and eight teeth by the time they are 1 year.

Sleep Patterns.   In the first months of life, babies spend most of their time sleeping. They wake up when they are hungry, they eat, play, or fuss for a while, and then go back to sleep. The average 1-month-old may be awake a total of 10 hours out of every 24. Some babies sleep more, others less.

Babies are "supposed" to sleep through the night by the time they weigh 11 pounds. Many parents, however, have children who do not follow this rule of thumb. Breast-fed babies, in particular, often demand a night feeding for several months.

As a rule, the older the infant, the less he or she sleeps. By the end of the first year, most infants' naps are limited to 1 or 2 hours in the morning or afternoon or both.

Motor Development.   The 1-month-old infant's movements seem clumsy and uncoordinated. Unsupported, the baby's head will flop forward or backward. The infant may grasp an object such as a rattle, but it

Your physician may use charts like those shown below to assess your baby's growth over a period of time.

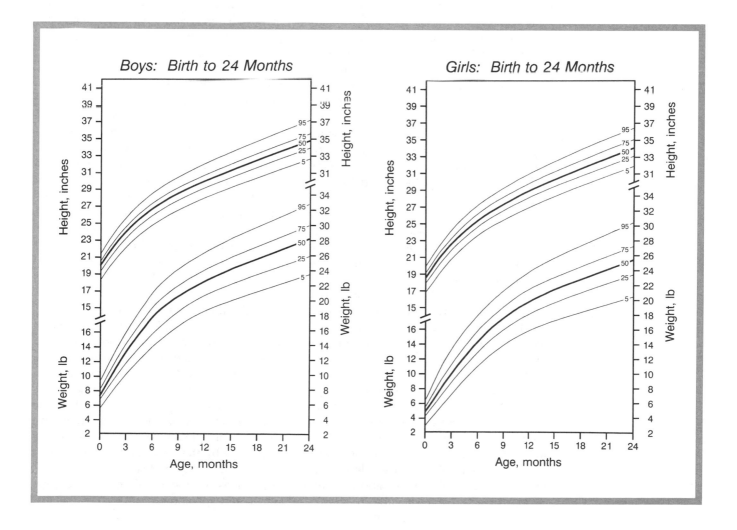

lets go quickly. The baby may stare at an object but does not try to reach for it.

Most 2-month-old infants can move their arms and legs smoothly, hold the head up at a 45° angle for a few minutes, and grasp an object briefly.

The 3-month-old can sit supported with minimal head bobbing. At this age, the baby may begin to swipe at objects, but often misses. The body now is less floppy.

A 4-month-old infant can sit with assistance for 10 or 15 minutes and maintain good control of its head. When on his or her stomach, your baby may rock, rolling from side to side. Some infants at this age can roll from their stomach or side to the back.

The 5-month-old can put its feet in his or her mouth and suck on the toes. The baby can now roll from stomach to back. When on the stomach, he or she can push with the hands and bring up the knees. When pulled to stand, the baby can move his or her body up and down and push down on one foot and then the other, as though walking. The baby may be able to hold a bottle, can swap objects from hand to hand, and can reach with accuracy.

A 6-month-old rolls from back to stomach. Some babies of this age can get up on their hands and knees and creep. The baby can sit in a chair and bounce and can play with his or her hands by touching them together.

At 7 months, your infant's ability to sit has improved and he or she may even be able to sit unsupported. The baby can use thumb and finger to grasp a block and bang together two objects.

The 8-month-old infant is trying to crawl. Some babies of this age can stand when leaning against something. The baby can hold a rattle for several minutes and tries to pick up small objects.

Many 9-month-old babies can crawl while grasping a toy in one hand. The baby may be able to stand alone for brief periods and can grasp small objects between the thumb and forefinger.

The 10-month-old infant may be holding on to your furniture to walk around the room. Most infants can walk at 10 months provided you hold onto both hands. Your child can climb up and down from chairs and carry two small objects in one hand.

The 11-month-old may be able to stand alone and wave, climb stairs, and squat and stoop. The child may be able to grasp a spoon and bring it to his or her mouth, make marks with a crayon, and pull off his or her shoes.

By the time many children have their first birthday, they are walking, although crawling still may be the preferred method of getting around. The child may be capable of climbing stairs and going down stairs and may be able to climb out of the crib. The child can point with the index finger and can take the covers off containers.

Verbal Development. The 1-month-old baby, besides crying, begins to make small throaty sounds. At 2 months, these sounds begin to sound like coos. The 3-month-old baby's verbal repertoire is expanded with squeals, chuckles, whimpers, and vowel-like sounds such as ooh, ah, and ae. Considerable cooing and gurgling take place during this time. Language comprehension is limited to responses to loud noises and familiar voices.

Between 4 and 6 months is the babbling stage—complete with sighing, grunting, gurgling, laughing, and crying differently for pain and hunger. Your child vocalizes for pleasure and displeasure.

Between 7 and 9 months your child repeats syllables, babbles in a singsong manner, and may produce as many as 12 different sounds, particularly the p, b, and m sounds. He or she may use different vowels. Your infant may use sounds as a means of play and may repeat the word mama. Toward the end of this period, actual imitation of intonation and speech sounds made by others can be heard. Your child will search for sources of sound, listen intently to speech and non-speech sounds, and recognize dada, mama and bye-bye. Your child may recognize his or her own name and is able to differentiate friendliness or anger from the tone of people's voices.

Between 10 and 12 months, the babbling may take on some of the melody of actual speech. Your child enjoys repeating sounds made by others. Considerable vocalization is used during play. Almost all of the consonant and vowel sounds are used. In some children, the first words emerge during this period. Your child's comprehension also is improved by this time, and he or she can respond to names and simple requests and recognizes the names of common objects and family members.

COMMON CONCERNS DURING INFANCY

As the parent of an infant, you may find yourself frequently wondering whether your baby is well. Is he or she gaining enough weight? Can he or she see and hear normally? Are the infant's difficulties with bowel movements cause for alarm? How do you know whether your fussy baby is really ill or simply having a bad day?

In this section we will provide you with information that will help you answer some of your own questions. Commonly expressed concerns during the first year of life include what to do about infant diarrhea, constipation, and rashes. Also, we will give you signs to look for to determine whether your baby is sick.

SIGNS OF ILLNESS

Illness in an infant may be difficult to detect initially. Unlike the older child, the 1-month-old infant cannot tell you that his or her head hurts. Your baby may cry more, but if he or she is a fussy baby anyway, the crying may not arouse your suspicions. Or, the child may—like most of us when we are sick—sleep more.

If your infant's eating and sleeping patterns abruptly change, it is reasonable to suspect that the baby may not be feeling well. Taking the baby's temperature is a good first step, although a baby might not have a fever when ill.

Remember, the most important factor is not how elevated the temperature is but how the baby is acting. A baby who has a normal temperature but is limp, lethargic, and refusing food or liquids is more likely to be ill than the bright-eyed, into-everything 8-month-old baby with a temperature of 103°F.

The following are some signs that may indicate illness.

Fever. A rectal temperature of more than 100.4°F is considered a fever, the body's response to infection. Fevers are common during childhood and usually are due to a viral infection. Most fevers less than 102°F do not cause symptoms, and contrary to popular belief, the seriousness of an illness is usually not related to the degree of fever.

Again, always ask yourself, "How is my baby acting?"

If a baby younger than 2 months develops a fever of more than 100.4°F, call your physician. A fever of more than 102°F in a child older than 2 months also warrants a call to your physician, as does one that has been present for 3 days or more.

Constant Crying. Babies, particularly those younger than 3 months, frequently cry for long periods. Although constant crying during early infancy usually is attributable to colic (see Excessive Crying, page 12), it also may be an indication that the child is ill. If your baby cries for a long period (2 or 3 hours) or is inconsolable, or if the cry sounds strange (unusually high-pitched or a weak moan), call the physician. If you are worried that your baby is sick, do not be embarrassed to call your infant's physician or to bring your child in to be examined.

Sleeping Problems. If your infant cannot sleep for more than 30 minutes at a time, does not awaken for feedings, or cannot be fully awakened, consult your physician (see page 88).

Breathing Problems. Your baby may catch a cold that interferes with his or her breathing. Removing mucus from the nose with a special rubber bulb (available at your local pharmacy) often enables your baby to breathe freely and may be all the treatment required. However, if your baby develops a raspy, harsh-sounding cough, begins to wheeze, has difficulty breathing, or turns bluish around the lips and mouth, call your infant's physician (see Common and Recurrent Colds, page 90).

Soft Spot (Fontanelle). For the first year and a half of life, your baby has a soft spot on the top front part of the skull where the bones have yet to grow together. Normally, this area is flat or may be slightly depressed. If, however, your baby is sick and its soft spot bulges or if it appears sunken, call your physician immediately. Note that the soft spot bulges out naturally with respiration or crying.

Vomiting. Most healthy babies spit up; some do it more than others. Spitting up is the effortless regurgitation of food or milk, and vomiting is the forceful exit of the stomach's contents. If vomiting continues for more than 12 hours or if there is blood in the vomitus, call your physician (see Vomiting and Spitting Up, page 14).

Diarrhea. The best indicators of the severity of diarrhea are its frequency and how sick your baby is acting. If the stool is green, it indicates the rapid passage of food through the intestines.

If your infant passes more than eight diarrheal stools in 8 hours, is also vomiting, or has blood in the stool, call your pediatrician or family physician.

Dehydration. The main danger of vomiting and diarrhea is a depletion of the body's fluids. Dehydration is potentially life-threatening and can occur in infancy after only a few hours of illness. Signs to look for include an absence of tears during crying, a dry mouth, the failure to produce a wet diaper after 8 hours, and a shrunken soft spot. If your child has any symptoms of dehydration, call your physician immediately. You may need to bring your baby in for an examination.

FAILURE TO GAIN WEIGHT

The vast majority of babies grow normally. There are differences, of course, from one child to the next in the achievement of specific weights and lengths—after all, some babies are born several pounds lighter or heavier than average.

In rare instances, an infant stops growing or grows unusually slowly. The most evident symptom of a child who is failing to thrive is a lack of weight gain or even weight loss. Moreover, many babies who fail to thrive show signs of developmental retardation and physical and emotional deprivation. They may be unwilling to make eye contact, apathetic, and withdrawn. Some may have gastrointestinal problems such as vomiting, diarrhea, and regurgitation.

Although failure to thrive can occur at any time during childhood, it is most common during infancy, particularly among babies who are reared in institutions. Babies who are mentally retarded or autistic or who have cerebral palsy are much more likely to display a failure to thrive.

The basic cause of failure to thrive falls into one of two categories: organic, which means there is a physical problem responsible for the infant's poor weight gain; and nonorganic, an indication that the cause is psychosocial or environmental factors such as feeding errors, the absence of care, or the lack of a nurturing emotional environment.

Approximately 70 percent of all cases of failure to thrive are of nonorganic origin, and in the remainder a physical cause for the problem is found.

Many physical problems can cause failure to thrive. Malabsorption disorders of the small intestine, liver disease, kidney disorders, chronic heart failure, malignancies, central nervous system abnormalities, cleft palate, and endocrine disorders are some of the ailments that can interfere with weight gain. When a specific physical cause is found, treatment of that disorder generally remedies the failure to thrive.

The solution to nonorganic causes of failure to thrive is often more complicated.

About half of the nonorganic cases of failure to thrive are due to psychological or physical neglect of the infant. Typically, the baby simply is not fed enough. The parent—usually a mother—may feel overwhelmed with responsibility, preoccupied with other problems, or depressed. Often, the pregnancy was unplanned. She did not want to be pregnant and now she does not want the baby. In addition to withholding food, the mother withholds love and affection. Babies treated in this way usually have not been kissed, cuddled, or played with. When the baby is held, it is often in a rough manner.

Babies who have failure to thrive because of neglect usually wear the signs of their neglect. They often have severe diaper rashes, uncut fingernails, untreated rashes, and dirty clothes.

Not all babies who do not have a physical cause for their lack of weight gain are neglected or abused. Sometimes parents make feeding errors that result in the baby not consuming enough calories. An inexperienced parent may, for instance, dilute the baby's formula. Or, the parent may not feed the baby often enough, or the feedings themselves may be too small.

What should you do if your infant fails to gain weight? Consult the baby's physician. During your infant's first year of life, he or she should be seeing a physician every month or two. At each checkup, the baby is weighed and measured and the weight and height are recorded (see Height and Weight Charts, page 63). If the baby is not gaining properly or is losing weight, the physician will question you about the baby's feedings and appetite and about whether he or she has had any vomiting or diarrhea.

Hospitalization may be necessary. During this time, your infant will be given unlimited feedings and his or her growth will be monitored. For cases in which the cause of failure to thrive is neglect or improper feeding, the infant, ravenous, usually gains a pound during a week in the hospital.

If evidence points toward an organic cause, tests will be done to confirm the diagnosis.

The outlook for babies who have nonorganic failure to thrive varies. About 75 percent of neglected babies return to the parents after hospitalization. These families typically require help, including precise feeding instructions and visits from a public health nurse or representative of some form of community service.

A small percentage of affected babies are not treated until it is too late to save them. Although poor weight gain and growth attributable to malnutrition can be reversed, an infant malnourished for more than 6 months may never achieve a normal-sized brain. Moreover, many of these children go on to have reading and language problems and exhibit antisocial behavior in later years.

CONCERNS WITH HEARING

In order to develop normal speech and language abilities, a baby must be able to hear.

Normally, babies are born with the ability to hear. But sometimes events that occur in or out of the womb can impair to varying degrees a baby's ability to hear out of one or both ears.

Infants at high risk for hearing impairment include those with severe birth asphyxia (oxygen deprivation) or bacterial meningitis, those who have infections in the womb or in early infancy, some head or neck defects, or severe jaundice requir-

ing exchange transfusions, or those who are born prematurely. It is also important to evaluate hearing if there is a history of hearing impairment in the family.

Hearing loss is an insidious problem and one that might go undetected until the child is 18 to 24 months of age, when concerned parents become aware that he or she is not developing normal speech. Unfortunately, at this point, the child has missed valuable stages that are critical for language and learning. Thus, all newborns considered to be at high risk for hearing loss should be tested within the first 6 months of life.

There are four types of hearing loss found in infants.

Conductive hearing loss occurs when something interferes with the reception of sound by the external ear or with the transmission of sound from the external to the inner ear. The most common causes of conductive hearing loss are structural abnormalities of the ear and chronic ear infections. This type of hearing loss often can be treated successfully.

Sensorineural hearing loss stems from abnormalities of the cochlear hair cells or the auditory nerve. More than half of the cases of sensorineural hearing loss are congenital, and the remainder are due to conditions such as birth trauma, intrauterine infections, certain medications, and other factors. Generally, sensorineural hearing loss cannot be reversed.

Mixed hearing loss occurs when the child has both a conductive and a sensorineural hearing loss. The hearing loss is often severe.

Central auditory disorders are a result of a problem with the central auditory nervous system. These problems can occur during pregnancy, birth, or early life.

Early detection of a hearing loss is critical for determining effects on the development of language and speech. Many children with hearing problems can be helped with medical or surgical treatments and hearing aids. Specific testing may be arranged for infants at risk for hearing problems and those with speech difficulties.

Moreover, if your baby is found to have a hearing loss, your physician may recommend a parent-infant program that will teach you to make the most of your child's hearing abilities.

YOUR CHILD'S HEARING PROGRESS

As a parent, there are certain developmental signs that you can watch for to determine whether your baby's hearing is within the normal range.

Hearing

A hearing problem that is not detected shortly after birth is usually not discovered until well into the child's second year, when it becomes apparent that his or her speech is delayed. By this time, a crucial point in language development has been missed.

Under normal circumstances, an infant is born hearing and may even have sound preferences. The 1-month-old often stops moving and appears to listen to a sudden sound. By 2 months, the child should appear to be listening to his mother or father. At 3 months, the baby should coo and gurgle in response to speech and look in the direction of the speaker. The child should startle to a clap within 3 feet.

The 4-month-old infant responds differently to angry and pleasant voices, the 5-month-old baby should begin to mimic sounds and respond to his or her own name, and the 6-month-old should be able to protest loudly and squeal with delight. The child should search (turn his or her eyes and head) in an attempt to find the source of sounds or speech.

Most babies at 7 months begin to make some word-like sounds and respond with gestures to simple words such as bye-bye. At 8 months your baby may stop activity when you call his or her name, at 9 months he or she stops an activity when you say "no," and he or she may begin to speak at 10 months. The 1-year-old baby should be able to answer simple questions by pointing to the named object (Where is your nose? Where is your hair?).

There is some normal variation in the development of hearing from one child to the next—but if you suspect that your baby's development is abnormally slow, consult your physician.

CONCERNS WITH VISION

Although your newborn probably keeps his or her eyes closed much of the time, the baby was born with the ability to see, albeit not too clearly. Your baby's vision responses and the interior of the eye (retina) are checked shortly after birth by your infant's physician.

In most infants, the ability to see things clearly rapidly progresses, and by the time most children are 3 years old or even younger, they have 20/30 or 20/20 vision.

Many normal babies also have difficulty coordinating their eye movements during the initial months. Hence, at times your baby may seem cross-eyed. In most cases, however, this appearance should not persist beyond the first few months.

Sometimes—for various reasons—a vision problem surfaces during infancy. As is so often the case, the earlier the diagnosis, the better the chances that treatment will be successful. For this reason, an eye examination should be a part of even the young child's routine examinations.

The following are some of the vision problems that may occur during infancy.

Amblyopia. This term describes subnormal vision in one or both eyes. There are numerous causes, including trauma to the eye, diseases of the eye, and disorders of vision such as the failure of the eyes to focus or align properly (lazy eye).

The most important factor in the treatment of amblyopia is early detection and prompt treatment. Typically, a child is most susceptible to amblyopia during the first 3 years.

Treatment involves providing the clearest vision possible and may include eye drops, glasses to correct a refraction error, or even surgery. Another crucial component of treatment is forcing the use of the amblyopic eye. This is usually done by putting a patch over the better eye to force the child to use the weaker eye. In some infants, amblyopia can be reversed within weeks of treatment.

Strabismus. Strabismus describes the inability of the eyes to align properly. When this occurs, a person is unable to integrate what he or she sees from both eyes into a single visual image, which is essential to develop normal depth perception.

In one form of strabismus, the eyes malalign only when the child is tired, under stress, or ill.

A child who has alternating strabismus learns to see out of one eye at a time. While one eye is being used to see with, the other one wanders. Because both eyes are used (at different times), vision develops in both, whereas a child who uses one eye exclusively may develop amblyopia in the other eye because it is used improperly.

Another type of strabismus is accommodative esotropia. This form of strabismus usually occurs when a child is between 2 and 3 years, but in some cases it surfaces during infancy. These children are typically farsighted (unable to see clearly objects close at hand) and cross-eyed. The crossed eyes may be most apparent when the child is looking at something close.

If your infant has strabismus, the first goal of treatment is to establish the best achievable vision and, when possible, equal vision in both eyes. Surgery is often necessary in children born with strabismus, and it should be done as soon as possible so that the infant will be able to develop normal vision. Sometimes several operations are necessary, but in most children with strabismus, one or possibly two operations are usually sufficient. Total correction, however, is not always possible (see Strabismus and Amblyopia, page 750).

'Cross-eye' is one form of a common eye disorder called strabismus. In any of its varieties, strabismus must be treated as early as possible to assure development of normal or near-normal vision.

DIARRHEA

Diarrhea—the frequent passage of abnormally loose or liquid stools—is one of the most common reasons for seeking consultation with pediatricians and family physicians. During the first 3 years of your baby's life, he or she probably will have from one to three severe episodes of diarrhea.

In infants, diarrhea usually is caused by a viral infection. In some cases, the offender may be a bacterium or toxin that invades the intestinal tract. Diarrhea also can be due to diet because loose stools often are noted with the introduction of new foods. Finally, diarrhea can be a symptom of chronic gastrointestinal diseases, anatomical defects, and congenital disorders.

In the formula-fed infant, the stools increase in frequency and go from formed to being mushy or watery, in some cases turning green.

Breast-fed babies, however, normally have stools the consistency of cream soup. Occasionally, the stools of a healthy breast-fed baby may be green. As for frequency, many breast-fed infants have a bowel movement after each feeding. So how do you know whether your breast-fed infant has diarrhea? One clue is the presence of blood, mucus, or a bad odor (the stools of a baby nourished exclusively at the breast do not

HOW TO DETERMINE WHETHER YOUR INFANT SEES PROPERLY

Although an important part of a newborn's initial physical examination includes a check for any apparent vision or hearing defects, it is not uncommon for some sensory problems to go undetected during early infancy. Often the problem is later discovered by the parents when the infant fails to develop speech or seems unusually clumsy.

As a parent, there are certain developmental signs that you can watch for to determine whether your baby's vision is indeed within the normal range.

Vision
When your infant is between 4 and 6 weeks old, try the following test. Bring your face within 20 inches of your baby's. This should elicit a smile. By the time your infant is 3 months, the baby should be able to visually follow a toy that is dangled in front of his or her face. The infant also should attempt to reach for a toy or rattle. A baby this age also can see objects at least several feet away.

By the time your infant is 4 months old, his or her vision capabilities—the ability of the eye to distinguish color, adjust itself to various distances, see one image instead of two, perceive depth, and orient itself to moving images—are on the way to reaching those of an adult.

Although there is some normal variation in development, if you suspect that your baby's development is abnormally slow, consult your physician.

have an offensive odor). An abrupt increase in frequency is another sign to watch for. When in doubt, ask yourself, how is the baby acting? Is he or she feeding poorly, acting sick, or feverish?

If your baby has diarrhea, what should you do? If the baby is acting normally, a change in diet is usually sufficient. If the baby's diarrhea is mild (mushy stools), try giving him or her extra fluids by mixing the formula or milk with 1 or 2 extra ounces of water in each bottle. If you are breast-feeding your baby, continue feeding as always. Simply offer the infant extra water or a commercial oral electrolyte replacement solution such as Pedialyte, Lytren, or Infalyte (several brands are available at your drugstore) between feedings.

If the baby with mild diarrhea has already been eating solids, offer only foods such as applesauce, bananas, boiled carrots, and rice cereal because these foods tend to firm the stool. If in doubt as to what to feed, consult your physician.

When diarrhea in a formula-fed infant is watery or frequent, everything but clear liquids should be eliminated for 24 hours. Give your baby an oral electrolyte replacement solution to help replace electrolytes lost in the diarrhea. Drinking fluids is important to prevent dehydration (depletion of the body's fluids). So encourage your baby to drink. When you begin feeding formula again, some physicians suggest trying a soy formula, which is less likely to cause diarrhea than one made with cow's milk. Mix the formula with 1 or 2 extra ounces of water until the stools look normal. Any solids should be restricted to the foods recommended above.

Anyone caring for a child with diarrhea should be reminded that diarrhea caused by a virus or bacteria is extremely contagious. Be especially diligent about hand-washing after diaper changes.

Although most cases of diarrhea are over within 72 hours and require no more than a diet change and an increased fluid intake, severe diarrhea—particularly in infants and young children—can be dangerous because of the possibility of dehydration. Babies who are dehydrated often require hospitalization, during which replacement fluids are infused into the child's body through a vein.

If your infant has diarrhea, watch carefully for the following signs:

No wet diaper for 8 hours or more;

Crying that produces no tears;

A dry mouth;

Depressed soft spot on baby's head;

More than eight diarrheal stools in 8 hours;

Blood in the stool;

Persistent vomiting of clear fluids three or more times with diarrhea; or

Actions that indicate the baby is very sick.

If your baby has any of these, call your physician immediately.

CONSTIPATION

Many parents assume that if their infant does not have a daily bowel movement, the baby is constipated. Constipation, however, is not marked by the frequency of bowel movements but by the consistency and effort required to pass the stool.

Constipation is uncommon in breast-fed babies. Typically, breast-fed infants have several loose bowel movements a day, often after each feeding; yet sometimes your baby may go several days without having a stool. The infant may grunt and push until he or she is red in the face. Yet when the movement is passed, it is not the hard stool associated with constipation.

The seemingly difficult passage of this loose stool may be due to the fact that the baby's intestines are not yet smoothly coordinating intestinal contractions with relaxation of the anus. Sometimes the gentle insertion of a rectal thermometer into the infant's anus will help expel the feces.

Some infants who are formula-fed do suffer from constipation. Sometimes an increase in the amount of fluids or other diet changes will alleviate the problem. If the infant is more than 4 months old, adding foods such as fruits or vegetables may help.

Consult your baby's physician for further specific advice on foods or before giving a suppository or enema.

If the constipation does not improve with these measures, check with your pediatrician or family physician, who may want to perform a rectal examination. Some congenital disorders can cause chronic constipation, as can small cracks (fissures) around the anus, which make having a bowel movement painful for the infant.

VOMITING AND REGURGITATION

Vomiting is the forceful ejection of a large amount of food from the stomach, occurring usually when your infant is sick. Vomiting is most often caused by a virus, although it can be the result of more serious problems. Regurgitation is the effortless spitting up of food or milk that frequently occurs in most healthy babies, usually after a feeding.

One episode of vomiting in a baby who otherwise appears healthy is not cause for alarm. However, if the vomiting continues in a sick infant, call your physician.

If your infant is vomiting, give the child an oral electrolyte replacement solution such as Pedialyte, Lytren, or Infalyte, available without prescription at any pharmacy. Use small amounts at first, perhaps a tablespoon at a time. Feed the baby cautiously in quantity and frequency until the vomiting ceases.

The solution will help replace electrolytes that are being lost in vomiting. Avoid milk or solids until the child has gone 8 hours without vomiting. Then, if the baby is eating solids, try easily digested foods such as bananas, applesauce, and rice cereal.

A baby who vomits repeatedly—especially if diarrhea is also present—is at risk for dehydration, the depletion of the body's fluids. Signs that should alert you to the possibility of dehydration include the absence of wet diapers for more than 8 hours, a shrunken soft spot on the baby's head, tearless crying, and a dry mouth. If the baby vomits clear fluids three or more times, call your physician immediately.

In contrast to vomiting, regurgitation—seen in more than half of all infants—is the gentle spitting up of small amounts of food or milk, usually shortly after eating. Regurgitation, also called gastroesophageal reflux, occurs because the upper end of the stomach has allowed food to travel back up the esophagus.

Regurgitation, especially for the first 6 months of life, is normal and nothing to be concerned about unless there is blood in the material or the infant is not gaining weight properly. In most infants, regurgitation improves as the child grows older.

Although nothing will completely stop a baby from spitting up, there are things you can do to improve the problem.

Because overfeeding worsens the problem, start giving the baby 1 ounce less per feeding. Limit the feeding time to less than 20 minutes, and wait at least 2½ hours between feedings.

Be diligent about burping. During pauses in the feeding, try to get the baby to burp so that he or she has several burps during a feeding.

After meals, do not immediately lay the baby down. Try to keep him or her upright in a backpack or frontpack or, if the child is 6 months or older, in a walker.

Avoid putting tight clothing on the baby or bouncing him or her after a meal.

RASHES

Rashes are common in infancy. Most rashes are not dangerous and often can be treated at home, but a rash also can be a symptom of an infectious disease (chickenpox or measles, for example) or of a serious disease such as allergic purpura (see Henoch-Schönlein Purpura, page 894).

As a general rule, if your baby suddenly develops a purple or blood-colored rash, develops a rash that looks like a burn, or seems to be acting sick and develops a rash, call your infant's physician immediately.

The following are common rashes that occur during infancy.

Diaper Rash. This rash is the result of prolonged contact with wetness, bacteria, and other waste products from the digestive tract. Diaper rashes occur more commonly in babies who wear disposable diapers.

The diaper area of a child with a diaper rash is covered with red, spotty sores that may smell of ammonia. *(See color photograph of diaper rash, page B-2.)*

To treat a diaper rash, leave your infant's bottom exposed to air as much as possible. Avoid plastic pants and, if possible, switch to cloth diapers or at least a disposable diaper that keeps wetness away from your baby's skin.

To clean the baby's bottom, use plain water, which is less irritating than baby wipes. Mild rashes do not require ointment unless the skin is dry and cracked. Baby powder such as cornstarch or talcum powder is generally to be avoided because of concerns that it can lead to coughing or choking if inhaled by your infant.

Most diaper rashes respond within 3 days of drying efforts. If your baby's rash does not improve, it could mean the child has a yeast infection, which may require a prescription medication. If the rash is so severe that it interferes with the child's sleep, if it is a solid, bright red, if it causes fever, or if the bottom develops blisters, boils, or drains pus, call your child's physician.

Cradle Cap.　If your baby has yellow, oily scales and crusts on the scalp, he or she has cradle cap (seborrheic eczema). Without treatment, cradle cap may persist for months. However, when properly treated, it usually resolves within a few weeks.

For cradle cap, wash your baby's hair with baby shampoo once a day. After lathering, massage the scaly scalp with a soft toothbrush for a few minutes. If the scalp is very crusty, you can rub in mineral oil an hour before you shampoo. However, if the oil is not thoroughly washed out, it will aggravate the problem. If the rash is red and irritated, you can apply a 0.05 percent hydrocortisone cream, available without a prescription. A particularly stubborn case should be evaluated by your infant's physician. (See color photograph of cradle cap, page B-2.)

WHAT TO DO IF YOUR INFANT HAS A SEIZURE

Seizures can be a frightening event for a parent. You are bound to feel helpless, especially the first time.

Remember, in the vast majority of cases, the child is fine after the seizure. The following instructions can help you deal with a seizure.

Febrile Seizure

If the infant with a fever has a seizure, the most important thing to remember is that the seizure usually stops by itself within several minutes. However, take steps to gradually bring down your baby's fever. Remove your baby's clothes and apply cool cloths to the infant's head and chest. Sponge the body with cool water. Never sponge with alcohol. Do not put the infant in the bathtub during the seizure because this can be dangerous.

If your baby begins to vomit during the seizure, place the child on his or her stomach or side, never on the back. If the child's breathing becomes labored, gently pull the jaw and chin forward by placing two fingers behind the corner of the jaw on each side.

After the seizure is over and your baby is awake, notify your physician, who will probably want to see the baby right away. If you are unable to contact your infant's physician, take your baby to a clinic or emergency room for examination.

Seizure Without Fever

The rules for handling this type of seizure are similar to those for a febrile seizure except that you do not have to worry about bringing down your baby's fever.

Do not try to move the baby or restrain any movements. Although the infant's breathing may stop for a moment, do not begin resuscitation; the child will begin breathing on his or her own. People are often concerned that someone in the midst of a seizure will somehow swallow or bite off his or her tongue. Although occasionally a child will bite the tongue, there is no way he or she will swallow it or inflict a severe injury. Keep your hands and other objects out of the baby's mouth.

Again, after the seizure has passed, call your baby's physician.

Infant Acne.　About a third of all infants develop acne, usually after the third week of life. The cause appears to be related to maternal hormones that cross the placenta before birth.

The presence of acne on an infant can be disturbing, but parents should know that it is only temporary. In some infants, the acne disappears within weeks; in others, it may persist for up to 6 months.

We recommend no treatment other than washing your baby's face with water and mild soap.

Drool Rash.　Many infants develop a rash on their cheeks and chin. The rash, which is caused by contact with food and stomach contents (regurgitation), comes and goes. The only treatment generally required is cleansing the skin after a feeding. Placing a diaper under your infant's face during naps to absorb the drool or regurgitated material also may help.

Milia.　These are small white bumps that are found on the faces of 40 percent of all newborns. These blocked skin pores generally open up and disappear by the time the infant is 2 months old. Treatment is not needed. (See color photograph of milia, page B-2.)

Heat Rash.　This rash of tiny pink bumps is usually found on the back of the neck and on the upper back and is the result of blocked sweat glands. Typically, the rash occurs during hot, humid weather, although an infant who is overdressed or who has a fever may develop a heat rash at any time.

Treatment involves cooling the skin. Let the skin dry on its own, and dress your infant in as few clothes as possible. Use a fan while the child is sleeping. Cool baths sometimes help. (For more information about rashes, see Chapter 37, page 1150.)

FEBRILE SEIZURES

A seizure (convulsion) occurs as a result of abnormal activity in the brain's nerve cells. Typically, the infant having a seizure suddenly becomes unconscious, with the arms and legs held rigid. After a few seconds, the limbs and face may begin to twitch rhythmically.

The majority of childhood seizures are related to fevers. When seizures are recurrent and not related to fever, a child is said to have a seizure disorder (see also Seizures and Tics, page 541).

A febrile seizure is triggered by a fever. Typically, a seizure occurs in a child between 6 months and 5 years of age who develops a sudden fever. The severity of fever does not necessarily correlate with the development of a febrile seizure. Sometimes a febrile seizure is the first indication that a child is ill. Between 4 and 5 percent of all children have at least one febrile convulsion; 50 percent have no recurrence after the initial episode.

Febrile seizures tend to be short—usually less than 5 minutes. Although it was once believed that a child who had a febrile seizure risked brain damage, this is rare. In febrile seizures, the cause of the illness is more important than the extent of the fever. For example, meningitis is far more serious than a simple febrile seizure (see also Febrile Seizure, page 543).

SUDDEN INFANT DEATH SYNDROME

Sudden infant death syndrome (SIDS) is the most common cause of death during infancy. It is commonly called crib death.

Typically, a seemingly healthy infant—most commonly between the ages of 2 and 4 months—is put to bed one night and found dead the next morning. Even if an autopsy is performed, the precise cause usually remains a mystery and the parents may be left trying to cope with guilt, wondering what they could have done to prevent their infant's tragic death.

In the United States, there is approximately 1 case of SIDS in 500 births. Among various ethnic groups, the incidence is lowest in Asians and whites and highest in blacks and American Indians.

The majority of infants who die of SIDS seemed healthy, but detailed investigations done after death often show evidence of heart, lung, and brain problems. Moreover, several genetic, environmental, and social factors have been associated with this syndrome. These include low birth weight for gestational age, premature birth, cold weather, a history of maternal smoking or drug abuse, history of a sibling with SIDS, and a history of near-miss SIDS (infant had stopped breathing but was found and resuscitated before death). Near-miss SIDS is now called acute life-threatening event (ALTE) to point out that such episodes are not necessarily related to SIDS.

This is not to say that all infants who die of SIDS fit into one of these categories. Many, in fact, are not considered high risk. Thus, even if all high-risk infants were stringently monitored, it may be impossible to prevent SIDS altogether.

Although the search for a single cause of SIDS has not been fruitful, researchers have found several physiological abnormalities that appear more commonly in many infants with this syndrome. Among them are central nervous system abnormalities, abnormal heart rates, muscle tone abnormalities, a defect in the autonomic nervous system, and abnormal breathing pauses (apnea) during sleep. An autopsy is often very helpful for determining whether a specific cause of death is present.

The prospect of SIDS is so frightening that many parents today inquire about monitoring their infant's heart rate and breathing at home. This is usually not recommended, however, unless the infant has been shown to be at high risk for SIDS. Your physician can give you information about the National SIDS Foundation. (For a detailed discussion of SIDS, see page 21.)

GENERAL INFANT CARE AND HYGIENE

Caring for your baby is certainly time-consuming, but it is not difficult.

One of the most important aspects of care falls under the realm of safety. Your infant—especially after he or she begins to crawl—is particularly susceptible to injury in the home. Thus, it is up to you to make certain that the child's environment is as safe as possible. This means childproofing your home and making sure that your infant's toys are both safe and appropriate from a developmental standpoint. It also includes being diligent about the use of a car seat.

In this section, in addition to safety, we discuss diaper care and what steps you can take to minimize the spread of disease.

SAFETY

Making your home as safe as possible for your infant is imperative during these early months when your baby has no sense of danger.

How can you make your baby's environment safe?

First, start with the baby's bed. Since 1974, the federal government has required that the spaces between crib bars be no more than 2⅜ inches. This precaution is important because it prevents an infant from getting his or her head stuck between the bars. If you are using an old crib, make certain that the bars are spaced in accordance with these specifications. Moreover, make certain that the mattress fits the crib snugly because babies have been known to get their heads caught in the space between the crib and the mattress. In either situation, a baby's breathing may be obstructed and he or she may die.

Make sure that any toys in the crib are soft, with no sharp edges that could hurt your baby. Remember to check stuffed animals for any loose buttons or parts that could find their way into baby's mouth and cause choking.

Another important safety rule is to *never* leave your infant unattended in the bath or on a bed or table. When bathing the baby, do not allow yourself to be distracted by the doorbell or telephone. Let it ring. All it takes is a second alone for a baby's head to become submerged under water.

Many parents have no qualms about putting a very young baby in the middle of a bed to nap. This practice can be dangerous because some infants will manage to roll off. Also, there is always the possibility that another child will push the baby off, so it is best to avoid this practice. If a crib is not available, put a blanket on the floor. The baby will be comfortable there. But select a location well away from stairs or adult "traffic."

A similar rule applies to infant seats: do not put your baby in a seat perched on a table or counter. One slight move is often all it takes to tip the carrier and the infant off the table or counter.

As your infant becomes more mobile, your child-proofing efforts will have to increase. If you have stairs in your home, make sure you have gates at the top and bottom of the stairway. Babies love to poke and prod, and electrical outlets are often a source of curiosity, so cover your unused outlets. You can purchase protective covers at many drugstores and at hardware and grocery stores that carry infant-related items.

An infant is forever mouthing anything he or she comes into contact with. Although it is impossible to keep the occasional bug or bit of dirt out of your baby's grasp, you must keep your child away from substances that can potentially cause harm. Make sure that all cleaning solutions, insecticides, and medications are stored well out of your infant's reach. If you do not have a high shelf or cupboard, you can buy locks that make it difficult for a child to open a cabinet.

Check your houseplants. Be familiar with the toxic plants in and around your home, and make sure that they are well out of reach of your baby (see Garden-Variety Poisonous Plants, page 302).

CAR SEATS

Install a car seat in your car before your baby has his or her first ride home from the hospital. In many hospitals, an infant will not be released to the parents unless they have a

For every car ride, your child must be safely buckled into a car seat that, in turn, is fastened to the seat of your car.

safety seat in their car. In all 50 states, the parent who does not strap a young child into a car seat is breaking the law.

If this rule seems extreme, consider the statistics. The major killer and crippler of young children in the United States is automobile accidents. Yet an estimated 80 percent of these deaths and serious injuries are thought to be avoidable if safety seats are used.

When shopping for your car seat, make sure it meets certain government standards. Since 1981, all manufacturers have been required to meet stringent specifications set down by the federal government. Somewhere on the seat you should see an indication that the seat has met Federal Motor Vehicle Safety Standard 213, which includes crash testing.

Two types of car seats are suitable for infants.

An infant safety seat can only be installed so that the baby faces the rear of the car. This seat can be used until the child weighs 20 pounds.

Most parents find a convertible safety seat more practical because it can be used until the child weighs 40 pounds. During early infancy, the convertible seat is installed so that the baby faces the rear; later, when the

infant weighs at least 18 pounds, it can be turned around so that the infant faces the front of the car.

No matter what type of seat you purchase, it will not provide optimal protection unless it is used properly. Here are some tips on proper use of car seats.

Install the seat in the back seat of the car, preferably in the middle.

Make sure the seat belt is fastened securely around the car seat.

Adjust the harness straps so that they fit snugly, and fasten all parts of the harness.

If the seat has a top anchor strap, make sure it is installed.

Always use the car seat. Even if you are just going a block down the road, do not assume your baby will be safe unless he or she is securely fastened in the seat. For more information about car seats, see page 324.

SAFE TOYS

Like the older child, your infant needs toys to keep him or her amused and stimulated and to learn. The key is finding appropriate toys—your 5-year-old's marbles and jacks could have disastrous consequences in the hands of a 6-month-old.

Always be on the lookout for toys that could be hazardous. Do not give an infant toys that contain small pieces that can easily be swallowed. Keep anything made of a material that can be broken, such as glass, away from your baby. Avoid toys with sharp edges or loose buttons. Discard objects painted with a lead-base paint because an infant gnawing on the toy can ingest enough lead to cause lead poisoning.

During the first 3 months, your baby needs toys that can be looked at (he or she is not yet adept at grasping). Babies prefer patterns over solids and bright colors over pastels. Look for interesting patterns in the bedding you use in the crib—and do not be surprised if your baby seems mesmerized. Buy a colorful mobile, one whose full impact is seen from the baby's position and not from the parent's upright view. Interesting pictures on the wall can capture a baby's attention. A mirror attached to the side of the crib, a music box or tape recorder playing a soothing lullaby, colorful plastic shapes hung on strings suspended between the crib rails, rattles your baby can shake, furry stuffed animals with which you can stroke the baby—these are all good toys for the young infant.

By the end of the fourth month, most babies have mastered the ability to grasp and can swipe at objects, although they often miss. At this age, your baby can appreciate rattles, clacking discs, and stuffed animals.

At 6 months, a baby's greatest pleasure is putting things in his or her mouth. Teething rings, cloth dolls, squeeze toys, and kitchen objects such as measuring spoons, plastic cups, and bowls are good toys.

An infant swing, jumper, bouncing chair, and walker also are appropriate toys at this age. For the older infant, a riding toy such as a small car is often a source of enjoyment, as are balls, blocks, and toy telephones.

When buying toys, read the description on the box to determine whether a toy is appropriate. Most major toy manufacturers indicate on the packaging the age range for which the toy is intended.

COMFORTABLE CLOTHING

When buying clothes for your infant, remember that what is important to your baby is comfort. Is the material soft? Does it feel good to the touch? Is it loose enough for the baby to move about in without feeling constrained? For your convenience and the baby's, is it easy to put on and take off?

In planning your infant's wardrobe, remember to buy larger sizes than your baby's age suggests. For example, most newborns can easily wear clothes made for a 3-month-old. And many 6-month-olds may be large enough to wear 9-month or even 12-month sizes. In the same vein, do not stock up on one particular size. Babies grow at an astonishing rate during the first year, and parents

---

LEAD POISONING

For generations, lead was used in plumbing pipes and paint. It was used in typesetting, in soldering, and for sash weights in windows. Its weight, malleability, and other characteristics also were adapted to numerous other products.

Today, we know that lead is poisonous. When ingested—whether in lead paint chips by children, in water supplies tainted by lead pipes, or in the air from auto emissions—lead can accumulate in the bone marrow, nerves, and kidneys.

In many cases, there are no symptoms of lead poisoning. However, such signs as irritability, weight loss, and sluggishness may occur, perhaps accompanied by vomiting, constipation, or stomach pain.

If you suspect lead poisoning in your child, consult your physician, who may prescribe chelation therapy, in which a drug called penicillamine is given. The drug binds to the lead and causes it to be excreted.

Prevention

The best approach to prevention is to inspect your home for potential sources of lead—and to eliminate them. If you live in an older home and the paint is flaking off as dust, consult your local health department and have the paint dust tested. Older homes should also be checked to determine whether any of the pipes are lead. Look for the main line where the water pipe enters your house: if there is a swelling at one of the joints, gently tap it with a hammer. If it dents easily, it is made of lead and you should have your water tested to determine whether it contains lead.

Beware of old lead toys or jewelry and fishing or curtain weights—do not let your children play with them. Do not store juices in earthenware jars because the glazes may be lead-based.

who buy too many clothes often end up with a drawer full of unopened packages.

The following are some basic guidelines for dressing your infant:

Knitted nightgowns and stretchies: During the first 2 or 3 months it is often easier to dress your baby the same during the day as you do at night. Knitted nightgowns and stretchies (which are usually made of a soft terry cloth material or cotton) are perfect for sleep and wakeful periods. Because many babies virtually live in these clothes, you should have several of each.

Underclothes: There are two styles of undershirts: shirts that are pulled over the baby's head and shirts with a snap closing, which are usually easier to use on a very young baby. Buy three or four in at least a 6-month size for the young infant.

Socks: Buy several pair. Booties, while cute, are not needed and often do not stay on. Shoes are not necessary until the infant begins to walk.

Sweaters: During cool weather, you may find that your baby needs a sweater for extra warmth over the stretchie. Usually made of acrylic, a sweater should fit loose around the neck.

Outerwear: If you are taking your baby out in cold weather, he or she will need some type of snowsuit or bunting. A bunting—a zippered bag in which the baby is encased up to the shoulders—is fine for the very young baby. However, once the infant is several months old, he or she will prefer the freedom of a snowsuit. The baby also will need a knitted cap that fits snugly over the ears. If the baby is going to be in the sun, a sun hat is great for protecting his or her skin.

Bibs: Once your infant begins to eat solids, make sure you buy several bibs. Forget the dainty little round bibs. You need bibs large enough to cover the entire front of your infant. Bibs made of plastic are good because they can be rinsed off.

Other clothes: Once your infant begins to move around, you will probably want to begin dressing him or her more for play and less for sleep. Jeans, cotton overalls with snaps along the legs and crotch, and knit pants and shirts are good choices. When the weather is warm, sunsuits, shorts, and T-shirts are appropriate clothing.

DIAPER CARE

Stringent care of the diaper area will help prevent diaper rash, a problem affecting most babies at least once during their diaper-wearing years. Follow these key preventive steps.

Check your infant's diaper frequently and change it if it is wet or soiled. In a 1-month-old infant, this sometimes means changing the baby before and after feeding. In the 10-month-old baby, it may entail checking every 2 or 3 hours.

After you remove a wet diaper, rinse the baby's bottom with a wet washcloth. When changing a soiled diaper, make certain you clean the area thoroughly with a mild soap and water. On a boy, pay particular attention to the scrotum; on a girl, separate the creases of the labia and gently wipe from front to back.

Disposable diapers currently are used widely and are convenient in our mobile society. There is, however, increasing discussion of the fact that disposable diapers are not biodegradable and contribute significantly to the growing problems with managing solid waste and other garbage. As a result, we are beginning to see a renaissance in the use of cloth diapers. In fact, cloth diapers are preferable to disposable diapers, although care must be taken to wash and dry them thoroughly.

A word of caution regarding disposable diapers: they tend to keep in warmth and moisture, which may dispose your child to diaper rash. The message is clear: change your infant's disposable diapers often (see Diaper Rash, page 16).

PREVENTING THE SPREAD OF DISEASE

Once one member of the family contracts an infectious disease such as a cold, preventing others in the household from catching the infection is usually difficult.

The following simple measures could reduce the spread of some infectious diseases in your home:

Hand washing is the most important thing you can do to help reduce the spread of disease. After changing your infant's diaper, using the bathroom yourself, or blowing your nose or wiping your baby's nose, make sure you thoroughly wash your hands with soap and water.

Avoid touching your mouth and nose.

Do not let your children kiss pets.

Never smoke at home. (Children who breathe tobacco smoke have a higher incidence of respiratory infection.)

Cook all poultry thoroughly and be sure you wash anything that comes into contact with uncooked poultry (such as knives or cutting boards) and poultry juice (foods stored beneath a leaky package of chicken in the refrigerator, for example).

Use a disinfectant in the kitchen, bathroom, family room, and nursery and on your infant's playthings (see Day-Care Centers, page 105).

DEVELOPMENT OF PERSONALITY AND BEHAVIOR

During the first 12 months of life, your baby works harder than at any other stage of his or her existence. In the course of this incredible first year, your infant goes from being totally dependent to walking, feeding himself or herself, and even speaking a few words. Bonds are formed, a routine is established, and, at some point early in the year, the parent notices a distinct personality emerging.

In this section, we examine normal development and we review milestones to look for. We also offer advice on handling sleeping problems that may arise.

NORMAL DEVELOPMENTAL MILESTONES

A momentous occasion during the early weeks of life is your baby's first smile. Although you often will see a smile on your newborn, an infant generally does not have what is called a social smile until after the first month, usually by the eighth week.

By the time your infant is *6 weeks* old, he or she may be showing a clear preference for family members over strangers. Smile at your infant and he or she may smile back. Watch your infant gaze at you intently while he or she is eating.

The infant at *2 months* smiles with his or her entire body. Watch your baby when you walk into his or her room. Your baby begins flailing both arms and legs in excitement. He or she gurgles and coos.

Your response to your infant's smiles during these early weeks is important. When you cuddle your infant, smile, coo, or attend to his or her needs, you encourage the smiles.

By the second month of life, your baby can differentiate between people and objects, with the former eliciting a much more immediate response. Your infant is beginning to recognize your voice. Thus, you may find that the baby who screams when with a babysitter calms immediately when a parent enters the room and talks in a soothing voice.

The infant at *3 months* can actually play for up to three-quarters of an hour. The infant at this age is more easily distracted and will even interrupt nursing to look at or listen to something that catches his or her attention. The baby will spend time staring at things—a picture, a mobile, or his or her own hand.

You may notice that your baby's memory seems to improve with each passing day. At this point, the infant may associate certain acts with rewards—for example, the sound of the refrigerator door closing and your footsteps with feeding. The baby may wait patiently for a moment or two anticipating your arrival. Should that arrival be delayed by a ringing telephone, he or she may erupt in a howl.

At *4 months* your infant is less interested in feeding than in the world around him or her. Hence, do not be surprised if it takes longer than usual to finish a feeding.

A milestone during this period—usually at around 20 weeks—is your baby's behavior in front of a mirror. Hold him or her in front of the mirror and watch the infant smile. When the image smiles back, the baby will get really excited and begin to babble. It will puzzle him or her to see two of you and he or she will repeatedly look back at you and then at the mirror.

At *5 months* your baby definitely knows the difference between his or her parents and strangers. For the first time, you may notice a real fear of strangers.

At this age, your infant has learned to identify and find objects. For example, if a toy drops to the floor, your infant will try to find it. Similarly, he or she will play with a stuffed animal, lay it down, and later come back to it.

A *6-month-old* infant is alert for half of his or her waking hours.

If you are bottle-feeding, your baby may insist on trying to hold the bottle. Some babies at this age are ready to start using a cup in conjunction with a bottle.

By this age, solid foods may be a part of the diet. Gone are the days when your baby was content to have you do the feeding. Now that the infant's dexterity is improved, he or she wants to pick up pieces of food and put them in his or her own mouth and anywhere else mood dictates.

Increased motor skills give the infant of *7 months* a taste of freedom. At the same time that your baby longs to test his or her wings, however, the infant only wants to do it within sight of your reassuring presence. Do not be surprised if every time you leave the room your baby cries. The infant who has been content up until now to spend time in a playpen may suddenly rebel unless you are in the same room.

The infant of this age loves to mouth things. Chewing on fingers, sucking a thumb, and nibbling toes are very satisfying activities. During feedings, the baby may be able to grasp a spoon.

The *8-month-old* baby is clearly attached to his or her mother. Separation anxiety often occurs at this age, and you may find that you cannot leave the room without sending your baby into a panic. Even the baby who previously was not bothered by strangers suddenly may fear the next-door neighbor or the physician. Or, the infant may cry uncontrollably when the babysitter arrives, even when the care-giver is someone the baby knows. This reaction is a normal part of development and is nothing to be concerned about. Simply cuddle the child and reassure him or her that you will return soon.

The infant at *9 months* is sophisticated enough to be bored. This is because his or her memory is more developed. Thus, the infant is constantly searching for new stimulation, and the nightly game that has amused him or her for the past month suddenly has become uninteresting.

Another stage to expect around this time is insecurity and even fears. Every time you turn on the vacuum cleaner your baby begins to cry. Or one day the beloved bath is shunned out of fear. With a little patience and understanding on your part, these fears usually are conquered within a month or so.

The *10-month-old* is capable of carrying two small objects in one hand.

During this time your baby's sense of identity within your family is emerging. His or her moods become more apparent. Scold your baby, and he or she looks sad; praise your infant, and he or she beams. Watch your child smack his or her lips after a good meal or light up when your spouse comes in the door after work.

Your baby may begin to say "no" at this age. Your child also is developing a sense of possession and may for the first time distinguish between baby's toys and those belonging to a sibling.

You also will notice how imitation plays a role in your infant's learning. During a meal, the baby may offer you bits of food; afterward he or she may attempt to wash your face and hands.

Although not always cooperative, your *11-month-old* baby seeks your approval and will try to avoid your disapproval. Still, the infant cannot avoid trying to test your authority. After you have put your son or daughter to bed, he or she may summon you every 5 minutes. At the same time, your every request is apt to be met with a resounding "no." At this age, "no" sometimes means "yes."

This negativism increases in the *12-month-old* baby. Some infants at this age begin to have tantrums; you should expect refusals (see Tantrums and Breath Holding, page 95). Appetite naturally begins to decrease, so do not be surprised when your eager eater suddenly becomes picky. This refusal also may extend to bedtime. Sleep problems are common at this age.

If you are concerned that your infant is not achieving these developmental milestones, see your child's physician.

SLEEPING PROBLEMS

Sleeping problems commonly occur during infancy and even throughout early childhood.

These problems often are brought about by well-meaning parents who believe it is somehow wrong to let their baby cry in bed. Your infant cries in the middle of the night, you rush in, pick the child up, give him or her a bottle, or play for a while. The pattern is set. Your baby has learned that it is okay to wake up at night and that when he or she does you will immediately arrive for company and entertainment.

The prevention of sleep problems is easier than the cure. Early infancy is the time to train your child that nighttime is for sleep.

Follow these guidelines:

By the time your baby is 2 months old, make sure he or she is out of your bedroom and into his or her own room.

At 2 months, begin to discourage middle-of-the-night feeding. Do not awaken your infant for this feeding. When the child does wake up, allow him or her to cry for 5 minutes—the infant may go back to sleep without eating. If this does not work, you may want to try offering your baby an ounce or two less than at daytime feedings or nursing for a shorter time than usual. Before feeding, hold your baby for a couple of minutes to see whether that is sufficient.

A 4-month-old infant does not need a 2 a.m. feeding. Infants who continue to demand food at this age may do so out of habit. If you do not eliminate this feeding by 4 months, it will be increasingly difficult to do so.

If your baby cries, go to the infant. Instead of picking him or her up, rub your baby's back for a moment and let your voice do the soothing. You need to help him or her understand that he or she belongs in the crib at night, not in your arms.

The infant at 6 months starts to have separation anxiety. Make sure your baby has a security object such as a blanket or stuffed toy that he or she can snuggle up next to every night. Leaving the door to the baby's room open is very reassuring for the child, as is providing extra affection during the day. A night-light is often helpful.

By the time your infant is 12 months old, he or she should have a consistent bedtime ritual. If your baby has a nightmare or nighttime fear, sit by the crib a few moments. Be reassuring.

SIBLING RELATIONSHIPS

If your infant has a brother or sister, he or she is indeed fortunate.

Much attention has been devoted to sibling rivalry—the hostilities and insecurities aroused in the older child by the birth of a baby (see page 110). But what about the infant and its relationship with big brother or sister?

Granted, life is not as cozy for the infant with a sibling. This baby is apt to be poked and jabbed more than once, especially as he or she becomes more mobile.

On the positive side, watch your 5-month-old's obvious delight when he or she is included in a game with an older sibling. Play with a sibling is so rewarding for the baby that he or she is willing to put up with even a little roughness. Of course, you have to monitor the play and make sure your infant is not put in a situation where he or she could be hurt.

Besides the simple enjoyment of having a brother or sister to play with, the baby develops mentally and socially from this exposure to an older child. The infant learns about self-protection, cooperation, and imagination and how to get along with others. Moreover, the bond between your children is developed and they grow to love each other.

Do not feel guilty that your second and subsequent children do not get undivided attention as did your first child. Remember, your first child did not reap the benefits of an older brother or sister. There will be times when your baby actually prefers a brother or sister over you, or when a sibling's request that baby eat his or her cereal is immediately granted—whereas your efforts were met with resolute rejection.

This is not to imply that the relationship is always going to be smooth. At around 9 months, some babies have trouble getting along with a sibling who only weeks before was an object of admiration. Babies this age are intent on battling their own insecurities and fears. An older sibling who loves to tease or assert authority is just too much sometimes. If this happens to your infant, do not worry. The stage will pass.

NUTRITION IN YOUR INFANT

One of the important decisions you will be making during your baby's first year regards nutrition. Which is preferable—bottle- or breast-feeding? When should I wean the baby? When is the best time to introduce solids? These are questions on every parent's mind.

The purpose of this section is to address the issue of infant nutrition. By the time your infant is 1 month old you have already decided whether you will nurse the baby, so we will not debate the merits of breast-feeding over bottle-feeding (see Bottle-Feeding versus Breast-Feeding, page 43). Rather, we will talk about what foods your infant needs to grow and remain healthy and when it is best to begin serving those foods. In addition, we will discuss common feeding problems during the first year.

FEEDING RECOMMENDATIONS

During your infant's first year of life, his or her birth weight may triple. It should come as no surprise, then, that eating will be an important part of your baby's day.

In the first few months of life, your baby's diet consists solely of breast milk or formula. Evaporated milk or cow's milk is not a replacement for formula. In fact, do not give your baby cow's milk until the infant is at least 6 months old and preferably 9 months old, because cow's milk does not provide proper nutrition for young babies.

In hot weather, you might offer your baby a bottle of water twice a day. Your baby's physician also may prescribe a general vitamin preparation. Also, if you are breast-feeding, your baby's physician may prescribe vitamin D for your infant (breast milk may be deficient in vitamin D). Although both breast milk and formula contain most nutrients, they lack fluoride, which aids in the prevention of tooth decay and is advised from the second week of life until age 12 years.

The frequency of feedings depends on your baby's needs and the method of feeding.

A baby between 1 and 3 months old probably will want between five and six feedings a day, usually eating every 3 hours, except for a longer stretch at night. As the baby grows, the number of feedings is reduced. Typically, a 5-month-old is down to four or five feedings, and by nine months the child has only three milk feedings. Remember, each infant is a distinct individual. Accept each one's differences in feeding behavior.

Breast-fed infants often require more frequent feedings because breast milk is digested more quickly than formula. During the first 3 months some infants want to nurse every 2 or 2½ hours.

Parents always ask when they should offer their baby solids. This is a difficult question and one that has no shortage of opinions. From a nutritional standpoint, your baby gets everything he or she needs from breast milk or formula for the first 6 months. Yet many physicians recommend starting babies, particularly formula-fed babies, on solids after 4 months. Moreover, if your infant is drinking a quart of formula a day and is still ravenous, or is nursing more often rather than less, your physician may recommend an early introduction to solids.

Before you introduce your baby to solids, consult your physician. He or she will be able to tell you whether the child is physically able to handle solid foods. For example, for several months the neuromuscular development of infants is geared only toward sucking and swallowing liquids. Until the child has the ability to recognize a spoon and his or her tongue and swallowing mechanisms can respond to solid food—usually between 3 and 6 months—the infant is not ready to expand his or her diet.

Once the decision to start solids is made, what foods should you introduce? Many physicians recommend starting the baby on a cereal. Precooked rice cereal (found in the baby food section of the supermarket) is often used as baby's first solid food because it is easy to digest. Mix a small amount (1 tablespoon) of cereal with 4 or 5 tablespoons of formula or breast milk. Initially, babies generally respond better to solids if the solid foods are thin rather than thick. Put some food on the tip of a small spoon and place it in your baby's mouth. Do not be surprised if it comes back out. Many babies take time to adjust to this new taste and consistency. Be patient. Do not put solids in a bottle or a syringe-type feeder; the former can encourage your baby to overeat; the latter can cause choking.

You have two basic options in feeding your baby: buy commercial baby food or prepare your own. Commercial baby food is certainly easier, but it is more expensive and may contain fillers or sugars, which add empty calories. If you decide to buy commercial baby food, make certain that you read the labels.

Making your own baby food is not difficult if you have a blender or food grinder. Cook meats, vegetables, and fruits (bananas do not need to be cooked) in a small amount of water. Remove fat, skin, and seeds and then puree the mixture in the blender until it is a suitable consistency. A little water aids in the blending process. From a nutritional standpoint, fresh fruits and vegetables are preferable. If you cannot obtain them, frozen produce should be your second choice.

After your baby is acquainted with cereal, your next step should be a fruit such as pureed bananas. Generally, fruits are popular with babies.

At 7 months, most infants are ready to try pureed vegetables and then meats. After 8 months most babies are able to eat small pieces of table food. Toast, bits of cheese, pieces of scrambled egg, dry cereals, crackers, mashed potato, french fries, pasta, and ground meat are good finger foods.

Avoid foods that could easily choke your baby. These include whole hot dogs (if you want to give the baby a hot dog, cut it lengthwise first and then into small pieces), grapes, popcorn, nuts, and raw carrots.

Some general rules are these:

Introduce only one new food at a time and never more than three a week.
Avoid seasoning, especially salt, and desserts.

Do not force your baby to eat. Spitting the food out, putting a hand over his or her mouth, turning his or her head, or fussing are all indications that your infant's appetite has been satisfied.

How much food should your baby be eating? By the time the infant is between 6 and 8 months old, he or she should be eating 3 to 4 ounces of solids at each of the three meals, or between 5 and 8 tablespoons of food per meal. A good diet for an infant of this age would be, for example, cereal and fruit for breakfast, meat and vegetable for lunch, and meat, fruit, and vegetable for supper. Most babies eating this diet reduce their milk consumption to about 16 ounces a day. Many babies also need a mid-morning and mid-afternoon snack, which should be something nutritious such as fruit or a cracker.

Sometimes your baby's diet needs to be supplemented with vitamins and minerals (see accompanying table). Consult your physician.

Once your child reaches his or her first birthday, the infant should be eating table food exclusively.

A note of caution: never allow your infant to have food away from the table and away from your watchful eye.

FEEDING PROBLEMS

Several feeding problems can be encountered during the first year of life. If your baby is not gaining adequately or seems to be gaining an excessive amount of weight, is colicky, is constipated, or has frequent diarrhea, consult your physician. A change in formula or in the amount the baby is fed may be all that is necessary to eliminate the problem.

The following are common feeding problems.

Underfeeding. A baby who is not getting enough to eat does not gain weight on schedule, is frequently restless, and cries often. The baby also may be constipated and have wrinkled, dry skin as a result of the loss of fat. Babies may be underfed deliberately (the parent withholds food) or as a result of the baby's own inability to

Vitamin and Mineral Supplements for Infants

Type of Feeding	Supplement			
	Iron	Vitamin D	Fluoride	Other
Breast	Additional iron from a supplement or an iron-fortified infant cereal is needed after 6 months of age	Vitamin D supplementation may be recommended if the infant has little exposure to sunlight	Fluoride supplementation may be recommended	None
Formula	Supplementation is needed by 4 months of age if the formula does not contain iron	No supplementation needed	Fluoride supplementation may be recommended, based on the fluoride content of the water supply	None
Cow's milk plus solid food (after 6 months of age)	Additional iron from a supplement or from an iron-fortified infant cereal is needed	No supplementation needed	Fluoride supplementation may be recommended	None

From: *Mayo Clinic Diet Manual*, sixth edition. By permission of Mayo Foundation.

consume adequate amounts. (See Failure To Gain Weight, page 66.)

Although the vast majority of women can successfully breast-feed, sometimes the infant may not nurse well enough to be satisfied. This problem is often temporary, and most women are encouraged to continue breast-feeding. Check with your physician for help with breast-feeding or supplementation with formula.

For bottle-fed infants who do not eat enough, sometimes the problem is solved by enlarging the holes in the bottle nipple. This enables the baby to take in more milk with less effort. You also can try increasing the number of feedings.

If these measures fail, your physician will want to determine whether an underlying disease may be causing the problem.

Overfeeding. A baby who eats too much or too often may have excessive regurgitation or even vomiting. Excessive weight gain, abdominal pain, and bloating are other symptoms of overfeeding.

Unlike adults, most babies stop eating when they have had enough. However, a parent who offers the bottle or breast every time the infant cries, is overzealous in pushing solids, or rewards an older baby with food may contribute to overeating.

Regurgitation and Vomiting. The spitting up of small amounts of food during or shortly after a feeding is normal during the first 6 months. Some babies are simply spitters. Although spitting up is impossible to eliminate totally, you can reduce the amount your infant regurgitates by trying to get the baby to burp frequently during a feeding, avoiding bouncing your baby after a feeding, keeping the baby upright for a while after eating, and reducing intake slightly (see page 14).

Vomiting, unlike regurgitation, is the forceful expulsion of most of the stomach's contents. It is a common complaint during infancy. The cause is most often a stomach virus or something the infant ate that disagreed with him or her. Frequent or prolonged vomiting, however, can be serious and needs to be investigated (see page 14).

Loose Stools and Diarrhea. A breast-fed baby normally has loose, curd-like stools. Actual diarrhea in the breast-fed infant, although uncommon, may occur as a result of an infection.

In the bottle-fed infant, however, firmer stools are the norm.

These mild digestive disturbances usually require no more than a temporary decrease in or cessation of feedings. If your infant is eating solid food, withhold all solids and eliminate one or more milk feedings for a day, substituting boiled water or an oral electrolyte replacement, such as Pedialyte, Lytren, or Infalyte. (They are available without prescription at most pharmacies.)

Constipation. Constipation rarely occurs in breast-fed infants or in formula-fed babies who get enough to eat. Do not assume that your infant is constipated if he or she goes a couple of days without a bowel movement (see page 70). Most babies have one or more bowel movements each day, but some frequently skip a day or two.

If your baby has difficulty passing a stool, your physician may want to check for any rectal abnormality. If your baby is eating solids, increase his intake of fruits (not bananas), vegetables, and cereals, which will add bulk to the stool and make it easier to pass.

Colic. A baby who has colic has abdominal pain that may last for hours. Typically, the attack begins suddenly, and the baby cries, draws his or her legs up, and clenches his or her hands. The infant's face may be flushed and pale and the feet cold. The attack may end when the baby cries himself or herself to sleep or with the passage of gas or a bowel movement.

The cause of colic is unknown. Although distressing for both the baby and the parents, colic is not dangerous and generally is over by the third month (see Excessive Crying, page 12).

CHAPTER 3

THE PRESCHOOL YEARS

AGES 1 THROUGH 5

CHAPTER CONTENTS

A TIME OF RAPID CHANGE

It may seem like only yesterday that you held your baby for the first time. After 9 long months, the waiting was over when the physician handed you a bundle of energy, tiny and helpless and giving little hint of what he or she was to become.

With each passing day a bit of the mystery was revealed—perhaps dark hair from the father's side or the mother's eyes or maybe a preference for rice cereal over oat cereal or for fruits instead of vegetables. Little by little, step by step, you became acquainted.

Now, having celebrated your baby's first birthday, you have a better idea of who this little person is. Although it has been only 365 days—barely enough time to alter your appearance beyond the deepening of a wrinkle or the addition of a few gray hairs— the changes in your baby have been phenomenal. Even so, most of the story of the development of your child has yet to be written. This chapter discusses changes you will see in your child from ages 1 through 5 years.

If you are the parent of a preschooler, you occasionally may have entertained thoughts of taking a permanent vacation. These years can be trying. Preschoolers are demanding and can consume your energy. Caught between wanting to "do it myself" yet longing for the safety net that only a parent can provide, the preschooler is often at odds with himself or herself and with everything that gets in the way.

Negativism, anxieties over monsters that hide under beds or in closets, temper tantrums, toilet training, and discovery of the genitals are among the issues brought to the forefront during ages 1 through 5.

Helping to offset these often difficult issues are the amazing developmental changes that occur during this time. The 12-month-old who knows a handful of words grows into the 2-year-old who proudly recites the ABCs and then becomes the 3-year-old capable of carrying on a conversation. This virtual explosion of language is indeed exciting for a parent, as is the determination with which many children this age approach a new task. Watch your child struggle to master a new toy or task. Even a temperamental 2-year-old will usually give it a good try before, out of frustration and disappointment, he or she bursts into a tantrum.

In this chapter we look at common problems such as toilet training, recurring colds and infections, and general care. A large segment is devoted to the psychosocial development of children in this age group. Elsewhere in this volume (primarily in Part IV, Human Disease and Disorders) are discussions of most of the disorders that commonly occur in this age group.

If the theme of this chapter can be boiled down into a single thought, it should be "enjoy these years." They are special. Although some days may seem endless when your life appears to revolve around temper tantrums and getting your child to the bathroom before an accident occurs, the time will pass quickly. Ask any parent whose children have moved beyond this stage. These are years to be savored.

NORMAL GROWTH AND DEVELOPMENT

THE 1-YEAR-OLD

The rapid weight gain of the first year levels off during the second, with an average gain of 5 to 6 pounds. Your child's physical changes involve a transition from the plumpness of babyhood to the leaner and more muscular body of a toddler.

This is an exciting time for you and your baby. Your 1-year-old begins to walk and talk. These skills, combined with a will of his or her own and a tentative sense of independence, produce a determined explorer.

Even though the 1-year-old does not have a large vocabulary, he or she develops an increasing ability to understand language. This so-called passive language lays the groundwork for the virtual explosion of language that occurs between ages 2 and 3. The average 18-month-old probably uses only about 10 words, but within a year he or she has a significant vocabulary and can speak in simple sentences.

A child of this age is constantly exploring by touching, holding, climbing, and mouthing. The 1-year-old will leave no wastebasket unturned nor drawer unemptied. Every corner is investigated. Safety becomes vitally important; the 1-year-old's world must be baby-proofed (see page 319).

THE 2-YEAR-OLD

At 2 years most children begin to communicate verbally. At some point after reaching 2 years, most children can tell you their name and the names of common objects. They can speak in three- to four-word sentences and even carry on brief conversations.

Two-year-olds are most famous for negative behavior. Temper tantrums—often out of frustration—are common (see Tantrums and Breath Holding, page 95).

Most 2-year-olds do not actively play with other children. Rather, they enjoy playing side by side with children their age. As the child approaches age 3, he or she will begin to become more interested in socializing.

The 2-year-old child is a great imitator. If you mow the lawn, your 2-year-old may want to follow behind with a miniature lawn mower. Or, your child will insist on his or her own broom and dustpan when you are cleaning house.

THE 3-YEAR-OLD

Your 3-year-old is more coordinated than he or she was at age 2. By age 3, most children can climb stairs with alternating feet, although most cannot descend in the same manner until age 4. The 3-year-old also can stand briefly on one foot.

Your 3-year-old's vocabulary and pronunciation continue to expand. A 3-year-old can tell you his or her age and sex, and crudely imitate simple drawings.

Emotionally, the 3-year-old loves his or her parents and wants to be just like them. Identification with these powerful role models is important in laying the foundation for your child's character.

THE 4-YEAR-OLD

The child of 4 speaks so well that strangers can understand him or her, and sentences are becoming increasingly complex.

GROWTH DISORDERS

There is a wide variation in height and weight during the preschool years. If you look at a growth chart, your child may fall in the bottom range for his or her age, in the middle, or near the top. The child's size generally depends on heredity; large parents are more likely to have a large child, and small parents typically have small children. Most children fall somewhere within the normal range (5th to 95th percentile) for weight and height (see height and weight charts, page 63).

So how do you know whether your child is "abnormal"? If your child is either substantially below or substantially above the range, there may be a problem.

There are many types of growth disorders, the most common of which we discuss below.

Nutritional Deficiencies

The most common nutritional disorder in American children is obesity (see page 117). Malnutrition, although less common, also occurs frequently, especially among lower socioeconomic groups. Malnutrition can be the result of diseases such as cystic fibrosis (see page 933) and celiac disease (see Malabsorption Problems, page 621).

Hormonal Disorders

Sometimes the pituitary or thyroid gland produces an insufficient or an excess amount of hormones, the result of which can be a growth disorder. These rare disorders include gigantism and dwarfism (see Pituitary Tumors, page 723) and hypothyroidism (see page 730).

Chronic Disease

Children with diseases such as congenital heart disorders (see page 54), chronic kidney failure (see page 909), and anemia (see Anemias, page 477) also may have impaired growth as a result of the primary disease.

What To Do

If you suspect a growth disorder, take your child to the physician. Depending on the physical findings, diagnostic tests may be necessary. These may include blood tests and x-ray studies of the bones.

Again, treatment depends on the specific problem. An obese child may be placed on a diet, whereas one who is malnourished may need high-calorie supplements and even hospitalization. Children with growth disorders due to a hormone deficiency may be helped by injections of the deficient hormone.

The imagination of a child this age is vivid, and the line between what is real and what is imaginary oftentimes becomes indistinct.

Some children at this age or even younger develop fears. Common fears of the 4-year-old include the fear of death, animals, and the dark.

THE 5-YEAR-OLD

A child of 5 is generally able to hop on one foot and even skip, can accurately copy figures such as a triangle, and continues to develop language skills.

Children this age have the coordination required to write, and many have learned to do so. Moreover, it is not uncommon for 5-year-olds to begin reading before starting school.

The 5-year-old is a social person. Unlike the younger child, when given a choice between spending time with his or her parents or the afternoon with a friend, the 5-year-old child will almost invariably choose the friend.

COMMON CONCERNS DURING THE PRESCHOOL YEARS

How do you know whether your fussy 1-year-old is sick or is simply having a bad day? Is it normal for a preschooler to have repeated colds? What is the best way to toilet train the resistant 3-year-old? How should you handle your 2-year-old's daily temper tantrums?

These are just a few of the common concerns expressed by parents of young children.

This section considers a wide range of these concerns.

SIGNS OF ILLNESS

As many parents can attest, preschoolers do get sick with amazing frequency. Some months you seem to be caught in a revolving door between home and the physician's office. No sooner is an ear infection cleared up than your child develops a cold. Before you know it, you are back to see the physician.

Most parents are understandably concerned when their young child seems to fall prey to every virus that hits the block. In the back of your mind, you may wonder whether there is something wrong—a serious underlying illness—that is interfering with your child's ability to fight these infections.

Almost always, these fears are groundless. If your child is active and gaining weight, there is probably nothing wrong with his or her health. It is a simple fact that young children are particularly susceptible to colds, ear infections, and gastrointestinal viruses. Your child's immune system must be exposed to many viruses before it fully develops its own resistance. Moreover, your child's habits, alone and with others, ensure this exposure. The way young children play and relate is not geared toward avoiding germs. A 2-year-old with a running nose does not worry about germs before handing a toy to a friend. A cold will not stop a 4-year-old from offering a bite of his or her cookie to a friend.

It is no wonder that the average preschooler has seven or eight colds a year and two or three bouts of intestinal flu. These illnesses may also provide means for our bodies to learn to recognize and fight infections. Many illnesses are actually better tolerated by a young child than by an adult. For example, chickenpox is a common and usually well-tolerated illness of childhood, whereas an adult who develops chickenpox may have a more serious illness. So, some of these illnesses not only may be common but also are an important, normal part of growing up.

In addition to the frequency of minor illness, another common concern is how to tell whether your child is ill. Unlike an older child, a 1-year-old does not have the verbal abilities to communicate distress beyond a cry or crankiness. And even though your 5-year-old can certainly tell you whether he or she is sick, your child may not be able to articulate anything more specific.

Keep in mind that certain common ailments tend to be seasonal in children, as in adults. Thus, if your child seems ill in late winter, the cause may be the flu (see Influenza, page 853). By the same token, chickenpox is most likely to strike in the spring; colds, ear infections, and croup in the winter; and certain viral infections, including meningitis, in the late summer or fall.

Here are some signs that will help you to determine whether your child is ill. Keep in mind, however, that there is often no substitute for a parent's intuition. Many parents simply sense that something is wrong with their child even before the child develops a fever or other symptoms. In the absence of obvious symptoms, trust your instincts; you will be surprised how frequently you are on target.

Fever. A rectal temperature of more than 101° Fahrenheit (F) or an oral temperature of more than 100°F is considered to be a fever (see also How To Take a Temperature, page 859). A fever is one of the body's ways of fighting infection. It is not automatically a cause for alarm, nor does it necessarily need to be lowered.

Children tolerate fever better than adults. If your child is responsive, continues to drink fluids, and wants to play, there probably is nothing to worry about. If you think that your child will be more comfortable with the fever lowered, you can use acetaminophen to help reduce it.

Extra fluids, minimal clothing, and, perhaps, a sponge bath with tepid water also may help. Do not use aspirin to lower the fever of a viral illness in children because aspirin has been possibly linked to Reye's syndrome, a potentially life-threatening illness (see Reye's Syndrome, page 531). Some authorities believe that aggressively lowering all fevers actually will blunt the body's immune response and possibly prolong some illnesses.

Decreased Appetite. A sick child often does not feel like eating. This is a normal response and nothing to worry about. However, even though it is not important that your child eat normal meals during an illness, an adequate fluid intake is important (although the risk of dehydration is very low in most minor illnesses). Do not insist that the child eat, but do try to coax him or her to drink liquids, whether in the form of water, juices, ice pops, or clear soups.

Increased Sleep. Another sign of illness may be that your child seems to be sleeping more than usual. This too is one way the body fights infection and speeds recovery. If, however, it becomes difficult to arouse your child or if your child appears to be confused and drowsy when awake, call your physician.

Lethargy. Surprisingly, even children with high fevers can have much energy. However, if your child is lethargic, does not re-

spond to you, or is limp and uninterested in playing or anything else, this is cause for concern. Call your physician.

Breathing Changes. Noisy breathing and coughing are common with an upper respiratory tract infection. If your child has difficulty breathing, breathes rapidly, or is wheezing, call your physician.

Diarrhea. Diarrhea is a frequent gastrointestinal disturbance. Mild diarrhea is the passage of a few mushy stools, whereas with moderate or severe diarrhea the frequency increases and the stools become more watery. Dehydration is the main danger because the body is losing so much fluid in the stools.

If your child does not urinate for about 8 hours and has a dry mouth and tearless crying, call your physician immediately. He or she may have severe dehydration. Blood or pus in the stool, severe abdominal pain, the passage of frequent diarrheal stools in a few hours, or the combination of watery diarrhea and frequent vomiting also may warrant a call to your physician.

Vomiting. Vomiting may or may not be associated with diarrhea. If your child is vomiting, avoid feeding solid foods for about 8 hours. Your child may try to drink small amounts of clear liquids or suck on ice pops. If there is no vomiting for about 8 hours, you can try such foods as soda crackers, white bread, or chicken soup. If you see blood in

---

WARNING SIGNS OF SERIOUS ILLNESS

The following signs and symptoms may suggest a serious illness. If your child has any of these, call your physician immediately:

Fever higher than 105°F;
Fever that lasts longer than 24 hours without any obvious cause (such as a cold or gastrointestinal symptoms);
Fever that lasts more than 72 hours;
Lethargy or no drinking of fluids;
Stiff or painful neck;
Such severe pain that he or she does not want to be touched;
Sudden inability to walk;
Breathing difficulty;
Difficulty being awakened;
Painful urination;
A convulsion;
Pain in the groin (boys);
Blue lips;
Profuse drooling;
Purple or deep red spots on the skin.

the vomitus or note that your child has severe abdominal pain or a swollen abdomen, if your child is delirious or is difficult to awaken, or if your child has signs of dehydration (no saliva or tears, absence of urination), call your physician immediately.

COMMON AND RECURRENT COLDS

The common cold is one of the most frequent illnesses of childhood—preschoolers, in fact, have an average of five to eight infections each year, often during the peak times for colds of early September, late January, and late April.

If your child constantly seems to have a congested head, to be sneezing, and even to have a fever and a sore throat, there are various possible causes.

The most common cause of a constant running nose is simply a recurring cold. A recurring viral upper respiratory tract infection is often found in children older than 6 months. A young child with a cold is generally sicker than his older counterpart or an adult.

Fever in the child younger than 3 is an early symptom. Irritability, restlessness, and sneezing usually follow. A few hours later a clear liquid begins to drip from the nose, which gradually changes to a thick mucus that makes it difficult to breathe through the nose. The virus irritates the throat and windpipe, causing a sore throat and cough. Other symptoms may include headache, lack of appetite, and muscle aches.

What can you do for a cold? In general, there is little anyone can do to make your child better rapidly. Usually, the child's temperature will return to normal in 1 to 3 days. All nose and throat symptoms will disappear within a week; however, the cough may persist for 2 to 3 weeks.

There is no magic potion for a cold, but there are some things you can do to make your child more comfortable.

1. If your child is too young to blow his or her nose, use a soft rubber suction bulb to remove mucus.
2. If the child's nose is stuffed, try administering nose drops 15 to 20 minutes before meals and at bedtime. You can use saline nose drops, which are available without a prescription. For the child who is too young to blow his or her nose, place three drops in each nostril. After waiting 1 minute, use a suction bulb to remove the loosened mucus. For the older child, put three drops in each nostril while the child is lying face-up on the bed with his or her head over the side. After a moment, have the child blow the nose. This can be repeated several times in a row until the nose is cleared.
3. When saline drops do not work, you can buy nonprescription nose drops that will shrink the mucous membranes, allowing your child to breathe easier.

   (Do not give nose drops for more than a few days. Prolonged use of these nose drops causes a rebound reaction and actually makes the congestion worse instead of clearing it up. Simply stopping use of the nose drops should clear up the problem; see also Beware: Nose-Drop Addiction, page 695. Discuss this with your child's physician. Many physicians recommend use of nose drops only in certain specific circumstances.)
4. If the child has aches or a fever of more than 102°F, you can give acetaminophen. DO NOT give aspirin, which has been possibly linked with Reye's syndrome, a life-threatening condition (see Reye's Syndrome, page 531).

In addition to an increased frequency of colds, preschoolers are more apt than older children to have complications from colds. The most common complication is an acute ear infection (otitis media) (see page 680). This occurs when bacteria infiltrate the space behind the eardrum.

Symptoms may include an earache (children too young to verbalize their pain may simply cry or pull on the infected ear). You may see a yellow or green discharge from the nose. Drainage from the ear means that the eardrum has ruptured. The rupture may relieve the pressure and the pain. See your child's physician. Another symptom may be a return of fever after the initial fever of the cold has already gone down.

Unlike a cold, an ear infection must be treated with antibiotics to clear the infection and to help prevent damage to the middle and inner ear and resulting hearing loss (see also Disorders of the Ear, page 676).

Other Possible Causes.   Another cause of nasal congestion in some children is environmental respiratory irritants. Air pollution, tobacco smoke, or sudden changes in the air temperature may cause a prolonged stuffy nose and sneezing.

Finally, your child may suffer from hay fever (allergic rhinitis). Usually, it takes several years before the child has been exposed to enough allergic substances to have a reaction to them; therefore, hay fever seldom occurs in children younger than 2 years. Your child will have symptoms that include a constantly running nose, with large amounts of clear, watery discharge, frequent sneezing, and an itchy nose. Antihistamines may relieve these symptoms. If not, your child's physician may want to obtain a consultation from a pediatric allergist (see also Common Viral Colds, page 860, Respiratory Allergies, page 461, and Prevention of the Spread of Disease in the Family, page 102).

CONSTIPATION AND DIARRHEA

Parents of young children are often overly concerned about their child's bowel movements. If the child skips a day, many assume he or she is constipated. Or, if the consistency of the stool is mushy, they may assume the child has diarrhea.

The characteristics of constipation and diarrhea are detailed below.

Constipation. Just because your son or daughter does not have a bowel movement every day does not mean the child is constipated. Although it may be normal for many people to have a daily bowel movement, others may have one only every second or third day.

The symptoms of constipation are the painful passage of the stool; the inability to pass a stool, even though the urge to defecate is strong; going more than 3 days without having a bowel movement; or passing a large, hard stool that may even plug the toilet.

If your child has the symptoms of constipation, they are probably the result of not getting enough fiber or fluid in the diet. Moreover, children may hold back their stool because it is inconvenient to go when the urge hits or as a response to toilet training (see Toilet Training, page 92). Some children hold in the stool because a previous passage of a hard stool created a tear (fissure) in the anal opening. It hurts when they try to have a bowel movement, so they try to avoid the pain (see Anal Fissures and Fistulas, page 645).

Treatment for constipation is generally dietary, including lots of fruits and vegetables, foods high in fiber such as wheat breads, legumes, and whole-grain cereals, and an increased intake of water and other fluids. Encourage your child to have bowel movements at regular intervals, perhaps after breakfast or supper. If this does not resolve the constipation, check with your child's physician.

Diarrhea. A child with diarrhea has a sudden increase in the frequency and looseness of the bowel movements. If the diarrhea is mild, the stools may only be loose; when it is moderate or severe, they may be watery, green, and very frequent. If your child has only a couple of diarrheal stools, it may be the result of something he or she ate. Diarrhea usually is caused by a virus or, less commonly, by bacteria or parasites.

Some young children develop "toddler's diarrhea." Typically, the child with toddler's diarrhea has several days of loose stools that are malodorous and runny. Some of these children are incredibly thirsty during this time. Despite the diarrhea, a child with toddler's diarrhea usually is very active, appears healthy, and does not have a fever. If the stool is tested for organisms, it almost always is normal. In the case of toddler's diarrhea, dietary restrictions usually do not make much difference.

If your child has diarrhea, take steps to avoid dehydration by increasing your child's fluid intake. Water, juices, ice pops, and broth are good choices. Do not use diet pop or diet juices. In addition, commercially available oral electrolyte replacement solutions, such as Pedialyte or Lytren, provide excellent replacement of what the body loses with diarrhea. They also help slow down the amount of fluid loss.

If your child is not hungry, there is a good reason, so do not force food. If he or she wants to eat, offer a general diet and a lot of fluids. Foods that contain bulk such as cereal, fruits, and vegetables are good because they usually make the stool firmer.

Diarrhea may last up to a week.

Although it is unnecessary to call your physician every time your child has a bout of diarrhea, consult your child's physician if any of the following symptoms occur:

Signs of dehydration (no wet diapers or urination for 8 hours, tearless crying, no saliva in mouth);
Bowel movement every hour for more than 8 hours;
Blood, pus, or mucus in the stool;
Abdominal pain lasting more than 12 hours;
Diarrhea that does not improve within 48 hours of dietary changes;
Mild diarrhea lasting more than a week.

TOILET TRAINING

The toilet training of a toddler can be a difficult time in the life of parent and child. Or, when handled properly, it can be simply one in a series of many milestones.

The first question most parents ask is, "When is the right time to attempt toilet training?"

That is not an easy question to answer because every child is different. Your first child may have been day-trained within 24 hours at 24 months, whereas the second one may still be balking at the approach of the third birthday. The readiness of one child for toilet training may be different from that of another.

Generally, most physicians advise never trying to train a child before 18 months, and many believe this is even too early except in rare cases. Unless a child appears extremely interested in being trained, most physicians today usually advise waiting until between 2 and 2½ years.

Control at night comes later. Most children continue to wear a diaper at night for several months after they are day-trained, which usually is accomplished by the time they turn 3. Even so, 40 percent of 3-year-olds wet the bed at least once a month.

There are signs that you as a parent can look for to determine whether the time is right to attempt training. Remember, no rule says that training has to be successful immediately. Try it for a few days, and if the child is clearly not interested or protests, put the plan off for a few weeks. Next time it may work. Signs of readiness include the following:

1. Your child has a vocabulary of bathroom words such as "potty," "pee pee," or "poo poo."
2. The child has watched others use the toilet.
3. The child indicates when he or she is wet or dirty and wants to be changed.
4. The child can briefly control the bowel and bladder; in other words, he or she can delay having a bowel movement or urinating until it is convenient.

Once you determine that the time may be right, you will need some supplies.

1. A small potty chair that sits on the floor. There are children's toilet seats designed to fit on a regular toilet, but many children prefer the floor type. This type not only allows the child to get on and off at will but also enables the child to push better because his or her feet are on the floor. Purchase the potty a few weeks before you are ready to begin training so that the child can become familiar with it.
2. Training pants, which are heavy, absorbent underwear.
3. Favorite treats and stars or stickers if you want to use tangible rewards in addition to your praise.

Now, you are ready to begin. Tell the child he or she is now going to wear underpants like the big boys and girls. Save the diapers for nap and bedtime.

There are various ways to go about toilet training. No matter which one you ultimately choose, make sure that you do not turn the bathroom into a battleground.

Many physicians suggest allowing the child to become trained according to his or her own free will. This means no coercion whatsoever. Ask the child if he or she wants to sit on the potty. If the answer is no, do not pressure the child. If your child sits a minute but does not do anything, let him or her get off the potty when ready. If your child urinates or has a bowel movement, be free with your praise. But when there is an "accident" (and there undoubtedly will be), do not scold or shame your toddler.

Other methods use similar principles but require more parental involvement. The parent takes the child to the potty at appropriate intervals and asks him or her to "pee pee." If the child is reluctant to cooperate, you can try entertaining your toddler with books or games. If the child does not go within 5 minutes, take him or her off and try later. When the child does go, offer praise. You can even try rewards such as nutritious snacks, stars, or stickers.

Several months after day-control is achieved, you can try putting your child to bed without a diaper. Although not necessary, taking the child to the bathroom just before he or she goes to bed may hasten night training.

For some children, bowel and bladder control occur simultaneously, whereas others achieve one before the other. In most cases, toilet training can be accomplished within 2 months. If not, it may be an indication that the child is too young, and you should probably try again in a few weeks or months.

If, however, the child is older than 2½ years and still is not trained after 2 months, he or she is resisting toilet training. The most common cause of this resistance is too much parental pressure. Often, these children have been reminded too much; some have been forced to sit for long periods on the potty. Hence, control of one's urine and bowels has become a political issue in the child's mind.

In trying to train the resistant child, shift the responsibility to him or her. Tell your child that you are not going to remind him or her to go to the bathroom and that he or she must decide when to go. Use positive reinforcement and incentives to reward your toddler for a day without wet or dirty pants. Try a reward system such as buying your child a calendar and awarding a star every time the toilet is successfully used. If your child has an accident, change him or her and then involve the toddler in cleaning up the mess. Again, do not punish or criticize. Above all, try to be patient, however difficult that may be.

Encopresis and Enuresis. The involuntary passage of feces far beyond an age at which most other children are toilet trained is called encopresis. It is not a disease, but it may be a symptom of constipation or emotional difficulties (there is rarely a physical cause) (see Encopresis, page 1016).

Bedwetting (enuresis) is also a common problem in preschool children (see Enuresis, page 1015).

TEETHING PROBLEMS

Many babies breeze through teething, the process during which the teeth erupt through the gums. Their only symptoms are increased drooling and an insatiable need to chew on things.

For others, however, the process is fraught with discomfort, daytime restlessness, and crankiness. Your child may take to thumb sucking as never before, rub his or her gums, and temporarily lose his or her appetite.

If your baby develops a fever or diarrhea, *do not* assume that it is due to teething. Teething, in fact, generally does not cause fever, diarrhea, sleep problems, seizures, bronchitis, or diaper rash. Seek appropriate care for such problems: do not assume that they are part of the normal teething process.

If your baby is among those with discomfort, there are some things you can do.

1. If your child allows, massage the swollen gum for a couple of minutes with or without a piece of ice. Some children, however, voluntarily or involuntarily tend to bite your fingers trying to relieve their discomfort.
2. A cold teething ring may help. You also may want to give the child some ice, an ice pop, or a slice of frozen banana to gnaw on. *Never,* however, tie a teething ring around the child's neck—this could cause strangulation.
3. Do not use lotions or ointments designed to reduce teething pain. These not only are unnecessary but also may contain benzocaine, an agent that could numb the throat and cause the baby to choke. Many of these products also have a bitter taste and your child may refuse to take them.
4. Acetaminophen can be used for a few days if the baby is uncomfortable.

SWALLOWING OBJECTS

Young children are naturally curious and are not averse to putting coins, safety pins, buttons, fruit pits, and other things into their mouths. Keep these and other small objects out of reach.

Large chunks of food such as hot dogs occasionally lodge in a child's throat; to minimize this risk, do not allow your preschooler to eat while walking or playing.

In addition to a penchant for small objects, some children chronically ingest non-nutrient substances such as dirt, plaster, clay, paint, and ashes. This habit, called pica, may occur during the first 2 years, when the child's natural curiosity compels him or her to sample everything. However, if your child persists with this practice, inform your physician.

A watchful parent may be able to retrieve an object before it is swallowed. When the child swallows the object, it usually passes through the digestive system uneventfully.

A good rule is that if a swallowed object passes into the stomach, it will pass the rest of the way through the intestines. However, objects can lodge in the esophagus. If your child has difficulty with swallowing, or if he or she is spitting up saliva, you might suspect that a swallowed object has become stuck in the esophagus. If this occurs, or if your child develops chest or abdominal pain or vomiting, call your physician.

Another exception is if your child swallows a button-sized battery such as those found in watches, pocket calculators, cameras, and hearing aids. If this occurs, contact your physician at once even if no symptoms are present (see also Children and Button Batteries, page 289).

The frightening possibility is that the swallowed object might become lodged in the windpipe, preventing your child from breathing, crying, or speaking. This is a true emergency. If the obstruction is not relieved within a few minutes, the child will become unconscious and may convulse due to a lack of oxygen. Death could follow.

If your preschooler stops breathing due to an obstruction, try the Heimlich maneuver and seek emergency help (see Choking, Breathing Emergencies, and Resuscitation, page 268).

EYE PROBLEMS

The preschool years, particularly between ages 3 and 4, are crucial for the detection and successful treatment of many eye problems, including the following.

Strabismus and Amblyopia. Strabismus occurs when the eyes are malaligned. Cross-eyes is a type of strabismus, for example. In some cases, one eye deviates only when the child is tired; in another form of the problem, both eyes alternate deviating. Treatment may require an operation. The earlier the condition is discovered, the better the chances of substantial improvement.

Amblyopia is subnormal vision in one or both eyes. It can be caused by many vision defects. Susceptibility to amblyopia is greatest within the first 3 years. Amblyopia can be treated. The most important factor in its successful treatment is early detection. Amblyopia, often called "lazy eye," frequently is a consequence of strabismus.

Although examination of the eyes should be a part of your child's regular checkups, a more thorough examination by your eye specialist ideally should occur when the child is 4 years old (see Strabismus and Amblyopia, page 750).

SLEEP PROBLEMS

Crying uncontrollably at bedtime, waking up frequently during the night, and getting out of bed and attempting to crawl in with the parents are common sleep problems found in the preschool age group.

If your child has a sleep problem, you are not alone. This is a frequent complaint of parents. Whether the problem is temporary or intermittent or has been occurring for months, a child who is awakening at night creates tired parents, not to mention a cranky child.

Causes vary, often depending on the age of the child.

If your child is between 12 and 24 months old and has always had problems sleeping through the night, you may have been too responsive to his or her night cries. Most babies older than 4 months awaken several times during the night but can put themselves back to sleep. However, if the baby has learned that Mom or Dad will come rushing every time he or she cries, the child becomes dependent on a parent to get back to sleep. The child, in essence, becomes trained to cry at night.

To assist your child in improving sleep patterns, avoid the following: nursing the child to sleep or giving him or her a bottle to take to bed, sleeping in the same room, rocking your child to sleep, entertaining him or her at night, letting your child nap more than 3 hours a day, or changing his or her diaper at night.

Then, try the following, whether for the child who protests going to bed or for one who wakes up at night. Although this approach may leave you wide awake for awhile, it will ultimately (usually within 2 weeks) improve the situation.

1. Put your child to bed awake, say goodnight, and leave the room despite the protests.
2. Do not go in immediately when your baby begins crying. Wait 15 or 20 minutes before checking on the child. Then, stay in the room for less than a minute. Do not turn on the light or pick the child up; simply reassure him or her that everything is all right and that it is time for sleep.

The first night your baby may cry for an hour, but generally the crying time will decrease each night when this method is used.

Some children have not been trained to cry at night but, because of a fear, they resist going to bed or awaken terrified.

If your young toddler's cries sound fearful rather than simply angry, go to him or her immediately. Seeing your face should calm the child, although after you reassure your toddler you may have to sit by the crib awhile. Do not play or talk. You do not want your child to think this is play time.

Older preschoolers also often develop nighttime fears that impede sleep. Again, be reassuring. Do not make fun of your child, be impatient, or try to argue him or her out of a fear. Leaving the door open or using a night light can work wonders.

If you find your child crawling into bed with you at night, gently but firmly take him or her back to his or her bed. In the long run, this is better for the child and the parents.

FEARS AND PHOBIAS

As your child grows, he or she inevitably will have certain fears, which will change with age. Such fears are normal and may even be necessary for psychological development.

Fear—the perception of a threat, whether actual or simply a possibility—is necessary to survival. For example, fear of a barking, snarling dog is normal. Your child perceives a real threat, and it is correct to be frightened and to try to avoid the danger. However, the child who continues to be terrified of the friendly, tail-wagging cocker spaniel who lives next door has an irrational fear or phobia.

Fears vary from child to child, but some appear more commonly in certain age groups. For example, a common fear between 1 and 2 years is of the bath. Often children this age are afraid of slipping under the water or of getting soap in their eyes. Toddlers this age also tend to be fearful of strangers. Fear of separation from the parents is another common fear in the child who is 2 or younger.

Fears in 3-, 4-, and 5-year-old children often revolve around the dark, animals, monsters, and death.

If your child is going through a fearful time, try to be supportive and encouraging. Do not force your child to confront the object of the fear. A parent who tries to make a child who is afraid of animals pet a dog will only complicate the situation.

Your reassurance in the form of a hug or kiss can be powerful medicine for the 2-year-old who is afraid of the dark. A nightlight is often helpful. Be creative in your quest for a solution. One mother whose 3-year-old girl was terrified that there were monsters lurking in her dark room initiated a nightly "monster check." At bedtime every night they would scour the room together in search of a monster. Reassured, the little girl went to bed and immediately fell asleep. Within a few weeks she stopped asking for the monster check.

When your child conquers even a tiny part of his or her fear, do not forget the praise.

Most fears resolve themselves in time. Those that do not or that incapacitate the child or the family may require some psychiatric counseling.

TANTRUMS AND BREATH HOLDING

Few children exit the toddler years without demonstrating temper tantrums.

Between the ages of 18 months and 3 years, negativism reigns. "No" (sometimes even when it means "yes") seems to be your child's favorite word. Sometimes everything you do, no matter how innocuous, seems to provoke your child. This stubborn, oppositional, and defiant behavior is simply a natural part of moving from total dependence to a taste of independence.

This time is not called the "terrible twos" because the time is easy. Nothing is more exasperating than when your child decides to throw a temper tantrum. Any parent who has been through one knows that it does not take much to drive a toddler to uncontrollable kicking, screaming, head banging, and even breath holding. Often, in fact, the temper tantrum has nothing to do with you but is your child's response to frustration.

When a child reaches this point, he or she is out of control and beyond reason. You talk or try to placate to no avail. Generally, a temper tantrum, once started, has to run its course.

What should you do?

Giving in is not the answer. If, for example, your 2-year-old has a tantrum because you deny a second cookie, you will be sending the wrong message if you suddenly reverse your decision. Once the tantrum starts, giving your child a "time out" is most helpful. Leave the room. Try to ignore what is going on (it will be difficult). Even if your child holds his or her breath, do not worry, because this is not harmful. As for any head banging, children hate pain as much as adults; when things get too uncomfortable, they know it's time to quit.

When to return to your child is variable. Some parents find that their child finishes the tantrum on his or her own; other children may need to be held for a moment before they can stop crying.

Although ignoring a tantrum is effective in most cases, sometimes other measures must be taken. Obviously, the child who decides to throw a tantrum in the middle of the supermarket cannot be left there to kick and flail, nor should a child who is physically aggressive toward someone else or toward property be allowed to continue unchecked. Take the child to his or her room or separate the child from others until his or her composure is regained.

WALKING AND FALLING

A frequent question is, "When will my baby walk?"

No one can answer this with precision.

One child may walk as early as 9 months and another may be content to crawl at 14 months.

The new walker is amusing to watch. On plump feet that look flat because of baby fat, your child will toddle about with the toes turned out. Many babies also may be bow-legged or knock-kneed. Virtually all these characteristics are normal and disappear on their own (see Flatfeet, page 99; Knock-Knees, page 100; and Bowlegs, page 100).

Do not expect the new walker to be graceful. One minute your 1-year-old will be making his or her way across the room and the next he or she will be lying in a heap on the floor. Falls can be frequent events at first and usually are no real deterrent to the determined baby. Falls are part of learning to walk.

For the parent, however, they should serve as a signal of things to come. The child that only weeks before had limited mobility now has discovered the ability to go where he or she wants to. By the time your "explorer" is 18 months old, he or she may be able to climb the stairs while holding your hand; at 20 months, your child can walk down the stairs, providing one hand is held. By 24 months, there is little stopping most children from traversing a steep stairwell except a safety-conscious parent who has installed a safety gate at the top and bottom of all staircases in the home.

SPEECH AND LANGUAGE DEVELOPMENT

Your child's speech and language development begins almost immediately upon entering the world and is not complete until age 6 or 7. Such development takes place in stages. Be aware that there are considerable developmental variations from child to child, even within the same family. Therefore, the following are to be regarded as no more than general guidelines.

During the *first 3 months* of life, beginning with what is called the "undifferentiated birth cry," your infant will experiment with making sounds, producing several consonants and vowels that have no meaning. Considerable cooing and gurgling take place during this time. Language comprehension is limited to responses to loud noises and familiar voices.

Between *4 and 6 months,* your baby

moves into the babbling stage, which is accompanied by sighing, grunting, gurgling, laughing, and crying differently in response to pain and hunger. Your child vocalizes for pleasure and displeasure.

Between *7 and 9 months,* your child repeats syllables, babbles in a sing-song manner, may produce as many as 12 different sounds, particularly the p, b, and m sounds, uses different vowels, uses sounds as a means of play, and may repeat the word "mama." You may hear your child utter sounds that mimic the letters m, n, t, d, p, b, z.

Toward the end of this period, actual imitation of intonation and speech sounds made by others begins. During this period your child searches for sources of sound, listens intently to speech and nonspeech sounds, recognizes "dada," "mama," and "bye-bye," recognizes his or her name, and is able to differentiate friendliness or anger from the tone of other people's voices.

At *10 to 12 months,* the babbling may take on some of the melody of actual speech. Your child enjoys repeating sounds made by others. Considerable vocalization is used during play. Almost all of the consonant and vowel sounds are used. In some children, the first true words can emerge during this period. Your child's comprehension is improved by this time. He or she responds to names and simple requests and recognizes the names of common objects and family members.

Between *13 and 18 months,* your child is using sentence-like intonations, continues repeating sounds made by others, and uses all the vowels and consonants. However, his or her language is basically unintelligible except for a few words, such as "mama" and "dada." During this time your child makes genuine efforts to name objects. Your child comprehends a few simple words, phrases, and commands, shakes his or her head appropriately in response to simple yes-or-no questions, and shows an interest in simple rhymes and songs.

Between the ages of *1½ and 2 years,* your child produces words that are more understandable. Jargon usually disappears by age 2. During this period your child may begin to use two-word phrases such as "more milk" and has a vocabulary of 10 to 20 words. Your child may still use jargon that sounds like sentences. Single words are used to express larger ideas, such as

"wawa" for "I want water" or "Look at the water." When your child is about 2 years old, you should understand about two-thirds of what he or she says. Your child can comprehend well enough to bring objects on command, to point to some body parts, to understand simple questions, and to recognize pictures, although he or she may be unable to name them.

Between *2 and 2½ years,* your child uses two- to three-word phrases, has a vocabulary of 50 or more words, begins to use words such as "me," "you," and "mine," and shows considerable substitution and omission of final consonant sounds. You can now understand about 70 percent of what he or she says. Your child ought to be able to point to body parts by this age, understand many complex sentences, and follow three or four directions in succession.

Between *2½ and 3 years,* your child still has many consonant omissions and substitutions, but you should be able to understand most of what he or she says. Your child is able to use three- to four-word sentences, may repeat words when excited or anxious, and comprehends most of what is said.

Between the ages of *3½ and 4 years,* your child is able to give his or her full name and age, can use the present and past tenses of verbs, and uses more complicated sentences. You can understand virtually all of what your child says. Your child may begin to use the plural forms of words. People outside the family understand most of what the child says. Your child often will talk to himself or herself. He or she begins to ask "what?" questions. Your child can understand a simple story, recognizes several colors, and can put foods and animals into their proper groups. Your child can understand the concept of time by this age.

Between the ages of *4 and 5 years,* your child is able to count to five, uses complete sentences, asks "why?" and "who?", uses four- to five-word sentences, uses 75 percent of all speech sounds correctly, enjoys naming objects, knows most colors, and understands the concept of the past, present, and future forms of verbs and the difference between single and plural nouns. Most of the time you can understand what your child says.

By now your child has a 2,500-word vocabulary and uses most consonant sounds consistently and accurately, although not in all words.

At ages *5 to 6 years,* a stranger can understand what your child says. Your child uses words such as "and" and "but," asks many questions, and uses five- to six-word sentences and grammatically different types of sentences. He or she is able to carry on a conversation and can define and explain words. Your child understands most of what is heard and can follow three directions given at the same time. By age 6, your child may have a vocabulary comprehension of about 13,000 words and understands such concepts as yesterday, tomorrow, more, less, some, many, several, few, most, and least.

By age *6 to 7 years,* all of the consonants and vowels should have been mastered. You should be able to understand everything your child says. Your child has a vocabulary comprehension of 20,000 words, understands time intervals and seasons of the year, can print the alphabet and write one-syllable words, can read approximately 10 printed words, and can count to 100.

If you think that your child's speech is not developing at an appropriate rate or if you are having trouble understanding your child's words, see your physician.

URINARY TRACT INFECTIONS

Urinary tract infection occurs when bacteria enter the bladder via the urethra (the channel leading from the bladder to the outside of the body). Under normal circumstances these bacteria are rinsed out of the body during urination. Urine itself has properties that inhibit the growth of bacteria. However, factors such as the virulence of the particular bacteria and anatomic abnormalities in the urinary system can increase the chance of a urinary tract infection.

Urinary tract infections are common in young children, particularly girls. Usually the infection is confined to the bladder and is called cystitis. In this situation, the child may seem as though she constantly has to go to the bathroom and complains of pain with urination. The urine may be foul-smelling; bed-wetting may occur in a child who had previously been night-trained. Fever, vomiting, and chills also may occur. In some cases the child has no symptoms.

Sometimes, however, the infection can travel from the bladder up the ureter to a kidney. Symptoms then may include a fever, chills, back pain, and vomiting. When this occurs, your child may have an acute infection of the kidney called acute pyelonephritis (see page 892). Unlike cystitis, a kidney infection may require hospitalization.

If your child has the symptoms of a urinary tract infection, your physician will collect a urine specimen to determine whether there are bacteria in the urine. If bacteria are seen by microscope examination, the urine is cultured to determine the type of bacteria. Although this test reveals whether there is infection, it is no indication of whether the infection is confined to the bladder or has invaded the kidney. For this, your physician must rely on an accurate description of your child's symptoms, your child's appearance, and a physical examination. A child with a kidney infection will appear more ill than one with cystitis.

If the child is having recurrent infections, x-rays such as an IVP (see page 885) and a voiding cystourethrogram (see page 885) may be obtained to determine whether there is an abnormality and whether there has been kidney damage as a result of repeated infections.

Most urinary tract infections respond promptly to antibiotic treatment. When properly treated, acute pyelonephritis rarely progresses to chronic renal disease. Urinary tract infections, however, should not be ignored. Untreated cystitis can involve the kidney, and a kidney infection that is not totally eradicated can recur, which may damage the kidney. Moreover, recurrent urinary tract infections can be a symptom of other diseases. One problem frequently associated with recurrent kidney infection is vesicoureteral reflux (see page 884), an abnormality in the ureter that allows urine to reflux back into the kidney. Thus, when the child's urine is invaded by bacteria and urine automatically flows up to the kidney, the result is a kidney infection (see page 889).

If your child has cystitis, he or she will be treated with antibiotics for 7 to 10 days.

For acute pyelonephritis, intravenous infusion of antibiotics may be necessary if the child is very ill.

The urine should be cultured again a week after any urinary tract infection to make sure that the medication has been effective.

Some children who have recurrent urinary tract infections need daily doses of an antibiotic for months or even years to keep their urine sterile. Some children should have urine cultures performed at regular intervals (even if they have no symptoms) to ensure that the urinary tract is free of bacteria.

When an abnormality such as reflux is responsible for the infections, an operation may be considered if there is concern about kidney damage.

ORTHOPEDIC CONCERNS

Beyond breaking a bone from time to time or pulling a muscle, most children do not have serious problems of their muscles, bones, and joints.

Yet a wide range of growth patterns can occur in the preschool-age child. Flatfeet or pigeon-toed feet, bowlegs, and knock-knees are all stages through which most children pass during the normal pattern of leg development. For example, the infant's toes tend to bend inward and the feet appear flat because of the abundance of baby fat. As the child slims down, however, the arches gradually become visible by the age of 5.

Likewise, the legs are ordinarily slightly bowed from birth until about 2 years of age. Then the toddler's legs often overcorrect in the opposite direction, giving a knock-kneed appearance by age 3. Normally the legs straighten by 7 years of age.

Even when these variations continue through the school-age years, they seldom require treatment. Only rarely are they caused by disease.

Flatfeet. Your child's feet are flat if the arches are not apparent. There is no reason to be concerned about flatfeet in infants whose baby fat always makes their feet look flat. However, if the arches do not become discernible by age 5 years, the child may have flatfeet which are either flexible or fixed.

Flexible flatfeet look flat only when the child stands up. When he or she stands on tiptoe or the foot bears no weight, the arch is restored. Flexible flatfeet tend to run in families and are more common in Jewish and black people. The feet are mobile and painless and have excellent muscle strength. Children with flexible flatfeet also tend to have toes that turn in (see Pigeon Toe, this page).

Usually, flexible flatfeet do not require treatment. However, if the feet are extremely flat, your child's physician may pre-

scribe an arch support in a firm shoe. Although this will not correct the foot, it can permit long walks without foot strain.

Fixed or rigid flatfeet are cause for more concern because they may occur with congenital bone malformations. Your child's physician will take x-rays to determine whether this is the case. An operation may be appropriate if the condition is not relieved by special footwear.

Pigeon Toe. In pigeon toe, the toes turn inward. Most newborns are pigeon toed as a holdover from their fetal position in the womb. They usually sleep with their toes pointed inward. Then, as they start to walk, their feet often turn inward to keep their balance and make up for such conditions as flatfeet, bowlegs, and knock-knees (see above).

The condition usually resolves spontaneously by age 5. If it persists, your physician will watch your child standing and walking and also may take x-rays. He or she will check for the presence of diseases that can cause pigeon toe, such as congenital bone malformations in which the bones of the thigh, shin, ankle, or foot turn inward. (Rarely, cerebral palsy is the cause.)

Malposition, such as sitting or sleeping on the in-turned feet, does not cause further deformity but may perpetuate the problem. If your infant's foot is flexible, stretching exercises may be advised. If the foot is fixed, a cast may be required.

Encourage your child to sit and to walk with his or her toes straight ahead or turned slightly outward. Have your child sit cross-legged rather than with the knees together and the lower legs flat on the floor and

Flatfeet are feet that have little or no arch. At left (top and bottom) is a normal foot and footprint. If your child's foot and footprint more nearly resemble the illustrations at right, then he or she has flat feet.

pointing outward. Severe cases of pigeon toe may require special shoes or a brace worn at night that consists of a pair of turned-out shoes with a bar between them.

An underlying structural malformation can be treated by putting the feet in casts and then in orthopedic shoes. If these measures do not work, an operation may be necessary but it usually is not performed before the child is 9.

If your child's toes seem to turn inward, this condition is termed pigeon toe. In most children, this condition resolves itself spontaneously by age 5. Severe cases of pigeon toe may require corrective shoes or shoes that are attached to a brace like the one shown here.

Knock-Knees. When a child with knock-knees stands up, the knees touch each other but the ankles do not. Knock-knees are more common in girls than in boys, partly because of their wider pelvises. They also occur more frequently in overweight children whose developing bones and joints are hard put to support their weight.

A knock-kneed appearance can persist after age 4, but most children's legs straighten by age 7. If the legs do not straighten or if the condition develops after your child is of school age, a physician may rule out diseases of the knee joint that can cause knock-knees, such as juvenile rheumatoid arthritis, rickets, and infections. An unrecognized injury or developmental problem can cause asymmetrical knock-knees. The physician measures the distance between the ankles when the knees are touching each other and takes x-rays to determine the severity of the condition.

Knock-knees are common, especially when they run in the child's family. In most cases the legs tend to straighten as the child grows, so treatment is seldom required.

Children with severe knock-knees often have flatfeet because the weight falls on the inner edge of the foot and ankle. If the child is overweight, this condition may strain the feet and require an arch support to relieve foot fatigue and to prevent the inner border of the shoe from wearing. Severe knock-knees also can be treated with braces worn at night. Occasionally, an operation is needed, but it should not be performed until the knees have been given a chance to straighten on their own—after age 10 for girls and 12 for boys, but before growth is complete.

Bowlegs. The legs are considered to be bowed if, when the ankles touch each other, the unbent knees do not. The legs are normally bowed at birth because of the way the fetus's legs are folded over each other in the cramped space of the womb. The legs often stay bowed for up to 2 years. If bowed legs persist or worsen after age 3, they should be examined by your child's physician.

The physician measures the distance between your child's knees when the ankles touch each other and takes x-rays to determine the severity of the bowing. Sometimes the legs merely appear bowed because of the distribution of the fat on the child's legs. When one leg is more bowed than the other, it may be the result of an injury or a growth problem. Persistently bowed legs usually straighten without treatment by age 8. Occasionally physicians prescribe night braces. Surgical correction is a possibility if conservative measures fail.

In rare cases, bowlegs are caused by disorders such as rickets (see Osteomalacia and Rickets, page 985) or Blount's disease. In Blount's disease, the shin bone curves out below the knee and is not securely inserted into the knee. Severe problems of the knee joint may develop. This disease tends to occur more often in children who are overweight or short or who walked at an early age. It is more common in girls than in boys. It can be corrected with an operation on the upper part of the shin bone.

CHILD ABUSE

In recent years, child abuse has been increasingly recognized as a problem in the United States. Each year an estimated 650,000 children in this country are reported to be abused or neglected. Because of the secrecy surrounding the issue and the difficulty in collecting information, this number may significantly underestimate the true magnitude of the problem. Children of all ages may be abused.

In most cases of child abuse, the abuser is related to the child and is involved in caring for the child. Parents who abuse their offspring come from all walks of life. Some are high-salaried professionals; others are unemployed. Abuse is seen in all educational backgrounds, from high school dropouts to people with advanced degrees. Child abusers are rich and poor, white and black, Hispanic and Asian, and of all faiths, economic strata, and political beliefs.

Abusing parents often tend to be lonely, angry, and very unhappy people who often are under stress with which they cannot cope. Many of them were physically abused when they were children.

With so much emphasis recently given to the problem of child abuse, some improvement has been made in identifying parents who are at risk of becoming abusive. This information may help prevent abuse before it takes place, but much more remains to be learned.

Although protection of the child is the most important objective, the goal of comprehensive treatment of the entire family is

Knock-knees are the reverse of bowlegs. When standing straight, the knock-kneed child finds his or her knees in contact but the ankles do not touch.

Most children are bowlegged as infants. If the legs are still bowed at age three, consult your child's physician.

for 80 to 90 percent of these families to remain intact and safe for the child, with the parents providing adequate care. Abused children who are returned home without intervention run a significant risk of serious injury or even death.

If child abuse is to be dealt with, everyone must help by reporting instances of suspected child abuse. Reports can be filed by contacting people who are trained in dealing with suspected abuse, such as local social service and law enforcement agencies. Further information and assistance may be obtained by talking to physicians, counselors, clergy, school professionals, or others who deal with child abuse or families with problems.

Parents who fear they have abused or may abuse their children are encouraged to contact these groups as well. In addition, self-help groups, such as Parents Anonymous, are available in many communities.

GENERAL CARE

Taking care of a preschooler is a full-time job. This section discusses some basic hygiene concerns. When should the child begin regular visits to the dentist? How can you help prevent diaper rash? Ways to minimize the spread of infectious disease in your household and how to prevent your child from bringing home every infection he or she is exposed to are presented.

This section also examines safety. These early years can be dangerous for the young child whose parents are not conscious of the safety risks. Young children are curious about everything. They have no qualms about tasting something—anything—they find in a container under your sink, popping beads or other objects into their mouths, or jumping off the edge of the pool. How can you make your home a safe place in which to live and play?

Many parents work; thus, we offer tips on what to look for in a day-care center. Care of the handicapped child is also addressed.

PREVENTION OF THE SPREAD OF DISEASE IN THE FAMILY

If you have a young child, you may notice that you have more colds and viral illnesses. Given the frequency with which young children contract these ailments and their high degree of contagiousness, this is not a surprise.

Infections that typically afflict the American family are spread in various ways.

Respiratory infections such as colds are most often spread through contact with secretions from the nose, mouth, or eye of the infected person. Toddlers are great at spreading colds because of their habit of touching and mouthing everything they come across.

Your child sneezes and a stream of infectious agents is released into the atmosphere. Although colds are spread less commonly in this manner, the infectious particles contained in a sneeze or cough can travel up to 6 feet.

Some infections such as diarrhea and hepatitis A are spread through contact with the infected person's feces, which are most often found on the hands of the infected person or on an object touched by the infected person.

Finally, sharing of combs, brushes, and hats can contribute to the spread of lice, ringworm, and impetigo.

Although it is impossible to totally halt the spread of contagious disease within a family, you can take measures to reduce its frequency. These measure are more successful in keeping gastrointestinal illnesses from making the rounds in your family, although they also may lower your incidence of colds somewhat.

1. Wash your hands. This is particularly important after using the bathroom, blowing your nose, or changing a diaper.
2. Do not smoke around your children. Passive smoking increases both the frequency and the severity of children's colds.
3. Discourage your child from touching his or her mouth or nose.
4. After an illness, throw out the old toothbrush. It may contain bacteria that can cause reinfection.
5. Use a disinfectant in the bathroom, kitchen, and diaper-changing area. Clean the areas frequently.

6. If you have pets, discourage your children from kissing them. Pets, especially puppies, can spread worms and other parasites.
7. To help prevent salmonellosis, a form of food poisoning, cook eggs and poultry thoroughly. And be sure that you carefully wash your hands and any object that comes into contact with uncooked food.

DIAPER CARE

Almost all children who wear diapers have diaper rash at some time. It develops when the skin is in prolonged contact with wetness, ammonia, digestive enzymes, and bacteria.

The following measures can minimize the chance of your child developing a diaper rash.

1. Check frequently for wetness. If a diaper is wet or dirty, change it immediately. Prolonged exposure to feces is particularly conducive to diaper rash.
2. Avoid use of plastic pants.
3. Cleanse the child's bottom with warm water and a mild soap after a bowel movement, and dry it thoroughly before putting another diaper on.
4. If you use cloth diapers, wash them with a mild detergent during the first cycle, then use a cup of bleach during the second cycle. This kills the bacteria. (See color photograph of diaper rash, page B-2.)

SAFETY AT HOME AND PLAY

The leading cause of death in young children is accidents. Preschoolers, especially those between 2 and 3 years old, are particularly vulnerable to accidents in the home, many of which prove to be fatal.

Even though certain precautions must be taken to ensure the safety of the young baby (see pages 74 and 319), safety should move to the forefront of parents' minds once the baby becomes mobile.

By the time the baby is 1 year old, your home should be childproofed. By age 1, most children are beginning to walk. Add to that the immense curiosity that often compels them to explore and their inability to comprehend the dangers of certain actions and you have a potentially hazardous situation.

As preschoolers grow up, they will be able to understand why they should not stick their fingers in an electrical socket, put buttons in their mouths, or play with matches. Even so, 4- and 5-year-olds at times do things that they know could hurt them. So even with the older preschooler, never take chances with safety.

The following are some of the more common accidents in the home or during play and tips on how to prevent them.

Burns. In young children, burns are the leading cause of accidental death in the home. Here are some tips for minimizing the chances that your child will be a burn victim.

1. Install smoke detectors on each floor of your home and test them periodically.
2. Have a fire extinguisher in your kitchen.
3. Never leave your child alone in the house.
4. Keep matches out of your child's reach.
5. When cooking, turn pot handles toward the back of the stove.
6. Do not use cloths or mats that a child can pull off the table.
7. Never drink hot beverages with a child on your lap or leave a cup of hot coffee near the edge of a table where a child might easily pull it off.
8. Place electric outlet covers on all unused outlets.
9. Turn down the thermostat on your water heater to between 120°F and 125°F. At 160°F a child can be scalded in less than a second.

For procedures to deal with burn emergencies, see page 266.

Drowning. After burns, drowning is the second most common cause of accidental death of young children in the home. Drowning is more common in hot climates, where people are more apt to have outdoor pools. To decrease the chance of drowning, follow these measures.

1. Never leave a preschooler alone in the bathtub.
2. If you have an outdoor pool, install a childproof fence around it.

3. Teach your child to swim.
4. Teach your child that he or she is never to swim without adult supervision.
5. When boating or around water, always have your child wear a life preserver. When boating, set a good example by wearing your life preserver.

For procedures to deal with drowning emergencies, see page 279.

Poisoning.   Another common cause of accidents at home is poisoning; a fifth of all accidental poisonings occur during the second year of life.

1. Keep all medicine in a high or locked cabinet.
2. Keep cleaning solutions out of reach of children. If you must keep them in a low cupboard, install fixtures that make it impossible for your child to open the cupboard door.
3. Do not store anything in the wrong container. For example, if you store paint thinner in a juice bottle, your child may take a drink, thinking it is juice.
4. Look around your garage for toxic chemicals that may be accessible to your wandering child.
5. Many common houseplants are poisonous when eaten. You can obtain a list of these plants from your local Poison Control Center. If you choose to have one of these plants in your home, keep it out of reach of your child. (See also Garden-Variety Poisonous Plants, page 302.)
6. Keep the number of the Poison Control Center next to your telephone and call the Center immediately if you think your child has taken a poison.
7. Keep a bottle of syrup of ipecac on hand to induce vomiting in case your child ingests something harmful. However, NEVER induce vomiting until you have been advised to do so by a Poison Control Center or your physician. Some substances can cause more damage coming back up the esophagus.

For procedures in dealing with poisoning emergencies, see page 299.

Falls.   Falls also are common during the preschool years. To protect your child from dangerous falls, follow these measures.

1. Keep the side rails up on the crib.
2. Install gates at the tops and bottoms of the staircases in your home.
3. Install a safety net or guard on outdoor decks or staircase openings where a young child could squeeze through.
4. Never let your child use a walker near a staircase.
5. Make sure your windows are locked or have window guards.
6. Do not put a child younger than 6 in the top bunk of a bunk bed.
7. Make sure your child is securely fastened in his or her stroller or carriage.
8. Always supervise outdoor activity.
9. Forbid use of home trampolines; these can result in serious injury even when a parent is supervising.
10. Serious accidents can occur at playgrounds. Before you let your child use play equipment, make sure it is adequately maintained, with no rust, sharp edges or protrusions, or loose nuts and bolts. The surface beneath swings or other playground equipment your child may climb on should not be concrete, asphalt, or packed dirt but rather should be an energy-absorbing material such as loose sand or wood chips to lessen the chance of injury should the child fall.

Choking.   Young preschoolers will put anything into their mouth. This can lead to choking.

1. Select toys appropriate for your child's age. A 1-year-old should not have a toy with small pieces that could be accidentally swallowed.
2. Make sure your preschooler's toys do not have loose buttons or sharp edges.
3. Avoid giving your child food that could get stuck in his or her throat. Such foods include, for example, whole hot dogs (cut them lengthwise and then into small pieces), popcorn, nuts, hard candy, and raw carrots.
4. Do not allow food to be in your baby's hand away from the table.

See also Swallowing Objects, page 93. For procedures in dealing with a choking emergency see Choking, Breathing Emergencies, and Resuscitation, page 268.

CAR SAFETY

When riding in the car, your preschooler must be strapped into a proper child car seat. After the child grows out of the seat (usually at about 40 pounds), he or she should always wear a seat belt.

CARING FOR YOUR CHILD'S TEETH

Eighty to 90 percent of dental cavities (caries) can be prevented by a combination of measures that include water fluoridation, sealants, brushing and flossing, good nutrition, and regular visits to the dentist.

Some parents assume that a child has to be a certain age before dental hygiene becomes necessary. In fact, once your baby has a single tooth, you need to begin a daily program of care. Many babies younger than a year will not stand for having a brush in their mouth, but you can at least wipe the tooth with a wet cloth after meals.

The following are the components of a sound oral hygiene program.

Fluoride. From the time your child is 2 weeks old until he or she is 12 years old, fluoride is an important deterrent to tooth decay. Fluoride, which helps make the tooth enamel cavity resistant, can reduce caries up to 25 percent. It is typically consumed either in drinking water or in a vitamin supplement. If you live in an area where fluoride is added to the water supply, your child must drink at least 1 pint of water daily to reap its full benefits. If your city water supply contains no fluoride or if you have a well, ask your child's physician or dentist to prescribe a supplement. The application of fluoride to the surface of the teeth also may be beneficial for some children.

Diet. Never let your child go to bed with a bottle. Sleeping with a bottle containing milk, juice, or anything other than water can cause severe decay, particularly in the front teeth. As for sugar, it is virtually impossible to keep children away from it altogether. Avoid sugary foods that stick to the teeth or stay in the mouth. These include, for example, hard candy and caramels.

Try to limit sugary treats to mealtime, and then insist that your child brush his or her teeth immediately after the meal. Some parents find that sugary treats can be limited to being an "award" at one certain time during the day, such as immediately after lunch, and be followed immediately by toothbrushing. "Smart snacks," such as vegetables and fruits, not only help minimize caries but also are nutritionally better for your child.

Brushing and Flossing. Before your child is 1 year old, buy him or her a soft-bristled toothbrush. Although it is fine to let the preschooler attempt to brush his or her own teeth, you will need to do it also to ensure proper cleaning. If the child is negative about brushing, make a game of it. Let your child brush your teeth while you brush his or hers. Whenever possible, teeth should be brushed after every meal. Even rinsing with water or drinking a glass of water after eating is helpful (see Proper Flossing and Brushing Techniques, page 395).

Floss your child's teeth, beginning at the time the molars touch.

The Dentist. Your child should begin to visit a dentist twice a year by age 3 years and sooner if the teeth appear abnormal or if he or she complains of toothache.

DAY-CARE CENTERS

Few issues are as relevant to working parents as that of day-care. Today, more than 50 percent of mothers with preschool children work outside the home. The need for day-care centers that provide a nurturing and educational environment has never been so great.

Day-care in the United States has become a multimillion dollar business. Still, there are not enough centers that provide high-quality care. Many families, especially those in the lower-income brackets, are forced to accept less-than-ideal conditions for their preschoolers. Many of the truly fine centers have such limited space that many parents put their unborn child's name on a waiting list in anticipation of the need a year down the road.

If you are about to begin the search for a high-quality day-care center, here are things to look for.

1. Make sure the center has been licensed by the state. This means that the center meets certain standards and must comply with various health regulations. Family day-care centers (those operated out of a private home) are often less expensive but may not be state-licensed. This means that they are not monitored by state authorities, as are the licensed day-care operations.

2. Visit several centers before you make your choice. A center should be open to parents at all times. Any center that requires a parent to call ahead before visiting should be suspect.

3. Once you think you have decided on a center, visit it again, preferably at a different time of day. Are the children happy and busy? Are there lots of things to do, or do the children appear to be at loose ends? Are the teachers warm, encouraging, and willing to hug a crying child? Are there adequate sinks and toilets for the children? Make sure there is a safe playground, with proper fences and equipment that is in good condition.

4. Interview the director of the center and the teacher who would be in charge of your child. Ideally, the staff-to-student ratio should be between 1:4 and 1:6, depending on the preschooler's age (the younger the children, the more staff is required). What is staff turnover? What education does the center require of its teachers? Is there a television set and how often are children allowed to watch it? (Television viewing should be minimal and selective, if at all.)

Once you find the center that is right for your child, spend some time helping your child adjust to it. For the child who is younger than 2½ years, separation from the parent can be painful and tearful, so plan on spending most of the first day with your child at the center. This may be unnecessary for the 4- or 5-year-old, particularly if the child is outgoing and has spent time in the homes of friends.

For the first week or until your child adjusts, avoid rushing off in the morning. Linger for 5 or 10 minutes, until your child begins to interact with someone else. Then, do not sneak away while his or her back is turned. Say "good-bye" and leave. You may find it helpful to let the child bring something from home such as a favorite blanket or a stuffed toy.

Every parent who has a child in day-care should expect the child to pick up his or her share of colds and viruses. All young children get sick from time to time, but the chances are that your child will have more bouts of illness during his or her time in day-care. In part, this increase is because these common illnesses are so contagious. In addition, children are often contagious before the outbreak of any symptoms, so a seemingly healthy child can infect an entire class. Thus, epidemics of childhood ailments in some centers are commonplace.

What can be done to help prevent the spread of infection in your child's day-care center? No practical measures can eliminate the spread of infection, but teachers or assistants can help by making sure they wash their hands thoroughly after changing diapers and before handling food.

As a parent, you can help by not sending your ill child to day-care. When is a child too sick to go? Each center generally has its own rules but, as a guideline, most centers do not want your child to attend if he or she has a fever of more than 100°F or is vomiting or has diarrhea.

As to when the child can return to day-care, it usually depends on how well he or she feels and whether the illness is contagious. Many cold symptoms persist for a week or more. Once the temperature is normal for 24 hours, your child probably can return to day-care even though he or she still has a slight running nose and cough.

The following is a guide to when a child with a contagious disease is no longer contagious:

Chickenpox: after all sores are crusted, usually 7 days.

Strep throat: 24 hours after treatment begins.

Conjunctivitis: 24 hours after treatment begins.

Head lice: after one treatment.

Diarrhea: after stools form again.

CARE OF THE HANDICAPPED CHILD

The care of a handicapped child involves a combination of family support, social and academic adaptation, adjustments in the physical environment to accommodate the handicap, and, often, special medical care.

Permanent handicaps in children can be severe mental retardation, conspicuous physical deformities such as the absence of a limb, or sensory defects such as blindness or deafness.

Whatever a child's handicap, it does not take him or her long to realize that he or she is different. Helping the child develop a sense of self-worth and the ability to get along in the world despite this difference is fundamental to the successful rearing of a handicapped child. This can be achieved, in part, by helping the child become as self-sufficient as possible and by creating an environment in which the child can develop to his or her potential.

Few things are as traumatic as the birth of a child with a major handicap. Some parents initially try to deny the reality of the situation, especially if the defect is not physically apparent. Guilt, anger, accusation, and fear about one's ability to cope with a handicapped child as well as anxiety over the child's future are all normal reactions.

In some severe cases, the question of institutional care must be addressed early. It used to be common to place severely retarded infants in institutions. Today, physicians know that infants and young children do better developmentally if they have a consistent parent figure in a nurturing home environment. Still, parents of handicapped children often come to the realization that they alone cannot care for their child, thus an institution is found. Even so, parents who at least attempt home care generally do not feel as guilty as those who institutionalize their child without making an effort.

If you have a handicapped child that you are attempting to rear at home, there are some things you can do to make your child as happy and well-adjusted as possible.

Treat the child as you do your other children. Some parents tend to tread softly around the handicapped child, which only serves to make the child feel more different than he or she is. Household rules should apply to everyone in the family. Like his or her siblings, your handicapped child should have certain responsibilities around the house and should be punished for breaking the rules (when he or she is capable of understanding the rules), just as any other child would be.

Be aware of the impact of your attitude. Children are amazingly deft at compensating for a defect. For example, a child born without one hand becomes very proficient with the other hand and, having known nothing else, does not miss the absent hand. However, if the parent is embarrassed about the deformity, the child will sense these feelings and probably become self-conscious.

Do not neglect your other children. The care of a handicapped child can be so time-consuming that other family members are ignored. Answer your other children's questions about their handicapped brother or sister honestly. Try to set aside time each week to be alone with each child.

Accept your child for what he or she is. Like any child, your handicapped child has both strengths and weaknesses. When your child accomplishes something, no matter how small, he or she should be praised and made to feel special.

Do not isolate the child. All children need friends. It is normal to want to protect your child from contagious illness and the potential cruelty of some children, but do not do it at the expense of your child's socialization.

Providing an education for handicapped children in the community school is a relatively recent concept. Handicapped children used to go to a special school with other handicapped children. Today, however, by law, most public schools must provide special education classes for handicapped children. And, in many cases, the children take some classes with those in the normal student population. Mixing handicapped persons with the rest of the class is beneficial for both groups.

Address your child's special needs. The child with a handicap has countless special needs, needs that may range from a specially designed house and van to home care by a trained nurse or weekly visits to a medical facility.

Remember, you are not alone. Many community resources can help you meet the needs of your handicapped son or daughter. Some agencies offer financial help for qualifying parents who cannot provide for the medical needs of their child. Others offer services such as transportation, counseling, psychological evaluation, babysitting, daycare, and play activities.

Your child's physician can be an excellent source of information in regard to available community resources. Public health nurses and social workers are familiar with local resources and are often a very useful source of information and support. In addition, there are parent organizations that can help. These groups give parents a chance to express their common concerns and share information. In recent years, these groups have organized and have become a force in influencing legislation that has expanded and improved opportunities for the handicapped.

PSYCHOSOCIAL DEVELOPMENT OF PERSONALITY AND BEHAVIOR

The development of your child's personality is as important as his or her physical development. During the preschool years, problems may emerge that can affect the way your child behaves around you and other people.

Some of these problems, such as mental retardation and autism, are severe. Others, such as negativism and sibling rivalry, are normal.

This section discusses normal behavioral development during the preschool years, including the development of imagination and sexual curiosity. Problems that cause abnormal development, such as hyperactivity, learning disabilities, and sexual abuse, also are explored.

NORMAL BEHAVIORAL DEVELOPMENT

During the 5 years that constitute the preschool period, your child goes through many developmental changes. In the course of these few years, your child's vocabulary goes from a few words to hundreds. The child at 1 year may be barely able to walk but at 5 years may be skipping rope. The 1-year-old who hides behind you when a stranger comes grows into the kindergartner who waves at you nonchalantly from the school bus.

The following are some examples of development that occur typically during these years. Keep in mind that the behavioral development of a child does not adhere to a strict schedule. Every child is different and develops according to his or her own schedule. Thus, these are only general guidelines of what to expect. If you think there is a problem with your child's development, consult your physician.

The 1-Year-Old. Your 1-year-old will hand you a toy when you ask for it. He or she can understand your gestures, obey your commands, and respond to his or her own name. Your child has learned to indicate a need or want in ways other than crying.

He or she is a bit of a "ham," never happier than when there is an audience. Your child sings, plays pat-a-cake, and loves to hide from you, although he or she always wants to keep mom or dad in sight. Although he or she still may fear strangers, your toddler is beginning to adjust to having a babysitter from time to time. He or she will hug or kiss either parent spontaneously or when requested and is beginning to show affection to stuffed toys or other objects.

The 1-year-old child loves to drop small objects into a container, dump them out, and then put them back in. He or she will combine objects with other objects to invent new ways of doing things, can retrieve a hidden toy, and is beginning to understand the concept of "up" and "down."

Your 1-year-old probably will insist on feeding himself or herself, can hold a cup with a little help, tries to use a spoon, may fight sleep, and cooperates when being dressed.

The 2-Year-Old. The 2-year-old child can be bossy. He or she has yet to learn to share although on rare occasions can put someone else's wishes above his or her own. He or she is able to communicate feelings, desires, and interests to others by using words or gestures.

By this time, most children have a vocabulary of 50 words or more, but they understand much more. Your 2-year-old is beginning to discover that everything has a name, can respond to commands such as "Point to your nose" or "Point to a dog in the book,'' and can locate items around the house. The child of this age likes to watch television and may be able to identify some cartoon characters.

By the second birthday, most children are becoming more negative. They are beginning to become more aggressive and may take their aggression out on siblings or playmates. They become more possessive of their toys and more self-sufficient and are more likely to challenge their parents' authority.

At play, the 2-year-old mimics parents' behavior, plays better with older children than with those of the same age, and is beginning to pretend.

The 2-year-old wants to do everything without help. He or she can verbalize toilet needs, although most children are not trained at age 2.

The 3-Year-Old. The 3-year-old is madly in love with his or her parents and wants to be just like them. Much of the hostility and negative behavior of the 2-year-old recedes into the background.

The 2-year-old may have picked up his or her mop every time you mopped the floor but the focus was on the mop, whereas the 3-year-old who engages in this imitative behavior is actually trying to be like you. The child this age loves pretend games. After a visit to the physician, your 3-year-old gets out the toy ''doctor kit'' and examines his or her sick teddy bear or sits in the car and pretends to be daddy driving. Dressing up in your old clothing is a favorite game. At this age, children become more interested in their peers and begin to interact, although side-by-side play is still common.

The 3-year-old can conduct a conversation and uses relatively complex sentences. Many children can recognize several numbers and letters.

At this age, many children develop sleep problems, often as a result of fears.

Most 3-year-old children are toilet-trained and are capable of helping you dress them.

The 4-Year-Old. Four-year-olds are extremely social creatures, capable of playing with several children at the same time. The 4-year-old has a vivid imagination, and frequent make-believe play reflects that.

Whereas 3-year-olds tend to be quite agreeable, some 4-year-olds are assertive, cocky, and loud.

The 4-year-old is capable of telling a story. He or she now has the ability to think about language, and his or her speech is intelligible even to strangers. A child this age can accurately count four pennies, pedal a tricycle, play games that require taking turns and following rules, can copy a cross and a square, and can draw a person with as many as four parts besides the head. Some children this age begin writing the letters of the alphabet.

The 5-Year-Old. Even more so than the 4-year-old, the 5-year-old delights in having other children around. Given a choice between doing something with a friend or with parents, the 5-year-old usually chooses the former.

The 5-year-old can get dressed alone (buttoning some buttons and perhaps even tying shoes). The child probably also wants to choose what to wear. The 5-year-old is extremely conscious of the differences between boys and girls. Children at this age often assert that they have a boyfriend or girlfriend whom they plan to marry.

Many children at 5 have been in nursery school for a year or two; some do not begin school until kindergarten. Depending on how much stimulation and exposure a child has had, it is not unusual for a 5-year-old to begin reading and writing and even to have some rudimentary skills in arithmetic.

NEGATIVISM

Between the ages of 18 months and 3 years, children go through a period when ''No'' is their favorite word. It matters not what you say to the child; most of the time it will be met by an emphatic ''No.''

''Do you want to stay in the bathtub?'' you ask your young daughter. ''No,'' she answers. ''Well, then, do you want to get out of the bathtub?'' ''No.''

Negativism (along with tantrums) is a normal part of the so-called terrible twos. Although it may seem as though your child is purposely trying to provoke you, he or she is not. This is simply one step down the long road toward independence.

Getting through this sometimes difficult phase of development requires lots of patience and a good sense of humor. If you are the parent of a child in the thick of the terrible twos, remember that every parent goes through this and lives to laugh about it later.

The following are some guidelines that may help make the road a little less bumpy.

1. Do not take your child's negativism too seriously.
2. Don't punish your child for saying "No."
3. Give your child choices: "Do you want to wear the red pants or the green pants?" Letting him or her choose between acceptable choices will give your child a sense of freedom and control and make him or her more likely to cooperate. (Be careful about asking a question when there is only one answer. For example, at bedtime, do not offer your child a choice between staying up and going to bed if you have no intention of letting him or her stay up.)
4. Give your child a transition time between activities. If, for example, your child is having fun but it is time to leave the playground, give him or her adequate time. "You can go down the slide three more times and then we have to go home."
5. Go easy on rules. Children this age are not likely to follow a long list of house rules. Avoid arguing about unimportant things such as whether your child should eat all the carrots on his or her plate. Make sure that your daily interactions with your child are weighted toward the positive, not the negative.
6. Try to avoid saying "No" yourself. You want the child to see you as an agreeable person, someone he or she can imitate.

IMAGINATION

Preschoolers live part of their lives in a rich, imaginary world where anything is possible. Play during these years often revolves around pretending. Sometimes it is difficult for a child to know where pretend stops and reality starts. Hence, you have the 3-year-old who explains to you that he or she was not the one who broke your bottle of perfume but that it was a little green man with a yellow hat. Your child is not lying, not in the true sense of the word. And you should not punish your child or make him or her feel guilty for making up stories like this from time to time.

However, some children seem to live in their imaginations most of the day. If your child seems to be spending too much time with an imaginary friend whom he or she truly believes in, you might ask yourself whether the youngster's real life is sufficiently interesting. A child who lives in his or her own private dream world may need to spend more time with friends or may not be getting enough attention from parents.

SIBLING PROBLEMS

Few things are as exasperating to parents as constant bickering among their children.

Problems between siblings can range from rivalry between the young toddler and the newborn to physical aggression to incessant quarreling.

Although these fights can make even easygoing parents wish they were rearing an only child, you should know that fighting and rivalry between siblings are normal. Although at times your children may seem to reside in enemy camps, on other days they may be the best of friends.

The following paragraphs describe some common problems between siblings and offer suggestions that may make them easier to live with.

Sibling Rivalry. Children can be jealous of a sibling at any age. One of the most common situations of sibling rivalry is the jealousy that older siblings feel toward a new baby in the family. The worst age for this rivalry is between 12 and 36 months.

A child who is jealous of a new brother or sister typically demands attention, may show aggression toward the infant, and often regresses (for example, he or she returns to thumb-sucking or wants to wear a diaper even though he or she is toilet trained).

Although you cannot totally eliminate these natural feelings, you can help prepare the child for the new baby by talking about the baby during pregnancy. Let the child help you get ready for the baby. If you need your child's crib, move him or her to a bed long before the baby is due. Praise the child for mature behavior.

At the very least, call your child each day that you are in the hospital. Preferably, your child should be allowed to visit and meet his or her new brother or sister.

When you get home, hand the baby to someone else and spend time alone with your older child.

Fighting. Children must be taught that they cannot kick, punch, or bite each other. When your children physically fight, separate them immediately. Send them to separate rooms for a few minutes.

Quarrels. Make it clear that the children have to settle their own arguments. Then, when they do argue, try to ignore it, even if you have to go into another room. Try to stay out of the argument. If they do bring it to you, help them clarify the problem—but let *them* find the solution. When they do settle it, praise them. Avoid showing favoritism.

Refusal To Share Toys. Some 3-year-olds will share toys, but many do not start sharing until months later. You cannot make your child share with a sibling. Do not punish your child for refusing to share. However, encourage sharing and praise the child when this occurs.

In the same vein, many young children frequently grab toys away from a sibling playing nearby. When this happens, take the toy away from the child and return it to the child who was using it. Always praise the child for asking to use a toy and for returning it on request (see also Difficulties With Sibling and Peer Relationships, page 129).

THUMB AND FINGER SUCKING

Thumb and finger sucking is common in infants. Only 6 percent of thumb- or finger-sucking babies continue doing so beyond their first birthday, and only 3 percent do it beyond their second birthday.

By the time most thumb or finger suckers are 4, they have given up the practice, except when the issue has become a power struggle between parent and child or when it has become a deeply ingrained habit.

Thumb sucking is not a serious problem. However, it makes the child appear babyish, which may subject him or her to ridicule from peers. Moreover, prolonged thumb or finger sucking can interfere with the normal alignment of the teeth, making orthodontic treatment necessary in later years.

If your child is younger than 4 and sucks his or her thumb, try to ignore or distract the child. Never punish, scold, or pull your child's hand out of his or her mouth. These methods can make the problem worse.

In the older preschooler, you can appeal to vanity. Show your child how his or her teeth are beginning to protrude and the wrinkled skin of the thumb. Remind your child gently when you catch him or her in the act, and lavish praise when you notice he or she is not sucking the thumb.

Because thumb sucking during sleep is involuntary, it ceases when your child's sleep deepens.

DELAYED PSYCHOMOTOR DEVELOPMENT

In most cases the development of gross and fine motor control proceeds smoothly. Sometimes, however, a child falls way behind his or her peers. For example, most children walk between 12 and 15 months. But what about the child who is not walking at 20 months? Is there something wrong?

There are several different types of delayed development in either fine (muscles used for hand dexterity) or gross (larger muscles used for walking, jumping, and skipping) motor function.

Some types of fine motor dysfunction may make it difficult for a preschooler to draw or color or may delay him or her in learning to tie shoes. Some of these children show impairments in hand-eye coordination. Some children with fine motor dysfunction are unable to hold a crayon correctly. Because of their problems with fine motor skills, these children often have difficulty when they enter school.

Children who are clumsy or who have delayed gross motor skills such as the inability to skip or jump often feel self-conscious and humiliated. These are the children who are always the last ones picked to be on the athletic team. Often they develop a poor self-image as a result.

The cause for delayed psychomotor development is generally unknown, although it may run in families.

If you suspect that your child may have a delay in psychomotor development, take your concerns to your physician. There are tests that can determine whether there is a problem.

If there is a delay in motor skills, your child may lose an important area from which he or she draws for building self-esteem. As parents you need to preserve your child's sense of self-esteem by being understanding and patient with his or her progress. If you are impatient, even though your child ultimately will "catch up," your child's self-esteem may suffer.

LEARNING PROBLEMS

Speech, hearing, and vision problems can affect a child's ability to learn. Many of these can be treated successfully or at least made less severe. Often, the key factor is early detection. A sensory problem discovered during the preschool years often can be resolved before it irreparably affects the child's intellectual development.

Thus, it is important that a young child's periodic examinations include vision and hearing tests. Even children with no history or indication of eye problems should see an ophthalmologist by age 4.

The following are some sensory defects that can cause learning problems.

Hearing Disorders. In order to develop speech and language, a person must hear. Therefore, even a mild loss of hearing or hearing loss in one ear during childhood can have a negative impact on a child's acquisition of language. The more severe the hearing loss, the greater the learning problem.

An estimated 4 percent of children younger than 5 have some hearing loss in both ears, and as many as 10 percent have a loss in one ear.

Four types of hearing loss are found in young children. *Conductive hearing loss* involves interference with the reception of sound from the external to the internal ear. *Sensorineural hearing loss* is the result of abnormalities of the cochlear hair cells or the auditory nerve. *Mixed hearing loss* occurs when both a conductive and a sensorineural hearing loss are present. *Central auditory disorders* are the result of a dysfunction of the auditory center in the central nervous system.

If your child was born totally deaf, the problem might be suspected within the first 6 months of life. If the deafness is partial, however, it likely will not be diagnosed until your child is between 12 and 24 months old.

At this point, your child has already missed critical stages for language development and learning. For these reasons, many infants thought to be at high risk for hearing loss (those with neonatal asphyxia, bacterial meningitis, congenital or perinatal infections, a family history of deafness, or birth defects of the head or neck or those who were severely premature) are often tested within the first 6 months of life (see Your Child's Hearing Progress, page 68).

The extent to which a hearing loss influences a child's ability to learn depends on the severity of the loss and the range of frequencies affected. Moreover, the outcome for the child's language development, learning, and future educational achievements depends on the age at which the loss occurs and how soon the problem is discovered and treatment begins.

Some hearing losses can be treated with medication. Others can be treated surgically. A hearing aid amplifies what hearing the child has and is considered the single most important tool toward allowing the child to function normally.

Some form of special education is generally required, even when the hearing loss is mild. This may be restricted to speech and language therapy if the loss is slight; in more severe cases, your child may require special education programs throughout his or her school career.

Finally, you should know that the parents of a child with a hearing loss are an important component to the child's future academic success. You will need to learn how to make the most of whatever hearing your young child has. Techniques such as lipreading and sign language can help. A class to learn such techniques may be available in your community.

Speech and Language Disorders. Certain illnesses can interfere with the normal development of articulation of words and sentences as well as with understanding language in your preschool child. The following paragraphs describe problems that can significantly delay development by a mild to a marked degree.

Severely delayed speech and language development that are part of an overall developmental retardation can play a part in a broader slowdown in reaching other developmental milestones such as sitting, standing, walking, and toilet training.

Hearing loss, caused by nerve deafness at birth or by middle ear infections during infancy and early childhood, can be a cause of speech and language disorders.

Neurological disorders involving a lack of muscle strength or coordination, either present at birth or acquired during early infancy or childhood, along with damage to language areas of the brain, also can cause impairment of speech and language.

Environmental deprivation of language and emotional stimulation due to parental conflict, separation, or child abuse may contribute to speech and language disorders.

If you are concerned about an apparent failure of normal articulation, language development, stuttering, or other deviations in your child's speech or comprehension, consult your pediatrician or family physician and a speech-language specialist for proper diagnosis and, particularly, therapy. This step can be important and profitable in many cases of childhood speech and language disorders (see also Speech and Language Development, page 96).

Vision Problems. The preschool years are crucial for the detection and treatment of many vision disorders, some serious and some, such as myopia, serious only in their ability to create a learning difficulty.

Children with abnormalities of refraction (conditions that require eyeglasses) may show a lack of interest in learning. The child who is farsighted may not want to look at books, and the one who is nearsighted may seem uninterested in any activity more than a few feet away. Squinting, eye rubbing, fatigue, and headaches are common manifestations.

These problems are easily rectified with prescription glasses. When caught in the preschool years, simple vision problems do not have an adverse effect on a child's learning (see Refraction Problems, page 739, and Strabismus and Myopia, page 750).

MENTAL RETARDATION

Mental retardation can range from a slight slowness that makes school a struggle to profound retardation requiring constant supervision. Children who are mentally retarded are slow in acquiring motor skills and language. They lack the social skills and emotional maturity appropriate to their age.

Some children who are otherwise normal may lag behind in one or another of these areas of development. This may represent a developmental lag in a child who will eventually catch up. Others have emotional or social immaturities that may indicate a disturbance (see also Mental Health, page 1011). However, the mentally retarded child is behind in all of these areas and will not catch up with his or her peers.

Mild forms of retardation may not become evident until the child begins school. Children with mild forms are able to learn academic skills but do so more slowly than the average child. They are identified as educationally mentally handicapped.

Children with moderate mental retardation are identified as trainable because they can learn self-care skills such as dressing and toileting. They have limited ability to benefit from academic school programs but can attend day activity centers and eventually can be trained to do certain simple jobs in sheltered workshops.

Children who are severely or profoundly retarded can learn minimal self-care skills and may become toilet trained but require almost total supervision and care. They learn little or no language.

In the past, most retarded children, even those with mild retardation, were institutionalized. Today the great majority live at home or in small group homes in their communities. Special education programs for slow learners are available in all school districts, and many resources have become available in communities to provide social and recreational opportunities for the more severely retarded children.

Even when there are some early signs, in many children mild retardation is not actually diagnosed until they begin school because it is then that they are being compared with large numbers of peers and their developmental differences become more apparent.

If your child is mentally retarded, the goal of treatment is to help your child reach his or her potential, whatever it may be, and to enable him or her to cope as well as possible with the handicap.

When the diagnosis is made in infancy, the baby and the parents sometimes can be enrolled in an infant stimulation program. Such a program offers multisensory stimulation in an attempt to facilitate emotional, intellectual, and physical development. It also helps parents to understand more about their child's strengths and weaknesses and offers parents support during what is usually a very difficult time emotionally.

Federal legislation has guaranteed an education to all retarded children in the United States, regardless of the severity of the handicap. Special education classes are taught in regular community schools. Some retarded children may spend part of the day in a class with other retarded children and then attend a class or two with children who are not handicapped.

Like any child, a retarded one needs friends. Despite the mixing (mainstreaming) of retarded with normal children in schools, the retarded are still not always accepted by these classmates. Thus, the parents must often take it upon themselves to plan social and recreational activities for their child. There are organizations for the retarded that offer various activities, including summer camps. These programs help the child both to become more comfortable in social situations and to increase his or her independence.

Finally, caring for a retarded child can leave little time for the rest of the family. However devoted, parents need a break. Because of the child's handicap, though, many parents who would leave a normal child with a babysitter are reluctant to do so with their retarded child. Many communities have recognized this need and opened respite centers where parents can temporarily leave their retarded child with a caregiver experienced in the needs of these children. If you are lucky enough to live in a community with this option, take advantage of it (see also Mental Retardation, page 113, and Infantile Autism, page 1017).

SEXUALITY IN THE PRESCHOOL CHILD

The preschool child has a natural sexual curiosity that manifests itself in various ways.

From birth, boys are capable of having erections, and the vagina of a newborn girl can become lubricated. By the first birthday, one-third of all children have been observed stimulating their genitals; boys typically pull at their penises, and girls rub their vaginas. Between the ages of 2 and 5, one-half of all boys and one-third of all girls masturbate.

Occasional masturbation is normal and nothing to worry about. The child stimulates himself or herself simply because it feels good. Some children masturbate because they are unhappy or are reacting to punishment to stop the practice.

If your child masturbates, try not to get upset. Masturbation does not mean your child will grow up to be promiscuous or sexually deviant. It is not physically harmful, nor does it cause emotional problems unless a parent overreacts and sends the message that sex is dirty and frightening.

Because it is difficult to stop a child from masturbating, it is best to simply accept it. However, it should be made clear to the child that although it is all right to masturbate in the privacy of the bedroom, other areas are off limits. If the child suddenly starts masturbating in the middle of a play group, try to distract him or her. If that fails, take your child aside and remind him or her that this is done only in the privacy of the bedroom or bathroom.

In addition to self-stimulation, many preschoolers are fascinated by their parents' bodies. A young child may want to touch the mother's breasts or father's penis. That same child may be found half undressed playing "doctor" with the child next door.

These behaviors are normal. Avoid showing shock or anger. Instead, stress that some activities are private and, although it is okay for the child to touch himself or herself, it is not okay for others, even friends, to touch them that way except in special circumstances, such as an examination by a physician. Then point out that this is true for adults as well as for children.

SEXUAL ABUSE

The sexual abuse of children has, in recent years, emerged from the proverbial closet. The problem certainly is not new—but our understanding of the extent of the problem surely is: as many as 1 in 5 girls and 1 in 10 boys will be victims of sexual abuse before reaching the age of 18.

Recognize the Signs.   Be alert for the following possible signs of sexual abuse in a child:

1. Sexually provocative behavior in a preschooler;

2. Withdrawal from friends, family, or school activities;

3. Unusually hostile or aggressive behavior.

There may be no physical signs of abuse, but a physician may identify evidence of trauma to the genital area or the presence of sexually transmitted infections (see also page 875). However, the absence of all of these signs is not necessarily proof that no abuse has occurred.

Why a Child Is Susceptible. Children need affection; depriving a child of healthy physical contact (such as hugging), in fact, is to risk significant problems in a youngster's psychological development. There is even a natural sexual aspect that is present from birth. Breast-feeding, for example, can prompt physiological changes of sexual arousal in infants.

Children often seek some sexual contact with their peers, but such experimentation is not sought with adults. If your child describes an experience in which he or she was touched by an adult in an inappropriate way, take it seriously.

What To Do. If you suspect that your child has been sexually abused, contact your physician or an official in your local child-protection system (child welfare worker, local public attorney, police, or sheriff). If you are tempted to keep the abuse a private or family matter, keep in mind that most perpetrators are involved with many children. Seldom is the abuser a complete stranger to the child. The welfare or even the life of your child may be at stake.

NUTRITION

Some days it may seem like your preschooler does not eat enough to keep an ant alive, and other days you cannot keep him or her away from the refrigerator. Such is the preschooler's appetite.

Unlike the infant, who tripled his or her weight during the first year and ate well, the 1-year-old child's rate of growth slows considerably, as does his or her appetite. Some preschoolers are reluctant to try new foods or expand their food repertoire beyond three or four old favorites.

If you have a preschooler with a finicky appetite, you may be worried about whether your child is being adequately nourished. Or, your child may be eating too much of the wrong thing and be overweight.

This section addresses these and other common nutritional issues.

NUTRITION IN THE PRESCHOOL CHILD

By the time a child enters the second year of life, he or she should be eating a diet that consists of the four basic food groups: milk products; meat, poultry, fish, and eggs; grains; and fruits and vegetables. The chart on page 116 suggests the approximate serving size and mix of foods that are appropriate for filling the preschooler's nutritional needs.

Keep in mind, however, that every child's energy needs are different. Your child is not growing at the same rate he or she was as an infant, so it will not seem as if the child lives for the next meal. Your child does not need or want the quantities of food that only a few months ago were consumed with relish.

Parents often fail to recognize this important fact and become concerned when the child is uninterested and picks at food. They often attempt to force the child into eating, which can create long-term feeding problems and make mealtime an unpleasant experience for the entire family.

While the preschooler advances to the point where he or she can start to assume the same pattern of eating as that of older siblings or parents—that is, a three-meals-a-day pattern—keep in mind that snacking is acceptable. The key point is that children should be encouraged to determine for themselves how much they need to eat. As parents, you cannot judge for your child how much food is necessary; your role is to offer your preschooler a variety of nutritious foods and to let him or her decide what he or she is going to eat and how much. Offering a variety of nutritious foods and setting a good example as a parent are good strategies to help the child formulate healthy eating habits.

Do not think that the dietary model has to be followed slavishly every day: a child does not have to eat two servings of vegetables 7 days a week. More to the point, your child, despite occasional daily slips in amounts and choices, should be getting an overall good selection of foods.

Allow your child to help design his or her own eating style. Although the basic three-meals-a-day approach is best, snacks are

THE BALANCED DIET FOR YOUR PRESCHOOL CHILD

The following mix of foods should form the foundation of your child's diet.

Milk Products
Milk, cheese, cottage cheese, and yogurt are excellent sources of calcium, which is necessary for building strong bones and teeth. We recommend four servings a day. For the 1-year-old child, a serving is one-half cup, and for older preschoolers the serving size may be as large as ¾ cup.

Meat and Eggs
This group includes beef, poultry, lamb, fish, pork, liver, eggs, and peanut butter. These foods are excellent sources of protein, which is necessary for the growth and repair of tissue cells. Your preschooler needs three or more servings a day. The serving size for a 1-year-old is 2 tablespoons and that for a 4- or 5-year-old is 3 tablespoons.

Fruits and Vegetables
Your child should have at least four servings a day from this food group. To obtain an adequate amount of vitamin C, one or more servings should be citrus fruit, berries, tomato, cabbage, or cantaloupe. The child needs at least one serving of a green or yellow fruit or vegetable, which are excellent sources of vitamin A. Two servings a day of potato, legumes, apple, or banana are recommended.

Grains
This food group includes whole-grain cereals, breads, rice, and pasta. We recommend four or more daily servings. The serving size for the 1-year-old is one-half slice of bread, one-half ounce of ready-to-eat cereal, or one-fourth cup of pasta. For the 5-year-old, one and one-half slices of bread, one ounce of ready-to-eat cereal, or one-half cup of pasta constitutes a serving.

These are the food groups necessary for a nutritionally balanced diet, but do not expect your preschooler to eat a completely balanced diet every day. When allowed to choose from a selection of nutritionally sound foods, most children tend to select diets that, over several days, offer the necessary balance. This may mean that one day your child is eating a lot of peanut butter sandwiches, oranges, and milk and the next it is hamburgers, french fries, and carrots.

In essence, the overall picture is more important than what he or she eats on any given day.

How Much and What Kind of Food Does Your Preschool Child Need?

Food Group	Daily Servings	1 Year	2 to 3 Years	4 to 6 Years
Milk	4			
Milk (whole, skim, dry, evaporated, buttermilk, yogurt, or pudding)		½ cup	½ to ¾ cup	¾ cup
Meat	3 or more			
Eggs		1	1	1
Lean meat, fish, poultry		½ oz (2 Tbsp)	½ oz (2 Tbsp)	¾ oz (3 Tbsp)
Peanut butter		None	1 Tbsp	2 Tbsp
Legumes (dried peas and beans)		None	½ cup	½ to ¾ cup
Fruits and vegetables	4 or more			
Vegetables		3 Tbsp	3 Tbsp	¼ cup
Fruits		3 Tbsp	3 Tbsp	¼ cup
Breads and cereals	4 or more			
Whole-grain bread		½ slice	1 slice	1½ slices
Ready-to-eat cereals		½ oz	¾ oz	1 oz
Cooked cereals		¼ cup	⅓ cup	½ cup
Spaghetti, macaroni, noodles, rice		¼ cup	⅓ cup	½ cup
Crackers		1 to 2	1 to 2	2 to 3

Amounts of foods such as fats, oils, desserts, and sweets should be determined by individual caloric needs.

good for children. In fact, we recommend them, especially for smaller preschoolers, who cannot eat enough to satisfy their energy needs all at once. Small amounts of nutritious foods eaten frequently over the course of the day as a snack are healthful and normal.

However, poorly chosen snacks or completely uncontrolled snacking can diminish your child's appetite for meals. If this pattern emerges, snacks made from the same sort of foods that could be eaten for meals (for example, slices of cheese, a slice of bread, yogurt, or raw vegetables) will provide your child the same necessary nutrients. As long as your child is given the right foods and an opportunity to eat them, the issue of a meal versus a snack really is not the important one.

Remember that a balanced diet may also include fats such as butter, margarine, mayonnaise, oils, and desserts. Fats should be consumed in moderation after the child's second birthday. Desserts should be restricted to one portion per day for the 1-year-old and to one and one-half portions for the older preschooler.

In recent years, Americans have become much more conscious of their diets. The excessive consumption of fat may contribute to later health problems—so excess fat should be trimmed from the preschooler's diet, too. However, the intake of fat or calories should not necessarily be limited: rather, *excessive* amounts of foods high in fat should be discouraged.

Testing your child's cholesterol concentration is probably unnecessary. Cholesterol, in fact, is important for growth; thus, such screening is necessary only if your family has a history of premature heart disease or high blood fat levels. If there is a family history and your physician finds an elevated value, take steps to reduce the cholesterol content of your child's diet. Consult your physician.

Nothing radical is needed. Just follow these guidelines when buying food and planning menus.

1. Buy 2 percent milk rather than whole milk for children older than 2.
2. Trim the fat off meats.
3. Serve more fish, poultry, and lean meats.
4. Offer low-fat cheeses, frozen yogurt, or light ice cream.
5. Serve cookies that are lower in fats, such as homemade oatmeal cookies, animal crackers, ginger snaps, vanilla wafers, or fig newtons; use skim milk to make pudding.
6. Limit the number of eggs to three or four a week.
7. Replace butter with margarine.

OBESITY

Some disorders can cause obesity, but if your child is overweight it is probably because he or she consumes more calories than are burned. However, obesity is more common during the first year of life, after age 5 or 6 years, and during adolescence than it is during the preschool years.

Not all children who are overweight are considered obese. Some children have larger-than-average body frames. These children tend to be stocky and look big, but they are not truly fat.

The obese child looks fat to the casual observer. The obese child is, in fact, more than 20 percent over what is considered his or her ideal weight.

Obesity is generally caused by a combination of factors. Heredity appears to play a role. If one or both parents are obese, their offspring is more likely to be fat than is the child of thin parents. In addition, overeating may be more common in households whose members are overweight than in those whose members maintain a normal weight. Lack of exercise also may be a factor. Finally, overweight persons tend to have more fat cells than their thinner peers, which may be a factor in converting food to fat rather than to energy.

If your preschooler is obese, now is the time to do something, while you still have some control over what your child eats. Once the child gets older and is more independent, dieting will be much more difficult.

Never put your child on a diet without consulting a physician or dietician. Any diet must take into account the child's nutritional needs. Fad diets are dangerous and should not be considered.

Of course, prevention is the best treatment. The time to be alert to obesity (especially if there is a family history) is during infancy.

Infant obesity has poor or little correlation with adult obesity, but family eating habits may persist into adolescence and adulthood (see also Obesity, page 1016).

CHAPTER 4

THE SCHOOL-AGE CHILD

AGES 6 THROUGH 12

CHAPTER CONTENTS

BEGINNING THE SCHOOL YEARS

Through the school-age years (ages 6 to 12), your child will gradually become a citizen of a larger world. In particular, peers and teachers become ever more influential as your child develops greater independence from the family. More relationships will be formed outside the home.

Age 6 marks the start of your child's formal education. Most 6-year-olds will already have attended kindergarten, and many will have gone to nursery school or day-care. These programs, however, tend to have less structured and more flexible settings. First grade is different.

Your child is required to adhere to the rules of an external authority and to devote almost all of his or her time to the work of learning. Suddenly your child has less time to play or to enjoy the informal learning that occurs throughout the preschool years. At school, your child is required to follow a rather fixed schedule. These new rules extend the limit-setting that you started in your child's preschool years.

As with younger children, those of school age are generally healthy, active, and enthusiastic. Not surprisingly, it is often hard for them to control their energy and exuberance enough to conform to rules of good behavior at home and at school. Trouble with hearing and seeing, learning disorders, attention deficits, and hyperactivity may become apparent. In the flexible atmosphere of the home—or even the day-care center—you may have been able to work around these problems, adapting the situation to your individual child. In the school setting, however, this is no longer possible. Such problems need to be identified and treated.

Witnessing your child's achievements and successful integration into this wider world can be a great source of pride. At the same time, your child's broad new horizons may provoke anxiety. As your child moves in directions that are new or unfamiliar or of which you do not approve, you may be frustrated by your waning control over him or her. Be assured that you still have a crucial role to play in guiding your child through these years of tremendous physical and psychosocial development.

The increasing independence of your school-age child may stand in welcome contrast to the continual demands of your preschooler. Although it may be easy to allow your increasingly independent child to occupy himself or herself, an open and trusting relationship must be nurtured if it is to be maintained during the turbulent adolescent years.

Seek your child's company. Discuss his or her interests; participate in activities, however mundane, together. The lines of communication you keep open during these critical formative years may prove invaluable in the future.

This chapter is designed to help you identify and play a significant role in your child's development as he or she moves through the school-age years to adolescence. It also outlines the normal growth and development of school-age children. Unlike the changes of puberty, the school-age child's physical, psychological, and social growth move forward in gradual and steady increments. Nonetheless, this is all previously uncharted territory. School, peers, and the advent of puberty all present fresh challenges.

NORMAL GROWTH AND DEVELOPMENT

Growth and development are slow and steady in the early school-age years, in sharp contrast with the rapid changes that occurred during the preschool years and those to follow during adolescence.

Your school-age child will gain about 7 pounds a year, and his or her height will increase by approximately 2.5 inches a year. The growth of your child's head also will slow down; head circumference increases from about 20 inches to 21 inches between the ages of 6 and 12. This is the time when your child's brain has almost reached its adult size.

Your child's motor skills also will be refined between the ages of 6 and 12. During this period, running, jumping, and throwing show steady improvement. To enhance this important process, encourage your child to be physically active.

You and your child may enjoy tracking his or her progress on a growth chart at home. Your child's physician also will keep a close watch on your child's height and weight. Growth charts can provide an opportunity to detect serious diseases. For instance, when children develop chronic illnesses their weight often stays the same or even decreases and their height does not increase at the expected rate.

During the period of rapid growth toward the end of the school-age years, children suddenly grow at dramatically different rates. If you think your child seems unusually short or tall, you can ask his or her physician about it. The physician may obtain an x-ray of a long bone. By reviewing this x-ray with a standardized set of tables, your pediatrician or family physician can determine whether the bone age correlates with your child's actual age.

School-age girls and boys have distinctly different growth patterns. There is a period during the late school-age years when girls are taller and heavier than boys because their growth spurt comes first (before the age of about 9½ years, average height is similar for both sexes). By the age of 13½ years, most boys have grown taller than girls. Girls tend to be lighter than boys until almost age 9 and after age 14, but they are heavier than boys between those two ages.

Toward the end of the school-age years, children begin to grow at a dramatic but highly variable rate. This pre-adolescent growth spurt is a part of puberty, which is a sequence of events that transforms a child into a young adult. Early puberty generally begins at about age 10 in girls and age 12 in boys. For a discussion of normal growth and development in the teenage years, see page 143.

Your physician may use charts like those shown below to assess your child's growth over a period of time.

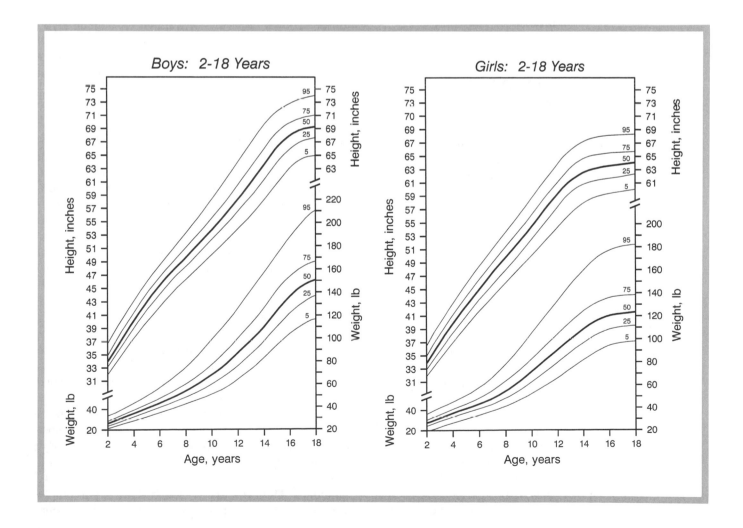

COMMON CONCERNS DURING SCHOOL-AGE YEARS

In this section we give guidelines for general care and nutrition. We also discuss the effects common diseases can have on your child. We emphasize features of these disorders that are unique to children of school age.

School-age children gradually become less prone to the common respiratory infections of the preschooler, including colds (see Common Viral Colds, page 860) and flu (see Influenza, page 853). Many school-age children commonly complain of recurrent stomachache or headache and growing pains. In the following pages we will review each of these concerns.

We cover many of the disorders that occur commonly in school-age children elsewhere in this book, specifically in Part IV, Human Disease and Disorders. Most disorders of school-age children do not have serious consequences. At this age children are extraordinarily resilient, and their young bodies easily recover from most common disorders.

GENERAL CARE

Immunizations. By age 6, your child should have completed the recommended schedule of childhood immunizations. Most states require that all children have a documented, completed series before entering kindergarten. Thus, your child will be immunized against diphtheria, tetanus, pertussis, measles, mumps, rubella, and polio before admission to kindergarten (see Immunizations, page 866).

Regular Checkups. In most schools, children are screened routinely for problems with hearing, vision, height, weight, and spine curvature (see Scoliosis, page 994). If the school health staff detects a disorder, they will tell you and urge you to consult a physician.

However, do not rely solely on the school to provide your child's health care. In addition, schedule occasional visits to your child's physician when your child is well. The physician will check your child's height, weight, posture, and blood pressure, among other things. Special problems may arise between these checkups. When they do, telephone the physician's office and describe the trouble. Together with the physician's staff, you can decide whether an office visit is warranted.

Infectious Diseases. At school, your child will come in contact with large numbers of other children. As in a day-care center, if one child in a school is carrying a contagious disease, it can spread easily to the other children. To help curb this spread, keep your child home from school whenever he or she has a communicable disease. Common examples include colds (see Common Viral Colds, page 860), flu (see Influenza, page 853), strep throat (see page 1295), and chickenpox (see page 864).

If you are not sure whether to keep your child home, check with his or her physician, nurse practitioner, or school nurse about whether the disease is communicable—and if so, for how long. It may be difficult if you must rearrange your schedule, get time off from work, or arrange for a sitter to stay with your sick child at home. However, a day at home may be best for the health of your child and his or her classmates.

Hygiene. Hand washing is the single most important way to prevent the spread of infectious diseases, including colds. As you started to do in the preschool years, continue reinforcing your child's good hand-washing habits. Insist that the child wash his or her hands after using the bathroom and before eating or preparing food, whether at home or in school. Your child should use soap and warm water to wash both hands thoroughly—including the palms and between the fingers.

Sleep Requirements. Another way to help maintain your child's health is to make sure he or she gets enough sleep. Your child needs more sleep than you do. At age 6, most children require almost 11 hours of sleep to feel their best. This amount declines gradually to just over 9 hours by the time they reach age 12.

Dental Care. One by one, your child's permanent teeth will make their debut during the school-age years. They come in, replacing the primary (baby) teeth, at a rate of about four a year. Because the permanent teeth will have to last a lifetime, it is imperative to care for them well. As you began to do in the preschool years, continue teaching your child to brush his or her teeth after each meal. It is also a good time to start demonstrating how to floss at bedtime (see Proper Flossing and Brushing Techniques, page 395). Schedule regular visits to your child's dentist at least twice a year.

As soon as the permanent back teeth have broken through, your child's dentist may cover them with a brush-on sealant. This will help protect them against tooth decay.

You can do your part to decrease the risks of tooth decay by limiting your child's consumption of sweets. If your water does not contain fluoride, your child's physician or dentist may prescribe fluoride as a supplement. If the teeth need straightening, orthodontic treatment is often started at this age (for a detailed discussion of dental care, see Tooth Care, page 393).

Accident and Injury. Normal behavioral and physical development increase the school-age child's susceptibility to accidental injury. You can minimize your child's risk by diligently taking precautions.

Car accidents are the most common cause of death in school-age children. The risk of these accidents is raised by the school-age child's natural inclination to experiment with adventurous behavior. It is extremely important to require that your child wear a seat belt for the entire duration of each automobile trip, regardless of how far you travel. Set a good example by wearing your seat belt, too.

Your school-age child needs plenty of exercise—he or she should spend more time after school in active play than in watching television. However, physical activity also increases the risk of injury and the need for supervision. Children age 6 to 9 have more control over their large-muscle groups than their small ones. This makes bicycle accidents more likely. You can help by stressing the traffic rules that apply to bicyclists (see Basic Bicycling Safety, page 124).

Peers play an increasingly important role in the life of a school-age child. More and more, your child will enjoy playing with a group and will develop steadfast loyalty to its members. In unsupervised situations he or she may follow the group's lead, no matter how dangerous. The influence of the child's peers tends to increase during the school-age years. Eventually, the peer group may demand that children of late school age (especially boys) perform daring, often hazardous, feats, simply to be accepted. This type of play can result in drowning, burns, and even shootings.

No parent can supervise every minute of his or her child's life. Yet it is possible—really essential—to instill in your child an idea of what is safe and unsafe. A certain amount of daredevil behavior is normal in the late school-age years. However, you may be able to minimize the danger to your child by promoting a positive self-image so he or she will not feel so much pressure to do what the group says.

Other basic precautions to be taken are ensuring that your child can swim, that guns in the house, if any, are kept under lock and key, and that your child follows the rules of pedestrian safety.

It is also important to find the safest possible facilities for your child to use for supervised recreation. Backyards, playgrounds, parks, and community centers are examples. Otherwise, they may choose to play in hazardous or poorly supervised places where the risk of injury is greater and the availability of help is less if an accident does occur. Organized activities such as youth baseball and soccer, under adult supervision, which emphasize the teaching of skills and the discipline of playing on a team rather than winning, are excellent activities for school-age boys and girls.

Healthful Lifestyles. School-age children can take increasing personal responsibility for their own health and can learn the foundations of a healthful lifestyle. This is the time to teach them about hygiene, nutrition, dental care, substance abuse, and accident prevention.

Accidents are a major cause of death and disability among school-age children. Sexual development and sexuality, for older children, may raise questions and concerns. Girls should be prepared for the onset of menses (menarche), and both sexes should be informed about normal sexual development.

Provide guidance for your child in development and socialization issues, such as discipline, school progress, and relationships

BASIC BICYCLING SAFETY

Bicycling is a wonderful way to build and maintain endurance while providing a means of transportation. But there are potential hazards. If your school-age child is a cyclist, share with him or her these tips.

Wear a Helmet

Three of every four bicyclists killed in crashes die of head injuries; most bicyclists' injuries involve the head. So wearing a helmet is a sensible precaution.

Ride With Traffic

Wrong-way riders are much more likely to be involved in accidents with motor vehicles. In addition, all 50 states require bicyclists to go with the traffic flow.

Stop at Stop Signs

Stop signs are there for bicyclists too, not just for cars.

Check for Traffic Before Turning

Always look back, signal, and check for traffic before turning.

Watch Out for Water

Remember that in wet conditions braking time is greatly increased. Watch out for wet leaves, too; they are slippery and hazardous.

Drive Defensively

Make eye contact with other riders, drivers, and pedestrians. Watch out for potholes, rubbish, sand, and other potential hazards. Know your own reaction time and other skills, and ride at speeds and with the care commensurate to your abilities.

---

with peers. Encourage your child's sense of personal responsibility for chores at home, for schoolwork, and for his or her own behavior.

GROWING PAINS

Many school-age children, particularly during the later years of this period, experience relatively severe, recurrent limb pain. These pains may come on at any time, but they seem to occur most frequently in the evening, particularly after a day of strenuous activity.

Usually these pains are located in the thighs or calves, and the pains leave after an hour or two. The children are otherwise healthy, and the results of physical examination, laboratory tests, and x-rays are always normal. Although these pains are probably not directly related to physical growth, the symptoms often are labeled "growing pains."

So-called growing pains have no known explanation and usually disappear over time without any lasting ill effects. Unless other associated symptoms develop, the best treatment for growing pains is sympathy and understanding and offering reassurance that the symptoms do not represent a health problem and will disappear with time.

RECURRENT HEADACHES

Although recurrent headaches are a common and usually not serious problem during late childhood and adolescence, the school-age child who complains of frequent headaches may have a serious underlying problem (see Headaches, page 545).

This is not to say that you have cause for alarm if your 7-year-old complains of headaches during a fever associated with the flu. Headache is a common symptom of fever and is associated with many viral illnesses.

However, if your child frequently complains of headache, even during times when he or she is otherwise well, consult your physician.

Migraine headaches may occur in children and, although rare, may be suspected if there is a family history of migraine. In children, this type of headache often is accompanied by vomiting, light sensitivity, and sleep. Recovery follows within a few hours (see Migraine Headaches, page 549).

RECURRENT ABDOMINAL ACHES

Stomachaches are common in children. Typically, the pains are nothing more than the result of eating something that does not agree with them or the beginning of a bout with a gastrointestinal virus.

Sometimes, however, a child complains of recurrent abdominal pains. These children may have intermittent or chronic diarrhea and abdominal pain, a condition known as irritable bowel syndrome if other disorders are not found to be the cause. The cause of irritable bowel syndrome is unknown. The two most prevalent theories are that the condition is related to stress or that there is a difficulty in the movement of food through the large intestine.

Irritable bowel syndrome is not a dangerous disease, but the pain that accompanies this syndrome can be very severe, at times even mimicking acute appendicitis. Constipation and the frequent passage of intestinal gas are also common.

Treatment with antispasmodics may benefit some children, as may the addition of fiber-rich foods to the diet. Psychiatric counseling may be helpful in exploring the emotional factors that often seem to precipitate the pain.

The prognosis varies. In some children the symptoms disappear, whereas others have recurrent bouts of pain throughout their lives (see also Irritable Bowel Syndrome, page 632).

Consult your child's physician if vomiting, fever, or loss of weight occurs or if your child refuses to participate in usual day-to-day activities because of such discomforts.

NUTRITION

By the time your child is of school age, his or her habits are well on the way to being established. The school-age years are a good time to continue the establishment of healthful eating habits that were initiated during the preschool years.

Offer a variety of nutritious foods. Emphasize foods that are low in fat and high in complex carbohydrates and fiber. For school-age children, we recommend consumption of between 1,650 and 3,000 calories daily for normal development. Equally important, promote regular physical activity to help maintain normal weight.

In general, the nutritional guidelines are the same for children and adults. Have your school-age child eat a variety of foods with nutritional value. Consult the chart below for an approximate guide to serving sizes and food varieties for your school-age child (see also Nutrition and Health, page 345).

At home, you can set basic eating patterns to guide what your child learns about nutrition. However, no matter how good and consistent your dietary example, your child will be receiving conflicting messages from the media, the lunch program at school (see School Lunch Programs, page 126), and the children with whom he or she plays and attends school. These outside influences become even stronger as your child matures. However, so too does your child's ability to make his or her own choices.

Help your child learn that breakfast is an important meal. It is worth getting the whole family up earlier to avoid having this meal cut short by school-bus schedules. After school, your child may need a snack to replace the energy used at school. However, you can control the amount and type of this snack. A good choice is a piece of fruit, a

How Much and What Kind of Food Does Your School-Age Child Need?

Food Group	Daily Servings	Size of Serving 6 to 10 Years	11 to Teen
Milk	4		
Milk (whole, skim, dry, evaporated, buttermilk, yogurt, or pudding)		¾ to 1 cup	1 cup
Meat	3 or more		
Eggs		1	1
Lean meat, fish, poultry		1½ to 2 oz	2 to 3 oz
Peanut butter		2 to 3 Tbsp	2 to 3 Tbsp
Legumes (dried peas and beans)		½ to ¾ cup	
Fruits and vegetables	4 or more		
Vegetables		⅓ cup	½ cup
Fruits		⅓ cup	½ cup
Breads and cereals	4 or more		
Whole-grain bread		1 to 2 slices	1 to 2 slices
Ready-to-eat cereals		1 oz	1 oz
Cooked cereals		½ cup	½ cup
Spaghetti, macaroni, noodles, rice		½ cup	½ cup
Crackers		3 to 4	3 to 4

Amounts of foods such as fats, oils, desserts, and sweets should be determined by individual caloric needs.
From: *Mayo Clinic Diet Manual,* sixth edition. By permission of Mayo Foundation.

whole-grain muffin, or some low-fat yogurt. This snack should tide your child over until dinner but should not replace that meal.

The most common nutritional problem in school-age children is iron-deficiency anemia (see page 478). However, your child will get enough iron, zinc, and other essential minerals if he or she eats low-fat dairy products, lean meats, whole grains, fish, beans, fruits, and vegetables.

If your child is involved in vigorous physical activity, he or she will need more calories. If heart disease or high cholesterol runs in your family, discuss this with your child's physician, who will determine whether the child's cholesterol concentration should be measured. If the value is high, your child's physician may recommend a diet that restricts fat, saturated fat, and cholesterol.

However, if your child's cholesterol value is normal, it is important not to overdo a low-fat diet. Your school-age child is still growing and needs a balanced diet to grow to his or her full potential. For this reason, it is unfair—and even dangerous—to impose any unusual diet on your child.

It is important for you not to use food inappropriately with your child. Do not use food as a means of controlling your child's behavior or as discipline, reward, or your primary form of affection.

As in the preschool years, feed your child in response to hunger or at mealtimes. When your child feels restless, encourage him or her to be active rather than giving more food. Remember, the best way to teach your child about good nutrition is by setting a good example in your own eating habits.

OBESITY

An increasing number of American children are overweight. Today, national surveys suggest that more than 50 percent of school-age children are overweight.

Being overweight can have various effects on a child. Social or emotional stresses may result from peers making fun of the child's excess weight. There are also potential health problems, including an increased risk of diabetes, high blood pressure, and cholesterol.

Contributing Factors. Overeating is not always the cause; often, however, eating too much of the wrong foods is. High-calorie snacks can be a significant factor in obesity.

Physical Inactivity. Weight control at any age is largely a matter of balancing the intake of calories with the amount of energy burned in everyday activities. If more calories are consumed than are burned, the pounds will add up. Especially in children, the cycle is more complicated than it may seem, however, because it is often difficult to determine whether low activity levels are the cause or the result of overeating.

Heredity. Studies of adopted children reveal that these children take on the weight

---

SCHOOL LUNCH PROGRAMS: DO THEY MAKE THE NUTRITIONAL GRADE?

The United States National School Lunch Program now serves many of the nation's children breakfast as well as lunch. The program supplies meals free or at a reduced rate to children. Menus and minimal portion sizes are revised periodically.

But are these programs adequate and appropriate? A 1987 study of school foods found excess fat and sodium (salt) in these meals. This finding is of concern because lifetime dietary habits of eating too much fat, sodium, and calories contribute to increased risks of heart disease, high blood pressure, and obesity.

In general, a school lunch—whether homemade or produced at the school—should offer at least five items: meat or other protein, fruit, vegetable, bread or some other form of starch, and milk. Each meal should provide about a third of a school-age child's recommended daily allowance (RDA) of various nutrients.

Recently, school lunch programs have made some improvements. Many schools have reduced the amount of fat, salt, and sugar and have increased fiber in the foods they serve. Some schools have expanded their offerings, providing children with more options.

Future changes will be limited by conflicting pressures on the school lunch program. One factor is economic: schools save money by getting about a fifth of their food from commodities provided by the federal government. When the agricultural surplus is heavy on processed cheese, ice cream, butter, and ground beef, these items will find their way into school lunches.

Ideally, the food offered in school should complement what your child is taught in school about good dietary practices. Health, social studies, and science programs can reinforce healthful eating habits.

characteristics of their biological parents and not of their adoptive parents. This occurred even though most of the children had been adopted before their first birthdays. Clearly, heredity is an important factor in obesity.

Controlling Your Child's Weight. Never put your child on a diet without consulting your child's physician or dietician. Any diet must take into account your child's nutritional needs. Fad diets are dangerous. Stay away from them.

Even an overweight child should not be put on a weight-loss diet during his or her growth phase. The goal is to slow the rate of weight gain and allow height (growth) to catch up. The result is the same as weight loss.

Overweight children have the same nutritional needs as other children. Do not restrict meeting these essential needs. Do not give your overweight child special meals; rather, give less total food.

Increase Activity Levels. Encourage physical activity. Plan family activities.

Never Criticize. Support your child: insensitive jokes, especially from one's parents and loved ones, can be devastating to children. Be patient: Do not attempt to solve the problem overnight. Achieving a more normal weight takes time.

MEMORANDUM: TO PARENTS AND SCHOOL OFFICIALS

Here are some steps for a healthier school lunch.

Reduce Fat

Use nonfat dry or low-fat milks. Serve ice milk, frozen low-fat yogurt, or sherbet rather than ice cream. Limit whipped toppings. Replace butter with margarine.

Use lower-fat (15 percent) ground beef and low-fat ham. Bake or broil rather than fry foods.

Increase Fiber

Use whole-wheat flour when baking. Add granola, bran, rolled oats, and cornmeal to quick breads.

Offer a salad bar regularly.

Reduce Sodium

Reduce salt in recipes; use fresh garlic or onion instead of garlic or onion powders. Remove salt shakers from the table. Serve soups lower in sodium.

Reduce Calories and Sugar

Use less sugar in recipes. Serve unsweetened fruit juice; serve fresh fruit whenever possible. Serve smaller portions of baked desserts.

PSYCHOSOCIAL DEVELOPMENT OF PERSONALITY AND BEHAVIOR

In contrast to your school-age child's relatively slow physical growth, his or her psychological and social development proceed at a rapid clip. Your child is busy mastering a host of psychosocial tasks. Impressive changes take place in his or her ability to reason, learn, act in a moral fashion, follow rules intelligently, and interact with adults and other children. Many of these changes may seem surprising or even shocking to you as a parent, so it is best to have some understanding of the normal course of events.

NORMAL PSYCHOSOCIAL DEVELOPMENT

Starting first grade can be scary, but most children proudly accept their new status.

The school places social and learning expectations on the child, and it can be quite a challenge to meet them.

At the advent of the school-age years, most children have just become able to think logically about concrete things that they experience directly in everyday life. Between ages 6 and 12, children's ways of thinking and remembering become much more sophisticated. They become better at classifying bits of knowledge, and their memories improve. Enhanced memory lets them keep several related ideas in mind while they solve more complex problems.

During the school-age years, most children also progress in their ability to take account of other people's perspectives. They learn to tailor their approach to the viewpoints of others and not to assume that everyone shares their knowledge and interests.

For the first time, they understand that mommy and daddy have other things in life that demand their time. This realization, in turn, hones their powers of persuasion. School-age children become more adept at drawing inferences from incomplete information. They also discover how to coordinate two different but related meanings—an important element in understanding jokes, metaphors, and certain grammatical rules.

Learning to read is the most important part of schoolwork, opening the door to the discovery of all other knowledge. Reading to your child may inspire him or her to want to read. Learning to read starts with reading aloud. Your child must discriminate the letters of the alphabet, then decode them into speech sounds and master how to pronounce common groupings of letters. Eventually, your child can skip these steps and read silently by processing sounds, words, and meanings simultaneously.

You can motivate your child by stimulating his or her desire to learn. Simply showing an interest in your child's performance in school or other activities and spending plenty of time actively involved with your child can help encourage him or her to try harder to learn or acquire skills.

Schoolchildren also tend to shift, gradually, from an impulsive learning style to a reflective one. The 6-year-old is more likely to blurt out a careless answer, whereas the 12-year-old will think about a question longer before answering.

Through the school-age years, children also learn about moral behavior—how to distinguish between what is right and wrong. Your child must learn how to balance his or her needs and wants with the requirements of the family, school, and society.

You can help your child develop a sense of duty, responsibility, and realistic accomplishment. Encourage your child to assume a helpful role in the family. It may help to assign reasonable household chores such as setting the table. As your child accomplishes the tasks you set, he or she will develop confidence in his or her abilities and a sense of responsibility regarding the task. This will also reinforce that he or she is an important part of the family.

Setting an example of moral behavior is also important. In addition, it is a good idea to limit and monitor your child's television watching and to keep to a minimum his or her exposure to violent and inappropriate sexual behavior.

If you consistently specify what behavior you are rewarding or punishing, and explain why you are doing so, your child will be more likely to develop internal control of moral actions (that is, a conscience). Less desirable are external controls, which influence behavior through fear of being caught or of displeasing parents.

Children who believe securely in their own worth tend to be more industrious, creative, and successful at school. They are also better at resisting pressure to conform to their peers, which is especially important when peers demand that they join in self-destructive behavior.

To help your child develop high self-esteem, it is necessary to show your child that you truly care for him or her. Your child generally wants to do well and will practice hard to do so. Your child will measure his or her performance by the response given by peers and "important" adults. Success at this stage is enabling your child to realize that he or she has strong points and some areas that need work—and that that is okay.

In contrast, low self-esteem often occurs in children whose parents are rejecting, overbearing, or distant. The child may feel inferior to others of the same age or may feel that he or she must be good at everything to be okay.

Set clearly defined limits for your child's behavior, and enforce those limits consistently. Parents who are too permissive may also convey that they do not care for their child. Your school-age son or daughter is becoming increasingly independent but still needs firm guidance and consistent boundaries within which to grow.

During the preschool years, children tend not to conform. Social rules may be confusing to them. The early school-age years mark a decided change in behavior. Children enjoy identifying with their peers and begin to be able to understand social situations. They often show a rigid conformity that makes them embrace each new social norm that they come to comprehend. You may have noticed that your child relishes some strict compulsion, such as never stepping on a crack in the sidewalk. This is one form of the child's temporary infatuation with arbitrary rules.

Toward the end of the school-age years,

most children become more flexible about social roles and norms. They gradually learn to reconcile conflicting value systems, such as the ones at home and those at school. They come to recognize that compromise is not necessarily a sign of weakness.

On the other hand, the later years of the school-age period are characterized by some degree of rigidity. Eleven- and 12-year-olds are often extremely concerned about acting and dressing like their peers and not being out of the mainstream.

At times, your child may have difficulty with learning at school, interrelationships with peers, or acquiring common exercise-related skills. Sometimes the difficulties arise from a child's unrecognized problems with vision or hearing. At other times unrecognized learning disabilities or attention-deficit disorders may be contributing to your child's inability to keep up with his or her peers. Emotional problems can also be both a cause and a consequence of learning difficulties.

Even if they are quite intelligent, children who are upset by family troubles can find it difficult to pay attention in school. Sometimes this takes the form of a school phobia, which may prevent your child from taking full advantage of his or her school environment. We discuss these disorders in the following section.

DIFFICULTIES WITH SIBLING AND PEER RELATIONSHIPS

Peers and siblings play important roles in the integration of your child into society. From their peers and siblings, school-age children learn a great deal about competition and cooperation as well as about conformity and independence.

The influence of other children can rival or even overtake that of adults. Part of the reason is that children play together as equals. It is easy for them to understand each other. Another child's perspective often provides an alternative to the prevailing wisdom that the child has been accustomed to hearing from his or her parents.

Conflicting behaviors may develop. Parents and siblings within the family may advocate different approaches than do teachers and peers at school. This conflict can pose problems for school-age children, who yearn to be liked and accepted by everyone they meet, including adults and other children. However, when sibling and peer norms conflict with those of adults, school-age children are often more inclined to follow their siblings and peers.

Elementary school is the first social world that most children have to deal with without direct help from the family. As school-age children become part of a peer group, new social traits become important to them, such as popularity and leadership. At this age, children are eager to be popular. They are concerned about being left out in the fringes of the group.

In addition to being peers, brothers and sisters may be rivals. A certain amount of rivalry between siblings is normal, and it even helps them learn how to interact with other people. There is not necessarily any reason for concern if your children compete, roughhouse, and bicker with each other. Despite the friction between them, most older siblings do contribute greatly to the education, socialization, and support of younger ones. Frequently, overt rivalry gives way to closeness by the end of the school-age years.

However, sometimes the discord between siblings is severe. If so, you may want to seek family counseling to identify how the trouble started and how it can be stopped. The underlying cause of sibling antagonism may be a family problem such as marital strain. Without realizing it, parents can cast a child in a role that enmeshes him or her in a conflict between the mother and father, and the other siblings react according to their sympathies.

The birth of a sibling can make a school-age child feel that his or her place in the family has been upset. Compared with the preschooler, the school-age child is usually better equipped to control his or her jealousy of a newborn sibling. Still, your school-age child may protest a decline in the amount of your attention that he or she receives by starting to act younger. It helps if you are sensitive to the school-age child's needs and reserve some time just for the two of you. School-age children often enjoy playing with and caring for "their" new baby. (See also Sibling Problems of the Preschool Years, page 110.)

If concerns about your school-age child persist, see your child's physician.

SEXUALITY IN YOUR SCHOOL-AGE CHILD

Through the school-age years, your child will continue to define his or her sexuality. This process is a vital part of your child's larger task of discovering and deciding whom he or she is. Your child may also make his or her first attempts to explore sexual activity before this period is over. As a result, this is a good age for sex education, if you have not already started it.

Most school-age children are already well on their way to reflecting the divergent sex roles that our society considers appropriate to men and women.

Perhaps you would prefer your child to feel free to express all aspects of his or her personality, including masculine and feminine ones. However, you may notice how often your efforts are thwarted by the startling array of overt and subtle sex-stereotyping pressures from other relatives, peers, teachers, television, and society at large.

Regardless of your own attitudes, your school-age child may choose not to embrace the role assigned to his or her sex. The girl may be called a tomboy and the boy, a sissy. Society and the family may tend to put more pressure on boys than on girls to conform strictly to a narrow sex role. Tomboys are often tolerated, whereas sissies are frequently rejected.

SEXUAL ABUSE

Sexual abuse of children involves an adult, usually a man, forcing or persuading a child, frequently a girl, to participate in a sexual act. The problem is not new—yet our comprehension of how widespread a problem it is surely is new: as many as 1 in 5 girls and 1 in 10 boys will be victims of sexual abuse before reaching the age of 18.

Recognizing the Signs
Be alert for the following possible signs of sexual abuse in a child:

Provocative or promiscuous sexual behavior;

Withdrawal from friends, family, or school activities;

Unusually hostile or aggressive behavior.

There may be no physical signs of abuse, but your physician may identify evidence of trauma to the genital area or the presence of sexually transmitted infections (see page 139). However, the absence of all of these signs is not necessarily proof that no abuse has occurred.

Why a Child Is Susceptible
Young people need affection. Depriving a child of healthy physical contact (such as hugging), in fact, is to risk significant problems in a youngster's psychological development. There is even a natural sexual aspect that is present from birth. Breast-feeding, for example, prompts physiological changes of sexual arousal in infants.

Children often seek some sexual contact with their peers, but such experimentation is not sought with adults. If your child describes an experience in which he or she was touched by an adult in an inappropriate way, take it seriously.

What To Do
If you suspect that your child has been sexually abused, contact your physician or an official in your local child-protection system (child welfare worker, local public attorney, police or sheriff).

If the sexual abuse involved rape, handle it as a specific type of aggression against the child. This will help to minimize the sexual significance of the trauma and to prevent lasting psychological reverberations. It is best for you and the child's physician not to dwell on the sexual nature of the assault. If you do, your child may become insecure and anxious, without clearly understanding what is going on.

Make sure that your child is safe from further harm. Report the attack to the police. As soon as possible, take your child to an emergency room at a hospital, preferably one that offers emergency and follow-up psychological support. The child will be checked and treated for any internal and external injuries. Later on, the child may be tested for sexually transmitted diseases (see Sexual Assault and Sexual Abuse, page 290).

Have your child talk with a sensitive professional who is experienced at counseling victims of child abuse. This counseling is particularly important if it was a family member or friend, not a stranger, who perpetrated the attack.

Do not keep the abuse a private or family matter. Most perpetrators are involved with several children. Seldom is the abuser a complete stranger to the child. The welfare or even the life of your child may be at stake.

If you are concerned that your school-age son is showing too much interest in playing with dolls or dressing up in girls' clothes, it is best to discourage him gently and not to show your anxiety. This type of behavior does not lead to homosexuality. Be reassured that a great many boys are taunted by their peers at some time or other for their lack of masculinity. It is also important to recognize that sexuality and sex roles are not static. They continue to evolve throughout childhood, adolescence, and even adulthood.

Most school-age children devote most of their attention to peers of the same sex. Many even develop "crushes" on their same-sex peers. However, it is also normal for them to explore the opposite sex tentatively. Curiosity and lack of understanding of social taboos are usually the reasons for their "playing doctor."

During the school-age years, most school-age children continue to play occasionally with their own sex organs, as they did in infancy and the preschool years. Masturbation generally should not be a cause for concern.

The onset of puberty provides a good opportunity to educate your child about sexual development, whether or not you have already done so. You can help prepare your child for the cascade of changes that his or her body will go through during the next few years. The goal is for the child to welcome these changes without shame or anxiety that they are occurring too quickly or too slowly.

Unfortunately, events often conspire against this goal. In the late school-age years, children's minds are most eager to conform. Yet this obsession with "normality" coincides with the time when their bodies are diverging most in their development. Even children who are right in the middle of the spectrum of physical maturity often feel they are developing too fast or too slow. You can help by reassuring your child that he or she fits well within the wide range of normal developmental timetables.

Do not worry if your child's puberty starts a little earlier or later than that of his or her peers. This is not a serious medical problem. However, your child may feel awkward and self-conscious about diverging from the average schedule. Be sensitive to these feelings. At the same time, reassure your child that he or she is fine. It may help to stress that every child, including your child and each of his or her peers, is traveling along the same road toward adulthood and that everyone takes a different amount of time to arrive (see also Sexual Precocity, page 139).

DEALING WITH PHYSICAL ILLNESS AND HOSPITALIZATION

The school-age years are a good time to instill attitudes of wellness and to promote a positive body image in your child. Of course, whenever your child becomes ill, you will want to make him or her as comfortable as possible. However, avoid rewarding your child for being sick, lest he or she gets to like being sick.

An acute illness can have psychological effects on both you and your child. If your child is in the early school-age years, he or she may respond to a mild acute illness with restlessness and hyperactivity. This behavior may frustrate you if you are trying to encourage your child to rest. It is usually best not to insist too strenuously on bed rest because for many disorders rest is not necessarily helpful.

If your child develops a severe acute illness, do not be surprised if he or she becomes listless and irritable. Disturbances in your child's sleeping and eating habits can appear and, if not deftly handled, they may persist long after recovery. Together with your child's physician, do your best to comfort and inform your child.

A chronic illness is even more likely than an acute one to alter your child's psychosocial development. His or her mood can easily be depressed by the social isolation of extended absences from school and spending much of the day indoors. This is particularly true in the event of a permanent disability. Your child can feel helpless and may start regressing to younger behavior. This can slow and change the evolution of your child's personality and role in the family and school.

Chronic childhood illnesses, if not handled adeptly, can sometimes foster the development of problems with school. For instance, if the family treats a sick child like a fragile flower, he or she is more likely to cling to the home and even suffer from school phobia (see page 137).

Some chronically ill school-age children become extremely dependent, anxious, passive, and withdrawn. Others tend to deny their illness and act too independently too soon. The best adjustment occurs between these two extremes in children who are able to accept their limitations realistically while finding other ways to achieve competence and self-confidence.

You can help your child find this middle road. However, this task may be too much to shoulder on your own. Accept support from your relatives and friends. Psychological counseling from health-care professionals may, at times, be helpful.

Your school-age child, unlike a preschooler, has the ability to understand disease. With this comprehension comes the opportunity to lessen the psychological burden of the disorder. You can help your child a great deal simply by answering questions in ways he or she can grasp. Your child may fear that the illness is a punishment for bad behavior, even if he or she does not state this fear. You can help by verbalizing such fears and reassuring your child that they are baseless.

Together with your child's physician, encourage your chronically ill school-age child to have an active role in gaining control over the disease. For instance, children with asthma can learn to recognize their symptoms (see Asthma, page 466). This allows treatment early in an asthma episode, before it becomes serious. Such an approach to a chronic illness can help set the stage for good control of the disease later on in adolescence, when refusal to cooperate with treatment is more often a problem.

If your child has a chronic disease, it is natural for you to be tempted to overprotect your child, to indulge him or her, and to stop setting limits. You may also find it hard to resist seeking out unproven "cures," which can raise false hopes and then dash them. Resist these temptations and encourage your child to live the most full, normal, active life possible.

Do not unnecessarily shelter your child from any activity, including school attendance and physical exercise. Talk with your child's teacher and school nurse to ensure that the child is included in all of the activities in which he or she wants and is able to participate.

In most cases, there is no justification for banishing your child to study hall while his or her peers enjoy themselves in the gym or on the playing field. It is not only the exercise that is missed. Your child also needs the social activity involved. If the group activities are too strenuous for your child, the gym teacher should be flexible enough to propose an individualized program for him or her. Even if your child does special exercises while the rest of the class pursues another activity, at least he or she will not feel so excluded.

Your child may have to spend some time in the hospital. You can help it seem like a less scary place. Beforehand, prepare your child for this new experience by discussing it thoroughly. Many children's hospitals offer pre-admission programs, orientation programs, and tours. Once your child is in the hospital, you can make the stay less threatening by bringing in a favorite toy, book, or picture. It is particularly important to stay with your child as much as you can.

If the treatment involves surgery, try to allay your child's fears about being marred. It is good for your child to get a chance to ask the surgeon and anesthesiologist questions in advance (see The Hospital Stay, page 1215).

As with adults, confronting and fighting an illness are more likely to be successful if the person with the ailment is a partner in his or her care. Even young children instinctively know when secrets are being kept from them. You do not need to discuss every medical detail. Still, your child is more likely to develop normally and to work harder toward recovery if he or she has some degree of control over decisions made about his or her care.

LEARNING DISORDERS

Your child's ability to learn depends on the mental processes that make learning possible and on his or her emotional comfort and overall health.

The following pages consider factors within the child that interfere with learning, but many other factors must be considered also. Illness interferes with learning when it leaves a child tired and listless; emotions interfere when a child is depressed or worried about himself or herself or about problems at home. Such worries or daydreaming in school distracts the child from schoolwork. Finally, a motivation to learn is necessary in order for the child to use his or her capacities.

Vision, hearing, and general health are evaluated by your child's physician. Intelligence is evaluated by psychological testing within or outside the school. When your physician suspects an emotional problem, he or she may refer your child to a child psychiatrist or psychologist.

Cognitive learning disorders are more difficult to diagnose than vision or hearing disorders and require specialists such as child psychiatrists and educational psychologists. These disorders of mental processing include problems with remembering, grasping patterns, focusing attention, writing, speaking, and interpreting written words. Sometimes they are caused by birth injuries. More commonly, however, they occur in children with normal health and intelligence.

If your child has a learning disorder, he or she may need help in learning how to learn. The following sections discuss the various cognitive problems and the kinds of special education needed to overcome them.

LEARNING DISABILITIES

Signs and Symptoms
- Significant problems in speaking, writing, spelling, or arithmetic;
- Inability to listen, read, or organize thoughts;
- Chronic impulsiveness, restlessness, or distractibility;
- Poor memory.

Children can have normal or high intelligence and still be unable to learn. Specific learning disabilities are not disorders of seeing, hearing, emotions, or mental capacity. They are mental process disorders in acquiring or expressing knowledge (cognition).

Your child may be unable to grasp overall patterns, remember what was said, write legibly, copy a drawing, relate printed text to spoken words, interpret written words (see Specific Reading Disability [Dyslexia], page 134), or speak coherently (see Speech Disorder, page 135). These mental process disorders relate to your child's use or comprehension of language and symbols. There are other reasons for some of these signs, such as impulsiveness and restlessness; therefore, the signs do not necessarily indicate the presence of a learning disability.

Another type of learning disability occurs when your child cannot pay attention for more than a minute or two (see Attention Deficit Disorder, page 136) or cannot exercise self-control over certain physical activities (see Hyperactivity, page 136). These conditions may be due to disorders in the normal process of ignoring distractions and focusing attention in a deliberate way.

Various causes have been cited for learning disabilities. In some cases, they may be genetic. Boys are affected 4 to 5 times more frequently than girls, and these disabilities can run in families. In other cases, there is evidence of a disorder in the way the brain functions, although no evidence of brain damage can be found.

Frequently, however, no specific cause for a child's learning disorder is found. Some experts in the field believe it may be due to developmental delays or immaturity.

Learning disorders are thought to occur in 5 to 20 percent of school-age children in the United States. This range is wide because many definitions are used and because no large-scale study has been done to determine the extent of the problem.

The Diagnosis. You may not become aware of your child's learning disorder until school failures start in the third or fourth grade. A complete diagnosis is essential for determining the specific disorder and ways to improve your child's education as soon as possible.

The basic diagnosis will require several types of examinations to evaluate your child's mental capacity, educational performance, eyesight, hearing, emotional status, and general neurological functions. Further testing may be necessary to identify particular disorders in reading, writing, listening, speaking, or understanding mathematics.

Various tests for the processes involved in learning have been developed in recent years, and it is now possible to obtain a very detailed diagnosis. Your child may need to visit a child psychiatrist, child neurologist, psychologist, or educational evaluation clinic for this testing.

How Serious Are Learning Disabilities?
Your child's learning disability can lead to chronic academic failure and to major social and emotional problems. Although children sometimes outgrow their disability, this may occur too late to prevent a severe limitation in future achievements and self-esteem.

The damage often is minimized by early diagnosis and treatment. Many children can overcome their disability and perform much closer to their potential with special education and tutoring. Your child can achieve most academic and occupational goals if the appropriate teaching method and motivation are found.

Treatment. The primary treatment may be a special education program tailored to your child's needs. Many methods are available, including techniques to help your child develop sound-symbol relationships, number concepts, eye-hand coordination, phonetic articulation, sense of time, and pattern recognition. The special education team in your school system or a private clinic may work with you and your child in using diagnostic results to select appropriate methods.

The educational objective is to help your child acquire the missing abilities and to apply them; in other words, your child must learn how to learn. Attendance in a separate class or school may be needed for awhile or your child may go to special education facilities during part of the school day. Additional tutoring and practice at home often are needed.

Counseling by a mental health professional may be necessary to help your child cope more effectively with his or her disability and to improve self-esteem. Your physician may prescribe medication if distractibility, poor attention, and hyperactivity interfere with your child's learning.

SPECIFIC READING DISABILITY (DYSLEXIA)

Signs and Symptoms
- Inability to recognize letters and words on the printed page;
- Reading ability much below the expected level for the age of the child.

Specific reading disability is often referred to as dyslexia. It is the most common learning disability, and it occurs in children with normal vision and normal intelligence. The child is unable to interpret written language, and reading is therefore difficult. Children with dyslexia usually have normal speech but often have difficulty with spoken language and with writing. The disorder is an impairment of the brain's ability to translate images received from the eyes into meaningful language.

The reading problem is characterized by a delay in the age at which a child begins to read. Most children are ready to learn this skill by age 6 years, but children with reading disability cannot grasp the basics of reading in first or even second grade. Reversal of letters ("b" for "d") and a reversal of words ("saw" for "was") are common among children with this problem. In normal children younger than 6 years of age, such reversals should not be of concern. With reading disability, however, the reversals persist.

The condition may also manifest itself by your child's trying to read from right to left, failure to see (and occasionally to hear) similarities or differences in letters or words, and inability to sound out the pronunciation of an unfamiliar word.

If you have a child with reading disability, you may find that his or her inability to read does not affect achievement in other school subjects, such as arithmetic. However, because reading is a skill basic to most other school subjects, a child with reading disability is at a great disadvantage in most classes.

Although the basis of reading disability is unknown, there is evidence that it is caused by a malfunction of certain areas of the brain concerned with language. A family history of language disorders also is frequently found. Reading disability affects boys more often than girls. Approximately 10 to 15 percent of school-age children have the disorder.

The Diagnosis. Reading achievement significantly below that expected for age is the key symptom of dyslexia. An evaluation of medical, cognitive, sensory processing, educational, and psychological factors will be required to plan treatment and follow your child's progress. Thorough vision, hearing, and neurological examinations are needed to verify that your child's poor reading ability is not due to another disorder.

A battery of educational tests, such as the Wechsler Intelligence Scale for Children (WISC), and academic achievement tests will be performed to help diagnose the problem. More importantly, an expert will analyze the process and quality of your child's reading skills.

How Serious Is Specific Reading Disability? Inability to read affects most aspects of school learning. If untreated, the disorder may lead to low self-esteem, behavioral problems, delinquency, aggression, and withdrawal or alienation from friends, parents, and teachers.

Reading disability varies in severity. Some children have a relatively mild form of the disorder, whereas some have a severe form.

Treatment. Treatment is by remedial education because there is no known way to correct the underlying brain malfunction that causes reading disability. Psychological testing will help your child's educators to design a suitable remedial teaching program. Techniques emphasizing many of the senses including hearing, vision, and touch are used to improve reading. Most important is frequent instruction by a reading specialist who uses both sight and phonic methods of teaching. It is important to provide emotional support and opportunities for achievement in areas other than reading.

If the reading disability is severe, effective tutoring for remedial reading usually requires several individual or small-group sessions each week. Progress is likely to be slow and laborious. Children with milder forms eventually learn to read well enough to get through school and to be able to read newspapers. Those with severe forms will never be able to read well and may need training for vocations that do not require good reading skills.

SPEECH DISORDER

Signs and Symptoms
- Failure to use speech sounds correctly;
- Speech that is hard to understand or scrambled;
- Slow speech development;
- Stuttering.

The critical period for your child's speech and language development is between ages 6 and 24 months, but occasional mispronunciations are normal up to age 7 years as long as your child's conversational speech is understood readily.

Some speech problems, such as a speech impediment (difficulty in articulation), stuttered speech, and voice problems, have no physical cause. Using one letter for another or leaving off the beginnings and endings of words are typical articulation problems. Stuttering is difficulty in getting the words out in a smooth flow. Voice problems include too soft a voice, a nasal voice, or a loud, booming voice.

Other speech disorders may have a recognizable cause such as cerebral palsy (see page 524), cleft palate or lip (see page 53), hearing loss or deafness (see page 67), mental retardation (see page 1017), brain damage, or autism (see page 1017).

Your child may be normal physically, emotionally, and intellectually but may have a speech disorder due to mental processing problems with spoken language. These speech problems are associated with learning disabilities (see page 133).

Your child may have difficulty receiving information and making sense of it. Sentences may come out scrambled or with one word substituted for another. The correct ordering of sounds may be impaired. Your child might be unable to tell the difference between two sounds or might have problems focusing on one specific sound or conversation while ignoring background noise.

Speech disorder is common. It occurs in about 10 percent of children younger than 8 years of age and in 5 percent of those 8 years and older.

The Diagnosis. Talk to your child's teacher or to your physician if you suspect that your child has a speech disorder. You probably need to seek help from a speech and language clinic. Most school systems offer these services. A speech pathologist will test your child's speech. A game with earphones may be used to check for hearing loss or deafness, and a complete physical and neurological examination may be needed.

How Serious Is Speech Disorder? Many children acquire vastly improved speech with proper professional therapy and help from you at home, but the disorder is likely to cause your child frustration. The social penalty can be costly if your child is taunted or rejected by other children at school. Early diagnosis and treatment are desirable before deep frustration and low self-esteem become part of the pattern.

Treatment. Children with speech disorders require speech therapy. This usually entails at least two sessions a week with a speech professional. Your child's speech therapist can explain what you should do at home.

ATTENTION DEFICIT DISORDER

Signs and Symptoms
- Habitual failure to pay attention;
- Excessive distractibility;
- Inability to organize;
- Impulsiveness;
- Restlessness and hyperactivity.

Your child's ability to learn depends on paying attention and remembering previous lessons. Many sights, sounds, memories, and other stimulating things compete for your child's attention. Sometimes they can cause any child trouble in paying attention.

Most school-age children, however, have developed the ability to focus their attention and to ignore distractions.

Attention deficit disorder is the habitual inability to pay attention for more than a minute or two despite repeated requests or even punishment. As a result of attention deficit disorder, your child may have problems with learning, following directions, and remembering information.

This disorder can have different causes. It has been attributed to heredity and to brain injuries during pregnancy, at birth, or after birth. Attention deficit disorder may not noticeably affect your child's intelligence or early development. It may become apparent only later as your child has increasing difficulty with learning after the second or third grade, when sitting still in class and paying attention become more important.

The Diagnosis. Your physician will need to observe your child's behavior and get a detailed history of early development. Early symptoms may appear during infancy, including problems with feeding, sleeping, and restlessness. Physical and neurological examinations are used to identify any sensory or neurological disorders. Your physician also may refer you to specialists for EEG (see page 1294), psychological, and educational testing.

How Serious Is Attention Deficit Disorder? Attention deficit disorder is a chronic problem that can continue through childhood and adolescence and into adulthood. It can damage your child's self-esteem and confidence, generate rejection and ridicule by other children, and cause academic failure. Treatment can help the child with learning, behavior control, and self-esteem.

Treatment. Your child may need a special education program (see Learning Disabilities, page 133). Children with attention deficit disorder often have behavior problems that require specialized counseling for the child and parents. This often is provided by child psychiatrists and psychologists.

Behavior modification techniques and restructuring home and school routines, avoiding overstimulation, and providing consistency may be effective for decreasing

---

HYPERACTIVITY

Hyperactivity, or extreme overactivity, is not a diagnosis and not a separate disorder. Rather it is a behavior that often accompanies the other symptoms of attention deficit disorder.

Children normally vary in their level of physical activity. Some youngsters are naturally much more active than others, and boys tend to be more active than girls. In general, young children usually are very active. These variations in activity are not abnormal.

However, a small percentage of children, more often boys than girls, are excessively active. Some seem to be in constant motion; others are erratically active. These children are not necessarily less coordinated or less intelligent than other children. The difference lies in how organized or purposeful the activity is and whether it can be stopped on request.

Hyperactive children tend to act without consideration for results, punishment, or other people's reactions. They cannot direct their activity, nor can you or their teachers. (For specific advice on treatment, see Attention Deficit Disorder, above.)

unacceptable behavior and rewarding good behavior.

Your physician may prescribe medications to help focus your child's attention and to reduce overactivity. The most common medications for this purpose are dextroamphetamine (Dexedrine), methylphenidate (Ritalin), and pemoline (Cylert). When taken by adults, most of these medications have a stimulating effect; they have the opposite effect on hyperactive children, and they improve attention. When the medication is carefully prescribed and when the child's progress is followed closely by your physician, it may be taken safely for as long as it is needed, even for years.

SCHOOL PHOBIAS

Signs and Symptoms

- Refusal to go to school;
- Stomach pain and sometimes fever beginning the day before or the morning school begins;
- Illness continues or worsens rather than disappearing after a day or two;
- No physical cause for the pain can be found.

School phobia or school refusal is distinguished by a cycle of physical symptoms and anxiety that gets worse instead of better. It is not the occasional stomachache or headache that disappears as soon as the school bus pulls away. In school phobia, no physical cause is found to explain the child's complaint.

School phobia actually is not a fear of school but a fear of separation from parents. Your child may be unwilling to sleep over at a friend's house. An older child is more likely to be afraid of something specific at school—a bully or a new class or getting picked on in the bathroom. These fears, unlike school phobia, are rational.

School phobia is a way of responding to overwhelming stress by substituting an acceptable and predictable pain for a situation the child is unable to control. Sometimes the disorder is triggered by the death or illness of a parent, a divorce, or entering junior high or middle school (where students have a variety of teachers, choices, and classmates). The disorder seems to run in families and is most common in the early school grades. It affects boys and girls equally.

Treatment. Sympathy or nurturing the child for missing school is only likely to reinforce the physical symptoms. However, if the parent becomes angry, the child's anxiety is likely to increase, raising the stress level and worsening the physical symptoms.

In children in kindergarten and first grade, the problem can usually be resolved easily by firmly expecting school attendance and providing emotional support for the child. Close cooperation between the parents and school personnel is essential. If the problem persists in an older child, evaluation and treatment by a mental health professional often are necessary.

SEXUAL DEVELOPMENT AND GYNECOLOGICAL DISORDERS

The onset of puberty occurs in both boys and girls in the later stages of the school-age years. The age at onset may be over a wide range of years. In general, puberty is thought to be premature if it occurs before age 8 in girls and before age 8 to 9 in boys.

In girls, the first sign of puberty is generally the development of the breast bud (thelarche). The onset of menses (menarche) then follows within several years.

In boys, enlargement or growth of the testes and penis is generally the first sign of puberty, to be followed by the appearance of pubic hair.

Several potential disorders concerning sexual development may occur during the school-age years, especially in girls. Premature puberty is far more common in girls than boys. We discuss this condition, along with other gynecological problems in school-age girls, in the following section.

BREAST ABNORMALITIES

The start of breast development in girls is known as thelarche. Thelarche signals the onset of puberty. Breast development may be the only indication of puberty for 6 months or so; it is not unusual for one breast to develop first and remain larger for months.

When the breasts commence budding in girls younger than 8 years, this sign of early sexual maturation is called premature thelarche. Most often, premature thelarche occurs between the ages of 1 and 3 years. If it is not followed by the other signs of sexual maturity (such as hair growth in the genital area), the girl's puberty is considered to be premature and incomplete.

The budded breasts often flatten within a year, but they may persist until the normal onset of puberty. The condition is harmless and seldom affects the girl's growth. Supportive counseling is usually all that is necessary to help her cope with her temporary difference from other girls.

Consult your physician for a full evaluation to differentiate premature thelarche from premature puberty (see Premature Puberty, below).

VAGINAL BLEEDING

Some school-age girls may have bleeding from the vagina before the expected age of menstruation. Consult your daughter's physician if this occurs.

The physician will first ascertain the source of the bleeding. Often the cause is not the commencement of menstruation but another cause such as vulvovaginitis (an inflammation of the genital and vaginal areas), genital tumor, trauma, or a foreign body lodged in the vagina.

In some cases, however, the cause is premature menstruation due to precocious puberty (see Premature Puberty, below).

ADRENARCHE

Adrenarche refers to activity in the adrenal glands. Premature adrenarche occurs most often in girls between ages 5 and 8 years. It is often accompanied by rapid short-term growth. The armpits may sweat and have hair. Pubic hair can develop (pubarche).

The physician may perform tests to determine whether the girl has a tumor or other abnormality of the adrenal glands, which can cause premature adrenarche in rare cases.

PREMATURE PUBERTY

Premature (precocious) puberty is rare. It is much more common in girls than in boys. In girls it can start at any time before 8 years of age. The events of puberty may proceed as usual but start earlier than normal. In normal puberty (and usually in premature puberty), the breast buds appear first, then pubic hair appears, and later menstruation begins, often with irregular cycles. Ovulation is uncommon but can occur.

Usually no underlying cause can be determined. However, the condition is known to involve early maturation of the ovaries, pituitary, or hypothalamus, which are hormone-producing glands.

Rarely, premature puberty results from a tumor of the brain or ovaries, so the child's physician may initiate studies to rule out these possibilities. The physician may also ask whether the girl has used any face creams or medications containing estrogens, which can also induce the disorder.

A potential long-term consequence of premature puberty is shorter height. It is usu-

---

GYNECOLOGICAL EVALUATION OF THE SCHOOL-AGE GIRL

Examination of a school-age girl's external genitalia should be a standard part of a routine physical examination. Your physician will be looking to identify physiological and anatomical abnormalities.

Normally, visual examination and palpation of the vaginal area are required. The physician may ask you to accompany your child during the examination to reassure her that the examination is appropriate. The examination is much less likely to scare, embarrass, or cause any pain if your daughter is relaxed and cooperative.

Rarely is any instrumentation required, but if abnormalities are observed, the physician will probably discuss the details of any possible additional tests with both you and your child.

The breasts will also be examined, especially when symptoms of a disorder of puberty are reported. The nipples and breast tissue will be examined visually and palpated to identify changes or abnormal masses.

ally associated with rapid short-term growth that stops earlier than normal.

Treatment may include psychological counseling for the girl and the family to deal with an appearance different from that of her peers. This problem should not be minimized. However, it is reassuring that by about age 10 most of the girl's peers will have caught up with her in sexual maturity, and she should not feel different anymore.

If your daughter undergoes puberty prematurely, it is important not to respond to her according to her physical appearance or to deny her hugs. Keep treating her like the little girl she is. Advise her teachers to do the same.

It is also imperative to guard the girl against sexual abuse and especially to prevent pregnancy. When puberty occurs very early, medication may be considered, but it has drawbacks. A progesterone-like drug can stop menstruation and reverse breast development. However, it does not prevent growth spurts or increase the height eventually attained, and it can cause undesirable side effects.

In boys, the onset, before age 9, of enlargement of the testes and penis, appearance of pubic hair, deepening of the voice, and accelerated growth may be signs of premature puberty. If your child develops these signs of advanced sexual development at an early age, see your physician. Studies may be done to rule out a tumor of the brain and nervous system, adrenal gland, or gonads. Approximately half of the time an identifiable cause is found.

Newer and better treatments such as luteinizing hormone (LH) analog therapy are being made available for premature puberty. If you are concerned about premature puberty in your child, consult his or her physician for a full evaluation.

GENITAL INFECTIONS IN YOUNG GIRLS

Genital infections (vulvovaginitis) can occur in girls not only after puberty but also before. The usual cause is inadequate bathing and toilet habits. A young girl may not wash her genitalia adequately. Or she may wipe herself from back to front after bowel movements, inadvertently picking up microbes

---

SEXUAL PRECOCITY

Like puberty, sexual behavior has been starting earlier in many school-age children in recent years. Because of the danger of pregnancy, it is particularly important to bolster your daughter's self-esteem and give her the strength to resist any pressure from her peers or older people to engage in sexual behavior before she is ready for it.

Premature puberty (see page 138) and sexual precocity are different problems. Precocious sexual knowledge and behavior, and preoccupation with sexual matters, can sometimes be signs that the child has been a victim of sexual abuse (see Sexual Abuse, page 114).

---

that normally live harmlessly in the intestines and spreading them to the genitalia.

Agents that can cause vaginal infections include yeast, parasites, bacteria, and irritants found in soaps and other toiletries. Yeast infections occur more commonly among girls who have diabetes or who have been taking antibiotics. Another possible cause is the insertion of foreign bodies into the vagina.

When sexual abuse has occurred, a sexually transmitted disease may also be the cause. Excessive masturbation or manipulation can also irritate the genital area.

Your daughter's physician will ask whether she has had any vaginal discharge, itching of the anus or vagina, other infections, or bedwetting. The physician will examine the area (see Gynecological Evaluation of the School-Age Girl, page 138) and may take a sample of vaginal discharge to examine for microbes. Pinworm, which commonly infects the rectums of school-age children, can also contaminate the vagina. Gonorrhea and other sexually transmitted diseases can cause vaginal infections in young girls. If the girl has one of these diseases, she may have caught it through sexual abuse (see page 114).

Many of these infections can be prevented—and treated—by teaching your daughter about her genital area and showing her how to wipe from front to back. When she bathes, encourage her to wash her genital area well and use no bubble bath preparations. Her toilet paper and underpants should be white, not colored, because dyes can irritate the skin. Her underpants should also be all cotton and changed once a day.

Discourage wearing clothing that increases moisture in the area—including such attire as tight-fitting jeans, nylon panties, and panties while sleeping.

Specific treatment for certain problems may involve taking oral antibiotics or applying an antibacterial or antifungal cream to the vagina or the genital area.

CHAPTER 5

THE TEENAGE YEARS

AGES 13 THROUGH 19

CHAPTER CONTENTS

ON BEING A TEENAGER

In chronological terms, the teenage years extend from age 13 through 19. During this time a child evolves into an adult. In biological terms, the time starts with puberty, the phase when sexual reproduction first becomes a physical possibility, and continues through the attainment of mental and social adulthood.

The growth during these years is perhaps most apparent in a physical sense. The teenage boy or girl becomes a taller and heavier person with a recognizably adult shape. Yet equally significant is the broadening of intellectual growth, providing new insights and abilities to understand more and more complex matters. In tandem, the child's psychological development helps integrate the multitude of changes into a better understanding of his or her physical and intellectual presence.

Often, the physical, intellectual, and psychological developments occur at different rates; in fact, the differences can lead to anxiety, insecurity, conflict, and other emotional hurdles. For example, in recent generations puberty has been starting earlier, whereas, ironically, graduation from adolescence, signaled by independence, seems to be attained later and later. The result is that the transitional period we call adolescence has been lengthening. In today's world, with drug use and sexual behaviors commencing earlier and earlier, the challenges of these years seem to grow continually.

Adolescence is the time when the ongoing tug-of-war between parents and children begins to be resolved. This struggle, which starts in infancy and continues through childhood and sometimes even into early adulthood, concerns the normal tension between the child's dependence on his or her parents and the growing independence from them.

Just as children are distinct from adults, so too are adolescents, and they are best understood as such: a teenage boy or girl is not an overgrown child or a miniature or immature adult. In the early teenage years, the adolescent begins forging an individuality that is separate from his or her parents. In middle adolescence, the 15- to 17-year-old is concerned with defining his or her sexual identity.

As this time of life gives way to young adulthood, perhaps at age 18, 19, or even later, the tension between parents and their children most often is resolved, with both generations learning to accept the new adult's independence. The teenage child continually strives to coordinate the physical, intellectual, and psychological growth and to develop a fully formed ego identity and sense of self.

During adolescence, the relationship between parents and children is challenged and stressed and gradually redefined. To ensure that a good relationship is maintained, it is crucial for both generations to communicate with each other as openly as possible. In part, this chapter is devoted to furthering this communication. Teenagers are profoundly influenced by the unique physical and mental changes of adolescence. In contrast with younger age groups, adolescents start to take responsibility for their own lives, including their own health care.

The pages that follow speak directly to teenagers and parents: our goal is to provide you—whether teen or adult—with the information you need to best cope with these uniquely challenging years.

PHYSICAL GROWTH

As an adolescent, your body grows and develops faster than at any other time except for the first year of life.

This growth occurs unevenly. Changes may occur relatively slowly during some of your teenage years and rapidly during the so-called growth spurt of preadolescence, which starts about 2 years earlier in girls than in boys.

It is not the actual stage of your physical growth that is of greatest importance at any one time. More important is how you *feel* about your body and how you are reacting to the changes you are experiencing.

You may expect or desire an ideal body, perhaps one like that of a much-admired peer or performer or even a parent or teacher. Rarely, however, is perfection achieved. More important, in fact, is that you accept and grow accustomed to the changes you are experiencing. At times you may feel as if things are happening to your body that are literally out of your control, especially during the growth spurt. You cannot expect to control the transformation, but you can attempt to understand, enjoy, and accept your body.

NORMAL GROWTH AND DEVELOPMENT

On average, the growth spurt begins at about age 10 in girls and 12 in boys, tending to reach its peak about 2 years later in both sexes. At the peak of this spurt, you grow between 3 and 4 inches per year. Most boys grow faster than girls. When the preadolescent growth spurt ends, you have nearly attained your adult height. If you have not started a conspicuous increase in growth by age 15, consult your physician.

If you grow and develop either slower or faster than average, you are not alone; it is also normal to feel somewhat insecure about yourself at this time. It is important to remember that there is no standard timetable for growth and development during adolescence. Entirely normal teenagers mature at such widely varying rates that even those whose growth rate falls in the middle may feel that they are the only ones going through such changes at that particular time. Your parents can help by providing love and reassurance, neither minimizing nor over-dramatizing your concerns.

The external changes caused by the pre-adolescent growth spurt are obvious: your body grows taller and heavier and its shape changes. Your bones grow too; even the facial bones change, sharpening your features and transforming your face into that of an adult.

The preadolescent growth spurt dramatically alters the composition of your body, accentuating the difference between the sexes. As the spurt starts, fat collects on the buttocks and around the abdomen in both boys and girls. During the course of the spurt, boys accumulate mostly lean tissue (muscle and bone), and girls add more fat, particularly on their hips and breasts. The result is that fat makes up 25 percent of the total body weight in girls and between 15 and 20 percent in boys.

By the time of a girl's first menstrual period or the end of a boy's growth spurt, fully developed adult proportions have been reached, with the distinctly different contours of men and women. The respective male and female sex hormones, along with family traits, account for most of this difference. These hormones are also responsible for the secondary sex changes, which usually begin about 1 year after the start of the adolescent growth spurt in boys and girls.

For a chart illustrating growth patterns and rates for teenagers, see page 121.

SEXUAL CHANGES IN BOYS

During the teen years, the child's body gains sexual maturity. Male changes include the appearance of hair in the pubic area, under the arms, and on the face, as well as deepening of the voice.

Your body prepares for sexual maturity by producing male hormones. These hormones cause your testicles to enlarge and your scrotum to darken.

The first male change you are likely to notice is the appearance of sparse, lightly pigmented pubic hair on the skin surrounding the base of your penis. Your sex changes are likely to be well under way before your growth spurt reaches its peak. Do not be worried if you happen to develop some breast tissue about this time. Only rarely is this change (called gynecomastia) due to any hormonal problem. The development usually disappears within a few months.

Your penis has been able to become erect since you were an infant. However, it is usually not until about 2 years after the start of puberty, and 1 year after your penis starts to lengthen, that you become capable of ejaculating semen for the first time. This may occur while you masturbate, spontaneously while you enjoy a sexual fantasy, or at night during a nocturnal ejaculation (commonly referred to as "wet dream"; see also Masturbation, page 154, and Sexual Fantasies, page 154).

Later, hair begins to appear under your arms and on your face. As your larynx (voice box) develops, your Adam's apple becomes more prominent. Your voice also starts to change, taking on a deeper tone. Occasionally, your higher, younger voice may still be heard, though fleetingly, when your voice "cracks."

Throughout this period of sexual maturation, which usually lasts 4 or 5 years, your testicles continue to enlarge and your penis gets longer and thicker. By the end of this period, your penis, testicles, and pubic hair are fully developed, and your mustache and beard hair has started to appear.

The period of sexual maturation usually starts a couple of years later in boys than in girls. Sexual changes in boys start anytime between age 9 and 14. If puberty starts outside that age range, it is considered either delayed or premature (see Premature Puberty, page 138).

SEXUAL CHANGES IN GIRLS

Female changes include the development of breasts and, as in boys, the appearance of hair in the pubic area and under the arms. In both girls and boys, the hormones surge with a flurry of preparatory activity well before you can see any of these changes.

The first visible change is either breast budding—that is, the beginning of breast development—or the appearance of sparse, lightly pigmented pubic hair. The activity of your sweat glands also increases. Do not worry if one breast happens to start developing before the other, even if the difference in size persists for many months.

About 1 year after your breasts begin to develop, your growth rate is likely to reach its peak, or fastest point. Within the year after the peak of your growth spurt, you will probably experience menarche—that is, your first menstrual period.

The advent of your first menstrual period means that it is now physically possible for you to become pregnant and bear a child. You can even get pregnant before then if you happen to ovulate (produce an egg) before your first period. If you are sexually active, find out about the various methods to prevent bearing a child as a result of sexual intercourse (see Contraception, page 153).

You may notice an intermittent increase in either white or yellow vaginal discharge during the months before menstruation starts. It is also normal for your first few menstrual periods to occur irregularly. However, within about a year they will start to appear more nearly on schedule. You will then experience a 3- to 7-day period about every 24 to 34 days.

Most girls start out using disposable, external pads to absorb their menstrual blood. However, because the hymen usually does not cover the vaginal opening you can use tampons instead, given a little practice in insertion. If you choose to use tampons, you should change them frequently to minimize the risk of toxic shock syndrome (see page 1061).

Painful menstruation (dysmenorrhea) is unusual during the first few menstrual periods but may occur in later periods during adolescence (see Dysmenorrhea, page 164).

As you experience your first menstrual periods, you continue to grow taller. Your breasts will also grow larger. More and more of your pubic and underarm hair appears. Your voice deepens, though not as much as that of a boy who is experiencing puberty.

It usually takes approximately 4 or 5 years for puberty to reach completion, resulting in full body development.

There is a wide range of normal ages for you to begin sexual maturation. When a girl's sexual maturation starts before age 8, it is considered premature (see Premature Puberty, page 138). If it begins after age 13, it is deemed delayed.

There is also a link between your nutrition and the timing of your puberty. Improvements in nutrition in recent decades explain why the onset of puberty occurs at younger ages in successive generations of young females in industrialized nations such as the United States. In addition, puberty tends to start earlier in girls who have more body fat and later in those who are thin (see also The Normal Menstrual Cycle, page 1058).

NUTRITION DURING THE TEENAGE YEARS

Don't believe the bad news. Too often teenagers receive a "bad rap" when it comes to eating smart. Parents sometimes are led to believe that teenagers, as a group, are nutritionally vulnerable. This thinking may be inspired in part by the ready availability of fast food and junk food and by reports that single out teenagers as people who do not eat properly.

This is not necessarily so. Teenage eating habits tend to reflect those of adults.

We know of very little data that suggest that the nutritional status of teenagers, as a group, is particularly poor. However, there probably is room for improvement. As a teenager, why is nutrition important to you?

You are growing and you are learning, and you are living in a competitive world. You need an edge over your competition in school, at work, and perhaps in athletics. Nutrition can help give it to you.

A balanced diet has practical advantages. It can help give you shining hair and a glowing complexion. If you are an athlete, it may help improve your performance.

Each day, you are faced with many decisions relating to what you eat. Remember this: each decision you make can have an effect on how you ultimately look and feel. Teenagers who are well nourished are people who make more good decisions than bad decisions when it comes to selecting food.

Almost all of us, from time to time, enjoy fast food. Occasionally, some of us are prone to indulge in junk food. Then we feel guilty about eating these foods. The guilt can lead to depression, which, in turn, can lead to overindulgence in the wrong kind of food. Do not fall into this trap.

Remember this: just about anything you eat has some nutritional value. That means that you can eat anything you want to eat as long as you refrain from overindulgence and take care not to allow the food to replace a consistently balanced diet. Instead of joining the crowd and eating poorly, you can join the crowd and eat smart by making appropriate food choices. The decision is up to you.

It is true that some teenagers consume amounts of calcium, iron, and vitamins A and C that are below the recommended daily allowances (RDAs) for these nutrients. Iron, for example, is a key ingredient during the teenage years. Ample iron is essential because of the expanding volume of blood in your body and the increase in muscle mass you will experience as you grow. Teenage girls are at particular risk for a shortage of iron because of significant iron loss through menstruation.

How can you ensure an adequate supply of dietary iron? Meats and grains are two excellent food sources.

As at any age, the key to good nutrition for you as a teenager is a variety of nutritious foods. Variety means choices from all four food groups: protein (meat, fish, poultry, and eggs); dairy products (milk, cheese, yogurt); fruits and vegetables; and complex carbohydrates (cereals, grains, potatoes, and rice). Like any health-conscious adult, you may want to make a special effort to eat foods with adequate fiber. Also, go easy on the extra salt and limit fat (especially saturated fat).

As busy as you are, try not to skip meals. In particular, eat a nutritious breakfast. Ideally, breakfast should be the main meal of your day.

Your growth and development require various nutrients and a certain number of calories. For example, depending on your height, frame, and level of activity, you may need from 1,200 to 3,000 calories each day if you are a girl and 2,100 to 3,900 if you are a boy. Under special circumstances, such as during intensive physical training for a sport, your nutritional needs are even higher.

If you are an athlete (male or female), a balanced diet is especially important to good performance. But this is not to say that you should "load up" on any particular type of food, drink, or supplement. In particular, skip the vitamin supplements that too often are highly publicized. They will not give you a competitive edge and may be harmful.

An equally important fact to remember is that when you perspire you are losing chiefly water but also some important nutrients. Specifically, there can be a significant decrease in your sodium, potassium, and magnesium levels.

To offset losses in sodium, some athletes take salt tablets. We do not recommend salt tablets. Unless there are unusual circumstances, the salt in your food should be sufficient. In fact, swallowing too many salt tablets can cause an upset stomach and further enhance dehydration.

Electrolyte-replacement beverages also are common and highly promoted. However, the sugar content of some of these solutions can interfere with the movement of fluid from your stomach into your intestinal tract. The sugar content should not exceed one-half teaspoon of sugar per half cup. Most electrolyte-replacement beverages have 2 to 3 times that amount (see Normal Athletic Eating, page 360).

It is important that you have an adequate intake of fluid, especially when you are perspiring heavily. Your best choice is the one that is most readily available and least expensive: water. Drink plenty of it before, during, and after competing.

For optimal performance, iron also plays an important role. It is an essential component of your blood's hemoglobin, which is necessary for transporting oxygen throughout your body. If you have an inadequate supply of iron, your endurance and ability to compete can be significantly reduced. Be sure to get an adequate supply of meats and grains. Also, you may want to discuss your potential need for an iron supplement with your team physician.

Remember that as physical training increases, your body spends more energy. Therefore, you will need more food than you would under normal circumstances.

The key to peak performance is a balanced diet with an adequate supply of foods and fluids.

Finally, a word to parents. You have a crucial role to play in setting a good example and taking time to prepare and serve wholesome family meals. Get the entire family involved in meal preparation. If family meals are not possible because of differing schedules, stock your kitchen with healthy, convenient snacks such as fresh fruits and vegetables, yogurt, milk, whole-grain bread, and popcorn.

Do not be too critical of your teenager. There is a place in the American diet for hamburgers and pizza. In fact, both of these foods have significant nutritional value. But again, the key is moderation and good judgment. Adults are no different from teenagers when it comes to making wise food choices. If we want to operate at peak efficiency, we need to make wise choices and exercise a reasonable amount of self-discipline.

INTELLECTUAL GROWTH AND DEVELOPMENT

During adolescence, your thinking process undergoes a transformation from childhood into adulthood, just as surely as your body does. It is important to realize, however, that your physical growth and intellectual growth may not be synchronized but may develop at distinctly different rates.

At the start of the teenage years, you are thinking like a child; by the end, your cognitive processes are those of an adult. Until about age 12, your learning primarily concerns understanding the logic of "concrete things," objects that can be seen and felt. The next step in your intellectual development is the achievement of abstract thought.

Throughout adolescence, you become increasingly adept at considering intangible ideas, including concepts that involve the past and the future. Your newfound abilities allow your thoughts to take wing, traveling through time, perhaps even speculating about what you and the world around you might become.

Along the way, the sudden expansion in your powers of thought may blur the boundaries between you and the world around you. As a young teenager, you may feel that you are at the center of the universe and that your power knows no limits. You may assume that others are thinking about you—positively or negatively—more than they really are. This feeling of being on stage also may make you feel self-conscious, essentially powerless, or lost.

You may go through periods when at one moment you believe that everyone thinks as you do, and the next second you may feel with great intensity that no one else in the world can understand your thoughts or feelings. Eventually, you will begin to realize that your thoughts are both distinct from yet similar to those of others. This realization also is accompanied by the knowledge that you are not the focus of everyone's attention.

Ultimately, your abstract reasoning becomes mature and comprehensive. You start to be capable of judging whether the relationships between two or more propositions are logical. You can solve increasingly complex problems. You become able to think like a scientist, conceiving of hypotheses and of ways to test them. In addition, you can also think reflectively, which means that you can think about thinking. For example, you can frame an argument for a discussion or debate and simultaneously make judgments about that argument's strengths or weaknesses.

The advances in your intellectual development change the way you think about the world and how you behave in response to it (see Development of Standards, page 149). You become able to discern much more clearly how past actions have affected what is happening now. You also become capable of predicting more accurately what implications your current actions or those of others will have for the future, even in the long term.

An important aspect of this concerns your health: you begin to appreciate the cause-and-effect relationship between destructive behaviors (such as drug abuse) and good health; on the other hand, the health benefits of good nutrition and ample physical activity also may begin to make sense to you. Your actions in these areas affect your future, and you may decide to act on this new understanding.

For the first time, you may be interested in discussing various serious subjects with your friends, family, and teachers. Topics may involve love, morality, work, politics, religion, and philosophy. By the time you complete adolescence, you, like most teenagers, probably will spend a great deal of time wrestling with such major questions as the purpose of life.

Your advancing intellectual development gives you the flexibility of formal thought that you will need to cope with change as you take your place in the world. This will help you make momentous decisions that will affect the rest of your life. Although you will probably still be guided by your parents, teachers, and other adults, your decisions can now be truly your own. For instance, you will decide whether to work or go to trade school or college after high school. You will choose which school to attend or which job to take.

In addition, you will make your choices among various possible career directions, religions, and political parties (see also Psychosocial Growth and Development of Personality and Behavior, below).

PSYCHOSOCIAL GROWTH AND DEVELOPMENT OF PERSONALITY AND BEHAVIOR

Much of your psychosocial development as an adolescent involves coping with the profound physical changes that your body is undergoing. You need to come to terms with your sexual development and the emotions that go with it. At the same time, you are developing an identity distinct from that of your parents and you are becoming independent of them.

Psychosocial development of adolescents is usually divided into three phases: early, starting at about 13 or younger; middle, at around 15 to 17; and late, extending to 19 or often well into the 20s or even 30s in some individuals. In early adolescence, the mental focus starts to shift from the family to peers. The middle phase may involve outright conflicts over independence. By the end of late adolescence, independence is virtually secured, parental advice can be taken or not, and body image and gender role definition are established.

These stages are not easy. The diverse aspects of your physical, psychological, and social development are not synchronized, and the progress is not smooth and easy. You may find yourself alternating between childish and adult behaviors.

Do not blame yourself for having a difficult time with your psychosocial development. You are not alone. When you face challenging situations, you may feel the need for adult guidance and support. For this purpose, many adolescents find themselves turning to an adult outside their family, such as a teacher or counselor. This compromise offers them needed guidance without falling back on the parental influences.

Part of your maturation process is developing and accepting a realistic image of your body. Difficulty with this image may manifest itself in eating disorders (see Anorexia Nervosa, page 1019, and Bulimia Nervosa, page 1020), particularly in girls. Because your body changes quickly during adolescence, you might start feeling uncomfortable with your physical self. You may be deeply concerned about whether your developing body is attractive or adequate. Your fears that you are physically imperfect may cause severe anxiety.

You may find yourself measuring the progress of your body against that of your peers. If you mature later or earlier than average—and many adolescents do—you may encounter trouble with your peers and your own image of your body. Often it helps to talk about these concerns with an understanding adult. Whether it is your physician, parent, or trusted teacher, this person can reassure you that your body is normal.

During the teenage years, you also will do a great deal of thinking about what kind of person you are and who you will become. You will muse, and then think seriously, about what you will do when you grow up. In early adolescence, you may set career goals that are idealistic, or even unrealistic beyond your given talents and abilities. You may imagine yourself as a rock star, airplane pilot, or investigative reporter. Later in adolescence, you may set your sights more practically, considering vocations that more immediately suit your abilities and interests. The merging of idle musings with practical planning is yet another part of the maturation process.

Because your psychosocial status is in such rapid flux, your role in society is extremely ambiguous. This presents complicated questions such as whether contraceptives should be prescribed for a teenager without parental consent. Generally, professionals in medicine, psychology, and social work will encourage you to involve your parents in your psychosocial concerns; however, they will not reveal your confidences, unless they perceive a serious danger to you.

The gradual changes of this time will enable you to develop a sense of who you are and to understand the nature of personal responsibility, both for yourself and for your actions. You begin to appreciate how what you do—what you eat and the activities you involve yourself in (playing on sports teams at school or pursuing risk-taking leisure-time activities such as illicit drug or alcohol or tobacco use)—has a major impact on your entire life. During these years you begin to take an active role in making countless decisions about what you do—and what you elect not to do. Good decisions can have a significant impact on your present and future health.

PSYCHOLOGICAL CHANGES

In early adolescence you may start to experiment with new ways of behaving and dressing at home. You may be seeking some approval from your family before you try anything out on the outside world. You may make a few tentative motions toward asserting your independence. You may become less interested in family activities and less willing to accept advice or criticism from your parents. You may find more social comfort in a close relationship with a best friend of the same sex.

As you start to break away from your family's influence, you begin paying more attention to your peers. For some time, they may even dominate your thinking and behavior. Your chosen peer group may be a club, team, gang, or other group of adolescents of about your age. At first, your peer group is likely to be restricted to members of your own sex. During adolescence, it usually shifts to a mixed group.

Your peer group may provide you with social status and a comforting sense of security: you have a place within the group, and you feel a sense of belonging there. In return, however, teenage cliques often demand conformity of behavior, attitudes, and dress.

Privacy becomes increasingly important to you. At home, you may ask for a room, or a part of one, to be yours alone. You may start keeping a journal or diary to record your private thoughts. This secrecy is important to you, and it deserves to be respected.

Your struggle for independence is often most overt in middle adolescence. You may start testing your parents' controls and discipline. You may decide that your parents' standards are unfair. You may develop your own value system, or adopt that of your peer group, and challenge your parents' and teachers' authority.

You and your peers may delight in playing pranks and practical jokes. Your peer group's behavior may involve rebellion (see Teenage Rebellion, page 154). You may feel intense peer pressure to take risks that pose dangers to you and others—for instance, experimenting with drugs, sex, or vandalism. Some teenagers carry this activity even further into negative behavior (see Bizarre Behavior, page 155). If you take it too far, your rebellion can get you into lasting trouble at home, at school, and even with the law.

By late adolescence or early adulthood, you have evolved a new way of thinking about your family. In your mind, you have become a separate entity from your family, even if you still live at home. Either you are financially independent, earning money to support yourself, or you will be soon. As you have become more comfortable with your own identity, you have started to break free of the values of your peer group.

Achieving independence does not mean that you cut yourself off from others. Rather, you have enough resources from your education, family, and community to allow you to start supporting yourself financially, emotionally, and socially. Part of this mature functioning is knowing when and how to use others for support when needed. You may even be able to appreciate your parents' values enough to seek their advice when you need it. Now that you are more your own person, you may no longer feel threatened that your parents are trying to control you or make you a child again.

Parents often have a difficult time coping with the psychological changes in their adolescent children. However, it is possible for your parents to ease your transition to independence. They can achieve a delicate, ever-shifting balance between their often-conflicting responsibilities: providing support and understanding while setting standards and limiting dangerous or harmful behavior.

When your parents disagree with what you are doing, they should seek to be firm without being harshly punitive. They should respect your sincere efforts to achieve independence. Gradually, they should let go of the control that they have exerted over you throughout childhood and trust that you will be guided by the self-control that they have helped to instill in you.

It is important to realize that parents are trying to make an adjustment from being providers and protectors to a less controlling role. The challenge that parents face is to relinquish involvement gracefully rather than abdicate their role.

DEVELOPMENT OF STANDARDS

Along with the psychosocial development of adolescence comes the evolution of standards. As you move from childhood to adulthood, your moral standards may progress in more-or-less distinct phases. At each stage, a different type of moral reasoning predominates.

As a child and young teenager, you may evaluate situations in a self-centered or opportunistic manner. When you judge whether an action is moral, the sole basis for your decision may be whether that action will help or hurt you. You may be concerned primarily with avoiding punishment and gaining rewards. Thus, most of the definition of your standards comes from outside yourself, not inside.

In middle adolescence, you may become more interested in conforming to legal standards. You start to realize that laws apply to everyone, including yourself. Accordingly, you may judge actions based on whether they are legal or illegal—not just on whether there is a risk of punishment.

However, teenagers do not always obey the law. Indeed, many adolescents go through a phase of rebelling, testing the limits of authority and sometimes even breaking the law. In a way, they may be asking to be disciplined, to experience tangible proof of the reality of the law. Ultimately, however, most teenagers progress beyond this testing phase. They decide that they should follow the law even if they are not likely to be punished for not doing so.

By late adolescence or adulthood, you start caring more about how your actions affect others. Your moral concerns may now extend to rules of human behavior beyond the letter of the law. You may follow standards based on broad ethical principles that in some cases may be even more restrictive than the law. You start to view real-life moral conflicts in abstract terms. You can recognize everyday examples of justice, equality, honesty, responsibility, cooperation, and reciprocity—and their opposites.

Eventually, your standards should evolve so that you become fully responsible for the morality of your own actions. Ideally, you develop your own detailed, individualized definitions of what your society deems as right and wrong. You follow this internalized personal moral code relatively independently of the endorsement or disapproval of others. If you ever violate your principles, you feel guilty and condemn yourself. You do not feel gleeful that you have gotten away without punishment.

Unfortunately, not everyone reaches the fruition of the development of their standards by the end of their adolescence. Even some adults never achieve it.

The evolution of standards is intertwined

with social interactions and intellectual development. Teenagers who participate in social activities have more opportunities to observe interactions. This experience may help them to form more mature moral judgments. An advanced level of abstract thinking may be needed to decipher the moral concepts that underlie everyday situations. Cognitive maturity also may aid in developing sensitivity to the roles, perceptions, and feelings of others. However, neither social nor intellectual prowess necessarily guarantees the development of high moral standards.

Your parents can encourage your development of standards by the example they set. Teenagers tend to develop more self-controlled behavior and make more mature moral judgments when their parents have followed a certain style of child-rearing. This style includes the following: consistent disciplining that involves reasoning and explanation; discussing how others feel about actions taken; and promoting democratic family discussions, in which even the young children can have their say. But parents do often set examples by their own values and lifestyles.

TEENAGE SEXUALITY

In the early teenage years, your closest relationship is usually with a best friend of the same sex. By the mid-teens, you may be most concerned with a larger group of peers, a group within which a natural process of social experimentation is occurring: in some sense, you all learn from and with each other.

Even if you choose a special friend of the opposite sex at this age, your choice is likely to be made with your peer group's acceptance uppermost in your mind. In the late teenage years, however, you may be ready to embark on an intimate relationship with another person. Compared with your earlier relationships, this one demands a different type of sharing and commitment.

Base your relationship with another person on mutual understanding and enjoyment rather than on the opinion of your peers. It is a mistake to get involved in such a serious relationship merely to impress your peers—or to annoy your parents.

THE ROLE OF PARENTS

Parents often feel perplexed and even threatened by their teenager's emerging sexuality. If you are the parent of a teenager, it is best for everyone if you can come to terms with your child's sexuality, show your trust, and give him or her any help needed.

Your child may receive education about sex, family life, and sexually transmitted diseases at school. However, do not rely on the school to explain all of the complexities of sexual relationships that you want your child to know. No matter how awkward it may be for you, you have a responsibility to know what your child learns about the facts of life. If you are unsure how to present the facts, it may help to consult a book or suggest one to your child to read. You can also ask your physician or other trusted persons for help.

If you are like most parents, you want your child to delay the start of sexual activity until after he or she has reached an adequate level of emotional maturity. This is a sensible goal. Unfortunately, however, it is not always achieved (see Sexual Activity, page 152). If your adolescent child becomes sexually active, denying or ignoring the fact will not resolve the conflict you have with the situation and with your son or daughter.

Well before your child starts sexual activity, he or she needs your support and assistance in understanding sexual feelings, defining sexual behavior, and learning to respect himself or herself as well as others. Ideally, your instruction about sex and family life should start when your child is a preschooler or even a toddler. Respond honestly and in a straightforward manner to your child's spontaneous questions, including where babies come from. If your child never asks any sex-related questions, do not assume that he or she is not interested. Bring up the subject if the opportunity presents itself.

All along the way, make an effort to gear your advice on sexual matters to your child's current phase of intellectual, psychosocial, and moral development. The younger your child is, the simpler the advice should be.

Do not use only scare tactics in discussing sexual behavior with your teenager. By doing this, you put your child at risk of having insufficient knowledge about sexual situations. A purely negative approach may be less likely to discourage a teenager from embarking on a sexual relationship than providing a basic understanding and perspective from which to make sensible and responsible decisions in sexual matters. In addition, scare tactics may cut off the parent as a source of information for the teenager.

Discuss contraception and sexually transmitted diseases frankly. Be sure your child understands your feelings and works to form his or her own attitudes on abortion, contraception, and teenage pregnancy (see Teenage Pregnancy, page 152).

Teach your child about the dangers of acquiring sexually transmitted diseases, including AIDS (acquired immune deficiency syndrome). The risk factors for these diseases include sexual activity (especially promiscuity and male homosexual activity) and sharing needles or syringes to inject drugs (see Sexually Transmitted Diseases, page 162, and AIDS, page 848). If your adolescent child is already sexually active, stress the risk of sexual exposure to people known or suspected to be infected with the virus (HIV) that causes AIDS. Explain that the risk of infection is increased by sexual contact with many partners or with a person who has had multiple partners.

To protect your adolescent child from AIDS, other sexually transmitted diseases, and also pregnancy, it makes sense to discourage your adolescent child from becoming sexually active until he or she is more mature. At the same time, however, it is important to emphasize that sex can be a joyous experience. Stress that when your child does start sexual activity, the regular use of condoms can reduce the risks of infection with the AIDS virus and other sexually transmitted diseases as well as help prevent pregnancy. Concurrent use of spermicidal foam may provide added contraceptive protection.

INITIAL SEXUALITY

As an adolescent, your sexual development has started. Along with it, your sexual feelings and fantasies increase. You may find it difficult to deal with these feelings, particularly if they seem to conflict with the attitudes that you have been taught about sex.

At first you may retreat from your emergence as a sexual being into the safety of friendships with members of the same sex. At the same time, you may find yourself intrigued by sexual matters and frequently seeking information about sex. Sometimes the emergence of sexual feelings in early adolescence is relieved through telling dirty jokes.

When your body first becomes capable of sexual intercourse and, if you are a female, of having a child, you are probably years away from being emotionally prepared for either event. However, you have likely started masturbating, or privately fondling your own sex organs for pleasure. This enjoyable and harmless activity may involve reaching an orgasm, or climax (see Masturbation, page 154).

In middle adolescence, you start feeling more aware of yourself as male or female. You become more interested in forming relationships with members of the opposite sex. Dating may start, as well as some sexual experimentation. This may involve kissing, fondling your partner, mutual masturbation, or even intercourse.

You may feel strong pressure from your peers to lose your virginity. Some teenagers react to this pressure, and to their own curiosity, by starting to have sexual intercourse at a very young age. Having a series of sexual partners may reflect emotional immaturity.

It is best to wait to have sexual intercourse until you have reasons other than peer acceptance and curiosity. Ideally, sexual intercourse is a joyous union of two people who love each other. Depending on your own moral and religious beliefs—and those of the adults you respect, including your parents—you may want to wait until you are married.

In the meantime, there are many other ways you can use to express your affection. You may enjoy intimate talks, long walks while holding hands, listening to music, and dancing together. Many adolescents give each other great pleasure through kisses and caresses.

By late adolescence, you become more secure about your sexual identity. You may then feel that you are emotionally ready to have sexual intercourse with someone you care about deeply. But you are unlikely to be prepared to become a parent. Therefore, whenever you start having sexual intercourse, use methods to prevent pregnancy and sexually transmitted diseases (see Contraception, page 153, Sexually Transmitted Diseases, page 162, and AIDS, page 848).

Regular use of a condom (rubber) can help protect you from both conceiving a baby and being infected with a sexually transmitted disease, including AIDS. If you are considering becoming sexually active, arrange in advance to use contraception and prophylaxis against sexually transmitted diseases (see also Contraception, page 153).

You might feel awkward about broaching the subject of contraception with your prospective partner. However, if the two of you are intimate enough to be thinking about making love with each other, you both should feel free to discuss these issues. If your prospective partner does not seem to care about the possibility of pregnancy or sexually transmitted disease, you may want to reevaluate your relationship.

SEXUAL ACTIVITY

If you have had sexual intercourse at least once, you are considered sexually active.

Male and female adolescents tend to report different reactions to their first experience of sexual intercourse. Girls more often say they were scared, guilty, worried, embarrassed, and curious. Boys, on the other hand, usually report feeling excited, thrilled, satisfied, happy, and grown-up.

The reality is that a wide range of experience is normal. You may not date at all in junior high or high school, or you may have a sole high school sweetheart. The most common pattern, though, is two or three close emotional commitments as a teenager, one after the other. During the course of each relationship, you and your partner will stay monogamous and, if sexual activity is part of the relationship, there will be no other sexual partners.

About 1 in 10 teenagers experiments with many sexual partners, including more than one at a time. These individuals are more likely to have psychological and physical health problems. They raise their risk of acquiring sexually transmitted diseases—including the fatal illness, AIDS (see Sexually Transmitted Diseases, page 162, and AIDS, page 848).

TEENAGE PREGNANCY

The United States has the highest rate of teenage pregnancy of any Western industrialized nation. More than 1 million American teenage girls become pregnant each year. More than a third of American girls become pregnant at least once during adolescence. Most of those who become pregnant carry their pregnancies to term. One-third of adolescent mothers get pregnant again before the end of their teenage years. Adolescent pregnancy and childbirth are a virtual epidemic in many inner-city communities.

Most of these pregnancies are neither planned nor wanted. They are a direct result of widespread ignorance about birth control along with denial of the risks of becoming pregnant. Two-thirds of the sexually active teenagers in the United States do not regularly use any form of contraception. Among the main reasons teens give for not using contraception are the following: they think it is the wrong time of the month to conceive; they do not know when to expect sexual intercourse; they think they are too young to become pregnant; they think contraception is wrong or dangerous; they do not have access to information about contraception; or they think they have intercourse too infrequently to become pregnant. In fact, having sexual intercourse just once can result in pregnancy. One-half of teenage pregnancies occur within 6 months of becoming sexually active.

If you are thinking about becoming sexually active, find out about contraception. As soon as your sexual activity starts—including the first time you have sexual intercourse—use contraception (see Contraception, page 153). Otherwise, you are likely to have an unwanted pregnancy.

If you have missed a menstrual period and you think you or your partner may be pregnant—tell your parents or another trusted adult immediately. The pregnant girl should see her physician as soon as possible. The sooner she seeks medical help, the more options are available.

Terminating the pregnancy may be a legal option. The earlier in pregnancy that abortion is performed, the safer it is (see Pregnancy Termination: Medical Problems and Personal Choices, page 199). If this route is chosen, the abortion should be done by a licensed physician in a hospital or clinic.

For many people, abortion is not a personal or practical option. The prospective mother may choose to carry the pregnancy to term, deciding either to give her child up for adoption or to raise it herself. Appropriate prenatal medical care is important to ensure the good health of the mother and the child (see Prenatal Care, page 184).

Raising a child is a serious responsibility that can last 2 decades. Most teenagers are not yet equipped, emotionally or financially, to make the necessary commitment. Some school districts have special programs that help pregnant adolescents continue their education, but having a baby is likely to put an end to your education, employment, and school friendships. It may force you into a strained, short-lived marriage.

It takes two to make a baby. The father bears just as much of the responsibility as the mother does. Just like adults, teenage fathers should participate in caring for their children and supporting them. Often, however, a teenage mother ends up having to raise her child under difficult circumstances, without any help from the child's father. There are not enough hours in the day for the mother to support herself and to care for her child alone. The children in such situations often face an uncertain future.

Despite these drawbacks, most pregnant teenagers carry their pregnancy to term and keep their babies to raise. Unfortunately, teenagers usually receive less medical care during pregnancy than more mature women do; however, they actually need more. Special considerations need to be taken to ensure a healthy mother and child when the mother-to-be is an adolescent who is still growing herself (see Concerns During Pregnancy, page 181).

CONTRACEPTION

If you are considering sexual intercourse, arrange in advance some method of contraception. If you are already sexually active, contraception is even more crucial.

Consult your physician or a reputable family planning clinic about contraception. Some schools have clinics that offer a range of health care, including counseling about contraception options.

Various methods of contraception are available, and they are discussed elsewhere in this book (see Pregnancy Prevention and Family Planning, page 175). Your choice of method may be affected by how motivated you are to avoid pregnancy and by how often you have intercourse.

However, it is important to remember that any contraception is better than none. Aside from the intrauterine device, all the contraceptive methods discussed, including birth control pills, are considered safe for teenagers. Your physician or family planning worker can help you decide what is best for you. Moreover, certain forms of birth control, such as oral contraceptives (the pill), do not offer any protection against sexually transmitted diseases (see page 162).

HOMOSEXUALITY

Intimacies often are exchanged between two or more boys or girls in early adolescence. They may try holding hands, kissing, fondling, or mutual masturbation. Participating in this kind of activity does not necessarily mean that you will be a gay man or a lesbian when you grow up.

Although it is estimated that almost half of American boys have one or more homosexual experiences, only about 1 of 10 men are homosexual. There is also a high incidence of early same-sex experimentation among girls and women, only female homosexuality is about half as common as that of males.

Some teenagers decide that they prefer members of their own sex. They may later become heterosexual adults or choose bisexuality, in which sexual intimacies are shared with members of both sexes. However, if their sexual identity is well defined in adolescence—or even in childhood—they may remain homosexual throughout adulthood.

If you are an openly homosexual teenager, you may face rejection by some of your peers, teachers, and family. If you are having difficulty adjusting to your sexual preference, or to others' reactions to it, psychotherapy may prove helpful.

If you are a male homosexual, your risk of contracting certain infectious diseases is raised. You are at even higher risk if you have experimented with several sexual partners. The potential infective agents include *Giardiasis, Chlamydia,* hepatitis B, and AIDS (see pages 619, 876, 650, and 848). Tell your physician about your sexual preference. Then, he or she can help you detect these illnesses early.

As a member of an acknowledged risk group for AIDS, get tested for the presence of antibodies to HIV, the virus that causes AIDS. Because AIDS is fatal, you might save your life by using a condom every time you have oral or anal intercourse.

SEXUAL FANTASIES

Daydreaming is an important part of adolescence, providing an outlet for your actively expanding imagination.

Do not be concerned if many of your daydreams have some sexual content. You also may have sexual fantasies at night. Sometimes you may conjure up hypothetical sexual experiences—or remember actual ones—while you masturbate alone. It is normal to have sexual fantasies. They may even be useful in the development of your sexual identity because they allow you to explore

sexual situations that would be unsuitable for you to act out in reality.

MASTURBATION

Masturbation, or stimulation of the genitals for sensual pleasure, is a normal and healthy activity. Some teenagers feel guilty about masturbating because of old, unfounded myths. No, masturbation will not cause you to go blind or to develop genital warts—there is no reason for fear.

There is nothing wrong with masturbating during your teenage years and beyond. You may even have started doing so in your school-age years or before. Masturbation provides a way for you to release sexual tension, give yourself pleasure, savor sexual fantasies, and even curb your impulses to engage in sexual activity with others that might be inappropriate. As long as you do not masturbate publicly, there is nothing at all unusual, harmful, or unacceptable about the practice.

PSYCHOLOGICAL AND BEHAVIORAL CONCERNS

Adolescence is often regarded as the worst of times—but it also can be the best of times. It is true that teenagers have to cope with dramatic physical and psychological changes. They sometimes feel confused, moody, or angry as they wrestle with the conflicts that seem to be heightened by the rapidity of all of these changes. However, it is important to remember that all of life, from birth to death, is a process of change.

Difficulties in adjusting to the changes of the teenage years occur in virtually all communities. No matter what their socioeconomic status, teenagers seem to encounter turbulent times, although children who grow up under deprived conditions and in single-parent families seem to be at greater risk. These children are more likely to fall victim to the three leading causes of death in adolescents—accidents, murder, and suicide. They may not receive the positive feedback needed to keep the psychological and behavioral problems of adolescence in check.

All these negatives should be balanced by positives. Developmental studies now show that most teenagers do not go through the turmoil and rebellion that we

used to think was the norm. Most teenagers enjoy their new skills, activities, friends, and opportunities.

TEENAGE REBELLION

A child who previously has been obedient and calm may become moody, inconsistent, unpredictable, and even rebellious in adolescence. Your adolescent child may bicker with you about a range of issues, large and small. They can include everything from what to wear and when to take out the garbage to when to come home at night and sexual activity.

A certain amount of teenage rebellion, risk-taking, and testing of authority is normal. Indeed, it may be an essential stage in the adolescent's process of separating from his or her parents and developing his or her own identity. However, most teenagers do not rebel greatly. A lack of rebellion should also not be taken to suggest unresolved problems that may surface in later years.

Rebellion can be seen as part of the process by which adolescents define their identities. They may take an action merely to see what reactions it provokes in the people around them. This is why you should not just give up on your rebellious teenager. Explain when his or her behavior exceeds the limits you have set. Eventually, he or she will learn from the consequences of the behavior and work toward the establishment of his or her own boundaries.

Mild rebellion is common and even normal in early and middle adolescence. By late adolescence, most teenagers are on their way to developing a sense of perspective. They have become better able to delay gratification, compromise on conflicting demands, and set limits. However, if rebellious behavior becomes more self-destructive or lingers into late adolescence, you should be concerned. Family problems may be causing or worsening the rebellion. Psychotherapy involving the whole family may help alleviate these problems.

If your teenage child is rebellious, hold your ground. Keep stating your concerns and setting reasonable limits. Do not threaten punishments that you will not carry out. In most cases, with your firm handling, your teenager will outgrow this rebellious phase without doing any lasting damage to himself or herself or others.

Even if your teenager has been rebellious, things usually change by the time he or she grows up and starts a family. Your child is likely to return to the viewpoints that he or she learned from you during childhood. With this in mind, try to prevent rifts during your child's adolescence that will stand in the way of later reunion.

As a parent, you remain the greatest influence on your teenager's beliefs and behavior, even more than his or her peers. Even when your child appears to be disagreeing with everything you say, he or she needs you to hold and defend your own reasonable and consistent view of the world.

BIZARRE BEHAVIOR

Sometimes rebellion becomes so marked that teenagers lose control over their impulses. They may feel all-powerful and immortal. Together, these characteristics can result in dangerous risk-taking behavior.

The teenager may alternate between self-consciousness and defiance. He or she may relish being dirty, messy, or even totally rejecting society. When teenage rebellion gets out of control, it can appear as bizarre (odd) behavior. Truly bizarre behavior may indicate mental illness, although many people term "bizarre" any behavior that is out of the ordinary.

Almost overnight your polite child who impresses all your friends and neighbors may seem to become a recalcitrant, stubborn irritant in your life. Your adolescent's new way of acting may appall you; in fact, it may well be calculated to do so. However, you should recognize that definitions of "odd" and "bizarre" often vary from one person to another. If your child "acts out" by dyeing his or her hair purple, you may be shocked, whereas your child's peer group (and perhaps even his or her teachers) may consider it normal. On the other hand, if your child is acting violently hostile, this behavior should be regarded as a serious problem by parents and peers alike.

The consequences of exaggerated teenage rebellion can be severe. It may contribute to the high rates of accidents, suicides, drug use, pregnancy, and sexually transmitted diseases in this age group.

Rebellion that is extreme may be seen in highly impulsive adolescents or when there is severe family conflict. Its causes are not always evident, but whatever its cause, bizarre behavior usually subsides with time. Decide which aspects of your child's behavior really matter and try to intervene only in those chosen areas. Individual and family psychotherapy may be needed.

Dropping out of social and sports activities, isolation from peers, and deterioration of schoolwork may be signs of drug use (see Drug Abuse and Addiction, below).

DRUG ABUSE AND ADDICTION

In the 1960s and 1970s, abuse of illegal drugs increased sharply among American teenagers. Drug abuse became a rite of passage in adolescence. Since then, the explosion of drug abuse has subsided somewhat. For instance, fewer adolescents smoke marijuana every day (see Medications and Drug Abuse, page 431).

In some ways, however, the problem has worsened. The age of first experimentation with marijuana has continually grown younger. Today, two-thirds of all teenagers have tried marijuana at least once before finishing high school, some of them during grade school. Also, the marijuana now on the market has higher levels of marijuana's active ingredient, tetrahydrocannabinol (THC). In addition, the "crack" form of cocaine is widely available at prices low enough for an adolescent to afford.

Alcohol also is a drug. Because it is legal for adults, it is easily accessible to teenagers. For most adolescents, experimentation with drugs starts with an alcoholic drink. Next usually comes smoking a marijuana cigarette (joint). Fortunately, relatively few teenagers "graduate" to trying harder drugs or using marijuana heavily or regularly over prolonged periods (see Marijuana Abuse and Dependence, page 440, and Street Drugs, page 441).

Some drugs, such as heroin, are physically addicting. Others, such as marijuana, can cause psychological dependence that is strong enough to approach a form of addiction. Adolescents are at high risk of psychological dependence on drugs because they are so vulnerable to peer pressure.

The teenage years should involve the evolution of independence, increasingly serious scholarship, and the formation of a sexual identity, among other processes. All this may be daunting enough when your adolescent child is clear-eyed. He or she may be tempted to use drugs as an escape from the difficult task of being a teenager. However, if your child is habitually drugged or drunk, the challenges of adolescence can be nearly impossible to meet.

Problems at school make teenagers more likely to abuse drugs; conversely, drug abuse can dampen the adolescent's motivation to do well in school. Drugs can impair the learning process, causing memory loss and shortening the attention span. Drug-abusing teenagers compromise their future outside school also. They may get into legal trouble for abusing illegal drugs, peddling them, or stealing to get enough money to buy them.

Drugs can disrupt the process by which your teenage child develops a secure sexual identity. They can cause sexual anxiety. They can also mar judgment and self-control. They release inhibitions and can make it easier for your child to do things that he or she would not normally consider doing. Some of these actions can have lasting effects. For instance, drugs might prevent your child from resisting sexual advances or from remembering to use contraception. An unwanted pregnancy could result. The adverse effects of maternal abuse of drugs—particularly alcohol—are well documented (see Smoking and Use of Alcohol and Illegal Drugs During Pregnancy, page 188).

Just like an adult who takes a drink to feel more comfortable at a party, an adolescent may take a drug to relax and join the crowd. For adults and teenagers alike, this is a counterproductive strategy. Social interactions are more successful when one is really one's self, rather than some other personality induced by a drug. Drugged or drunk people often withdraw socially and become depressed. Likewise, depressed adolescents may abuse more drugs in a vain effort to improve their mood.

Most seriously, drug abuse raises the risk of death during adolescence. The three leading killers of teenagers—accidents, murder, and suicide—are more prevalent among drug abusers.

The senses are distorted by drugs. This effect interferes with motor coordination and raises the risk of accidents. It is dangerous to operate machinery or even play sports while under the influence of drugs. Advise your child against the use of drugs. Insist that your child not drive a car while drugged (or drunk).

When adolescents share needles and syringes used to "shoot up" drugs intravenously, they are at high risk of getting AIDS. If they engage in this high-risk behavior, they should be tested for the virus that causes this fatal disease.

The most effective way to discourage your teenage child from abusing drugs—or alcohol or tobacco—is to gear your message to his or her level of intellectual and moral development (see Intellectual Growth and Development, page 146, and Development of Standards, page 149). Particularly in early and middle adolescence, your child may be less impressed by the long-term health effects of these substances than by their immediate social consequences.

Even more important than delivering an anti-drug message is to set a good example. Addictive behavior often repeats itself in successive generations of a family. Particularly if your child is abusing drugs and others in your family have been alcoholics or drug users, family therapy can help break this cycle. It also helps to build your child's self-confidence, so that he or she can better resist peer pressure to abuse drugs (see Teenagers and Drugs, page 437).

SEXUAL ABUSE

Sexual abuse can occur in adolescence or even earlier in childhood (see Sexual Abuse in the Preschool and School-Age Years, pages 114 and 130). It can include incest and rape.

Rape usually involves force or the threat of force. However, rape also includes situations in which the victim is unable to give consent because of being drunk, drugged, or mentally ill or retarded. Almost half of reported rape victims are adolescents. Most sexual abuse of teenagers involves girls, but the rate of assaults on boys may be increasing.

Incest is sexual contact between close relatives. It can occur between a teenager—or a younger child—and a member of the family. Most often, it involves a father and daughter, uncle and niece, or brother and sister. However, the perpetrator can be anyone perceived to be a family member, even if that person is not related to the adolescent by blood or marriage. Examples include the boyfriends of an adolescent's mother or a foster parent. Even when it does not involve blood relatives or any threat of force, incest is a betrayal of trust.

Rape and incest are devastating events. It is no wonder that sexual abuse often leaves psychological trauma in its wake. Rape is hostile and dehumanizing, and it can have lasting effects on the victim's self-worth and identity. This is especially true for adolescents, who are still figuring out who they are, including trying to forge a sexual identity. If rape is a teenager's first sexual experience, future sexual adjustment can be threatened.

After being raped, the victim may go through rapid mood swings, feeling alternately degraded, angry, guilty, and helpless. The sense of equilibrium is disrupted. The victim may be plagued for a long time by fears, nightmares, and disturbed sleep. The victim's relationships with peers and consensual sexual partners may suffer. Fearing retaliation from the attacker, the victim may act withdrawn and develop ritualistic behavior as a defense.

Counseling can help the victim and family to cope with long-term effects of the sexual abuse. You may want to seek professional guidance from an established rape crisis center. Unfortunately, some parents reject their children who have been victims, while others overprotect them. You can help your child come to terms with the sexual abuse and then proceed with life by neither denying nor overreacting to the sexual abuse.

The psychological ramifications of incest can be even more complex than those of rape. Fearing that reporting the incest will disrupt the structure of the family, the victim may be too frightened to tell anyone about it. Thus, the incest may occur repeatedly. The incestuous relative may invoke family authority to keep the victim from reporting the abuse. As the incest continues unreported, the victim may feel increasingly helpless, ashamed, guilty, and even responsible.

More cases of incest are thought to be kept secret than disclosed. Serious consequences can occur when adolescents do not have the opportunity to disclose incest, end it, and learn to cope with its aftereffects. They are at high risk of drug abuse, promiscuity, running away, or even suicide. In contrast, professional treatment can deal with incest. Sometimes the abusive relative is rehabilitated. However, temporary or permanent breakup of the family and foster placement may be necessary.

When adolescents are victims of rape or incest, they are sometimes blamed for provoking the sexual abuse. Teenagers experiment with provocative modes of dressing and behavior. However, these experiments are just steps along the road to the creation of a personal sexual identity. In most cases, to say that an adolescent asked for sexual abuse is to perpetuate a cruel myth (see Sexual Assault and Sexual Abuse, page 290).

SCHOOL PROBLEMS

School problems during the teenage years include school phobia, truancy, school failure, learning disabilities, and, occasionally, consequences of chronic illness. School problems can also result from rebellion, bizarre behavior, drug abuse, sexual abuse (see above), depression, anxiety disorders, or alcohol use.

School phobia is an irrational, persistent fear of attending school. The child actually fears leaving home rather than fearing school. This condition most often appears when a student first begins school. Less often, it may accompany entry into junior high or high school or transfer to an unfamiliar school. School phobia can respond to treatment (see School Phobias, page 137).

Truancy involves not going to school. Unlike the teenager with school phobia, the truant is not afraid of school but does not want to attend school and is not fearful of leaving home. Truancy can start with cutting an occasional class and then escalate into prolonged absences. It can result from conflicts within the family, parental expectations that are too high or low, and peer pressure to drop out. Truants are often rebellious teenagers who are in trouble not only at school but also at home and elsewhere.

Sometimes truancy can be reversed with an educational plan that emphasizes behavior management and involves the family, school, and medical personnel. Individual and family psychotherapy also may help. If the teenager still does not start attending school regularly, it may be possible to work out an educational alternative. Examples include early graduation and special programs such as work-study and independent study.

School failure can result from truancy. It is difficult for your child to know what is going on in class if he or she does not attend. Some schools have policies that automatically drop students who have been absent more than a certain amount of time. A host of other problems may be involved in school failure among adolescents. High school dropouts face a bleak employment future, so it is important to prevent school failure.

Failure in school can be caused by problems with peers or behavior, not only by an inability to achieve academically. For instance, sometimes a young adolescent starts to separate from the family without succeeding in finding an alternative support group of peers. This can create a social void that results in problems at school. In addition, underachievement can result from problems with an overdemanding teacher, parent, or school.

Alternatively, the cause can be the student's failure to learn up to his or her potential. This does not necessarily spring from lack of intelligence or hard work. Learning disabilities and attention deficits can cause teenagers to perform below average in school, regardless of intelligence (see Learning Disorders, page 132). Undetected problems with hearing and vision also can interfere with learning at school.

If your teenager has had a chronic illness through childhood and adolescence, such as asthma or cystic fibrosis, he or she may often have had to stay home from school during acute episodes of the disease. Too often, these absences pave the way for school failure. Your child may need extra encouragement and support to enable him or her to make up the missed schoolwork. As parents, do not support frequent school absences for minor physical complaints. Work with your child's physician, teachers, and school nurse. Together, you can help your child to keep achieving in junior high and high school.

DEPRESSION AND SUICIDE

Transient moodiness in response to a difficult situation is normal in adolescence, even more so than at other times of life. However, prolonged periods of profound unhappiness indicate depression, which can often be treated.

Once it was thought that only adults got depressed. Now, depression is being recognized increasingly in teenagers and even in younger children.

Symptoms of depression may include complaints of insomnia, fatigue, headache, stomachache, weakness, and dizziness. Your child may "act out" with unusual behavior, find it difficult to concentrate, and feel isolated from his or her family and friends. Your child may feel hopeless, expressing inner turmoil, chaos, and worthlessness. He or she may start abusing drugs or alcohol, trying in vain to feel better. Each bout of depression can last longer than 2 weeks. Often, the episode of depression is accompanied by a lack of interest in food and resulting weight loss or failure to gain.

If you think your child may be depressed, seek professional help. Professional treatment can help the depressed adolescent regain hope. He or she can realize that things will get better and problems will be overcome. Treatment involves individual psychotherapy or family therapy, sometimes with antidepressant medication. Hospitalization may be appropriate for a particularly long and severe bout of depression.

Especially if your child has mentioned suicidal thoughts, do not try to take care of his or her depression yourself. However, you do have an important role to play at home. Because depressed adolescents often feel that their families do not understand them, make a special effort to bridge this communication gap. Your understandable hopes for your child's happiness, strength, and success should not stand in the way of your accepting his or her revelations of frustration, weakness, or failure.

Ask your child how he or she feels—and listen. Check how long the mood lasts, and how intense it is. You can help by offering your support and concern. You can also remind your child that he or she will not feel so bad indefinitely. Each episode of depression ends eventually. However, a teenager who is feeling deep depression for the first time may not recognize this.

Sometimes, depressed teenagers' lives become so painful that they feel they have nothing to live for. They may try to take their own lives. Most adolescents who attempt suicide are depressed. However, others may be motivated by other triggers, such as the breakup of a relationship, the death of a friend or family member, psychological problems within the family, chronic physical illness, drug abuse, or physical or sexual abuse. There are many reasons why teenagers attempt suicide. Sometimes they give no warning and the attempt cannot be predicted.

The rate of suicide among teenagers, young adults, and even young children is rising rapidly. An estimated 500,000 teenagers survive suicide attempts each year in the United States. Suicide is now the third leading cause of death among American adolescents. In young adults, suicide is the second leading cause of death. The suicide rate may be even higher because many suicides are likely reported as accidents.

When male adolescents attempt suicide, they are more likely to use guns and to succeed in killing themselves. In contrast, female teenagers more often use drugs, which are not as reliably lethal.

If your child confides that he or she has considered suicide, take this admission seriously and seek counseling for him or her immediately. Even if it does not mean your child is really going to kill himself or herself, it is a cry for help that deserves to be heeded.

CAUSES OF DEATH IN TEENAGERS

Largely because of violent deaths, adolescents are the only group in the United States whose death rate is actually increasing. The three major causes of death in teenagers are accidents, murder, and suicide. Together, these three causes of death account for three-quarters of the deaths that occur in adolescents.

Most of the accidental injuries that kill adolescents occur in car crashes. Many of these deaths could be prevented if teenagers wore seat belts and did not drive after drinking alcohol or abusing drugs. Other commonly fatal accidents include drowning, poisoning, burns, falls, and guns going off unexpectedly.

Many of these accidents do not occur randomly. Factors that raise the risk of death in adolescents include poverty, stressful family situations, and risk-taking behavior.

For further information, see Adolescent Depression (page 1018), Teenage Suicide (page 1019), Warning Signs of Potential Suicide (page 1040), and Depression and Mood Disorders (page 1037).

ANXIETY AND PANIC ATTACKS

Anxiety can be a helpful defense against stress. However, when it becomes overwhelming and incapacitating, it is considered a disorder. Anxiety disorders can involve fears (phobias), obsessive-compulsive behavior, posttraumatic stress disorder, and panic attacks.

Panic attacks are episodes of extreme fear and anxiety. Treatment involves medications and psychotherapy (see Anxiety Disorders, page 1033).

EATING DISORDERS

Anorexia nervosa is severe food restriction, and bulimia is binge eating, with or without alternating cycles of purging (by self-induced vomiting, fasting, or abuse of laxatives, diet pills, or diuretics). Anorexia nervosa and bulimia are now regarded as different poles in the spectrum of many different eating disorders that occur most often in teenage girls and young women under age 25. Most individuals with eating disorders recover with treatment. Rarely, the disorders prove fatal (see Anorexia Nervosa, page 1019, and Bulimia Nervosa, page 1020).

One hallmark of anorexia nervosa is that the girl perceives her body as fat, even if she is emaciated. Many individuals with anorexia indulge in compulsive, excessive exercising. It is often impossible for these individuals to confront—or even recognize—their conditions.

If your daughter's growth chart shows that she is failing to gain weight, or even starting to lose it, her physician may suspect anorexia nervosa. Unfortunately, bulimia does not send off such clear-cut signals. Depending on the frequency and timing of the binges and purges, some girls with bulimia maintain their normal weight, whereas others lose or even gain weight. But one telltale sign of bulimia—not seen in every case—is weight that fluctuates wildly.

Girls with anorexia nervosa often lack body fat. Without much development of breasts, thighs, or waistline, they often maintain the appearance of small children.

USE OF ALCOHOL

Most young people try at least one alcoholic drink during their teenage years. Alcohol is widely available, and many adolescents start unfortunate patterns of excessive drinking (see also Alcohol Abuse, page 417).

Alcohol can be thought of as a potentially addicting drug—and an illegal one for most teenagers. Many of the issues that pertain to drug abuse apply to alcohol use also (see Drug Abuse and Addiction, page 155). Most important, alcohol plays major roles in depression and in the leading causes of death among teenagers—accidents, murder, and suicide (see Depression and Suicide, page 158, and Causes of Death in Teenagers, page 159).

USE OF TOBACCO

Tobacco use can be an expensive, long-term, potentially life-threatening addiction that often is extremely difficult to overcome. Thanks to widespread public information about the health hazards of smoking, cigarette smoking among teenagers is decreasing, especially among boys. However, the rate of decline has been slower among girls. In addition, male adolescents seem to be using more smokeless tobacco (chewing tobacco and snuff). Rather than being a safe alternative to cigarette smoking, smokeless tobacco can cause mouth cancer, throat cancer, and gum disease (see Tobacco, page 407).

COMMON CONCERNS OF THE TEENAGE YEARS

Adolescence has the reputation of being the healthiest of times, and most teenagers are healthy and robust. However, many adolescents do have significant health problems. Because it is normal for them to rebel and to question authority to some extent, they may find it difficult to comply with the treatment for these problems. They may resent any diagnosis that sets them apart from their peers—and any treatment that makes them feel dependent.

In addition, teenagers are bombarded by temptations to experiment with risk-taking behaviors that pose grave threats to their health, including abusing drugs and alcohol. At the same time, adolescence is also a key opportunity for preventive care because it is the last chance to establish a healthy lifestyle that can be carried into adulthood.

Therefore, it is a matter of concern that this age group receives the least medical attention. The childhood illnesses have passed and the health problems of the adult have not yet developed. The annual rate of visits to a physician is less for teenagers than for all other ages. In fact, adolescence is no time to skimp on checkups. Routine visits should be scheduled at least every 2 years. Among other things, these visits provide the opportunity to keep up with immunizations. Adult-type combined tetanus and diphtheria toxoids should be given at age 14 to 16 and again every 10 years after that (see Immunizations, page 867). Routine examinations also allow teenagers to seek professional guidance regarding their health-related concerns.

The promotion of good health habits and healthy lifestyle behaviors should be a major focus of these medical visits. In addition, school-based health education and health-care programs, with the active participation of physicians and other health-care professionals, should be actively encouraged. This is a critical time for teenagers to begin taking responsibility for their health and health-care decisions.

The teenage years are a time for identifying risk factors for cardiovascular disease, such as hypertension and elevated serum cholesterol (see also page 789). In addition, diabetes mellitus often is identified during adolescence. So if you are a teenager, heed our recommendation and schedule a health checkup.

Your physician or other health-care professionals can counsel you if you smoke or use alcohol or street drugs. Because motor vehicle accidents also are a concern, you will be encouraged to use seat belts regularly and especially warned against use of alcohol or drugs while driving. In addition, this is the time to receive counseling regarding sexual activity, the use of nonprescription and prescription birth control devices, and the option of postponing sexual activity.

If you have questions about the cause and spread of AIDS (see page 848) or other sexually transmitted diseases (see page 875), ask your physician about this. If you are sexually active, you need to protect yourself against exposure to these infections.

If you are an athlete, ask your physician about nutrition (see page 360) and about anabolic steroids (see page 439). Before you compete, be sure your physician checks you for problems that could predispose you to an injury or health risk.

ROUTINE EXAMINATION

As the years pass and you mature in your teenage years, you will become increasingly independent from your parents and the rest of the world; and the medical office is no exception. Ideally, your physician should see you separately from your parents for private discussions at each office visit. Privacy is important because your concerns often are not the same as those of your parents.

Many teenagers are reluctant to discuss health-related problems that concern them most—problems such as acne, contraception, depression, drugs, being overweight, sexual practices, sexually transmitted diseases, and getting along with parents and other adults. This reluctance can prompt a teenager to make an appointment ostensibly for a sore throat when the true problem centers, for example, on how to cope with depression. Physicians understand this reluctance. Often, it takes time, privacy, and special skill for a physician to draw the teenager out about his or her true concerns.

In the interest of effective communication, try to understand any tendency you may have to be reluctant and avoid it. Be direct and honest when discussing your health problem with your physician. You may want to involve your parents, whose support can be a great help. But remember this: your physician will respect your right to confidentiality unless suicide or some other potentially fatal emergency is threatened.

Your physician will appreciate an opportunity to discuss the issue of confidentiality with you. In most cases, physicians will seek your permission before communicating with parents, schools, other institutions, or previous physicians concerning your personal medical history.

Strive to achieve a comfortable relationship with your physician. You should know each other well. Sometimes teenagers continue consulting the pediatrician they have visited throughout childhood. Other adolescents prefer a general or family practitioner who serves the whole family. Either way, select a physician in whom you can place your confidence, one who will respect your desire to be treated seriously and confidentially. In late adolescence, some young women consult an obstetrician/gynecologist for all their routine health concerns. Teenagers with chronic acne may select a dermatologist for this purpose.

As in other age groups, the routine physical examination you will receive involves a review of your skin, head, eyes, ears, nose, mouth, glands, chest, lungs, abdomen, musculoskeletal system, neurological system, and external genitals. A good physician is gentle and sensitive when examining all patients, and you should expect no less. If you would prefer to involve a parent in your examination, your physician should not object to this. Also, your physician should explain the goals of the examination and provide you with a clean gown and ample time to disrobe privately.

Checkups for teenagers offer an opportunity for early detection of chronic conditions that could stand in the way of a healthy adulthood. For example, your physician will measure your blood pressure at each routine visit. As you grow, your blood pressure will increase. This is normal. Because teenagers grow at varying rates, height tends to be a better determinant than age for deciding whether blood pressure is normal. But if you do have high blood pressure, early identification is important. Your physician can intervene and perhaps prevent consequences of high blood pressure over an extended period of time.

Although the main purpose of a health examination relates to the physical condition of your body, this also can be a helpful learning experience for you. For example, if you are a female, your physician can teach you how to perform your own breast self-examination (see Breast Self-Examination, page 1076). This is something you should begin to do on a regular basis during your teenage years. Also, your physician can answer any questions you may have about your menstrual cycle (see The Normal Menstrual Cycle, page 1058).

Adolescent girls generally start having pelvic examinations by at least age 18. If you are sexually active and need contraception, if you have symptoms that suggest a possible problem in your urinary tract or reproductive organs, or if you just want reassurance that your anatomy is normal, request a pelvic examination even if you are younger than age 18 (see The Pelvic Examination, page 1055). Again, you can expect your physician to be gentle and thorough in explaining what is happening.

As part of your examination, your physician may ask about family practices and attitudes that could lead to health problems. For example, do your parents use alcohol? What are their views toward use of recreational drugs? Is there a history of physical or sexual abuse in your family?

Your physician should know about any diseases that run in your family. For example, has a parent or grandparent had a heart attack or cancer? To answer these questions, you may need help from your parents.

If you have a chronic disease such as diabetes or asthma, keep this principle in mind: You should be given as much responsibility for managing your personal health problem as you can handle. Learn everything you can about your ailment and how it is to be managed. You may want to keep a journal of chronic symptoms and treatment methods to help determine what treatment works best.

By accepting any potential disability realistically and by taking charge of your ailment, you will come to feel that you have, to the best of your ability, mastered your body and your unique circumstances. Over the long term, this can enhance the effectiveness of treatment and the outcome of your disease.

SEXUALLY TRANSMITTED DISEASES

Signs and Symptoms
- Sores, lumps, bumps, or warts on or around the genitals;
- Genital or anal itching;
- Discharge from the vagina, penis, or anus;
- Burning during urination;
- Sore throat;
- Swollen lymph glands;
- Pain in the upper thigh (groin) or lower abdomen;
- Skin rashes, especially on the soles of the feet or palms of the hands.

Sexually transmitted diseases are spread from one person to another during sexual contact. Usually that contact is sexual intercourse, but sometimes it is oral or anal sex or some other sexual activity. These diseases are called STDs for short. An older term is venereal disease (VD). Each type of STD is caused by a different infectious agent. The most common STDs are gonorrhea, chlamydiosis, syphilis, trichomoniasis, and genital herpes. In addition, AIDS is becoming more widespread.

STDs occur most commonly among teenagers and young adults. Part of the reason may be the increase in sexual activity and experimentation in this age group. Unfortunately, most adolescents' decision-making and communication skills are still being developed and do not keep pace with this activity. The lack of adequate sex education may also play a role.

If you are sexually active, you are at some risk of contracting an STD. The more sexual partners you have, the higher your risk of catching one of these diseases.

The Diagnosis.   It is important to note that symptoms do not always accompany STDs.

When no symptoms are present, you and your partner have no reason to believe that anything is wrong, and the infection can easily be passed on. Because of this, if you are a sexually active teenager you should be tested and examined regularly for the common STDs. This step can be part of your routine checkups.

As a first step in determining whether you have an STD, your physician will perform a physical examination, including a pelvic examination (see page 1055) if you are female. The next step is taking samples of your blood, urine, or genital discharge, which can be tested for the presence of either an STD-causing infectious agent or antibodies to such a microbe.

Abstain from sexual contact if your sexual partner tells you that he or she has an STD. If you think you have one, abstain from sexual contact until your STD is cured. Consult a physician immediately. You can visit your own physician, a clinic that specializes in STDs or birth control, or a hospital emergency room. Whatever your choice, your visit will be kept strictly confidential. Do not worry that your parents will be notified. If you do not want them to be, your request will be honored. However, physicians are required by law to report many STDs to state health authorities.

Whenever an STD is diagnosed, it is important for all sexual partners to be examined and treated. Do not feel guilty for revealing the identities of your partner or partners to your physician. Again, this information will be kept confidential.

How Serious Are Sexually Transmitted Diseases? Most STDs can be cured with medications. AIDS, which leads to death, is the exception (see AIDS, page 848). Before effective treatment for syphilis was developed, it was also fatal.

The longer you delay treatment, the more difficult your STD will be to control. Sometimes, STDs are left untreated for so long that they lead to lasting complications. For instance, repeated bouts of pelvic inflammatory disease (see page 1104) can leave a young woman infertile (incapable of having a baby). Teenage girls tend to be at extra risk of complications of STDs.

Treatment. *Medication.* Various antibiotics are available to cure STDs and kill the microbes that cause them.

Prevention. You can avoid contracting an STD by abstaining from sexual activity. If you are sexually active, you can minimize your risk of STDs by being selective about your sexual partners and using a condom. Condoms are relatively effective—although not foolproof—at blocking the spread of infectious agents, including AIDS. Such precautions allow what is termed "safer sex." When used together with a condom, contraceptive foam offers added protection against the spread of STDs (see also Sexually Transmitted Diseases, page 875).

ACNE

Signs and Symptoms
- Numerous pimples, which come and go, appearing as red lumps, whiteheads, or blackheads.

Pimples result from inflammation of the follicles from which your body hair grows. This inflammation is usually caused by over-production of oil (sebum) by the sebaceous gland in each hair follicle. The oil can block the follicle and predispose it to bacterial infection and inflammation. When a pimple is plugged with white pus, it is called a whitehead. If this plug extends to the skin surface and is exposed to air, it turns black and is called a blackhead.

Acne is so common in adolescence that almost all teenagers have it to some degree. Acne usually starts around puberty and disappears by the end of the teenage years. It is somewhat more common in boys than in girls. When girls have acne, it tends to worsen around the time of their menstrual periods. In both boys and girls, it is caused by surges in production of hormones. These hormones (called androgen hormones) occur normally in both sexes, although to different extents. They make the sebaceous glands produce extra oil (see Acne, page 1158).

INFECTIOUS MONONUCLEOSIS

Infectious mononucleosis is caused by the Epstein-Barr virus. The virus can be transmitted by coughing and sneezing, not only by kissing; but it is not highly contagious. Most children between 4 and 15 become infected with the virus. However, their initial infection usually results in only mild symptoms— short-term fever and tiredness. Later in adolescence and young adulthood the virus can cause a prolonged, exhausting illness. Symptoms of infectious mononucleosis include long-term fever, swollen glands, sore throat, and fatigue. Rest is the main treatment (see Infectious Mononucleosis, page 852).

URINARY TRACT INFECTIONS

The most common infection caused by bacteria multiplying in the urinary tract is cystitis, which is inflammation of the bladder. Cystitis occurs often among teenage girls.

It usually results when traces of stool contaminate the urethra, the canal that transports urine from the bladder out of the body. It can be worsened by frequent sexual intercourse, which can irritate the urethra. The symptoms can include urination that is frequent, urgent, and painful, as well as foul-smelling urine and fever (see Cystitis, page 892).

IRON-DEFICIENCY ANEMIA

Iron-deficiency anemia is most common in young children between 6 months and 3 years old. Its prevalence increases again in the teens.

Iron deficiency tends to be more common in males than in females during adolescence, unlike in other age groups, because the male teenager has higher iron and hemoglobin needs as a result of his astounding increase in muscle mass. You can prevent iron deficiency by eating plenty of meat and green vegetables (see Iron-Deficiency Anemia, page 478).

DYSMENORRHEA

Dysmenorrhea, or painful menstruation, tends to be most common in adolescence. As a woman matures—and particularly after pregnancy—the problem usually subsides. At some time, more than half of all teenage girls and young women experience dysmenorrhea (see Dysmenorrhea, page 1063).

MIGRAINE HEADACHES

Migraine headaches are repeated attacks of intense, throbbing head pain lasting at least an hour each. They are often accompanied by nausea, vomiting, loss of appetite, and sensitivity to light. They usually occur for the first time in early adolescence, although they can also appear in young children and in adults. They are more common in girls than in boys, and they tend to run in families (see Migraine Headaches, page 549).

SCOLIOSIS

Scoliosis is a lateral (sideways) curvature of the spine. It is most commonly detected in girls who are 10 to 14 years old. Screening for scoliosis is performed routinely at many schools. Some cases of scoliosis are too slight to need treatment. In other cases treatment is needed with special braces, exercises, or surgery; if untreated, the scoliosis may worsen rapidly and become permanently disabling. If scoliosis is identified before it progresses, bracing and exercises can be started early, and surgery can often be avoided (see Scoliosis, page 994).

EPIPHYSITIS

Epiphysitis is inflammation of an epiphysis, the wide end of a long bone such as the shin bone (tibia), thighbone (femur), or upper arm bone (humerus). The epiphysis is considered distinct from the thin length of the bone, the shaft. Rapid growth, as occurs during adolescence, can place extra stresses on the epiphyses and predispose them to epiphysitis.

The most common type of epiphysitis is Osgood-Schlatter disease, a painful inflammation of the epiphysis of the shin bone. It is caused by overuse in activities that place repeated stress on the top of the shin bone, where the tendon of the kneecap inserts. The major symptom is knee pain, which is worsened by activity and relieved by rest. Treatment involves resting and avoiding activities that place prolonged stress on the flexed knee. These activities include bicycle riding and playing basketball. When growth of the affected bone ends, the pain usually subsides on its own (see Osgood-Schlatter Disease, page 999).

SPORTS INJURIES

Many competitive sports that teenagers pursue in high school can cause injuries. Most sports injuries are minor sprains (injuries to the ligaments) and strains (injuries to the muscles). However, some can cause permanent disability. The more direct physical contact that the sport demands, the higher the risk of serious injury. The sports most often involved are football, wrestling, soccer, and basketball. However, even noncontact sports such as cross-country running, swimming, and tennis carry some risk of injury. Part of the reason for the high rate of sports injuries among adolescents is that individual teenagers vary greatly in their weights, strengths, and stages of development, yet they all play together.

You can minimize your risk of injury by wearing the protective equipment designed for each sport you play and by appropriate physical conditioning. Before you start any organized sports program, get a pretraining physical examination to confirm that the program will be safe for you.

VISION PROBLEMS

The rapid growth of adolescence involves the whole body, including the eyes. Sometimes a teenager's eyes change their shape as well as their size. As a result, problems with vision acuity often develop during adolescence. The most common problem is the development of or worsening of nearsightedness (myopia), which can be corrected by prescription glasses or contact lenses (see Refraction Problems, page 739).

Teenagers are also prone to injury-related vision problems. Most of these problems can be prevented by wearing protective goggles, masks, or other headgear during sports (see Protecting Your Eyes, page 748).

At school, you may be screened for vision problems and hearing disorders. At routine visits, your physician will also check your eyes and ears. If you notice any difficulty seeing or hearing, tell your parents and your physician.

HEARING DISORDERS

Sometimes teenagers develop a permanent high-frequency hearing loss—that is, it becomes more difficult for them to hear sounds that are higher than 4,000 hertz. You can help prevent this hearing disorder by avoiding extended exposure to loud noises such as the sound of loud amplified music, subway trains, and heavy machinery. Such loud sounds can damage your inner ears (see How To Protect Your Ears, page 679).

CHAPTER 6

YOUNG ADULTHOOD

AGES 20 THROUGH 39

CHAPTER CONTENTS

THE TRANSITION YEARS

Becoming an adult is one of life's greatest transitions. The fundamental change from dependency on one's parents—in financial, emotional, and other terms—to independence usually occurs shortly before or after the age of 20.

Part of this change involves the switch from being a student. The world of the student is defined by expanding horizons and new worlds to investigate. Alternatively, having a job implies a wide range of new disciplines and responsibilities.

Working should, of course, offer stimulating challenges and the opportunity for accomplishments. Yet an ex-student who starts work suddenly may face specified hours, the need to master teamwork skills, and a boss whose role is unlike that of any parent or teacher.

For most young Americans, career choices are made in their third decade of life, but that is only one of several major adjustments. Many young adults also come to grips with their sexuality during this period. Relationships are established and some are cemented. For some this may be a time of experimentation with numerous sexual partners, alcohol, or drugs.

For the most part, these years are a time of good health: our bodies change relatively little during the third and fourth decades, and concerns of aging seem some distance in the future. Nevertheless, it is a time to develop good habits: healthful exercise patterns and a good nutritional regimen can help make the passage to middle and later years healthier and happier (see Exercise and Fitness, page 377).

BECOMING A PARENT

Today, many couples delay until the late 20s or 30s the inevitable question of whether to have children (for some, of course, the question is answered earlier). An increasing number of women and men are asking another question: whether to end childbearing years with permanent sterilization.

How does a man or woman maintain sexual and reproductive health? The time to begin is before damage has been done. Be aware of sexually transmitted diseases that could impair your ability to have children (see also page 875). Take the time to practice self-examination, whether it be breast examination by women (see page 1076) or testicle examination by men (see page 1116); the earlier a cancer is found, the better the chance of cure. Also, have medical checkups regularly (see Periodic Medical Examinations: How Often Should I Consult My Physician?, page 1210). For a woman in her childbearing years, a Papanicolaou smear (Pap test) (see page 1096) should be a part of the regular examination.

Prevention of pregnancy is a major concern of many young adults. You can minimize the chances of that happening to you by avoiding intercourse or by practicing birth control. Today, couples have more birth control options than ever before, some of which are more effective for preventing pregnancy than others. This chapter explains the options, risks, and benefits of birth control. It also discusses permanent sterilization techniques for both men and women.

Today, more and more often, couples postpone pregnancy. People marry later. More women than ever before are working, many in fulfilling and demanding careers. Inevitably, though, couples must acknowledge the biological clock. Those in their 30s must realize that if they are to have a child, the years of postponement are nearing an end.

When is the best time in the menstrual cycle to plan intercourse to achieve pregnancy? What happens when the egg and sperm meet? What are the symptoms of pregnancy? These and other concerns are covered in the following pages.

Unfortunately, drug and alcohol abuse are major health and social problems. Some women continue to drink excessively or to use drugs even after they learn they are pregnant, and their infants often pay a price. A section in the chapter discusses the use of alcohol, drugs, and cigarettes during pregnancy.

Although most women are not drug users or alcoholics, many do take prescription drugs, even during pregnancy. Is this safe? In some cases these drugs can harm the developing baby. Never take a medication unless your physician recommends it (make sure any physician you consult knows you are pregnant). A list of some prescription medications known to cause birth defects or other medical problems is included in the chapter.

Most pregnancies are medically uneventful; only a small percentage of women have complications. Complications—such as diabetes, preeclampsia, hypertension, and hemorrhage—are discussed in this chapter. Factors that increase the risk of problems for either you or your baby also are discussed; these include poor diet, advanced age, and the use of alcohol and cigarettes.

Many women wonder what is involved in, and to some extent fear, the culmination of pregnancy. What are the signs of true labor and false labor? What are your pain relief options? What are the indications for a cesarean section and what should you expect if your physician deems it necessary? You will get answers to these questions in the pages that follow.

Finally, the chapter discusses concerns during the postpartum period. These can be trying weeks. A husband who is used to his wife's undivided attention may feel resentful when her energies become consumed by the new family member. The wife may be exhausted and suffering from postpartum depression, a not uncommon affliction. To worsen the situation, the couple must avoid intercourse, so both may feel some sexual frustration. Although time usually resolves these problems, this chapter offers advice on getting through the often difficult postpartum period.

The childbearing decades can be packed full of life. In this chapter you will find much guidance about your overall and reproductive health—and also about the new-life process, from conception to birth.

THE MALE REPRODUCTIVE ORGANS

Unlike the female, whose reproductive abilities usually come to a halt in midlife, the male is capable of fathering a child well into old age.

A man's sperm is produced constantly. Each time a man ejaculates, millions of microscopic spermatozoa are propelled in a pool of semen. Whether or not one will fertilize an egg depends on several factors, including how well the male reproductive system is working.

The following is a description of the components of the male reproductive system.

The *testes* function as a sperm and hormone production center. Each testicle contains coiled tubes, called seminiferous tubules, in which sperm are made. Normally, a male child is born with two testicles. While the fetus is in the uterus, the testicles are located near its kidneys, but they gradually work their way down into the scrotum, the sac-like structure below the penis. Premature infants sometimes are born with an empty scrotum because the testicles have not had time to descend. Full-term infants also may have undescended testes, and treatment with hormones or even an operation may be needed (see Undescended Testicle, page 1118).

Within the testes, the cells whose job it is to make sperm are extremely sensitive to heat. Thus, exposure to excessive heat can interrupt production of sperm.

The *scrotum* protects the testes. It is a highly efficient air conditioner, maintaining the temperature of the testes about 6 degrees below the normal body temperature. When the weather is cold, the scrotum shrinks to maintain heat; in hot weather, it becomes larger and flaccid in order to expose a larger area for heat loss.

A single human *sperm* is made up of a head, containing the nucleus (center) of the cell, a body, and a tail. A sperm is about 1/600th of an inch long. The mechanism that propels the sperm is in the tail. Depending on whether a woman's vaginal mucus is watery or thick, a sperm can swim an inch in 4 to 16 minutes in the vagina.

Semen is the ejaculated fluid that contains the sperm. It is produced by the prostate and the seminal vesicles. The amount of semen depends to some extent on the amount of time between ejaculations. The average amount of semen ejaculated varies from ½ to 1½ teaspoons. The average ejaculation contains a half billion sperm.

The *epididymis* is a long, coiled tube above each testicle through which sperm is propelled by contractions on its way to the *vas deferens,* a tube that runs from the upper scrotum to the seminal vesicles and the urethra at the base of the penis. The vas deferens is the body's warehouse for sperm as well as the conduit that carries the sperm from the epididymis to the urethra. Millions of sperm enter the vas deferens daily.

The *penis* is the organ through which sperm are released into the vagina. Normally, the penis is soft and flexible. However, when a man is sexually aroused, the spongy tissue of the penis becomes engorged with blood because the exit valves of the penile veins close. The result is an erection. The penis becomes firm, expanding in length and circumference.

The *prostate* is a gland surrounding the urethra, the tube through which urine passes from the bladder. The prostate and the seminal vesicles are sources of the semen.

Hormones are chemical messengers produced in various parts of the body. Testosterone, the important masculinizing hormone, is produced within the testicles. It influences body shape, voice, body hair, sexual drive, and the ability to have an erection.

The first step in reproduction is sexual desire (libido), which is regulated by a combination of psychological factors and sexual hormones. When a man is sexually stimulated, an erection occurs. During intercourse, the sexual excitement intensifies to the point of orgasm. It is during orgasm that ejaculation occurs. It begins at the base of the bladder and in the prostate and seminal vesicles. The muscles go through a series of involuntary contractions, resulting in the sudden propulsion of semen through the

From the testes, sperm are moved by contractions through the epididymis and the vas deferens to the seminal vesicles. Fluids are added in the seminal vesicles and prostate gland. Semen is comprised of these fluids and sperm. Following sexual stimulation, the semen is ejaculated at orgasm through the urethra.

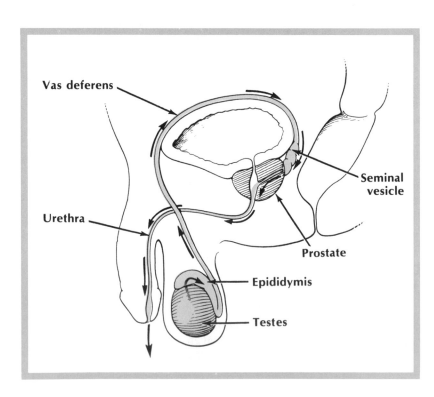

Vas deferens

Urethra

Seminal vesicle

Prostate

Epididymis

Testes

urethra. This fluid traverses the length of the penis and is released into the vagina.

The vagina is flooded with millions of sperm, swimming in all directions in search of an egg. Most never reach the cervical canal but die within the vagina. Of those that make it to the 1-inch cervical canal, most get sidetracked and never go farther. A few reach the uterus and successfully make the 2-inch journey to the openings of the fallopian tubes.

Out of an average of 400 million sperm, only a few reach the fertilization point—midway down the fallopian tube that contains an egg. The sperm that ultimately fertilizes the egg has overcome enormous odds.

SEXUAL FUNCTION

In men, the ability to function sexually depends on psychological, hormonal, neurological, and vascular (blood vessel) factors.

The sexual sequence in the male involves five steps: stimulation, erection, ejaculation, orgasm, and detumescence (loss of erection).

Sexual desire (libido) is governed by hormones and psychological factors. The ability to have an erection is controlled by both the nervous system and the vascular system. Ejaculation is controlled by a part of the nervous system. Orgasm is purely a psychological phenomenon that includes the sensation caused by the ejaculation, and detumescence probably is under the control of the vascular system.

Sometimes problems occur. Some neurological disorders and diseases of the urogenital system directly interfere with sexual performance (see Sexual Problems of Men, page 1127). Many chronic diseases impede a man's ability to perform sexually because of their debilitating effect on overall health. The use of alcohol or other drugs also may impair sexual function.

For a detailed discussion of the most common forms of male sexual dysfunction, see Health Problems of Partners, page 1129.

PREVENTION OF PREGNANCY

Throughout history, men and women have attempted—not always successfully—to prevent pregnancy.

More than 1,500 years ago, the Talmud recommended that couples drink a "cup of roots" to prevent pregnancy. The American Indians brewed a special tea for those who wished to avoid conception. As early as the 16th century, Arabs were inserting crude versions of today's intrauterine device inside their camels to prevent an increase in the herd.

Today, most couples in the United States use some form of birth control.

Two methods of temporary contraception depend primarily on the man: condoms and coitus interruptus; the former is both more effective and more sexually satisfying.

Condoms are used by approximately 10 to 15 percent of all couples practicing birth control. The condom is a thin rubber sheath that the man places over his erect penis just before intercourse. When the man ejaculates, the semen remains inside the condom and is not released into the vagina.

When used correctly, condoms almost always are effective for preventing pregnancy. Moreover, if intact and properly used, condoms help to protect each partner from venereal diseases, AIDS, and infections such as trichomoniasis.

One reason for the popularity of condoms is that they are easy to obtain. Condoms are available without prescription in drugstores and can be purchased in vending machines in some men's restrooms. They are available in various materials, ranging from rubber to animal skin, they come with or without a lubricant, and they are packaged in small and large quantities. Packaged condoms are good for at least 2 years.

If you want to try a condom, make sure that after you unroll the condom down over the penis, you leave room at the tip for the ejaculate. If you are uncircumcised, make sure the foreskin is pulled back before you put on the condom.

After intercourse, the penis should be withdrawn from the vagina, and then the condom is removed and disposed of.

Condom "accidents" can occur during intercourse, usually as a result of rupture. The chance of an accident can be lessened by always allowing extra room at the tip for ejaculate and by using a lubricant on the condom, especially if your partner's vagina seems dry. Finally, the risk of pregnancy when using a condom is reduced further when a spermicide is inserted into the woman's vagina before intercourse.

About ¹⁄₆₀₀th of an inch long, the human sperm is made up of a head, containing the nucleus or center of the cell, a body, and a tail that propels it.

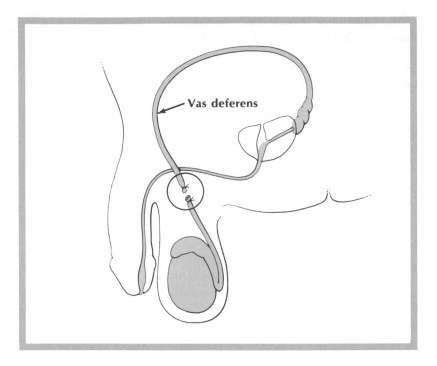

Vas deferens

In performing a vasectomy, the surgeon cuts the vas deferens, thus closing off the path taken by sperm to the outside.

trol, and it is used throughout the world more extensively than any other form of contraception. In the United States, however, fewer than 3 percent of adults use it as their primary method of contraception.

Although some couples have used coitus interruptus effectively, most physicians do not recommend it. Aside from being frustrating for both partners, coitus interruptus requires that the man maintain stringent control. Even the smallest leak of semen into the vagina can result in pregnancy.

A *male birth control pill* has been talked about for years. In fact, some hormonal treatments have been tested and they do render the male temporarily infertile. Unfortunately, they also take away sexual drive and the ability to maintain an erection. Thus, at this time, there is no male birth control pill on the market.

VASECTOMY

The most common complaints associated with condoms are not that they are ineffective but that they dull sensation for the man, thus diminishing sexual pleasure. Some couples also complain that spontaneity is lost.

Coitus interruptus is the withdrawal of the penis from the vagina before orgasm. It is probably the oldest method of birth con-

At some point, many couples decide that they do not want any more children. For these couples, permanent sterilization may be the answer.

Many couples opt for male sterilization simply because the procedure is less physically traumatic, is less expensive, and involves less time away from work and home than does the counterpart for women, tubal ligation (see page 179). Vasectomy is a relatively simple operation that can be done in a urologist's office or in an outpatient surgical setting.

Vasectomy involves cutting and sealing the vas deferens, the tube that carries sperm to the urethra in the penis. The procedure in no way interferes with a man's ability to maintain an erection or reach orgasm. Nor does it impede the production of male hormones or of sperm in the testicles. The only change is that the sperm's link to the outside has been severed permanently. After a vasectomy, you continue to ejaculate about the same amount of semen because sperm account for only a small part of the ejaculate.

If you have a vasectomy, you will be given an injection of anesthetic in the scrotum to numb the area so you will not feel pain. After your physician has located the vas deferens, a pair of small cuts are made in the skin of the scrotum. Each vas deferens is then pulled through the opening until it forms a loop. Approximately a half inch is cut out of

REVERSING A VASECTOMY: THE VASOVASECTOMY

Always consider a vasectomy as permanent sterilization.

However, circumstances do change. Maybe your financial situation suddenly has taken a turn for the better and you and your partner decide you want another child. Or perhaps you are widowed or divorced and on remarriage you and your spouse want a child.

It is possible to reattach the vas deferens once it has been severed. Unlike the initial operation, however, the vasovasectomy requires the skill of a

surgeon trained to work under the magnification of a powerful microscope. Moreover, this is not an office procedure but requires 2 to 3 days in the hospital.

Approximately 80 to 90 percent of men who have their vasectomies reversed do ejaculate sperm. However, only 30 to 40 percent father children after the reversal. The reason for this discrepancy may be that as a result of vasectomy many men develop antibodies that fight their sperm.

Consult your family physician or urologist for referral to a surgeon experienced in this procedure.

each vas deferens and removed. The two ends of each vas deferens are closed by stitches and are placed back in the scrotum. The incisions are closed with stitches.

The operation takes approximately 20 minutes, after which you will be asked to stay for an hour for observation. After a vasectomy, refrain from any strenuous activity for at least 48 hours. However, if your work does not involve hard physical labor, you can return to your job as soon as you feel like it. The stitches generally are of a type that dissolves in 7 to 10 days.

You may notice some swelling and discomfort in the scrotum for a few days. However, if the pain persists for more than a few days or becomes severe or if fever develops, call your physician.

The failure rate for a vasectomy is less than 1 percent. But your vasectomy is no immediate guarantee against pregnancy be-

---

SELF-EXAMINATION

Many diseases of the male genitals—cancer being the most serious—when detected early, have an excellent cure rate. Therefore, all men should examine their genitals routinely for any suspicious changes.

For a detailed discussion of Self-Examination of the Testicles, see page 1116.

---

cause of the sperm stored above the point where the vas deferens was tied. Thus, your physician will want to test your ejaculate for sperm. Generally, in most men the semen becomes sperm-free after 8 to 10 ejaculations following the vasectomy. Until your physician has determined that your ejaculate does not contain sperm, you should continue to use contraception.

THE WOMAN OF CHILDBEARING AGE

If you are a woman between the ages of 20 and 39, many of your health concerns are related to sexual and reproductive health.

THE REPRODUCTIVE SYSTEM

The organs of the female reproductive system are the two ovaries, the fallopian tubes, and the uterus. The vagina is a tubular structure that extends from the lower portion of the uterus (the cervix) to the external genitalia.

The *ovaries* are situated in the lower part of the abdomen and produce and store eggs and also feminizing hormones. While it is still in the uterus, the female fetus contains hundreds of thousands of eggs, many of which disappear before birth. Later, some of the eggs are surrounded by cells that begin to form a capsule (follicle) around individual eggs. As a girl reaches puberty, a substance called follicle-stimulating hormone (FSH) is secreted by the pituitary gland. As a result, fluid develops within some follicles. Some grow fat and bulge; others shrivel and die. Every month after puberty, one or sometimes two of these fluid-filled follicles (graafian follicles) grow larger until another pituitary substance called luteinizing hor-

mone (LH) stimulates the follicle, which then bursts through the surface of the ovary into the pelvic cavity and eventually enters the fallopian tube. This process is called ovulation.

The *fallopian tubes* are two thin 5-inch-long tubes that lead from near the ovaries to the uterus. It is within a fallopian tube that

Every month, one of the eggs present at birth in the ovary is released during ovulation. The egg travels down the fallopian tube, where fertilization may occur. The fertilized egg implants itself in the lining of the uterus. If fertilization does not occur, the egg, along with the lining of the uterus, is shed during menstruation.

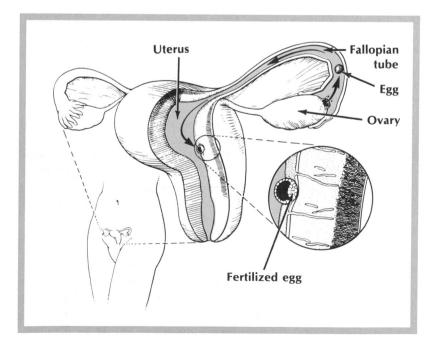

Uterus

Fallopian tube

Egg

Ovary

Fertilized egg

fertilization occurs. In any given cycle, ovulation occurs from only one ovary.

The *uterus* is a pear-shaped muscular organ. The uterus receives the egg after its journey down the fallopian tube. If the egg has been fertilized, it implants itself within the wall of the uterus and begins to grow into a baby. If it is not fertilized, the egg and the lining of the uterus are shed, the result of which is menstruation.

Reproduction depends on several factors.

Timing is critical. To result in pregnancy, intercourse must take place within the 72 hours before the egg enters the tube or within the 24 hours after it enters the tube. A sperm cell is capable of fertilizing an egg for only 72 hours after ejaculation, and an unfertilized egg survives for only about 24 hours after its release from the ovary. Your best chance of becoming pregnant is on the 13th or 14th day preceding the onset of your period.

Even perfect timing, however, does not guarantee a pregnancy. Healthy male and female reproductive systems are necessary. In a woman, irregular ovulation patterns hinder the chance of fertilization. Moreover, the fallopian tubes must be open and receptive to the egg and sperm. Women whose tubes contain scar tissue may require an operation to achieve pregnancy. Another factor that can inhibit the chance of pregnancy is cervical mucus. If a woman's mucus is too acidic, the vaginal environment may be hostile to sperm, which thrive in alkaline surroundings.

Finally, a man must produce not only an adequate number of sperm but the sperm must be healthy (see Infertility, page 1131).

COMMON CONCERNS

Questions that often are asked concerning reproductive health include the following: How often should I have a pelvic examination? What is the correct way to perform a self-examination of my breasts? How safe is the birth control pill if I smoke and am over 35 years old? What are the risks of permanent sterilization? If I do not have orgasms, do I have a sexual problem?

The following section addresses some of these concerns, including ways in which you can spot potential health problems, the benefits of exercise for every woman, common breast problems, and family planning.

For detailed discussions of the most common forms of female sexual dysfunction, see Health Problems of Partners, page 1129.

SEXUAL AND REPRODUCTIVE HEALTH

Most women ages 20 through 39 are basically healthy. Thus, the major thrust of health care for this age group is prevention rather than treatment.

You can play an active role in helping to ensure your future sexual and reproductive health. This is not to imply that serious diseases of the reproductive organs do not occur in women who take good care of themselves. Unfortunately, they do. However, you can reduce the likelihood of a serious problem or at least discover the problem in its early stages, when it is more easily treated, by following a few simple rules.

1. Beginning at age 18 years, every woman should have a yearly pelvic examination (see page 1055). For sexually active teenagers, annual pelvic examinations should start earlier. The examination may be part of a routine examination by your internist, family physician, or gynecologist. (See also Selecting a Gynecologist, page 1056.)

   The pelvic examination is important in that any abnormalities such as cysts, tumors, and infections, or problems such as muscle weakness that cause the uterus or vagina to sag, can be detected. If you have a suspicious discharge, your physician can obtain a sample of the material to be analyzed to identify the cause. (See also The Pelvic Examination, page 1055.)

2. An important part of the pelvic examination is the Papanicolaou (Pap) smear. This simple and painless test is done by removing a few cells from your cervix with a spatula, brush, or swab. The Pap test is used to detect cervical cancer, a disease that occurs more often in women older than 40 years. It is also useful for detecting precancerous conditions.

   Starting at age 18 years (earlier if the teenager is sexually active), every woman should have a Pap test at least every 3 years. Because it is inexpensive and painless, many physicians recommend a yearly Pap test. (See also The Pap Smear, page 1096.)

3. Examine your breasts monthly. This enables you to become acquainted with the topography of each breast so that you will be able to detect any change, lump, bump, or thickening.

   Remember, the sooner breast cancer is discovered, the better your chance of cure. Ninety percent of breast masses are found by women, either accidentally or during self-examination. (See also Breast Self-Examination, page 1076.)

4. Mammography is an x-ray study of the breasts that can detect tumors long before they are large enough to be felt.

   There is debate over who should have mammography. In general, women older than 50 years who have no symptoms should have it annually. For women thought to be at high risk of developing breast cancer (those with prior breast cancer or whose mother or sister had the disease), annual mammography is recommended after age 40 years. If you are between the ages of 40 and 50 years and have no family history of breast cancer, have mammography every 2 years. (See also Mammograms, page 1080.)

5. Today, many women are postponing pregnancy well into their 30s and even 40s, only to discover that they cannot get pregnant. A frequent cause of female infertility is pelvic inflammatory disease, a condition that ultimately can scar the fallopian tubes. This disease usually occurs when bacteria—often those that cause gonorrhea—are introduced into the vagina during intercourse. It occasionally may occur after abortion, miscarriage, or insertion of an intrauterine device.

   This disease most often is found in young, sexually active women. Thus, particularly if you have multiple sex partners, be aware of the risks.

The use of condoms is generally effective for preventing pelvic inflammatory disease, venereal diseases such as herpes, syphilis, and gonorrhea, and AIDS because bacteria or viruses are not allowed to pass from one partner to the other.

If you have pelvic pain, tenderness in your lower abdomen, fever, or an unpleasant-smelling vaginal discharge, you may have pelvic inflammatory disease. See your physician immediately. Early treatment with antibiotics is necessary to minimize damage to your fallopian tubes (see Pelvic Inflammatory Disease, page 1104, and Toxic Shock Syndrome, page 1061).

BREAST DISORDERS

The female breasts are often the site of various disorders, ranging from annoying to fatal. You have access to your breasts, unlike your internal organs. You can see them, feel them, and notice change. Thus, the importance of monthly self-examination cannot be emphasized enough.

Until puberty, the female breasts are basically the same as the breasts of a boy. At some point—usually between the ages of 9 and 13—female hormones are released by the hypothalamus, pituitary, ovaries, and adrenal glands in increasing amounts, the result of which is increased female hormone concentration and the beginning of breast development. Often, this is the first concrete sign that a girl is approaching puberty.

A woman's breast is made up of as many as 20 groups of milk-producing glands housed in fatty tissue. Each gland group contains a milk duct that runs to the nipple. Surrounding the nipple is a dark area (areola).

For a detailed discussion of Problems of the Breast, see page 1072.

PREGNANCY PREVENTION AND FAMILY PLANNING

A healthy woman who becomes sexually active in her teens and uses no birth control whatsoever may have 30 to 35 years of reproductive life. Today, thanks to several effective contraceptive methods, women can choose whether they want to become mothers and, if so, when. Popular birth control methods that depend primarily on the woman are described below (for the options for men, see Prevention of Pregnancy, page 171).

Natural family planning encompasses several methods that rely on a woman's menstrual cycle to determine what days are safe for intercourse. They are variations of the so-called rhythm method.

Each of the approaches in natural family planning involves a conscientious awareness of when you can become pregnant, which is but a brief span approximately in the middle of each menstrual cycle—from about 72 hours before ovulation to about 24 hours after ovulation. The key is to determine when these days are and then to avoid having intercourse during that time.

Overall, these methods are less than 80 percent effective for preventing pregnancy. Predicting ovulation is often difficult because a woman's cycle may vary. If you decide to try natural family planning, keep records for several months to establish a pattern for your cycle. There are four ways to calculate the time of ovulation: the temperature method, the calendar method, the mucus inspection method, and the mucothermal method.

The temperature method involves determining when you have ovulated. Most women have a slight rise in body temperature just after ovulation. To detect a temperature change, take your temperature every day when you wake up. A special thermometer designed to record small changes is used. Once you have determined your time of ovulation, refrain from intercourse for 3 days before ovulation and 3 days after to avoid pregnancy.

For the calendar method, you need to keep a record of your cycle for a year. Subtract 18 days from the number of days in the shortest cycle (14 days from ovulation to your period, and 4 days for the average life of sperm) and 10 days from the longest cycle (14 days from ovulation to your period, minus 1 day for the lifespan of an egg, and minus 3 days for a margin of error). The numbers you calculate are the first and last days of your cycle during which you can become pregnant.

For example, if your shortest cycle is 24 days and the longest is 35 days, then the time during which you can become pregnant is between 24 days minus 18 days (or the 6th day) and 35 days minus 10 days (or the 25th day). Thus, in this example, during the 6th through the 25th days of each cycle you could become pregnant.

The mucus inspection method depends on the fact that about 4 days before the release of an egg, your vaginal mucus becomes thin, clear, runnier, and profuse. To prevent pregnancy, avoid intercourse from the time the mucus appears until 4 days after it becomes thicker and drier.

The mucothermal method is a combination of the temperature method and mucus

inspection. It is the most reliable natural method.

Birth control pills are used by one out of every four American women younger than 45 years. The pill is the most effective method of contraception. *If used correctly,* only 1 out of 1,000 women on the pill should become pregnant per year.

The most commonly prescribed pill, and the most effective, is a combination of synthetic estrogen and progestogen; its actions are the same as the two naturally occurring hormones produced by the body. Some women take the so-called mini-pill, which contains only progestogen. Although less effective than the combination pill, it is believed to be marginally safer for women older than 35 years and for those with problems such as hypertension and diabetes.

Birth control pills work by preventing the hypothalamus (a gland in the brain) from instructing the pituitary gland to mobilize follicle-stimulating hormone and luteinizing hormone. If these hormones are suppressed, you simply do not release an egg.

Moreover, the pill also prevents the cervical mucus from becoming watery, as it normally does during ovulation. Instead, the mucus for the entire cycle is scant, making it difficult for sperm to reach the fallopian tubes.

The pill does not suppress menstruation, but the flow is generally not as heavy (in some women the flow may be so light they wonder whether they are even having a period) and does not last for as many days as normal menstruation. Most women on the pill do not experience cramps before and during the menses.

If you want to begin taking the pill, you will need a prescription from your physician. Begin taking the pill on the fifth day of your period. Get in the habit of taking your pill at the same time every day to lessen the chance that you will forget to take one. You continue to take a pill for 21 days, after which you do not take one for 7 days. About 3 days after you take the last pill, your period will start. (Note, however, that some prescriptions come in packages with 21 pills that contain hormones and 7 pills that have no active ingredient; thus, the daily pattern of taking a pill is not interrupted. You simply finish one package and start another the following day.) Sometimes a woman will not have a period. If this happens to you, simply begin your new pills 1 week after you finish the previous pack. If you miss a second period, consult your physician.

Even though birth control pills are effective and easy to use, they have some side effects, most of which are minor. Weight gain, nausea, vomiting, and a sense of fullness in the breasts and pelvis may occur. Some women also have spotting or breakthrough bleeding.

The most serious side effect is a tendency to develop blood clots in the veins, which can be fatal if they dislodge and travel to the lungs. The incidence of blood clots is slightly higher in women who take the pill than in those who do not. Those who take pills high in estrogen seem to be at the most risk.

In addition, a small percentage of women who take the pill develop significant high blood pressure. Strokes and heart attacks that are due to the pill are rare, as are gallbladder problems.

Smoking increases the risk of many of these side effects, especially for women older than 35 years.

The pill does not seem to increase the incidence of cancer in the reproductive organs. In fact, there is good evidence that oral contraceptives may decrease the risk of ovarian and endometrial cancer. In addition, the pill is beneficial for reducing the risk of ovarian and breast cysts, the anemia that results from excessive menstrual flow, and the incidence of rheumatoid arthritis and pelvic infections. Whether the pill increases your chance of breast cancer has not been determined.

How do you know whether the pill is safe for you? It probably is safe if you are younger than 40 and a nonsmoker. If you smoke, you probably should not use the pill after age 35 years. Women who have had certain forms of blood vessel disease, heart problems, or some types of cancer should find another method of birth control. If you have migraine headaches, hypertension, sickle cell anemia, or diabetes, or if you are about to undergo operation, the pill may increase your risk of complications. You and your physician must weigh the risks. In general, the risks of the pill are significantly less than the risk of pregnancy itself.

Intrauterine devices (IUDs) are 95 to 98 percent effective for preventing pregnancy.

The IUD is a small piece of plastic inserted into your uterus by your physician, usually during your menstrual period when the cervix is more open. The device has a small string hanging from it. The string makes it easy for the physician to remove the device. Also, the wearer can use the string to make sure the IUD is in place.

The IUD prevents pregnancy by creating changes in the lining of the uterus that make it difficult for a fertilized egg to implant and grow.

The most common side effects of an IUD are increased bleeding during your period and increased menstrual pain. Sometimes the device can be expelled during a menstrual period, so it is important that you periodically check the string to make sure the device is still in place.

The most serious side effects are pelvic infection and ectopic or tubal pregnancy (see page 202). Severe pelvic infection can render a woman sterile.

Today, most manufacturers have suspended production of IUDs because of the proliferation of lawsuits by women who developed severe infection or uterine perforations as a result of using the device.

Most physicians no longer recommend the IUD unless a woman already has been using one and has had no problems with it.

Barrier methods of contraception block the sperm from access to the egg. There are both physical barriers, such as the diaphragm, vaginal sponge, and cervical cap, and chemical barriers (spermicides) in the form of creams, jellies, foams, and suppositories. The effectiveness of these methods is enhanced greatly when a physical barrier is used with a spermicide.

The *diaphragm* is the most effective barrier method for women and has a success rate of 98.5 percent when used consistently and correctly. The diaphragm always should be used in conjunction with a spermicide.

Developed more than 100 years ago, the diaphragm is a rubber cap that is inserted into the vagina to cover the cervix. If you want to use a diaphragm, you must see your physician to be fitted for one. Proper fit is essential because the diaphragm must cover the entire cervical opening to be effective. If you gain or lose a large amount of weight, you may require a diaphragm of a different size.

Before intercourse, insert your diaphragm with about a teaspoon of spermicidal cream or jelly, spread around the edge and in the

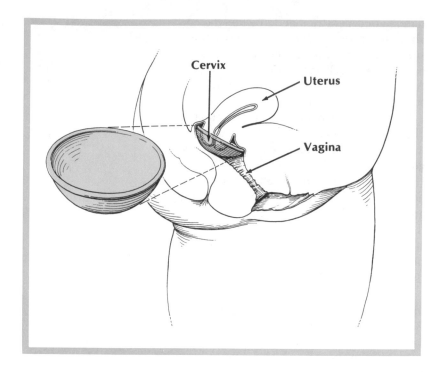

Cervix

Uterus

Vagina

The contraceptive device known as a diaphragm is a rubber cap that is inserted into the vagina to cover the cervix, which is the opening to the uterus.

center of the device. After intercourse, wait at least 6 hours to remove the diaphragm. If you have intercourse again within the 6 hours, you must apply more spermicide.

Clean your diaphragm with soap and water. Periodically check for holes or thinning; if either occurs, you need a new diaphragm.

There are no side effects unless you are allergic to spermicide. The most common complaint is that having to interrupt sex to insert a diaphragm interferes with enjoyment.

The *vaginal sponge* is the newest barrier method available and is less effective than the diaphragm. Unlike the diaphragm, it is available without a prescription and does not require a special fitting.

The sponge is inserted deep into the vagina, much like the diaphragm. The significant difference is that the sponge contains spermicide that is released continually for 24 hours. During that time, you can have repeated intercourse without worrying about adding more spermicide. After intercourse, the sponge must remain in the vagina for 6 hours before removal.

The *cervical cap,* a plastic cap designed to fit snugly over the cervix, is similar to the diaphragm in that it must be fitted by a physician. Unlike the diaphragm, however, the cap is difficult for many women to insert because it needs to be placed deeply within the vagina. Thus, the tendency is to leave

the cap in for extended periods. Many physicians, however, recommend against this because it can become a breeding ground for toxin-producing bacteria.

The cervical cap is about 85 percent effective for preventing pregnancy, a rate far below that with the diaphragm or vaginal sponge.

SEXUAL DYSFUNCTION

If you find sexual intercourse either painful or uncomfortable, if you do not become sexually aroused even when your partner is patient and loving, or if you cannot achieve orgasm, you may have a sexual dysfunction.

Sexual dysfunction is not uncommon among either sex. Do not feel embarrassed or ashamed to seek professional help.

The cause of a woman's inability to respond sexually may be organic (that is, there is a physical reason for the dysfunction). For example, diseases such as diabetes and multiple sclerosis cause nerve damage, which may prevent you from becoming sexually aroused. Similarly, pelvic infections or endometriosis (see pages 1104 and 1101) can make intercourse painful.

The more common cause of sexual dysfunction, however, is psychological. Traumatic events such as rape or incest, the perception that sex is "dirty" and not to be enjoyed, guilt over sexual enjoyment, a poor self-image after a hysterectomy or mastectomy, depression, chronic fatigue, and marital problems all can cause sexual problems.

To understand how sexual problems occur, you need to understand how the normal woman responds to a sexually exciting situation. When you are sexually aroused, the glands in your vagina secrete a lubricant to facilitate entry of the penis. For this to take place, your vaginal tissues must be functioning properly and there must be adequate sexual stimuli. The next stage of sexual response is known as orgasm. This is a series of involuntary contractions of the muscles of the pelvis and is controlled by a specific part of your nervous system. For orgasm to occur, the clitoris generally must be stimulated, either directly or indirectly.

Sexual dysfunction can occur at any point during intercourse. The following are the types of sexual dysfunction that can occur in women.

Painful intercourse (dyspareunia) can be due to psychological or physical causes (see Vaginal Pain, page 1088).

A rare cause of painful intercourse is vaginismus. If you have vaginismus, the natural lubrication of your vagina is not activated when you are sexually aroused. At the same time, the muscles surrounding the entrance to the vagina contract, making intercourse difficult if not impossible.

The cause of vaginismus may be psychological, perhaps as a response to a traumatic sexual experience. If you have vaginismus, consult a physician or therapist trained in treating sexual disorders. Treatment often combines marital counseling with progressive vaginal dilation. Your physician or therapist will prescribe several tubes or dilators of various sizes. You begin by inserting the smallest into your vagina. Once you can tolerate that one without pain, you insert the next size and so on until you can insert a penis-size dilator without pain.

Infections of the vagina and vulva can make intercourse painful. Genital herpes, cysts, rashes, or allergic reactions make the vulva extremely tender and unable to tolerate the friction during intercourse. A bladder infection (cystitis) or an infection in your urethra (urethritis) also can make intercourse uncomfortable (see pages 1109 and 1108). Diseases of the reproductive organs (such as pelvic inflammatory disease, see page 1104, or endometriosis, page 1101) can make intercourse painful, especially when your partner thrusts deeply. Occasionally you may notice blood after intercourse (postcoital bleeding). This can result from a lack of lubrication in your vagina. See your physician in order to eliminate other causes.

These causes of painful intercourse are treatable. When the medical problem is eliminated, so is the pain during intercourse. (See also Sensation Disorders in Women, page 1138.)

The lack of a sexual response may be a psychological problem, although it can occur after a disease or as a result of medications. The blame may rest with a selfish and unresponsive partner, a faltering marriage, or other stressful situations.

However, if you are in a loving relationship with a caring partner who takes the time to stimulate the sensitive areas of your body before intercourse and you still cannot respond, you may want to explore emotional or psychological factors.

Often the cause for a lack of sexual response is unknown. Identifiable causes may include guilt, an inner conflict over sexuality, fear, anxiety, or shame, any of which can block a woman's sexual response.

If you are concerned about being sexually unresponsive, seek help. Often a combination of psychotherapy with a psychiatrist or psychologist and sex therapy can alleviate the problem. (See also Desire Disorders in Women, page 1137.)

Failure to reach orgasm differs from a lack of sexual responsiveness in that a woman remains sexually responsive. The vagina is lubricated and ready for intercourse and lovemaking is enjoyable.

Sometimes a woman's failure to achieve orgasm can be resolved by a frank discussion with her partner. More foreplay, a change in positions during intercourse, or physical stimulation of the clitoris may help.

Occasionally, however, the problem requires therapy. Your physician may suggest sexual exercises that can be done at home with your partner. These, together with psychotherapy, can be beneficial. (See also Orgasm Disorders in Women, page 1139.)

STERILIZATION OPERATIONS

Sterilization in the female is accomplished by interrupting the fallopian tubes so that the egg cannot travel down the tubes and the sperm cannot move upward. Hence, contact between egg and sperm is avoided.

Female sterilization—tubal ligation—is highly effective for preventing pregnancy. Of 100 women who have the operation, 99 will not get pregnant.

Many women opt to be sterilized immediately or shortly after giving birth. This is a good time for a tubal ligation because the abdominal wall is relaxed and the top of the uterus is near the navel, the entry point of operation. Minimal anesthesia is usually all that is necessary, and the procedure does not alter the duration of the postpartum hospital stay. When the abdomen is open for a cesarean birth, a tubal ligation can be performed in a matter of minutes.

The most common method of sterilization is tubal ligation. This procedure can be done in a hospital or in an outpatient clinic. It can be done with a general anesthetic (which means you will be asleep), or a local anesthetic can be injected into the operative site.

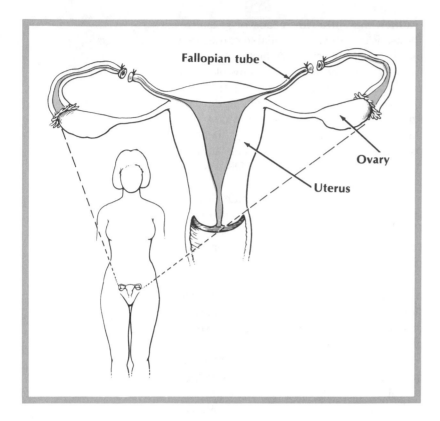

Fallopian tube

Ovary

Uterus

In performing a tubal ligation, the most common surgical procedure to sterilize a female, the paths normally taken by eggs is interrupted by cutting and sealing off the fallopian tubes.

If you choose to have a local anesthetic, you will be given medications to relax you but you will remain awake.

A small incision will be made in the skin near your navel. A harmless gas will then be pumped into your abdomen to distend it so the abdominal wall is away from your internal organs. A thin, telescope-like instrument (laparoscope) is then inserted into the opening, allowing your physician to see your reproductive organs clearly. The physician then inserts a small instrument either through the original incision or through a second tiny opening. Using this instrument, the physician then seals the tubes by using an electric current, a clip, or a band. The gas in the abdomen is then released, and the small incisions are closed with a couple of stitches (see page 1297).

Most women go home either the same day or the next day.

After the procedure you may have some abdominal pain for a few days. Dizziness, fatigue, nausea, and bloating are not uncommon. Most women resume their normal schedules within a few days.

About 1 in 1,000 women will have a serious problem after sterilization. Infection, bowel injuries, bleeding, burns (when the tubes are cauterized), and complications from the anesthesia occasionally occur.

Unlike male sterilization, tubal ligation is immediately effective for preventing pregnancy.

Some women who have been sterilized later decide they want to become pregnant. Operation to reverse the tubal ligation can be done, but fewer than half of the women who have reversal procedures bear a child. Moreover, the risk of an ectopic pregnancy is increased (see page 202). For these reasons, physicians stress that before you undergo sterilization be very sure that you do not want to become pregnant.

PREPARATION FOR PREGNANCY

Before attempting to become pregnant, see your physician for a thorough physical examination. This is important because many conditions that are initially without symptoms can complicate pregnancy. Diabetes, high blood pressure, pelvic tumors, and anemia are just a few common conditions that can be detected easily during a physical examination. If your physician discovers a health problem, in most cases it does not mean you cannot have a child. But you will want to have the disease under control before attempting pregnancy. Some pregnant women with chronic diseases such as diabetes may be best cared for by an obstetrician who specializes in high-risk situations.

A particular disease or genetic abnormality may run in your family. Or you may be older than 35 years, considering a first pregnancy, and worried about the possibility of having a child with Down syndrome or another birth defect. This is a good time to inquire about genetic counseling. A frank discussion with an expert can provide helpful information about your chances of having a healthy baby (see page 45).

Once your physician determines you are healthy, you may want to examine your lifestyle before giving up contraception. If you are overweight and want to reduce, do it before you become pregnant. Pregnancy is not the time to begin a diet.

Moreover, if you are a cigarette smoker, quit smoking or, at the very least, drastically cut down before you attempt pregnancy. Women who smoke during pregnancy tend to have babies of lower birth weight than nonsmokers, and these babies may have developmental problems. In addition, smokers have a higher incidence of miscarriages and stillbirths. For help quitting smoking, see page 412.

If you take drugs, prescription or otherwise, stop using them before you try to become pregnant. If you need a particular medication for a health problem, inform your physician of your plans. He or she will know whether the medication could be harmful and if there is a safer drug that can be substituted.

Avoid alcohol during pregnancy, although infrequent small amounts probably are not harmful.

If you have difficulty becoming pregnant, you or your partner may have a fertility problem.

For a detailed discussion of Infertility, see page 1131.

CONCERNS DURING PREGNANCY

Pregnancy is a natural condition for which your body was constructed. Most women come through pregnancy and birth uneventfully. Occasionally, however, there are complications.

This section discusses many of these problems. Some are concerns such as morning sickness, heartburn, and backache that make you uncomfortable but generally do not threaten your or your developing baby's health. Problems such as diabetes and hemorrhage are more serious and can have dire consequences for mother or child.

Also covered in this section are ways in which you can help ensure that you and your baby are healthy during pregnancy, the most important being regular visits to your physician, a proper diet, and the elimination of potentially harmful substances such as cigarettes, alcohol, and drugs.

Today, most obstetricians or family physicians who deliver babies would think something was wrong if you did not ask questions—lots of them. You and your partner are expected to be active participants in your pregnancy and the birth of your baby.

FERTILIZATION

The process of fertilization begins with the penetration of the female egg by a single male sperm, one out of the hundreds of millions that traveled up the female reproductive system.

It is not completely understood how the minute sperm penetrates the firm capsule (zona pellucida) of the egg. Swimming in an indirect path, the sperm attacks the egg with the side of its head. Several sperm may begin to enter the outer egg capsule, but ultimately only one will enter the egg itself. Approximately 266 days later, a baby will be born.

The egg and the sperm each bring to the union 23 chromosomes containing thousands of genes. This produces a new individual with 46 chromosomes, the correct number for a human being. It is this genetic material that determines sex, physical characteristics such as eye, hair, and skin color, body size and type, facial features, creativity, and, to a large extent, intellectual capabilities and even personality. After the sperm penetrates to the center of the egg, sperm and egg merge to become a one-cell embryo (zygote) and fertilization is complete.

Multiple births result either from the fertilization of two or more eggs or from a single egg being fertilized and then splitting to form two or more embryos.

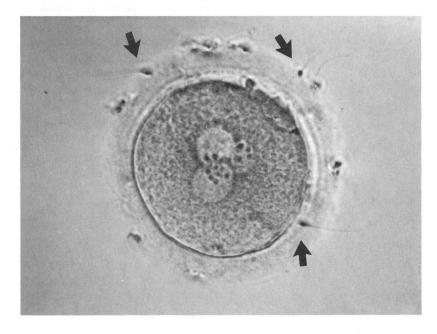

Recently fertilized ovum in early stages of cell division. Arrows reveal sperm that entered the capsule but did not penetrate the egg.

The next step in the process is cell division. Within 12 hours, the new cell has divided into two cells, which then become four cells, and so on, with the number of cells doubling every 12 hours.

The new egg continues to make its way slowly down the fallopian tube to the uterus, regularly doubling its cell number and becoming not larger but more complex. Within 4 to 5 days after fertilization, the egg, by this time made up of 500 cells, reaches its destination inside the uterus.

By the time the egg reaches the uterus, it has changed considerably from a solid mass of cells to a group of cells arranged around a fluid-filled cavity. This is called a blastocyst. One section of the blastocyst contains a compact mass of cells that will ultimately produce an embryo. The outer layer of cells, called the trophoblast, will produce the placenta, which provides nourishment.

While all this has been taking place, the rest of the female reproductive system has not been idle. The ovaries have been secreting the hormone progesterone into the bloodstream. The result of this hormonal surge is a uterine lining that is swollen with blood, the perfect environment for implantation to take place.

Initially the egg does not dig deeply into the uterus. It clings to the surface of the uterus for a few days. Then the egg releases an enzyme that eats away at the lining of the uterus, allowing the egg to drop deeper into the lining, where it is surrounded by a pool of the mother's blood. Eight days have passed since fertilization took place. By the 12th day, the egg will be firmly embedded in its new home.

At this point, you are pregnant, although it is too early for you to have missed a period or to have any other symptoms of pregnancy. In the initial days and weeks after fertilization, miscarriage is common, often before a woman knows she was pregnant. In fact, an estimated 50 percent of fertilizations end in miscarriage.

PRENATAL DEVELOPMENT

The average time from fertilization to the birth of a baby is 266 days. Compared with the duration of gestation in most other species, that might seem an incredibly long time; when you consider the magnitude of this creation, it is a wonder it does not take longer.

It is difficult to comprehend how something as complex as a human being can emerge from a single cell. What is equally perplexing is the seemingly effortless development of this microscopic speck. Every aspect of this process, from the creation of the smallest fingernail to the brain itself, is set into an exquisitely scripted timetable that rarely falters. If it does, the result can be a miscarriage or a birth defect.

The following is an overview of the development process during the three trimesters of pregnancy. The two methods used to measure the duration of pregnancy are gestational age and fertilization age.

Gestational age is measured from the first day of your last menstrual period, which is about 2 weeks before actual fertilization. Thus, a pregnancy calculated by this method is about 280 days (9.3 months). Fertilization age is measured from the time of fertilization. Thus, the duration of pregnancy calculated with this method is 2 weeks shorter than with the other method.

Usually, obstetricians or family physicians calculate the duration of your pregnancy on the basis of gestational age, so this section will also.

The First Trimester. The first 3 months of fetal development are in many ways the most important. During this time, all the major organs in the body are formed. By the end of this period your baby is not more than 3 inches long and weighs little more than 1 ounce.

The time from fertilization of the sperm and egg to implantation in the uterus is about 5 to 7 days. After burrowing deep within the uterus, the egg begins to grow, doubling in size every day. By now, the placenta has begun to form. In another week, the rudiments of a spinal cord are evident and, within days, five to eight vertebrae are in place. In addition, the eyes and heart have begun to form.

It is during the third week after fertilization that the embryonic period begins. Before this, the products of conception are referred to as an ovum. This is about the time that an expected period does not happen. If you have a pregnancy test, the results probably will be positive.

Over the next few weeks the components of a human being develop, although at first the human baby is similar in appearance to the developing babies of some other mammals. The head begins to form, as does the intestinal tract.

At the end of the sixth week the brain becomes more noticeable, and arm and leg buds begin to appear. Cells that will later become either an ovary or testes have appeared.

By the seventh week, the chest and abdomen are fully formed and the lungs are beginning to develop. The embryo measures slightly more than one-half inch and weighs a fraction of an ounce.

Your baby's face and features are forming in the eighth gestational week. Fingers and toes are beginning to develop, as is the ovary or testis. If the embryo is a male, his penis begins to appear at this time.

At the end of the second month of pregnancy, your baby looks like a human infant, albeit in miniature.

By the 10th week, your baby's face, with the exception of the jaws, is very developed. The heart has four chambers and beats at 120 to 160 beats per minute. At this point, the embryo is considered a fetus.

By the end of the first trimester, the fetus has a head that is disproportionately large compared with the rest of its body.

PREGNANCY TESTS

The earliest way to know for sure whether you are pregnant is to have a pregnancy test.

The fertilized egg at 4 days old begins to secrete a hormone called human chorionic gonadotropin (hCG). This hormone spreads in body water to the body's tissues. Initially it can be detected in the blood, and shortly thereafter it is detected in the urine.

Most pregnancy tests are conducted with a sample of urine, which is obtained more easily than a sample of blood.

Many types of urine tests are used to detect the presence of hCG. Most depend on a reaction between the hCG and an anti-hCG antibody. A second reaction is then needed to determine whether the first reaction has taken place. Often that is a color change.

Some women use home pregnancy tests. These testing kits can be purchased at most drugstores and other retail outlets. Most contain a solution that is mixed with urine in a test tube. After a specified amount of time—anywhere from a few minutes to a couple of hours, depending on the test—a dark ring forms if you are pregnant. In some brands, a color change indicates pregnancy.

If you decide to use a home pregnancy test, follow the instructions precisely. Moreover, any pregnancy test, whether done at home or in the physician's office, is more accurate if you use your first urine of the day.

How accurate are urine tests? Their accuracy depends on how closely you follow the instructions, which can be complicated. First-time users or inexperienced users are less likely to get an accurate test result, and no test is foolproof. Also, pregnancy tests, particularly when done in the early days of pregnancy, may indicate you are not pregnant when in fact you are. This is because early in pregnancy the levels of hCG are low and may go undetected. For this reason, negative results from any pregnancy test are less reliable than a positive result.

Home pregnancy tests should be considered screening tests. If your test result is negative but you have the symptoms and signs of pregnancy (see Early Pregnancy: The First Trimester, page 198), consult your physician. If the result is positive, see your physician for confirmation and prenatal care.

About three-fourths of the time, results of a urine test done in a clinic or at your physician's office will be positive if you are pregnant and your period is 4 to 7 days late. When your period is 2 weeks late, the accuracy is close to 100 percent. The results of home pregnancy tests are about 95 percent accurate 10 days after a missed period.

Urine pregnancy tests are the most frequently used, but in some cases a blood test may be indicated because it is more accurate and can detect pregnancy earlier. In the case of an ectopic pregnancy—in which the egg begins to grow in the fallopian tube or someplace other than the uterus—a woman may have all the signs of pregnancy, despite negative results of urine pregnancy tests (see Ectopic Pregnancy, page 202). This occurs because hCG levels are not high when the egg is not in the uterus. The blood test, however, is more sensitive and could detect the pregnancy. Because ectopic pregnancy is a potentially life-threatening condition, this information could ultimately help save the mother's life.

The Second Trimester. During the second trimester the fetus grows and the organs that formed during the previous weeks mature.

At 13½ weeks the fetus has tiny fingernails. The genitals are fully formed, and the sex can be determined with certain prenatal tests (see page 200). The fetus can kick and move its toes. The mouth can open and close, and the fetus is capable of bending its arms and of making a fist.

By the end of the fourth month, the heartbeat can be detected with a stethoscope (other specialized instruments can detect a heartbeat much earlier). You are also likely to feel the first signs of life in your abdomen. The fetus's skin at this point is slightly pink and less transparent than it was previously. Fine hair covers the entire body. The first eyelashes and eyebrows begin to appear.

One month later, the fetus may have hair on its head. Fat deposits begin to appear beneath the wrinkly skin. The fetus is now 12 inches long and weighs about 1 pound. If it is born at this time, it will attempt to breathe but probably will not be able to survive.

The Third Trimester. The fetus takes on most of its weight during its last 13 weeks of development. At the beginning of this last phase of development the fetus weighs slightly more than a pound. The average baby is born 3 months later weighing 7½ pounds.

When you are 28 weeks pregnant, your baby is covered with a thick white protective coating called vernix. The infant's eyes are open, and a baby born at this time can cry weakly and move its limbs. Although an infant at this stage weighs only 2 pounds, two out of three babies born at this stage survive because of recent advances in the care of premature and ill newborns, although they may experience significant medical problems.

One month later the male infant's testicles descend into the scrotum. The infant now weighs 3 pounds 12 ounces. The vast majority of these infants are also capable of surviving with proper care.

The infant born at term or at 40 weeks after the mother's last menstrual period has a more rounded body and is less wrinkly than babies born earlier. The skin may or may not still be covered with vernix. Most of the body hair is gone, although the shoulders and arms may still have a light covering. The fingernails and toenails may extend beyond the fingers and toes.

PRENATAL CARE

One of the most important things you can do for yourself—and your baby—is to seek prenatal care as soon as you suspect you may be pregnant.

By the time many women call for an appointment with an obstetrician or other physician who provides prenatal care, they already know they are pregnant. They have all the symptoms and a pregnancy test that they performed at home was positive for pregnancy (see Pregnancy Tests, page 183). If your pregnancy has not been confirmed by a test, you can have one done at your physician's office.

Most physicians advise that as soon as you have missed a period—especially when you are trying to get pregnant—seek prenatal care. At the very latest, wait no longer than two missed periods.

During your first visit you will fill out a detailed health form and your physician will ask you many questions about your family history and overall health to determine whether there are any preexisting conditions that may cause problems or call for special measures during the pregnancy.

It is important to determine when you conceived, so the physician will ask you about your menstrual history to try to pinpoint when the baby will be born. This is only an approximation, however. Most babies are not born on the precise date they are expected. It is perfectly normal for a baby to be born anywhere from 2 weeks before to 2 weeks after the due date.

After taking your medical history, your physician will perform a physical examination and a pelvic examination (see The Pelvic Examination, page 1055). Typically, after this first visit a pelvic examination usually is not done again until the last weeks of pregnancy, and then it is done to determine whether labor is imminent. Blood and urine tests are done during the first visit.

The visit usually concludes with the physician discussing pregnancy with you, advising you on nutrition, weight gain, and exercise, and alerting you to potential complications such as vaginal bleeding.

Most physicians see their pregnant patients once a month for the first 7 months, twice during the eighth month, and then weekly.

After the initial visit, your regular visits usually begin with your weight and blood pressure being determined, and you also will be asked to submit a urine sample for testing. Your physician also will want to know whether you are having any problems such as headache, altered vision, abdominal pain, nausea, vomiting, swelling of the legs or feet, or vaginal bleeding. Write down any questions that have occurred to you during the past month so that you remember to ask your physician.

After about 10 to 12 weeks' gestation, an exciting part of the visit is listening to your baby's heartbeat, which can be detected with a Doppler instrument (a means of amplifying sound).

Your physician will feel your abdomen to determine whether the baby is growing properly. Sometimes there is a discrepancy between when you thought the conception occurred and the size of the fetus. When fetal age is in question, your physician may request that an ultrasound examination be done (see page 1286) to determine whether the fetus is indeed older than was believed. This is a painless test that uses high-frequency sound waves to record a picture of the fetus, allowing the physician to measure the width of the baby's skull. The fetus usually can be seen with this test, also called ultrasonography, 7 weeks after the last menstrual period.

The ultrasound test has had a major impact on the practice of obstetrics in that it can supply vital information about the health of the fetus without invading the body. In addition to its use in determining fetal age, it can clearly show whether you are carrying more than one baby, whether the infant has all its parts, whether it is growing properly, the position of the placenta, and, in some cases, the sex of the child.

Some physicians have small ultrasound devices in their offices and use them during prenatal visits to reassure the mother that the baby is alive and active. These units generally, however, cannot provide much detailed information about the fetus, so most

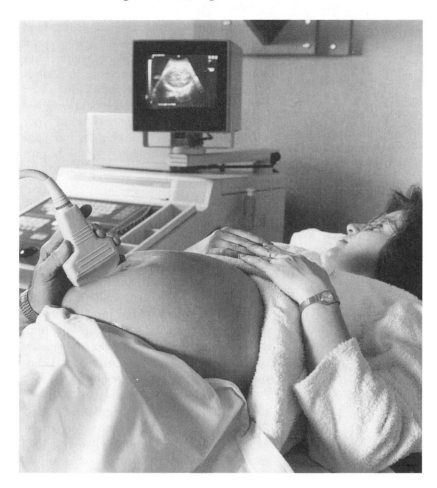

ultrasound studies are done in hospitals or radiology offices.

NUTRITION AND WEIGHT CONTROL DURING PREGNANCY

Pregnancy is not the time to start a diet. On the other hand, it is not the time to eat to excess. Women who do that often end up with extra pounds that do not automatically melt away with the birth of the baby.

Instead, concentrate on eating healthful and well-balanced meals. Do not deprive yourself, but try not to overindulge either. Do not skip meals. If you feel like having a snack between meals or at bedtime, go ahead; but avoid snacking on foods that are high in calories but low in nutritional value.

Remember, what you eat also affects your baby.

Most obstetricians recommend a weight gain of somewhere between 20 and 30 pounds, with the average gain being 24

Ultrasound examination painlessly reveals shape of fetus within uterus. By measuring width of the skull, fetal age can be determined.

pounds. Of this, about 20 pounds is gained simply as a result of your baby's weight and the changes that take place within your body. The average baby weighs 7½ pounds at birth, the placenta and membranes weigh 1½ pounds, and the amniotic fluid weighs 2 pounds. In addition, the weight of your uterus increases by 2½ pounds and your breasts by 2 pounds, and your body produces about 3½ pounds of extra blood and fluid.

The bulk of your weight gain probably will occur toward the end of your second trimester and throughout the third trimester, although this can vary.

As a general rule, what you eat during pregnancy will affect the health of your fetus. If your nutrition is inadequate, your newborn may suffer from growth retardation, a condition that can cause long-term development problems. Also, pregnancy can be complicated by excessive food consumption and excessive weight gain.

The average pregnant woman needs between 2,200 and 2,400 calories a day. Those who are especially active need more. Many physicians prescribe a vitamin supplement that, unlike ordinary supplements, will include folic acid. Iron supplements also may be included.

The following are basic elements of a well-balanced diet. Some pregnant women are so concerned about eating right that they weigh their food to make sure their servings conform with dietary standards. Such efforts usually are not necessary. When considering what to eat, common sense generally is sufficient.

Protein is important, and you can get it in meat, poultry, fish, eggs, milk, and dried beans, to name a few good sources. Protein is necessary for the repair of your body and for the growth of your baby. Two or three servings a day are adequate.

Carbohydrates are good sources of energy. They include breads, noodles, rice, potatoes, and pasta. We recommend four or more servings a day.

Minerals are found in the foods we eat. The only mineral usually needed as a supplement in the diet of a pregnant woman is iron because most women do not have sufficient iron stores to supply the amount needed for the demands of pregnancy. Still, too much iron can be harmful to your health. Discuss iron supplementation with your physician.

Calcium helps in the formation of strong bones and teeth. Milk and milk products such as yogurt, cottage cheese, hard cheese, and ice cream are excellent sources. We recommend three or four servings a day.

Vitamins are organic compounds contained in food. They are essential to the growth and maintenance of your body. If you are eating a balanced diet, you probably are getting the necessary vitamins. Nevertheless, many physicians prescribe a supplement. Fruits and vegetables are good sources of vitamins. We recommend four or five servings a day.

In addition to the foods you should eat, there are foods you should avoid.

Caffeine, a stimulant found in coffee, tea, cola, and chocolate, should be used only in moderation. Both ordinary and decaffeinated coffee may aggravate heartburn (see page 190), a common concern of pregnancy. Shun alcohol during pregnancy (see Smoking and Use of Alcohol and Illegal Drugs During Pregnancy, page 188).

EXERCISE IN PREGNANCY

Today, an increasing number of health-conscious women are exercising throughout their pregnancies.

This is not to say that pregnancy is the time to embark on a vigorous fitness regimen, especially if you have never done as much as a knee bend in your life. However, if you have been exercising regularly before pregnancy, you probably can continue unless your physician advises against it. Many physicians even recommend that previously sedentary patients slowly begin some form of mild exercise during pregnancy.

The long-term benefits of a regular exercise program for men and women are well known. What impact, however, does exercising by an expectant mother have on the fetus? Studies have shown that exercise probably does not have any impact, negative or positive, on the developing fetus. However, it may increase maternal stamina.

The result of this increased stamina may be a shorter and easier labor. Some speculate that this effect may be due to increased cardiorespiratory fitness and better endurance. The latter characteristic of the physically fit mother is particularly valuable when she is to push the baby out during delivery. Women who exercise regularly often can push for longer periods without succumbing to fatigue.

Although the possibility of an easier and shorter labor may entice you to try exercising, proceed with caution. Because of hormonal changes in your body, you are more vulnerable to injury. Your joints are more unstable and easily injured because your connective tissues now stretch more easily. Moreover, as you become larger, your center of gravity shifts and you may find yourself losing your balance.

Thus, deep bending or any movement that stretches your joints too much is not recommended, nor are high-impact aerobics or any other jerking movements. In addition, caution is indicated because of the danger of falling. Do not play games such as tennis and racquetball. The abrupt changes in direction during these games can cause joint damage.

After about the fourth month of pregnancy, avoid exercises that require you to lie on your back because of the possibility of interrupting blood flow to the fetus.

Avoid strenuous and potentially dangerous activities such as horseback riding, mountain climbing, scuba diving, and water skiing. Do not do any downhill skiing for the duration of your pregnancy. Pregnancy is not the time to take up marathon running, although some long-distance runners have completed marathons during pregnancy with no adverse consequences to themselves or their babies.

Despite these few exercise restrictions, there are many sports and exercises that are suitable for a pregnant woman. One of the best exercises during pregnancy is swimming. It provides a good cardiovascular workout; there is no risk of injury to your joints because of the water's buoyancy.

Low-impact aerobics are fine, and in many communities there are low-impact aerobic classes geared for expectant mothers. Jogging and cycling also are good if you enjoyed these exercises before conception. You may need to decrease your activity level if you find yourself becoming more fatigued than usual. Walking during pregnancy is often recommended, and it is usually the first exercise advised for the previously inactive pregnant woman who wants to begin exercising.

No matter what exercise you choose, check with your physician before you begin. Although it is safe for most women to exercise during pregnancy, some pregnant women have medical problems such as hypertension that make exertion dangerous.

Never exercise to the point of exhaustion. Drink plenty of fluids to prevent dehydration during a workout. If the weather is hot and humid, delay your run or walk until a cooler day.

THERAPEUTIC DRUGS IN PREGNANCY

Almost any drug you take during pregnancy affects your baby too. Even a seemingly innocuous over-the-counter drug such as aspirin travels through the placenta to your baby.

Thus, avoid taking medication unless it is approved by your physician. If you have a condition for which medication is necessary, your physician will select a drug that will help your problem without jeopardizing your baby unnecessarily.

Sometimes the effects of exposure of the fetus to a drug do not appear for many years. Such is the case with the female offspring of women who took diethylstilbestrol (DES). This drug commonly was prescribed for women who were thought to be in danger of miscarriage or who had a history of miscarriage. In the 1970s, many adolescent girls and young women were found to have unusual vaginal, cervical, and uterine changes. The one thing they had in common was that their mothers had taken DES while pregnant.

Drugs that are known to affect the fetus adversely are called teratogens. In general, the most dangerous time to take medication is during the first trimester of pregnancy because that is when most fetal development occurs and when the fetus is most vulnerable to injury. However, some drugs, such as aspirin, are more dangerous later in pregnancy.

Most drugs should be avoided during pregnancy unless they are absolutely necessary to treat a medical condition, but in a few cases a drug helps rather than hurts the fetus.

Some abnormalities in fetal heart rate can be treated with cardiac drugs through the mother, even though she does not have a heart abnormality. Similarly, if your physician anticipates that labor will have to be induced before 32 weeks' gestation, because of a medical problem, the infant can be given corticosteroid medications before labor that may enable the infant to breathe better after birth.

Sometimes drugs cannot be avoided during pregnancy. Some women have chronic diseases such as diabetes or hypertension that necessitate medication. Many pregnant women develop urinary infections that re-

quire antibiotics. And often physicians recommend that their pregnant patients with a high fever due to a viral illness take acetaminophen because a prolonged high fever is potentially dangerous to the fetus.

The following are some drugs that are known to cause or are suspected of causing birth defects.

Isotretinoin (Accutane) is a drug used for acne. It can cause heart disease and severe facial and ear abnormalities.

The antibiotic streptomycin can cause deafness when used by a pregnant woman

SMOKING AND USE OF ALCOHOL AND ILLEGAL DRUGS DURING PREGNANCY

Pregnant women who use illegal drugs, smoke, or drink large amounts of alcohol are gambling with the future health of their unborn child.

If you use illegal drugs, drink, or smoke cigarettes, the time to quit is before you get pregnant and not after, when it is possible that your habit has already done some irreparable damage to your developing baby.

Smoking is a difficult habit to break, but it is not impossible, as millions of Americans can attest. Why should you stop smoking if you are pregnant or contemplating pregnancy?

Studies show that mothers who smoke a pack or more of cigarettes a day consistently produce smaller babies than do nonsmokers. A small baby is generally weaker and more vulnerable to illness than one of average size. Moreover, smokers are more apt to have their pregnancy end in miscarriage or stillbirth. (For help in stopping smoking, see page 412.)

Alcohol can be a dangerous drug when used during pregnancy.

If you are an alcoholic or heavy drinker, your infant may be born with fetal alcohol syndrome. This syndrome, found in 1 to 2 infants out of every 1,000, is characterized by prenatal and postnatal growth retardation, facial abnormalities, heart defects, joint and limb problems, and intellectual handicaps.

The more alcohol you drink, the greater the chances of producing a child with fetal alcohol syndrome or at least some congenital defects. For example, up to 33 percent of infants whose mothers are heavy drinkers have some congenital abnormality, whereas fewer than 5 percent whose mothers did not drink during pregnancy have a congenital abnormality.

The question that most women ask their physicians is whether it is safe to drink socially during pregnancy. Many physicians allow their pregnant patients to have a glass of wine or beer once or twice a week. Other physicians are more strict and advise against any alcohol consumption because no one has ever quantified the amount of alcohol it takes to inflict damage on the fetus. Ultimately, it may be less than some physicians think.

Illegal drug use is becoming more common, with the result

that more infants are being born with both drug addiction and severe health problems.

If you are using heroin or another addictive drug such as cocaine, amphetamines, or barbiturates, your infant is 2 to 6 times more likely to be born prematurely or to be retarded in growth than a baby whose mother does not use drugs. Moreover, your pregnancy is apt to be complicated by hypertension and hemorrhage.

Approximately half of the infants born to addicted mothers also are addicted. Generally, within the first day of life the heroin-addicted infant becomes irritable and has convulsions, congestion, vomiting, diarrhea, and fever. Sedatives such as phenobarbital frequently are given to the baby and then slowly withdrawn. The withdrawal must be slow or the infant may experience convulsions.

Because of the ease with which cocaine or crack (cocaine that is smoked) can be obtained, in some areas of the country mothers of as many as one in four new babies are users (see also page 441). A significant percentage of their infants are born prematurely or with brain damage.

for a long time; and tetracycline can lead to retarded bone growth and damage to tooth pigmentation.

Dicumarol is an anticoagulant used by some patients with heart disease or excessive blood clotting. Abnormal facial features and mental retardation are associated with its use.

Dilantin, an anticonvulsant used for seizure disorders (epilepsy), can cause tumors, retarded growth, and other abnormalities.

Diuretics, used when water retention is a problem, can interfere with fetal nutrition if used in excess.

Methyltestosterone can cause masculinization of the female fetus.

Tranquilizers may produce tremors that continue for months after birth.

Valium may cause depression.

This is not a complete list. Always check with your obstetrician before taking *any* medication.

TRAVEL DURING PREGNANCY

Travel does not induce labor, miscarriage, or any other pregnancy complication.

Thus, there is no medical reason why you cannot travel during your pregnancy unless your physician advises against it.

Before you contemplate a cross-country car trip or a 2-week cruise, however, consider how you are going to feel. Many women, particularly during the first 3 months of pregnancy, have frequent bouts of nausea or morning sickness (this is a misnomer because the nausea can occur morning, noon, or night). Travel during this period may make the nausea worse.

Another consideration is the proximity to your due date. Most physicians advise against traveling during the last weeks of pregnancy, particularly if you have a history of premature labor. Many airlines will not allow you to fly if you are close to your due date.

If you are feeling well, have plenty of time before the baby is due, and feel like taking an airline trip, go ahead. Make sure, however, that you get up from your seat every 2 hours and walk around.

When traveling by car, remember to always wear your seat belt. A lap belt should be fastened below your uterus, and a shoulder harness should be adjusted between your breasts and to the side of your abdomen.

You may find it is helpful to put a pillow in the small of your back to prevent low-back pain. Also, stop periodically (every couple of hours) to get out and walk.

COMMON DISCOMFORTS DURING PREGNANCY

Although most women have pregnancies uncomplicated by serious medical problems or emergencies, few escape without at least some discomfort. Some problems, such as morning sickness, are more common during the early weeks of pregnancy and usually subside by the end of the third month. Others, such as hemorrhoids, may worsen as your pregnancy advances.

Morning sickness is the term used to describe the queasiness, nausea, or vomiting that about half of all pregnant women have during the first 12 weeks of pregnancy. Although morning sickness tends to be worse in the morning, some women complain of bouts of nausea throughout the day.

It is not understood why some women have nausea and vomiting. Hormonal changes may be responsible. Although morning sickness is certainly unpleasant, it is rarely dangerous.

If you have morning sickness, there are certain things you can do to minimize your nausea and vomiting, although nothing is 100 percent effective. Many women find that the nausea is worse when their stomachs are empty. Thus, they make it a point to eat several small meals a day. Some keep crackers next to their bedside and find that they feel better when they nibble a few before rising in the morning.

You may find the smell of certain foods brings on the nausea. If this happens, avoid that particular food. If you feel nauseated, stick to a bland diet, avoiding spicy, rich, and fried foods.

Drink lots of fluid, especially if you are vomiting. If plain water upsets your stomach, try crushed ice, fruit juice, or Popsicles.

Some drugs are effective for eliminating the problem. However, many physicians are reluctant to prescribe a medication for nausea unless the problem is severe.

Occasionally, however, vomiting may be serious enough that a pregnant woman becomes dehydrated. This condition usually requires hospitalization, during which anti-vomiting drugs are administered and lost body fluid is replaced intravenously.

Constipation is a common problem during pregnancy. If you usually are constipated, you may find the problem worsens during your pregnancy. It probably occurs because of decreased intestinal contractions and diminished ability of the bowel to expel its contents because of the pressure from the enlarged uterus.

There are things you can do to alleviate the problem. Drink plenty of fluids, exercise daily, and make sure your diet contains several servings of fruits (prunes are particularly good), vegetables, and grains such as whole wheat and bran. Bulk formers that contain psyllium (available without a prescription) are often helpful.

Do not take a laxative unless you check with your physician.

Heartburn has nothing to do with your heart. Rather, the burning sensation in the middle of your chest and the sometimes bad taste in your mouth are the result of stomach acid flowing upward into your lower esophagus (see page 593).

This problem occurs in about half of all pregnant women when the muscle that closes off the stomach from the esophagus becomes lax, allowing stomach juices to flow back up and irritate the esophagus. It often worsens with advancing pregnancy because the stomach is moved out of position by the expanding uterus, which delays the emptying of its contents.

If you have heartburn, try eating smaller meals at more frequent intervals, which will keep food in your stomach to soak up the excess acid. Eat slowly and avoid greasy foods. Both regular and decaffeinated coffee may aggravate heartburn. Because heartburn is often worse when you lie flat, your physician may suggest sleeping with the head of your bed on 4- to 6-inch blocks. Also, avoid eating during the 2 or 3 hours immediately preceding bedtime.

If these practices do not help, consult your physician, who may recommend an antacid.

Backache is common in pregnancies.

Often backache occurs when you are tired or have been bending, lifting, or walking too much.

When you are pregnant, your ligaments are more elastic, which allows your pelvis to expand during the birth of your baby. Although this is necessary, its negative effect is that your joints are more prone to strain and injury. During pregnancy, as your center of balance changes, so does your posture, inflicting more strain than ever on your already vulnerable back.

Usually the pain is in the lower back. Some women get sciatica (pain that radiates down the legs). Most women also have pain in the abdomen because of the stretching of abdominal ligaments by the expanding uterus; called round ligament pain, it is generally worse during the second trimester.

Try not to gain more weight than is recommended because weight places stress on your back. Backache usually can be relieved by eliminating as much strain as possible. Sometimes a maternity girdle can help. Your physician also may recommend exercises to relieve the pain. If the pain is severe, your physician may recommend an orthopedic examination to determine whether there is an underlying problem.

Varicose veins usually become worse in later pregnancy and are more pronounced in women who stand for long periods and in older mothers. Heredity also plays a role in whether you get varicose veins.

As many as 20 percent of all pregnant women have varicose veins. The condition tends to appear earlier and is more pronounced with each pregnancy.

When you are pregnant, your blood vessels must accommodate an increased blood volume to supply the needs of your baby. Your uterus enlarges and the flow of blood from your leg veins to your pelvis decreases. This combination causes the veins in your legs to become swollen and uncomfortable or even very painful.

If you have varicose veins, keep off your feet (and elevate them) as much as possible. Do not wear clothing that is tight around the legs or waist. Support hose can help relieve the pain and swelling. Many physicians recommend that you put your support hose on first thing in the morning and not take them off until just before you go to bed.

Surgery to treat varicose veins generally is not recommended during pregnancy. Rarely, the problem is so severe that it becomes necessary.

Hemorrhoids occur when the veins at the anal opening become enlarged due to pressure. When you strain during a bowel movement, the veins may protrude through the anus and cause pain and itching. Generally, they become worse during pregnancy and often occur in conjunction with constipation.

Prevention is the best treatment. Avoid becoming constipated and straining at stool (see Constipation, page 190).

If you notice pain during a bowel movement and feel a swollen mass near your rectum, you probably have a hemorrhoid. To ease the discomfort, take frequent warm water baths. A cotton pad soaked with cold witch hazel cream applied to the hemorrhoidal area also may help.

Sleeping problems often occur during the later months of pregnancy. The frequent urge to urinate contributes to lack of sleep; the movement of your baby also may keep you awake. Some women simply have so much on their minds that sleep eludes them.

What should you do if you find yourself staring at the ceiling half the night?

Avoid coffee, tea, or cola drinks because they contain caffeine, which can keep you awake. Also, do not eat a huge meal just before bedtime.

Some physicians recommend exercising a little more so you will be more tired and more apt to fall asleep. For some pregnant women, a warm bath helps. If nothing seems to work, get up; read a book, pay some bills, or catch up on household tasks. Try sleeping later.

If the lack of sleep becomes significant, consult your physician. Some physicians will prescribe sleeping pills when a woman is exhausted from lack of sleep. Do not, however, take any pills unless recommended by your physician.

Anemia occurs when your hemoglobin—a protein in blood that carries oxygen throughout the body—falls below an adequate amount. A small decrease in hemoglobin is normal during pregnancy.

Usually, anemia in pregnancy is due to an iron deficiency or an inadequate supply of folic acid.

If you have mild anemia, you may have no symptoms and the condition may be discovered accidentally during a routine blood test. With more severe anemia, symptoms include fatigue, breathlessness, fainting, palpitations, and pallor.

Unlike other problems discussed in this section, anemia can be risky for both mother and child. Should hemorrhaging occur, the anemic mother is less able to cope with blood loss than one with adequate hemoglobin.

Most physicians prescribe iron and folic acid supplements to prevent anemia. You also can help prevent anemia by eating a diet rich in iron, which is found in foods such as liver, eggs, dried fruit, whole grains, and beef. Green vegetables are a good source of folic acid.

If you do develop anemia, your physician will determine what type of anemia is present and prescribe appropriate treatment. Most often, this will include iron and folic acid supplements. (See also Anemias, page 477.)

Edema (swelling) is common during pregnancy because of accumulated fluid in body tissues.

Approximately one-quarter of your weight gain during pregnancy is fluid, which tends to congregate in various parts of your body, including the lower legs, feet, and hands.

You may notice swelling in your legs, ankles, and feet after you have been standing for long periods. The problem usually is worse at the end of the day and in warm weather. After a night of rest, the legs and feet return to their normal size in most women.

The fingers also are a common site for swelling. You may wake up in the morning with your fingers so stiff that you cannot button your clothing. Your fingers also may be puffy. Cold water compresses help relieve the swelling.

Some women notice facial swelling. If your face becomes extremely swollen, especially around the eyes, this may be a sign of toxemia, a serious medical condition (see page 207). See your physician immediately.

Use diuretics only at your physician's direction. Often a low-salt diet will prove helpful. Lying down and elevating your legs for an hour in midafternoon also may reduce the swelling in your legs.

BLEEDING DURING PREGNANCY

Bleeding from the vagina during pregnancy often is an indication that something is wrong. Notify your physician immediately.

In the first 20 weeks of pregnancy, bleeding is often associated with miscarriage. Bleeding during a miscarriage may be slight or heavy. There may be no warning, or you may first notice some brownish discharge.

During the first days of pregnancy when the egg is implanting itself within the uterus, you may have some spotting. Moreover, approximately 20 percent of all pregnant women have some bleeding in early pregnancy that does not result in miscarriage. So *do not* necessarily assume the worst, but *do* check with your physician.

After the 20th week of pregnancy, bleeding is called antepartum hemorrhage. This is much less common than early pregnancy bleeding, affecting less than 2 percent of all women. There are many causes of antepartum hemorrhage, including placenta previa (see page 209), tubal (ectopic) pregnancy (see page 202), miscarriage (see page 199), or the onset of premature labor (see page 204).

In most cases the bleeding is mild. However, a severe hemorrhage can endanger your life and your baby's.

If you begin bleeding after the first months of pregnancy, see your physician immediately. You may require hospitalization and tests such as ultrasonography to determine the cause of your bleeding. If the hemorrhage is severe, blood transfusions may be necessary. In the worst cases, labor is induced or a cesarean section is performed.

INTRAUTERINE GROWTH RETARDATION

An infant who is born extremely small for its gestational age—usually below the 10th percentile—is considered to be growth retarded.

Intrauterine growth retardation occurs when the fetus does not get adequate nourishment from the mother via the placenta. An infant born growth retarded does not have the amount of body fat that a normal-size newborn does. Thus, the infant has difficulty maintaining a normal body temperature and blood sugar level. Moreover, many growth-retarded infants grow slowly throughout at least early childhood. There also may be some delayed intellectual development.

Many conditions and life-style characteristics can produce intrauterine growth retardation. A woman who smokes, uses illegal drugs, or drinks large amounts of alcohol is more likely to produce a small infant. A mother who is malnourished or fails to gain adequate weight also is in danger of giving birth to a small infant. Certain chronic diseases also place you at risk.

Conditions related to pregnancy can cause growth retardation. These include abnormalities of the placenta and cord, fetal infections or malformations, and the presence of more than one fetus.

If your physician suspects intrauterine growth retardation, he or she probably will ask you to have an ultrasound examination.

When the fetus is not growing at a proper rate because you are smoking, drinking, using drugs, or not eating properly, sometimes a change to a healthier life-style can help.

Often, however, labor must be induced or a cesarean section performed. If the fetus is still far from term, the risk of such early delivery must be weighed against the risk of leaving it in the womb and further malnutrition.

INFECTIOUS DISEASES DURING PREGNANCY

Some common diseases that seem to do little more than make a pregnant woman miserable can, in fact, do irreparable damage to the fetus, depending on when in fetal development they strike.

German measles (rubella) is usually a mild disease that causes a mild, itchy rash and fever. If contracted during the first 10 weeks of pregnancy, however, the virus can cross the placenta and infect the fetus. More than half of the infants born to women who have rubella during early pregnancy have congenital malformations such as eye cataracts, deafness, hernias, heart defects, and defects of the central nervous system. (See page B-1 for color photograph of rubella rash.)

When contracted in later pregnancy, rubella does not cause congenital defects but the infant is born with the virus, which can cause serious illness. Many of these babies later develop diabetes.

Your best defense against rubella is immunization. If you have not had German measles, ask your physician about immunization before you become pregnant. (See also page 862.)

Chickenpox (varicella) may be a serious disease in pregnant women. It sometimes can be dangerous for the infant as well. (See page B-1 for color photograph of chickenpox rash.)

If you have chickenpox during pregnancy, the virus may also infect your developing infant either while it is in the uterus or during delivery. The infant in the uterus actually develops pockmarks. If there is sufficient time before delivery, the pockmarks generally heal and the infant is born without skin blemishes.

The greatest risk seems to be exposure to the virus just before delivery. If the infant is delivered before receiving your antibodies against the virus, he or she may develop the disease. Unless the infant immediately is given a shot of zoster immune globulin, the baby may die from complications of the virus. (See also page 864.)

Toxoplasmosis is a disease due to contact with the parasite *Toxoplasma gondii.* It is contracted by eating infected undercooked meat or through contact with infected cat feces, or it can be passed from an infected pregnant mother to her baby. If you are pregnant, do not handle untested cats or empty their litter boxes.

As many as 25 to 45 percent of American women of reproductive age carry the organism, although they may not have symptoms. It is estimated that 1 fetus in every 800 to 1,400 pregnancies acquires toxoplasmosis.

The symptoms of toxoplasmosis are fatigue and muscle pain. You may feel like you have the flu. Some women have no symptoms. The disease cannot be confirmed unless you had a test for toxoplasmosis early in pregnancy and did not carry the antibodies. The infection in the mother can be treated with medication.

If you contract the infection early in pregnancy, you may have a miscarriage.

Most infants born with toxoplasmosis do not immediately show evidence of having been infected, but many physicians advise treatment anyway. In addition, most infants are not infected despite maternal infection. Of those who are, most have only minor symptoms. A few, however, eventually develop neurological problems and partial blindness. A small percentage of these infants die from the disease.

Genital herpes is a sexually transmitted disease that appears as painful blisters on the genitals. The cervix or upper vagina also may have blisters, which may not produce symptoms. In the newborn, herpes can cause serious damage to the eyes and central nervous system or death.

There is no cure for genital herpes. After one attack it may be a month or years before the next attack. Some women carry the virus but never have symptoms.

If you have confirmed herpes or suspect you have the virus, tell your physician. There are tests that can be done to determine whether you have any active lesions.

The danger to the baby is generally thought to be exposure to the virus as it travels down the birth canal. Thus, if tests confirm that you have active herpes near your delivery time, your physician will want to deliver the baby by cesarean section. (See also page 877.)

Hepatitis B is a liver infection caused by the hepatitis B virus (see page 650); it is transmitted in much the same manner as the AIDS virus (see page 848). If you have this virus, it can be transmitted through the placenta to your fetus. Also, your newborn baby can become infected by the virus from contact with you.

This virus can cause liver failure. The risk of premature birth also is higher among women who have hepatitis B.

If your physician suspects that you have hepatitis B, he or she will test your blood for the presence of antibodies to the virus. If you have hepatitis B, your infant will be given an injection of antibodies against the virus after delivery.

Because the hepatitis virus also may be found in breast milk, a mother with hepatitis B should not breast-feed.

Group B streptococci are bacteria that can be transmitted to the fetus during childbirth. As many as 40 percent of pregnant women tested in the last trimester of pregnancy harbor these bacteria in their vagina.

Many infants are born with this bacteria, but only 2 or 3 per 1,000 develop infection.

An infant with group B streptococcal infection usually shows symptoms within 48 hours after delivery. Symptoms include breathing problems and shock. Occasionally an infant will be a week old before there are symptoms, which then usually appear as meningitis.

Immediate treatment with antibiotics is necessary for infants with this infection. Even so, the mortality rate is high.

Syphilis is a serious sexually transmitted

disease that can be passed from a pregnant mother to her baby.

If you have syphilis, you may see one or more lesions, called chancres, on your genitals, although sometimes they may go unnoticed. They occur 10 to 90 days after exposure.

About 6 weeks later you may notice a rash.

During your first prenatal visit you will be tested for syphilis, as required by law. The disease can be treated easily with penicillin.

At birth, your infant will be tested. If the baby has syphilis, treatment will be initiated immediately. (See also page 876.)

Gonorrhea is another sexually transmitted (so-called venereal) disease. It can be treated effectively with antibiotics. However, if you have gonorrhea, your infant can also contract the infection as it moves down the birth canal.

Infection with gonorrhea may result in damage to your baby's eyes. For this reason, all newborns receive preventive treatment immediately after birth. This consists of an antibiotic ointment applied under the baby's eyelids.

A discharge of pus from the baby's eyes may be a sign that the infant has gonorrhea. If you have gonorrhea, your infant will be treated with penicillin (see also page 875).

Chlamydial infection, another sexually transmitted disease, can cause conjunctivitis (an eye infection, see page 759) in the newborn. This usually appears during the second week of life. When treated with antibiotics, it does not have any long-term adverse effects.

Cytomegalovirus is the most common virus affecting the fetus; an estimated 2,500 to 7,500 babies are born infected by this virus each year. It can cause death during the newborn period or numerous birth defects such as blindness, seizures, anemia, and neurological disorders. Some women carry the virus in their urine or cervix during pregnancy, but few pass the disease to their infants. There is no effective treatment.

Papilloma appears as warts on the skin. The type of warts usually found on the genitals is called condylomata or venereal warts. These are highly infectious, sexually transmitted, and often painful. The warts tend to grow faster during pregnancy. Usually, treatment during pregnancy is not effective. Rarely, the application of a topical medication has proved fatal to the fetus. Sometimes the warts grow so large that they interfere with the baby's passage down the birth canal, necessitating a cesarean section. (See also page 879.)

AIDS (acquired immune deficiency syndrome) is a fatal disease (see page 848). A pregnant woman can be infected by the AIDS virus through sexual intercourse with an infected man, by blood transfusion, or by injecting drugs with dirty needles (as drug addicts often do), or the virus can be passed through artificial insemination with semen containing the virus.

To date, more than 70 percent of the babies born with AIDS were infected by mothers who used illegal intravenous drugs. Another large percentage were born to mothers whose partners were intravenous drug abusers, and many of the others were born to women whose partners were bisexual.

If you have AIDS, you can pass the disease to the baby you are carrying. There is no cure for AIDS. Babies born with the disease usually do not live more than a few years. Therefore, if you have the AIDS virus, do not become pregnant. (See also AIDS, page 848.)

MEDICAL PROBLEMS OF PREGNANCY

Most women go through pregnancy without any major complications.

For a small percentage of women, however, this 9-month experience is not without problems. If you have a chronic disease such as diabetes or hypertension, take extra care throughout your pregnancy to ensure your health and that of your baby. Then, too, pregnancy does not make a healthy woman immune to disease. Some women who were healthy before becoming pregnant develop disease over the course of the 9 months.

This section explores some of the more common medical problems that complicate pregnancy.

Diabetes does not preclude a woman from becoming pregnant, although before the introduction of insulin in 1922, most diabetics were too ill to conceive. Those who did become pregnant often aborted or died during pregnancy. Even years later, when the outcome for diabetic women was not so bleak, their infants still did not fare well.

Today, if you are a diabetic you have an excellent chance of having a healthy baby, provided your blood sugar concentration is kept stringently under control through careful measurements of its value and appropriate adjustment of insulin injections (see page 715). If not, the excess blood sugar will travel through the placenta and cause an increase in the fetus's blood sugar concentration. This, in turn, activates the fetal pancreas to produce insulin, which acts as a growth hormone. Babies born to mothers whose diabetes is out of control often are extremely large, a characteristic that complicates labor and delivery. They tend to have more congenital defects and are predisposed to diabetes. Moreover, some of these babies die before birth because of metabolic problems.

For the diabetic mother, the risks associated with the disease include infection, postpartum hemorrhage, heart and lung problems, and a 4-fold greater risk of preeclampsia than in nondiabetic mothers (see Preeclampsia and Eclampsia, page 207).

Ordinarily, diabetes occurring at an age when a woman can become pregnant requires insulin therapy.

Sometimes nondiabetic women develop what is called gestational diabetes during pregnancy. This form of diabetes also requires careful control but may not require insulin injection; it usually goes away after the baby is born.

If you are a diabetic, seek the care of an obstetrician who specializes in high-risk pregnancy. If you previously had an infant who weighed more than 9 pounds, have a history of stillbirth, have family members with diabetes, or have sugar in your urine, your physician will do a test for diabetes.

The diabetic pregnant woman must adhere to a strict diet to keep her blood sugar under control. If this is not effective, insulin shots are required. Blood tests now available allow your physician to determine how well your diet and blood sugar are being controlled. With strict control of your diabetes, the infant is more likely to be nearly normal in size. Sometimes an early delivery by cesarean section is necessary because of the infant's large size or because the environment of the womb is becoming detrimental to the baby (see Cesarean Section, page 214, and Diabetes Mellitus, page 707).

Hypertension (high blood pressure) is a common and potentially dangerous problem during pregnancy. Infants born to hypertensive mothers tend to be small and have small placentas. The incidence of fetal death also is higher than in the general population.

Some women are naturally hypertensive; in others the pregnancy is responsible for this sudden elevation in blood pressure.

You may have hypertension but not have symptoms. The condition is detected easily during the routine blood pressure check that is a part of every prenatal visit.

Some women with mild hypertension have no major problems during pregnancy. In others the blood pressure continues to increase, fluid begins to accumulate in their body, and protein is detected in their urine. This is called preeclampsia and usually occurs after the 20th week of pregnancy. Convulsions (eclampsia) can follow (see Preeclampsia and Eclampsia, page 207). This is an extreme emergency and can result in death for the mother and child.

Thus, it is important that your hypertension be controlled. This means frequent examinations, blood and urine tests to determine whether your kidneys are functioning properly, and possibly repeat ultrasound examinations to ascertain whether your baby is growing properly.

Sometimes bed rest is advised. If your blood pressure is extremely high, medication may be prescribed (see High Blood Pressure, page 796).

Asthma is a chronic respiratory disease that afflicts about 3 percent of adults.

The course of asthma during pregnancy is difficult to predict. In some women the disease becomes worse with pregnancy, in others it seems to improve, and in others it remains the same.

If you have asthma, you may be more prone to respiratory infections during pregnancy. The emotional stress of pregnancy may make your attacks more intense. However, most asthmatic women can carry a baby to term safely.

Many women with asthma require medication. Most asthma medication is safe to use during pregnancy. However, avoid taking medication that contains large amounts of iodide; when taken over a prolonged period, this can cause problems with your baby's thyroid gland. (See also Asthma, page 466.)

Heart disorders occur in about 1 percent of all pregnant women. Although they are a potentially serious complication, many women with heart disorders have successful pregnancies and healthy babies.

Pregnancy makes your heart and other organs work extra hard. Thus, if you already have a heart disorder, this extra load can cause heart failure. If you have a heart problem, particularly one involving the valves (see Disorders of the Heart Valves, page 822), make sure you discuss the risks of pregnancy with your physician before becoming pregnant.

Generally, if you are in good health otherwise and have no evidence of heart failure, you probably will have a successful pregnancy and a healthy baby.

Excessive weight gain, abnormal retention of fluid, and anemia can be particularly dangerous for a woman with a heart disorder, and every effort should be made to avoid these problems. In some cases, bed rest for part of the pregnancy may be recommended.

Seizure disorders (epilepsy), if controlled with medication, generally do not affect pregnancy. However, severe nausea and vomiting during early pregnancy may interfere with your ability to take your anticonvulsant medication. This can increase the risk of seizures.

Rarely, medications to control seizures can cause birth defects and increase the risk of prematurity, low birth weight, and infant death. Some drugs are worse than others, so if you have a seizure disorder and are contemplating pregnancy, make sure you consult a physician who has experience in treating such disorders.

Skin problems, while a nuisance, usually do not pose a risk during pregnancy. Pruritus (itching), when it occurs, is generally all over the body. One form of pruritus appears as small red patches that usually are found around the abdomen and then spread to the buttocks, hips, thighs, and upper arms.

If you have pruritus, avoid scratching, which may cause infection. Wash the area with a mild soap. If your symptoms are severe, your physician may recommend a cortisone cream (see Itching, page 1162).

Pruritus is more likely to appear in first pregnancies.

Pigmentation changes often occur during pregnancy. You may notice brownish spots on your face or on other parts of your body. The discoloration on your face is sometimes called the mask of pregnancy.

These spots of pigment usually, but not always, disappear after the baby is born.

RISK FACTORS AND PREGNANCY

There are never any guarantees, but the vast majority of pregnant women deliver healthy, normal babies at or near term.

Some factors, however, tend to increase your chances of pregnancy complications such as miscarriage, stillbirth, intrauterine growth retardation, and premature birth.

Some of these factors—such as age—are to a large extent beyond your control. Others, including smoking and the consumption of alcohol and illegal drugs, are dangerous practices that you should avoid.

Age is especially worthy of some attention today because so many women are delaying pregnancy until their 30s and even 40s. How safe is this? Again, the vast majority of healthy women older than 35 years tend to have uneventful pregnancies. Because many of these women have planned their pregnancies, they are often highly motivated and take especially good care of themselves.

There is, however, an increased risk for mother and child.

Women older than 35 tend to develop diabetes and hypertension more frequently than younger women. The rate of miscarriage and stillbirth also is slightly higher. Placenta previa, an uncommon condition requiring premature delivery, is more common among older mothers (see page 209).

Labor also tends to be slightly longer in older first-time mothers.

Teenagers also are at higher risk for complications of pregnancy. The risk may not be so much age-related as the result of the youthful mother being uninterested in taking care of herself. These young girls may have inadequate diets and little or no prenatal care, which may result in a higher frequency of preeclampsia and eclampsia—often called toxemia (see page 207), a potentially fatal condition. Pregnant teenagers also have higher rates of miscarriage, intrauterine growth retardation, stillbirths, and premature births than women a few years older.

An *inadequate diet* increases your risk of giving birth to a low-birth-weight infant, which makes the infant more vulnerable to infection, disease, and death. Failure to gain an adequate amount of weight can affect your baby adversely. Most physicians recommend a weight gain of between 20 and 30 pounds, with the average being 24 pounds. If you have been poorly nourished most of your life, the effects may be felt by your baby despite improved nutrition during pregnancy.

Smokers tend to produce smaller infants. Moreover, a woman who smokes is slightly more likely to have a spontaneous abortion (miscarriage) or stillbirth than a nonsmoker.

Alcohol can produce abnormal changes in the developing infant. Fetal alcohol syndrome most often occurs in the infants of alcoholics and heavy drinkers, although it has been known to occur in babies whose

RHESUS (Rh) INCOMPATIBILITY

During childbirth, some of your baby's blood can escape into your bloodstream. If your blood and that of your child are compatible, this is not a problem. However, if they are incompatible, you can develop antibodies that could be a threat to subsequent pregnancies.

Blood groups are determined by whether or not a person has certain protein molecules on the surface of his or her blood cells. The Rh factor is one of these blood groups. Eighty-five percent of whites are Rh positive, which means they have the Rh component on their blood cells. Among blacks, the percentage is slightly higher, and virtually all American Indians and Orientals are Rh positive.

About 15 percent of whites and 7 percent of blacks are Rh negative. If you are Rh negative, you do not have a potential problem unless the father of your baby is Rh positive. If the baby has inherited the father's Rh-positive blood, the blood of the baby is incompatible with your blood (see also Blood Groups, page 500).

In most cases, the first child is not at risk even if it is Rh positive because your Rh-negative blood has not had prior exposure to Rh-positive blood. Thus, you have not been sensitized, meaning your body has not yet begun to develop the antibodies that would attack

the fetus. However, if you become pregnant again and the fetus is Rh positive, these antibodies can pass through the placenta and harm the developing baby. The risk increases with each Rh-incompatible pregnancy.

Rh disease is not the problem it once was because of more thorough screening techniques, use of a serum that prevents the Rh-negative woman from developing antibodies, and more effective therapy for infants who are affected.

If you are pregnant, your physician will do a blood test that will determine whether you are Rh negative or Rh positive. If you are negative, the baby's father will be tested also (unless you already know his Rh status).

If the father's blood is Rh positive, regular blood tests will be required throughout your pregnancy to check for development of antibodies. Although this is unlikely to occur during a first pregnancy, it is not unheard of. If you have ever had an abortion or a miscarriage, it is possible that some of the fetus's blood cells entered your body and triggered the development of antibodies. Moreover, there is always the possibility of small leaks of fetal blood during pregnancy.

Physicians now give all their pregnant Rh-negative patients a shot of Rho immune globulin at 28 weeks' gestation to prevent sensitization should there be some early leakage of fetal blood. This serum destroys any fetal red blood cells that have entered your circulation before your body has time to marshal its forces against them.

In the end you may discover this precaution is unnecessary if the baby you deliver is Rh negative. But because there is no risk from the shot itself and because of the possibility of injury to the baby without it, the choice seems clear.

When you deliver an Rh-positive infant, you will be given another dose of Rho immune globulin within 72 hours after the delivery. This will enable you to enter the next pregnancy without having been sensitized.

If you have been sensitized and your baby is being affected, an early delivery may be necessary. Some infants die in the uterus because of severe anemia as a result of this blood incompatibility. The infant may be given a blood transfusion while still in the womb. This is done to "buy time" until the baby's lungs are developed enough so that it can withstand an early delivery.

After birth, a baby with Rh disease is severely anemic and jaundiced. Exchange transfusions will be necessary. This involves slowly removing the infant's anemic Rh-positive blood and replacing it with Rh-negative blood. The outlook for these infants has improved markedly over the years.

mothers have told their physicians that their drinking habits are more moderate. These infants have facial abnormalities and limb and heart defects. Some are growth retarded and also mentally retarded.

Caffeine is a stimulant found in coffee, tea, chocolate, and cola. Women who consume an excessive amount of caffeine tend to have babies who are slightly smaller than average. However, because these women also often smoke, it is not known whether caffeine is responsible for the low weight (see page 359).

Radiation from x-rays can damage the fetus. Therefore, avoid x-rays directed at the abdomen if at all possible.

Physicians now are clearly aware of the potential risks of x-ray to a fetus. Moreover, equipment has improved so that less radiation is needed. These factors combine to make x-ray examinations relatively safe when a pregnant woman has a medical condition that requires them.

If you are pregnant, it is safe to have an x-ray of your teeth, head, or extremities. Modern techniques protect your abdomen, and the only part of your body exposed to radiation is the area on which the x-ray is focused.

Congenital defects occur in about 2 to 3 percent of all newborns. Some defects correlate with the age of the mother. For example, if you are 30 years old, your chance of having a baby with Down syndrome is 1 in 885, but if you are over 40 the incidence is 1 in 109 births.

The risk of congenital defects is known to be increased by some drugs taken by the pregnant mother (see Therapeutic Drugs in Pregnancy, page 187), diseases such as diabetes, intrauterine infections, and alcoholism (see Pregnancy and Alcohol, page 429).

EARLY PREGNANCY: THE FIRST TRIMESTER

The first trimester of pregnancy can be difficult for an expectant mother and is without doubt the time when a developing embryo is most vulnerable.

Virtually every organ in your baby's body is being formed during the first 3 months of pregnancy. Thus, the embryo is particularly sensitive to assaults from the outside. If you take drugs, prescription or otherwise, drink alcohol, or are exposed to toxins or improper use of x-rays, this development can go awry and the result can be birth defects.

Miscarriage also is more likely to occur during this critical first trimester. Often this is nature's way of dealing with an abnormal embryo that could not have lived a normal life had the pregnancy been brought to term.

For you, the first 3 months of your pregnancy can be like riding a roller coaster. You are delighted and yet have some fears. If the pregnancy was unplanned, you may be losing sleep considering your options (see Pregnancy Termination: Medical Problems and Personal Choices, page 199). Physically, you may feel drained and find yourself napping whenever you get the opportunity. In many women the first trimester of pregnancy is marked by bouts of nausea and vomiting.

If you are considering becoming pregnant, think you may be pregnant, or are already in the early stages of pregnancy, rest assured that these weeks will pass quickly and so will most of the symptoms.

What are the symptoms of pregnancy? How do you know whether you are pregnant?

The first sign for most women is a missed menstrual period. If your periods are usually regular and suddenly you are a week late and you have had intercourse during your cycle, have a pregnancy test. Sometimes a woman will have what appears to be a period even though she is pregnant; however, this bleeding usually is scant.

Many pregnant women complain of breast tenderness. Your breasts may seem fuller and tingle. The nipples are often extremely sensitive. Sometimes the breasts actually hurt.

Morning sickness refers to the queasiness, nausea, and vomiting that are common during the first trimester. These problems, which often do not confine themselves to the morning, range from a slight upset stomach to incessant vomiting. This often begins a few days after a missed period.

Fatigue is common during early pregnancy. If you are home during the day, you probably find yourself lying down for a nap.

Women who work outside the home often arrive home so tired that they cannot wait to get into bed.

Frequent urination is another sign of pregnancy. This occurs initially because of the hormonal effects on the bladder and later because of the growing uterus exerting pressure on the bladder. As the size of your uterus begins to increase in your abdomen, this symptom will diminish. However, in the final weeks of pregnancy it returns, and many women find themselves unable to sleep through the night because of the urge to go to the bathroom.

When you have missed a period and have some of these other symptoms, see your physician. He or she will confirm your pregnancy with a pregnancy test (see Pregnancy Tests, page 183). Most women receive prenatal care from an obstetrician, a physician specially trained in the care of pregnant women and the delivery of babies. Some family physicians, especially in small towns, also offer this service to their patients. In some communities, licensed certified nurse midwives also provide maternity care.

Aside from the initial discomfort of pregnancy, the greatest threat in this first trimester is miscarriage (spontaneous abortion). *Miscarriage* and *abortion* refer to the termination of a pregnancy before the time the fetus can survive even for a few minutes outside the womb. This generally occurs after the 20th week after conception. If the abortion occurs spontaneously (spontaneous abortion), it is also known as a miscarriage. (Any fetus born dead after the 20th week is termed stillborn.)

About 50 percent of all fertilized eggs spontaneously abort, most of them before a woman has any idea she is pregnant. The percentage of miscarriages in women who know they are pregnant is about 10 percent. Three-quarters of these miscarriages occur in the first trimester, most between the 9th and 11th weeks of gestation.

Conditions associated with miscarriage include age (women older than 35 years), difficulty in becoming pregnant, and a history of miscarriage.

In the first trimester, miscarriage almost always occurs after the death of the embryo or fetus. Why does an embryo die in the uterus? The most common cause of miscarriage—an estimated 60 percent—is an abnormality in development, usually as a result of extra chromosomes. Other possible causes include chronic infections, unrecognized diabetes in the mother, and defects in the uterus.

Women who suffer a miscarriage (spontaneous abortion) tend to blame themselves. "I exercised too hard." "The stress at work caused it." "The fall off my bike caused me to lose my baby." It is natural to seek an explanation when this sad event occurs. However, rarely is it the result of stress or trauma. So try not to blame yourself.

The first symptom of a potential miscarriage is usually vaginal bleeding with or without cramping. An estimated one in five

PREGNANCY TERMINATION: MEDICAL PROBLEMS AND PERSONAL CHOICES

Therapeutic and elective abortions present an intensely politicized and personal dilemma in our nation. Since the Supreme Court ruled in 1973, in the landmark *Roe* v. *Wade* decision, that abortions were legal up to the 24th week, speeches, demonstrations, and even violence have been associated with the issue.

Elective Abortion
Resolution of the moral and ethical issues concerning abortion is an intensely personal decision among you, your physician, the father of the baby, and perhaps other counselors. At this time, however, if you do not want the fetus you are carrying and do not want to carry the fetus until birth, abortion is a legal means of terminating your pregnancy.

In most states, the decision is solely yours until the 12th week of pregnancy; some states have laws that affect the decision after that time. The choice to abort also may be made on the basis of information discovered through prenatal testing about the health of the fetus (for example, the finding that the fetus has Down syndrome or spina bifida).

Therapeutic Abortion
Abortions are performed not only as a matter of choice but also for medical reasons. For reasons of the mother's health, either physical or mental, a physician may recommend that an abortion be performed. Termed therapeutic abortion, it is done when the physician judges that the mother's life is endangered by the pregnancy.

The Procedures
There are different procedural options for terminating pregnancy. One, called vacuum suction, involves the insertion, into the cervix, of a tube attached to a suction device that removes the fetal tissue. Another procedure, called dilation and curettage (D & C) is described in detail on page 1066.

Pregnancy can be terminated after the 24th week, but the process involves inducing labor artificially through the use of drugs.

women have some vaginal bleeding or bloody discharge during the first trimester, and more than half of these women do not lose their babies. However, if you have any bleeding, call your physician immediately. Special precautions such as curtailing exercise, staying off your feet as much as possible, and avoiding intercourse may be necessary for several weeks.

When the embryo or fetus dies, miscarriage is inevitable. An inevitable miscarriage usually is accompanied by pain in the lower abdomen or back. The pain may be dull and relentless or sharp and intermittent. Bleeding may be heavy. Some clot-like material may emerge from your vagina. This is the embryo and placenta; if possible, save it and give it to your physician, who can examine it to try to determine the cause of death.

Sometimes only some of the products of conception are expelled. When this occurs it is called an incomplete abortion and the pain and bleeding can continue for several days.

If neither the fetus nor the placenta is expelled but the fetus has died, it is termed a missed abortion. You may not have any bleeding or pain during a missed abortion, but the symptoms of pregnancy will disappear soon. Your physician may suspect miscarriage when your uterus fails to grow.

Little can be done to prevent an inevitable, incomplete, or missed abortion. Usually a surgical procedure called a dilation and curettage (see page 1066) or a vacuum suction procedure is done to empty the uterus of any fetal remains. This is usually done in the hospital.

Most physicians recommend waiting a few months before trying to conceive again.

PRENATAL DIAGNOSIS

Recent years have seen a virtual revolution in the field of obstetrics. Today, physicians have the technology and the skill to examine

PRENATAL TESTS

Tests to determine whether the fetus has a congenital defect are becoming increasingly common, particularly for women older than 35 years.

Here are some of the prenatal tests now in use.

Genetic amniocentesis is performed early in the second trimester of pregnancy, usually between the 16th and 18th weeks of gestation. It is recommended for women 35 or older, for those who have a family history of congenital abnormalities such as Down syndrome or spina bifida, and for women who have previously given birth to an abnormal child.

During amniocentesis, your abdomen is anesthetized with a local anesthetic and the physician, guided by ultrasonography, inserts a long, thin needle through it into your uterus. This punctures the amniotic sac in which the fetus floats. A small amount of amniotic fluid is drawn into the needle,

which is then removed and sent to the laboratory for tests.

This fluid contains valuable genetic information about your growing baby. After a few weeks in a culture medium, the cells can be studied for chromosome distri-

bution. The presence of Down syndrome, indicated by the presence of an extra chromosome, can be successfully diagnosed with amniocentesis. In addition, other defects such as neurological problems, kidney diseases, and

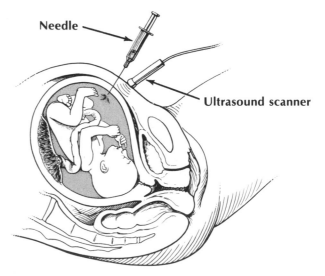

Needle

Ultrasound scanner

Amniocentesis involves removal of a small amount of amniotic fluid from the sac containing the fetus. Guided by an ultrasound image, your physician inserts a long, thin needle to withdraw fluid. Laboratory analysis of the fluid can reveal such things as your baby's sex, development, and overall health.

metabolic disorders may be diagnosed. Your baby's sex also can be determined, which can be helpful if there is a risk of a sex-linked disorder.

Amniocentesis also can be used later in pregnancy to detect Rh disease (see Rhesus [Rh] Incompatibility, page 197) or to ascertain whether the lungs are developed enough to withstand an early delivery.

Amniocentesis is usually safe for mother and child, but there is a slightly increased risk of miscarriage after the procedure.

Chorionic villus sampling is similar to amniocentesis in that it is an invasive technique that can detect many genetic abnormalities, including Down syndrome. A big advantage is that it can be done between 6 and 8 weeks of gestation. Thus, if a defect is found, you have the option of terminating the pregnancy in its early stages.

During chorionic sampling, a small piece of the placenta supporting the embryo is removed. Using ultrasonography, the physician inserts a catheter or small tube into your cervix. A suction procedure is used to suck the tissue into the catheter. You may feel slight discomfort but little more than is normally felt during a pelvic examination.

The removed tissue contains the same chromosomes as your developing baby. After an analysis of the membrane, your physician can determine whether your child has Down syndrome or other chromosome diseases. The test also can determine sex. Chorionic villus sampling is not as effective as amniocentesis for detecting some disorders, however. Sometimes amniocentesis is used after chorionic villus sampling, especially when it becomes important to rule out one of these defects.

Like amniocentesis, chorionic sampling slightly increases the risk of miscarriage. Moreover, the risk of intrauterine infection is greater than that associated with amniocentesis.

The maternal alpha-fetoprotein analysis is a noninvasive blood test that is useful for detecting defects in the nervous system, sometimes Down syndrome, and some other chromosome abnormalities.

Because the test carries no risk to mother or baby, many physicians recommend that all their pregnant patients undergo the test for alpha-fetoprotein at 16 weeks' gestation.

Alpha-fetoprotein is a protein made by every fetus. Normally, a small amount crosses the placenta and can be detected in the mother's blood. When it is found at higher than normal amounts, however, the fetus may have a neurological defect such as spina bifida (open spine) because large amounts of alpha-fetoprotein are allowed to leak into the amniotic fluid. These defects are rare, occurring in an estimated 1 to 2 babies out of 1,000.

Your physician will draw blood from your arm for this test. To enhance the accuracy of the test, it should be done around your fourth month of pregnancy. If the test results are negative, the chances are that your baby does not have a neurological defect, although the test is not an absolute guarantee.

Approximately 50 women out of 1,000 have positive results. If this should happen to you, do not assume the worst. This finding may mean the fetus is simply older than was thought, that you are carrying twins, or that something else increased the alpha-fetoprotein level in your blood. A second blood test is then warranted.

When two blood tests are positive, an ultrasound examination usually is done. If this test fails to find a defect, amniocentesis is the next step.

Of 50 women with positive test results, only 1 or 2 will be carrying a child with a defect of this kind.

Percutaneous umbilical cord sampling tests fetal blood from the umbilical cord for the prenatal diagnosis of some genetic disorders. It is done most easily in the third trimester. This technique also has been used to determine oxygen and carbon dioxide levels in the blood, which may help diagnose growth retardation.

(See also Antenatal Testing, page 206.)

your baby in the womb without causing discomfort to you or your baby.

The advent of ultrasound examination (see page 1286) has made it possible to visualize the embryo as early as 7 weeks after you have missed a period. This noninvasive and painless diagnostic tool has proved invaluable in many cases, although some physicians believe that the ultrasound examination has become too commonplace.

Ultrasound examination is effective for determining whether you are carrying more than one baby. It allows a physician to monitor your baby's rate of growth to determine whether it is normal for gestational age. With ultrasound examination, it may be possible to tell whether the fetus has kidney disease or an intestinal obstruction or is missing an arm or leg. The tiny fetal brain can be examined for a few abnormalities. When there is a question about whether the fetus has died in the uterus, ultrasound examination usually can provide the answer.

With a simple blood test done at 16 weeks' gestation, it is now possible to tell whether your baby may have a defect such as spina bifida (see page 56). Many physicians are routinely doing this test (alpha-fetoprotein test) or at least are offering it to all their pregnant patients (see page 201).

Many women are delaying motherhood to an age at which genetic abnormalities are more likely. A few years ago, these women had to wait 9 months to know whether their child had an abnormality. Now, women 35 years or older, as well as those with a family history of certain abnormalities, can know earlier in the pregnancy whether the fetus they are carrying has a birth defect. In addition, physicians can determine fetal sex (see Prenatal Tests, page 200).

Not only can problems be diagnosed in the womb but also a few can be treated. Using ultrasonography to visualize the fetus, physicians can perform surgery through the womb to alleviate problems such as urinary obstruction and hydrocephalus (the accumulation of cerebrospinal fluid in the head). This type of intervention can sometimes prevent irreparable damage.

ECTOPIC PREGNANCY

Signs and Symptoms
- Vaginal bleeding.

Ectopic pregnancy occurs when the fertilized egg implants itself anywhere other than in the uterus. The fertilized egg may become implanted on the ovary or in the abdominal cavity, but in 95 percent of all ectopic pregnancies the egg is implanted in the fallopian tube. Thus an ectopic pregnancy is sometimes called a tubal pregnancy.

This is an extremely dangerous condition that, when not detected early, can have dire consequences. It is a leading cause of pregnancy-related death.

Normally, the egg and sperm meet in the fallopian tube, where fertilization then takes place. The fertilized egg, which rapidly is becoming a more complex mass of cells, then travels to the uterus, where it implants itself in the lining of the uterus. The interior of the fallopian tube is not unlike a maze, with twists and turns and folds. Sometimes, for various reasons, the fertilized egg becomes stuck and implants in this unsuitable environment. This growing egg immediately begins to produce human chorionic gonadotropin (hCG), a hormone associated with pregnancy (see Pregnancy Tests, page 183). The growing embryo then begins to secrete other hormones, which cause an increase in the tube's blood supply. As the embryo continues to drill into the tube, vessels begin to bleed.

Unlike the uterus, the tube was not made for pregnancy. As the embryo grows, the tube becomes stretched beyond its capacity. Hemorrhage often occurs. If the pregnancy continues long enough the tube will rupture, a potentially life-threatening situation.

The frequency of ectopic pregnancy has increased in recent years. It now occurs in about 1 out of every 100 pregnancies.

No one is certain why ectopic pregnancy has become more common. Some speculate that an increase in the incidence of pelvic inflammatory disease may be at least partially responsible. It is known, however, that some medical conditions tend to be associated with a higher risk of ectopic pregnancy. These include abnormalities of the tube, tubal adhesions caused by infection, appendicitis, endometriosis, and the absence of one ovary.

The Diagnosis. If you have an ectopic pregnancy, initially you may not know that anything is wrong. Despite a missed menstrual period, results of a urine pregnancy test may be negative. This occurs because hCG (a hormone found in pregnant women's urine) is present in much higher amounts when the pregnancy is uterine.

Potentially life-threatening, an ectopic pregnancy occurs when a fertilized egg implants itself in the fallopian tube rather than the uterus. As the embryo develops, it causes the tube to expand beyond its capacity, producing hemorrhage and potentially serious medical consequences.

Fallopian tube

Uterus

Thus, if you have the symptoms of pregnancy but the pregnancy test is negative, your physician will probably order a blood test, which can detect hCG at lower levels.

As the embryo continues to grow and exert pressure on the walls of the tube, you will begin to have abdominal pain. You may have some vaginal bleeding, which is usually scanty and dark brown. The pain and bleeding will get worse as the pregnancy progresses. During bouts of internal bleeding, you may have severe cramping. If enough blood leaks into the abdominal cavity, you may have the sudden urge to urinate or have a bowel movement. Dizziness and fainting also are associated with ectopic pregnancy when the internal hemorrhage becomes severe.

Treatment. Report any of these symptoms to your physician immediately. If your physician suspects an ectopic pregnancy, he or she will first do a pelvic examination to detect any abnormalities. An ultrasound examination (see page 1286) or laparoscopy (see page 1297) may be done to confirm the presence of a mass.

There is no chance you can carry this pregnancy to term or to a point at which the fetus has a good chance of surviving. Ectopic fetuses seldom develop beyond 3 months.

The treatment is immediate operation. If the embryo is still small and the fallopian tube has not been ruptured, the embryo may be squeezed out without further injury to the tube. Some physicians favor removing the injured part of the tube and rejoining the ends.

When there has been massive hemorrhage, blood transfusion may be necessary. In such a case, the physician will have to stop the internal bleeding by clamping off blood vessels. Often the removal of a tube and even of an ovary is necessary.

If you have had an ectopic pregnancy, what are your chances of having a normal pregnancy later? In women who have had an initial ectopic pregnancy, about 10 percent of subsequent pregnancies will be ectopic pregnancies. Once you have had two ectopic pregnancies, your chances are less than 50 percent of ever having a normal pregnancy. If the ectopic pregnancies have significantly injured both fallopian tubes, in vitro fertilization (see page 1135) may be the only option left if you still want to try a pregnancy.

MID-PREGNANCY: THE SECOND TRIMESTER

For most women the second trimester of pregnancy is less eventful than the first trimester.

The fatigue is lessened. The nausea and vomiting decrease or are absent. And you no longer have frequent urination.

Your abdomen is growing slowly and you start to wear maternity clothes. Your body is becoming rounder around the middle and probably at the hips, too, but it is not yet unwieldy.

In short, you feel great.

For most women, the 4th, 5th, and 6th months of pregnancy are uneventful and even enjoyable.

At this stage, you are still seeing your physician once a month, unless you have a medical condition that warrants more frequent visits. You are taking an iron and folic acid supplement, and you should be making an effort to eat a balanced diet containing several servings each day of protein-rich foods including milk products, fruits, vegetables, and grains (see Nutrition and Weight Control During Pregnancy, page 185).

You probably did not gain more than a few pounds during your first trimester but now notice your weight starts to increase. This is not uncommon; many women gain the bulk of their weight during the second trimester.

If you have been contemplating travel, now is probably the best time during pregnancy to take a trip. You are feeling better than during the earlier months, and as your due date approaches your increased size will tax your energies and you will be better off staying close to home.

Although the second trimester is the easiest part of pregnancy for most women, it is not without risks. Miscarriage is not the risk that it was during the first 3 months, but some labors commence during the second trimester. A fetus delivered this early is not yet mature enough to survive. Although premature labor most often occurs later (third trimester), defects of the uterus can lead to this early labor during mid-pregnancy.

This section explores some of the medical complications of this normally uneventful part of pregnancy.

PREMATURE LABOR

Signs and Symptoms
- A gush of fluid escaping from your vagina;
- Abdominal contractions.

Normally, labor occurs about 40 weeks (280 days) after the first day of your last period. If your baby is born between 38 and 42 weeks, delivery is considered at term.

Sometimes, for various reasons, labor—the signal that your baby is about to be born—begins before term. The less time your infant has had in your womb, the less its chances of survival. Thus, premature labor can be an ominous sign. In some cases, however, an early labor may be induced by your physician if the uterine environment appears to be becoming increasingly harmful to the fetus and its chances of survival are better outside the womb.

What are the symptoms of premature labor? The membranes that surround the baby may rupture. If that occurs, you will feel a gush of fluid escape from your vagina. This usually occurs when labor is in progress, but occasionally it is the first step. You also may feel some contractions in your abdomen, which may go from mild to severe. Generally, if you have contractions that last for at least 30 seconds and occur every 10 minutes, you are probably in labor.

What causes a woman to begin labor weeks or even months too soon? Most often the precise cause is never determined. However, the following conditions are associated with premature or preterm labor: spontaneous rupture of membranes (see page 208), incompetent cervix (see page 205), abnormal uterus, hydramnios (see page 205), abnormal fetus or placenta, placenta previa (see page 209), retained intrauterine contraceptive device, preeclampsia and eclampsia (see page 207), death of the fetus, and history of premature delivery, multiple fetuses, cigarette smoking, hemorrhage, and serious maternal disease. Teenagers and women older than 40 are more likely to have premature labor.

Treatment.   The treatment for premature labor varies, depending on the age of the fetus.

Initially, many physicians prescribe bed rest and observation. This precaution alone is sometimes successful for stopping contractions. Tranquilizers may be given to ease your anxiety.

Thus far there is no specific drug that is always successful for stopping premature labor. However, several therapies have had some degree of success.

Magnesium sulfate may be effective for stopping labor. If your physician prescribes this drug, you will be monitored in the hospital very carefully because magnesium sulfate can cause breathing problems. Moreover, the drug does pass through the placenta, and it also may affect your newborn's respiratory movements.

Another group of drugs that has had some success in arresting labor are the beta-mimetics. These drugs, which must be given in the hospital where you can be monitored closely, mimic the effects of epinephrine, the hormone the body secretes in response to danger (it is well known that fright can delay or halt labor). These drugs will temporarily stop labor and relax the uterus. If you are given one of these drugs, your heart will beat faster, you may feel shaky and anxious, and your blood pressure and blood sugar concentration will increase. Other possible side effects include fluid in the lungs and chest pain. Like magnesium sulfate, the beta-mimetics cross the placenta, and as a result your baby experiences similar symptoms.

If your premature labor is determined to be the result of a defect in your uterus, sometimes an operation can be done to forestall labor. One procedure, called "cerclage," involves placing surgical stitches (sutures) around the cervix so the infant can stay in the womb until term (see Incompetent Cervix, page 205).

In recent years, major advances have been made in the care of seriously ill or premature infants. Babies as small as 1 pound now have a chance of survival when they are cared for in specialized neonatal units. However, most infants born before the third trimester of pregnancy do not survive (see Premature Babies, page 19).

HYDRAMNIOS

Signs and Symptoms
- Breathlessness;
- Indigestion or nausea;
- Abdominal distention and accompanying intense pain;
- Premature labor (see page 204).

Hydramnios refers to a condition in which there is an excessive amount of amniotic fluid around the baby.

In most cases the swelling is slight and harmless; in about 1 out of 1,000 pregnancies, however, the condition is severe enough to cause symptoms. Diabetic women and those carrying multiple fetuses have a higher incidence of hydramnios than other pregnant women.

Normally, the fetus begins to urinate and to swallow amniotic fluid in the second trimester of pregnancy. Later in the pregnancy these functions may help control the amount of fluid in the womb. Hydramnios often is associated with birth defects, particularly with malformations of the central nervous system and gastrointestinal tract. Some of these defects prevent the fetus from swallowing amniotic fluid, and others may cause it to excrete an excessive amount of urine. When hydramnios occurs in a woman who is carrying twins, one fetus perhaps takes over most of the circulation meant for both babies. The result is an increased urine output for this twin.

Some women with slight hydramnios have no symptoms or the gradual onset of breathlessness, indigestion, and a distended abdomen. Rarely, the swelling causes severe abdominal distention, nausea, and intense pain. These effects can lead to premature labor.

Treatment. If your physician suspects hydramnios, he or she probably will want you to have an immediate ultrasound examination. If the hydramnios is not severe, no treatment other than resting a little more than usual may be prescribed. If the pain is severe, hospitalization and sedation may be necessary. You may be given drugs to relax your uterus to reduce the chance of premature labor. Sometimes amniocentesis is used to release some of the excess fluid. Although this relieves pain, it must be repeated often and it can initiate premature labor.

INCOMPETENT CERVIX

If you have an incompetent cervix, the mouth (lower portion) of your uterus opens during the second trimester or early part of the third trimester. The result is a miscarriage or premature delivery.

A woman with an incompetent cervix usually has a history of miscarriage, typically in the second trimester of pregnancy. The cervix usually does not open before the 4th month of pregnancy because the fetus is not sufficiently large to dilate it.

The cause of incompetent cervix is unknown, but the condition often is associated with trauma to the cervix after procedures such as dilation and curettage and with abnormal development of the cervix (such as occurs with exposure to the synthetic estrogen hormone diethylstilbestrol, see page 1092).

If your medical history indicates a possible incompetent cervix, surgery can be done to close your cervix during pregnancy. Called cerclage, the procedure is performed while you are under a general anesthetic, usually after the first trimester. Using strong thread, your physician will actually stitch around your cervix to close it to prevent you from expelling the fetus. After the operation

If the lower portion of your uterus, your cervix, opens during pregnancy, a surgical procedure may be done to prevent premature delivery of your baby. Called cerclage, this involves stitching the cervix closed to prevent expulsion of the fetus from the uterus.

ANTENATAL TESTING

Life in the uterus is not without risk.

Sometimes, for various reasons, there is cause to suspect that the fetus may be in danger. Perhaps a previously active baby suddenly ceases to move, or blood tests reveal that an Rh-negative mother is developing antibodies against her Rh-positive fetus. Whatever the reason, if your physician suspects something is wrong, several techniques can be used to evaluate fetal health, the goal being to find any sign of distress before irreparable damage has been done. The following are commonly used methods.

The ultrasound examination (sonography) has had a major impact on the practice of modern-day obstetrics. The use of high-frequency sound waves seems to be safe for both mother and baby. Moreover, it is not invasive or painful (see also page 1286).

In addition to its applications in early pregnancy, it is often used to ascertain whether the fetus has intrauterine growth retardation, to determine the infant's position in the womb, to locate the position of the placenta if placenta previa (see page 209) is suspected, and to detect hydramnios (see page 205).

Doppler studies are done to detect the action of the fetal heart. These can be done by the 12th week of pregnancy. Using ultrasound, these studies are particularly useful for determining whether a fetus has died in the uterus when the heartbeat cannot be heard with a stethoscope.

Electronic fetal nonstress and stress tests evaluate the fetal heart rate to determine whether there is a problem and whether the infant will be able to withstand a normal labor and delivery. These tests often are used when a woman notices a marked reduction in the amount of movement of the fetus. They also often are prescribed for women with the symptoms of pre-eclampsia (see page 207), for women with a history of stillbirth, for diabetics, for sensitized Rh-negative mothers, and when fetal growth rate seems to be abnormally slow.

The first step is often the nonstress test. During this test, you lie on your back and a recording device connected to an electronic monitor is attached to your abdomen. Fetal heart rate, uterine contractions, and fetal movements are recorded.

Contraction stress testing is done when the results of the nonstress test are abnormal. If your physician prescribes this test, you will be given a drug that stimulates contractions. The effect of the contractions on the fetus is then monitored. This test can help your physician determine whether your infant is in fetal distress. If so, a decision to induce labor may be made if the fetus is old enough to survive. The test also can help the physician determine whether the infant is able to withstand a normal labor and vaginal delivery or whether a cesarean section should be done (see also Prenatal Tests, page 200).

you will be given drugs to reduce the chance that the procedure could have stimulated premature labor.

Cerclage is successful in 85 to 90 percent of cases. The thread is cut in your 9th month of pregnancy.

LATE PREGNANCY: THE THIRD TRIMESTER

During the third trimester of pregnancy, what seemed so far off just a few months ago is now within reach—almost.

No matter how well you have felt, this is probably the point when you ask, "When will it be over?" Your maternity clothes are getting tight. Your walk has given way to the pregnant waddle. You may notice stretch marks on your breasts and abdomen. Your feet and ankles may be so swollen that your shoes do not fit.

You may be exhausted. Somehow you cannot seem to get comfortable at night, and when you do the baby starts kicking you.

Finally, the kicking stops and you sleep an hour or two and then wake up with the uncontrollable urge to urinate. You awake the next morning, looking as though you have been up all night. But it is hard to find time to sleep. The easy days of middle pregnancy are over.

Many couples attend classes in preparation for childbirth; these often are taken during your last trimester of pregnancy. There you are taught about the birth process, given exercises to strengthen your pelvic muscles and to enable you to push more effectively, and taught relaxation and breathing techniques that may help to relieve some of the pain. Many physicians recommend these classes even for women who know they want to use an anesthetic during labor and delivery.

Many women, particularly those who have previously miscarried in early pregnancy, understandably are relieved to reach the late stage of pregnancy. With proper treatment in a specialized neonatal unit, even babies born early in the third trimester have a good chance of survival. However, barring any maternal disease that can make the environment of the womb harmful, there is no substitute for a full 9-month pregnancy. Thus, one of your physician's goals is to prevent premature labor whenever possible.

Your visits to the physician will be more frequent during the final trimester. Up until now, you probably have been seeing the physician once a month, unless you have a medical problem that warrants more frequent visits. After the 30th gestational week, your physician probably will want to see you every 2 weeks until the 36th week, when you will begin weekly visits. Toward the end of your pregnancy, your physician may perform a pelvic examination to see whether your cervix is beginning to dilate in preparation for labor.

The vast majority of women deliver near term and have no major complications. The problem of premature labor may occur in the third trimester as well as in the second (see page 204); but the later in pregnancy it occurs, the better the outlook for the infant. However, there are some serious conditions associated with late pregnancy. Preeclampsia and eclampsia are dangerous conditions that, when not detected early, can cause both fetal and maternal death (see below). Other problems that your physician will be watching for include hemorrhage (see page 208), placenta previa (see page 209), premature rupture of membranes (see page 208), intrauterine death (see page 209), and intrauterine growth retardation (see page 192).

PREECLAMPSIA AND ECLAMPSIA

Signs and Symptoms
- High blood pressure;
- Increased amounts of fluid (edema) leading to puffiness of the face and hands;

- Seizures;
- Unconsciousness.

Preeclampsia is a serious disease of late pregnancy. The symptoms include hypertension, protein in the urine, and fluid retention that causes the face and hands to become puffy.

Eclampsia is the next stage of the disease, occurring when the preeclamptic symptoms are not brought under control. Warning signs of eclampsia include pain in the upper right side of your abdomen and seeing flashing lights. A pregnant woman with eclampsia has severe convulsions, followed by unconsciousness. Eclampsia is one of the most dangerous conditions of pregnancy, and it can be fatal for both the mother and her baby.

Neither of these conditions is as common as they once were, presumably because of improved prenatal care. Preeclampsia occurs in about 5 percent of all pregnancies, and the overall incidence of eclampsia is about 1 in 1,500 pregnancies.

Preeclampsia and eclampsia are called the toxemias of pregnancy, although thus far no one has been able to identify a toxic substance in a pregnant woman's blood that can cause these conditions. Hence, the cause remains unknown. As a result, there is no treatment that is universally effective.

Physicians do know, however, how to diagnose the conditions and that some women appear to be at higher risk. Teenage mothers, women older than 40 years, women in their first pregnancy, women with a history of high blood pressure, and women who are carrying twins all are at higher risk for preeclampsia and eclampsia.

The Diagnosis. If preeclampsia develops, you will know it. Initially you may feel normal because hypertension and protein in the urine usually do not cause pain (this is one of the reasons why it is so important to keep your prenatal appointments). However, other symptoms occur as the preeclampsia progresses. They include facial puffiness, particularly around the eyes, sudden and excessive weight gain, severe headaches, and vision disturbances.

Treatment. If you have very mild preeclampsia, your physician may prescribe medication to control your blood pressure, instruct you to eat a low-salt diet, and tell you to rest in bed, lying on your left side as much as possible to take the weight of the uterus off your major blood vessels. These precautions will improve blood flow to your kidneys. Sometimes this is all the treatment that is necessary.

However, you may require hospitalization, during which you will be given medications for your hypertension and to remove excess body fluid. The goal in treating preeclampsia is to keep it from progressing to eclampsia. The best treatment for severe preeclampsia is delivery of the baby. If you are near term, your physician may induce labor or perform a cesarean section. If the fetus does not have a good chance of surviving at this stage in its gestation, many physicians will try to forestall labor if the preeclampsia is not too severe. You and your baby will both be monitored continuously to make sure neither of you is in distress.

After delivery, the symptoms of preeclampsia usually become less severe, although in some women eclampsia develops during the first 24 hours after delivery.

Eclampsia is not the problem it once was. However, if eclampsia does occur, your physician will want you to deliver at once. Because of the availability of improved prenatal care, the vast majority of women with preeclampsia never progress to eclampsia.

ANTEPARTUM HEMORRHAGE

Signs and Symptoms
- Vaginal bleeding that occurs after the fifth month of pregnancy.

Many conditions can cause antepartum (pre-birth) hemorrhage in middle or late pregnancy, including placenta previa (see page 209), cervical damage, separation of the placenta from the uterine wall, and a burst varicose vein in the vagina.

Most often, antepartum bleeding is mild and no damage is done. However, when this bleeding becomes heavy, it can be dangerous for both you and your baby.

Treatment. Report any bleeding during pregnancy to your physician immediately. Your physician will want to determine the cause of the problem. You may need to be hospitalized and have an ultrasound examination and blood tests.

When there is substantial blood loss, blood transfusion is often necessary.

Sometimes, when the hemorrhage poses a threat, early delivery of the infant—either by inducing labor or by cesarean section—is warranted.

PREMATURE RUPTURE OF MEMBRANES

Signs and Symptoms
- A gush or a constant dribble of fluid from the vagina.

Normally, the membranes that surround the fetus rupture either just before labor or during labor. Occasionally, however, these membranes rupture weeks or months before the anticipated delivery date.

When this occurs, there is a high risk that your labor will also begin within a few days—this is a dangerous prospect if you are in the middle of your pregnancy. Moreover, there is a risk of infection once the membranes have ruptured.

The cause of ruptured membranes usually remains a mystery.

The Diagnosis. If your membranes rupture, you may feel a sudden gush or a slow

WHAT IS FALSE LABOR?

Many women have one or more bouts of false labor before real labor begins.

False labor is more likely to occur in the final weeks of pregnancy and in women who have already borne a child.

How can you distinguish false labor from true labor?

With false labor you will have contractions, but they will be irregular and will not increase in frequency and intensity, as true contractions do. Moreover, the pain will be in the lower abdomen and groin, whereas true labor pains begin higher in the uterus and then radiate throughout the abdomen and lower back.

When your labor is false, walking may stop the contractions, whereas with true labor, walking generally has no effect.

If you suspect you are in labor, call your physician. A pelvic examination can ascertain whether your cervix is beginning to dilate, a sign of true labor.

Above all, do not dismiss your symptoms without seeking medical advice. Many pregnant women have postponed going to the hospital, convinced it was only a false alarm, only to end up giving birth before reaching the hospital.

trickle of fluid from your vagina. Call your physician immediately. You probably will be hospitalized. Amniocentesis (see page 200) may be done to determine whether your infant's lungs are mature enough for it to survive an early delivery. If the lungs are mature, labor may be induced with drugs.

Treatment.   If your infant is too immature to have a good chance of survival outside the womb, your physician may give you drugs to relax the uterine muscles to decrease the chance of early labor. This can be successful, but the risk of serious infection remains, so your condition must be monitored closely.

PLACENTA PREVIA

Signs and Symptoms
- Painless bleeding from the vagina.

In placenta previa, the placenta is not implanted high in the uterus but is located partially or completely over the cervix. Late in pregnancy as the uterus prepares for labor, the cervix expands and any placenta near it is torn loose. The result is a raw area that bleeds.

Approximately 1 in 200 pregnancies that go beyond the 7th month have placenta previa. Uncommon in first pregnancies, placenta previa is more likely to occur with each subsequent pregnancy. Older mothers tend to be more at risk, as are women who have had cesarean sections.

The Diagnosis.   The most common sign of placenta previa is painless hemorrhage, usually at the end of the second trimester or later. Often the hemorrhage first occurs at night when you are asleep. You may awaken to find yourself in a pool of blood. Usually the bleeding stops on its own.

Treatment.   If your physician suspects placenta previa, he or she will ask you to have an ultrasound examination. If you are close to your delivery date, your physician may want you to undergo a cesarean section to prevent further bleeding from the placenta, which can cause fetal brain damage or even death. Blood transfusions may be necessary if the hemorrhage is severe.

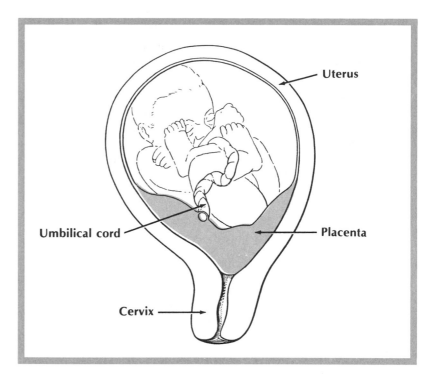

INTRAUTERINE DEATH

Most fetal deaths occur as miscarriages in the first weeks of pregnancy. Occasionally, however, a fetus will die after the 5th month of gestation.

There are several conditions that are responsible for intrauterine death. These include preeclampsia and eclampsia (see page 207), maternal diabetes (see page 24), antepartum hemorrhage (see page 208), postmaturity (see page 210), Rh disease (see page 197), and severe congenital abnormalities.

Usually the death of a fetus is silent. One day you may notice that you do not feel the baby move like you used to. When the physician fails to detect a heartbeat, monitoring techniques will be used to determine whether the fetus is still alive (see page 200).

Most often, labor begins within 2 weeks after fetal death, although it may be longer in middle pregnancy. If your labor does not begin on its own, you will be given drugs to induce it. There is concern that if your labor is too overdue, you may develop blood clotting abnormalities that can set the stage for a life-threatening hemorrhage.

In most cases, the outlook for future pregnancies is the same as for first pregnancies. The biggest hurdle is the grief that every couple must work through after an intrauterine death.

If the placenta is located over the cervix (placenta previa), painless hemorrhage may occur. If this happens, see your physician immediately.

TWINS AND MULTIPLE PREGNANCIES

What are the chances that you are expecting twins? If you are Oriental, you are much less likely to have a multiple birth than if you are black. A teenager has a 1 in 167 chance of having twins, while the rate for a 40-year-old woman is 1 in 55. The more children you have, the greater your likelihood of producing twins. Finally, fraternal twins simply run in some families.

Twin pregnancies account for 1 in 90 births in the United States; triplets occur in 1 of 8,000 pregnancies.

A multiple pregnancy occurs when either more than one egg is fertilized or the one egg splits after fertilization. Seven of 10 pairs of twins are fraternal, meaning they came from two eggs and two sperm.

In about 7 of 10 cases, your physician will discover you are carrying multiple fetuses before labor. Abnormal weight gain or size, an excessive amount of movement, and the detection of two heartbeats are common clues. If your physician suspects twins, he or she will order an ultrasound examination.

If you are expecting twins, you need to take extra good care of yourself. Try to increase the amount of rest you get, take in more calories, and be diligent about your prenatal visits; adherence to your prenatal checkup schedule is especially important because the incidence of preeclampsia and eclampsia (see page 207), placenta previa (see page 209), and hemorrhage is higher when you are carrying multiple fetuses.

Multiple pregnancies tend to be shorter, an average of 21 days shorter for women delivering twins. Unless there is a medical reason to indicate cesarean section, twins can be delivered vaginally. And a woman who wants to breast-feed can do so.

POSTMATURITY (PROLONGED PREGNANCY)

Signs and Symptoms
- Labor and delivery that fail to occur by the 42nd week of pregnancy.

"Postmaturity" means a pregnancy that is prolonged beyond 42 weeks (the average pregnancy lasts 40 weeks from the onset of the last menstrual period).

As with prematurity, postmaturity can be dangerous. The overdue infant is living in an aging placenta that often fails to provide adequate oxygen. Moreover, the infant may be getting larger than a newborn is supposed to be, which may make delivery extremely difficult. Or fetal growth may be halted altogether by the increasingly harmful womb environment, and the infant may be literally starving to death.

As a result, the stillbirth rate of these babies is twice that of those born after a pregnancy of normal length.

Treatment. If your pregnancy continues after 42 weeks, your physician probably will induce labor, provided he or she is sure that the baby is indeed overdue and there has not been a mistake in calculating the time of conception. If the baby is very large, forceps may be needed during the delivery or a cesarean section may be performed.

LABOR AND DELIVERY

How will I know when my labor begins?

That is sometimes a difficult question because each woman and each pregnancy are different. Maybe this is your first child, and you are confused by friends and relatives who tell you that labor will be the toughest hours of your life or that it will not be so bad. Perhaps you have already borne a child and you expect this labor to be similar to your previous one. Whatever you expect, expect the unexpected.

Every labor is slightly different. But there are some good indicators that labor is beginning or about ready to begin.

1. A few days or hours before labor actually begins, you may have what is called "bloody show." This is the discharge of a small amount of blood-tinged mucus. Actually, it is the mucus plug that formed the barrier between your uterus and your vagina during your pregnancy.

2. The membranes that surround the amniotic fluid may rupture at the beginning of labor or as the labor progresses. If the membranes fail to rupture during labor, the physician ruptures them. When your membranes (sometimes called "bag of waters") rupture, you may feel a gush of fluid from your vagina or simply a slow trickle.

3. Contractions may or may not be a sign that you are in labor. Throughout pregnancy, you may have noticed your uterus

contracting. These are called Braxton Hicks contractions, and they usually do not cause discomfort until the last weeks of pregnancy. Many women then have these contractions and believe they are in labor. It is often difficult for pregnant women to distinguish between these Braxton Hicks contractions (false labor) and those of real labor (see page 210). As a rule, the contractions of real labor occur at regular intervals. The period between contractions slowly begins to get shorter, and the contractions become longer and more intense. The pain usually begins high in the uterus and then radiates down the abdomen and to the lower back. If walking makes the contractions stop, they are generally false labor (see What Is False Labor?, page 208).

If you have any of these signs, notify your physician. Your physician may want to examine you to see whether your cervix is dilating and thinning (effacing), signs that the baby is getting ready to be born. If your membranes rupture, your physician probably will want you to go to the hospital immediately.

How long will I be in labor? That is a common question and one that is impossible to predict with any accuracy until your physician can determine how quickly your cervix is readying itself. As a rule, labor usually is longer with first babies. The uterus and birth canal of a first-time mother are less flexible, and as such it takes longer for labor and birth. A first-time mother generally can expect about 13 hours to pass between the time she goes into active labor and the birth of her baby. Some women, however, are in labor much longer. For a woman who has previously given birth, the average time is between 4 and 8 hours.

There are three stages of labor.

During the first stage your cervix opens so that the baby can pass into the birth canal. Think of the uterus as a large, upside down, elastic bottle. When labor begins the cervix is about ½ inch long and almost closed. It would be impossible for a baby to pass through such a small opening, so somehow the cervix has to open. Contractions cause the cervix to open (dilate) by creating pressure within the uterus. This force is tremendous and is directed against the uterus in two ways. During a contraction, the infant is sub-

jected to an intense pressure that forces it against the cervix. These repeated attempts eventually will stretch the cervix open. The cervix is said to be fully dilated when it is open to a diameter of 4 inches. At the same time, the contractions cause the cervix to become thinned (effaced) or to merge with the uterine walls.

During the first stage of labor, your contractions will become more frequent and last longer. You may be attached to a machine that monitors your infant's heart rate and charts the onset and cessation of each contraction. Your physician or a nurse periodically will do a pelvic examination to determine how you are progressing. When the contractions are not forceful enough to open the cervix, a drug may be given to make your uterus contract.

Some women go through the entire labor with no pain medication. These women usually have taken classes in prepared childbirth and learned breathing techniques. Many women find that they need some pain relief, however, particularly as they get closer to full dilation. If you need something for the pain, do not be afraid to ask your physician.

The second stage of labor is when your baby is born. Your cervix is now fully dilated and effaced. This is the baby's signal to start the 5-inch journey down the birth canal. Now that the cervix offers no resistance, each contraction serves to propel the infant downward. You may feel a tremendous urge to push, almost as though you want to have a bowel movement. You must wait, however, until instructed to do so by your physician or nurse. Sometimes this urge to push comes before the cervix is fully dilated.

Push only when you are having a contraction. In this way two forces—that of the contraction and your pushing—combine to move the baby, which conserves your energy.

Both the first and the second stages of labor are longer for first-time mothers. On the average it takes about 1 to 2 hours to push a first baby out, whereas women who have previously given birth complete the second stage in anywhere from 15 to 40 minutes.

As you push and the baby begins to move, the vaginal opening becomes more and more dilated and begins to bulge. At this point you might be moved from the labor room to the delivery room. In some hospitals, all stages of labor and delivery occur in

PROCEDURES YOU MAY ENCOUNTER DURING LABOR AND DELIVERY

Electronic Fetal Monitoring

Electronic fetal monitoring is commonly used to record the unborn baby's heartbeat during labor.

Fetal monitoring also may be done before labor when the mother has a medical problem that may jeopardize the fetus (see page 192).

As the uterus contracts during labor, there is a temporary reduction in the flow of blood through the placenta. This can place stress on an infant who has been weakened by disease. Thus, many physicians use fetal monitoring during all labors as a precautionary method to help ensure the safety of the unborn infant.

During labor, an electrode may be inserted through your vagina onto the baby's scalp. This is done after the membranes have ruptured. At the same time, an electrode is attached to your abdomen. Your contractions and the response of the baby's heart to these contractions are then recorded.

If the baby's heart rate indicates possible distress, your physician may decide it is safer to deliver the infant immediately by cesarean section.

Fetal Blood Sampling

Another method of helping to identify a fetus in distress during labor is by extracting a sample of fetal blood and measuring its alkaline or acid content (pH). If your physician suspects your baby is getting an inadequate amount of oxygen, he or she may perform this test. A tube called an endoscope will be inserted through your dilated cervix to the baby's skin, usually the scalp. A couple of incisions are then made in the skin and a small amount of blood is drawn into a tube. The pH in the blood is measured. If the pH is lower than normal, you may need an immediate cesarean section.

Induction of Labor

Sometimes it is necessary to start (induce) labor.

Although there are cases in which labor is induced because of convenience—either the physician's or the mother's—this is not recommended. Most labor inductions occur because the mother, baby, or both are in danger if the pregnancy continues.

The most common medical reasons for inducing labor include preeclampsia and eclampsia (see page 207) and premature rupture of the membranes, which makes infection a risk (see page 208). Labor also may be induced when the fetus is in distress as a result of its mother's preeclampsia, eclampsia, or diabetes or when the baby is overdue.

If your physician recommends that your labor be induced, he or she may first rupture your membranes if your cervix shows no sign of dilation. Sometimes this will bring on labor. At other times, drugs such as oxytocin may be used after rupture of the membranes to bring on or enhance contractions. Another method involves the insertion of prostaglandin suppositories into the vagina.

Episiotomy

An episiotomy is an incision made just before delivery that widens the vagina so that the mother's tissues are not damaged.

This surgical procedure is often done with first pregnancies, during premature labor, and when a forceps delivery is necessary.

If your physician believes your vagina will be torn during delivery, he or she will inject a local anesthetic into the area between your vagina and rectum. An incision is then made just before the emergence of the baby's head.

After the delivery, the incision is sutured with stitches that will dissolve. You may have some pain for a while; this can be relieved with hot baths or ice packs, pain medication, and sprays that contain a local anesthetic.

Pain Relief

Everyone's pain threshold is different. Some women are able to withstand the pain of even a difficult labor and delivery with no pain relief; but others cannot.

Gone are the days when women routinely were given general anesthetics and woke up hours later to be told they had had a boy or girl. Today, most women want to be awake and alert for the birth.

Four basic types of anesthesia are used during labor and delivery.

Narcotics such as meperidine can be given to help a woman in labor relax and tolerate the pain better. They do not totally eliminate pain but may enable you to rest between contractions. Usually given by injection, these drugs pass through the placenta. In high doses they can slow down both the mother's and the baby's breathing. Therefore, they usually are not given close to delivery.

Epidural anesthesia is the most popular method used in obstetrics. It is safe for both the mother and the baby, and it allows the mother to be alert for labor and delivery.

If you choose to have an epidural anesthetic, an anesthesiologist will inject a drug into your spine. A thin tube is then inserted so that medication can be given as needed.

In this method, the anesthetic cannot be given until labor is well under way, with the cervix dilated 1 to 2 inches.

One advantage of epidural anesthesia is that if it is allowed to wear off gradually as the delivery approaches, you feel enough sensation to be able to push the baby out.

For *spinal anesthesia,* like the epidural, an anesthetic is injected into your spine. It does not interfere with your alertness. However, it usually is given just before delivery.

Because most women prefer the continuous pain relief of epidural anesthesia, the popularity of spinal anesthesia is waning. Today, it is used mainly for cesarean sections.

General anesthesia involves the injection or inhalation of drugs that will make you sleep. This method was popular a generation ago. Now it is mainly used in emergency cesarean sections or when there is a breech birth, a retained placenta, or a need to turn and deliver a twin baby.

Forceps

Forceps are two blunt blades that resemble a pair of tongs. They are used to pull the baby out of the vagina when the delivery is not progressing as it should or when there are signs of fetal distress.

Reasons for using forceps include an umbilical cord that has preceded the baby down the birth canal, an infant who is too large to pass through the birth canal unaided, a breech birth (see below), or signs of asphyxia (oxygen deprivation). Sometimes use of forceps may be necessary when a woman does not have the strength to push the baby out.

If a forceps delivery is necessary, you will have an episiotomy (see page 212). You also will be given an anesthetic.

Complications from forceps deliveries are relatively rare. Occasionally, temporary bruises to an infant's face and nerve damage occur. However, when used by a skilled obstetrician or family physician, forceps have saved the lives of many babies.

Vacuum Extraction

The vacuum extractor was designed as a gentler method to replace forceps.

A metal cup is fitted over the baby's scalp. The vacuum extractor then relies on a pump to attach it to the baby's head. Using the handle on the cup, the physician can then move the baby's head to a better position. The baby then can be pulled out of the birth canal. Occasionally there is some bruising under the infant's scalp; this resolves in several days.

specially equipped rooms called birthing rooms. If the vaginal opening does not provide adequate room for the baby to be born and it appears that your tissues may tear, your physician may give you a local anesthetic and then make an incision (an episiotomy) at the opening of the vagina. This will create a larger opening for delivery of the infant (see Procedures You May Encounter During Labor and Delivery, page 212). After you have pushed the baby's head out, you will be instructed to stop pushing for a moment while your physician clears the baby's airway. A few more pushes and your baby is born.

The umbilical cord that connects the baby to the placenta is cut and your baby is examined, weighed, and cleaned.

The third stage of labor is delivery of the placenta. Your uterus will continue to contract to expel it, but you should not feel any great pain.

ABNORMAL FETAL POSITIONS

Most babies are born head first, with the face toward the mother's back. This position is called occiput anterior. It allows for the easiest passage through the birth canal.

An estimated 4 percent of babies, however, enter the world in other positions, some of which are potentially dangerous and warrant special measures during labor and delivery.

Breech presentation is the most common of the abnormal positions. If your baby is breech, it is positioned with its buttocks near your cervix. Thus, either the buttocks or feet emerge first instead of the head.

Breech births are particularly common in premature infants because many babies do not assume the correct position until the last few weeks or even days of pregnancy. Other factors that predispose some women to breech birth include multiple fetuses, uterine abnormalities, tumors, hydramnios (see page 205), and placenta previa (see page 209).

If your infant is in the breech position in the last weeks of pregnancy, your physician may attempt to turn the baby. If the baby does not turn before labor, most physicians perform a cesarean section, which usually results in a healthier infant but offers a slight increase in risk to the mother.

CESAREAN SECTION

Shakespeare was familiar with cesarean section: it was basic to the plot of the play *Macbeth*. Macbeth had been told by an apparition that "none of woman born shall harm Macbeth"—but he later learned that Macduff had been "from his mother's womb untimely ripp'd." Thus, he became Macbeth's slayer.

Although for many centuries it was an accepted procedure for attempting to save the baby after the mother's death, it was not until anesthesia and aseptic surgery were developed in the 19th century that cesarean section became feasible as a means of saving both the baby and the mother in a difficult childbirth. In fact, although childbirth through cesarean section was once an operation of last resort, today it accounts for more than 20 percent of all births in the United States.

Even though many critics think the pendulum has swung too far, there is no doubt that many women and babies are alive today because this alternative to vaginal delivery was available.

A cesarean section is a surgical procedure that involves incisions through the abdomen and into the uterus. The infant is then lifted out.

When Is a Cesarean Section Necessary?

Many conditions call for a cesarean section. Some premature infants tend to have a better chance of survival when delivered in this way. Infants in breech or other abnormal positions (see page 213) more often than not are delivered by cesarean section. When the infant is too large or the mother's birth canal is unusually small, a cesarean section is the only safe way of delivery. Sometimes abnormalities of the uterus or vagina obstruct the birth canal and necessitate this

operation. If a mother has preeclampsia, diabetes, genital herpes, or hypertension, a cesarean section may be indicated. Placental abnormalities such as placenta previa often require cesarean section. In the event of twins or multiple fetuses, many physicians advise this procedure. When labor is prolonged because of insufficient uterine contractions, many physicians believe a cesarean section is better for both the mother and the baby.

Some believe that the procedure is done too often and that physicians do a cesarean section whenever they are faced with the possibility of a difficult birth, just to make sure that all precautions have been taken. Some of this so-called defensive medicine is practiced, but the threat of a lawsuit is not the reason for most cesarean sections.

Improved fetal monitoring techniques now provide vital information about the health of the fetus and its ability to withstand labor and delivery. If it appears that the fetus may be jeopardized, most physicians are quick to perform a cesarean section. At the same time, improvements in the operation itself, in anesthesia, and in antibiotics make the procedure safer for the mother than it once was.

In addition, more women are postponing pregnancy until later in life. These women and their infants are at higher risk of medical complications than their younger counterparts. Hence, cesarean births in this group are more common.

The Procedure

If you need a cesarean section, you will be given an anesthetic. Unless the procedure is being done because of an emergency—in which case you will be put to sleep with a general anesthetic—you will have either epidural or

spinal anesthesia (see page 1218), which allows you to remain awake without feeling pain. Most hospitals now allow your partner to be in the operating room, unless you are having an emergency cesarean.

It takes a little less than an hour to perform a cesarean section. Two types of incisions into the abdomen can be used. One is the so-called bikini cut, which is a horizontal incision near the pubic hair line. The other is a vertical cut from the navel to the pubis.

Once the incision reaches the uterus, one of two commonly used incisions can be made. The most common method is a horizontal incision in the lower part of the uterus called a lower uterine transverse incision. This incision heals better and is associated with less chance of uterine rupture. On occasion, your physician will use a vertical incision to open the uterus. This incision allows more access to your uterus and is used, for example, when an infant is large or when an infant is known to have an abnormally large head (see Hydrocephalus, page 535).

After the uterus is opened, the physician may use a forceps to extract the baby from the womb. The placenta also is removed, and the wound then is stitched closed.

The Complications

Although cesarean section is safer than it used to be and most women recover well, there can be complications. It is a major operation and, as with any other one, there is a risk of infection at the surgical site as well as bladder and kidney infections. Hemorrhage is rare, but when it does occur it can be severe.

The death rate for women who have a cesarean section is 2 to 4 times higher than that for women who have a vaginal delivery.

Many of the women who die, however, were ill before the operation.

The Recovery
From an emotional standpoint, a cesarean section can be difficult because it can impede bonding with your new baby. Initially you will feel groggy and be in pain, and so you are less likely to want to spend time with the baby.

After the procedure, you will be encouraged to try to move around your room on the same day. You can eat a regular diet when you have an appetite. You can hold your baby and begin breast-feeding whenever you feel well enough.

The average hospital stay after a cesarean section is between 5 and 6 days.

Future Pregnancies
Women who have had a cesarean naturally wonder about the next pregnancy. Formerly, once you had a cesarean, you always had one for subsequent births. This was done because of the risk of the uterine scar rupturing during labor, which occurred in about 2 out of 100 births.

Now, however, as many as 60 percent of women who have had a cesarean section may be able to have a vaginal delivery subsequently. This depends on the initial reason for the operation and on whether the condition is still present. For example, if the cesarean section was done because of fetal distress, your next baby may be able to withstand labor and a vaginal delivery. Alternatively, if your pelvis is unusually small, all your future deliveries probably will have to be by cesarean section.

The other factors that determine whether you can try a vaginal delivery are the type of uterine incision that was made and whether the postoperative course for the first cesarean section was free of infection. If your uterine scar is the horizontal type (lower uterine transverse incision), you may be a candidate for vaginal delivery.

Occiput posterior position is when the infant's head is positioned near the cervix but its face is toward the mother's front. This presentation makes it difficult for the infant to travel down the birth canal.

This position can delay labor, especially if the infant is large. Forceps often are used for an occiput posterior presentation. Sometimes a cesarean section is necessary.

Transverse presentation occurs when the long axis of the infant's body is at right angles to the long axis of the mother's body, usually with the shoulder over the birth canal.

This presentation is more common in women who have had four or more children. Prematurity and placenta previa are other conditions associated with the transverse presentation.

Vaginal delivery is impossible when a live infant is in the transverse position. There is a real danger that the umbilical cord will become obstructed and cut off the infant's oxygen supply. Moreover, an infant in this position cannot move through the birth canal.

Cesarean section should be performed either before active labor begins or just after. If a woman is allowed to labor too long, both she and her baby are at increased risk because of uterine rupture and the chance of cord damage.

PROLONGED LABOR

Sometimes a labor drags on without much progress.

When this occurs, it is usually because the contractions are poorly coordinated, the contractions are not strong enough, or there is some obstruction.

If the cause is inadequate contractions, the uterus can be stimulated to contract by the intravenous infusion of a medication. This is successful in most cases. In some cases, a cesarean section is necessary.

Conditions that obstruct delivery include a head that is too large to pass down the birth canal or a fetal position (such as bottom first) that makes delivery difficult. In these cases, either a cesarean section or a vaginal delivery with forceps usually is done.

POSTPARTUM HEMORRHAGE

Signs and Symptoms
• Continued heavy vaginal bleeding after delivery.

Postpartum hemorrhage is the excessive loss of blood after delivery. This is the most common type of serious obstetrical hemorrhage.

At the time of delivery, the normal position for the unborn baby is head first (A), with the face toward the mother's back. This position is called occiput anterior. Other presentations include breech (B), transverse (C) and occiput posterior (D).

A

B

C

D

One of the most common causes of postpartum hemorrhage is the inability of the uterus to contract firmly enough to control the bleeding that occurs when the placenta separates from the uterus. This inability often is the result of uterine muscles being exhausted or weak. Other causes of postpartum hemorrhage include trauma to the vaginal wall from an episiotomy or lacerations, uterine rupture, and retention of part of the placenta. The risk of postpartum hemorrhage increases with the delivery of an excessively large baby or more than one infant, a forceps delivery, vaginal delivery after a previous cesarean section, several previous deliveries, labor that has been induced with drugs, and hydramnios (see page 205).

How Serious Is Postpartum Hemorrhage?

If you have postpartum hemorrhage, the bleeding may be massive or just a steady seepage over a period of hours. Sometimes the blood does not escape through the vagina but collects inside the uterus, causing the uterus to become distended.

Treatment.   Postpartum hemorrhage usually can be controlled with drugs that make the uterus contract. If this does not stop the bleeding, your physician will do a pelvic examination. Any torn tissues will be repaired after a local anesthetic is administered.

When the bleeding cannot be brought under control, the body's ability to form clots may be jeopardized. You may be given medications that help your blood clot.

An abdominal operation may be necessary if no cause can be found. The first step is tying off the major blood vessels that feed your uterus. If this is successful, the bleeding will stop and your ability to have more children will not be hampered. If the hemorrhage continues, the uterus must be removed.

RETAINED PLACENTA

Signs and Symptoms
• A placenta that does not emerge from the birth canal within 30 minutes of the delivery of the baby.

A retained placenta is one that is trapped in the uterus after delivery, often because it has not separated completely from the uterine wall.

Normally, the placenta is delivered after the baby. The physician presses on your abdomen and pulls on the umbilical cord to expel the placenta. If the placenta is not delivered within 30 minutes after your baby's birth, you have a retained placenta.

Treatment. Sometimes the physician has to peel the placenta from the uterine wall manually; if you are not already under anesthesia, you will be given something so you will not feel pain. After any delivery, it is important that the uterus remain contracted because of the possibility of hemorrhage. Techniques such as uterine massage through the abdomen and breast-feeding help the uterus contract. When these measures are insufficient, certain drugs help stimulate uterine contractions.

AFTER PREGNANCY

No doubt you will feel a great sense of relief after giving birth to a healthy baby. Accompanying that relief, however, is a whole new set of responsibilities and worries. There are decisions to make and no doubt more than a few problems and hurdles to deal with during the ensuing months.

In the chapter titled "Newborn: The First Month of Life," many of the health matters concerning your baby are discussed in detail (see page 3). However, you also may confront a few matters pertaining largely to your health. You may experience postpartum depression, you may still be unsure about whether to breast-feed or bottle-feed, and you may have questions about sexual activity after birth. These and other matters are discussed in the following pages.

BREAST-FEEDING

The feeding of your newborn baby occupies a considerable portion of your time. The first chapter of this book, "Newborn: The First Month of Life" (see page 3), discusses breast-feeding and bottle-feeding. The section that follows here discusses what you will experience when you nurse.

The vast majority of women are physically capable of breast-feeding. Some small-breasted women automatically assume they will not be able to produce enough milk for a baby. This is not true, because breast-feeding has nothing to do with breast size.

During pregnancy your breasts are preparing to produce milk. The hormones estrogen and progesterone are produced by the placenta and promote the growth of special breast tissue designed to produce milk. At the same time, these hormones suppress the release of prolactin, a hormone produced by the pituitary gland. Your breasts will slowly increase in size, and the nipples will change, becoming thinner, darker, and more prominent.

After the delivery of the placenta, release of the hormone prolactin is triggered. The result of this surge is the production of colostrum, a thin, sticky fluid that fills the breasts.

Besides being a wonderful way to begin bonding with your baby, breast-feeding has another advantage. The colostrum contains antibodies to resist viruses and bacteria. By nursing, your infant gets the benefits of your body's immune system.

After your baby is born, you probably will be able to breast-feed immediately. The baby's suckling stimulates production of the pituitary hormone oxytocin, which helps contract the uterus. The result is that your uterus returns to its normal size more quickly than usual. Nursing also can help prevent postpartum hemorrhage of the uterus.

NUTRITION AND LACTATION: WHAT YOU EAT AFFECTS WHAT YOUR NURSING BABY EATS

Adequate milk production can be maintained over a wide range of the mother's eating practices—but it is true that what you eat influences the amount and quality of the milk you produce. If you have gained an appropriate amount of weight during the pregnancy and if the baby was of normal weight, the chances for successful lactation are good.

What You Should Do

You need to consume extra calories in order to provide for the calories lost from your body in the form of milk. Consume perhaps 500 to 800 calories more than you would otherwise require. This will help guarantee good milk production, and you will either lose weight slowly or maintain your weight.

Avoid going too long between meals. Three regular meals and a bedtime snack are advisable.

Select the foods that will replenish the nutrients that go into the manufacture of the milk. Additional protein is needed, and this can be obtained in the form of more generous servings of meat, milk, eggs, or cheese. Additional calcium can be obtained in the form of 2 cups of milk daily, and your vitamin D needs will be met by the vitamin D in fortified milk and by your exposure to ordinary amounts of sunlight.

Your physician may direct you to continue taking the calcium and vitamin supplements you were using during the pregnancy. An iron supplement is usually prescribed for the first 3 months after delivery to replenish your iron stores. Even if your body has sufficient iron, fluoride, and vitamin D, these nutrients in the milk may not be adequate for the infant's needs, and your family physician or pediatrician may advise giving supplements of these directly to the infant.

What You Should Not Do

Avoid trying to lose weight too quickly after your baby's birth. If you radically reduce the calories you consume, both the amount and the quality of the milk your breasts produce will be affected.

You cannot increase the milk volume by drinking more water, so you will do best to drink only when you are thirsty. Your body will tell you when you have had enough water.

Avoid caffeine while nursing. Caffeine will pass into the milk and may make the infant irritable and wakeful. Alcohol passes into the milk in the same concentration as in the mother's blood, so it is best to avoid too much alcohol consumption while nursing. Some drugs also are passed from the mother's blood into the milk. Check with your physician to see whether any of the drugs you may have been prescribed or that you may want to obtain over the counter will harm the baby.

The oxytocin also stimulates contraction of the muscles that surround the milk ducts, and this contraction pumps the milk into storage areas behind the nipples. This is called the "let-down" reflex.

About 2 days after delivery, your milk comes in. Initially your breasts may feel uncomfortable. They will be much larger than usual, tender, and hard. You may notice prominent veins appearing. These are normal changes. The best cure for this discomfort is a hungry baby.

As your baby nurses more and empties your breasts, the breasts are stimulated to produce more milk. However, before long a balance is achieved, and the overproduction that causes your discomfort ceases.

If you are uncomfortable for the first few days of nursing, try putting ice packs on your breasts. You also can use mild pain relievers. Nursing your infant will help ease the discomfort of engorged breasts. A bra that offers good support is a necessity. These same rules apply if you do not want to nurse. Although there are some drugs that can suppress the production of milk, most of them have side effects such as high blood pressure. Most physicians advise their non-nursing patients to put up with a couple of days of discomfort. The breasts will feel full for days after the discomfort is gone, but gradually milk production will cease because there will be nothing stimulating it.

Because your baby eats and drinks what you do, avoid drugs and excessive amounts of alcohol. If you need to take a prescription medication, make sure your physician is aware that you are nursing (see also Nutrition and Lactation: What You Eat Affects What Your Nursing Baby Eats, this page).

The initial days and weeks of breast-feeding can be trying under the best of circumstances.

Many women find it difficult to relax during nursing. Sometimes this can interfere with the "let-down" reflex. The milk is in the breast but it does not come out easily when the baby sucks. If this seems to be happening to you, do not hesitate to discuss the problem with your physician. A quieter and more relaxing environment may be all that is necessary.

If milk production fails, consult your physician. Chances are that it is easily corrected. If not, your physician may want to do diagnostic tests to determine whether there is a problem with your pituitary gland.

Unlike a mother who bottle-feeds her child and knows exactly how many ounces her infant took at the last feeding, a woman who breast-feeds cannot determine the amount her baby is getting. It is not uncommon for a new mother to wonder whether she is producing enough milk for her baby. You probably are. If the baby is gaining weight, has at least six wet diapers during a 24-hour period, and sleeps well after a meal and if the time between feedings gradually increases rather than decreases (see page 42), you can assume that the amount is adequate.

At some point you will begin to think about weaning your baby, or one day your infant may make the decision for you when he or she pushes your breast away.

The best way to wean—from an emotional and a physical standpoint—is gradually. Cutting the baby off abruptly will result in unhappiness for the baby and discomfort for you. Start by eliminating one feeding for a few days. This will signal your breasts to cut down production. Then skip another one and so on.

BREAST PROBLEMS

During the postpartum period you may have problems with your breasts. These are some that you may encounter.

Engorgement is often a painful condition that occurs a few days after delivery when your milk comes in. Your breasts will probably become swollen, unusually hard, and sore.

If the engorgement is severe, you may have to use a breast pump or express your milk manually for a few days because it will be difficult for your infant to nurse. Have your physician or a trained nurse practitioner show you how. If nursing is possible, this should ease some of the discomfort.

Wear a bra that offers optimal support during this time. It should be worn even while sleeping. Ice packs may alleviate some of the swelling. If the pain is very severe, your physician may prescribe pain medication.

Cracked nipples are more common among women who breast-feed. The nipples may even bleed. Nursing the infant may be painful.

Moist nipples are more apt to crack than dry ones, so it is important that you keep your nipples as dry as possible. Some physicians recommend drying them with a hair dryer after nursing. Exposure to air also is helpful.

If you have a cracked nipple, call your physician, who will probably recommend a soothing cream such as lanolin that you can apply several times a day (not before nursing). This should help the nipple heal within a few days.

A *blocked milk duct* appears as a small, hard lump in your breast. Sometimes the lump will disappear on its own, or you can try massaging the breast and using hot water compresses.

If the lump persists, you may have an abscess (a pus-filled infected area of tissue; see page 1076).

Infectious mastitis occurs when a bacterium, most commonly *Staphylococcus aureus,* enters the breast, usually through a crack in the nipple. Part of the breast becomes red and is hard and hot. You may feel unusually tired and have joint pains, chills, and a high fever.

Your infant, although not sick, may have boils or a rash.

If you have infectious mastitis, you will be given antibiotics. Continue nursing to empty your breasts. The antibiotics you are taking will not hurt your infant, although you may notice a change in the color of the baby's stool.

With treatment, mastitis usually clears up within a few days. If it is untreated, an abscess may form, which will require surgical drainage. (See also Breast Infections, page 1076.)

POSTPARTUM DEPRESSION

You have the baby you have looked forward to for 9 months. Your husband or partner has been attentive. Family and friends have come to see the baby. The pain of labor and childbirth has receded quickly into a memory. You are finally home, surrounded by the people and things you love.

So why do you feel so awful?

You are not the first woman to have postpartum depression or the "baby blues." Many women feel depressed—some more than others.

Postpartum depression most commonly occurs a few days after delivery. Most women are home from the hospital when it

SEX AFTER BIRTH

Most couples want to know when they can resume sexual intercourse after the birth of a baby.

There is some variation, but most physicians recommend not resuming intercourse too soon. The vagina of a woman who has just given birth has been through some trauma. It has been stretched, cut, and possibly torn. Under the best of circumstances, it is bound to be tender.

Thus, many physicians recommend waiting 3 or 4 weeks before having intercourse. Some ask their patients to wait until after their postnatal examination, which generally occurs 6 weeks after birth. During this time you and your physician can discuss contraceptive methods so that you are not faced with an untimely pregnancy.

Even though a month or 6 weeks may seem like a long time to wait, you may not feel very much like having sex during the first weeks after delivery.

Your vagina is apt to be sore, especially if you have had an episiotomy or if your tissues were torn during the birth. Time for healing is needed. Gently clean the area daily. Hot baths may help ease the discomfort.

When you do begin having intercourse, you may find it painful at first. This is often an indication that more time is needed for healing. Hold off for a few more days and try again. If it is still uncomfortable, see your physician. You may have an area of raw skin in your vagina or a stitch from your episiotomy that has not disappeared.

Some women find that childbirth makes the vaginal muscles less elastic, which may make intercourse less pleasurable for both partners. Many physicians recommend exercises to restore vaginal elasticity. You can begin these vaginal exercises immediately after delivery.

A very good—and easy—muscle tightener is called the Kegel exercise. You simply tighten your vaginal muscles as you would if you needed to stop urinating in midstream. Hold it for a few seconds, release, and repeat several times. This exercise is both effective and easy to do. And no one but you knows what you are doing, so you can do this when you are driving, doing dishes, eating dinner, or watching television.

Even after intercourse is no longer uncomfortable, many women find they have no sexual desire. The care of a newborn is extremely tiring, both physically and emotionally. After a day of walking the floor with a colicky baby, there is often little energy left for sex. Unfortunately, this is a time when men—particularly new fathers—may feel the need for extra love and affection. Many men feel left out after the birth of a baby. Suddenly your life revolves around the baby and meeting its constant needs.

A woman should not be solely responsible for the care of the child. This not only is unfair to her but also makes her partner feel left out.

In the initial weeks and even months after the birth of a baby, both partners have to make an effort to communicate their love and continuing need for each other.

hits. You may find yourself bursting into tears over nothing. One minute you feel fine and the next you are sobbing.

For the woman who has gone through it before, postpartum depression may be easy to dismiss. For the first-time mother, however, it is both confusing and frightening.

Many factors combine to produce postpartum depression.

An important element is the abrupt hormonal change your body undergoes after the birth of a child.

Then, too, there is something of an emotional letdown after a baby is born. For 9 months you have focused on this one event. You may have feared it, looked forward to it, even dreamed about it. Now it is over. The attention that once was focused on you is now shifted to your baby. Suddenly you feel inadequate. You wonder how you are ever going to care for such a helpless creature.

Add to this the general fatigue that most new mothers feel. Your body has been through a lot and you are tired. But with a new baby to care for and several night feedings, there is not much opportunity to get the rest you so badly need.

If you are used to working and are now staying home, you may be in for a shock. The house seems so quiet—except when the baby is crying. You feel like having a conversation with an adult, but it seems as though everyone in the world but you is at work.

Finally, the way you look may add to your depression. You feel fat and you have not had a chance to shower today and it is almost time for dinner. How, you wonder, will your husband ever be attracted to you again?

In most cases, postpartum depression is over within a few weeks. Most women with postpartum depression simply ride out the storm. Some with severe depression may require professional help.

There are some things you can do, however, to help you get through this difficult time.

One of the most important things you can do for yourself is to get as much sleep as possible. If you are bottle-feeding, arrange for your partner to take one or more night feedings so that your sleep is not interrupted. If you are nursing, you may want to consider pumping your breasts before you go to bed so that your partner can give the baby a bottle of your milk.

This is not the time to worry about an immaculate house or gourmet dinners every night. Nap when your baby naps if you do not have other children to take care of.

A supportive partner can go a long way toward helping a mother weather postpartum depression. Often, all it takes is some reassurance that she is still loved and desired.

If you suspect that your depression goes beyond what is normal, consult your physician. Your physician may prescribe counseling and an antidepressant drug. In severe or prolonged cases, hospitalization for more intensive psychiatric treatment may be suggested.

STERILIZATION

If you are certain you do not want any more children and are thinking about permanent sterilization, an ideal time for the procedure is soon after childbirth.

Although sterilization of the female—most commonly tubal ligation—can be done at any time, the period immediately after the birth of a baby is the safest and easiest time because the abdominal wall is relaxed and the top of the uterus is near the navel.

When your infant is delivered by cesarean section, your abdomen is already open and the sterilization takes a matter of minutes. Moreover, your hospital stay should not be increased as a result of the sterilization.

If you are pregnant and considering sterilization, discuss the options with your physician. Some physicians perform the tubal ligation immediately after childbirth, but most prefer to wait at least 12 hours. There are two reasons. The likelihood of a postpartum hemorrhage is reduced greatly after this period. In addition, if your infant has a life-threatening condition that could jeopardize survival—and that could change your mind about sterilization—it probably has been detected by this time.

During the tubal ligation you will be given an anesthetic so that you do not feel pain. You will receive either a general anesthetic, which puts you to sleep, or a local anesthetic. The latter method deadens the area but does not bring on sleep.

There are various ways to perform a sterilization, the most common being to interrupt the passage of the egg through the fallopian tubes.

A common method in the woman who recently has had a vaginal delivery is to make a small incision below the navel. The tubes are found easily. A knuckle of tube is raised and the base is tied with sutures made of catgut. The knuckle is then cut off, and the two ends are rejoined.

Generally, this technique is effective for preventing pregnancy. One in 350 women who have it soon after childbirth eventually will become pregnant. For some unknown reason, the failure rate is slightly higher when the procedure is done immediately after a cesarean section.

Another method of sterilization uses a laparoscope. This is a thin instrument that is inserted through a small incision below the navel after the abdomen has been inflated with gas. The instrument has a viewing scope through which the physician can see the reproductive organs. Using operating instruments through either the same incision or a second one, the physician locates the tubes and either cauterizes them or attaches plastic clips to them.

As with any operation, tubal ligation is not without risks. Complications include reactions to the anesthetic, pelvic infection, and accidental injury to blood vessels in the abdomen. Most women, however, have no major complications.

After a tubal ligation, you may be given pain medication for your sore abdomen. Within 8 hours, most women can walk around, eat a regular diet, and care for their infants.

Hysterectomy—the removal of the uterus—should not be done for the sole purpose of sterilization. It is too risky to justify doing unless there are medical conditions that warrant it. (See also page 1100.)

CONTRACEPTION

Some new mothers—particularly those who breast-feed—think they are somehow protected from pregnancy. Do not make this mistake; just because you have recently had a baby, do not think that you cannot get pregnant right away.

It is true that breast-feeding does temporarily impair fertility to some degree and that many breast-feeding mothers do not menstruate for several months or even until the baby is weaned, but breast-feeding should not be relied on to prevent pregnancy—unless you do not mind having another baby soon. So, even if you are breast-feeding, you will want to use some form of contraception.

The options for contraception are basically the same after delivery as they were before pregnancy (see Pregnancy Prevention and Family Planning, page 175). However, factors such as nursing, irregular periods, and a change in vaginal size may necessitate a change in your method of contraception.

One purpose of your postpartum examination (usually done about 6 weeks after delivery) is to discuss your contraceptive options and preferences.

If you have used a diaphragm and want to continue, do not assume your old one will do. Many women require a slightly larger diaphragm after giving birth. Take your pre-pregnancy diaphragm with you to your postpartum examination. Your physician can check whether it still fits and, if not, refit you.

Although the popularity of the intrauterine device has diminished because of serious side effects, which have led most manufacturers to cease production, many physicians will still fit former wearers with the device. If you want to use this method again, wait at least a month after the birth of your baby to have one inserted. If it is inserted before the uterus is firm, it may fall out.

Many women want to resume taking birth control pills, the most effective contraceptive available. Is it safe for a nursing mother? There is no doubt that the use of some pills, most often the combination of estrogen and progestogen pills, will somewhat reduce the milk supply in as many as a third of women who use this method. The reduction, however, is usually only temporary, and it is not thought to be a major deterrent to using the pill. Moreover, if you take the pill, your baby also is getting some of these hormones. Again, the amount is thought to be insignificant. The low-dose pills do not tend to reduce the milk supply. However, they are not as effective a contraceptive as the combination pills.

If you are nursing but want to take the pill, ask your physician about this. If you have no medical problems that increase the risk of complications, most physicians will prescribe the pill.

There are several natural methods of contraception that depend in part on a regular menstrual cycle. Even if you were using these methods before you became pregnant, you should use another method for the first few postpartum months because your cycle may be irregular for awhile. Consult your physician if your periods fail to return 3 to 4 months after delivery of your baby.

CHAPTER 7
THE MIDDLE YEARS
AGES 40 THROUGH 65

CHAPTER CONTENTS

WHY CALL THEM MIDDLE YEARS?

To some people, the term middle age has a negative meaning. In our youth-oriented culture, a middle-aged person occasionally is viewed as an individual past his or her prime years.

This, of course, is not true. For most of us, the midlife period is our most productive and fruitful time. In fact, in the United States, people of this age group are the mainstream—demographically, culturally, economically, and in a host of other ways.

We deliberately chose not to use the term middle age in the title of this chapter because, apart from its negative associations, it means different things to different people. For some, middle age begins in the 50s; for others, in the 40s (or even with their 40th birthday). To the healthy 60-year-old at the height of his or her career, however, the notion of middle age may seem laughable. To make matters more complicated, the changes and events we describe in this chapter sometimes occur much earlier or later, well beyond what people sometimes refer to as middle age.

For our purposes, the term middle years simply means the years that lie approximately in the middle of the human lifespan, ages 40 to 65.

During the middle years, some people barely notice changes in their bodies. Most of us, however, start to realize that we are getting older. Some of us need to modify our lifestyle. Fairly minor problems can be corrected before they develop into more serious ones that can affect life after the middle years.

For convenience, this chapter groups the problems and challenges of the middle years into two broad categories: those that concern issues of life and lifestyle, and those that are manifested by health changes.

LIFE IN THE MIDDLE YEARS

In the middle of our lives, several transitions occur. Children may grow up and leave home. Spouses may enter or reenter the work force. Some people change jobs. Others begin to think of retirement or actually do retire. Divorce is as common during the middle years as during other times. Some of us experience a "midlife crisis" (see Midlife Crisis, page 227). Such changes can present great challenges and opportunities.

Think about this time of life as the "sandwich years." Two key responsibilities often dominate these decades. The first involves children: they have not quite left the nest to start their lives on their own, a transition that may involve substantial financial as well as emotional and logistical adjustments. The second is dealing with aging parents and the impact of changes in their lives—illness, retirement to nursing homes or other care facilities, or even death.

FAMILY LIFE

The middle years are a time of change for your family. The children, on whom so much parental attention has been focused, may be leaving the home for further schooling or to begin new lives.

Although not unique to this period, changes in your relationship with your spouse or the need to deal with the loss of a parent, spouse, or loved one occur more frequently and require adjustments in your life.

Retirement, once thought of as so far away, is now rapidly approaching. Plans to ensure financial stability and protect your future need to be well in hand. The care of aging parents may be a part of your responsibilities.

In addition, you and your spouse may have more time to focus on each other as you begin to plan the "golden years."

Parenting.   At times, it can seem that children are the whole point of a marriage or of a parent's life. Certainly, they are an important part. So much time, energy, financial resources, and love are spent on them. But during the middle years, children often leave home.

In addition, you will have more time, as well as space and perhaps financial resources, than when your children lived at home.

Neither of these changes is negative. The sense of loss that we feel when children first leave is lessened if we realize that this is a brief and transitional period. Our parenting relationship will continue, although on a new footing, after the quite normal event of their leaving the nest to live their own lives.

It is wise to think a bit about the children's departure ahead of time. For example, how much more time will you have when you no longer need to do many of the things that raising your children necessitated? Everything is easier—shopping, doing the laundry, cooking, going out, taking trips. This extra time is an asset—plan what to do with it.

The middle years are the time for developing interests that you did not have time for before, or for discovering new ones.

Divorce. Today, divorce is very frequent in all periods of life, including the middle years. Going through a divorce and adjusting to the new circumstances that follow the separation and legal proceedings can be among the most stressful events that take place during a person's lifetime. In most divorces, both members experience a decline in financial resources. Adjustments in lifestyle may be needed.

As with other events of the middle years, it is important to keep the events associated with divorce in perspective. First, preventing the breakup may be possible. If you and your spouse fail to set your relationship back on the right track, a marriage counselor may be able to help. Couples are often reluctant to visit marriage counselors. However, these professionals have seen a great many marriages in trouble and often have practical advice about your conflicts.

If you are getting divorced, the clear-headed approach is to plan for the events of your future life—which may include entering or reentering the work force, moving, and perhaps even starting to date again.

There are two key rules about life after divorce or after any change in lifestyle: one change almost always begets others, and it is always a good idea to try to pace yourself. Too much change too fast can be stressful; a more considered, one-day-at-a-time approach usually is the healthiest approach.

Loss of a Parent. For many of us, in the middle years we see the death of one or even both of our parents. This is upsetting and can be devastating, triggering depression or a midlife crisis (see pages 227 and 1037).

One reason the loss of a parent can be so upsetting is that it reminds us of our own mortality. As we get older, so do they, but often we do not think about this and its inevitable consequence—that one day our parents simply will not be there.

Of course, as adults in our middle years, we are competent to live without parental intervention. Losing parents is inevitable. Grieving for lost parents is natural and beneficial. However, if grief gets you down for too long, seek help (see Grief Responses, page 1027).

Loss of Spouse. Statistically, about three of every four wives will outlive their husbands.

As with other changes in family life, loss of a spouse needs to be dealt with in more than one way. First, there is the sense of personal loss and grief. Depending on the closeness of the relationship, this can seem quite devastating. It may take time to regain your footing. A period of grieving is normal and healthy. However, if you cannot proceed on to other things, talk to your physician. Depression could be part of the problem (see page 227).

Second, it will be necessary to restructure your life in some respects once your spouse is gone. This may entail economic difficulties, at least temporarily. If you have not been working outside the home, there may be a need to reenter the work force. It may mean learning to do things yourself that your spouse did with you or for you. In time, friendship with those of the opposite sex may take on a new dimension.

WORK

The middle years may afford an opportunity for career shifts or realignment. You may feel that your occupation no longer offers the satisfaction or rewards it once did. While it may be unrealistic to do a complete about-face, it may be appropriate to evaluate exactly where you are and compare what you see with what you would like to see.

For some parents of grown children, this may be the time to enter or reenter the work force. Such a change in one's life can seem like a dismaying prospect. Counseling regarding job choices often is helpful. Most communities offer courses that can help you regain old skills or learn new ones.

Another work problem is being laid off or in some other way phased out of a job. During the middle years, this can take on a special urgency. The classic and quite legitimate concern of anyone in their 50s who suddenly is unemployed is that other potential employers might want a younger person.

First, realistically evaluate your strengths and experience. Typically, you have more of these than you realize. Second, reassess your financial needs. If your mortgage is paid off or your children grown, you may need less money than before. On the other hand, with the need to put children through college, to pay for the care of an aged parent, or to support yourself after a divorce, financial needs may be greater. This is also an appropriate time to begin to plan for your retirement, in terms of both finances and living arrangements. Third, having recognized your strengths and determined your needs, you need to match them with a specific job or career objective.

Honest self-assessment can work, or seek help from an established career counselor. The important thing is to deal openly with change. Don't be frightened by the prospect of change.

Entering or reentering the job market, or changing careers, is made easier by some of the flexible work arrangements now available. Many jobs offer schedules such that strict adherence to a five-days-a-week, 9-to-5 schedule is not required. Part-time work is also available. Work during different shifts, temporary work, and job-sharing also are possible. Some people even can work at a computer terminal at home.

Midnight Shifts. Some jobs entail working night shifts on a regular basis. Others rotate shifts: for example, you might work 3 p.m. to 11 p.m. one week, 11 p.m. to 7 a.m. the next, and 7 a.m. to 3 p.m. the one after that.

To remain healthy, you will require a sound diet, exercise, and enough sleep. As a young person, you may have gotten away with temporarily shortchanging yourself on one of these—such as subsisting on nothing but coffee and doughnuts for an entire day, or skipping sleep altogether to finish a school project.

During the middle years, however, our bodies are not as forgiving of mistreatment as they once were. The potential results of not enough exercise or inadequate sleep are lessened vigor and poor health. Poor diets, erratic meals, eating under periods of stress, or eating too rapidly or to excess also may cause immediate problems.

Assuming that you do get enough sleep, however, there is still a problem in working shifts that change from week to week. Bodies get accustomed to a particular rhythm of waking and sleeping. Changing this rhythm—switching shifts—requires a period of adjustment while the body experiences something like jet lag. If your job entails the constant changing of shifts, as you get older your body will have more difficulty adjusting and readjusting than it did during your younger years. This opens the way for health problems.

Suppose you feel that you can handle any shift arrangement. One objection remains. Midnight shifts are not conducive to family life. You will be better able to deal with family problems if you are awake when your family is.

Planning for Retirement. The events of the middle years often seem to creep up on one. Nowhere is this so true as in regard to retirement. There are at least two reasons why.

The first is economic: we need to establish how we will live. Old age—which seemed a distant possibility not so long ago—now is not far over the horizon.

The second reason is that we need to have, or to develop, a full range of interests that we can pursue during retirement. For the sake of our physical, mental, and emotional well-being, retirement needs to be an active time. It is also a time of opportunity, a time in which to pursue interests and goals that we may not have been able to pursue before.

The possibilities are endless: new interests, volunteer work, consulting, travel. One person may take drawing classes and move on to painting; another might serve as a consultant for businesses starting up or take on a new, less-demanding but productive job; a third may travel to places he or she had always intended to go.

Some of us are happy during our working years: we feel important or necessary and enjoy being at the center of activity. When we retire and no longer receive this daily boost to the ego, it is easy to feel useless. We may turn this resentment against our former workplace and bosses, feeling that they should continue to keep us a part of their activities. Thus, it is important to anticipate and to prepare for a good life without work.

Keep in mind, however, that the more interests and skills you have prior to retirement, the more you will have to build on. Such lifestyle retirement planning is often overlooked and should not be.

DEPRESSION

Everyone feels depressed from time to time. The feeling may be one of sadness at a particular event or turn of circumstances, or just a general "out-of-sorts" mood for no reason in particular. Usually the feeling passes on its own.

Sometimes it does not. This is the situation physicians speak of as depression. Sometimes they even call it a major depression, to distinguish it from the occasional "blues." It is common among adolescents, people in their middle years, and the elderly.

Signs and Symptoms
- Generalized sad or numb feeling such that you do not enjoy normal activities;
- Loss of appetite;
- Difficulty in sleeping;
- Physical signs such as dizziness, headaches, or impotence;
- Irritability, crying for no evident reason, difficulty making decisions;
- Withdrawal from contact with others;
- Decreased sexual interest.

Events that are common in the middle years—such as loss of a loved one, work problems, or a perceived failure to reach a particular goal—can trigger depression, as can physical illness. At other times, depression just appears.

If you have occasional episodes of this sort in your life, which pass in a few days or even weeks, then depression is not a major problem. But when an episode does not pass or is more severe than usual, you need help.

DRUG AND ALCOHOL ABUSE

The abuse of drugs, including alcohol, is not limited to any particular age group. The middle years are a time when what was only a tendency toward substance abuse earlier in life can "blossom" to the point such that it throws a life completely into turmoil.

For example, if you rely on tranquilizers to get through difficult periods you may find yourself addicted to them in earnest if the going gets even more difficult during the middle years. If you enjoy a drink to relax before dinner you may find that this method of lightening life's load is gradually inducing an alcoholic haze at the advent of midlife crisis.

The abuse of prescription or nonprescription drugs, alcohol, or controlled substances will not solve the personal or physical problems associated with the middle years; it can only aggravate them. If you think you may have an addiction problem, see your physician or call an alcohol or drug abuse hotline for referral to an appropriate support group (see Alcohol Abuse, page 417, and Medications and Drug Abuse, page 431).

The severely depressed individual sometimes has suicidal feelings.

It is important to seek help. Others who care about you—even your physician—may not be able to recognize your depression unless you tell them how you are feeling. The outward signs of depression may appear to be nothing more than silence or boredom.

Help for the depressed person comes in the form of counseling from a psychiatrist, psychologist, or social worker and may result in the prescription of a mood-altering drug or some other form of therapy.

Do not consider depression, at any time in life, to be the normal state of events. You can get over it if you seek help (see Depression and Mood Disorders, page 1037).

MIDLIFE CRISIS

What constitutes a midlife crisis? Does everyone go through it? Is it possible to emerge from it unscathed, or even better off? The midlife crisis is as confusing as it is commonplace.

Childhood is a period of preparation to be an adult. As a young adult, we start making our own way through life, exploring alternatives and perhaps striving to reach certain goals. By the middle years, our earlier activi-

SUICIDE

The events that can trigger depression can cause some people to consider—and even attempt—suicide. Adolescence, the middle years, and old age are times when a life is full of transitional events, some of which can be very disturbing.

In the 50s, for example, a person may lose a spouse or a parent, watch his or her children leave the family home, or find out that he or she has some chronic disease. If such events happen, usually they do not happen all at once. Yet, on occasion these events can be all-consuming and provoke a serious depression. At other times, depression occurs without an identifiable cause. For whatever reason, life may seem to be not worth living.

Some people think of suicide. If you have such thoughts, it is important to communicate them clearly to someone and to seek help. Although it may be very hard to recognize, just talking about your problems to an understanding listener can make you feel better.

If a spouse or friend communicates to you a thought of suicide, even casually, take it seriously. For example, sometimes a person may say in passing, almost jokingly, that he or she sometimes thinks of ending it all. Do not ignore such a remark. Assist that person in seeking help.

The bulk of suicide attempts in fact amount to a cry for help gone unheeded. Many suicide attempts fail; some do not.

Help comes in the form of professional counseling, drug therapy, and, occasionally, temporary hospitalization (see also Warning Signs of Potential Suicide, page 1040.)

---

ties have led to results in areas such as marriage and work.

We may not have reached the goals of our youth, but we have constructed a life as a result of our efforts and choices, and this life generally has a measure of stability. The middle years are a productive period, a time during which people in many walks of life achieve their greatest accomplishments. To the person in the middle years, life may seem comfortable and indeed almost to run itself, with adequate personal and financial resources and a certain well-worn sense of familiarity.

Where, then, is the crisis? "Stability," "comfort," perhaps even "success" are not words that describe a crisis.

If it occurs at all, the crisis may involve the other side of the coin. A lot happens during the middle years. In this chapter, we have discussed major shifts that occur in work, marriage, and parenting as well as problem situations that can arise such as drug or alcohol abuse, depression, suicide, divorce, and loss of a parent or spouse or both. In addition, during these middle years we become aware that retirement and old age are not far away.

Changes in our bodies make it clear that we are no longer as young as we once were. We have wrinkles; we worry that we are no longer attractive to the opposite sex. We may consider turning to cosmetic surgery to retrieve our lost youth (see Cosmetic Surgery, page 232). If we have not reached the goals of our youth or learned to modify them along the way, we may be considering ourselves failures. In short, it takes considerable personal stability to cope with the full array of problems and changes that the middle years can provide.

You may end up asking questions such as, "Is this where I want to be?" "What did I do to deserve this?" or "Why do all these things happen to me?"

Not everyone goes through a midlife crisis. Self-doubt may be a key feature of the midlife crisis, and behavior during the crisis period often includes sudden job changes, extramarital affairs, obsession with aging and mortality, and depression.

However, the word "crisis" probably does not best describe any but the most problematic situations because taking stock of where we are headed is a positive thing to do at any age. The situation becomes a crisis only when we feel unable to cope with all the changes or with the possible need to shift directions in our life based on new priorities and goals. It also becomes a crisis when we react to our analysis of the situation in unproductive ways—for example, if there are significant problems in our marriage or if we feel unsure of our physical attractiveness as we age, having extramarital affairs often can be a harmful way to come to terms with the situation.

If you experience a midlife crisis, you can emerge from it better off—more aware of yourself as an individual and better able to direct your life under new and challenging circumstances. If you get bogged down in the challenges of the middle years rather than coming to terms with them, seek help from your spouse or other family member, a marriage counselor, your family physician, or a psychologist or psychiatrist (see page 1026).

PHYSICAL AGING

We have a finite lifespan. The upper limit is around 100 years; only a few human beings live a century or a little longer.

For years scientists have wondered why aging occurs. Some of our cells are continually replaced with new ones; others are not. The existence of a biological "clock," specific to humans, that runs down with time has been postulated; others believe that with aging there is subtle damage to cells that impairs their efficiency. But no one knows for sure why we age.

As we age, changes take place in our organ systems and in their appearance. The middle years is the period when most people begin to notice some changes; during the later years (the topic of Chapter 8) the cumulative effects are more noticeable. Good health, sound nutrition, and regular exercise tend to delay and minimize the changes associated with aging. Many changes occur without being visible to others, and some we barely notice ourselves. Conversely, poor nutrition, stress, and an inactive lifestyle accelerate the changes and hamper our ability to fight disease or to recover from injury.

This section groups the normal physical effects of aging into those affecting the cardiovascular system, digestive system, bones and joints, skin and hair, and reproductive system.

CARDIOVASCULAR SYSTEM

Your heart and blood vessels change as you age, even in the absence of any disease process. The muscle of the heart becomes less elastic, and your body's metabolic processes may produce less of the energy that the heart needs. The heart becomes a less efficient pump, working harder to do the same job. Your heart may atrophy with age and therefore weigh less than it did when you were young. There also may be some loss of the pacemaker cells that control your heart's activities.

In addition to these changes in your heart, your blood vessels become less elastic with age. Arteriosclerosis may make the passageway through your vessels narrower (see page 786). This makes it necessary for your heart to work harder to pump the blood through the more resistant network of vessels.

Less elasticity in the walls of your arteries and atherosclerosis may cause high blood pressure, which makes your heart work even harder. The arteries supplying the heart itself (coronary arteries) may narrow. The result of this is less oxygen reaching your heart, which may cause angina or heart attack (see pages 803 and 809).

A mild increase in blood pressure with age is normal. Blood pressure readings beyond this, however, are cause for concern. Prolonged high blood pressure (called hypertension) can precipitate a heart attack or stroke (see page 796).

Despite such general age-related deterioration in your cardiovascular system, your heart is strong enough to meet the needs of your body. However, as your body ages, your cardiovascular system has much less reserve capacity for overcoming injury or handling the sudden demands placed on it by stress or illness.

Such changes in the cardiovascular system occur gradually rather than overnight. By the middle years, the process already may be well along. The middle years see many heart and blood pressure problems, particularly in men. People now seem to be more conscious of death due to cancer or AIDS, but heart attacks kill as many people as cancer, AIDS, and all other diseases combined.

Activity level and diet play significant roles in keeping your cardiovascular system healthy. An aerobic exercise, such as vigorous walking or running for at least half an hour a day on at least three days a week, places demands on your cardiovascular system that sitting at a desk does not. Your body responds to the demands of exercise by increasing its capacity to pump blood. This increased capacity is healthy, becomes a characteristic of your body, and stays with you when you are not exercising (provided, of course, that you keep up the exercise program).

Especially important is the fact that, in situations of physical exertion, the extra capacity is there; also, exercise may slow or even prevent the progression of atherosclerosis (see page 803). You cannot stop the effects of aging altogether, but you can greatly minimize them and thus increase the odds of having a healthier life.

Exercise programs should be phased in gradually to avoid injury. If you have been inactive, contact a physician before embarking on an exercise program (see Cardiovascular Fitness, page 793).

Another way to help your cardiovascular system is by following a low-fat low-cholesterol diet. A principal effect of a healthy diet is to slow the process of atherosclerosis, the process by which fatty deposits accumulate in your blood vessels. Atherosclerosis occurs in nearly everyone, narrowing the openings in the blood vessels and thereby increasing the resistance to the heart's pumping action (see Heart Disease, Controllable Risk Factors, page 787; and Coronary Artery Disease, page 801).

DIGESTIVE SYSTEM

With age, several changes take place in your digestive system. They are subtle. You may not notice them until you are past the middle years.

The swallowing motions of the esophagus become somewhat slower. This change is too slight to be noticeable. Similarly, the motions that automatically move digested food through the intestine also slow down. The amount of surface area within the intestine diminishes slightly because of changes in the shape of the ridges of the intestine. The flow of secretions from the stomach, liver, pancreas, and small intestine that aid digestion may lessen. These changes generally are inconsequential and do not disrupt the digestive process. Adding vitamin or mineral supplements generally is not necessary unless your physician finds a specific deficiency.

Constipation may occur with more frequency. Often this is related to a lack of water intake rather than to problems with the intestine itself. Increasing your daily consumption of water and adding fiber to your diet are helpful approaches. But avoid long-term use of laxatives (see pages 241 and 633.)

Older people have more illnesses of the digestive system than do younger people. If you see evidence of blood in your stool, experience abdominal pain, or start losing weight or if your bowel habits undergo a dramatic change, consult your physician. If the problem is serious, the earlier it is treated the better.

BONES AND JOINTS

Although we tend to think of bones as hard, rigid, and unchanging, living bones constantly are undergoing renewal and respond to the demands placed on them. For example, a person who does a lot of heavy, physical work using his or her arms not only will develop larger and more powerful arm muscles than someone who does not but also will develop larger bones in the arms.

A natural consequence of aging is that the bones get slightly smaller as well as less dense. Your bone mass reaches its maximum between ages 25 and 35. During subsequent years, your bones decline slightly in size and density. One consequence is that during the middle years or after, your height may decrease slightly. Another consequence is that your bones are more brittle than those of a younger adult. This renders you more vulnerable to fractures in the event of a fall or other injury.

Sometimes the decrease in the size and density of the bones reaches a point such that it becomes a true health hazard. This condition is called osteoporosis. If you have osteoporosis, your bones are much more brittle and they fracture or break more easily. This means that even a slight fall or injury can break a bone.

Osteoporosis also makes bones more susceptible to being distorted under the pull or weight of particular muscles on the body, which leads to the severely stooped backs sometimes seen in the elderly. This disorder especially affects women after menopause. Men also lose bone density with aging, becoming more vulnerable to hip and other fractures, but because they start with a larger bone mass they are much less likely to have difficulty from osteoporosis. Osteoporosis is one of the most serious health hazards that the elderly face (see Osteoporosis, page 982).

Aging eventually renders joints a little stiffer and a little slower in their movements. This change may not show up until after the middle years. Beyond the normal stiffening, however, there is arthritis, a familiar problem with joints that often begins during the middle years.

Most arthritis (osteoarthritis) is a simple deterioration of a joint. Heredity, diet, and previous injuries and diseases in our joints are possible causative factors, but everyday use also is a factor, which is why osteoarthritis is also known as the wear-and-tear disease.

Arthritis usually starts in the larger joints that bear the weight of your body, such as the hips, knees, and spine. Arthritis also shows up elsewhere, such as in the knuckle joints (see Osteoarthritis, page 995).

During the middle years, osteoarthritis develops in at least one joint in most people. The symptoms of arthritis are intermittent pain, stiffness, and occasional swelling in the joint. Sometimes there are no symptoms. If present, the pain is usually a minor discomfort, although in some cases it is severe. Because our natural response to a painful joint is to move it less, the muscles in the area are used less frequently, and they start to shrink in size and strength. This can produce a destructive cycle that increases the degree of disability. Arthritis in hips and knees can substantially affect how you walk.

Arthritis is a process that does not go away, but it can be treated effectively. Describe your symptoms to your physician. He or she generally can diagnose arthritis quite easily, although sometimes an x-ray and other tests are needed. If you are overweight, losing weight (so that less is carried by those joints) can help. Exercise can help, as can physical therapy, and your physician can suggest appropriate pain reliever drugs.

As with all of the physical changes associated with the middle years, you may experience less change and fewer associated problems if you follow a regular exercise program and avoid joint-damaging activities.

SKIN AND HAIR

As you get older, your body's largest organ, your skin, loses some of its elasticity and its natural oils, and it becomes a little thinner as well. The skin starts the wrinkling process that in old age will produce deep creases and furrows in some places. During midlife, portions of your skin may begin to droop a bit. You may keep some muscles firm and taut, avoiding a "spare tire" around your stomach, for example, but in some places (as on your face) the skin will sag anyway.

The skin also becomes drier. Thinner skin means that veins or discolorations beneath the surface show through more clearly than they used to. Also, you perspire less.

How fast your skin ages depends on many factors. One is how much unprotected exposure to the sun you have had over the years, as well as now. The more sun, the more aging your skin is likely to reveal. Other environmental factors also play a role, but the sun is the most important (see also Senile Skin, page 1167).

Whether or not you are physically fit and eat well also matters. The skin, like other organs, benefits from sound nutrients and a good blood supply provided by a healthy diet and regular exercise.

Although you may enter this period of life with virtually no wrinkles, by the end of the middle years you can expect to have a fair number. This is a natural consequence of aging; it can be postponed but not reversed. Cosmetic surgery (see page 232) is sometimes used in an attempt to counteract the effects of aging.

Age spots (sometimes called liver spots) may appear on your skin as you age. These are flat patches of increased pigmentation that range from the size of a freckle to a few inches across (see Liver Spots, page 1169; *see also page B-4 for color photograph of liver spots*). Although age spots are not dangerous, see your physician whenever anything new appears on your skin, just to be sure that it is not skin cancer (skin cancers and other diseases of the skin are discussed beginning on page 1170).

Tiny blood vessels just below the surface of the skin may become fragile, break, and bleed. This causes superficial bruising, a condition called senile purpura and which is seen mainly on the forearms.

Hair changes with age too, although individual variations are greater here. On average, by about age 50, half of us will be about 50 percent gray. Graying usually begins at the temples and slowly works its way up the scalp. The hair elsewhere on your body, such as underarm hair and pubic hair, may or may not turn gray.

Hair also thins with age, in both women and men. Thinning affects hair on the head and sometimes elsewhere on the body. In addition, baldness affects men, with about 60 percent of men showing some baldness by age 50.

Baldness is genetically determined and is not a sign of premature aging. Medications have been used to stimulate growth of hair on bald patches, and hair follicles have been surgically transplanted from other parts of the head. Toupees are another option.

Graying is not a sign of premature aging; it is considered attractive by some and unattractive by others. How it is viewed is largely a matter of personal preference, cultural background, and fashion. It is fairly easy to alter hair color temporarily with rinses and dyes.

With the hormone alterations that occur after menopause, the facial hair in some (but not all) women coarsens and may start to

---

COSMETIC SURGERY

Some people use the term cosmetic surgery synonymously with plastic surgery. However, these terms are not synonymous. Cosmetic surgery refers specifically to an attempt to improve on an appearance that already is within the limits of normal. Plastic surgery is a much broader term that includes reconstruction of all surface parts of the body, correction of congenital malformations, reconstruction after severe trauma or burns, removal of skin cancers, and other types of reconstructive procedures with the goal of returning a patient to a more normal state.

Cosmetic surgery is concerned almost entirely with aesthetics and has become a sizable business in the United States. If you are considering cosmetic surgery, here are answers to a few possible questions.

What can it do?
For the person with facial wrinkles, the classic facelift operation can tighten the skin, which eliminates at least the coarser wrinkles and restores a younger appearance. For finer wrinkles around the mouth, on the forehead, and, to a lesser extent, around the eyes, a chemical peel or dermabrasion may be carried out. Noses can be reshaped, puffiness under the eyes and redundant skin above the eyes can be corrected, and a

receding chin may be augmented. In short, most features of the face can be altered, and the effects of time and aging can be markedly diminished in most people.

Cosmetic surgery is not limited to the face. A common example elsewhere on the body is enlarging a woman's breasts when there is underdevelopment. A breast that is too large can be decreased in size, although this is not generally considered to be cosmetic surgery.

Recently, another form of cosmetic surgery, known as liposuction or suction lipectomy, has been widely used to remove excess fatty deposits from certain areas of the body. It is not generally suitable as a means of decreasing massive or generalized body fat deposits.

How is it done?
Cosmetic surgery often involves removing excess skin and underlying tissue from affected areas of the body with consequent tightening and smoothing of those areas. For example, a facelift involves incisions in the area of the sideburns, just in front of the ear, and behind the ear in the hairline with minimal visible scars. Subcutaneous fat in the area of the chin often is removed. Chemical peel or dermabrasion minimizes fine wrinkling, essentially by achieving a very superficial surface burn.

A brief hospital stay often is required for cosmetic surgery, although many procedures can be done on an outpatient basis. This varies with the individual surgeon and with the patient.

Is it dangerous?
Cosmetic surgery generally is not hazardous, although it is subject to complications as is any other type of surgery. Included among these complications are infection, swelling, injury to nerve structures, and, if general anesthesia is used, the risk of anesthesia itself. Before undergoing cosmetic surgery, make sure that your expectations are realistic. Such surgery can achieve a definite improvement, but it is not at all the "fountain of youth."

How long must I hide?
After cosmetic surgery of the face, it usually takes 2 to 3 weeks before the bruising and swelling largely disappear.

How long do the results last?
The results of cosmetic surgery can be expected to last from a few to many years. After that, the procedure may have to be repeated.

Who pays the bill?
As a rule, you do. Cosmetic surgery is expensive and is not covered by most health insurance policies.

grow. This facial hair can be removed. Such removal does not stimulate further growth (for more detailed discussions of healthy hair and baldness, see page 1181).

MENOPAUSE

Menopause is the end of menstruation in women. (The word is derived from the Greek words *men* for monthly and *pausis* for cessation.) With menopause, the possibility of bearing a child ends.

Menopause does not affect sexual desire. It need not alter your sexual life, and it does not spell the end of your desirability to the opposite sex. Because you may have heard folk wisdom stating the opposite, it is important to know what menopause really is and what it is not. Menopause can be an active and fulfilling phase in a woman's life.

For a detailed discussion of Menopause, see page 1067.

MALE MENOPAUSE

Menopause has no functional counterpart in the male. With aging, the production of testosterone, a male hormone, gradually lessens but does not cease. In the absence of disease, men continue to produce sperm and to remain sexually potent well into their 80s or beyond.

However, men do undergo sexual changes with age. There is a gradual lessening of sexual desire in many men. Some might call this a focus on quality rather than on quantity. In addition, after about age 50, sexual arousal often takes longer than it previously did. A man who used to attain erec-

tions without partner involvement may find that stimulation by the partner is now necessary. During ejaculation, less semen may be expelled, and with less force, than previously.

These changes do not lessen the sexual pleasure that either partner experiences. A man's sexual performance does not diminish with age. On the contrary, although it may take a little longer to achieve an erection, older men can also maintain an erection longer than younger men, who may ejaculate prematurely (see page 1144).

Impotence can affect men at any age, including the middle years. The important thing to realize about impotence is that a passing instance or two does not constitute a problem and should not be mistaken as some signal that your sex life is about to end. The middle years do not spell an end to desire or performance for either sex. Such an expectation is detrimental because it can become self-fulfilling. A few episodes of impotence should simply be taken in stride, with the expectation of a more successful sequel at another time.

Impotence that is not transient can be caused by various physical and psychological factors; in addition, some medications can contribute to or cause impotence. Stress also ranks high on the list of possible causes. The middle years—with the numerous transitions and potential problems that they entail—can be a time of high stress. If you experience impotence that is not confined to an occasional episode, the chances are excellent that, regardless of the cause, it can be cured. However, beware of claims that suggest that taking testosterone tablets can restore virility. Discuss the problem with your physician (see also Impotence, page 1141).

CHAPTER 8

THE LATER YEARS

AFTER AGE 65

CHAPTER CONTENTS

THE AGING PROCESS

The aging process begins the moment you are born, and it never ceases. By age 65, however, people vary a great deal in how old their bodies appear and how much they have changed. There are 65-year-olds who look like 45-year-olds and 65-year-olds who look like 85-year-olds.

These differences occur because people differ greatly in their genetic makeup, in their health history, and in their environments, including personal nutritional and exercise habits and patterns of stress.

It is not possible to predict what will happen to *you* in your 60s, 70s, and 80s because you are different from your spouse, your parents, your neighbors, and everyone else. On the other hand, we can develop a description of the typical human lifespan by examining statistics concerning older people. The next few pages will do that as well as characterize the physical changes that are to be expected during this period. Finally, we will take a look at independence and consider how it can be maintained for maximum health of mind and body.

STATISTICS ABOUT AGING

There always have been elderly people. We know this from ancient writings as well as from skeletal remains. Until fairly recently, however, there were not many elderly people. Disease was rampant, medicine was primitive, and nutrition was poor, so many people did not even live through what we call the middle years (40 to 65), let alone beyond age 65.

A woman born in 1841 could expect to live to age 42 years; for a man born the same year, the life expectancy was 41 years. A woman born today can expect about 76 years of life, and a man can expect 72. These are overall average numbers that include deaths in infancy, young adulthood, the middle years, and the elderly years.

It is more meaningful to look at the lifespans of people who reach age 65. The maximum human lifespan seems to be about 100 years, with a few exceptional cases recorded and verified up to about 115 years. A man who is 65 years old today can expect about 13 more years of life; a 65-year-old woman can expect about 18 more years.

If a woman is age 75 today, she can expect to live about 12 more years; a man at age 75 can expect to live about 9 more years.

On average, women live longer than men. This seems to be due to a combination of biological, genetic, and environmental factors that are not fully understood. Because women tend to live longer, the proportion of women among people 65 and over is greater than it is in younger population groups.

Many people now reach the later years and continue to thrive in them. In the United States, each day about 5,000 people reach age 65 and about 3,600 people age 65 and over die. The net increase of 1,400 people a day is changing the makeup of our society. And among these elderly, the group over 75 years of age is growing the fastest of all.

In the United States there now are 24 million people at age 65 or older—1 person in 10. This segment of the population is increasing twice as fast as the rest of the population. Today we have one-fourth more people age 65 or over than we had as recently as the 1970s. When compared with 1950, we have twice as many.

The United States has neither the highest nor the lowest proportion of older people in the world. Europe has a larger proportion of the elderly than the United States does. Japan has a slightly lower proportion than the United States does. Developing countries have far lower proportions; in Egypt, for example, only about 6 percent of the population is age 60 or above; in Nigeria, the figure is only 2 percent. A little over a century ago, the proportion was 2 percent in the United States.

At least in industrialized societies, we can expect the increase in the proportion of elderly in the population to continue. Even if we assume that medicine will make no advances in prolonging the lives of this age group (an unlikely assumption), a large segment of the existing population is about to reach their later years. In 2011, the postwar "baby boomers" will start turning 65. In that year, and for each of the 20 years that follow, we can expect our elderly population to increase by about 1 million people each year. This means that we will go from about 24 million elderly people today (11 percent of the population) to 51.5 million people (17 percent of the population) in the year 2030.

By the year 2000, the number of Americans over age 85 is expected to triple. By the same year we should have 100,000 people at 100 years of age or older.

In other words, you could say that it is "in" to be 65 or older. If you are over 65, you are a member of a growing group, and you will have more company than ever before in history. Society also shows some signs of gearing up to accommodate the greater numbers of elderly.

With the increasing proportion of our population in their later years and the greater frequency of illness in this group than in younger age groups, medicine (except for pediatrics and obstetrics) is dealing with older persons. Your physician has become accustomed to dealing with the problems of the elderly and is helped by a large and on-going body of scientific research that almost daily is discovering more about the aging process and how to go about living a longer, healthier life.

PHYSICAL CHANGES

The old saw that "you are as young as you feel" has a great deal of truth to it. As people age, in the absence of serious diseases or other crushing problems, they "feel" just about like they did when they were young. The essence of a person does not change; the body does.

The degree to which the body changes varies enormously. Men and women in their 60s and early 70s may participate regularly in vigorous exercise. Conditioned older athletes have hearts, lungs, and muscles that are in better shape than those of many much younger people. Moreover, they have a lot more vigor than someone years younger who has let his or her body get badly out of condition.

In the later years, healthy living with regular exercise, weight control, adequate rest, a balanced diet, avoidance of tobacco, and moderation in consumption of alcoholic beverages can produce a feeling of well-being and vigor that surpasses that of an overweight, sedentary, 30-year-old smoker.

Good health also helps ensure a satisfying sex life in the later years.

What are the general body changes in the later years? The changes that started during the middle years (described in Chapter 7) continue. Your heart, lungs, stomach, and other internal organs become somewhat less efficient. Regardless of conditioning, even the best of athletes lose some of the physical abilities they enjoyed in those earlier years. Your muscles lose tissue and strength, and your bones get a little lighter and smaller. Bones that are less dense break more easily, and recovery from illness and injury takes longer. You may move more slowly.

Your hair may turn gray and become thin, and your skin—which has protected you from the environment for decades—shows the effects of this battle, with more wrinkling and a bit of sagging as elastic tissue is lost. Eyesight and hearing often begin to fail, and illness is more common. Prostate problems in men, support of pelvic organs in women, and incontinence in both sexes are common concerns that must be dealt with.

LOSS OF INDEPENDENCE

One of the toughest adjustments to make in the later years is the loss of independence that some people experience. However, most do not lose it or do not lose all of it.

Moving into a nursing home has come to symbolize loss of independence. More than 1 million Americans who are 65 or older live in nursing homes. This is only about 5 percent, or 1 out of every 20, of those in this age group. Even among people age 85 or over, only about 1 in 5 lives in a nursing home.

When you find that you need a little help doing things or that your present living arrangements do not quite work, there are a lot of choices. Here is just a partial list:

1. Move to a smaller place all on one floor, if possible.
2. Outfit your home with special equipment to help prevent falls and make life easier.
3. Use home health services, including housekeeping, visiting nurses, and Meals on Wheels.
4. Move to a retirement community with congregated dining and convenient services.

5. Arrange for a companion to live with you and help you do things.
6. Move to special housing for the elderly that offers temporary or permanent nursing care, depending on need. These apartment communities often have arrangements from complete independence to skilled nursing care, all in one location.
7. Use the services of medical day-care, day hospitals, or adult day-care (all are described later in this chapter).
8. Move in with your family, or have them join you.
9. Hire help.
10. Join forces with another older person or share your home with a younger person. Placement services are now available at many senior citizen centers throughout the country.

These are not all the possibilities. Situations vary just as needs vary. For one person, being independent means having time to read and a ready supply of good books. To another, it means the chance to play golf several times a week. To another, it means not having to take orders from anyone. To most, it means the freedom to get up, move about, do things, have friends in, make telephone calls, go places, and pursue activities they deem to be important.

Before you make changes in your living situation, think about what the word "independence" means to you. You may be able to adapt your present way of life, perhaps with a little change, to accommodate to getting older and still keep your independence. On the other hand, if a lot of nursing help is required, especially constant care, then someone does have to provide it. This may limit your independence, but it may be the only wise thing to do.

Take nursing homes, for example. In the past, admission to a nursing home was regarded as the "last stop." Today, physicians often recommend a stay in a nursing home during recovery from a stroke, hip fracture, or other mishap; 25 percent of these people leave the nursing home after they complete their rehabilitation.

Nursing homes vary in the amount of independence they provide. If a nursing home is in your future, temporarily or permanently, try to pick one that suits your expectations, your personality, and your budget. (See the information on nursing homes later in this chapter.) If you cannot actually see the different nursing homes yourself, have someone else go and ask your questions for you.

Another threat to your independence is the possibility of no longer being able to drive. As you grow older, your reflexes become slower. Even more important, you lose the ability to deal quickly with two or more problems that occur simultaneously—to handle the most urgent first and the less urgent later. As a result, you become less able to react to traffic situations. This may be coupled with decreased visual acuity and problems with night vision (see Problems in Night Vision, page 240).

At some point, you stop driving at night; then, you stop driving on the highway, and, finally, you even give up driving around your neighborhood. Senior safety programs are an excellent way to relearn defensive driving and may restore your confidence behind the wheel.

However, at some point your enemy on the road may become yourself. For many people, turning in the car keys seems like giving up on life altogether; but if your skills have eroded dangerously, doing so may avoid a lawsuit or a tragic traffic death.

SPECIAL PROBLEMS OF THE ELDERLY

Although health problems can occur at any age, some are more common among older people. They include Alzheimer's disease and other disorders of the mind, eyesight and hearing problems, and impaired mobility. For women, support of pelvic organs and postmenopausal bleeding are discussed; for men, prostate problems are described. Also covered are incontinence, constipation, loss of sexual drive, voice changes, skin problems, and abuse of the elderly.

This is not a list of things that will happen to everyone. Aging is a time when the body reveals its wear and tear, but the odds are high that you will avoid some of these problems. And often, those that occur are easily managed and not disabling.

COGNITIVE DISORDERS

"Cognitive" means thinking, perceiving, and remembering. A cognitive disorder means that there is a problem in these areas.

People at any age sometimes have trouble remembering things. During the middle and later years, everyone experiences a slight loss of memory. Just as your body works a little more slowly, your mind becomes a little less reliable. The term cognitive disorder does not mean this normal condition of getting older.

With a cognitive disorder, a person has so much trouble thinking or remembering or is so apathetic that he or she cannot carry out normal daily activities. In extreme cases, a person cannot carry on a normal conversation, recognize familiar people, or express basic needs. The individual is no longer in control of his or her environment.

Cognitive disorders most often occur in people who are more than 80 years of age. However, 1 person in 10 above age 65 has a cognitive disorder of some kind. There are dozens of possible causes. In addition to Alzheimer's disease (described on page 516), which accounts for over half of the cases, the causes include depression (see page 243), strokes (see page 508), head injuries (see page 536), hypothyroidism (see page 730), pernicious anemia (see page 479), toxic reactions to prescriptions, nutritional deficiencies or excessive supplementation, or other chronic conditions.

For detailed discussions of Alzheimer's disease and other degenerative brain disorders, see page 516.

FAILING EYESIGHT

Signs and Symptoms
- Difficulty in focusing on objects;
- Blurring of the central portion of the field of vision;
- Clouding of vision in one or both eyes;
- Double vision;
- Difficulty driving at night due to glare from oncoming headlights.

ABUSE OF THE ELDERLY

In this context, abuse means anything from a consistent pattern of harsh words and marked unfriendliness to slapping, pushing, hitting, and sexual molestation, at times by the people on whom these victims are dependent. According to the American Medical Association, about 10 percent of people age 65 and over suffer some kind of chronic abuse.

Frequently the pattern emerges gradually, beginning with verbal abuse and progressing to physical abuse. Since 1981, there has been an increase in cases reported each year, to about 100,000 a year. In other words, abuse of the elderly is a common problem but is only beginning to be recognized.

Who is most likely to be abused? Those who are age 75 or older and who are dependent on others for basic care such as bathing, dressing, and eating are the ones most likely to be abused. Abuse is 3 times more likely among the elderly who live with someone. Although men are more often the victims, abused women suffer more physical harm. Abuse seems to occur in all economic and ethnic groups.

Who are the abusers? In about half of the cases they are the children of the victims or other younger relatives. About 40 percent of the time, the victim's spouse is the abuser. Other care-givers, as in institutions, also may be abusers. The abusers may be reacting to stress and exhaustion. They may have psychological or drug abuse problems. Some were abused themselves as children.

What can be done? If you are being abused, first realize that this kind of treatment is not acceptable. Your dependency on another person does not give that person the right to mistreat you. Call the police yourself or ask a visiting nurse to assess the situation and contact the authorities. Your local senior citizens center can provide help. Physicians and social workers also can help.

Remember: in order to get help from someone, you very likely will have to ask for it. Talking with the abuser about the problem is not likely to help.

Like the rest of your body, your eyes age. As a result, they become less "elastic." This change most often affects the lens, resulting in difficulty in focusing on nearby objects (called presbyopia, see page 743). If you do not need glasses at least some of the time after age 65, you are the exception.

When these changes become more pronounced, something other than normal aging is frequently at work. Glaucoma, the buildup of fluid within the eyeball to an abnormally high pressure, narrows the field of vision and can lead to blindness if not diagnosed and treated appropriately. Most persons have no symptoms, although occasionally glaucoma can cause pain, redness of the eyes, and seeing colorful halos around lights. About 3 percent of people over age 65 have glaucoma. Cataracts (clouding of the lens) blur the field of vision, may cause double vision, and typically create problems in night driving. Macular degeneration, possibly caused by a diminished blood supply to the macula (the center of vision), can affect reading acuity and visual sharpness.

These illnesses can affect one or both eyes. They generally come on gradually and are usually painless and so are often mistaken for the normal effects of aging on the eyes.

The Diagnosis. It is important to visit an ophthalmologist promptly when a vision problem occurs. If left untreated, some eye disorders can cause you to lose a substantial part of your eyesight or even to go totally blind. The tests that an ophthalmologist performs are generally painless.

How Serious Is Failing Eyesight? The moderate degree of eyesight failure that is normal to aging is not serious and can be corrected with eyeglasses. Diseases of the eyes and cataracts are serious because they have the potential for significant loss of vision.

Cataracts and glaucoma usually can be treated. Macular degeneration is sometimes treated with laser therapy, although the results often are disappointing.

For more detailed discussions, see Cataracts, page 768; Glaucoma, page 765; or Macular Degeneration, page 771.

INCONTINENCE

At any age and whether it involves urine, stool, or both, incontinence usually is caused by an underlying illness or ailment. Elderly people are more vulnerable to incontinence than are younger people. As you age, the muscles and ligaments that control urination and defecation become somewhat less efficient and thus are more readily disturbed by a physical ailment. However, incontinence is not an inevitable part of getting older.

For detailed discussions of urinary incontinence in women, see Urine Incontinence and Other Urine Loss Problems, page 1109; in men, see Urinary Incontinence, page 1123. For a discussion of Fecal Incontinence, see page 648.

IMPAIRED MOBILITY

There is a saying that "Once you're over the hill, you start to pick up speed." Unfortunately, at least when it comes to physical mobility, this is seldom true. Muscles, tendons, and joints generally lose a certain amount of their strength and flexibility, and the metabolic "power plant" that provides the energy for your body burns a little slower. You do not move as fast as you once did.

If you have had an active life, by age 60 your muscles will have lost little or none of the strength they had in your youth. However, you will have less flexibility, your reflexes will be slower, and your coordination will be poorer. With advancing age, and especially with lack of regular strenuous physical activity, muscles may lose some of their strength.

PROBLEMS IN NIGHT VISION

Night vision refers to how well you see in poor light or in the dark. With age, healthy eyes become a little less adept at night vision. A common, and potentially dangerous, consequence is difficulty in driving at night. For example, your eyes may not be able to recover as rapidly from the momentary blinding caused by the glare of oncoming headlights.

There are other causes of diminished night vision. Vitamin A is vital to night vision; a diet poor in vitamin A or a disease process that results in a vitamin A deficiency can all but eliminate night vision.

Today, vitamin A deficiency severe enough to impair vision is rare.

In addition, other problems with the eyes, such as cataracts and glaucoma, can cause difficulty with night vision (see pages 768 and 765).

If you have a night vision problem, consult your eye specialist. Never assume that a vision problem is simply something you have to put up with as you age. It may be caused by an easily treatable condition. A delay in seeking help could jeopardize your sight.

Finally, if night driving bothers you, reexamine your need to drive at night. For safety's sake, it may be wise to avoid such trips.

If you have a disease that saps your energy or an ailment that affects a body part involved in locomotion—such as hip, knee, ankle, or back—then you experience greater impairment. Arthritic changes in joints slow the movements of millions of Americans. Occasionally, medications have the same effect.

What Can Be Done? If you have a disease that affects your movements, it should be treated. But what about the usual slowing down that comes with age or with deterioration of a joint?

First, take a little more time to get where you have to go. In particular, avoid falls. The possibility of a fall represents a special danger. As you age, your bones become more brittle (especially in postmenopausal women who may have some degree of osteoporosis; see page 982). A fall that you would have easily walked away from as a younger person may cause a fracture. And certain fractures, such as those of the hip, may end your independence or even your life. However, surgical procedures now available may provide good recovery of joint function if you are in good health (see Joint Replacement, page 998).

Do not live your life in fear of falling, in part because the best single strategy to avoid many of the problems of aging is to keep yourself in good general health. This requires regular exercise—especially walking. Among the elderly who have accidents, those who are in good physical condition before the accident recover the most quickly and completely after the accident. Stay active. Be sensible. But think prevention.

CONSTIPATION

Signs and Symptoms
- Hard and occasionally painful bowel movements;
- Diminished frequency of bowel movements;
- Difficulty in evacuating stool.

Many people define constipation as not having at least one stool per day. This simply is not true. The range of normal stool patterns varies widely from individual to individual. For one individual, it may be one

---

SPECIAL NUTRITIONAL CONCERNS

Is there a single "old-age" diet that can help all elderly people live longer, healthier lives? No. But we can offer some nutrition strategies.

The maladies you accumulate as you age are unique to you. If you have hypertension, you will be advised to avoid salt. People with diabetes are told to avoid simple sugars.

Although there is little evidence that your need for vitamins changes as you age, other nutritional needs do change. For example, there is reason to believe that requirements for protein increase. At the same time, your need for energy may decrease. Thus, if you do not reduce the calories in your diet, you probably will gain weight. Obesity, in turn, puts you at risk for many ailments such as diabetes. So it is important to work at maintaining proper weight, especially as you age.

Nutrition Strategies
Variety and moderation are the keys to a healthful diet—at any age. A balanced diet ensures proper intake of vitamins, minerals, proteins, carbohydrates, and other food elements. Moderation controls calories and is especially important with regard to consumption of alcohol.

Drink plenty of water. Insufficient intake of water is a common cause of constipation.

If you have specific ailments, your physician or registered dietician will provide dietary advice tailored to your needs. Follow it. Sometimes these recommendations require changes in life-long habits or food preferences. Be assured that the self-discipline required is well worth the effort. It may enhance your health and even add years to your life.

---

bowel movement one to three times a day, while for another it may be only once every 2 or 3 days. Constipation means a change in the frequency of your normal bowel habits. In addition, with constipation, stools often tend to be harder in composition and the act of defecating occasionally may be painful. There may be difficulty in evacuating stool, or there is a sense of incomplete emptying of stool from the rectum.

Constipation can be caused by an improper diet, changes in your diet, dehydration, medications, or inactivity. Sometimes it is a symptom of an underlying disease such as cancer of the colon, hypothyroidism, or depression. You do not necessarily get constipated more frequently as you age.

What Can Be Done? The vast majority of cases of constipation are not serious. If the signs and symptoms described above are of recent onset, see your physician. He or she will review your medications and dietary habits to see if they are the cause. Your physician may perform an examination, obtain appropriate laboratory tests, and probably recommend examination of your colon (see pages 613 and 641).

If these studies do not reveal any significant abnormality, minor dietary modifications may be helpful. These include increased consumption of water or other fluids in your diet. In addition, include fresh fruits and vegetables to supply fiber in your diet. Your physician's recommendations might also include the use of fiber or bran in your breakfast cereal. At times, your physician might recommend a bulk former that contains psyllium. This is nothing more than a vegetable fiber ground into a powder. Mix it thoroughly with water or other liquids and drink it once or twice a day. Continue to be as active as you can. Avoid commercial laxatives because, over time, they can aggravate your constipation.

For a more detailed discussion of constipation, see page 633.

LOSS OF SEXUAL DRIVE

Signs and Symptoms
- Diminished sexual desire;
- Absence of sexual desire;
- Problems in sexual performance (such as impotence or painful intercourse).

Once, sex after age 70 was a nonissue; at least, it was thought to be an improper one to discuss. Now we recognize that intimacy remains important to a relationship throughout life.

Changes in sexual desire are common as one ages. The desire for intercourse may decrease. However, this varies greatly from one individual to another. In addition, longer foreplay may be required to stimulate either partner prior to arousal. It also may take longer to achieve orgasm.

These changes are normal consequences of the aging process. They do not necessarily make sex any less enjoyable (some, in fact, argue to the contrary).

Difficulties in sexual performance, such as painful intercourse or impotence, usually are secondary to some other problem. Painful intercourse in women is common after menopause because of the lessening of lubrication within the vagina (see page 1088). Impotence can result from stress, depression, or disease. Both of these conditions, and others, can be treated.

Complete absence of sexual desire is rare, except with disease, a disability, marital discord, or depression. At age 80, about 70 percent of men are impotent; at age 60 less than 20 percent are. In many cases, impotence is reversible at either age. A shift in focus sometimes occurs later in life, during which time affection and companionship supplant the physical aspects of intercourse.

HOW TO AVOID FALLS

Falls often have disastrous consequences for elderly people. Among those age 65 and over, falls are the leading cause of death from accident or injury.

Yet falls are not inevitable. According to the Public Health Service, up to half of such falls could be prevented by changing the home environment. Here are some things you can do:

Throughout Your Home. To help prevent tripping, remove raised thresholds in doorways or cover them with carpet. Move electric cords away from where you walk. Avoid using throw rugs, replace frayed rugs, and use tape or tacks to fasten area carpets to the floor. Repair or discard rickety furniture. Use bold colors on your walls and floors to improve depth perception. Avoid rugs with zigzag patterns, particularly on steps.

Stairways. Be sure they are well-lighted. Install handrails. If you have trouble seeing, apply bright tape to the first and last steps.

Bedrooms. Avoid having to cross a room in the dark to turn on a light. If necessary, have the light switch moved so that it is by the door. Obtain and use a good night light to avoid even momentary confusion or disorientation if you awaken at night. Night and day, keep furniture out of your walking path. Use beds and chairs of a height such that when you sit, your feet touch the floor with your knees comfortably bent.

Bathrooms. Install safety rails at the bathtub and grab-handles by the toilet (never use towel bars for this purpose). Place nonskid mats in and in front of the bathtub. Use shower chairs and bath benches. Don't forget that a fall in the shower can also lead to a burn injury if you fall against the water mixer or faucet. Adjust the temperature in your hot water tank to the lowest temperature that will provide satisfactory bathing (approximately 120°F).

Kitchens. Use extension tongs or a small stepladder (never a chair) to get into hard-to-reach cabinets. Stop using the highest shelves. Clean up spills promptly. Use nonskid floor wax.

How Serious Is Loss of Sexual Drive?
Loss of sexual desire or ability is serious only if it diminishes the quality of your life or your partner's. There are no negative physical effects.

For more detailed discussions, see Loss of Sexual Desire in Women, page 1140, and Loss of Sexual Desire in Men, page 1145.

HEARING LOSS

Signs and Symptoms

- Increasing difficulty in hearing well;
- Difficulty in hearing a conversation when surrounded by other noises.

Although some people retain perfect hearing throughout their lives, most lose some hearing sensitivity gradually, starting in the 20s. This normal hearing loss begins with the higher frequencies and, by age 65, generally has started to affect the lower frequencies as well.

Hearing impairment associated with aging is caused by changes that occur within the inner ear or in nerves attached to it. Wax in the ears, ear injuries caused by excessive exposure to noise, and various diseases also can impair hearing.

How Serious Is Hearing Loss?   Hearing loss can be serious in that it can interfere with your safety as well as your social life.

Treatment. *Hearing Aids.*   Many types of hearing impairment can be treated by use of a hearing aid. Ask your physician to recommend a hearing specialist who can test you and prescribe an aid tailored to your needs. If you buy a hearing aid without good advice, you may end up with one that does not do the job properly.

Surgery.   Some types of hearing impairment and loss are treatable by surgery.

See also Hearing Loss and Hearing Aids, page 686.

VOICE CHANGES

The characteristic sound of a person's voice can change. Three causes of voice changes are throat infection, stroke, and cancer.

Throat infections sometimes cause hoarseness. Most often, treatment is not required. If the hoarseness is severe, medications are available. Stroke sometimes affects the voice. Speech may become slurred and slow. After a stroke, the voice usually recovers on its own. Many physicians recommend speech therapy to help recovery (see also Stroke, page 508).

Hoarseness can be a symptom of cancer of the larynx. With early detection and prompt, appropriate treatment, this potentially fatal illness often can be controlled or even cured. Cancer of the larynx is associated with smoking and excessive use of alcohol. It affects men more often than women (see Cancers of the Throat, page 702).

If you experience rapid or chronic changes in the quality or loudness of your voice, consult your physician.

DEPRESSION

Signs and Symptoms

- Loss of interest or pleasure in usual activities;
- Feeling sad or "blue";
- Poor appetite;
- Sleep disturbance;
- Loss of energy, fatigue.

Sometimes people become depressed over specific events, such as the loss of a spouse or friend or the course an illness has taken, or they just may have a general "out of sorts" mood for no reason in particular. This second type of depression generally passes on its own.

When the feeling does not pass, physicians describe the condition by the term "major depression." It is common among people of all ages. Among the elderly, it is sometimes mistaken for Alzheimer's disease, which can have the same symptoms of withdrawal and apathy. However, there is no connection between the two.

One feature of depression in the elderly is an obsession with mortality. Depressed people often think they are about to die, or they dwell on the inevitable approach of death. Some consider suicide (see Warning Signs of Potential Suicide, page 1040).

For a more detailed discussion, see Depression in the Elderly, page 1021.

SKIN PROBLEMS

Age brings changes in your skin. It becomes more wrinkled, thinner (so that the veins are more apparent), and less supple than it was in youth. Also to be expected as a part of the aging process are blotches and spots on the skin. Your skin probably also perspires less as you age.

Some of these changes are caused in part by dryness of your skin, which can be minimized by good skin care throughout life (see Proper Skin Care, page 1153). Your skin also will benefit from sustained, sound nutrition. Also, avoid excessive exposure to the ultraviolet rays of sunlight (see also page 1167).

If you are white, age spots (also known as liver spots) probably will appear on your skin as you age. These small, flat patches look like freckles. Their color ranges from light brown to black. Their cause is unknown. They may be cosmetically troublesome but are medically insignificant. In particular, they have nothing to do with the liver and never become cancerous. Most people do not seek treatment for liver spots (see also page 1169).

Another skin condition that sometimes occurs is asteatosis. This is characterized by intense itching on your back, lower legs, hands, or elsewhere. It is caused by a loss of natural skin oils, which produces scaly skin that, in some cases, cracks deeply. See your physician about itchy skin because it may be caused by some other underlying condition. Asteatosis is often treated by commonsense measures such as restricting the frequency of baths, not wearing wool, increasing the

---

PROBLEMS RELATED TO TOO MANY MEDICATIONS

In your later years, you may be at risk for problems with the medicines you take. Older Americans take a disproportionately high percentage of the prescription drugs sold. Because they tend to have more than one health problem, they often find themselves taking several different medicines at various times of the day or night. This can be risky.

It is easy to forget a dose or mistakenly take an extra dose or two. In addition, aging alters the ways your body absorbs, metabolizes, and excretes medications.

The Risks

Many medicines can cause sedation or confusion. Many can cause stomach distress or other gastrointestinal problems. Some combinations of drugs can interfere with the action of your heart or other organs.

For many medicines, an occasional skipped dose or a double dose makes little difference. However, with some, precise dosage and timing are of great importance.

The Pill-Box Strategy

To organize your drug-taking, use a pill box with multiple compartments. If you miss a dose, the omission will be apparent. For example, if you think you forgot to take the pills scheduled at your previous meal, the empty compartment will indicate that you actually did take the medicine at the proper time.

Drug Interactions

The action of one drug can sometimes be altered by the action of another drug. The effects of anticoagulant medications, for example, can be influenced by over-the-counter drugs such as aspirin. Nonprescription drugs indeed can be potent. Some cause serious reactions when mixed with prescription medications.

Ask your physician to determine the proper dosage of the over-the-counter drugs you take. The amounts recommended on the package may be too great, especially for older people or when mixed with prescription medications.

It is essential to notify your physician if you have conditions such as heart disease, high blood pressure, or glaucoma or if you are allergic to certain drugs. In such cases, a standard prescription could threaten your life.

Our recommendation: List for your primary-care physician all the medications you take, even over-the-counter drugs such as laxatives and hay fever products. Then, follow your physician's instructions carefully and inform him or her of any side effects. If you take many medications, your physician might arrange a medicine calendar for you. This is a compilation of your drugs with directions for what and how much you should take throughout the day or night (see The Modern Pharmacy, page 1225).

humidity of dry rooms in winter, and applying oils to the skin.

Skin cancer, which can appear as various types of spots or growths, usually can be cured if found early. The appearance of any sore that does not heal is a good reason to consult your physician (see Skin Cancers, page 1170).

SUPPORT OF PELVIC ORGANS IN WOMEN

As women age, sometimes support of the organs in their pelvic area weakens. This is especially true in women who have borne children. Childbirth, particularly repeated childbirths, can stretch the supporting muscles and ligaments of the abdomen, and the results of this show up later in life. In addition, the aging process itself sometimes weakens these tissues.

The conditions that occur include cystocele, rectocele, enterocele, uterine prolapse, and urinary incontinence. Although such problems are not an inevitable consequence of aging, you should be aware of them so that you can recognize their symptoms and know the treatment options.

For detailed discussions of these problems, see Health Problems of Women, page 1053.

COMMUNITY SERVICES

If you, or a relative or friend, need a little help getting through the day, what can you do? If you require periodic or around-the-clock nursing attention, where can you best get it?

Today, only a minority of the people in their later years live in nursing homes. If you need help, several options are available. Some make it possible for you to remain at home.

HOME HEALTH CARE

Many hospitals or other health agencies offer home health services. A nurse or nurse's aide will come to your home and provide nursing services. For example, these services may include giving injections, changing bandages, or help with speech or physical therapy. Other services may include helping you bathe, dress, and even cook meals. Depending on the service and arrangements, care is provided for a portion of every day or for several days a week. Medicare, Medicaid, private insurance, and other programs sometimes pay for some or all of such care, even for extended periods. Home health care and other types of community facilities can be especially helpful if you live alone.

Other options include adult day-care, respite care programs, day respite care programs, and nutrition services.

ADULT DAY-CARE

Adult day-care is available in some communities. In this service, an older person who cannot function independently is looked after in a supervised setting during the day. Transportation to the day-care center usually can be arranged and, depending on the program, people can attend for part of a day, a day or two each week, or even daily. This type of program often is appropriate for people mildly incapacitated by a stroke or for those who have either physical or mental handicaps.

The services provided are useful but limited. A midday meal often is served. Contact with others is possible and, in some cases, organized activities are arranged. Medical and nursing attention are not provided.

RESPITE CARE PROGRAMS

People who need limited nursing or medical care often can check into a hospital or nursing home for a limited period of time during which they receive specific services. The help commonly offered includes rehabilitation programs such as physical or speech therapy after a stroke. After the service is provided, the patient returns home. This may occur within a week or two or for a month or more. Repeat or regular visits can be arranged.

To see if these services are available, check with your local hospital or nursing home.

DAY RESPITE CARE PROGRAMS

This is similar to the respite programs described above but the services are more limited. Again, you can visit the facility (a hospital or nursing home) on an as-needed basis for some particular medical procedure, nursing care, or therapy. Generally, the visit would be limited to several hours or perhaps once or twice a week.

NUTRITION SERVICES

The Meals on Wheels program changed life for the elderly in America. It delivers hot meals, generally one meal a day, to older people in their homes, sparing them the chore of cooking for themselves or the unhealthy option of skipping meals altogether.

The program receives some public funding; the cost charged for meals is nominal. Programs similar to Meals on Wheels also are offered by volunteer groups and churches, particularly in larger cities.

Congregate dining (dining with others) also is commonplace at senior citizens centers and at housing designed specifically for older people. The meal and the social gathering can become the high point of your day. More meals can be served with greater economy to senior citizens this way than by home delivery programs.

NURSING HOMES

More than 1 million Americans age 65 or older now reside in nursing homes. This is about 5 percent, or 1 out of every 20 people in this age range. Among people age 85 or older, approximately 20 percent live in nursing homes. About three-fourths of all nursing home residents are women.

In the past, admission to a nursing home was considered to be the "last stop." This is not necessarily the case today. Many physicians recommend a stay in a nursing home to recover from a stroke, a hip fracture, or some other mishap. Once rehabilitated, nursing home residents often return to independent living.

Among the common problems that lead to nursing home admission are incontinence, thinking disorders, stroke, a bone fracture, walking disabilities, general debility, loss of spouse or care-giver, and terminal illness.

Selecting a Good Home. In selecting a nursing home, the first person to turn to for advice is a social worker or hospital dismissal planner. These experts often deal with people who need nursing home accommodations. They are excellent sources of information on nursing homes. In addition, they will be familiar with entry criteria and options for different levels of care within the nursing home.

Service agencies funded by your county or the United Way are another source of help, or ask a member of the clergy, a friend, or your physician. Nursing homes are listed in the yellow pages of your telephone directory. Your state or county social services agency, health department, or county medical society can provide a list of nursing homes. They also may have information on how best to evaluate and select a home.

Most nursing homes now are termed skilled-care homes; so-called intermediate-care homes are being phased out in most areas. In a skilled-care home, you get 24-hour nursing service as well as restorative, physical, occupational, and other therapy.

If deciding between skilled-care and intermediate-care homes, take into account your future as well as your present health needs.

To select a nursing home, visit several. Before you go, however, prepare yourself for the visits. Write down the things you want to find out. Here are four suggestions:

1. **Atmosphere.** Are the staff members qualified? Friendly? Caring? How about the residents? Ask some residents what they think about the home. Also consider the facilities. Luxury is not necessary, but basic hygiene is. Notice odors. A pervasive urine smell suggests neglect or bad ventilation. Find out how hair care and personal laundry are handled.
2. **Food.** Ask the residents how they rate the food. Look at a menu. If you have special dietary needs, ask if the home can accommodate them. Do residents get help in eating if they need it? If possible, time your visit so you arrive at mealtime.

3. **Activities.** Ask about the home's activity program. A skilled-care nursing home must post its activity program; take a look at it. Is there anything going on that interests you? Can you pursue your own hobbies and interests in the home? Can you leave the home to go out and shop or just take a walk? Is it easy to get to a telephone? Can you have a say in choosing roommates?

4. **Medical Care.** Usually your physician will continue to take care of you after you enter a nursing home. However, see what medical care the home itself offers. Can it meet needs for physical or occupational therapy? Can it handle your specialized needs?

Paying the Bill. The cost of nursing home care can be high. However, financial assistance is available from Medicare, Medicaid, private health insurance policies, the Veterans Administration, trade unions, and fraternal organizations. Federal, state, and local governments pay for more than half of the nursing home care provided in the United States. Individuals and their families fund a little under half. Private insurance pays for less than 5 percent of the long-term nursing home care costs in the United States.

Reimbursements change and vary widely from state to state, so check current state and federal programs locally. A hospital social worker can help you.

Other Alternatives to a Nursing Home.

Do not forget retirement communities and special housing designed for the elderly. There are more options today than ever before. If you do not require constant or extensive care and help, an alternative to a nursing home often can be appropriate. (See also page 1203.)

WHEN IS A NURSING HOME APPROPRIATE?

It is not a matter of course that everyone who is old or who has a chronic illness has to enter a nursing home. Individual circumstances vary considerably. In addition, admission to a nursing home is getting more difficult.

The single most important reason for entering a nursing home probably is the need for intensive care. Nursing home residents receive help with many of the routine activities of daily life. Eighty-five percent need help bathing, 70 percent need help dressing, more than 50 percent need help going to the bathroom, and more than 30 percent need help eating. The average nursing home resident also has several chronic illnesses that require medical attention. More than half of all nursing home residents have Alzheimer's disease or some other mental impairment.

If you are able to get along pretty much by yourself, you may be able to find the help that you need without going to a nursing home. People who need a great deal of help with daily activities or a lot of nursing or medical attention, however, will not find such arrangements satisfactory. For them, a nursing home is preferable for the sake of safety or even survival.

Families often care for elderly family members who do not live alone. How much care a family can offer depends on many factors. If a household consists of two working parents and children in school, no one is around during the day to provide care to an elderly parent. Some mentally disoriented elderly people can pose a hazard to themselves and to others when left unsupervised.

If you have an elderly family member in your home, balance his or her care needs against the well-being of the rest of your family. Someone who needs long-term help in eating, dressing, bathing, and going to the bathroom can wear an entire family down. Families sometimes recruit temporary help for part of the day or for relief in order to shop, take a vacation, or pursue their own interests. Care provided at home should be shared by family members so that it does not all fall to one person, and it should lie within the limits of a family's physical, emotional, and financial resources.

When care at home is not feasible or threatens to destroy the fabric of a family, a nursing home should be considered. If the elderly person is physically able to visit prospective nursing homes and psychologically fit to help make the decision, then he or she should participate in the selection process.

PART II

THE WORLD AROUND US

In the following chapters, you will find guidance in the event of an emergency. In addition, there are discussions of key issues about the world we live in and, in particular, its risks—along with advice on recognizing and preventing them. A variety of concerns are discussed, ranging from radon in your home, to immunizations you may need for a trip abroad, to methods of making your home safe for your children or grandchildren.

CONTENTS

CHAPTER 9

FIRST AID AND EMERGENCY CARE

CHAPTER CONTENTS

FOR IMMEDIATE REFERENCE

COMMONSENSE MEDICINE

There's been an accident.

Someone—you, a companion, or another person—has been injured or is suddenly very ill. You must do something, but what?

In this chapter we will discuss dozens of common emergencies and suggest appropriate procedures for dealing with them. Some commonsense ground rules to follow in addressing an emergency medical problem, whether it's major or minor, are listed below.

Keep calm. Try not to panic: you may experience an overpowering sense of fear, but keep control. Often, a few deep breaths will help.

Reassure the victim. If it is another person who has sustained the major injury, reassure the person. A hand on the shoulder or a light, reassuring touch may help. Make the person as comfortable as possible.

Do no harm. Do not move someone who has been injured, who has seemingly lost consciousness, or who complains of neck pain. He or she may have an unstable injury such as a neck fracture.

If in doubt, call for help. It's human nature to want a problem to be small, even to resolve itself. Sometimes the temptation with a minor injury or illness is to say, "Oh, you'll be okay." That prediction may be so, of course, and lots of unnecessary trips are made annually to the nation's emergency rooms—but, as the cliché says, "It's better to be safe than sorry." (See Emergency Warning Signs, below.) If in doubt, make the call. In many communities, the emergency call number is 911.

Making the call. When you summon emergency assistance, speak clearly. As calmly as you can, give the emergency dispatcher the key information. This includes the victim's location ("He's at 111 Old Farm Road, in the big red barn, just beyond the house"), the nature of the problem, and your and the victim's name. Do not hang up until the dispatcher has all the required information; he or she will probably also need your telephone number and perhaps directions to the scene.

Be prepared. Keep the numbers of emergency services posted near your telephone. Although you can find some or all of them printed on the back cover or on one of the opening pages of your telephone book, it is better to have them always in view by or on the telephone.

Take a class in first aid. Your local branch of the American Red Cross or YMCA or other civic organization probably offers such a course for a nominal fee. Instruction in cardiopulmonary resuscitation (CPR) may be invaluable if someone in your family is at risk of heart attack. CPR courses are also generally available and inexpensive, and they require only a few hours.

In the emergency room. Patients are treated in the emergency room according to need: it's not first come, first served, it's a who-needs-help-now priority. A member of the emergency care team will evaluate the extent of the injury or illness.

The examining physician will need to know the circumstances of the injury; the symptoms as they developed; the person's medical history and what medications he or she uses, especially if they bear directly on the situation; and whether treatment or medication for the emergency has been administered.

Before you go home. Make sure when the physician or nurse releases you or the person being treated that any follow-up instructions are clearly understood. These may include advice on rest, exercise, medication, or scheduling further medical consultations, perhaps with a specialist or your family physician.

EMERGENCY WARNING SIGNS

Any of the following warning signs, compiled by the American College of Emergency Physicians, suggest an immediate trip to your physician's office or emergency room:

Sudden pain at any location in your body. Chest pain or pressure in the upper abdominal area, for example, can signal a heart attack.

Sudden dizziness, headache, or change in vision.

Weakness or faintness.

Difficulty breathing or shortness of breath.

Severe or persistent vomiting or diarrhea.

Suicidal or homicidal feelings.

Significant bleeding, whether or not accompanied by pain.

The presence of one or more of these symptoms suggests that you should seek immediate medical help.

BASIC FIRST AID SUPPLIES

Always keep your medicine chest or first aid kit well stocked—emergencies do not occur on a schedule.

Include the following basic supplies:

Adhesive or gauze wrappings or pads in several sizes
Bandages or surgical tape (Steri-Strips)
Soap
Sterile gauze
Absorbent cotton
Adhesive tape
Tweezers
Sharp scissors
Cotton-tipped swabs
Tissues
Thermometer
First aid manual

Aspirin or acetaminophen
Syrup of ipecac
Antiseptic solution (such as hydrogen peroxide)
Antiseptic cream (such as bacitracin)
Hydrocortisone cream (for bites and stings)

If a member of your family reacts to bee or insect stings (anaphylaxis, see page 307), have a kit containing a syringe with epinephrine (adrenaline) readily available.

Other medications you may want to have on hand include antihistamine tablets, an anti-diarrheal medication, insulin and a simple sugar (for diabetics), and reserve supplies of medications required by your family members.

Terms of the trade. An "emergency" is a general term describing any situation in which immediate care is required. The term "trauma" implies an injury, such as a burn, wound, or broken bone. The terms are often used interchangeably, but the distinction is a useful one.

Steri-Strip bandages can be used to effectively close a superficial cut if the cut has edges that can easily be drawn together.

Be ready. Have a proper stock of first aid materials on hand.

CARE OF MINOR WOUNDS

Everyday cuts, scrapes, or wounds often do not require a trip to the emergency room. Yet proper care is essential to avoid infection or other complications. The following guidelines can help you in caring for simple wounds.

Stop the bleeding. Minor bleeding from a cut or scrape usually will cease spontaneously within a few minutes. If it does not, apply pressure, using a gauze pad or clean cloth.

Emergency bleeding. If bleeding is persistent—if the blood spurts or continues to flow after several minutes of pressure—emergency care is called for. *Seek immediate medical assistance* (see also Bleeding Emergencies, page 261).

Keep the wound clean. Wash the area with mild soap and water, being sure to remove any dirt or grit (if dirt or other material is embedded in the wound, consult a physician). Pat the wound dry with a clean cloth. If you want, apply an over-the-counter antibiotic cream. Cover the wound with a protective bandage unless the cut or scrape is on the face; if the wound is facial, leave it unbandaged, but apply a thin layer of antiseptic or antibiotic cream.

Does it need stitches? A deep, gaping, or jagged-edged wound may require stitches to hold it together for proper healing. A strip or two of surgical tape (Steri-Strips) may close a minor cut, but if the mouth of the wound is not easily closed, *seek a physician's care.* Proper closure also will minimize scarring.

Follow-up care. Change the dressing at least once a day, taking care to keep the area of the injury clean and dry.

Danger signs. If any wound becomes inflamed—that is, tender to the touch and reddened—or if it oozes pus or other fluids, *consult your physician.* There may be an infection that requires additional treatment (see Wound Infections, page 1180).

CARE OF MINOR ILLNESSES

Everybody gets sick from time to time. The problem may be familiar, such as a cold or flu virus, or it may be a seemingly mysterious ailment. Most often, recovery from the common minor illnesses is a matter of time and commonsense treatments. For everyday minor complaints, follow these guidelines.

Take it easy. If you do not feel well, the first rule is to get some rest—or at least slow your usual pace. If you have the flu, bed rest, proper nutrition, and lots of liquids may help you recover more quickly (see Influenza, page 853). For a cold, patience is the first treatment: it will take a few days to recover. If you feel poorly, stay home and take it easy. However, if you feel up to it, go about your business (see Common Viral Colds, page 860).

Monitor the symptoms. Whatever your ailment, pay attention to what your body tells you. The familiar running nose, minor cough, and stuffed-up head of a cold usually come and go without the help that modern medicine can offer. However, a seemingly trivial ailment that persists for more than a week or two may actually be something more serious.

The following are a few symptoms that normally accompany minor ailments. However, they also can be danger signs to keep in mind when assessing that "minor ailment" from which you are suffering—just in case it is something more serious.

Pain. Acute pain (that is, pain that arrives suddenly) is usually a warning. If you experience a sudden, severe pain you have not had before, *consult your physician.*

Fever. Many minor ailments commonly are accompanied by fever. Elevated body temperature is your body's way of fighting infection and certain diseases. A fever also increases fluid loss from the body. Therefore, adequate water intake is important when fever is present.

Although your body temperature normally varies during the day (it is lower in the morning and higher in the afternoon), a low-grade fever (when measured with a thermometer placed beneath the tongue) is usually classified as a temperature between 99.5°F and 101.5°F.

Consult your physician if a temperature of 101°F or more persists for more than a day or two, if your temperature is higher than 103°F, if a fever persists for more than 3 days, or if a child 3 months or younger has a temperature of 100.5°F (see Fever: When Is It An Emergency?, page 285). A tempera-

---

A SHOT IN THE ARM: THE TETANUS IMMUNIZATION

A cut, laceration, bite, or other wound, even if minor, can lead to a tetanus infection. The result, days or even weeks later, can be "lockjaw": literally, a stiffness of the muscles of the jaw and other muscles. This may be followed by a range of other symptoms, possibly culminating in convulsions and an inability to breathe.

The Source of Infection
The tetanus bacteria usually are found in the soil but can occur virtually anywhere. If their spores enter a wound beyond the reach of oxygen, they germinate and produce a toxin that interferes with the nerves controlling your muscles. A tetanus infection is serious and can result in death if you have not been immunized previously (see Tetanus, page 857).

Treating the Wound
The good news is that tetanus infection is avoidable, given proper preventive steps. *Consult your physician immediately* if you sustain any cut or puncture wound and have not had a tetanus shot in the past 10 years. If you have had a series of tetanus shots many years ago, your physician probably will give you a booster shot of the vaccine. Your body will quickly manufacture the needed antibodies to protect you against tetanus.

If you have not had tetanus shots previously, your physician may administer tetanus immune globulin, which gives immediate protection but only for a few weeks. Your physician may decide to cleanse the wound carefully, cutting away dead tissue and leaving it open without stitches and only a light gauze dressing so that air can reach all parts of the wound. Several antibiotics can help eliminate the tetanus bacterium, but there is no substitute for proper care of the wound and use of a booster shot or the immune globulin (see also Care of Minor Wounds, page 254, and Immunizations, page 867).

Prevention
Active immunization is vital for everyone in advance of any injury. The tetanus vaccine usually is given to children as a DPT shot, in which diphtheria and pertussis (whooping cough) vaccines are given with the tetanus vaccine. Tetanus booster shots should be given every 10 years or at the time of a major injury.

---

ture of more than 103°F can, in an adult, confuse the mental processes.

Cough. A cough due to a cold is normal. However, a cough that persists for more than 2 or 3 weeks or one that produces bloody sputum is reason to *consult your physician.*

Persistent Diarrhea or Vomiting. The loss of body fluids can, if severe, be life-threatening, especially in children. *Consult your physician* if you or your child is unable to retain fluids. If watery diarrhea or vomiting persists longer than 2 or 3 days or is associated with a sensation of faintness when standing, see your physician.

BITES AND STINGS

A dog, a bee in a flowering bush, a spider or a snake, or even another person can deliver potentially dangerous bites. Every such injury must be treated promptly and properly in order to minimize the risks of infection, allergic reaction, or other complications.

The following pages discuss animal and human bites; bites by scorpions, spiders, and other insects; bee stings; snake bites; and stings by jellyfish.

ANIMAL BITES

Domestic pets are the cause of most animal bites. Dogs are more likely to bite than cats. However, cat bites are more likely to cause infection. For these reasons, the best treatment for an animal bite is prevention.

Teach your child from an early age not to approach strange animals. If you have a dog, obey the leash law in your town, and insist that your neighbors do the same. If an animal bites you or another person without provocation, report it to the local authorities. Animals that habitually bite should be constantly restrained or destroyed.

The vast majority of animal bites are inflicted by household pets, but strays and wild animals such as skunks, raccoons, squirrels, bats, and others also bite thousands of people each year. Animals living in the wild are especially dangerous because they may carry rabies, but any animal that

THE RISK OF RABIES

Bats, foxes, squirrels, and other wild animals may carry rabies—but so can the usually friendly pooch next door, especially if it runs wild in the woods from time to time.

Rabies is a virus that affects the brain. Transmitted to humans by saliva from the bite of an infected animal, the rabies virus has an incubation period (the time from a bite until symptoms appear) of between 3 and 7 weeks (although it can be much longer) (see Rabies, page 858).

The Symptoms

Once the incubation period is over, a tingling sensation usually develops at the site of the animal bite; a more generalized skin sensitivity may occur and changes in temperature become very uncomfortable. As the virus spreads, foaming at the mouth may occur (a consequence of excess saliva that cannot be swallowed). You may choke when you attempt to swallow even a small quantity of liquid. Uncontrolled irritability and confusion may follow, alternating with periods of calm. Convulsions and paralysis leading almost inevitably to death will result if the rabies virus is untreated. In the later stages, the virus is found in the person's saliva and could infect others.

Observe the Animal

In the event of an unprovoked bite by a domestic dog, cat, or farm animal, the animal should be caught, confined, and observed by a veterinarian for 7 to 10 days. If a wild animal has bitten you, the animal should be killed. Do this in such a way that the animal's brain is not crushed or damaged. Notify your local health department. They will be able to assist in testing the animal for rabies. Wild raccoons, skunks, bats, coyotes, and foxes, if not caught, are generally presumed to have rabies.

Treatment

Extensive cleaning of the wound with soap and water followed by a second scrubbing with antiseptics should be carried out as soon as possible after the bite. Your physician must decide whether to treat you for rabies. Treatment consists of a passive antibody, half injected directly into the wound and half injected into the muscle, and a vaccine, usually given in five injections over 28 days.

Consult Your Physician

If circumstances suggest you may have been exposed to rabies, consult your physician immediately.

bites a human should be impounded and checked for rabies (see The Risk of Rabies, page 256).

Emergency Treatment. *Minor Bites.* Treat a minor bite (one in which the skin is broken but not torn and bleeding is limited) as you would any minor wound. Wash the wound thoroughly with soap and water, and apply an antibiotic cream to prevent infection (see Care of Minor Wounds, page 254).

Establish whether the person who was bitten has had a tetanus shot within the past 5 years; if not, *seek medical care* from your physician or local emergency room.

Serious Bites. If the bite results in a deep puncture wound, if the skin in the bitten area is badly torn, or if bleeding persists, apply pressure to stop the bleeding (see How To Stop Severe Bleeding, page 262). Then *seek emergency medical assistance.* Your physician will examine, wash, and treat the wound; he or she also may give a tetanus shots (see A Shot in the Arm: The Tetanus Immunization, page 255.)

Indications of Infection. Whether the wound is superficial or more serious, watch for any signs of infection in the hours and days after the bite. Swelling, redness, pus draining from the wound, or pain should be reported immediately to your physician.

Certain diseases also can be transmitted through bites and scratches. In addition to swelling or soreness at the site of the wound, accompanying symptoms may include fever, headache, and other flu-like symptoms. Again, *consult your physician immediately.*

HUMAN BITES

Human bites are of two kinds. The first is what we usually think of as a bite: an injury that results from flesh being caught between the teeth of the upper and lower jaws. The second kind, called a fight bite, occurs when, in the act of striking another person, an assailant cuts his or her knuckles on the opponent's teeth. (See page B-13 for color photograph of human bite.)

Human bites are the most dangerous of mammalian bites—in part because people frequently delay seeking treatment out of embarrassment or fear of legal action. Human bites are also dangerous because of the considerable risk posed by the bacteria found in the human mouth. Carried by the saliva, the bacteria enter the tissues at the site of the bite and can lead to serious infections. There is also the obvious risk of injury to tendons and joints when the cut extends below the skin.

Emergency Treatment. If you sustain a human bite of either kind, *seek emergency medical assistance.* Do not treat a human bite yourself. A serious infection could put you at risk of a prolonged hospital stay, permanent joint stiffness, and even amputation if not appropriately treated.

Stop the bleeding by applying pressure, wash the wound thoroughly with soap and water, and bandage the wound. Then visit your physician or an emergency room. In addition to examining and treating the wound, your physician may prescribe antibiotics to prevent the development of infection.

INSECT BITES AND STINGS

The symptoms of an insect bite result from the injection of venom or other agents into your skin. With minor bites, the reaction is temporary and local: a bump rises on your skin at the site of the bite, the area may itch for a few hours, and then over a period of days the skin irritation and discomfort disappear. Typically, the bites of mosquitoes, fleas, flies, bedbugs, ants, and chiggers follow this course.

However, your entire body can be affected if the venom is potent, as is the case with certain spiders and scorpions, or if you are hypersensitive, as some people are, to bee, wasp, and yellow jacket stings.

Spider Bites. The black widow spider *(Latrodectus mactans)* is shiny and black and about a half-inch long, usually with an hourglass-shaped splash of red on its stomach. The brown recluse spider *(Loxosceles reclusa)* has long legs, and its body is roughly three-eighths of an inch long. Both the black widow and the brown recluse spiders usually are found in dark places; the black widow likes dampness (stumps and woodpiles provide excellent hiding places),

In the illustration below, distinctive marks of individual insects are emphasized to simplify identification; however, the insects are not drawn to scale. The deer tick, for example, is in reality only about the size of a sesame seed.

and the brown recluse likes dry environments. Both are most common in the southern United States.

The bite of the black widow spider is little more than a pinprick-like sensation—some victims are not even aware of the bite. At first there may be only slight swelling and faint red marks. Within a few hours, however, intense pain and stiffness begin. Other symptoms may include chills, fever, nausea, and severe abdominal pain. The bite is rarely lethal.

The bite of a brown recluse produces a mild stinging followed by local redness and intense pain within 8 hours. A fluid-filled blister forms at the site and then sloughs off to leave a deep, growing ulcer. Your body's reactions can vary from a mild fever and rash to nausea and listlessness. (See page B-14 for color photograph of brown recluse spider bite.)

Scorpion Bites. Scorpions are found in the southwestern United States. About 3 inches long, they have eight legs and a pair of crab-like pincers. At the end of their narrow tail is the stinger.

Some scorpions have a potentially lethal venom that is injected by a sting. They live in cool, damp places: basements, junk piles,

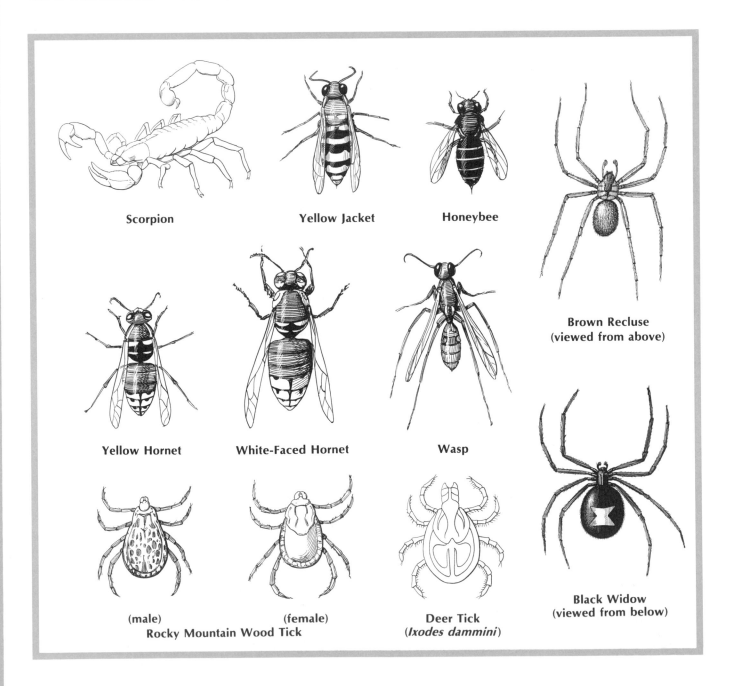

Scorpion

Yellow Jacket

Honeybee

Brown Recluse
(viewed from above)

Yellow Hornet

White-Faced Hornet

Wasp

(male)   (female)
Rocky Mountain Wood Tick

Deer Tick
(*Ixodes dammini*)

Black Widow
(viewed from below)

and woodpiles are favored locations. They tend to be nocturnal, and they are most likely to sting in the cool of the evening.

Because it is difficult to distinguish the highly poisonous scorpions *(Centruroides sculpturatus)* from the non-poisonous scorpions, all scorpion bites are to be treated as medical emergencies.

Bee, Wasp, Hornet, Fire Ant, or Yellow Jacket Stings. Perhaps 1 person in 10 is allergic to the venom injected by insects in the Hymenoptera family. For such sensitive individuals, being stung by a bee or other Hymenoptera insect can be a life-threatening emergency, called an anaphylactic reaction.

Symptoms of such a reaction after a bee sting may include swelling around the eyes, lips, tongue, or throat; difficulty in breathing, coughing, or wheezing; and widespread numbness or cramping. Hives may appear on the skin. Speech may be slurred, and anxiety, mental confusion, nausea and vomiting, and unconsciousness may occur. (See also Insect Bite Allergies, page 472, and Anaphylaxis, page 307.)

Tick Bites. Ticks live like fleas in the fur or feathers of many species of birds and animals. The principal risk usually is not from the tick bite itself but from a bacterium carried by the insect, which can cause Lyme disease. Lyme disease manifests mainly as a form of arthritis but, in addition, may cause a wide variety of symptoms (see Lyme Disease, page 854).

If you have a circular skin eruption when you have been in an area where ticks may live (mainly underbrush or tall grass), you may have had a bite by a tick carrying the infectious agent. This may occur even though you may not have seen this very small tick at that time.

(See page B-14 for color photograph of Lyme disease rash.)

Emergency Treatment. *Mild Insect Bites.* If the stinger from a bee or other insect remains in your skin, it must be removed carefully. Remove bee stingers, particularly the tip of the stinger, so as not to inject more venom. Mild insect bites can be treated with an application of a paste of baking soda, a cold, wet cloth, or ice cubes to reduce pain. You also may apply a hydrocortisone cream (purchased without a prescription) or calamine lotion to reduce itching and inflammation.

If you react more severely to minor bites, consult your physician.

Poisonous Stings. If bitten by a black widow spider, brown recluse spider, or scorpion, or if you are allergic to insects in the Hymenoptera family (such as bees and wasps), *seek immediate emergency medical care.*

Before seeking emergency care, however, take the following steps:

1. If the bite is on an arm or leg, snugly bandage the limb above the bite (between it and the heart). This will slow or halt the movement of the venom. The bandage should be tight enough to slow the flow of blood at skin level but not so tight as to halt all circulation in the arm or leg.
2. Apply a rag dampened with cold water or lined with ice to the bite.
3. Remove the bandage after 5 minutes, but keep the arm or leg dangling down.
4. Seek emergency medical assistance.

If you know you are sensitive to bee stings, your physician may provide you with a special emergency kit containing a hypodermic syringe with epinephrine (adrenaline). Keep this kit handy, especially at the time of the year when, or in situations in which, you are at risk of being bitten by an insect in the Hymenoptera family. A person who loses consciousness after a bee sting should be treated for shock (see Anaphylaxis, page 307).

Tick Bites. If you find a tick crawling on your skin, carefully remove it. Do not crush it between your fingers; drop it in a fire or smash it between two rocks. Wash your hands afterward.

If the tick has already bitten you and is holding on to your skin, *do not pull it off.* Cover it with oil (any kitchen or machine oil will do). The film of oil will make breathing difficult for the tick, so it will relax its clamp on your skin. When it is free, remove the tick with tweezers.

After the tick has been removed, wash the area thoroughly. Watch the area carefully for the next week or two for signs of Lyme disease (see page 854).

SNAKE BITES

Most snakes are not poisonous. However, because a few are—including rattlesnakes, coral snakes, water moccasins, and copperheads—avoid picking up or playing with any snake unless you have been trained in distinguishing and handling snakes. If you are bitten by a snake, it is important to be able to determine whether the snake is poisonous. Most poisonous snakes (including the rattlesnake, copperhead, and water moccasin) have elliptically shaped, slit-like eyes. Their heads are triangular in shape, with a depression or "pit" midway between the eyes and nostrils on both sides of the head (thus the collective name for these snakes, pit vipers). Rattlesnakes are also distinguished by a rattling sound made by the rings at the end of the snake's tail.

The water moccasin has a whitish, cottony lining in its mouth, and the coral snake has red, yellow, and black rings along its length.

Emergency Treatment.   If the snake was not poisonous, wash the bite thoroughly, cover it with an antibiotic cream, and bandage it. In general, such a snake bite is more scary than dangerous.

If, however, you suspect the snake was poisonous, follow these steps:

Many poisonous snakes, including the rattlesnake, copper-head, and water moccasin, are known as pit vipers. These snakes have triangularly shaped heads, elliptically shaped (slit-like) eyes, and a depression (pit) midway between the eyes and nostrils.

1. Remain as quiet and still as possible after the bite. Lie down quietly and, if possible, keep the bitten area lower than the level of the heart. This position will limit circulation of the venom.
2. If the area changes color, begins to swell, or is painful, the snake was probably poisonous. If the bite is on an arm or leg, tightly bandage the limb a few inches above the bite (between it and the heart). This will also help slow the movement of the venom. The bandage should be tight enough to slow the blood flow at skin level but not so tight as to halt all circulation in the arm or leg. Do not remove the band: the physician will do that.
3. If you are positive the snake was poisonous, you are more than 2 hours from a hospital, and the bite occurred in the previous 15 minutes, make a one-quarter-inch-deep cut with a sterile razor blade or knife over each fang mark. Be sure to make the cut along the length of the limb (do not cut across the leg or arm). *If it was a coral snake, do not make these incisions.*

    Suck out the venom, either orally or with a suction device if one is at hand. Spit out the venom.
4. *Seek emergency medical assistance immediately.*

JELLYFISH STINGS

Several aquatic organisms, including the jellyfish and the Portuguese man-of-war, carry venom in their tentacles. Their venom can be discharged on contact, in some cases even after they are dead.

Stinging and pain are the key symptoms, along with a red, hive-like line of lesions. If a considerable amount of venom is injected, shortness of breath, nausea, stomach cramps, and emotional upset also may occur.

More severe stings can lead to muscle cramps, fainting, cough, vomiting, and difficulty in breathing. In rare cases, a potentially fatal reaction (see Anaphylaxis, page 307) may occur.

The Portuguese man-of-war is found in the waters of the Atlantic Ocean, ranging from Canada to the West Indies and the Mediterranean Sea. They also live in the Pacific Ocean near Hawaii and southern Japan.

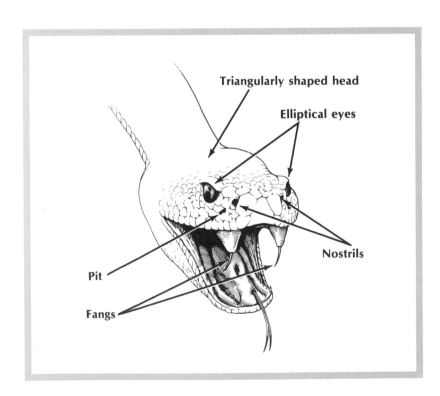

Triangularly shaped head

Elliptical eyes

Nostrils

Pit

Fangs

(See page B-13 for color photograph of man-of-war skin reaction.)

Emergency Treatment. If you are bitten by a jellyfish or Portuguese man-of-war, do the following:

1. Get out of the water: pain and cramps can be disabling and drowning could result.
2. Inactivate the stinging: sprinkle the area with meat tenderizer, vinegar, salt, sugar, or even dry sand; gently rub the material into the wound. This step often offers quick relief.
3. Cleanse the wound: after waiting 15 to 20 minutes, gently wash the area with sea water. Do not use fresh water and do not rub the skin because either action could trigger discharge of more venom.
4. Remove the stinging tentacles: apply a paste made of sea water and sand (or baking soda, talcum powder, or flour). Scrape the residue with a knife or other sharp object, such as a clam shell. It is best to wear gloves or use a towel when removing the man-of-war debris.
5. Apply 0.5 percent hydrocortisone cream (available without a prescription) to reduce redness and swelling. A local anesthetic ointment (such as benzocaine) helps relieve pain, and a calamine-type lotion lessens itching. Mild analgesics, such as aspirin and acetaminophen, are often used, but prescription pain killers may be necessary after severe stings.

BLEEDING EMERGENCIES

When an injury results in bleeding (hemorrhage), steps must be taken to stop the loss of blood. If substantial amounts of blood are lost, shock (see page 303), unconsciousness, and death can result.

Most bleeding injuries are not life-threatening, although appropriate care must be taken not only to stop the bleeding but also to avoid infection and other complications. The pages that follow discuss appropriate emergency procedures to accomplish these ends.

It is often useful to distinguish the kind of bleeding that was sustained. The three main classifications are capillary, venous, and arterial.

Capillary bleeding: The capillaries are the most numerous and the smallest blood vessels in the body. When a minor cut or skin scrape opens some capillaries, the bleeding is usually slow. The body's clotting action is generally sufficient to stop the bleeding in a matter of minutes.

Venous bleeding: Deep cuts often open veins, releasing blood that is on its way back to the heart. Having delivered its load of oxygen to the cells, the blood is dark red. It flows steadily but slowly. Placing pressure on the wound will usually stop the blood flow.

Arterial bleeding: The least common but most serious type of bleeding involves the opening of an artery. The blood that is released is bright red and often spews forth in rhythmic spurts that coincide with the contractions of the heart. If a major artery is severed and not treated promptly, it is possible to bleed to death in as little as a minute. In most cases, however, direct, firm pressure on the wound will stop arterial bleeding.

The location and nature of the wound itself also have an impact on the choice of treatment. The following pages discuss wounds to the skin, bleeding from the mouth or other body openings, and bleeding or severe bruising beneath the skin.

BLEEDING FROM A WOUND OR INJURY

Bleeding from the surface of your body can range from very minor—the prick of a sewing needle can produce a droplet of blood—to major, as with a deep gash in which an artery is severed and blood gushes forth in rhythmic spurts. All wounds, however, require appropriate care and treatment; inadequate care can result in serious infection (see Wound Infections, page 1180).

Cuts. If you sustain a small cut that bleeds only slightly, wash the cut thoroughly with mild soap and water. Apply a bandage to keep it clean.

If your cut is more serious—that is, the bleeding does not cease on its own in a short time or the cut is large, deep, or rough on the edges—*consult your physician*. But first stop the bleeding by applying pressure directly to the injury, using a sterilized gauze pad or clean cloth. Maintain pressure on the wound until the bleeding stops.

For severe bleeding, see How To Stop Severe Bleeding, page 262.

HOW TO STOP SEVERE BLEEDING

To stop a serious bleeding injury, follow these steps:

1. Lay the affected person down. If possible, the person's head should be slightly lower than the trunk of his or her body or the legs should be elevated. This position reduces the chances of fainting by increasing blood flow to the brain. If possible, elevate the site of bleeding; for example, an injured hand can be held up, over the level of the heart, in order to reduce blood flow.

2. Remove any obvious debris or dirt from the wound. Do not remove any objects impaled in the person. Do not probe the wound or attempt to clean it at

To stop bleeding, apply pressure directly to the wound, using gauze or a clean cloth.

this point. Your principal concern is to stop the loss of blood.

3. Put pressure directly on the wound with a sterile bandage, clean cloth, or even a piece of clothing. If nothing else is available, use your hand.

4. Maintain pressure until the bleeding stops. When it does, bind the wound dressing tightly with adhesive tape. If none is available, use a piece of clean clothing.

5. If the bleeding continues and seeps through the gauze or other material you are holding on the wound, *do not* remove it. Rather, add more absorbent material on top of it.

6. If the bleeding does not stop with direct pressure, you may need to apply pressure to the major artery that delivers blood to the area of the wound. In the case of a wound on the hand or lower arm, for example, squeeze the main artery in the upper arm against the bone. Keep your fingers flat; with the other hand, continue to exert pressure on the wound itself.

7. Immobilize the injured body part once the bleeding has been stopped. Leave the bandages in place, and get the injured person to the emergency room as soon as possible (see also Traumatic Amputation, page 312).

If bleeding continues despite pressure applied directly to the wound, maintain pressure and also apply pressure to the nearest major artery.

Arterial pressure points

Bruises.   Bruises (contusions) usually result from a blow or a fall. Bleeding beneath the skin then occurs, producing an accumulation of blood (hematoma).

When the skin is not broken, a bandage is unnecessary. However, elevating the injured area and periodically applying ice or cold packs for 30 to 60 minutes to the area for a day or two after sustaining the injury may reduce discomfort and swelling.

Punctures.   A puncture wound—stepping on a nail is a common example—does not usually result in excessive bleeding. Often, in fact, little blood will flow and the wound will seem to close almost instantly. These features, however, do not mean that treatment is unnecessary.

Puncture wounds are dangerous because of the risk of infection. The object that caused the wound, especially if it has been exposed to soil, may carry spores of the tetanus or other bacteria. These can result in serious infections (see A Shot in the Arm: The Tetanus Immunization, page 255).

If you sustain a puncture wound, stop the bleeding, if necessary, by applying pressure with a sterile gauze pad or clean cloth. Then *seek emergency care* for appropriate treatment to prevent tetanus or other infection.

Soft Tissue Injuries.   Another kind of injury that may involve considerable bleeding is termed a soft tissue injury. The skin is damaged, as are underlying tissues such as muscle, supporting structures, and blood vessels. Such injuries can occur when an area is struck (contusions), when an area is badly cut (lacerations), when skin is separated from the underlying tissues (degloving injuries), or when areas of skin are forcefully torn away (avulsions). Soft tissue injuries require special treatment once you reach the emergency room, but they are to be given emergency medical care like other bleeding incidents.

Abdominal Wounds.   Because of the presence of numerous internal organs, a wound that penetrates the abdominal wall is a potentially serious injury. *Seek professional emergency care* immediately by calling the emergency telephone number in your community (911 in many areas) or your local ambulance service if such a wound is sustained.

Before moving someone with an abdominal wound, position the person on his or her back. If no internal organs protrude through the wound, use a gauze pad or sterile cloth and exert pressure on the injury to stop the bleeding. When the flow has stopped, tape the bandage in place.

If organs have been displaced by the wound, do not try to reposition them: cover the injury with a dressing, and do not apply more than very gentle pressure to stop the bleeding.

BLEEDING FROM BODY OPENINGS

Internal bleeding may accompany seemingly superficial injuries: for example, a blow to the head that produces minor bleeding from the skin may result in much more dangerous internal bleeding. In some cases, internal injury may produce no signs of external bleeding; in others, the person may vomit blood or have bleeding from the mouth, anus, vagina, or penis.

Internal bleeding, especially in the abdomen, head, or chest, is extremely serious and can be life-threatening. Blood loss can be considerable—even if there is no evident external bleeding.

If the person has sustained a traumatic injury—an injury sustained during a fall, automobile accident, or other event involving an external force or violence—suspect internal bleeding (see Detecting Internal Bleeding, page 265).

Vomiting of Blood.   Hematemesis is the medical term for the vomiting of blood. This can occur as the result of injury to or disease of the throat, esophagus, stomach, or initial portion of the small bowel (duodenum).

Seek emergency assistance. While waiting for help to arrive, keep the person lying down with his or her legs elevated, if possible. An ice bag may be applied to the site of the internal bleeding (if known), but the person should be kept quiet and calm. The person should not attempt to eat or drink anything, even if he or she complains of being thirsty.

Coughing of Blood.   The medical term for the coughing up of blood is hemoptysis. The source of the blood is usually the lungs or windpipe. The blood that appears is usually frothy, is bright in color, and has a salty taste. Some possible causes include bronchial or lung infection, blunt injury to the chest, and lung cancer.

Summon emergency assistance immediately if the person coughs up large amounts of blood. While waiting for emergency help to arrive, the person who is coughing up blood should be lying down with his or her head elevated slightly and supported by pillows. Loosen clothing that is tight around the throat and chest. Keep the person warm, quiet, and as comfortable as possible. If the person complains of thirst, small amounts of crushed ice or sips of water may be given.

Rectal Bleeding.   Bleeding from the anus can be the result of various causes. Hemorrhoids can produce bleeding, a relatively minor event that produces bright red blood in the toilet bowl or on the toilet paper. Black, tarry stools, maroon stools, or bright red blood in the stool may suggest the presence of considerable bleeding in the gastrointestinal tract. (Note that the use of bismuth or iron-containing preparations also may cause black stools.) If you observe rectal bleeding of unknown cause, consult your physician.

If rectal bleeding occurs in moderate to large amounts, *seek immediate emergency care.*

Vaginal Bleeding.   Vaginal bleeding is a normal part of menstruation; however, bleeding from the vagina also may signal a wide range of medical and gynecological difficulties. *Consult your physician immediately* if you experience any unfamiliar bleeding, especially if you are pregnant.

Blood in the Urine.   Blood in the urine, termed hematuria, may be frightening. A relatively small amount of bright red, fresh blood in the toilet may make the bowl appear to be full of blood. The chances are high that relatively little blood has been lost. Nevertheless, *seek your physician's guidance* because the cause could be a tumor, infection, kidney disease, or other serious medical problem.

If the blood precedes the flow of urine and is bright red, it probably is coming from the urethra. Blood that seems to have been

---

DETECTING INTERNAL BLEEDING

In the event of a traumatic injury, such as might be experienced in an automobile crash or a fall, internal bleeding may not be immediately apparent. However, because of the dangers of internal bleeding, suspect it if you observe any of the following signs:

Bleeding from the ears, nose, rectum, or vagina, or the vomiting or coughing up of blood;

Bruising on the neck, chest, or abdomen;

Wounds that have penetrated the skull, chest, or abdomen;

Abdominal tenderness, perhaps accompanied by hardness or spasm of the abdominal muscles;

Fractures.

Internal bleeding may produce shock: the volume of blood in the body becomes inadequate and the person may feel weak, thirsty, and anxious. His or her skin may feel cool. Other symptoms of shock that may indicate the presence of internal bleeding include shallow and rapid breathing, a rapid and weak pulse, trembling, and restlessness.

The person may faint and lose consciousness when standing or seated but recovers when allowed to lie down. Elevating the legs may be of additional help.

Emergency Treatment

If you suspect internal bleeding, *request immediate emergency assistance* by calling the emergency number in your community (often 911) or by summoning your local ambulance. Treat the person for shock (see Recognizing and Treating Shock, page 304). Keep him or her lying quietly and comfortably. Loosen clothing, but do not give the person anything to eat or drink, even if he or she complains of being thirsty. If internal bleeding is in an extremity (as with a fracture or evident bruise on an arm or leg), apply pressure directly to this area or manually compress the major artery above the fracture or bruise to stop the bleeding (see How To Stop Severe Bleeding, page 262).

---

well mixed with the urine suggests that the source is the bladder or kidneys.

NOSEBLEED

This common condition involves sudden bleeding from one nostril. It may result from trauma (the most common example being a punch in the nose), from breathing dry air, from allergies, or for no apparent reason.

Most nosebleeds begin on the septum, the cartilage that separates the nasal chambers and is lined with fragile blood vessels. This form of nosebleed is not serious and is usually easy to stop.

In some people, nosebleeds may begin deeper in the nose. These nosebleeds, which are less common, are often harder to stop.

Emergency Treatment.   Stop the flow of blood from a common nosebleed using the following steps:

1. First, sit or stand upright. The upright positions slow the flow of blood in the veins of the nose. *Do not* tip your head back.
2. Pinch your nose with your thumb and index finger; breathe through your mouth. Do this for 5 or 10 minutes; this should stop the flow of blood.

If you succeed in stopping the flow of blood, there is no need for professional medical assistance. However, if the bleeding proves hard to stop, seek emergency medical assistance (see also Nosebleed, page 692).

BURNS

Burns are classified according to the degree of damage to skin and body tissue.

Burns can be caused by fire, the sun, chemicals, heated objects or fluids, electricity, and other means. They can be minor medical problems or life-threatening emergencies.

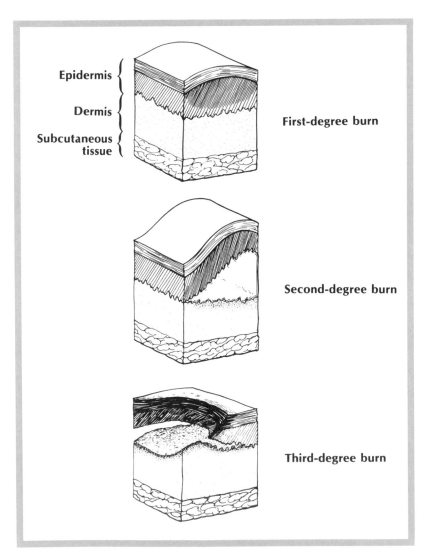

Epidermis
Dermis
Subcutaneous tissue

First-degree burn

Second-degree burn

Third-degree burn

BURN CLASSIFICATIONS

Distinguishing a minor burn from a more serious burn involves determining the degree of damage to the tissues of the body. The following are the three classifications physicians use.

First-Degree Burns.   The least serious burns are those in which only the outer layer of skin (epidermis) is burned. The skin is usually reddened and there may be swelling and pain. However, the outer layer of skin has not been burned through. Unless such a burn involves substantial portions of the hands, feet, face, groin, buttocks, or a major joint, it is to be treated as a minor burn (see Treating Minor Burns at Home, page 267). If the burn was caused by exposure to the sun, see Sunburn, page 276.

Second-Degree Burns.   When the first layer of skin has been burned through and the second layer of skin (dermis) is also burned, the injury is termed a second-degree burn. Blisters develop, and the skin will take on an intensely reddened appearance and become mottled. Severe pain and swelling are accompanying symptoms.

If a second-degree burn is limited to an area no larger than 2 to 3 inches in diameter, see Treating Minor Burns at Home, page 267; if the burned area of skin is larger or if the burn occurred on the hands, feet, face, groin, buttocks, or a major joint, see Treating Major Burns, page 267.

Third-Degree Burns: The most serious burns involve all layers of skin. Fat, nerves, muscles, and even bones also may be affected. There are usually areas that are charred black or that appear a dry white. There may be severe pain or, if nerve damage is substantial, no pain at all (see Treating Major Burns, this page).

ELECTRICAL BURNS

Any electrical burn should be examined by a physician. An electrical burn may appear minor, but the damage can extend deep to the tissues beneath the skin. A heart rhythm disturbance, cardiac arrest, or other internal damage can occur when the amount of electrical current that passed through the body was large.

Sometimes the jolt associated with the electrical injury can cause the person to be thrown or to fall, resulting in fractures or other associated injuries. For first aid measures to institute before reaching the emergency room, see Treating Major Burns, this page.

CHEMICAL BURNS

To treat chemical burns, follow these steps:

1. Make sure the cause of the burn has been removed. Flush the chemicals off the skin surface using cool running water for 20 minutes or more. (If the burning chemical is lime, brush the lime off the skin before flushing.)
2. Treat the person for shock if he or she is faint, pale, or breathing in a notably shallow, hurried fashion (see Recognizing and Treating Shock, page 304).
3. Remove clothing or jewelry from the victim that has been contaminated by the chemical.
4. Wrap the burned area with a dry sterile dressing (if possible) or clean cloth.
5. If the victim complains of increased burning after you have washed the area, rewash the burn with water for several more minutes.
6. Minor chemical burns will usually heal without further treatment. However, if

---

TREATING MINOR BURNS AT HOME

To treat minor burns (see Burn Classifications, page 266), follow these steps:

1. If the skin is unbroken, run cool water over the area of the burn or soak it in a cool water bath. Keep the area submerged for 2 to 5 minutes. (Note: If the burn occurred in a cold environment, do not apply water.)
2. After flushing or soaking for several minutes, cover the burn with a sterile bandage (if available) or clean cloth.
3. Aspirin or acetaminophen may help relieve the pain and swelling.
4. Minor burns will usually heal without further treatment. However, if a second-degree burn covers an area more than 2 to 3 inches in diameter, or if it occurred on the hands, feet, face, groin, buttocks, or a major joint, see Treating Major Burns, below.

TREATING MAJOR BURNS

In treating major burns (see Burn Classifications, page 266) *immediately request emergency assistance.* While waiting for professional medical assistance to arrive, follow these steps:

1. Make sure the cause of the burn has been extinguished or removed. If clothing is on fire, do not let the person run—that will only feed the fire. Put out the flames with water or roll the person in a blanket or coat on the ground. Do not remove burnt clothing, but do ensure that the victim is not still in contact with smoldering materials.
2. Make certain the burn victim is breathing; if breathing has stopped or you suspect that the person's airway is blocked, see Choking, Breathing Emergencies, and Resuscitation, page 268.
3. If breathing is not a problem, cover the area of the burn with a cool, moist sterile bandage (if available) or clean cloth (do not use a blanket or towel; a sheet will do if the burned area is large). Do not apply any ointments. Avoid breaking burn blisters.
4. Await the arrival of emergency medical assistance.

---

the chemical burned through the first layer of skin and the resulting second-degree burn covers an area more than 2 to 3 inches in diameter, or if the chemical burn occurred on the hands, feet, face, groin, buttocks, or a major joint, *seek emergency medical assistance.*

Chemicals in the Eyes. If chemicals have splashed in the eyes, the eyes should be flushed with water immediately. Any source of clean drinking water will do—it is more important to begin the flushing than it is to find sterile water.

Continue to flush the eyes with running water for at least 20 minutes. After washing the eyes thoroughly, close the eyelids and then cover them with loose, moist dressings. *Seek emergency medical assistance.*

CHOKING, BREATHING EMERGENCIES, AND RESUSCITATION

Choking results from a blockage of the respiratory passage in the throat or windpipe. The flow of air to the lungs is blocked; in turn, the circulation of fresh oxygen to the brain and other cells ceases. If the choking is not dealt with promptly, unconsciousness and death may result.

Choking, heart disease, or other causes may also result in the stoppage of the heart and breathing. In such an emergency, breathing and blood circulation must be restored if the life of the injured person is to be saved. Resuscitation is the appropriate means of restoring breathing (mouth-to-mouth resuscitation), perhaps with simultaneous pumping of the heart (cardiopulmonary resuscitation).

On the following pages you will learn the basics of determining the nature of the emergency at hand—that is, is your dinner partner having a heart attack or choking on a piece of steak? In addition, you will learn how to react to and deal with the medical emergency, including techniques for dislodging an obstruction in the airway and the skills of mouth-to-mouth and heart-and-lung resuscitation.

RECOGNIZING AN OBSTRUCTED AIRWAY

Choking is often the result of inadequately chewed food becoming lodged in the throat (pharynx) or windpipe (trachea). Most often, solid foods such as meats are the cause.

Commonly, persons who are choking have been conversing while simultaneously chewing a chunk of meat. False teeth may also set the stage for this problem by interfering with the way food feels in the mouth while it is being chewed. Food cannot be chewed as thoroughly with false teeth as with one's natural teeth because less chewing pressure is exerted by false teeth.

Panic is an accompanying sensation: the choking victim's face often assumes an expression of fear or terror. At first, he or she may turn purple, the eyes may bulge, and he or she may wheeze or gasp.

COUGHING VERSUS CHOKING

If a morsel of food "goes down the wrong pipe," often the coughing reflex will resolve the problem. In fact, a person is *not* choking if he or she is able to cough freely and has normal skin color. However, if the cough is more like a gasp and the person takes on a bluish tinge, the individual is probably choking.

If in doubt, ask the choking person whether he or she can talk. If the person is capable of speech, then the windpipe is not completely blocked and oxygen is reaching the lungs.

The universal choking sign is a hand at the throat with fingers and thumb extended.

THE HEIMLICH MANEUVER

You have seen it on television and on posters: but do you remember how to do it? Here's how.

1. The choking person may be standing or sitting. Stand behind the victim, and wrap your arms around his or her waist. Tip the person forward slightly.
2. Make a fist with one hand and position it slightly above the person's navel.
3. Grasp the fist with the other hand, and press hard into the abdomen. A quick, upward thrust—as if you were trying to lift the person off the ground—works best.
4. If necessary, repeat the Heimlich maneuver until the food or other blockage is dislodged. This technique is named after the physician who devised it.

If help is unavailable, you can perform the Heimlich maneuver on yourself. With clenched hands positioned slightly above your belly button, thrust your hands upward or drape your body over a chair or rail or some similar object.

Using It on Yourself

You can use a variation of the Heimlich maneuver if you begin

The Heimlich maneuver

to choke. Place a fist above your navel. Grasp your fist with the other hand, and bend over a hard surface (a countertop or chair will do). Shove your fist inward and upward.

For a Pregnant Woman or Obese Person

The abdomen of a pregnant woman or the flabby stomach of a very overweight person can prevent the effective use of an abdominal

thrust. However, a variation of the Heimlich maneuver may be used.

Position your hands higher on the victim's trunk: rather than just above the navel, grasp the victim at the base of the breastbone, just above the joining of the lowest ribs. Proceed as for the Heimlich maneuver, pressing hard into the chest with a quick, upward thrust. If necessary, repeat the maneuver until the food or other blockage is dislodged.

THE UNIVERSAL SIGN

A person who is choking is unable to communicate except by hand motions. Often the hand and arm motions are uncoordinated. As a potential affected person or rescuer, it is important to remember that the universal signal for choking is *a hand clutched to the throat, with thumb and fingers extended.*

CLEARING AN OBSTRUCTED AIRWAY

There are several techniques for opening an obstructed airway. First, determine that the

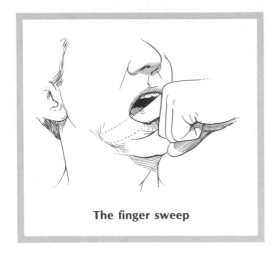

The finger sweep

individual is unable to breathe: if so, the person will be unable to speak, and his or her skin, if white, will be taking on a blue, gray, or ashen color.

The Heimlich maneuver is perhaps the best-known technique (see page 269), but there are several other options for certain situations, as follows.

To clear the airway of an unconscious, supine victim, kneel over the individual and apply thrusts to the upper abdomen.

The Finger Sweep.   The simplest method involves reaching a finger into the back of the throat. If you can see into the person's mouth, can you see the cause of the blockage? If so, sweep a finger into the back of the mouth to clear the airway.

This method works only if the blockage is at the very back of the mouth or high in the throat. *Be very careful not to push the food or object deeper into the airway.* Do not perform a finger sweep in children unless an object is visible.

The Unconscious Victim.   If the individual has collapsed, position the person on his or her back. Kneeling astride the person, place your hands at the base of the rib cage. The heel of one hand should be down, the fingers of the upper hand between those of the lower, grasping the palm. Deliver 6 to 10 quick thrusts to the abdomen, remembering to be more gentle with a child.

The Choking Child.   Assume a seated position. Hold the child face-down across your lap, with his or her upper trunk hanging off the side of your knees. Thump the child gently four times firmly on the middle of the back using the heel of your hand: the combination of gravity and the blows to the back should release the object blocking the airway.

A baby or very small child may be held by the ankles, head down. Thump the youngster's back more gently than you would an adult's but hard enough that the blockage may be jarred free.

Mouth-to-Mouth Resuscitation.   If one of these techniques opens the airway but the victim does not resume breathing, perform mouth-to-mouth resuscitation (see Cardiopulmonary Resuscitation, page 270).

CARDIOPULMONARY RESUSCITATION

This lifesaving technique is applicable to a range of emergencies, including heart attack, choking episode, and drowning. Each, however, has key components in common: the person is unconscious and has ceased breathing.

Death comes quickly when the heart stops: the absence of fresh oxygen can cause irreparable brain damage in only a few minutes, and death can occur in 8 to 10 minutes. Time is all-important when you are helping an unconscious person who is not breathing. Thus, the first rule is to begin cardiopulmonary resuscitation immediately.

Before proceeding with resuscitation, you must ascertain that the person is actually unconscious and has stopped breathing.

The American Heart Association, which sets standards for cardio (heart)-pulmonary (lung) resuscitation (CPR), distinguishes the three parts of the CPR process with the familiar letters ABC: A is for airway, B is for breathing, C is for circulation. Let's take the steps in order.

Clear the Airway. *Are You Okay?* The first step in dealing with an unconscious person is to be sure that he or she is not simply resting or sleeping. Ask the question: "Are you okay?" Firmly shake or tap his or her shoulder and ask, "Are you okay?"

Summon Assistance. If you get no response, *immediately call for help.* If you are alone at home, call your local emergency number (in many communities the number is 911) or your local ambulance service.

Position the Victim. Lay the person on his or her back. If necessary, roll the person over so that he or she is face up. Position yourself at a right angle on your knees, perpendicular to the person's neck and shoulders.

Head Tilt/Chin Lift. This is the primary maneuver for opening an airway. Position your palm on the person's forehead and push backward. This alone may open the

Left, **A gentle slap on the back can help clear the airway of a choking child.** *Right,* **To clear the obstructed airway of an infant, hold the child upside down and gently slap the back.**

Tilt the head (*left*) and lift the chin (*right*) to open the airway.

Left, **Look and listen for indications of breathing.** *Right,* **Mouth-to-mouth resuscitation.**

Check for a pulse at the carotid artery on either side of the person's neck.

airway. If necessary, place the second, third, and fourth fingers of your hand along the side of the person's jaw and lift the chin forward to further open the airway.

If you suspect a neck injury, a chin lift (without head lift or jaw thrust) may be used.

Examine the mouth to make sure no foreign material is present. If present, use a finger sweep to clear it.

Check for Breathing.   Check for breathing, positioning your ear immediately over the person's mouth. Look across the person's chest for the rise and fall of breathing. If no breathing is evident, begin mouth-to-mouth resuscitation immediately.

Breathe for the Person.   In the ABCs of CPR, "B" is for breathing. In the absence of emergency equipment or professional medical help, the restoration of the flow of oxygen to the lungs is best done by mouth-to-mouth resuscitation.

The basis of mouth-to-mouth resuscitation is simple: you are to provide breathing for the victim. You are to expel breath from your lungs into the victim's through that person's nose or mouth.

Deliver Two Slow Breaths.   Position yourself at a right angle to the person's shoulder. Use the head tilt/chin lift maneuver and pinch the person's nose closed using your thumb and forefinger.

Take a deep breath. Open your mouth wide, and place it tightly over the victim's mouth. Exhale into the victim. Remove your mouth from the victim's, inhale, and do it again. Deliver two big breaths. Observe the person's chest with each breath to note whether the air you are breathing into the person is actually causing his or her lungs to expand.

Check for a Pulse.   After you have delivered two breaths, position two fingers just to the side of the victim's Adam's apple. If the heart is pumping, the carotid artery on either side of the neck should be pulsating. If you do not feel it immediately, move your fingers a fraction of an inch up or down to be sure you are in the right place.

If There Is No Pulse.   If there is no pulse, cardiac compressions are necessary to circulate blood to the brain (see Cardiopulmonary Resuscitation, page 270).

Continue Breathing. If the person has a pulse but is not breathing, continue mouth-to-mouth breathing. Using the same technique, blow a big breath into the victim every 5 seconds (12 breaths per minute). Take your mouth away between breaths. Listen for signs of breathing and watch chest movement.

If the victim is breathing but the breaths are notably weak, shallow, or labored, mouth-to-mouth resuscitation may still be appropriate. However, coordinate your breathing assistance with the victim's breathing: deliver a breath when he or she inhales, and allow the person to exhale before you breathe for him or her again.

Continue to breathe for the person until he or she breathes on his or her own or until professional medical help arrives.

Restore Circulation. "C" is for circulation: the blood flow must be restored in order to deliver oxygen to the brain. Without oxygen, brain cells will die and, in a matter of minutes, irreversible damage can result.

If you are unable to find a pulse in an unconscious person, heart compressions are necessary to restore circulation. Also called closed heart massage, the heart compressions must be coordinated with mouth-to-mouth resuscitation: the breathing delivers the air to the lungs, then the heart massage pumps the oxygenated blood to the brain and other parts of the body.

Just as you are to act as a breathing machine for the lungs when you perform mouth-to-mouth resuscitation, performing a heart massage means you are artificially pumping the heart muscle.

Position Your Hands. Work from a kneeling position at right angles to the victim's chest. Find the base of the breastbone at the center of the chest where the ribs form a V. Position the heel of one hand on the chest immediately above the V; with the other hand, grasp the first hand from above, intertwining the fingers.

Lock Your Elbows. Shift your weight forward and upward so that your shoulders are over your hands; straighten your arms and lock your elbows.

Pump the Heart. Shift your weight onto your hands to depress the victim's chest (it

should fall about 1½ to 2 inches in an adult). Count aloud as you do it five times in a slow, even rhythm: one-thousand-one, one-thousand-two, and so on. Repeat the pattern three times for a total of 15 chest compressions.

Breathe for the Victim. You must also give the person oxygen. Use the same technique outlined above for mouth-to-mouth resuscitation. Use the head lift/chin tilt maneuver to open the airway. Pinch the nose closed with the thumb and forefinger. Take a deep breath, then cover the victim's mouth entirely with yours. Exhale into the victim. Repeat.

Heart compression (massage) must be coordinated with mouth-to-mouth resuscitation.

Use mouth-to-nose resuscitation if injury to the mouth or face makes mouth-to-mouth resuscitation difficult. First, hold the victim's mouth closed by lifting the chin. Then, cover his or her entire nose with your mouth and blow into the nose. After breathing, remove your mouth from the area to allow air to escape. Until help arrives, repeat these steps in a steady, rhythmic breathing pattern.

PERFORMING CPR ON AN INFANT

Cardiopulmonary resuscitation may also be used on infants (babies up to 12 months of age). The techniques are different but the goal is the same as with an older child or an adult victim: you need to restore oxygen and blood flow to the baby's brain.

Does the Baby Need Help?

Be sure that the baby is not simply resting or sleeping. Shake the child: is there a discernible response? Does breathing seem to have stopped? *Summon assistance immediately.*

Position the Baby

Put the baby on its back on a table. The floor or ground will do, too. Using the head tilt/chin lift maneuver described on page 271, gently tip the head back. This opens the airway.

Before giving mouth-to-mouth resuscitation to an infant, tilt the child's head back to open the airway (top). Then, if visual inspection reveals a foreign object in the infant's mouth, remove the object with a sweep of your finger (bottom). Be careful not to push the food or object deeper into the child's airway.

Examine the mouth to make sure no foreign material is in the mouth. Check for breathing, positioning your ear immediately over the baby's mouth and looking at the chest for the rise and fall of

Mouth-to-mouth resuscitation of a baby.

breathing. If no breathing is evident, begin mouth-to-mouth resuscitation immediately.

Deliver Two Gentle Breaths

Cover the baby's mouth and nose with your mouth. Using the strength of your cheeks rather than your lungs, breathe two times slowly—the breaths are more like puffs than deep exhalations. (Too much air can result in a distended stomach and vomiting, an unneeded complication.)

Check for a Pulse

After you have delivered two breaths, check for a pulse on the inside of the baby's upper arm. If no pulse is evident, begin chest compressions (see below). If there is a pulse, continue mouth-to-mouth breathing, delivering a breath every 5 seconds.

Continue to breathe for the baby until it breathes on its own or

Check for a brachial pulse on the inside of the baby's upper arm.

until professional medical help arrives.

Cardiopulmonary Resuscitation

To pump the baby's heart, position your index and middle fingers on the baby's breastbone. Compress the chest (no more than ½ to 1 inch: be gentle).

Count aloud as you pump in a fairly rapid rhythm. You should pump roughly 1½ times a second, or about 100 times a minute. Breathe for the baby gently on every fifth compression.

To perform cardiopulmonary resuscitation on an infant, alternate compression of the baby's chest with gentle breaths from your mouth while covering the baby's mouth and nose.

BREATHING DIFFICULTY DUE TO CROUP, EPIGLOTTITIS, OR BRONCHITIS

Several disorders of the upper respiratory tract can produce difficulty in breathing, especially in children. In most cases, the appropriate treatment is to keep the person with the ailment breathing moistened air, consuming plenty of fluids, and resting in bed.

These illnesses most often are temporary, but occasionally they can lead to extreme swelling in the airway, which produces labored breathing.

Croup

This infection is most likely to affect children 8 years or younger. The symptoms are fever, sore throat, hoarseness, and cough. The cough often sounds distinctly like a bark (see Croup, page 863).

Epiglottitis

The epiglottis is the lid-like cartilage that covers the windpipe. When it becomes inflamed, the condition is termed epiglottitis; its symptoms include sore throat, fever, difficulty swallowing with drooling, and hoarseness (see Epiglottitis, page 699).

Bronchitis

Characterized by a soreness and feeling of constriction in the chest, bronchitis is a common viral infection of the bronchi and the trachea, the principal air passages in the chest. Accompanying symptoms are cough, chills, an overall malaise, and slight fever (see Acute Bronchitis, page 916).

Wheezing, the sound made by air passing through narrowed breathing passages, may be common to all three of these conditions. Wheezing induced by these three conditions may sound similar to the wheezing of asthma. In fact, many individuals with asthma can develop severe asthma attacks with upper respiratory infections or bronchitis.

Emergency Treatment

If your child has any of these ailments, observe his or her breathing carefully. Croup, epiglottitis, and bronchitis, along with asthma, can lead to an obstructed airway because of the swelling of the tissues in the airway. Either a bathroom with warm humidified air from a tub full of hot water or, in the winter, the cold air outside may cause airway symptoms to improve.

Seek immediate emergency assistance if breathing becomes labored. Perform mouth-to-mouth resuscitation if breathing stops (see Cardiopulmonary Resuscitation, page 270).

Alternate Pumping and Breathing. Pump the person's chest 15 times, then breathe for him or her twice. Establish a regular rhythm, counting aloud. If help does not arrive in 1 minute and a phone is readily available, call for an ambulance immediately—then resume CPR.

Performing CPR on a Child. The procedure is essentially the same. However, keep in mind that you must be gentler with a child and that the number of compressions is greater. Use only one hand for chest compressions and breathe for the child more gently (see also Performing CPR on an Infant, page 274).

Two-Person CPR. The principles of two-person (two-rescuer) CPR are similar to those of one-person CPR with the exception that one person provides breathing assistance while the other pumps the heart. The heart is pumped at a rate of 60 to 80 times per minute. After each five compressions, a pause in pumping is allowed for a breath to be given by the second resuscitator. As with one-person CPR, it is important that an ambulance be called immediately.

SEVERE ASTHMA ATTACK

In people with asthma, occasional or even frequent asthma attacks occur. Usually the key symptom is a difficulty in breathing, accompanied by a tightness in the chest and coughing that may bring up excess mucus. Wheezing will be more pronounced when breathing out than when breathing in. Your physician's treatment strategy will be aimed at minimizing or eliminating these breathing difficulties (see Asthma, page 466).

Occasionally, however, more serious or even life-threatening asthma attacks may occur. Symptoms of a serious asthma attack may include extreme difficulty in breathing, a bluish cast to the face and lips, severe anxiety, an increased pulse rate, and heavy perspiration. Severe asthma attacks also may occur in a non-asthmatic person exposed to something that causes severe difficulty in breathing, such as croup or insecticide sprays.

Emergency Treatment

1. Establish that the problem is not a choking emergency: asthmatics, like the rest of us, choke on food or other foreign objects that block the airway. If the incident occurs during a meal, see Recognizing an Obstructed Airway, page 268.
2. Keep calm and try to reassure the asthmatic person having the attack.
3. Call the person's physician; if you are unable to reach the physician, call the emergency room at your local hospital.

Before you call, have any asthma medications being taken by the person at hand. When speaking with the physician, identify the person with the asthma attack by name and age. Describe the symptoms being experienced and other details about the person's recent medical history. Tell what medications and what dosages the person has been taking.

Follow the physician's instructions: he or she may suggest you go immediately to the hospital or may send an emergency vehicle. In some cases, the recommendation may be that you stay calm, medicate the person with doses of the drugs on hand, and allow the episode to pass.

ENVIRONMENTAL EMERGENCIES

The world around us presents a range of hazards to our health. For example, the sun warms us, but it also can burn our skin or cause our bodies to overheat (see Heat Stress, page 277). In a similar way, overexposure to cold and damp can also produce medical emergencies (see Hypothermia, page 278, and Frostbite, page 279).

In the following pages we discuss these environmentally induced emergencies and others as well, including near drowning (see page 279), electrocution (see page 280), smoke inhalation (see page 281), and carbon monoxide poisoning (see page 281).

SUNBURN

Prolonged exposure to the sun's ultraviolet rays produces red, tender, swollen skin. The skin also may develop water blisters. In severe cases of sun and heat exposure, fever, chills, nausea, or delirium also may result and require emergency medical care (see Heat Stress, page 277).

The symptoms of sunburn do not appear until a few hours after exposure, but the painful, hot-to-the-touch quality of sunburned skin is unmistakable. The swelling and redness are due to inflammation of the skin.

The effect of sunburn is like that of any burn, but its development is relatively slow, rather than rapid as from a heat burn. With mild sunburn, there may be only redness and mild pain on touching the sunburned skin. With more severe sunburn, there may be swelling, blisters, severe pain, and an overall sensation of illness.

Emergency Treatment. *Mild Sunburn.* Most cases of sunburn can be treated adequately at home with a cool bath or shower followed by the application of hydrocortisone cream several times a day. Do not break the water blisters: leaving them intact will speed healing. However, if they break on their own, remove the skin fragments and use an antibacterial ointment on the open areas. Dress them with clean gauze to promote healing.

Taking aspirin several times daily will help alleviate the general discomfort and may reduce swelling.

Severe Sunburn. If you have received a severe sunburn (after falling asleep in the sun, for example), contact your physician even before the sunburn is fully developed. Your physician may elect to give you an oral corticosteroid and thereby decrease the reaction and prevent some of the symptoms. Once the sunburn develops, treat it as you would a minor burn.

Prevention. Sun exposure in general is discouraged by most dermatologists: damage to your skin cells from recurrent sunburn is cumulative, and continued overexposure to ultraviolet radiation produces long-term effects. These can include skin discolorations, actinic keratosis (see page 1169), and

SKIN EMERGENCIES

Hives and Angioedema

Hives (urticaria) are raised, red, often itchy welts of various sizes that appear and disappear at random on the surface of the skin. Hives tend to occur in batches rather than singly; they may last a few minutes or for several days.

Angioedema consists of large welts below the surface of the skin, particularly around the eyes and lips. Angioedema also may occur on the hands and feet and within the throat.

Both hives and angioedema result from a bodily reaction to foods, drugs, pollen, animal dander, insect bites, infections, illness, cold, heat, light, emotional distress, or other, unclear factors. In most cases, hives and angioedema are harmless, leave no lasting marks, and sometimes are not even uncomfortable. Taking cool baths or showers, wearing light clothing, and minimizing vigorous activity often will speed recovery. An antihistamine prescribed by your physician also may help relieve itching and assist in your recovery.

Characterized by swelling that does not itch, one rare, hereditary variety of angioedema produces such symptoms as abdominal cramping and diarrhea and can cause fatal obstruction to the breathing passages (see page 474). When angioedema affects the throat or tongue, causing the air passage to be blocked, it can be life-threatening.

Seek emergency medical assistance if you experience serious angioedema, especially if it makes breathing difficult. If a companion experiences a stoppage of breathing or unconsciousness, resuscitation must be performed (see Cardiopulmonary Resuscitation, page 270).

Severe Contact Dermatitis

The term dermatitis simply means an inflammation of the skin. Contact dermatitis is the term used to describe such inflammation when redness and itching and, in severe cases, blisters and weeping from the sores occur after contact with a causative agent.

In sensitive individuals, the causes can include poison plants such as poison ivy, oak, or sumac; certain metals found in rings or other jewelry; household products; or certain cosmetics.

(See page B-3 for color photograph of contact dermatitis.)

In contact dermatitis, only the areas of skin contacted by the offending substance will react, and those areas with the greatest exposure will react first.

It is rare for contact dermatitis to be more than a discomfort and an inconvenience. However, if extreme swelling, redness, and inflammation occur, especially around the eyes or in the area of the throat, or if the amount of dermatitis is extensive, consult your physician (see Contact Dermatitis, page 457).

Contact dermatitis usually can be treated by cleansing the affected area with a mild soap and water and applying 0.5 percent hydrocortisone cream (which can be obtained without a prescription) up to four times daily. An antihistamine, in a dose prescribed by your physician, may relieve the itching.

---

skin cancer (see page 1170). Chronic sun exposure also prematurely ages your skin and increases wrinkling (see also Wrinkled Skin, page 1167).

For detailed strategies to prevent sunburn and protect your skin, see How To Avoid Sunburn, page 1165.

HEAT STRESS

Under normal conditions, a healthy body temperature is maintained by mechanisms involving your skin and perspiration. However, if you are exposed to high temperatures for prolonged periods, particularly where there is little breeze and high humidity, the normal control mechanisms may fail to dissipate the heat. The ability to tolerate high temperatures may be increased somewhat by being in warm surroundings for a few weeks (acclimatization).

Heatstroke.   Elderly and obese people are particularly at risk of heatstroke. Other contributing factors can be dehydration, alcohol consumption, heart disease, certain medications, and vigorous exercise.

The ability to sweat is your main protection against heatstroke. A few people are born with impaired ability to sweat and are particularly at risk. A few drugs may impair sweating and render you more vulnerable. Examples are medications for motion sickness or depression.

The key indication of heatstroke is a fever of 105°F with hot, dry skin. Other signs include rapid heartbeat, rapid and shallow breathing, and either elevated or lowered blood pressure. Often, the level of consciousness also may be altered, resulting in confusion or delirium. In extreme cases, seizures or even coma and death may occur.

Emergency Treatment. If you suspect heatstroke, get the person out of the sun and into a shady spot. A cool, air-conditioned location is best.

Summon emergency medical assistance immediately. Extreme elevation of temperature is a medical emergency requiring professional treatment to cool the victim, replace lost fluids, and monitor heartbeat and breathing.

While you are waiting for the emergency vehicle to arrive, cool the person by covering him or her with damp sheets or spraying with water. Direct air onto the person, either with an electric fan or by fanning with your hands or a newspaper. If possible, monitor the person's temperature with a thermometer. Stop attempting to cool the person when his or her temperature is normal. If breathing ceases, start cardiopulmonary resuscitation (see page 270).

Heat Exhaustion. Heat exhaustion can be thought of as a failure of your heart and vascular system to respond properly to high external temperatures. It often occurs in elderly people taking diuretics. Heat exhaustion is different from heatstroke in that it involves more than an elevated temperature. It sometimes occurs after excessive perspiration, coupled with inadequate consumption of water or other liquids to replace lost fluids. Symptoms often begin suddenly, and hence the term heat collapse is sometimes used. The symptoms resemble those of shock (see page 303), including faintness, rapid heartbeat, low blood pressure, an ashen appearance, cold clammy skin, and nausea.

Emergency Treatment. If you suspect heat exhaustion, get the person out of the sun and into a shady spot. A cool air-conditioned location is best. Once you get the person out of the sun into a cooler, shady location, lay the person down and elevate his or her feet slightly. Loosen or remove most or all of the person's clothing. Give the person cold (not iced) water to drink, but first stir in a teaspoon of salt per quart.

If signs of heatstroke appear—in particular, confusion, delirium, and a temperature of more than 102°F—*seek emergency medical assistance.*

Heat Cramps. Heat cramps consist of painful spasms of muscles, usually experienced after vigorous exercise, along with profuse perspiration. These do not always have to occur in very hot surroundings. The muscles most affected are usually the ones you use during the exercise or your abdominal muscles.

Emergency Treatment. Brief rest and ingestion of water with a teaspoon of salt per quart usually will resolve the symptoms. Often salt can be taken more conveniently in the form of a salty food, such as salted nuts.

HYPOTHERMIA

Under most conditions, your body is able to maintain a healthy body temperature. However, when exposed for prolonged periods to cold temperatures or a cool, damp environment, particularly if clothing is wet or damp, your body's control mechanisms may fail to keep your body heat normal. When more heat is lost than your body can generate, hypothermia can result.

Falling overboard from a boat into cold water is a common cause of hypothermia. An uncovered head in winter is another frequent source of heat loss.

The key symptom of hypothermia is a body temperature that drops below 94°F. Other signs include shivering, slurred speech, an abnormally slow rate of breathing, skin that is cold and pale, a loss of coordination, and feelings of tiredness, lethargy, or apathy.

The onset of symptoms is usually slow; there is likely to be a gradual loss of mental acuity and physical ability. The person experiencing hypothermia, in fact, may be unaware that he or she is in a state requiring emergency medical treatment.

The elderly, the very young, and very lean people are at particular risk of hypothermia. Other conditions that may predispose you to hypothermia are malnutrition, heart disease, and excessive consumption of alcohol or other drugs. Contributing medical factors may include untreated hypothyroidism (see page 730), hypopituitarism (see page 725), and diabetes mellitus (see page 707).

Emergency Treatment.   If you suspect hypothermia, get the person out of the cold. Change him or her into warm, dry clothing. If going indoors is not possible, get the person out of the wind, cover his or her head, and insulate the person from the cold ground. If at all possible, get the person inside to an area at room temperature and cover him or her with warm blankets.

Seek emergency medical assistance.

Monitor the person's breathing and pulse: if either has stopped or seems dangerously slow or shallow, initiate resuscitation immediately (see Cardiopulmonary Resuscitation, page 270).

In extreme cases, hemodialysis given in the same manner as for kidney failure (see page 906) is sometimes used to restore normal body temperature quickly.

Do not give the victim alcohol. Do give the person warm nonalcoholic drinks (unless he or she is vomiting). In most cases of hypothermia, warm baths are helpful for warming the person.

FROSTBITE

When exposed to very cold temperatures or cold temperatures with a low wind chill factor for a prolonged period, the skin and the underlying tissues may freeze. This condition is called frostbite. The areas most likely to be affected are the hands, feet, nose, and ears. While anyone can get frostbite given extended exposure to cold conditions, people with circulatory problems such as atherosclerosis are at greater risk (see Atherosclerosis: What Is It?, page 786).

Frostbite is distinguishable by the hard, pale, and cold quality of the skin that has been exposed to the cold for a length of time. The area is likely to have a definite lack of sensitivity to touch, although there is probably a sharp, aching pain. As the area thaws, the flesh becomes red and painful.

In severe cases, the flow of blood to the affected area actually stops and the blood vessels sustain damage. Immediate treatment is necessary if there is to be a chance of reversing the damage.

Emergency Treatment.   A person with frostbite on the extremities may also be subject to hypothermia (lowered body temperature): check for hypothermia and treat those symptoms first (see Hypothermia, page 278).

The Warming Process.   If your fingers, ears, or other areas are frostbitten, get out of the cold. Warm your hands by tucking them into your armpits; if your nose, ears, or face is frostbitten, warm the area by covering it with dry, gloved hands. If the skin tingles as it warms and there is a burning sensation, the circulation is returning. However, if numbness remains during warming, *seek professional medical care immediately.*

Do not rub the affected area. If the feet are affected, do not walk on them: allow them to dangle and wait for help to arrive.

If you are unable to get immediate emergency assistance, warm severely frostbitten hands or feet in warm—not hot—water (the water should be between 100°F and 105°F). Do not apply other heat sources (such as a heating pad) because the tissue, although desensitized because of the cold, can still be burned by temperatures that are comfortable for you to withstand under normal conditions.

Do not smoke cigarettes (nicotine causes your blood vessels to constrict and may limit circulation).

Prevention.   Wear proper clothing when in cold conditions. Upon arriving in a cold climate from a warmer one, allow your body to adjust to the change. Be sure to protect your hands, feet, nose, and ears, and avoid consuming large amounts of alcohol before and when you are exposed to prolonged cold (see also Frostbite, page 842).

NEAR DROWNING

The principal reason people drown is lack of oxygen (asphyxia). However, drowning is actually a complex process.

When a person inhales (aspirates) fresh water, red blood cells are destroyed and the blood is diluted. If this occurs, the resulting lack of oxygen also may lead to a heart arrythmia called ventricular fibrillation (see page 818). In addition, inhalation of salt water may cause damage and fluid accumulation (edema) in the lungs (see Pulmonary

Edema, page 808), and the blood becomes concentrated, which may contribute to death.

Your first and most immediate priority when trying to save the life of a drowning person is to get the person to a place where you can help him or her.

Get the Person Out of the Water. If the person is still floundering in the water and you believe you are strong enough and sufficiently well trained in swimming and water rescue to get him or her out, do so immediately. However, if you are not a swimmer or are unsure that you can manage the person by yourself, summon help.

Other options include using a throw rope attached to a buoyant object such as a life ring or life jacket. Toss it to the floundering person, then pull him or her to shore. Using a rowboat or canoe to reach the person is another option; the person can then cling to the side of the craft while you row or paddle to shore. Unless there is an access ladder, do not encourage the person to try to climb into the boat, however, because the boat might capsize and you will both be in the water.

Emergency Treatment. If the drowning person's breathing has stopped, begin mouth-to-mouth resuscitation as soon as you can safely help him or her. This means starting the breathing process even before

the person has been positioned on shore: clear the airway and deliver two quick breaths while in shallow water. Continue to breathe for the person every few seconds while moving him or her ashore.

Do not waste time trying to drain the person's lungs of water. Begin immediately to breathe for the person, hard if necessary. The air should still reach the lungs.

For step-by-step instructions on resuscitation, see Cardiopulmonary Resuscitation, page 270.

Summon emergency medical assistance. Near drowning can lead to various medical complications; thus, emergency medical care is required.

ELECTRICAL INJURY

Most of us experience minor electrical shocks now and again. They are usually more surprising than they are dangerous, because a reflex action almost instantly jerks our hands or other parts away from the source of electricity. For most of us, there is less pain from the stinging sensation than there is fear.

Under certain circumstances, however, even small amounts of electricity can be life-threatening. A substantial electrical current passing through the body can physically throw a person through the air, but even

Use a nonconducting object (such as a tree branch or wooden broom handle) to pull or push a victim of electrical shock away from the live electrical source.

lesser amounts for a sustained period can produce unconsciousness, cardiac arrest (see page 821), and a cessation of breathing. Electrical shocks also can produce serious, deep burns and tissue injury, although often even a serious electrical burn appears as only a minor mark on the skin.

Get the Person Away From the Electricity. If you find a person who you think has been electrocuted, *look first—do not touch.* He or she may still be in contact with the electrical source, so touching him or her may only pass the current through you also.

Turn off the power if the fuse box or circuit breakers are nearby; often, simply turning off the appliance itself will not stop the flow of electricity.

Move the source of the electricity away from you and the affected person. Use a nonconducting object: cardboard, plastic objects, or wood (a broom handle, for example) are best. Do not use a metal implement that will conduct the electricity and also endanger you.

Emergency Treatment. Once the victim is free of the source of electricity, check the person's breathing and pulse. If either has stopped or seems dangerously slow or shallow, initiate resuscitation immediately (see Cardiopulmonary Resuscitation, page 270).
Summon emergency medical assistance.

Treat for Shock. If the person is faint or pale or shows other signs of shock (see Recognizing and Treating Shock, page 304), lay the person down, with the head slightly lower than the trunk of his or her body and the legs elevated.

Treat any burns (see Treating Major Burns, page 267) and wait for emergency medical assistance to arrive. Remember, have a physician see any person with a significant exposure to an electrical current, even if he or she is not unconscious or lethargic, to verify that no internal injury has occurred.

SMOKE INHALATION

In addition to the risk of burns, fire presents another deadly danger: smoke inhalation. All combustion produces smoke that contains poisons. When burned, plastics and other synthetics, wood, chemicals, and other flammable materials can produce carbon monoxide and fumes that can irritate the eyes, burn the skin, and result in breathing problems when the lungs and airway are smoke-damaged.

The key symptoms of smoke inhalation usually appear in the victim's eyes and breathing pattern (the victim may gasp for breath). The eyes are likely to be irritated. Treat the eyes as you would if a foreign object were lodged there by flushing with quantities of clean water (see Foreign Bodies in the Eye, page 747). There also may be associated burns, which should be treated appropriately (see Burns, page 266).

Emergency Treatment

1. Move the victim to a smoke-free area a safe distance from the fire or source of smoke. In doing so, be careful to avoid flames and smoke. Keep as low to the floor as possible (the hot smoke rises, so the air at floor level is less toxic). If the smoke is especially dense, do not enter the area without a proper breathing apparatus, and leave the lifesaving to the professional rescue personnel.

2. Once the person is clear of the smoke, check for breathing and heartbeat; if they are not apparent, begin resuscitation (see Cardiopulmonary Resuscitation, page 270).

3. If the person is breathing, loosen any tight clothing and make the person as comfortable as possible. *Summon emergency medical assistance*—even if the person seems recovered.

4. Treat for shock (see Recognizing and Treating Shock, page 304).

CARBON MONOXIDE POISONING

A by-product of combustion is carbon monoxide. If inhaled in quantity, the carbon monoxide will take the place of oxygen in your bloodstream and reduce the supply of oxygen to your body's cells.

Typical symptoms of carbon monoxide poisoning are headache, nausea, vomiting, and confusion. Seizures and death may occur when levels of carbon monoxide in the blood become very high. One of the characteristic signs of carbon monoxide poisoning is the cherry-red color of the skin and lips.

If you wake up at night with a headache—especially if another member of your family complains of headache and is hard to arouse—get out of the house immediately. Go to a neighbor's home; also, seek emergency medical care. Inadequately vented furnaces and wood and coal stoves, among other things, can result in carbon monoxide accumulation in your home.

Emergency Treatment. Treat the person with carbon monoxide poisoning as specified for smoke inhalation on page 281. Administer oxygen as quickly as possible and transport the individual to an emergency facility.

FAINTS, SEIZURES, AND STROKES

Sudden loss of consciousness is among the most worrisome of medical emergencies. Fainting spells are generally the least serious of such events—some perfectly healthy people faint at the sight of blood, for example, only to recover completely in a matter of minutes. But all faints, seizures, and strokes must be treated as potentially serious medical emergencies. The unconscious individual should receive immediate and appropriate care.

FAINTING SPELLS

The medical term for fainting is syncope. It occurs when the supply of blood to the brain is momentarily inadequate. The person becomes pale as too little oxygen reaches the head, and consciousness is temporarily lost.

In syncope, the loss of consciousness is by definition brief: usually within a minute of lying flat, blood flow is restored and the individual who fainted is again aware of the world around him or her.

Fainting spells can occur as a result of various causes. Several medical disorders, including heart disease, severe coughing spells, and circulatory problems, can produce syncope. Some people, however, faint when they are extremely tired, when they receive news that is emotionally upsetting, or simply at the sight of blood: the heart slows, the blood vessels dilate, and blood pressure falls.

A fainting episode can have no medical significance or it can be a symptom of a serious disorder. No matter how trivial the cause, however, loss of consciousness is to be treated as a medical emergency until the symptoms are relieved and the cause is known.

Emergency Treatment. *If Lying Down.* If a fainting spell results in the person slumping to the floor, position the individual on his or her back. Be aware that people who lose consciousness frequently vomit: the airway must be watched carefully.

Check for vital signs. Is the person breathing? Position your ear over the person's mouth to listen for breathing sounds. Can you feel a pulse? It may be weak and slow, so check carefully. If breathing and heartbeat have ceased, the problem is more serious than a fainting spell and CPR must be initiated (see Cardiopulmonary Resuscitation, page 270).

Raise the legs above the level of the head. If the person is breathing, position the individual's legs on a chair or other object. This position allows gravity to increase blood flow to the brain. Loosen belts, collars, or other constrictive clothing. The person should revive quickly.

If Seated. If you feel faint or if a companion complains of faintness or dizziness while sitting, lie down. If there is not space to do so, then remain seated but position the head between the knees. This will help increase circulation to the brain. If a person faints, yet remains seated, quickly lay him or her down on the floor.

Take It Easy. After a fainting spell, the person's facial color should return to normal. Often, however, the person will continue to feel weak for a short time after fainting, so lying down quietly for a few minutes is advisable.

Check for Other Symptoms. Is chest pain present? Does the person complain of head pain? Is there apparent breathing difficulty? Does the person complain of numbness or continuing weakness? These may be signs of underlying medical problems. *Seek emergency medical assistance.*

Provide First Aid for Injuries.   If the person was injured in a fall associated with the faint, treat any bumps, bruises, or cuts appropriately (see Care of Minor Wounds, page 254).

Seek medical assistance immediately if: This is the person's first fainting spell;

The symptoms mentioned above are present on awakening;

The person has sustained an injury during the faint.

SEIZURES

Normally, the brain cells produce various coordinated electrical discharges. If, however, the electrical discharges by the brain cells become disorganized, a seizure occurs.

A seizure (also called a convulsion) is an involuntary episode of alternating muscular contractions and relaxations with loss of consciousness. Epileptic seizures are perhaps the most familiar variety of seizures, but several other disorders also can produce them. These include uremia (kidney failure, see page 907); meningitis (see page 527); toxemia of pregnancy (see page 207); withdrawal from benzodiazepines (such as Valium), barbiturates, or alcohol; or intake of certain poisons or street drugs. Rarely, a seizure may be the first manifestation of a brain tumor (see Seizures and Tics, page 541).

Emergency Treatment.   *During the Attack.*   When a seizure occurs, the principal strategy is to try to keep the person experiencing the seizure from injuring himself or herself. If possible, insert a soft pad (*not* a tongue depressor or stick) between the teeth to reduce the risk of the individual biting his or her tongue or cheeks. If vomiting occurs, try to turn the head so that the vomitus is expelled and is not aspirated into the lungs or windpipe. Frequently urine or stool will be involuntarily released during a seizure.

To reduce the risk that the individual will injure himself or herself in uncontrolled movements, clear the area around the person of furniture or other objects.

Do not try to limit the movements of a person having a seizure.

Although the person may cease breathing (and occasionally turn blue) for a part of a minute, breathing almost invariably returns without the need for CPR (see Cardiopulmonary Resuscitation, page 270).

If poisoning is suspected, attempt to determine the poison consumed. *Call for immediate medical assistance.*

In an infant or child, if the seizure seems to be the result of high fever (and your child is awake), cool the child gradually, using a dampened sponge or cool compress and tepid water. An appropriate dose of acetaminophen may be used. Do not, however, immerse the child in a cold bath (see Febrile Seizure, page 543). *Seek immediate medical assistance.*

After the Attack.   If the person has never had a seizure before, if the episode lasts more than a few minutes, or if the seizure recurs, *seek professional medical care.* Call for an ambulance.

Once the seizure is over, position the person on his or her side. This position will allow normal breathing and any vomitus or fluids to drain from the mouth and airway. Frequently, a person will have blood coming from the mouth from biting his or her tongue or cheek.

If the person injures himself or herself in a fall associated with the seizure, treat any bumps, bruises, or cuts appropriately after the seizure (see Care of Minor Wounds, page 254).

Record details of the attack for the physician. Important observations include the duration of the seizure, which extremities were involved, any apparent precipitating factors, the nature of the seizure (were the arms flailing about or was there generalized rigidity?), and any other characteristics you noticed.

STROKES

A blockage of blood flow or bleeding (hemorrhage) in the brain can result in a medical condition called a stroke. Symptoms of stroke may include:

Deterioration in vision, speech, or sensation over minutes to hours;

Sudden weakness, loss of sensation, or partial or complete paralysis in one limb or in an arm *and* a leg, with or without involvement of the face;

Acute onset of double vision, slurred speech, vertigo (a sensation of either you or your surroundings spinning), incoordination, vomiting, or swallowing difficulty;

Headache (accompanied by the above symptoms);

Abrupt loss of consciousness (not due to injury).

Seek immediate medical assistance. If you suspect you or someone else has experienced a stroke, summon emergency assistance immediately.

Emergency Treatment. While you are waiting for an emergency vehicle to arrive, you (or the person with the stroke) should lie down. Watch the person suspected of having a stroke: if breathing ceases, CPR is necessary (see Cardiopulmonary Resuscitation, page 270). Minor breathing difficulty may be alleviated by positioning the head and shoulders on a pillow. Watch for vomiting and potential aspiration of vomitus into the lungs. If vomiting occurs, turn the head to the side.

Do not allow the person to eat or drink anything. If paralysis is present, protect the paralyzed parts.

For a detailed discussion of Stroke, see page 508.

HYPERTENSIVE CRISES

High blood pressure is a common ailment—perhaps one in four Americans has high blood pressure (also known as hypertension). It is a serious but treatable ailment (see High Blood Pressure, page 796). However, a hypertensive crisis is a medical emergency.

Hypertensive crisis is extremely uncommon. It occurs when the blood pressure in your arteries rises to a dangerously high value (more than 140 mm Hg diastolic; see Normal Blood Pressure, page 797). Among the possible causes are stroke (see page 508), toxemia of pregnancy (see page 207), kidney failure (see page 906), and drug interactions. The cause also can be simpler: if a person with hypertension forgets to take his or her medication, blood pressure can become dangerously high.

In addition to a very high blood pressure, the following symptoms may indicate hypertensive crisis:

Severe headache, accompanied by confusion and blurred vision;

Chest pain;

Nausea and vomiting;

Seizures.

Emergency Treatment. If the above-listed symptoms occur, *seek emergency assistance.* While waiting for help to arrive, the person experiencing the symptoms should lie down and be encouraged to rest quietly. No food or fluids should be given.

In the event of seizures, care for the person as outlined above (see Seizures, page 283).

DIABETIC EMERGENCIES

People with diabetes may experience one or more of several different emergencies characteristic of their disorder. Among them are the insulin reaction, coma caused by ketoacidosis, and hyperosmolar coma.

For a detailed discussion of Diabetes Mellitus, see page 707.

Insulin Reaction. An insulin reaction is sometimes known as insulin shock or hypoglycemia (low blood sugar). An insulin reaction is most likely to occur in a middle-aged or younger person who is taking insulin for his or her diabetes. Some older diabetic persons also take insulin and are vulnerable to this problem. At times, an individual who is not known to have diabetes also may experience an insulin reaction.

An insulin reaction is most likely to occur several hours after eating. Exercise also can cause an insulin reaction unless the person with diabetes takes less insulin or extra food before exercising.

Symptoms vary, but they usually consist of nervousness, feelings of hunger or apprehension, confusion, cold and clammy skin with sometimes profuse perspiration, loss of consciousness, or a seizure. This progression of symptoms may take place rather quickly, usually in less than an hour. The individual may be wearing a bracelet that identifies him or her as an insulin-taking diabetic. It is also possible for a diabetic taking one of the oral hypoglycemic tablets to have a mild reaction, but this is unusual. If it occurs, usually the symptoms are less severe.

Once you recognize the problem, give the person some kind of carbohydrate or sugar. He or she may stubbornly resist taking the food because the thinking process has become affected by the low blood sugar. Fruit juices, candy, or sugar-containing carbonated drinks are effective. If the person vomits, wait a few minutes and then give small amounts of the carbohydrate cautiously. If the person is unable to cooperate in swallowing, a teaspoon or so of a syrup can be placed in the cheek at intervals of a few minutes. There often will be a period of 15 to 30 minutes from the time the sugar is administered until symptoms abate. Call a physician if recovery is not prompt. Administration of glucose in a vein or glucagon given just under the skin (subcutaneously) may be needed to reverse the symptoms.

Someone responsible should remain with the person for an hour or so after apparent recovery because full mental function sometimes does not return promptly.

Diabetic Ketoacidosis. Diabetic ketoacidosis (diabetic coma) tends to occur in middle-aged or younger persons, but older persons can also be affected. It usually is the result either of omission of or too small a dose of insulin in a person known to have insulin-dependent diabetes. In some cases, it may be the clue that leads to the identification of previously undiagnosed diabetes.

Symptoms begin more slowly than in an insulin reaction and usually will progress over several hours or days before becoming severe. Nausea, vomiting, weakness, thirst, warm and dry skin, increased rate and depth of breathing, and gradual alteration of consciousness culminating in coma are characteristic symptoms.

Treatment is directed by a physician. If you are uncertain initially whether impaired consciousness in a diabetic results from an insulin reaction or from ketoacidosis, give sugar by mouth (treat as an insulin reaction). If there is not an improvement in the person's condition, *seek immediate medical assistance.*

Hyperosmolar Coma. This condition tends to occur in older diabetic persons who do not require insulin injections. The most common sequence is an illness, such as gastroenteritis or stroke, that interferes with the person's ability to drink water or perceive thirst. The combination of the stress of the illness and the inability to consume enough water to maintain normal hydration leads to a progressive elevation of blood sugar to very high levels and a gradual loss of consciousness.

Hyperosmolar coma can be prevented by ensuring that older persons with diabetes consume generous quantities of water and by treating the precipitating illness promptly. Once consciousness is altered, this condition requires emergency evaluation.

FEVER

Fever is one of the body's reactions to infection. Although the mechanism is incompletely understood, a fever apparently plays a role in the way the body adjusts to and fights off many infectious diseases. Fever also can occur as a result of a reaction to a medication or for no apparent reason.

WHEN IS IT AN EMERGENCY?

Your body temperature normally traces a definite pattern. Low in the morning, it gradually rises during the course of the day and reaches its maximum during the late afternoon and evening. Ordinarily, body temper-

ature varies 1°F or 2°F over the course of the day, and it usually does not exceed 99°F.

Thus, the value of 98.6°F, generally considered normal body temperature, is only a general guide. Values somewhat above this are not necessarily abnormal; elevated body temperature usually does not become dangerous until it goes above 105°F to 106°F (see Heat Stress, page 277).

What Is a Fever? When fever is present, the mechanisms that control body temperature are simply set a few degrees higher. The new set point may be, for example, 102°F instead of the normal 97°F to 99°F. As fever begins, the body seeks to elevate its temper-

USING A THERMOMETER

There are three ways to take your temperature, all of which require use of a thermometer. Oral and rectal thermometers are glass tubes containing a column of mercury. The mercury expands, moving up the column in response to heat from your body.

Oral thermometers, which have a long, slender bulb at one end that contains mercury, are used for taking temperatures orally or under the armpit (axillary temperature). A rectal thermometer, which has a shorter, stubby bulb of mercury at one end, is used for taking a child's temperature from the rectum. Electronic and temperature strip thermometers are also available. When you are purchasing a thermometer, look for one that is easy to read and with degrees that are clearly marked.

Before taking a temperature, make sure that the mercury is down near the bulb. Holding the thermometer firmly, shake it with several abrupt downward flicks of your wrist. Then wash the thermometer in cold water. To read the thermometer, hold it near the light and rotate it slowly until you see the silver column of mercury.

In adults and in children older than 7, the temperature is taken orally. The bulb end of the thermometer is inserted under the tongue and the person closes his or her mouth. After 2 or 3 minutes, you can remove the thermometer and read it.

In children younger than 7, the temperature can be taken by placing an oral thermometer in the armpit and having the child cross his or her arms across the chest. After 3 minutes, remove the thermometer, read the temperature, and *add* 1°F for an accurate measurement. You also can use a rectal thermometer in young children. Insert the bulb end of the thermometer about an inch into the child's rectum, while holding the child down with your arm, if necessary. Never let go of the thermometer while it is inside your baby because one squirm may push it deeper into the rectum and cause an injury. After 2 or 3 minutes, remove the thermometer and *subtract* 1°F.

After taking someone's temperature, rinse the thermometer in cold water or alcohol.

When using a rectal thermometer to take a newborn's temperature, insert the thermometer approximately 1 inch. Never let go of the thermometer while it is in the child.

ature and you feel chilly and may shiver to generate heat. You may be more comfortable wrapped in a blanket and huddled with a heating pad: these methods will help your body gain heat and reach the new set point. Then, when the temperature reaches that new set point (for example, 102°F) you will no longer feel cold and will stop shivering and not need the blanket and heating pad.

If the cause of the fever disappears, or if you take aspirin or acetaminophen or another medication to reduce the fever, the set point will return toward the normal range and you will feel warm. You may seek cooler surroundings and have profuse perspiration, both of which tend to dissipate body heat.

What Is a Fever Emergency?   In the following situations, seek professional medical assistance.

In a Newborn.   In babies 3 months or younger, any temperature of 100.5°F is reason to *call the baby's physician immediately.*

High or Prolonged Fever.   A child with a temperature of 103°F or more must be given the emergency treatment discussed below. In an adult, *consult your physician* if you have a temperature of 101°F that persists for longer than 3 days or if your temperature is 103°F or more.

Severe Headache, Stiff Neck, Severe Swelling of the Throat, or Mental Confusion.   If any of these symptoms accompany a fever, consult your physician immediately.

Unexplained Fever.   In an adult, call your physician if you have no apparent symptoms except a temperature of 101°F that lasts more than 3 days or a low-grade fever that lasts for several weeks.

Other Symptoms.   Fever that accompanies sore throat, the aches and pains of the flu, coughing, and other symptoms suggests the presence of infection. Consult your physician and discuss your symptoms with him or her.

TREATMENT OF FEVER IN A CHILD

Dress a child with a fever in light clothing and, at most, cover with a sheet or light blanket.

Follow your physician's instructions about giving the child acetaminophen or other medication. Ordinarily, a child does not need acetaminophen for a temperature less than 102°F. A child with a temperature of 102°F to 104°F should be given an appropriate dose of acetaminophen. Do not give aspirin to a child with any unidentified or viral illness (such as influenza or chickenpox) because it can increase the risk of Reye's syndrome (see page 531).

A child with a temperature of 104°F or higher should be cooled gradually with a sponge bath of lukewarm water and be given an appropriate dose of acetaminophen. Check the child's temperature every 30 minutes; when the temperature drops below 102°F, stop the sponging. If your child has a temperature of more than 104°F, contact your physician.

If the fever does not moderate or if seizures occur, *seek immediate medical assistance* (see Febrile Seizure, page 543).

FOREIGN BODIES

Children and adults alike occasionally get foreign objects in their eyes, ears, noses, or other body orifices. You can take appropriate steps in some cases to remove the object; in other situations, the care of your physician or a visit to an emergency room is required. (If the foreign body is caught in the throat, see Choking, Breathing Emergencies, and Resuscitation, page 268.)

Foreign bodies in the vagina (such as a retained tampon), rectum, and urethra always require the evaluation and treatment of a physician. In such circumstances, *seek immediate medical attention.*

IN THE EYE

Often, the eye will clear itself of an airborne object: involuntary blinking and tearing will wash the particle out. If these natural mechanisms do not remove the foreign body, however, the eye must be treated with prompt and proper care because vision can be threatened by trauma, infection, or exposure to chemicals or particulate matter (dense smoke).

Emergency Treatment. *Clearing Someone Else's Eye.* Follow these emergency steps. (The same procedure applies if you think the object has been removed from the eye but redness and pain persist.)

1. Do not rub the eye. Wash your hands before examining the eye. Seat the person in a well-lighted area.

2. Locate the object in the eye visually: is it embedded in the eyeball? Examine the eye by gently pulling the lower lid downward and instructing the person to look upward. Reverse the procedure for the upper lid: hold the upper lid and examine the eye while the person looks downward.

If you find that the foreign object is embedded in the eyeball, cover the person's eye with a sterile pad (if available) or a clean cloth. *Do not try to remove the object.*

If the object is large and makes closing the eye difficult, cover it with a paper cup

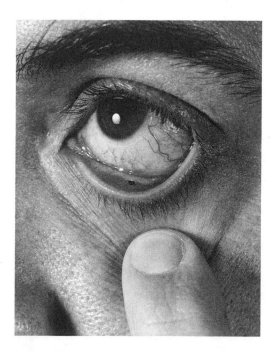

Examine the eye for foreign objects.

and tape the cup to the face and fore-head. *Seek emergency medical assist-ance immediately* (see also Trauma to the Eye, page 747).

3. If the object is floating in the tear film or surface of the eye, you may be able to flush it out or remove it manually. While holding the upper or lower lid open, use a moistened cotton swab or the corner of a clean cloth to remove the object. If you are unable to remove the object easily, cover both eyes with a soft cloth and *seek emergency medical assistance.*

4. If you do succeed in removing the object, flush the eye with an ophthalmic irrigating solution or with clean, lukewarm water.

5. If pain, vision problems, or redness persist, *seek emergency medical care.*

Clearing Your Own Eye.   The procedures outlined above are very difficult to follow when examining your own eye because involuntary blinking and tearing may make it impossible to see clearly.

If no one is nearby to help you when you get a foreign body in your eye, try to flush the eye clear. Using an eye cup or small juice glass, wash your eye with clean water. Position the glass with its rim resting on the bone at the base of your eye socket and pour the water in, keeping the eye open. If you do

To remove a small object from your eye, flush the eye with a small amount of clean water.

not succeed in clearing the eye, seek emergency medical help.

IN THE EAR

Children often insert objects into their ears; sometimes an insect or airborne object will accidentally enter the ear.

Emergency Treatment. If an object becomes lodged in the ear, follow these steps:

1. Do *not* attempt to remove the foreign object by probing with a cotton swab, matchstick, or any other tool. To do so is to risk pushing the object farther into the ear and damaging the fragile structures of the middle ear.

2. If the object is clearly visible, is pliable, and can be easily grasped with tweezers, gently remove it.

3. Try using the pull of gravity: tilt the head to the affected side. Do not strike the victim's head, but shake it gently in the direction of the ground to try to dislodge the object.

4. *If the foreign object is an insect,* tilt the person's head so that the ear with the offending insect is upward. Try to float the insect out by pouring mineral oil, olive oil, or baby oil into the ear. It should be warm but not hot. As you pour the oil, you can ease the entry of the oil by straightening the ear canal: pull the ear lobe gently backward and upward. The insect should suffocate and may float out in the oil bath. Do not use oil to remove any object other than an insect.

5. If these methods fail and the person continues to experience pain in the ear, reduced hearing, or a sensation of something lodged in the ear, *seek emergency medical assistance* (see Foreign Objects in the Ear, page 677).

IN THE NOSE

If an object becomes lodged in the nose, try the following procedures.

Emergency Treatment

1. Do *not* probe at the foreign object with a cotton swab, matchstick, or other tool.

To do so is to risk pushing the object further into the nose. Do not try to inhale the object by forcefully breathing in: in fact, you or the person with the foreign object lodged in the nose should breathe through the mouth until the object is removed.

2. Try gently blowing your nose to try to free the object. However, avoid blowing the nose hard or repeatedly.

3. If the object is clearly visible, is pliable, and can be easily grasped with tweezers, gently remove it.

4. If these methods fail, *seek emergency medical assistance.*

INHALED FOREIGN OBJECTS

When accidentally inhaled, some objects can lodge in the windpipe (trachea) or lungs (bronchial passages). If an inhaled object causes choking, the Heimlich maneuver and immediate medical intervention may be required (see Choking, Breathing Emergencies, and Resuscitation, page 268).

In some cases, however, the foreign bodies that become lodged in the trachea or a bronchial passage do not inhibit breathing—but they do constitute a hazard to the health of the inhaler. If you or your child inhales a foreign object, consult your physician.

Your physician may order an x-ray to establish the presence and location of the object. A procedure involving a bronchoscope (see Bronchoscopy, page 940) may be performed, in which a hollow tube that contains an optical system is introduced through the throat into the bronchial airways to find and remove the object from your windpipe or bronchi.

SWALLOWED FOREIGN OBJECTS

Occasionally children swallow non-food objects such as coins, pins, buttons, fruit pits, safety pins, and other household ob-

---

CHILDREN AND BUTTON BATTERIES

Increasingly, button-sized batteries are used in portable electronic equipment—cameras, pocket calculators, watches, hearing aides, and other items. To a curious young child, these shiny objects can be most intriguing. They are also most dangerous when swallowed.

These batteries contain dangerous alkali fluids; some also contain potentially life-threatening amounts of mercury. If released into the stomach or intestine, the battery fluid may eat through the lining, producing symptoms such as abdominal pain and tenderness, constipation, vomiting, and fever.

If your child swallows a button-sized battery, *seek the care of your child's physician immediately.* Surgery may be required.

Prevention
Parents and grandparents should consider this hazard in childproofing a house. Store unused batteries out of the reach of children. When disposing of exhausted batteries, do not toss them into a wastebasket that a toddler can easily explore.

---

jects. These foreign bodies usually pass through the digestive system uneventfully, but some can lodge in the esophagus. In adults, especially those who have esophageal disorders or chewing problems, there is also the risk of esophageal blockage.

If any swallowed object lodges in the throat and blocks the airway, it is a medical emergency requiring immediate intervention. The Heimlich maneuver may dislodge an offending piece of food (see The Heimlich Maneuver, page 269).

If you swallow a non-food object or if your young child seems to have difficulty with swallowing, or if he or she is spitting up saliva, especially if abdominal pain or vomiting occurs, call your physician. The object may be blocking the entrance to the stomach and may have to be removed with an endoscope, a hollow tube that contains an optical system. The endoscope may be introduced through the throat and then into the esophagus. It is used to find and remove the object from the esophagus (see also Foreign Bodies in the Esophagus, page 599).

GENITOURINARY EMERGENCIES

Medical emergencies involving the genitalia and urinary tract may produce intense pain in the groin (as occurs with testicular torsion or trauma to the penis or testicles), difficulty with urination, or inability to urinate. Sexual, violent, or abusive crimes to the genitalia constitute a medical emergency that requires appropriate and immediate care.

Pain in the flank or scrotum, especially when accompanied by blood in the urine, may be a consequence of trauma, kidney stones, or a tumor of the genitourinary system. If these symptoms occur, *seek emergency medical evaluation.*

Painful or burning urination may suggest an infection of the urethra, bladder, or kidney. If these symptoms occur or if you experience a sudden difficulty in urinating, obtain prompt medical evaluation.

SEXUAL ASSAULT AND SEXUAL ABUSE

When an act of sexual assault, violence, or abuse occurs, the physical injuries are often less significant than the emotional damage that may have been inflicted. However, if serious physical injury has been sustained, treat the injury with appropriate emergency measures (see Bleeding Emergencies, page 261; Choking, Breathing Emergencies, and Resuscitation, page 268; or Shock, page 303).

The victim of a violent crime, physical abuse, or sexual assault (forced sexual activity in which the person has not consented to the sexual act performed upon him or her) must be approached with care and consideration. Make sure the person understands that you are not going to hurt him or her. Do not ask lots of questions. Try to provide emotional support and reassurance. A child, in particular, may be distracted from the situation by talk of other matters.

Sexual crimes and crimes of abuse and violence, even if the associated physical injuries are minor, should be treated. Many major hospitals have sexual assault treatment centers and are accustomed to dealing with the legal and emotional as well as the medical manifestations of crimes of violence and abuse. Your regular physician is another option.

If you are uncertain where to go, look in the telephone book under "rape," "sexual assault," or "child abuse": there may be a special hot line with trained operators to provide advice about a physician to see as well as other help, including personal support and legal advice.

In the case of sexual assault, call for emergency assistance immediately. Do not wash or change clothing before being examined by a physician. Your physician will treat any injuries and provide psychological support. He or she also will be concerned with assembling evidence that can be used to prosecute the attacker. (For more information on sexual abuse in the preschool years, school-age years, or teenage years, see pages 114, 130, and 157.)

TESTICULAR TORSION

A sudden, severe pain in one testicle may be a condition called testicular torsion. This uncommon problem occurs when a testicle twists on its spermatic cord, cutting off the blood supply to the testicle. Testicular torsion sometimes occurs without any apparent cause, even during sleep. It also may follow strenuous physical activity.

Accompanying symptoms may include nausea and vomiting, abdominal pain, faintness, and fever. This condition is more likely to occur in teenagers around the time of puberty, but it may occur in younger and in older males. Epididymitis (see page 1115) is also a frequent cause of a painful testicle.

Emergency Treatment. *Consult your physician immediately.* Whenever you or a friend or family member experience pain in the testicles, seek immediate medical help. In cases of testicular torsion, if the testicle is not untwisted and returned to its normal position within a few hours—and often surgery may be required to do so—it will atrophy due to lack of a blood supply and will have to be removed from the scrotum.

Keep the person with testicular torsion as comfortable and still as possible while seeking professional help. For a detailed discussion of this condition, see Testicular Torsion, page 1113.

TRAUMA TO THE EXTERNAL GENITALIA

The male genital organs are not protected by being inside the abdomen, so the penis and testicles are prone to injury. The pelvis and thighs usually prevent injury to the external genitalia, but when injury does occur, it can be an intensely painful and dangerous injury.

Emergency Treatment. If the injury involves bleeding, use direct pressure to control it (see How To Stop Severe Bleeding, page 262). After bleeding has been controlled, the entire genital region should be protected with a large, triangular dressing applied like a diaper, and emergency medical assistance should be sought. When the genitalia are struck a hard blow but no bleeding results, an ice pack and firm support by a soft athletic supporter may be used to lessen severe pain in the testicles.

If the testicles have been struck by a blunt object or are injured in a fall and if the pain and swelling of the scrotum lessen within about an hour, there is probably no serious damage.

However, *seek emergency medical assistance* if the scrotum remains swollen, if it is bruised, if the pain persists, or if the penis or scrotum are seriously cut and bleeding.

If the scrotum is struck and penetrated by a sharp object, immediate emergency care is required.

INTOXICATION AND BEHAVIORAL EMERGENCIES

Intoxication, emotional difficulties, and behavioral disorders are common and require professional intervention. In the following pages we will discuss alcohol intoxication, drug intoxication, sudden personality changes, and suicidal thoughts and behavior, the most common signs of emotional and mental distress for which emergency care is appropriate.

ALCOHOL INTOXICATION

Alcohol is a drug, a central nervous system depressant with a range of effects depending on the amount consumed and the condition and metabolism of the person drinking the alcohol. Abuse of alcohol can result in short- and long-term illness, unpredictable behavior, and even death.

Recognizing Alcohol Abuse. The signs of acute alcohol intoxication range from slurred speech, uncoordinated movements, and loud and unruly behavior to vomiting, lethargy, and unconsciousness. The person may appear flushed and there may be a noticeable odor of alcohol about the person.

Recognizing Alcohol Withdrawal. When a habitual drinker suddenly ceases to drink, physical symptoms of withdrawal may occur. Delirium tremens (DTs) may result, in which the person hallucinates, acts strangely, is confused or restless, and may have a noticeable shaking of the hands (see Alcohol Withdrawal and the Dreaded DTs, page 422).

Emergency Treatment. Establish that the cause of the condition is alcohol consumption (or withdrawal): ask the person about the cause of his or her condition. Do so in a nonthreatening, calm way: you are more likely to get a candid answer to a gentle

query than if you appear to be menacing or challenging.

Look for the symptoms cited above, but also ask the person whether any medications have been taken while drinking. Mixing certain drugs, legal and illegal, and alcohol can be lethal, and such an interaction may be the cause of the symptoms.

Monitor breathing and other signs. If vomiting occurs, be sure the person does not inhale (aspirate) vomitus into the lungs. Keep the person leaning over or, if lying down, with the head turned to one side.

If the person has sustained any injuries in falls or other accidents, treat the injury to stop bleeding or immobilize fractures. Ask the person whether he or she has injuries of which you are not aware. (Remember: alcohol can be a strong painkiller, so the person may not be aware of the severity of an injury.)

Most episodes of alcohol intoxication result in little more than a few hours of nausea and a morning-after headache. However, if you observe any of the following circumstances, *seek emergency medical assistance:*

If the person is withdrawing from habitual alcohol use;

If there is no evidence of alcohol consumption but behavior is unusual;

If the person loses consciousness or aspirates vomit;

If there is evidence of both drug and alcohol consumption.

(See also Drug and Alcohol Abuse, page 1020, Alcohol- or Drug-Induced Psychosis, page 1043, and the chapter Alcohol Abuse, page 417.)

ACUTE DRUG INTOXICATION

Few drugs have no side effects; most can, in certain sensitive individuals, produce dangerous, strong reactions that require emergency medical care. Drug interactions also may produce adverse effects: that is why it is essential that you list for your physician any and all drugs you are taking and whether they were prescribed by a physician or purchased over the counter.

Legal Drugs. If on consumption of a medication you (or a friend or family member) experience severe headache, confusion, emotional instability, anxiety, vision problems, skin rashes, loss of consciousness, coma, or seizures, immediately stop taking the drug and *consult your physician or seek emergency assistance.*

Illegal Drugs. The signs of illegal drug use vary with the type of drug used. With a drug such as marijuana, the effects may be minor, and you may observe dilated pupils or redness about the eyes of the user. The person may have speech patterns that are exaggeratedly fast or slow and confused.

In the case of acute drug intoxication, however, the symptoms are likely to be more serious (see Marijuana Abuse and Dependence, page 440).

Mind-Altering Drugs. LSD and other street drugs may produce rapid pulse rate, dilated pupils, and a flushed complexion. The person may talk incoherently and "see" or "hear" things that you cannot (hallucinations). Some people experience great anxiety and fear. Paranoia, aggressive behavior, or extreme withdrawal also may occur (see pages 441 and 1049).

Uppers and Downers. The so-called uppers produce excitement, physically stimulating the body to increase the rates of heartbeat and breathing. Rapid speech, dilated pupils, perspiration, and sleeplessness also may occur. The effects of downers are the opposite, with reduced rates of heartbeat and respiration and stumbling or slurred speech patterns (see Drug Dependency, page 1046).

SUDDEN PERSONALITY CHANGES

Emotional problems, poisonings, alcohol or drug abuse, head injuries, insulin reactions, high fever, stroke, or other problems can result in various personality changes, ranging from disorientation or delirium to violent or self-destructive behavior. Intense stress can sometimes be overwhelming and result in disorganized and, at times, aggressive outbursts.

Reassure the Person

If you find yourself dealing with a person who is acting or talking in an unpredictable, bizarre, or "crazy" fashion, begin by trying to talk calmly to that person. Try to reassure him or her that you are there to help. Listen and respond gently; with eye contact and a nonthreatening manner, try to establish some kind of interaction with the person.

Safeguard the Person and Yourself

If the person has threatened suicide or harm to others, make certain the person is not armed. Do not try to deal with someone who has a weapon and has threatened to use it: the threat may be very real indeed, a danger to both you and the person. *Summon the police or other law enforcement authorities.*

Do not try to restrain a person unless you have proper training. Doing this puts you and the person you are trying to help at risk of physical harm. A person in a disturbed state turned violent can be more dangerous and stronger than you may imagine.

Seek emergency medical assistance if the person is disoriented, incoherent, or agitated or poses a danger to himself or herself or others; also seek assistance if you are

unable to communicate with the person.

While you are waiting for help to arrive, continue to try to reassure the person. Do not make jokes: humor may be misconstrued under such circumstances. Do not make threats: ask the person whether he or she is hurt or in pain or whether you can help in any way.

A person who is on a "bad trip"—regardless of whether it is the result of drug use or emotional stress—needs, for his or her own safety, to be isolated in a safe, quiet environment and accompanied by someone who will provide firm reassurance.

For guidance in dealing with these specific emergencies (each of which may be accompanied by strange behavior), see page 710 for Hypoglycemia and the Insulin Reaction, page 420 for Alcohol Intoxication, and page 293 for Suicidal Thoughts and Behavior.

Narcotics. As with downers, pulse and breathing patterns are likely to be reduced. The skin may be cool, although perspiration may be apparent. Sleepiness and even unconsciousness result from overdoses (see Street Drugs, page 441).

Emergency Treatment. *Seek emergency assistance* if you suspect a person has consumed an overdose of drugs. Emergency signs include loss of consciousness, breathing that seems dangerously slow or to have stopped (respiratory arrest), or aggressive, panicky, hostile, delusional, violent, or fearful behavior after use of a street drug.

If you believe that the overdose was taken orally within the past hour, it may be appropriate to induce vomiting (see Handling Poisoning Emergencies, page 299).

Drug Withdrawal. If a person abruptly stops the chronic use of alcohol or certain drugs, drug withdrawal may occur: the chronic alcoholic or drug abuser is in danger of seizures or delirium tremens (DTs) or even death if detoxification is not carried out in a systematic manner. Other complications may occur with cessation of the habitual use of benzodiazepines, barbiturates, heroin, morphine or other opioids, and alcohol.

Proper detoxification often requires a week or more of treatment, ideally in a hospital. *Seek emergency medical assistance* if you find someone experiencing signs of acute drug withdrawal (see Detoxification, page 1048).

SUICIDAL THOUGHTS AND BEHAVIOR

Conventional wisdom asserts that people who talk about committing suicide do not do it. Do not believe it: that old cliché simply is not true.

Recognizing the Signs. No two suicidal people are alike, but often potentially suicidal people do manifest similar behavior: withdrawal from the world around him or her, moodiness, the advent of a sudden life crisis or trauma with which the person has difficulty, an overnight personality change, a state of depression, and aggressive behavior in which respect for his or her own life and

for other lives is lacking: all these behaviors may indicate a suicidal state. (See Warning Signs of Potential Suicide, page 1040, and Teenage Suicide, page 1019).

Dealing With a Potential Suicide. If a friend or family member talks of suicide or behaves in a way that leads you to believe suicide is on his or her mind, treat the person with respect and seriousness. It is not unreasonable to ask the person if he or she is contemplating suicide.

Watch the person closely to prevent him or her from finding the opportunity. Seek professional help as soon as possible. Begin by calling your local suicide hot line or local physician, psychiatrist, or emergency room. These sources will be able to suggest where immediate help is most easily available.

Dealing With an Attempted Suicide. If you encounter a person who has attempted suicide, treat the situation as a medical emergency and get help as quickly as possible. If the person has stopped breathing, resuscitation must begin immediately (see Cardiopulmonary Resuscitation, page 270); if the person is bleeding, see How To Stop Severe Bleeding, page 262; if the person has taken an overdose of pills or poison, see Handling Poisoning Emergencies, page 299.

HYPERVENTILATION

Hyperventilation means over-breathing: too many breaths or breathing too deeply. Paradoxically, it leaves you with the sensation of not being able to get enough air.

This condition may be characterized by spasms of the hands in which the fingers are extended while the thumb and fifth finger are drawn together. The feet also have similar spasms. Hyperventilation usually stems from anxiety or panic attacks (see page 1034) and can be identified by simply observing the person's breathing.

Treatment of hyperventilation consists of reassuring the person and persuading him or her to breathe more normally. Sometimes breathing into a paper bag, so that the person is rebreathing the air from his or her lungs (the bag should expand and collapse if this is done properly), will be helpful.

PAIN EMERGENCIES

The single most common symptom reported to almost every physician is pain. "My head hurts." "It's my left leg." "It comes and goes, especially at night." In an average of one out of two office visits, the principal complaint is pain.

Pain can have many causes; consequently, there are many kinds of pain. *Chronic* (long-term) pain can be constant or intermittent; *acute* pain tends to occur suddenly, often as the result of a specific event, and may last minutes to hours. *Local* pain occurs in a relatively small, confined area of your body; *generalized* pain is spread over a larger area. When describing symptoms to your physician, identify the nature of your pain using these terms. The pain of arthritis, for example, which may endure for decades, is chronic pain; the brief but intense pain of a minor injury such as a burn, scrape, or abrasion is acute, localized pain.

In the following pages, we are concerned with distinguishing pains that signal medical emergencies. Certain chest pains, for example, may signal a life-threatening heart attack; others are the result of indigestion and are no more than a minor gastrointestinal discomfort. Because someone's life may depend on the availability of proper medical assistance in treating heart attack or some other serious medical emergency, distinguishing minor and transient discomforts from serious signs and symptoms is essential.

HEAD PAIN

We have all had a headache at one time or another. Most headaches are minor, passing discomforts that are usually forgotten after the pain has faded—and often a headache disappears almost as quickly as the discomfort arrives.

However, a headache can also be a symptom of a more dangerous and serious medical problem. Discuss with your physician any persistent headache or a headache that you would describe as "my worst ever." Some of the most common causes of head pain are discussed below.

Migraine Headache. An intense head pain, often predominantly on one side of the head and perhaps accompanied by nausea and vomiting, may be the result of a migraine headache. A migraine headache is often throbbing in character and may last from a few hours to a few days. Another common symptom of migraine headache is sparkling lights or black spots in your field of vision. You may want to avoid bright lights.

Migraine headaches can interfere with your activities and are painful, but they are not life-threatening and there is no indication that they lead to other disorders. However, if you suspect you have migraine, *seek your physician's guidance* in order to rule out other, more serious ailments. Your physician may devise a program of treatment to prevent them or to be used in the event of future episodes (see Migraine Headaches, page 549).

Meningitis. The presence of severe headache accompanied by fever, vomiting, confusion, or drowsiness, and perhaps by a stiff neck, may indicate meningitis. This dangerous disorder is an infection or inflammation in the lining that surrounds your brain tissue.

ABRUPT ONSET OF SEVERE PAIN: WHEN TO BE CONCERNED

Pain is part of your body's warning system. When you experience an intense pain, it usually means some tissues have been irritated or damaged: you may have burned yourself on the stove, or perhaps you sprained your ankle in a fall.

If you experience sudden, severe pain of no known cause that you have not had before, seek your physician's guidance. Infection or internal disease could be the cause, and it may require immediate and appropriate treatment. If the cause is known to you, it may still be appropriate to seek professional help, as is the case with an injury or discomfort after surgery.

Long-term pain from conditions such as arthritis or a back ailment may become a fact of life and something you learn to live with. Your physician may refer you to a chronic pain center for help in dealing with your pain (see Chronic Pain Centers, page 1052). However, if the nature of the pain suddenly changes, seek your primary physician's advice. For your own health and safety, do not try to "tough it out." Disregarding a serious, unfamiliar pain can put you at risk of unnecessary complications and even death. Seek prompt medical assistance.

Because long-term damage may occur if you go untreated, *seek emergency care immediately* (see Meningitis, page 527).

Cerebral or Subarachnoid Hemorrhage. Bleeding in the brain may be signaled by a range of symptoms. These include:

Sudden, severe headaches, frequently accompanied by vomiting;

Deterioration in vision, speech, or sensation over minutes to hours;

Sudden weakness or loss of sensation in one limb or in an arm *and* a leg, with or without involvement of the face;

Acute onset of double vision, slurred speech, vertigo (the sensation of either you or your surroundings spinning), incoordination, or difficulty swallowing;

Loss of consciousness shortly after onset of headache.

Summon emergency assistance immediately (see Stroke and Vascular Disorders, page 507).

Dental Abscess. If you experience persistent throbbing pain in a tooth, find chewing painful, or have sensitivity to liquids or hot or cold foods, you may have an abscessed tooth.

You also may have a slight fever and swollen neck glands and feel generally unwell; a pus-filled boil may develop on the gum near the sore tooth. At some point, this may burst, releasing foul-tasting and foul-smelling pus into your mouth and relieving the pain.

Left untreated, the pain will probably go away over time, but the infection will remain, slowly destroying the bone. If you experience these symptoms, *see your dentist immediately.*

Acute Ear Pain. If you experience pain in an ear with a sense of fullness and diminished hearing in the ear that is not due to trauma or a foreign object, the cause may be a middle ear infection (otitis media; see page 680).

Ear infections can be intensely painful. In the case of outer ear infections, called external otitis, there may be itching, hearing loss, and an oozing of yellowish, foul-smelling pus.

Infants are likely to cry often when they experience ear infections; they also may tug at their ears.

Consult your physician without delay. Ear infections are relatively easy to treat. In

---

IS IT A HEART ATTACK?

A heart attack is characterized by the following signs and symptoms:

Intense, prolonged chest pain, often described as a feeling of heavy pressure or heaviness. The pain may extend beyond your chest, radiating to your left shoulder and arm, to both arms, to your back, and even to your teeth, jaw, and neck. At times, the pain may occur in the upper abdomen and be described as akin to severe indigestion. Sometimes the pain occurs suddenly; sometimes it does not.

Nausea, vomiting, shortness of breath, and intense sweating.

Weakness, restlessness, and anxiety.

If you experience these symptoms, *summon emergency medical help immediately.*

---

most cases, permanent hearing loss is unlikely. However, consult your physician for appropriate antibiotic or other treatment.

To relieve the pain of an ear infection before seeing your physician, place a warm (not hot), moist cloth over your ear. Taking aspirin or another analgesic may also relieve the discomfort. Do not use ear drops before being evaluated by a physician.

CHEST PAIN

Pains in the chest are among the most difficult of symptoms to interpret. Simple indigestion can result in chest discomfort, especially when coupled with a growing anxiety that a heart attack might be the cause.

Chest pain can result from excessive sneezing or coughing brought on by allergies. If severe enough, the coughing can actually fracture a rib. The muscles between the ribs can become sore from prolonged coughing. Stress also can produce a tightening in the chest that resembles the pain of a heart attack.

Heart Attack. A heart attack occurs when an artery that supplies oxygen to the heart muscle becomes blocked. The heart attack may be preceded by chest pain (angina pectoris), for days or weeks, after exertion or even at rest, or it may occur in the absence of any previous pain.

During a heart attack, the heart muscle gradually dies, producing the signs and symptoms listed in Is It a Heart Attack?, page 295.

By definition, a heart attack is a medical emergency: if you think you are having a heart attack or are with someone who is, get immediate medical attention. If your companion's heart attack has caused him or her to cease breathing, resuscitation must be initiated immediately (see Cardiopulmonary Resuscitation, page 270).

Do not delay in seeking medical help: that mistake takes thousands of lives every year. If you experience symptoms that resemble those listed on page 295, telephone your physician or call an ambulance. If you think you are having a heart attack, do not try to drive to the hospital yourself.

Pulmonary Embolism.   Another medical emergency frequently signaled by chest pains is a pulmonary embolism. An embolus is a small accumulation of foreign material (usually a blood clot) that blocks an artery. Tissue death (infarction) occurs when the tissue supplied by the blocked artery is damaged by the sudden loss of blood. When a clot (usually from the pelvis or lower extremity) lodges in the lung, it is termed a pulmonary embolism.

The symptoms of a pulmonary embolism are these:

- Sudden, sharp chest pain that begins or worsens with a deep breath or a cough (pleurisy), often accompanied by shortness of breath;
- A cough that may produce blood-streaked sputum;
- Rapid heartbeat;
- Anxiety and excessive perspiration also may be accompanying symptoms.
- *Seek help immediately.* As with a suspected heart attack, seek emergency medical help immediately (see Pulmonary Embolism, page 947).

Pneumonia With Pleurisy.   The term pneumonia actually identifies a wide range of infections, each of which affects tissues of the lungs. A frequent symptom of pneumonia is chest pain (together with chills, fever, and a cough that may bring up bloody or foul-smelling sputum). When pneumonia is accompanied by an inflammation of the membranes that surround the lung (pleurisy), the accompanying chest discomfort upon inhaling may be considerable.

One sign of pleurisy is that the pain is usually relieved temporarily by holding your breath or putting pressure on the painful area of the chest; the same is not true of heart attack (see Pleurisy, page 925, and Pneumonia, page 917).

Seek your physician's care. If your chest pain is accompanied by a cough and fever or chills, consult your physician. Appropriate antibiotics and other treatment may be required.

Other Causes.   Chest pain also may be the result of other causes. For example, a dissecting aneurysm (tearing of an artery due to a weakness in its wall) that occurs in the main artery leaving the heart (the aorta) may produce severe chest pain (see Aortic Aneurysm, page 837). This is a medical emergency requiring immediate treatment.

Heartburn (esophageal pain) tends to occur more frequently when lying down or bending over. Often it is associated with an acid or sour taste in the mouth and generally can be relieved by belching or use of liquid antacids. Sometimes the pain of heartburn is confused with signs and symptoms of a heart attack.

Another form of chest pain that can cause needless worry is called a precordial catch. This is a sharp, recurring pain under the left

---

CHEST WALL PAIN

One of the most common varieties of harmless chest pain is called chest wall pain. Sometimes known as Tietze's syndrome or costochondritis, it consists of pain and tenderness in and about cartilage that connects your ribs to your sternum (breastbone).

Often, pressure over a few points along the margin of the sternum will demonstrate remarkable tenderness limited to these small areas. If your pain is duplicated by the pressure of the examining finger, you probably can conclude that a serious cause of chest pain, such as a heart attack, is not responsible.

This discomfort generally lasts only a few days. Use of aspirin or some other type of analgesic can help alleviate symptoms.

Other causes of chest wall pain include strained chest wall muscles from overuse or excessive coughing and muscle bruising from minor trauma. These pains tend to be worsened by chest wall movement and will usually resolve in several days with rest, heat, and use of aspirin or acetaminophen.

breast. Usually it is brief in duration but severe, making breathing painful.

This pain most often occurs in healthy young adults, who wonder whether it signals serious trouble. Although the cause of this common pain is unknown, it is apparently harmless.

As with other sudden, unexplained pain, all chest pain may be a signal for you to seek medical help.

ABDOMINAL AND PELVIC PAIN

For purposes of identification, the trunk of your body is divided into three main areas, the chest, abdomen, and pelvis. The chest is defined by the rib cage and contains the heart and lungs; the abdomen and pelvis contain digestive and other organs, including the stomach, large and small intestines, liver, gallbladder, pancreas, spleen, appendix, and the reproductive and sexual organs.

Given this number of organs, the potential sources for pain and medical problems are many and varied. If you experience intense, persistent pelvic or abdominal pain, *go to the emergency room or seek your physician's guidance.* The following medical emergencies may possibly be the cause of acute pains in the abdominal or pelvic area.

Perforated Peptic Ulcer. If a peptic ulcer, usually located in the lower part of the stomach or in the initial portion of the duodenum, erodes completely through the wall, it is said to have perforated.

A perforated peptic ulcer is a potentially life-threatening complication of an ulcer. The symptom is intense pain, generally in the upper abdomen. Leakage of stomach or duodenal material into the abdominal cavity may cause peritonitis (see page 642) and shock (see page 303). Emergency surgery to close the leak is usually required.

Gallstones. An intense and sudden pain on the upper right side of the abdomen that moves up to the right shoulder blade may signal gallbladder or bile duct disease. A small, stone-like accumulation of cholesterol or calcium salts, gallstones result in pain that may last for hours and be followed by general abdominal soreness. Nausea, loss of appetite, and sometimes fever and chills may be accompanying symptoms.

If you develop these symptoms, seek your physician's guidance (see Gallstones, page 661).

Pancreatitis. Intense, constant abdominal pain lasting many hours or even days may signal an attack of pancreatitis. The pain may radiate straight through to the back and chest; it may begin after the consumption of a large quantity of alcoholic beverages. Other symptoms may include fever, bulky stools that float, nausea or vomiting, clammy skin, abdominal distention, and an increase in pain on lying on your back.

Pancreatitis is an inflammation of the pancreas, the gland located just below and behind the stomach. The pancreas secretes enzymes essential to digestion in addition to the hormone insulin.

If you develop these symptoms, *seek your physician's guidance* (see Acute Pancreatitis, page 667).

Gastroenteritis. Also known as a stomach virus or flu, gastroenteritis is a common—and uncomfortable—ailment. Characteristic signs include nausea or vomiting, diarrhea, abdominal cramps, and bloating. A low-grade fever may accompany the other symptoms.

In the adult, gastroenteritis will usually last no more than about 36 hours. If the symptoms persist longer than 36 hours, consult your physician (see Gastroenteritis, page 305).

Appendicitis. A small appendage attached to the large intestine, the appendix has no known function. However, when the appendix becomes inflamed, it is a medical emergency requiring immediate treatment. The symptoms are a dull pain around the navel, gradually followed by a tenderness in the lower right side of the abdomen. Often a fever, lack of appetite, nausea, and occasionally vomiting and constipation accompany the pain.

If you suspect you or your child has appendicitis, *seek emergency medical treatment* (see Acute Appendicitis, page 624).

Diverticulitis. A severe, cramping pain, usually more severe on the left side of your abdomen, may indicate the presence of an infection or inflammation in the lower portion of your large intestine (colon).

Seek your physician's guidance if you experience such a discomfort (see Diverticulosis and Diverticulitis, page 631).

Ruptured Ectopic Pregnancy. Ectopic pregnancy (sometimes called tubal pregnancy) occurs when a fertilized egg begins to grow in the fallopian tube or someplace other than the uterus. The result is abdominal pain or cramping and, commonly, vaginal bleeding. Dizziness and the urge to urinate or have a bowel movement also may occur.

This is a potentially life-threatening condition that requires prompt surgical treatment. *Seek your physician's guidance immediately* (see Ectopic Pregnancy, page 202).

Ovarian Cysts. Most ovarian cysts are minor problems that present only minor discomfort and difficulty. In occasional instances, however, sudden, severe pain may occur in the abdomen, accompanied by fever and even vomiting. Consult your physician if such pains and symptoms occur (see Ovarian Cysts and Benign Tumors, page 1105).

Kidney and Ureteral Stones. If you experience flank pain on urination, blood in the urine, or a severe pain that moves downward from the flank to the groin, vulva, or testicle, you may have a stone in your kidney or ureteral tube. This intensely painful kidney condition usually is resolved when the stone is passed into your bladder or out of your body (sometimes there are several stones).

If you develop these symptoms, *seek your physician's guidance* (see Kidney Stones, page 898).

Cystitis. Painful urination, a frequent need to urinate, blood in the urine, a sensation of not being able to empty your bladder, and lower abdominal pain may indicate cystitis (an inflammation of the bladder). *Consult your physician:* this problem usually can be treated routinely, but it should be properly diagnosed to be sure that no other underlying cause is present (see Cystitis, page 1119).

Pyelonephritis. If the symptoms of cystitis are accompanied by pain in the flank and fever, an infection may be present that involves the kidney and ureter as well as the bladder. Symptoms may be accompanied by severe chills, followed by high fever and even shock (see page 303). Severe pyelonephritis often is associated with an extension of the infection from the kidney into the bloodstream (septicemia).

Consult your physician (see Acute Pyelonephritis, page 892). Hospital admission and administration of antibiotics and fluids through a vein may be required.

PAIN IN THE EXTREMITIES

Sudden, unexplained pain in the arms, legs, hands, and feet may be indications of medical problems requiring treatment. Among the potential causes are the following conditions.

Acute Arterial Occlusion. Sudden and severe pain accompanied by paleness and coldness in an arm or leg may indicate the presence of a blocked (occluded) artery.

The blockage commonly is the result of

ACUTE JOINT PAIN

Gout
If you experience a sharp, intense pain in a single joint that is not the result of a blow or other injury, you might have gout. Gout most often strikes the so-called bunion joint at the base of the big toe.

A type of arthritis, gout also produces swelling and redness in the painful joint. Although gout pain usually will disappear of its own accord over a period of days, *consult your physician.* He or she may prescribe medications to relieve your discomfort and to help prevent future occurrences (see Gout, page 1003).

Joint Infections
Pain and stiffness in one joint, typically a knee, shoulder, hip, ankle, elbow, finger, or wrist, accompanied by the warmth and redness of inflammation and perhaps chills, fever, and weakness, may mean a joint infection. This can be the result of a recent wound in which the infecting agent entered your tissues, or there may be no evident cause. *Contact your physician or visit your emergency room immediately* (see Infectious Arthritis, page 1002).

Other Possible Causes
Joint soreness after a period of exercise may result from several causes (see Runner's Knee, page 964, Acute Painful Shoulder, page 1004, and Bursitis, page 1006); but any intense, continuing pain in a joint is cause for consulting your physician.

atherosclerosis (see page 786), with a clot (embolism) of fragments of atherosclerotic plaques lodging where a major artery divides into two smaller ones. This most often occurs at the level of the knee. Because diabetes seems to accelerate the process of atherosclerosis, diabetic persons are more vulnerable.

Because of the risk of gangrene (see page 835) and the possible need for amputation, *seek emergency care immediately.* Protect the leg from both cold and heat. Wrap it in soft cloths or sheeting while getting the affected individual to the hospital (see page 835).

Thrombophlebitis. When a blood clot occurs in a deep vein in an extremity (usually a leg), there may be tenderness, pain, and swelling in the thigh or calf. Fever also may be present.

Because of the risk of pulmonary embolism (should the clot break loose and travel to the lung) and other complications, *seek emergency medical assistance* (see Thrombophlebitis, page 838).

POISONING EMERGENCIES

Any substance that is swallowed, breathed in, injected, or absorbed by the body and that interferes with the body's normal functioning is, by definition, a poison. Some poisons are familiar: pesticides, animal poisons, and cleaning and other household chemicals bearing printed warnings are obvious examples.

In fact, however, almost any non-food substance is poisonous if taken in large doses. Aspirin is a case in point: this useful medication is found in most homes and is ordinarily safe. Yet each year more children die of aspirin overdoses than from overdoses of any of the more familiar poisons.

Be aware of poisons in and around your home. Take steps to protect young children from toxic substances (see Preventing Poisonings, page 301). Keep the number of the Poison Control Center near your telephone (see page 300). Know the procedures to follow in case of a poisoning emergency.

Be familiar with plants in your home, yard, and vicinity: keep your children informed too (see Garden-Variety Poisonous Plants, page 302). If you are concerned that industrial poisons might be polluting nearby land or water, report your concerns to your local health department or to the state or federal Environmental Protection Agency.

HANDLING POISONING EMERGENCIES

Recognize the Problem. The poisoning may be obvious: there's no denying the child seated on the floor, surrounded by aspirin tablets, some of which are half-chewed in his or her mouth. Alternatively, some guesswork may be involved. Look for these signs if you suspect a poisoning emergency:

Burns or redness around the mouth and lips—they can result from drinking certain poisons;

Breath that smells like chemicals (perhaps gasoline or paint thinner);

Burns, stains, and odors on the person, his or her clothing, or on the furniture, floor, rugs, or other objects in the area in which the person was playing or working;

Difficulty breathing, vomiting, or other unexpected medical symptoms.

Note, however, that many conditions mimic the symptoms of poisoning, including seizures, alcohol intoxication, stroke, and insulin reaction. If you can find no indication of poisoning, do not treat the victim for poisoning. However, *summon emergency assistance.* Meanwhile, make the person as comfortable as possible. Treat for shock (see Recognizing and Treating Shock, page 304) or begin resuscitation if breathing slows or ceases (see Cardiopulmonary Resuscitation, page 270).

Emergency Treatment. If you conclude that a poison has been consumed, take the following steps:

1. Give the person a glass of water or milk to drink. The liquid will slow the rate at which the poison is absorbed by the body. However, if the person is very weak, lethargic, unconscious, or having

seizures, do not force the liquid on him or her.

2. Call your local poison control center. In most communities, the number is listed on the inside cover of the telephone book (see Poison Center Resources, below). If it is not, find the number and write it down near or on your telephone *before* you need it.

The person who answers will ask, in brief, the following questions.

What happened? "I came back inside and found Johnny with a bottle of laundry detergent. He had some of the blue fluid on his lips and was crying."

Who are you? "My name is Jane Doe. I'm Johnny's mother."

Where are you? "I'm calling from 555-5555. The address is 111 Anywhere Lane, Middletown."

Who is the victim? "Johnny is my son. He is 4 years old."

Is he conscious? Has he vomited? "He's crying, but he's okay, I think. He's not vomiting or unconscious."

What was the poison? "It was this de-

tergent. Here, I'll read you the label . . . ."

You will be asked other questions too, such as *How much was consumed?* and *What have you done so far?* and *When did this happen?*

3. Do not hang up. After consulting reference materials, the person will tell you what to do.

4. Should you induce vomiting? Certain poisons should be vomited up; others, such as petroleum products, acids, and alkalis, should not (see Acids and Alkalis, page 301). If you *do not* know the identity of the substance swallowed, *do not* induce vomiting.

If you are told to induce vomiting in the person who has swallowed poison, follow these instructions. Insert a finger into the person's mouth and touch the back of the throat (it may be easier for the poisoned person to do this himself or herself if he or she is old enough). Another technique is to use a glass of warm water containing 3 teaspoons of salt or 1 spoonful of dried mustard. If you have syrup of ipecac at hand (and every household with children should), use it. Ipecac is an emetic (an agent that causes vomiting) that can be used to eliminate poison from the stomach.

Whether vomiting is induced or occurs naturally, make sure that the person does not inhale (aspirate) the vomitus into the lungs. A small child can be held over your knees, face down. A larger person should bend way over or lie down, hanging the head off the side of a bed. In any case, the chin should be held lower than the level of the hips.

After the person has vomited, give additional milk or water.

5. Monitor vital signs. Be alert for changes in the person who has been poisoned. If breathing stops, CPR must be performed (see Cardiopulmonary Resuscitation, page 270). Treat for shock (see Recognizing and Treating Shock, page 304).

6. If the poison has spilled on the person's clothing, skin, or eyes, remove the clothing and flush the skin or eyes with water. You may need to hold the person's eyelids open while flushing.

7. Go to an emergency room immediately. If you are unable to transport the poisoned person, summon an ambulance. Be sure to take the container or packag-

POISON CENTER RESOURCES

A poison control center is not a hospital or treatment center—it is essentially a library staffed by persons familiar with poisonings. The information it can offer may be crucial to delivering prompt and proper treatment in a poisoning emergency.

In an Emergency
In a poisoning emergency, call the Poison Control Center in your area. The telephone number is usually listed inside the front cover of the white pages of the telephone directory; call the operator if you are unable to find it. Post it on or near the telephone *before* you have to use it.

Poison Control Centers operate 24 hours a day. They

need to know circumstances—who you are, who the poisoned person is, his or her condition, your location, and, most importantly, exactly what was swallowed.

Have the Substance at Hand
When you call, have the poison that has been consumed at hand. In order to analyze the poison and recommend treatment, the control center will need to know the name of the substance or product and any chemical description found on the label.

Poison Control Centers often are associated with large hospitals or emergency rooms. Each meets the standards for reference material and staff established by the American Association of Poison Control Centers.

PREVENTING POISONINGS

Small children are at special risk of poisoning: their curiosity is boundless and their bodies are small enough that relatively little poison can be harmful. Also, most small children put whatever they find into their mouths.

Keep Poisons Out of Reach

Seemingly innocent products such as shoe polish, nail polish, and nail polish remover can be hazardous. Make it a rule in your home that all hazardous items are to be kept in high cupboards, on tall shelves in closets, or in locked cabinets. Designate such an area in your kitchen or utility room for household cleaners, another in your garage for garden or automotive poisons, and another in your bathroom. Garden sheds, cellars, and other areas where such goods are stored require similar precautions.

Household Goods

Here is a sampling of common, potentially dangerous household poisons: alcohol of all kinds; virtually all cleaning products, especially those that contain chlorine bleach, ammonia, and detergents; toilet and drain cleaners (the latter often contain lye); cosmetics; paint and paint products such as turpentine and paint thinner; and furniture and floor polishes.

Garden and Garage Aids

Many of us use chemicals to control pests in or around our homes. Roach powders, rat pellets, rose dust, and other home, yard, and farm chemicals are common and, when used as directed, quite safe. However, when swallowed, virtually all are dangerous poisons, as are fuels and oils (including gasoline and kerosine); weed killers; flower, garden, and shrub sprays; and roach, rat, and other poisons.

Medications

Aspirin, acetaminophen, prescription medications, cough medicine, cold pills, and all other drugs can also pose a danger.

Label All Poisons

Label all poisons. If you store any poison in a container other than the one in which it was originally packaged, be sure to label the can or bottle clearly: the word "POISON" should be prominently printed. Never use baby food bottles or other familiar food containers to store poisons. Young children are likely to assume they contain food and may help themselves.

ACIDS AND ALKALIS

In high school chemistry, we learned that acids turn litmus paper red and that alkalis turn litmus paper blue. The chemical distinction between acid and base (alkali) is fundamental: in chemical interactions, the acids give up hydrogen ions and alkalis accept hydrogen ions.

Acids and alkalis are identified by their pH values, in a range from zero to 14. Acidity is expressed in pH values, weakest to strongest, by numbers that range from less than 7 to zero; alkalinity increases from 7 to 14. A substance is neutral—that is, neither acid nor base—at 7.

Many substances we eat and drink are slightly acid or base, as are our body fluids: urine from a healthy person typically is slightly acidic (pH 6), and blood is alkaline (pH 7.4). Gastric juices are very acidic (pH 1.5), and bile and pancreatic juice are alkaline (pH 7.5 and 8.5, respectively). Common acids include the innocent vitamin C (ascorbic acid) to hazardous hydrochloric acid and others. Ashes are high in alkalinity, as is bicarbonate of soda.

Acid and Alkali Poisons

Highly acidic and highly alkaline substances are, when swallowed or exposed to our skin or eyes, poisonous. Acids produce pain and corrosion of the tissues with which they come into contact. Difficulty in swallowing, nausea, intense thirst, shock, difficulty in breathing, and death can result from acid that is taken internally. The effect of alkalis varies, but the symptoms are similar—pain in the mouth, throat, and stomach as the alkalis damage the tissues of the gastrointestinal tract.

Emergency Treatment

Treat acid and alkali poisonings as you would any poisoning emergency: give the person fluids to drink, and call the Poison Control Center for specific instructions. However, do *not* induce vomiting.

ing in which the poison was stored with you. If the identity of the poison is unknown but the person has vomited, take a sample of the vomitus for analysis.

MEDICATIONS AS POISONS

Lifesaving medications also can be killers: overdoses of seemingly harmless medications such as the common painkillers aspirin and acetaminophen take many lives each year. Numerous other over-the-counter drugs are dangerous if taken in large doses, especially by a child or elderly person. Prominent on the list are sleeping medications, antihistamines, and vitamin supplements.

Follow the Instructions. Children are not the only ones at risk: anyone who fails to obey dosage instructions is in danger of overdose. *Read the label carefully; follow the instructions given there, or given by your physician.* If you are taking numerous medications daily, extra care and record keeping may be necessary (see The Hazards of Multiple-Drug Use, page 1231).

Prevention Is Best. Keep all your prescription and nonprescription drugs stored out of the reach of children. Do not take them for granted and absentmindedly leave them available to a toddler on a kitchen counter, bedside table, or pocketbook. Buy childproof packages. If you have medications that must be refrigerated, put them on a high shelf out of the reach of children. If medications are placed in drawers, lock them or install a latch that only an adult can use.

Drug Allergies. Some people have allergic reactions to medications: even a proper dosage taken at the recommendation of your physician can, in a sensitive person, produce hives, facial swelling, wheezing and difficulty breathing, various rashes, itching, and even shock. These reactions are not common, but *consult your physician immediately* if you suspect a drug allergy (see also Drug Allergies, page 471).

Emergency Treatment. If a child or adult takes too much of an appropriate or any of an inappropriate medication, give the person a glass of water or milk to drink and call the Poison Control Center (see Handling Poisoning Emergencies, page 299).

POISONOUS PLANTS

Many attractive plants—both cultivated and wild—are potentially poisonous if swallowed. Be aware of plants in your home, garden, and neighborhood. Instruct your children never to eat unfamiliar berries and plants.

Emergency Treatment. If you or your child consumes a poisonous plant, among the symptoms that may occur are a burning

---

GARDEN-VARIETY POISONOUS PLANTS

Plants are essential sources of food—but many are also poisonous. Did you know that apple seeds, potato vines, and tomato leaves are poisonous?

Do Not Eat Any Unfamiliar Plant
Beware of unidentified berries: they may be poisonous. Most mushrooms are edible and, to some people, great delicacies; but some are deadly. Do not experiment with the unknown in the woods, and do not encourage your children to do so either.

Be Careful at Home
Lilies of the valley make lovely borders—but they are poisonous, as are daffodil bulbs in the garden, buttercups in the field, the jack-in-the-pulpit on the forest floor, and the holly (berries) and poinsettia in your house at Christmas. Do not eat what you do not know about.

Skin Reactions
Certain poisonous plants, including poison ivy, poison oak, and poison sumac, produce an itchy rash and blisters in sensitive people after contact with the resin of such plants (see Skin Allergies, page 457).

Amanita mushroom

Common Plants To Avoid

Name	Poisonous Parts
Cherry	Pits
English ivy	Entire plant
Holly	Leaves and berries
Jimsonweed (also known as thorn apple)	Entire plant
Lily of the valley	Entire plant
Mistletoe	Berries
Mushrooms (especially amanita)	Entire plant
Potatoes	Sprouts, roots, and vines
Rhododendron	Entire plant
Rhubarb	Leaves

pain in the mouth and throat; swelling in the throat that may lead to difficulty in breathing; vomiting, abdominal pain, or other gastrointestinal distress; and hallucinations, seizures, and unconsciousness.

Seek emergency assistance. With a sample of the plant on hand, call your local Poison Control Center for instructions (see Handling Poisoning Emergencies, page 299).

FOOD POISONING

Food poisoning can cause various ailments, often distinguishable by the types of poison consumed. Among them are the following.

Gastroenteritis. Unwashed or improperly handled food of almost any sort, raw fish or meats, or contaminated water can lead to food poisoning. A good example is the potato salad left unrefrigerated for too long at the family picnic.

If you become ill after eating such food, your physician probably will call the condition gastroenteritis. Typically, within 1 to 6 hours of consuming food or water contaminated with staphylococcal bacteria, abdominal cramps and pain, diarrhea, and vomiting occur. The symptoms usually are gone in about 12 hours (see Gastroenteritis, page 305).

Botulism. Botulism is a potentially fatal food poisoning. It results from the ingestion of a toxin formed by certain spores in food. Botulism toxin is most often found in home-canned foods.

Symptoms usually begin 12 to 36 hours after eating the contaminated food; they may include headache, blurred vision, muscle weakness, and eventually paralysis. Some people also have nausea and vomiting, constipation, urinary retention, and reduced salivation. These symptoms require

---

HERBS AND HERB MEDICINE

Long before the founding of modern medicine, early health-care practitioners prescribed herbs and herb extracts. Some of these medicines worked—to this day, in fact, the valuable heart drug digitalis is extracted from the foxglove plant.

Most of the early remedies, however, have since been proved to have dangerous side effects. Some can kill, induce violent vomiting or seizures, or cause liver or other organ damage. Many are simply of no value.

Consult Your Physician
Never try to brew or mix your own herb remedies. Be suspicious of herbalists' claims for their wares. Before you take any herb medications, consult your physician.

---

immediate medical attention; a person with botulism needs to be hospitalized (see Botulism, page 534).

FOOD ALLERGIES

Some people are allergic to certain foods. After consumption of a food to which the person is allergic, symptoms such as abdominal pain, diarrhea, nausea or vomiting, hives, swelling of the lips, eyes, face, tongue, and throat, and nasal or respiratory congestion may occur.

For most people, food allergies are uncomfortable, often extremely so. Responses vary from minor sniffles and a cough to abdominal cramps, vomiting, and even (rarely) anaphylaxis (see Anaphylaxis, page 307). When a person reacts severely with an anaphylactic response—narrowed air passageways, rapid pulse, fall in blood pressure, cardiovascular collapse, and shock—food allergies can be life-threatening. In such cases, *summon emergency treatment immediately* (see also Food Allergies, page 469).

SHOCK

The name itself only vaguely suggests the nature of the problem—only rarely does shock result from an electrical current. In fact, a wide range of incidents or problems can cause it. Shock is a common complication of injury, infection, burns, and other conditions. It is *not* a consequence of emotional stress such as the sudden death of a loved one.

Shock is a condition in which there is a slowing or diminution of the flow of blood around your body (peripheral circulation).

This produces a decrease in your blood pressure and an inadequate volume of red blood cells. The result: the supply of oxygen to tissues falls below normal amounts. This decrease may produce various symptoms (see below).

Seek emergency assistance if you recognize the signs of shock. Shock is a medical

RECOGNIZING AND TREATING SHOCK

The following symptoms indicate the presence of shock in an ill or injured person:

Skin: it may appear pale or gray, and it is cool and clammy to the touch.

Pulse and breathing: the heartbeat is weak and rapid and is accompanied by a shallow, hurried breathing pattern. Blood pressure is reduced, perhaps below measurable values.

Eyes: the eyes are lusterless, staring, perhaps with dilated pupils.

Alteration of consciousness: the shock victim may be unconscious, but even if still awake he or she is likely to be faint, confused, or weak. Sometimes a person in shock becomes anxious and excited.

The person must be treated for shock immediately. *Summon professional emergency assistance:* this is a medical emergency.

Treatment
Serious injury, especially one that involves considerable blood loss, is likely to be accompanied by shock. Immediate first aid treatment for shock is essential. Even if a person who has been hurt seems alert and in control, treat him or her for shock.

Get the Person To Lie Down
Lay the person down, face upward, with the head below the level of the feet. This position will help maintain blood flow to the brain and may relieve symptoms of faintness. Elevating the feet on a chair, cushions, or another avail-able prop is usually the easiest means to establish this position. However, if the person has sustained an injury in which raising the legs will cause him or her pain, leave the person flat on his or her back.

Keep movement to a minimum.

Keep the Person Warm and Comfortable
Loosen tight collars, belts, or constricting clothing. Cover the person with a blanket if the air is cold; if the ground is cold, put the blanket beneath the victim. If it is hot outside, position the person in the shade if possible, on top of a blanket or coat or other material. Even if the person complains of thirst, do not give him or her anything to drink.

If the Person Is Vomiting or Bleeding From the Mouth
Position the person on his or her side. This position will help prevent choking or inhaling (aspirating) the vomitus or blood and make the person more comfortable.

Treat Injuries Appropriately
If an injury has occurred, stop any bleeding (see Bleeding Emergencies, page 261), immobilize any fracture (see Fractures, page 308, and Sprains, page 310), or take other appropriate first aid steps. Handle potential spinal injuries with special caution (see also page 309). The pain from a fracture that is not immobilized can worsen shock.

Get Hospital Care as Soon as Possible
Shock in each of its forms is potentially life-threatening. Care by medical professionals with appropriate equipment is essential. *Summon emergency medical assistance immediately.*

Keep the shock victim warm. Elevate legs and feet above the level of the heart to maximize flow of blood to the head.

emergency that requires appropriate and immediate care. You can take certain simple steps to help alleviate the symptoms, but summon professional medical help immediately.

THE KINDS OF SHOCK

Shock—insufficient blood flow and oxygen deficiency for normal functioning—can result from serious bleeding injuries (see Loss of Blood, below), major trauma, or dehydration resulting from losses of fluids due to vomiting or diarrhea (see below). This type is called *hypovolemic shock* because it results from too little blood volume (*hypo* comes from the Greek word for below; thus, below-volume shock).

Cardiogenic shock results when the heart does not pump effectively. Causes may include heart attack or heart arrhythmias (see page 817).

When blood vessel size or tension is affected, *vasogenic shock* (*vaso* for blood vessel) can result. Causes include insect and bee stings (see Anaphylaxis, page 307) or infection (see Septic Shock, page 306, and Toxic Shock Syndrome, page 307).

LOSS OF BLOOD

Excessive loss of blood can produce hypovolemic shock, in which the volume of blood falls below *(hypo)* a healthy amount. A traumatic injury can result in shock, whether the bleeding is external (as with a severe cut) or internal, as with a fractured pelvis or from the rupture of an internal organ or vessel. Bleeding (hemorrhage) due to a lesion in the gastrointestinal tract or heavy vaginal bleeding also can result in hypovolemic shock.

The symptoms will resemble those for other kinds of shock (see Shock, page 303). The skin will be pale and cool and clammy to the touch. The heartbeat will be weak and rapid, accompanied by a shallow, hurried breathing pattern, and blood pressure may have fallen below a measurable level. The person may be anxious and restless and complain of thirst. The skin at the knees and elbows may be mottled.

Emergency Treatment. *Seek immediate emergency care.* Hypovolemic shock can

be fatal, and emergency medical care must be initiated. Summon help immediately. When the emergency medical team arrives, oxygen may be administered, along with intravenous fluid replacement. Specially designed (shock) trousers, which divert blood from lower extremities to vital organs, may be applied.

While waiting for help to arrive, reassure the victim and make him or her as comfortable as possible. Treat as for other sorts of shock (see Recognizing and Treating Shock, page 304). If he or she stops breathing, perform resuscitation (see Cardiopulmonary Resuscitation, page 270).

DEHYDRATION

When the body's supply of fluids falls below certain amounts, hypovolemic shock may result. The loss of fluids usually will be known because the person will be aware of persistent vomiting, diarrhea, or loss of fluid through the urine. The other symptoms are similar to those for other kinds of shock (see Recognizing and Treating Shock, page 304).

The skin will be pale and cool and clammy to the touch. The heartbeat is weak and rapid, accompanied by a shallow, hurried breathing pattern, and blood pressure may have fallen below measurable levels. The person may be anxious and restless and complain of thirst. The skin at the knees and elbows may be mottled.

Emergency Treatment. *Seek immediate emergency care.* Hypovolemic shock can be fatal, and emergency medical care must be initiated. If the person stops breathing, initiate mouth-to-mouth resuscitation (see Cardiopulmonary Resuscitation, page 270).

Potential Causes. Some of the ailments that can result in extreme fluid losses and hypovolemic shock are discussed below.

Gastroenteritis. Gastroenteritis is an infection or inflammation of the gastrointestinal tract. It is frequently called stomach or intestinal flu, and it is usually caused by a virus or bacterium that irritates the lining of the intestine.

These common infections usually last no more than 36 hours. Particularly in children and the elderly, however, the severe loss of fluids that can result from gastroenteritis can produce hypovolemic shock. In such cases, *seek your physician's guidance* (see Infections of the Gastrointestinal Tract, page 617.)

All of the following ailments are to be regarded as medical emergencies. (See also Diabetic Ketoacidosis, page 285.) Seek emergency care immediately if you suspect that you or a member of your family suffers from any of them.

Cholera. This acute infection results from the consumption of water or foods contaminated by human wastes infected with the cholera bacterium. Vomiting and severe diarrhea are the major symptoms of cholera and can result in dehydration, hypovolemic shock, and death.

Addisonian Crisis. When the adrenal gland fails to produce the quantities of the steroid hormones your body needs for normal functioning, the disorder is termed Addison's disease. When the shortage of hormones becomes acute, adrenal failure (addisonian crisis) can occur.

There is loss of salt through the urine, and this leads to hypovolemic shock. Fortunately, this syndrome is rare. It may be suspected if the person looks deeply tanned without having been exposed to sunlight (see Addison's Disease, page 720).

Excessive Use of Diuretics. Among the most commonly prescribed drugs, diuretic medications stimulate your body to increase the rate and volume of urination and the loss of salt and potassium in the urine. Used in treating many ailments (including hypertension, certain liver disorders, and heart failure), they are valuable, often lifesaving medications.

However, you must monitor use of diuretics carefully. Overmedication combined with zealous adherence to a low-salt diet can result in fluid depletion. In extreme cases, shock can result.

HEART-RELATED SHOCK

Certain cardiac events and disorders can result in a decrease of blood flow. Heart-related shock occurs when the supply of blood to the tissues falls below certain levels due to inadequate pumping strength of the heart.

This condition is also called cardiogenic (or cardiac) shock.

Heart attack (myocardial infarction; see Heart Attack, page 809), heart failure (see page 807), heart arrhythmias (see page 817), or cardiac tamponade (see Pericarditis, page 832) can result in your heart's inability to pump sufficient blood to supply the cells of your body with enough oxygen for normal functioning. Shock can result.

The symptoms will resemble those for other kinds of shock (see Recognizing and Treating Shock, page 304). The skin will be pale and cool and clammy. The heartbeat is weak and rapid and is accompanied by a shallow, hurried breathing pattern, and the blood pressure may have fallen below measurable levels.

Emergency Treatment. *Seek immediate emergency care.* Cardiac shock is often fatal, so initiate emergency medical care immediately. When the emergency medical team arrives, oxygen may be administered, along with medication to control chest pain, if present.

While waiting for help to arrive, reassure the affected person. Make him or her as comfortable as possible. Treat as for other sorts of shock (see Recognizing and Treating Shock, page 304). If he or she stops breathing, initiate resuscitation (see Cardiopulmonary Resuscitation, page 270).

SEPTIC SHOCK

If an infection enters the bloodstream and circulates around your body, your body fights back. The unwanted bacteria are killed, but substances called endotoxins are also released.

The presence of endotoxins in your bloodstream can produce symptoms, which may include reddened, flushed skin that is warm to the touch, chills and fever, rapid heartbeat, and shallow breathing. Typically, these symptoms last from 30 minutes to a few hours and then give way to cool, clammy skin, a drop in blood pressure, extreme thirst, shortness of breath, and even respiratory failure. In many cases, an infection such as a kidney infection is known to the person before septic shock results: it is the spread of that infection to the bloodstream that produces septic shock.

Emergency Treatment. *Seek immediate emergency assistance.* Septic shock is a life-threatening emergency requiring a range of medical care. Summon professional help, and while waiting for an ambulance to arrive, keep the person lying down, warm and comfortable (see Recognizing and Treating Shock, page 304).

Medical professionals may administer oxygen, intravenous fluid therapy, antibiotics, and perhaps other drugs to fight the infection. The blood may be cultured before antibiotics are given so that the nature of the problem can be identified.

ANAPHYLAXIS

Anaphylaxis is a severe allergic reaction. Certain people react more strongly than others to certain allergens, and the introduction of the allergen into their systems can produce anaphylactic shock.

Anaphylaxis most often is experienced by people who have a history of allergies. It is to be suspected if symptoms develop within minutes after the person is bitten or stung by a bee or insect, has ingested a causative food, or begins taking a new medication. There are also other possible causes, but they typically occur while the person is under the immediate care of a physician. In sensitive individuals, these causes include the introduction into the body of certain vaccines, anesthetic agents, or the dyes used in certain diagnostic tests. A blood transfusion occasionally can produce anaphylactic shock.

The usual symptoms of anaphylactic shock are the following:

The skin is warm to the touch. There is also a notable redness to the skin (erythema), perhaps over much of the body in raised blotches (hives).

The person usually wheezes and has difficulty breathing.

Accompanying symptoms may include nausea, vomiting, abdominal cramps, increased pulse rate, and a sudden drop in blood pressure.

Without prompt and proper treatment, loss of consciousness and, eventually, death can result.

Death from anaphylactic shock is most commonly due to severe breathing difficulty. Swelling of tissues in the throat may result in the airway becoming blocked.

Emergency Treatment. *Seek emergency medical assistance immediately.* Summon emergency medical assistance or rush the person to an emergency room. If the person stops breathing, perform mouth-to-mouth resuscitation (see Cardiopulmonary Resuscitation, page 270).

If the cause was a bee sting, remove the stinger if it is still attached to the site of the sting. Apply an ice pack or a cold, moist cloth.

Prevention. If you or a member of your family have severe allergic (anaphylactic) reactions to stings, keep a properly equipped emergency kit available. Your family physician can advise you on its contents, but it may include epinephrine (adrenaline), to be administered with a hypodermic needle in case of an anaphylactic emergency.

Be careful when bees are around. Wear long-sleeved shirts and trousers. Avoid bright colors. Do not wear perfumes or colognes. If a bee hovers nearby, *do not panic.* Move away slowly and avoid wildly slapping at the bee or other insect (see Anaphylaxis, page 474).

TOXIC SHOCK SYNDROME

Toxic shock syndrome is a rare but dangerous disorder associated with the use of tampons, especially by women younger than 30. Typical symptoms may include a sudden fever of 102°F or higher; vomiting or diarrhea; dizziness, weakness, fainting, or disorientation; and a rash resembling a sunburn, which may appear even on your palms and the soles of your feet.

Summon emergency help immediately. If you or another female member of your family experiences the preceding symptoms, especially if they occur during menstruation and tampons are being used, summon emergency help. (Even before you call, remove the tampon.) Tell the physician what the symptoms are, how long they have been apparent, and when menstrual bleeding began.

Toxic shock syndrome can cause blood pressure to plummet, resulting in a state of shock (see Recognizing and Treating Shock, page 304, and Toxic Shock Syndrome, page 1061).

TRAUMA EMERGENCIES

A trauma wound is an injury sustained as a result of external force or violence. A broken bone, a severe blow to the head, a knocked-out tooth—all are trauma emergencies.

Fractures are among the most common trauma emergencies. A fracture is, simply, a broken bone; it results when the forces exerted on the bone are greater than the bone can withstand. The term sprain is frequently used to identify a wide range of injuries, but a true sprain involves damage to the ligaments that connect the bones.

Fractures, severe sprains, dislocations, and other serious bone and joint injuries usually require professional medical care: you risk permanent disability, deformity, and, in the case of skull, neck, and spinal injuries, even death if proper care is not given promptly. Likewise, eye injuries, tooth avulsion, and head trauma must be given appropriate emergency treatment. Each of these emergencies is discussed in the pages that follow.

In the case of blunt trauma to the chest or abdomen (as may occur in an automobile accident), *seek emergency medical attention.* Internal injuries can be sustained in such accidents, and even in the absence of apparent bleeding, life-threatening complications can result.

In all instances of trauma emergencies, the principal objective is to seek immediate medical assistance and to get to an emergency medical facility as quickly as possible.

FIRST AID FOR FRACTURES

If you suspect a fracture, the proper approach is to protect the affected area from further damage. Do not try to set the broken bone: reduction (the medical term for the process of setting the bone) is to be left to a physician.

Emergency Treatment. *Immobilize the Area.* Before the person with the broken bone is transported to a hospital, the bone should be splinted to prevent movement. Keep joints above and below the fracture immobilized. A splint will stabilize the damaged parts and prevent unwanted movement of the parts that could aggravate tissue damage. Proper splinting may reduce pain.

Splinting depends on the location of the break (see Limb Fractures, below, Spinal Injuries, page 309, Hip or Pelvic Fracture, page 310, and Other Broken Bones, page 310).

Stop the Bleeding. If the broken bone is a compound fracture (that is, the broken bone protrudes through the skin) or there is other bleeding associated with the injury, apply pressure to stop the bleeding.

The site of the fracture should be elevated. (For example, a broken arm can be held up, over the level of the heart, in order to reduce blood flow.)

Put pressure directly on the wound with a sterile bandage, clean cloth, or even a piece of clothing. If nothing else is available, use your hand. Maintain pressure until the bleeding stops (see How To Stop Severe Bleeding, page 262).

Treat for Shock. If the person is faint, pale, or breathing in a notably shallow, hurried fashion, treat the person for shock. Lay the person down, with head slightly lower than trunk and legs elevated (see Recognizing and Treating Shock, page 304).

Limb Fractures. If the fracture occurred in the hand, wrist, arm, thigh, or lower leg, a

If professional help is unavailable, immobilize an upper arm fracture with splint and sling.

Left, **A rolled newspaper or magazine can serve as an effective temporary splint for a fracture of the lower arm.** *Right,* **A simple sling can effectively immobilize an injured elbow.**

rigid splint should be used. Apply the splint after bleeding (if any) has been stopped, the wound has been bandaged, and the victim has been treated for shock.

Splints can be made of wood, plastic, metal, or other rigid material. Pad the splint with gauze, then apply it to the limb. The splint should be longer than the bone it is splinting and extend below and above the injury.

Pad the splint wherever possible. Pads make the splint more comfortable and help keep the bones straight.

Fasten the splint to the limb with gauze or strips of cloth, string, or other material. Start wrapping from the extremity and work toward the body. Splint the limb firmly to prevent motion but not so tightly that blood flow is stopped.

Arm Fractures. Rolled magazines or newspapers can be tied around a broken lower arm.

A sling over the shoulder and band around the sling can help keep an elbow still.

Leg Fractures. If a lower leg is broken, place the entire leg between two splints. If no splints are available, the healthy leg can be used as a splint to limit movement of the broken one.

A broken thighbone requires that the hip joint also be immobilized.

Spinal Injuries. If you suspect a spinal injury (back or neck), *do not move the af-*

fected person. Permanent paralysis and other serious complications can result from moving a person with a spinal injury.

Assume the person has sustained such an injury if:

There is evidence of a head injury;

There is severe pain in the neck or back;

An injury exerted substantial force on the back;

The person complains of weakness, numbness, or paralysis or lack of control of the limbs, bladder, or bowel;

The neck or back is twisted or positioned oddly.

Summon emergency assistance immediately. Keep the victim still: do not try to move the person unless he or she is choking or in immediate danger.

A leg splint can effectively immobilize a fracture of the lower leg.

Fracture of a thigh-bone requires splinting of the trunk and lower leg.

If the person must be moved, gently reposition him or her on a rigid board (a tabletop or door will do). Make sure the neck is stabilized: use a heavy towel or scarf, pocketbook, or other soft, bulky material to prevent the head from rotating while the person is being moved. Get several people to help, and make sure that the person's neck, head, and spine are held firmly in alignment.

Neck and back injuries require special precautions. If professional help is unavailable and the victim must be moved, recruit several people to help. Neck and back injuries can lead to permanent paralysis; therefore, special precautions are required. Proper use of a back board immobilizes the victim's head, neck, and spine. (See Spinal Injuries, page 309.)

Hip or Pelvic Fracture.   Hip or pelvic fractures usually occur as a result of falls or accidents, but in some elderly people whose bones have thinned from osteoporosis (see page 982), such breaks can occur spontaneously.

Suspect a broken pelvis or hip if the person complains of:

Pain in the hip, lower back, or groin area;

Pain in these areas that worsens with movement of the leg.

As with a spinal injury, do not try to move the victim. *Summon emergency medical assistance immediately.*

If the person must be moved, immobilize him or her on a board or tabletop as for a spinal injury (see Spinal Injuries, page 309). Do not attempt to straighten an injured leg or hip that seems oddly positioned.

Other Broken Bones.   In the case of broken bones in the fingers, toes, rib cage, or face, splinting is not usually necessary. Stop the bleeding and treat the victim for shock (see Recognizing and Treating Shock, page 304), then seek emergency treatment.

SPRAINS

A sprain occurs when trauma such as a violent twist or stretch causes the joint to move outside its normal range of movement and ligaments are torn. The usual indications of a sprain are the following:

Pain and tenderness in the affected area;

Rapid swelling, sometimes accompanied by discoloration of the skin;

Impaired joint function.

Emergency Treatment.   For most minor sprains, you can probably treat the injury

RECOGNIZING FRACTURES

A fracture usually occurs as a result of a fall, blow, or other traumatic event. Obvious signs may include:

Swelling or bruising over a bone;

Deformity of the affected limb;

Localized pain that is intensified when the affected area is moved or pressure is put on it;

Loss of function in the area of the injury;

A broken bone that has poked through adjacent soft tissues and is sticking out of the skin.

In identifying types of fractures, your physician will use the following terms:

Simple fracture: A fracture in which the broken bone does not protrude through the skin.

Compound fracture: The broken bone protrudes from the skin. This may allow entry of bacteria from the environment, which increases the risk of infection.

Complete fracture: Fracture in which the bone snaps into two or more parts.

Incomplete fracture: The break is limited to a crack (the bone is not separated into two parts).

Impacted fracture: One fragment of bone is embedded into another fragment of bone.

Pathological fracture: A bone break in a person with bones weakened by disease. Bone cancer (see page 988) or a bone disorder such as osteoporosis (see page 982) can result in weakened bones that fracture spontaneously or when only minor stresses are exerted on them. Such breaks are termed pathological fractures because a principal cause is an underlying disease.

Regardless of type, treat all suspected fractures with proper first aid (see page 308), then consult a physician (see also Fractures, page 955), who may x-ray the bone to evaluate the extent of the injury.

Compound **Simple** **Greenstick** **Transverse** **Oblique** **Comminuted**

yourself. The combination treatment approach is termed P.R.I.C.E., for protection, rest, ice, compression, and elevation. Here are the steps.

Protection. Immobilize the affected area to encourage healing and to protect it from further injury. Use elastic wraps, slings, splints, crutches, or canes as necessary.

Rest. Avoid activities that cause pain or swelling; rest is essential to promote tissue healing.

Ice. Apply ice immediately to decrease swelling, pain, and muscle spasm. Ice packs, ice massage, or slush baths are all useful applications. Reapply the ice periodically for the first day or two.

Compound fractures break through the skin; simple fractures do not.

Compression. Swelling can result in loss of motion in an injured joint, so compress the injury until the swelling has ceased. Wraps or compressive (Ace) bandages are best.

Elevation. Raise the swollen arm or leg joint above the level of your heart to reduce swelling. This is especially important at night.

Serious Sprains. If an audible popping sound and immediate difficulty in using the joint accompany the injury, seek emergency medical care. If you suspect bone or serious ligament damage in the joint or if the pain and difficulty in moving the joint do not recede within 2 or 3 days, *seek professional medical care.* Your physician may order an x-ray to look for a fracture (see Sprains, page 960).

DISLOCATIONS

A dislocation is an injury in which the ends of bones are forced from their normal positions. In most cases, it is a blow, fall, or other trauma that causes the dislocation, although in some cases an underlying disease such as rheumatoid arthritis, a congenital weakness, or a joint weakened by previous dislocations can be the cause.

The usual indications are as follows:

An injured joint that is visibly out of position, misshapen, and difficult to move;

Swelling and intense pain.

Emergency Treatment. Have a physician examine and x-ray any suspected dislocation as soon as possible. In the case of a suspected neck or back injury, however, do not move the injured person (see Spinal Injuries, page 309).

The dislocation should be treated as quickly as possible: if it is not treated within half an hour, the swelling and pain are usually such that treatment without an anesthetic is more difficult. However, *do not* try to return the joint to its proper place unless you have had training in how to do it. Further damage can result from improper attempts at joint manipulation (see page 957).

Splint the affected joint in its fixed position; treat it as you would a fracture (see Limb Fractures, page 308). *Seek immediate medical attention.*

TRAUMATIC AMPUTATION

An amputation is the removal, usually by surgery, of a limb, part, or even organ. When an amputation occurs as the result of injury, as when a finger, toe, or larger body part is severed, it is an emergency requiring immediate medical attention. There are various attendant risks, including loss of blood, shock, and the risk of infection.

Emergency Treatment. *Stop the Bleeding.* The first goal of emergency treatment is to stop blood loss. If the amputation involves a small amount of tissue (a fingertip, for example), it may be sufficient to apply pressure on the wound with a sterile bandage, clean cloth, or a piece of clothing. When the bleeding is under control, wrap the wound with additional layers and bandage.

Treat the Victim for Shock. The victim should be lying down, if possible, with his or her head lower than the heart and the area of the severed part elevated slightly (see Recognizing and Treating Shock, page 304).

If the Bleeding Continues. If a hand, foot, leg, or arm has been amputated, the bleeding may be difficult to stop. First, apply pressure to the artery that feeds the area (see How To Stop Severe Bleeding, page 262). If that fails, a tourniquet may be necessary.

Applying a Tourniquet. This is a last resort because tissue damage may result that will make reattaching the amputated part difficult or impossible. Wrap a necktie or other piece of cloth around the tissue immediately above—but not touching—the wound. It must be long enough to wrap around the area twice with enough material left for a knot. Tie a half knot first, then place a screwdriver, stick, dowel, or a similar object on top of the knot and tie the second half. Twist the screwdriver to tighten the tourniquet.

Tighten the cloth only as much as is required to stop the flow of blood. Note the time at which you applied the tourniquet.

Tie the tool in place with the cloth once bleeding has stopped.

Treat Other Injuries.   Once you have the bleeding at the site of the amputation under control, examine the person for other signs of injury that require emergency treatment. Treat fractures, additional cuts, and other injuries appropriately.

Seek Immediate Emergency Assistance. Once the bleeding has stopped and you have made the person as comfortable as possible, get emergency medical care immediately.

Save the Severed Part.   Once the amputation victim is stable and you have requested emergency assistance, carefully seal the amputated part in a clean plastic bag (if one is not available, wrap it in a clean cloth). If ice is at hand, put the bag with the part in it inside a second bag containing ice. Avoid putting the ice in direct contact with the amputated part. Do not use dry ice. If ice is not available, use very cold water.

Remarkable advances have been made in recent years in reattaching fingers, hands, and even severed limbs. The results depend on many factors, but if you pay proper attention to caring for the severed body part and

a qualified surgeon is readily available, the chances are good that a reattachment is possible (see Absence or Loss of a Limb, page 969).

HEAD TRAUMA

Most head injuries are minor: the skull provides the brain with considerable protection from injury. Only about 10 percent of all head injuries require hospitalization, and simple cuts and bruises can be treated with basic first aid techniques (see Care of Minor Wounds, page 254). However, *seek emergency medical care* if any of the following symptoms are apparent:

Severe head or facial bleeding.

Change in level of consciousness—if the injured person is confused, lethargic, or experiences even temporary loss of consciousness as a result of a head injury. Even if the person regains consciousness quickly, emergency care should be sought.

Cessation of breathing—if the person stops breathing or if no pulse is found, CPR is essential (see Cardiopulmonary Resuscitation, page 270).

In all cases of worrisome head injury, do not move the neck because it may have been injured. Among the potential complications of a head injury are concussion, intracranial hematoma, and a skull fracture.

If all other methods to stop bleeding fail, apply and tighten a tourniquet. (See Applying a Tourniquet, page 312.)

Concussion. When the head sustains a hard blow as the result of being struck or from a fall or other cause, a concussion may result. The impact creates a sudden movement of the brain within the skull.

Usually a concussion involves a loss of consciousness, either temporary or for a longer time. Amnesia (loss of memory), dizziness, and vomiting also may occur. Partial paralysis and shock are other possible symptoms.

During the 24 hours after the injury, headache, vomiting, increased pulse rate, and anxiety may occur. A concussion requires immediate emergency monitoring and care (see Concussion, page 535).

Intracranial Hematoma. An intracranial hematoma occurs when a blood vessel (either an artery or a vein) ruptures between the skull and the brain. Blood then leaks between the brain and the skull and forms a blood clot (hematoma) that compresses the brain tissue. Symptoms occur from a few hours to several weeks or more after a blow to the head.

Intracranial hemorrhage is caused by injury to the head, often as a result of automobile or motorcycle accidents. There may be no open wound, bruise, or other outward sign.

In intracranial hematoma, pressure on the brain mounts, producing such symptoms as headache, nausea, vomiting, alteration of consciousness, and pupils of unequal size. As more and more blood floods into the narrow space between brain and skull, there is progressive lethargy, unconsciousness, and death if the condition is not treated. Immediate emergency care is required (see Extradural Hemorrhage, page 515, and Subdural Hemorrhage, page 511).

Skull Fracture. When trauma to the head results in skull fracture, the injury may be apparent, as when bleeding or bone fragments are seen. However, if any of the following signs are apparent, there may also be a skull fracture:

Bruising or discoloring behind the ear or around the eyes;

Blood or clear, watery fluids leaking from the ears or nose;

Unequal size of pupils;

Deformity of the skull, including swelling or depressions.

A skull fracture is a medical emergency and must be treated to help avoid potential permanent brain damage and even death.

Emergency Treatment. If a concussion, intracranial hematoma, or skull fracture is suspected, *summon immediate emergency assistance.* Keep the person who sustained the injury lying down and quiet in a darkened room, with head and shoulders slightly elevated, perhaps on a pillow or blanket.

Observe the person for vital signs: if he or she stops breathing, CPR is essential (see Cardiopulmonary Resuscitation, page 270).

Stop any bleeding with a gauze band or clean cloth (see Bleeding Emergencies, page 261).

EYE EMERGENCIES

There are several common eye injuries and ailments. The following are those that you are most likely to encounter, and appropriate emergency treatments are described for each.

Corneal Abrasions. The cornea is the clear membrane at the center of your eye that functions to refract light from the front of your eye to the retina at the rear of your eye, where visual images are transmitted to your brain. The cornea is easily injured—a speck of sand or even a contact lens worn for too long can scratch (abrade) its fragile tissues. This injury also can result from prolonged exposure to bright light outdoors or in a tanning booth.

Instantaneous pain at the moment of the injury and the persistent pain and redness that follow are the key symptoms of a corneal abrasion (although in occasional cases the pain develops over a period of hours).

If eye pain persists after cleansing the eye to remove any foreign object (see Foreign Bodies in the Eyes, page 747), close your eye and cover it with soft gauze or an eye patch. *Seek emergency medical care* to be sure that the foreign body has been removed and that no serious abrasion requiring surgery or other treatment has occurred.

Blood in the Eye. Blood visible in the front chamber of the eye is a condition called hyphema (see page 749). It can result from a blow to the eye, an injury that perforates the eye, or certain medical conditions.

In most cases, the bleeding, whatever its cause, is completely absorbed within a few days. However, a more serious eye injury may be apparent. *Seek the care of an ophthalmologist or see your personal physician.*

Eyelid Laceration. If the eyelid is cut or damaged, loosely apply clean gauze to the eye. Do *not* apply pressure. *Seek emergency medical care* for the person with the injury.

Retinal Detachment. Your retina is a thin, transparent membrane located in the back of your eye. The retina contains cells (rods and cones) that are sensitive to light. It is attached to a layer of tiny blood vessels that provide oxygen and necessary nutrients.

If the retina separates from the layer of blood vessels, the condition is termed retinal detachment. There is no pain associated with the condition, but symptoms may include sensations of lights flashing and of many tiny floating objects in the eye. Vision may be blurred or double, and there often seems to be a shadow over a portion of your field of vision.

Retinal detachment is a medical emergency requiring immediate treatment in order to avoid permanent vision loss or damage. *Seek emergency ophthalmic care.* It is unnecessary to cover the affected eye unless the visual disturbance is uncomfortable (see also Retinal Detachment, page 772).

Central Retinal Artery Occlusion. When one or more of the blood vessels that serve the retina become blocked, you may experience a sudden blurring or loss of vision in a portion or all of the visual field of one eye only.

If you experience acute blurring of vision or partial blindness, *seek emergency medical care.* Contact your ophthalmologist or personal physician or go to a local emergency room immediately (see also Retinal Vessel Occlusion, page 774).

Acute Glaucoma. The symptoms of acute glaucoma are a red, painful eye, blurred vision, and often the appearance of halos around lights. It occurs when the pressure of the fluids inside the eye becomes too great.

This is a medical emergency requiring *immediate medical care.* Contact your ophthalmologist immediately (see also Glaucoma, page 765).

Orbital Cellulitis. An infection of the eye socket, orbital cellulitis may produce pain in the affected eye, decreased vision, fever, swelling of the eyelid, and a general malaise.

If your eye becomes swollen and painful or there is pain with movement of the eye, this is a medical emergency requiring that you *seek immediate medical care.* Contact your ophthalmologist or personal physician immediately (see also Orbital Cellulitis, page 761).

Acute Iritis. An inflammation of the iris, iritis and its associated disorder uveitis can result in redness of the eye, blurred vision, and a sensitivity to light.

Seek emergency medical care (see also Uveitis and Iritis, page 760).

Acute Conjunctivitis. Often referred to as pinkeye, conjunctivitis is an inflammation of the transparent membrane (the conjunctiva) that lines the eyelids and the eyeball up to the margin of the cornea. It is usually caused by a virus.

A highly contagious disorder common in children, its symptoms include redness, itching, and a gritty feeling about the eyes. There also may be a discharge in the eye that forms a crust (matting) during sleep. Blurred vision and sensitivity to light also may result.

In most cases, conjunctivitis is irritating but harmless to your vision. However, because it is extremely infectious, take special steps to prevent conjunctivitis from being communicated to others. Avoid sharing eating utensils. Wash your hands thoroughly and often (see also Conjunctivitis, page 759).

Emergency Treatment. If you have redness and matting of your eyes and you suspect pinkeye, irrigate several times daily with artificial tears, which you can purchase without a prescription. This may relieve the symptoms, which generally last less than 5 to 7 days. You can place a cool compress (washcloth) over the closed eyelids to help relieve any itching or swelling.

If your symptoms do not improve or if you have difficulty with vision, seek medical attention. Rarely, conjunctivitis may be due to bacteria, which may respond to specific treatment. If the conjunctivitis occurs in an eye with a contact lens, see an ophthalmologist immediately.

TOOTH AVULSION

When a tooth is accidentally knocked out (avulsion), it is an event requiring appropriate emergency medical care, whether a child or an adult is involved. Today, permanent teeth that are knocked out sometimes can be reimplanted, but only if you act quickly. A broken tooth, however, cannot be reimplanted.

Emergency Treatment. If a permanent tooth is knocked out, save the tooth and consult your dentist immediately. If it is after office hours, call your dentist at home. If he or she is unavailable, go to the nearest hospital.

Successful reimplantation depends on several factors: prompt reinsertion (within 30 minutes if possible; no longer than 2 hours after avulsion) and proper storage and transportation of the tooth. Keeping it moist is essential.

Here is what to do if a tooth is knocked out:

1. Handle the tooth by the crown only.
2. Do not rub it or scrape it to remove dirt.
3. Gently rinse the tooth in tap water, but not under the faucet.
4. Try to replace the tooth in the socket and bite down gently on gauze or a moistened tea bag to help keep it in place.
5. If the tooth cannot be replaced in the socket, immediately place it in milk, your own saliva, or a warm, mild salt water solution.

CHAPTER 10
SAFETY

CHAPTER CONTENTS

THE SAFER WAY

Today, a great deal of time, money, research, and personal effort is being invested in prevention of disease. Perhaps you, like millions of others, are increasingly conscious of improving your diet, getting proper exercise, and using other methods to help ensure the continued good health of you and your family.

All too often, however, we overlook the more obvious risks that confront us daily. Nearly 1 in every 20 deaths in the United States results from accidents. Accidents are the most common cause of death in persons under age 35. Half of all childhood deaths are due to accidents. On the highway, in the workplace, and at home, accidents injure or disable tens of millions of Americans annually.

Many of these accidents could be avoided. In the following pages, we offer various safety tips. This information is not comprehensive, but it may alert you to other potentially dangerous circumstances in your everyday life and during leisure activities.

HOME, SAFE HOME

Every year, tens of thousands of Americans die of injuries sustained in their own homes. Fire is a leading cause.

Most fires in homes result from carelessness and can be prevented with a few simple precautions and a little common sense. Here are guidelines to follow in trying to decrease the risks of personal injury and property damage from fires in your home.

Install Smoke Detectors. Smoke detectors are relatively new and invaluable safety devices. Every home should be equipped with them. Locate your smoke detectors on the ceiling between the sleeping areas of your home and the areas where fires are most likely to start (the kitchen or garage). Have a detector on each floor and in each bedroom area of your home.

Place the smoke detector at least 6 inches from where the wall joins the ceiling (the dead air space in a corner could prevent smoke from reaching the detector immediately). Keep the detector away from shower areas because steam can set a detector off.

Keep a Fire Extinguisher on Hand. Have a fire extinguisher and fire blanket in the kitchen; if you have a garage, have another set there, too. Be sure family members are familiar with the operation of the extinguishers.

Establish Escape Routes. Be sure there are alternative escape routes from every room; if needed, purchase fire ladders or other means of escaping from upstairs windows. Rehearse with your family procedures to follow in the event of fire.

Keep stairways and halls uncluttered. Never padlock an exit door.

Beware of Wood and Coal Stoves and Other Space Heaters. Be sure that the area around an open-flame space heater in your home is properly fireproofed. Building codes vary, but for most space heaters the walls around them must be a specified distance away from the stove, or insulated with a fireproof material. The floor beneath and, if the stove opens from the front, in front, also must be insulated with a nonflammable material (see Keep Fireplaces and Chimneys Clean, page 319.)

Keep kerosene or other free-standing heaters out of frequently used traffic paths in your home and away from hallways and stairways in particular. Many fires are started when such heaters are knocked over, spilling fuel and igniting nearby furniture and surfaces.

Maintain Electrical Equipment. Make sure that the wiring in your home is up-to-date and in good order. If it is not, hire a qualified electrician to make the necessary repairs.

Do not overload wall outlets with adapters. Never increase the size of a fuse or circuit breaker as a means to sustain service of a line that is overloaded. If you do not increase the capacity of the wire in the line itself, it could heat up and start an electrical fire in the walls of your home.

Do not run extension cords across floors or under rugs or carpets. You can easily trip over exposed extension cords (especially at night). Over time, the wear and tear on a cord beneath a carpet can damage the insulation and lead to overheating and a fire hazard.

Keep Fireplaces and Chimneys Clean. Use a screen in front of your fireplace to prevent sparks from jumping out of the firebox. Never leave an open fire unattended.

Clean your chimney regularly. If you vent a woodstove into your chimney, clean the chimney twice a year. If a wood fire in your fireplace is only an occasional event, an every-other-year chimney cleaning may be sufficient. If you use your fireplace or wood-burning stove at all, however, have your chimney inspected for a buildup of creosote (a flammable resin that is a by-product of wood fires). Be sure that the chimney lining is intact. Do not postpone chimney repairs.

Never Smoke in Bed. Careless smoking leads to the greatest number of deaths by fire in the United States. Keep cigarettes, cigars, or pipes out of your bedroom. When disposing of butts and ashes, be sure no embers remain.

Remove Flammable Materials. Store newspapers, other paper refuse, and any flammable trash away from heat sources. Locate paints and other household chemicals on a shelf that is both out of reach of little hands and away from any risk of exposure to sparks or heat.

Dispose of rags or papers contaminated with paint remover or other chemicals immediately; spontaneous combustion can occur, producing dangerous fumes and fire.

CHILD-PROOFING YOUR HOME

Accidents are the leading cause of death among children. Indeed, about one of every two children who die does so because of an accident.

Making your home safe for youngsters is an important priority, whether your child is very young and has no sense of danger or

---

BEWARE OF FIREWORKS

The brilliant illumination and resounding bangs and pops of fireworks provide thrills and excitement for young and old. But to avoid being an injury statistic, take care when using fireworks. Remember, one of every three fire-related injuries is caused by fireworks.

The Risks
When stored in your home, fireworks are a potential fire hazard. When put to use, they are even more dangerous. The potential risks include vision and hearing loss (about 1,000 people annually sustain permanent eye injuries from fireworks). Fingers and hands are often burned by carelessly used fireworks, which ignite at temperatures up to 1,000°F. Hearing loss is a common fireworks-related injury.

Preventing Problems
The first and most important advice we can give is this: be familiar with and obey laws that govern the purchase and use of fireworks in your state.

Second: supervise your child if he or she is using fireworks. Never expect any child to read and follow safety instructions.

Use fireworks outdoors only, and in an open area. Stay a discrete distance from them after they are lit. Locate fireworks on level ground.

Allow no horseplay. These devices are especially dangerous if tossed at a person or pet.

Never relight a dud. Douse it with water and discard it. Do not explode fireworks in a bottle, tin can, or clay pot, and never tamper with or disassemble fireworks.

Have a pail of water or hose on hand to douse the fireworks area when you're finished.

---

old enough to experiment deliberately with the hazards of your home.

Protecting Your Baby. Today, beds for babies must meet federal standards. Space between crib bars can be no more than 2⅜ inches. This prevents infants from getting their heads stuck between the bars. If you are using an old crib, make certain that the bars are spaced in accordance with these specifications.

The crib should have no sharp edges. A locking mechanism should keep the sides up. The distance from the top of the rail to the mattress should be at least 26 inches when the mattress is at its lowest level. The mattress should fit snugly. Use bumper pads to prevent your baby from banging against the sides. A pillow is unnecessary and should not be used.

One potential danger of an old crib is that it may be painted with a lead-based paint.

Infants sometimes chew the slats of their cribs and, if consumed, lead-based paint is poisonous.

Keep plastic bags away from your infant. Young children can suffocate while playing with such bags.

Select blankets and pajamas that are fireproof.

If there is a mobile over the crib, make sure that it is firmly secured and positioned well above the crib. If your child can reach the mobile, remove the mobile.

Toys in the crib should be large and soft, with no sharp edges that can hurt your baby. Avoid stuffed animals or other toys with buttons or parts that can be swallowed.

Remember that every moment of the day, *you* are your child's protector. Be alert for hazards until your child learns safety rules (see Safety, page 74).

When Your Child Begins To Crawl. Before your baby reaches 6 months of age, child-proof your home. This gives you a chance to practice safety measures before your child becomes mobile. Protect your infant not only from risks within immediate reach but also from hazards to which your baby might crawl. Remember that almost overnight, your child's universe will expand from a crib, baby seat, and playpen to the entire house (see Safety, page 74).

Place gates at the tops and bottoms of staircases in your home. Make sure to lock or guard windows that may be accessible to your child. If your child is under age 6, he or she should not be in the top bunk of a bunk bed. Make sure your bunk bed has sturdy safety rails.

Electrical outlets are often a target of curiosity, so cover unused ones; inexpensive plug covers are available at most hardware stores.

Young children are forever experimenting, putting into their mouths whatever comes to hand. Keep substances that can hurt children (such as cleaning solutions, insecticides, and medications) stored well out of their reach. You may need to buy fixtures that make it difficult for a child to open lower cabinets.

Never store toxic substances in the "wrong" container. For example, if you store paint thinner in a juice bottle, your child may take a drink, thinking it is juice.

Identify toxic plants in and around your home. Keep them well out of reach of your baby (see Garden-Variety Poisonous Plants, page 302).

Keep matches out of your child's reach. In the kitchen, keep pot handles pointed toward the back of the stove. Do not use cloths or mats that your child can pull off the kitchen or dining room tables. Never leave a hot beverage near the edge of a table. Your child might pull the beverage off. Do not drink hot beverages with your child on your lap.

Keep the thermostat on your hot-water heater between 120°F and 125°F. At 160°F, a child can quickly scald himself or herself.

In the bathroom, keep toilet seats covered. Use no-slip tub mats. Never leave your infant unattended in the bathtub, no matter how little water is present.

At Play. In laying out an outdoor play area for your child, locate it so that you can monitor activities from inside your home. Position equipment on grass, wood chips, sand, or other soft surfaces to reduce the risk of injury from inevitable falls. Anchor the equipment below the ground to prevent it from tipping.

Make sure that the equipment is safe and in good condition. Plane or sand rough wood to prevent slivers; file metal burrs smooth to avoid scrapes. Discard equipment that is fragile or worn out.

Establish rules: one person on the swing at a time; hold on with both hands; no standing or kneeling allowed.

At the playground—whether it is a public facility or in your backyard—supervise your young child's activity constantly.

HOUSEHOLD SAFETY: A CHECKLIST

There is no such thing as an accident-free home. Accidents happen even to the most conscientious and careful people. However, you can decrease your risk of accident and injury at home. Here are some suggestions.

The Kitchen. Clean up spills promptly. Water, foods, or other substances on a hard-surfaced floor can cause slips, falls, and injury.

Use a step stool to reach high shelves; do not stand on a chair or countertop.

Keep your kitchen knives stored out of the reach of children, perhaps on a wall rack.

When using them, hold the food you are cutting with your hand curled, not with your fingers extended.

Position pot and pan handles toward the back of the stove or counter. If they protrude over the front, a careless movement or a curious child could spill hot liquids or foods and cause burns. Always use a potholder or insulated gloves when handling heated pots, pans, trays, or other food containers.

Be careful to keep grease and drippings away from open flames. Keep curtains away from the stove.

In case of a small kitchen fire, use salt or baking soda to extinguish the flames. Do not throw water on them. Keep a fire extinguisher on hand for more serious fires.

Unplug appliances that are not in use; in particular irons, toasters, and food processors. Before inserting tools into a toaster, be sure it is unplugged. Before washing or cleaning any electrical device, unplug it.

Iron clothes on a well-balanced, sturdy surface covered with a fireproof material. Never leave a hot iron unattended.

Never leave small children alone in your kitchen.

Keep matches out of reach.

Store cleaning fluids and other chemicals in a high or locked cabinet.

Make it a habit to keep drawers and cupboards closed.

Be sure that all poisons are safely stored and clearly marked.

The Living Room. If you have a fireplace, use a fire screen to prevent sparks from flying into the room.

Make sure no electrical cords cross the room. They can trip you or, if worn, can cause a fire.

If you have a humidifier to moisten the air in your home, wash the water reservoir thoroughly on a regular schedule (at least once every 2 weeks during the heating season and when it is emptied for the summer). Bacteria and fungi can grow in such moist environments and create a health hazard for you and your family. Fungicide tablets are available to help prevent this.

The Bathrooms. Never turn electrical switches on or off while you are in the bathtub or shower or standing on a damp floor. Do not use electrical appliances such as hair dryers or electric shavers when you are wet or in the shower or bathtub. Electrical shock or death from electrocution can result. Change all conventional bathroom outlets to ground-fault outlets. Building codes in many states require them in new construction.

Use nonslip mats in and adjacent to the shower or bathtub to prevent slips and falls. Grab rails also can prevent falls.

Never leave your baby or young child alone in the tub. He or she can drown in only a small amount of water.

Install a night-light in or adjacent to the bathroom.

Keep all medicines safely out of the reach of children.

Avoid discarding razer blades, hypodermic needles (for insulin or other shots), or other potentially dangerous goods into wastebaskets to which your child has access. Flush expired medications down the toilet.

The Bedrooms. Have a lamp within reach on your bedside table. Keep your glasses at hand, too. A telephone within reach may be useful in an emergency, especially if you have a heart or other potentially debilitating chronic ailment. A special communication system also may be appropriate.

If young children visit your home, keep medications securely out of reach. For your own safety, and to avoid confusion, keep no more than one medication at your bedside.

Keep house keys on your bedside table or in an easy-to-reach, familiar place. Shoes and robe, too, should be easily available in the event you must leave quickly (such as in case of fire). This is also good practice when staying in a hotel or motel.

Never smoke in bed. Smoking in bed is particularly hazardous after drinking alcohol or when you are tired.

Unplug appliances (heating pads or electric blankets) when they are not in use.

Entrance and Stairway. All stair treads should be in good repair; replace broken or cracked stairs outside and within your home.

Fasten carpeting on stairs securely.

Every stairway should have a sturdy railing.

Stairway and entryway lighting is very important: if the light is not bright enough to read in, improve the lighting. Place a switch at the bottom and top of each set of stairs.

To help prevent falls, never leave objects on stairs. Do not wax stairways or stair land-

MICROWAVE OVEN SAFETY

Are microwave ovens safe to use in your home? Yes they are, so long as they are well maintained and used properly. In general, the risk from microwave radiation itself is relatively small. On the other hand, shocks, fires, and burns can result from improper or careless use of your microwave oven.

Electrical shock perhaps is the most common danger. Be sure your oven is properly installed and grounded. Periodically examine the electrical cord to be sure it is in good repair.

Fire can occur when food placed on paper or plastic becomes overheated.

An explosion can occur if you use glass containers not designed for your microwave oven. Be sure that dishes are designed for use in your microwave.

Burns can also occur. If you cover food containers to help hold in moisture (plastic wrap is commonly used for this purpose), beware of steam. During the heating process, steam can build up. When you remove the covering, a gush of steam can leave you with a serious and painful burn. Therefore, for safety's sake, remove such covers carefully with a long-handled wooden spoon.

Microwaves heat your food, but your dishes usually remain cool. Nevertheless, use a hot pad to take containers out of your microwave oven. Be careful with the first few bites. You may be lulled into a false sense of confidence by a dish that is not hot to the touch.

Baby bottles warmed in a microwave oven present the same danger: *always* test the milk temperature to prevent burning your baby's mouth.

Finally, there is some risk of microwave radiation if the door, seal, or hinges are damaged. If you suspect any such damage, consult a qualified service person.

---

ings. Falls are of special concern to the elderly (see How To Avoid Falls, page 242).

The Basement, Garage, and Utility Room. Proper lighting is essential. Install appropriate lighting fixtures near the washing machine and dryer, workbench, and entrance areas.

Have your washing machine and dryer installed and serviced by a qualified electrician or technician. Follow factory instructions for use. Make sure that your dryer is vented. Both machines should be grounded; the area must not be damp or have standing water.

Keep cleaning fluids, paints and additives, and fuels and oils labeled and well out of the reach of children. Never reuse food containers to store toxic liquids; your child might take a sip out of a pop bottle that now contains paint thinner or some other poison.

If you have a workshop, keep it neat and organized. Wood shavings on the floor are a potential fire hazard. A clutter of tools and materials can result in falling or stumbling, doubly dangerous events in the presence of tools.

Wear proper attire when working. Safety glasses, earplugs, and protective clothing (including work shoes or boots) may help you avoid injury. Never wear a scarf or a shirt with sleeves that can become entangled in power tools.

Do not allow children to handle tools until they are old enough to understand and obey instructions regarding safe use. Limit use of most power tools to people over age 18.

Keep tools in good repair with blades sharp, cords intact, and guards in working order.

Place a fire extinguisher in the basement, workshop, or utility room. Check it periodically to make sure it is fully charged. Be familiar with instructions for its use.

GUNS IN YOUR HOME

If you have a rifle or shotgun for sporting purposes, make sure that it is stored *without* ammunition and in a locked storage cabinet. If you keep a weapon for security reasons, be sure it is stored out of the reach of children.

Maintain the weapon carefully. Periodically, remove it from its place of storage and make sure that it is clean and working properly. Reacquaint yourself with the weapon's safety and with loading and unloading procedures.

(Note: We do not recommend the use of handguns or any other potentially lethal weapons for the purpose of home security.)

SAFETY OUTSIDE THE HOME

More accidents occur in the home than anywhere else; not far behind, however, are accidents in the workplace, on the highway, and during recreation. Consider the following recommendations for safer practices at work, in traveling, and at play.

SAFETY IN THE WORKPLACE

In recent years, the Occupational Safety and Health Administration (OSHA) and state and local agencies have made important gains in eliminating hazards in the workplace. Yet many potential dangers remain. Be on the alert for such dangers and protect yourself and others by following these safety rules and commonsense guidelines.

Protective Eye Wear. If your job carries a risk of eye injury, your employer is required by law to provide you with protective glasses, and you are required to wear them. If you think they interfere with your efficiency, try another design; many safe and practical varieties are available. Wear them whenever you are operating machinery or exposed to fumes or particles in the air that could endanger your eyes (see Protecting Your Eyes, page 748).

Protection From Noise. If your workplace is so noisy that you have to shout to make yourself heard, the noise level is great enough that it can permanently damage your hearing. Under such conditions, your employer should decrease the noise or provide a protective device.

Specially designed earmuffs are available. Some types close out the outside world; others are fitted with earphones and a microphone that enables you to communicate with other workers. Commercially available earplugs made of foam, plastic, or rubber or custom-molded plugs also effectively decrease your exposure to excessive noise. Cotton balls are not adequate and can get stuck deep in your ear canal (see Foreign Objects in the Ear, page 677). (See also Noise and Sound Levels, page 679, and Occupational Hearing Loss, page 678.)

Fumes, Smoke, Dust, and Gas Hazards. A wide variety of respiratory symptoms can result from exposure to toxic fumes, gases, particles, and smoke in the workplace. The exposure may be long-term with low levels of chemicals; accidental exposure also may occur in which high levels of industrial toxic chemicals are inhaled for a short time.

A sampling of dangerous chemicals includes ammonia, cyanides, formaldehyde, acid fumes, hydrogen sulfide, diazomethane, halides, nitrogen dioxide, isocyanates, ozone, phosgene, phthalic anhydride, and sulfur dioxide. The processing of metals such as cadmium, chromium, nickel, beryllium, copper, magnesium, and zinc can produce dangerous fumes. Dust diseases (pneumoconiosis), including asbestosis (from asbestos), silicosis (from silica), byssinosis (from cotton), and miners' disorders like black-lung disease, also result from long-term inhalation of dust particles (see Occupationally Related Lung Disease, page 941). Workers who use high levels of heat, such as welding, brazing, smelting, pottery making, and furnace work, also are at risk.

If your job involves any of these potential dangers, be sure to obey safety precautions posted in your workplace. Be especially careful if handling hazardous materials such as asbestos. Wear proper clothing, air-filtration masks, eye gear, and other appropriate protection. Be sure ventilation is adequate.

If you are pregnant or are trying to become pregnant, avoid any exposure to hazardous chemicals.

If you suspect that there may be dangerous smoke, fumes, dust, or chemical exposure in your workplace, discuss the matter with your physician. Remember that many permanent respiratory ailments develop slowly as a result of industrial exposure over a period of years. Small exposures that may seem harmless can result in chronic disease. If you think that you or your co-workers are at unnecessary risk (see Occupationally Related Lung Disease, page 941), consult OSHA or a state or local agency charged with workplace safety, your employer, or your union.

Medication, Drug, and Alcohol Use. Do not consume alcohol before or during working hours. Never use illegal drugs. Do not operate machinery when you are taking medications that might make you drowsy. Always ask your physician or your company or plant physician or nurse about the effect a medication may have on you.

Working Shifts. If your job requires that you work night shifts on a regular basis or if you rotate shifts from one week or month to the next, your health may suffer.

Changing your normal rhythm of waking and sleeping, as a result of switching shifts, requires a period of adjustment. If you have ever flown across multiple time zones, you know what can happen when your body's internal clock is disrupted. Insomnia, mental and physical fatigue, indigestion, and an overall feeling of ill health are common side effects. Business people commonly refer to this condition as jet lag.

If your job entails constant changing of shifts, your body will have more difficulty adjusting and readjusting as you get older. Some studies suggest that too frequent shift changes over a lengthy period of time can put you at an increased risk of coronary artery disease or peptic ulcer. Also, fatigue can lead to injury and error in the workplace.

There are no clear-cut solutions to this "occupational jet lag," but there are some strategies you might try.

Work a shift for 3 weeks rather than rotating to a different schedule every week.

Change the sequence. Research suggests that a more normal sleep pattern results when the shift sequence is day-evening-night rather than the more usual day-night-evening sequence.

Tolerance to shift rotation varies widely among people. If you have difficulty making the adjustment, consider changing your job. If you experience severe insomnia your physician may consider prescribing a short-acting sleeping pill that you can take for a few days after each shift change (see Insomnia, page 1028).

SAFETY ON THE ROAD

Approximately 50,000 people die on our roads and highways every year. Many more are severely injured. This terrible toll is more often the result of alcohol or carelessness than it is of mechanical failure. To help ensure your safety, follow these suggestions.

Always Wear a Seat Belt. Seat belts save lives. Wear one every time you get into a car, even if you are traveling only a short distance. Make sure your passengers wear seat belts too. Most accidents occur within a few miles of home.

Car Seats. In most states, children who weigh less than 40 pounds must ride in specially designed car seats. Even if your state does not have this law, buckle up your baby or young child when traveling by auto—always.

Infant safety seats are designed for babies weighing less than 20 pounds. This type of seat is installed so that your baby faces the rear of your car. The seat can be placed on a back or front seat. Many parents, initially at least, put the seat in front. This enables mom or dad to observe the baby while driving. A convertible seat can be used from birth until the child is approximately 40 pounds. This seat can be converted from the reclining, backward position (for an infant) to an upright and forward position (to accommodate a heavier child). Also, do not use shoulder harnesses for children less than 40 pounds. If worn by small children, shoulder harnesses can be hazardous.

When you begin shopping for a safety seat, look for one that conforms to the Federal Motor Vehicle Safety Standard of 1981

VDTs: SENSIBLE PRECAUTIONS

Video display terminals (VDTs) are the screens that more than 15 million Americans look at for hours each day. Also occurring daily are questions about the potential health risks of these helpful new devices.

Among concerns raised are the potential risks posed by the electrical fields and radiation produced by screens of VDTs. To date, however, these risks are discounted by experts as being insignificant. The exposure levels from the screens are well below currently acceptable levels. In addition, no major health risks have been found. However, eye and hand (musculoskeletal) strains have been reported.

Avoidance Strategies
If you work at a VDT daily, try these strategies to minimize eye and hand strain.

Position the screen at eye level, between 22 and 26 inches from where you are seated.

Keep your neck relaxed and your head facing forward.

Locate the keyboard so that your elbows are bent at 90°. You should not have to bend your wrists to type.

Pick a chair that offers ample back support, and position it about an arm's length from your terminal. Your feet should rest on the floor or on a footrest so that your thighs are parallel to the floor.

There are no proven long-term health risks from VDTs but research is continuing. In the meantime, follow the above suggestions. In addition, take a 15-minute break every 2 hours if your workload is moderate; do it every hour if your workload is heavy.

and has been crash tested (see Car Seats, page 74).

Drive Defensively. Driving legally and sensibly is not enough. If other drivers are not capable or careful, they can be the cause of an accident. Never assume that other drivers will drive responsibly. Driving defensively means that you are aware of other cars at all times and are prepared to take evasive action. Try to anticipate what other drivers are going to do. Be prepared to react promptly if another driver suddenly makes an unexpected maneuver.

Do not follow other cars too closely. For every 10 miles per hour of speed, allow one car length between you and the car in front (thus, at 50 mph, five car lengths or about 100 feet should separate you from the car ahead).

Make sure that at all angles your visibility is clear. Do not allow accumulation of toys or other objects to block your rear view. Make sure that your windows and mirrors are clean. Turn your head and use your eyes (in addition to rearview mirrors) to verify the presence or absence of other cars when changing lanes, pulling out from the curb, or turning.

Pedestrians, bicyclists, animals, runners, and motorcyclists all require special caution. Learn where the "blind spots" are in your car.

Consider the Weather. When it is snowing or raining or visibility is reduced for any reason, slow down. If conditions become severe, do not travel until they improve.

Be ready for the unexpected. In very cold weather, carry food, blankets, and cold-weather clothing. Keep your gas tank as full as possible. You may need to run your engine and heater in the event your auto becomes stalled in a blizzard. Do not leave your car in such an emergency. If your engine is running, roll windows down an inch or two to help avoid a potentially fatal buildup of carbon monoxide fumes.

Driving While Impaired. Do not drive after consuming alcoholic beverages or when you have taken medications that make you drowsy or impair your reaction time. If you feel especially tired or ill, someone else should be behind the wheel.

Avoid Distractions. Control the behavior of children in your car. Do not let them get too animated while you are driving. Also, do not let the radio, an interesting conversation, or a roadside attraction distract you from your driving.

Proper Maintenance. Keep your car properly serviced at the recommended intervals (at least every 6 months or 7,500 miles, whichever comes first). Keep your tires (including your spare) in good condition. Make sure your lights, brakes, windshield wipers, and steering work properly. Have a first aid kit (see page 254), flashlight, and emergency flare in your car. Obeying proper maintenance schedules can help ensure that a mechanical failure will not cause a highway mishap.

HOTEL FIRE SAFETY

Most hotels and motels are safe, protected by sprinklers and other precautions required by law in most states. But the unexpected can happen. Thus, take a few simple precautions.

Upon arrival, find the two exits nearest your room. Determine where they go and make sure they are unlocked. Locate the fire alarm nearest your room, too.

Once inside your room, familiarize yourself with its layout. If it ever were to become smoke-filled, you would not be able to see clearly. Review the hotel's fire safety information (often, it is fastened to the back of the door or is in a special brochure).

Never smoke in bed. Keep your room keys on your bedside table.

If you smell smoke or see flames, call the fire department directly and activate the hotel fire alarm.

If the fire alarm sounds, feel your door *before* you open it. If it is hot, do not open it; telephone for help. If your door is cool, open it slowly. Be alert for smoke and flames in the hall, and go to the nearest exit. Take your room key with you. If smoke or flames block your exit, you may have to return to your room. Your room may be the safest place.

If the fire is nearby and you are forced to stay in your room, telephone for help, turn off all air-conditioning and heating systems, and open your window slightly for ventilation. If smoke seeps into your room, soak sheets and towels and stuff them under and around the door to block out heat and smoke. Get as close as you can to the floor (for freshest air) and hold a wet washcloth over your face to keep cool and to filter out smoke particles.

Do not attempt to run through smoke or flames.

Never use elevators during a fire.

WATER AND BOATING SAFETY

Rule number 1 of water safety is that everyone, young and old, should know how to swim. It is never too late to learn. Classes are readily available in most towns and cities.

Going for a Swim.   If you have an outdoor pool, there must be a child-proof fence around it. Never let a child play alone at the edge of a pool, pond, or any body of water.

Never swim alone, not even if you are an excellent swimmer. Teach your child that he or she is never to swim without adult supervision.

Know your limits. Do not try to swim too far or in hazardous conditions (such as in areas with a strong undertow).

Teach your child to swim. Check out local classes *before* you enroll your child to make sure that the instructors are qualified and experienced.

Floating devices on arms can be used for toddlers. Avoid flotation vests on toddlers; these actually can cause drowning. Never leave your child unattended. Know the basics of cardiopulmonary resuscitation (see Cardiopulmonary Resuscitation, page 270).

Do not go swimming when:

You have been consuming alcoholic beverages;

A storm threatens, especially a lightning storm;

Boats or fishermen are operating in the immediate vicinity.

Boating Safety.   Know and obey the rules when using any boat—rowboat, powerboat, or sailboat. Keep your boat properly equipped and maintained. Never consume alcoholic beverages while boating.

Wear a life jacket. When you are in a boat, have as many life jackets as there are passengers. Adult nonswimmers and all children should wear life jackets at all times; it

is a good idea for adult swimmers to wear them, too.

Do not overload your boat. Be sure that the operator of the boat is familiar with its workings and is qualified to drive it. Know the boating rules and obey them. Stay off the water in dangerous weather conditions.

If your boat capsizes, stay with it until help arrives. Do not try to swim to shore.

IN A DROWNING EMERGENCY: For procedures to deal with drowning emergencies, see Near Drowning, page 279.

SAFETY ON THE FARM

Today's farmer works long hours and uses complex, potentially dangerous machinery. However, with proper precautions, the potential for an accident can be reduced or eliminated.

Operate Machinery With Care.   Half of all serious farm injuries involve mechanical equipment. Tractors, power take-offs (PTOs, which provide power from tractor shafts to other equipment), hay balers, augers (corkscrew-like devices used to move grain into storage bins), and corn pickers are highpowered devices that, if not used properly, can cause serious injury or death.

Never take your machinery for granted, especially if you use it every day. Never reach into equipment while parts are moving; turn the equipment off before making repairs. Do not remove safety shields or guards. Service the equipment at appropriate intervals.

When at work, never wear baggy clothing (loose shirttails, long sleeves, scarves) that can get caught in moving equipment (such as PTOs) and pull you into the mechanism. Use safety glasses, noise protection, and other precautions including masks when using chemicals and pesticides (see Safety in the Workplace, page 323).

Children on the Farm.   Supervise children at all times. Assign them only tasks within their level of competence and appropriate to their ages.

Do not allow youngsters to play with farm equipment. Children should never get the impression that tractors and other farm machinery are toys. This equipment is too dangerous to risk a child's misuse when you are not present to supervise.

Pesticides, Fuels, and Fire Risks. Store poisons and toxic materials in a safe, secure location. Keep flammable materials in fireproof areas away from barns and fodder storage.

Make sure that wiring is properly maintained. Keep fire extinguishers at hand for use in the event of fire. Enforce "no smoking" rules in areas where flammable goods are stored.

SAFETY WHILE HIKING AND CAMPING

The outdoors can be a wonderful place for exercise, fun, and experiencing nature firsthand. Without proper consideration of the risks, however, a casual hike in the woods can be a dangerous or even life-threatening activity.

Recognize Your Limits. Suit your outdoor activity to your physical condition. A newborn baby or an elderly person with a heart condition probably does not belong on a trek into the wilderness. Match the recreational activity to the capabilities of the campers.

Plan Ahead. If you are visiting an unfamiliar area, map your route in advance. Take the map with you, and locate your position on it from time to time. Know the weather forecast in advance, and monitor changes as you travel (see Safety and the Elements, page 328).

Dress for the Occasion. Sturdy shoes are important for the hiker. If you are hiking up a mountain, be prepared for climate changes. It probably will be cooler or damper on top.

Carry Appropriate Equipment. Know your needs. Plan ahead, and be sure that you have what you need for your outdoors adventure. Tents, sleeping bags, food, extra clothing, insect repellent, matches, flashlight, and other goods may be required.

Always carry first aid supplies when camping (see Basic First Aid Supplies, page 254).

Watch, Don't Touch, the Animals. Beware of wild animals. If they are acting oddly, rabies may be the cause; check wildlife conditions with the Forest Service before going in. Do not approach a young animal; a protective mother may be nearby. Do not keep food in your tent because it may attract unwanted animals. Instead, hang it from a tree nearby.

Beware of Bites and Blisters. Carry insect repellent with you if the area has mosquitoes, flies, ticks, or other insects (see Lyme Disease, page 854). If there is risk of an allergic response, consult your physician first because immunization may be appropriate. Watch out for resinous plants such as poison oak and sumac (see Contact Dermatitis, page 457).

Don't Drink the Water. Never drink the water unless you know it is clean. An important risk is giardiasis, infestation by a tiny

---

BASIC BICYCLING SAFETY

Wear a Helmet

Three of four cyclists killed in cycle-related accidents die of head injuries; the majority of bicyclists' injuries involve the head. So, wearing a helmet is a sensible precaution.

Your helmet should have a durable outer shell and a polystyrene liner. Adjustable foam pads should help ensure a proper fit at the front, back, and sides, and the straps should hold it snug. Check for a sticker from the American National Standards Institute or the Snell Memorial Foundation, the two groups that have established voluntary testing standards for bicycling helmets.

Ride With Traffic

Wrong-way riders are much more likely to be involved in accidents with motor vehicles. In addition, all 50 states require cyclists to go with the traffic flow.

Stop at Stop Signs

Stop signs are there for bicycles as well as autos. Look both ways before proceeding.

Check for Traffic Before Turning

Always look back, signal, and check for traffic before turning.

Watch Out for Water

In wet conditions, braking ability is greatly decreased. Watch out for wet leaves in the fall; they can be slippery and hazardous.

Bicycle Defensively

Make eye contact with other riders, drivers, and pedestrians. Watch out for potholes, rubbish, and other hazards. Know your own reaction time and other skills. Ride with care at speeds commensurate with your abilities. Beware of motorists who may be inclined to make a right turn into or in front of you.

parasite that produces diarrhea, abdominal cramps, and bloating. Even if the water looks crystal-clear, it may be contaminated. In fact, rushing mountain streams are more likely to infect you than placid lakes, because the parasites cannot settle to the bottom (see page 619).

Boil any water for a minimum of 3 minutes before drinking it. Adding halazone tablets (which contain iodine) to the water will also kill disease-producing bacteria.

Various types of lightweight, portable filters are available to remove *Giardia* from water, but do not rely on them. Experts disagree on their effectiveness.

Don't Pick the Berries.   Do not eat berries, mushrooms, or other plants unless you are positive that they are edible.

Douse Your Campfire.   Never risk the safety of other campers and animals by failing to drown your campfire.

SAFETY AND THE ELEMENTS

In our daily lives, we develop strategies to minimize the impact of weather on our normal activities. Most of us take for granted our ability to deal with rain, snow, or other challenges of climate. A word to the wise: never underestimate climate as a potential hazard to your health.

Thunder and Lightning.   In the event of an electrical storm, take appropriate precautions. Avoid the tallest object in the area, such as an isolated house on a hill or a single tree. Avoid *being* the tallest object, too: never carry your golf clubs or fishing rod in an open area during a storm. Go indoors and close windows and doors. Do not use your telephone, bathtub, or shower.

Get away from open water, tractors, or metal equipment (motorcycles, scooters, golf carts, bicycles). Avoid metallic structures (fences, clotheslines, pipes, rails) that can carry electricity to you from a distance. Your car, with windows and doors closed, is a safe place.

Intense Cold.   Dress for the cold. Many layers of thin clothing that trap insulating air between them are better than a single, bulky covering. For example, to keep your upper body warm, wear a T-shirt, a long-sleeved shirt, a sweater, and then a parka over everything. Add another layer if you get cold.

Always wear a hat to conserve body heat. Also wear mittens or gloves. Boots should have room for two pairs of warm socks.

Do not drink alcohol or smoke cigarettes before going out in extreme cold. Nicotine decreases circulation to your extremities, the areas most susceptible to cold injury. Alcohol enhances the removal of heat from your body, making you vulnerable to hypothermia. Adequate nutrition is especially important in cold weather. People with diseases that limit the blood supply to their extremities are especially at risk.

If you or a companion experience frostbite or hypothermia (significant decrease in body temperature), seek immediate emergency treatment (see Frostbite, page 279, and Hypothermia, page 278).

Protection From the Sun.   Exposure to the sun can damage your skin. Take precautions, especially if you will be exposed to the sun's rays for long periods or at the hottest part of the day (10:00 a.m. to 2:00 p.m.). Wear appropriate sunscreens such as those containing *para*-aminobenzoic acid (PABA) or benzophenone on your face, lips, and any other exposed skin. A rating of 15 is appropriate for most people (see How To Avoid Sunburn, page 1165).

If you are exposed to sun for long periods, especially when there is little breeze and high humidity, heat stroke or heat exhaustion may result. Heat stroke and heat exhaustion are emergencies and require immediate care (see Heat Stress, page 277).

Avoid the risk of heatstroke or heat exhaustion by staying out of the sun for extended periods (see page 277). Do not consume alcoholic beverages on hot, humid days when you are outside. Drink plenty of water. Wear a hat with a wide brim to protect yourself from sun exposure. Wear lightweight, loose-fitting clothing; light-colored clothing will reflect the heat. Frequent cool showers or baths may be helpful. Never leave children or pets unattended in a car in the sun—not even for a few minutes.

Sun Exposure in Children.   A very young child should not be exposed to more than 2 minutes of sun on the first day of exposure. Then, increase exposure by no more than 2 minutes on successive days. Always use sunscreens and hats.

CHAPTER 11
THE ENVIRONMENT

CHAPTER CONTENTS

In the last quarter century, Americans have made environmental matters a priority. Some rivers that were unswimmable 2 decades ago have regained recreational usefulness. The creation of the Environmental Protection Agency, the passing of the Clean Air Act of 1970, the establishment of a toxic waste "superfund," and various other private and governmental efforts are making a difference in the quality of the air we breathe and of the water we drink.

The job is far from complete. As a member of the general public you may be concerned that further steps be taken to address continuing and new pollution problems. In your own home, too, there are everyday concerns to be addressed to ensure that you and your family avoid exposure to dangerous and even potentially cancer-causing pollutants. In the following pages, we consider some of these concerns.

DRINKING WATER

In recent years, we have developed a new consciousness of the cleanliness of our water supply. Once, we regarded clean water as automatic because public health programs early in our century had greatly decreased the risks of cholera, typhoid, and other diseases caused by contaminated water.

Today, the risks are different. Infectious disease no longer is our greatest concern. Now the presence of heavy metals, polychlorinated biphenyls (PCBs), pesticides, and other contaminants in drinking water is of greater concern.

Landfills, especially those in which hazardous wastes have been discarded, are potential sources of contamination. Outmoded or improperly maintained tanks at gas stations and fuel oil depots also may contaminate ground water and wells. Runoff from agricultural lands that have been treated with certain chemical fertilizers and pesticides may contaminate rivers, streams, lakes, and ground water, as can industrial pollution. Septic tanks for homes in rural and semirural areas may contribute to ground water pollution.

Among the most serious potential risks are the following.

Trihalomethanes. Chlorine, the chemical responsible for clearing our drinking water of infectious microbes, can undergo chemical reactions in the presence of water pollutants. The resultant chemical compounds, the trihalomethanes (THMs), are potentially cancer-causing (carcinogenic) as demonstrated by tests on experimental animals.

Nitrates. Nitrate contamination as a result of runoff from fields poses an immediate danger to infants. In adults as well as children, ingested nitrates can result in the exposure of your digestive system to nitrosamines, potentially potent carcinogenic compounds.

Asbestos and Heavy Metals. Cadmium (from old galvanized pipes), lead in old homes (from lead-based paint and pipes), and asbestos (from asbestos-cement water pipes and other sources) are potentially dangerous substances (see Asbestosis, page 942).

SOLUTIONS

Using bottled water may or may not be the answer. It is expensive, and often the water in these bottles is no better than water from your tap. Boiling water is another option if your water is contaminated with bacteria, but this will not remove lead and cadmium. Commercially available filters may be of help, although claims made for them sometimes exceed their actual usefulness.

More important, if your water comes from a well, test it every year for pollutants. Find out when the last sampling and sanitary testing was done and what was found. You then can take steps to solve any problem found.

The Environmental Protection Agency and local and state organizations are responsible for monitoring public water supplies.

CANCER PREVENTION

The causes of the diverse group of diseases we call cancer remain largely unknown. Medical science continues to add new clues to our understanding of cancer, but much remains to be learned (see The Biology of Cancer, page 1239).

We do know that many cancers occur as a result of exposure to certain substances called carcinogens. These cancer-causing agents include cigarettes, asbestos, certain food substances, and various household and industrial chemicals.

Common sense suggests you should identify carcinogens to which you or members of your family are exposed and then devise strategies to eliminate them. These risk factors include the following.

Passive Smoking. It is not just smokers themselves who are at increased risk of cancer from tobacco smoke—anyone nearby who inhales the smoke also is at risk. In fact, the so-called sidestream smoke from a cigarette (that which curls up from a lighted cigarette in an ashtray) contains twice as much tar and nicotine as the inhaled smoke does, 3 times as much of a compound called 3,4-benzpyrene, a cancer-causing agent, 5 times as much carbon monoxide, and possibly 50 times as much ammonia.

In addition to quitting smoking yourself, convince other smokers to do the same. Parents who smoke put the health of their children in jeopardy (see How To Stop Smoking, page 412).

Diet and Cancer. The relationship between diet and cancer is under close scrutiny. Recent reports suggest a link between certain foods and some forms of cancer (see Diet and Cancer Protection, page 369).

Sun Exposure. Do not get burned by the sun. Chronic exposure to the ultraviolet rays of the sun is the major cause of skin cancer. Use sensible strategies to limit your exposure. Wear long-sleeved, loose-fitting clothes and a hat or bandanna. Use sunscreen (one with a 15 rating will block out most of the sun's ultraviolet rays). Stay out of the sun at the hottest time of the day, between 10:00 a.m. and 2:00 p.m. (see How To Avoid Sunburn, page 1165).

Industrial Exposure. Certain chemicals, the processing of certain metals, and the inhalation of some fibers and dusts have been linked to the occurrence of certain cancers. If you work with hazardous substances, follow instructions about protective clothing or equipment, including goggles, masks, gloves, and overalls (see Safety in the Workplace, page 323).

AIR POLLUTION

The air we breathe often is not clean. Industry, automobiles, and other sources, in combination with weather factors, can decrease air quality to the point that it can be hazardous to your health, especially if you have heart, lung, or other chronic disease.

Key sources of the potential air pollutants include the following.

Motor Vehicle Exhaust. Cars and trucks release a range of pollutants including carbon monoxide, oxides of nitrogen, and lead.

Industrial and Power Plants. Factories and power plants that burn fuels (such as oil or coal) that contain sulfur are the principal industrial polluters. They send oxides of sulfur into the air. Oxides of nitrogen (mostly from car exhaust) and oxides of sulfur are the principal causes of acid rain.

Chlorofluorocarbons. Scientists believe that the ozone (an atmospheric layer that protects us from the sun's ultraviolet rays) is gradually being depleted. Chlorofluorocarbons, which are used in refrigeration systems (air conditioners and refrigerators), dry cleaning chemicals, and numerous other products, are thought to be causing this change in the atmosphere of the earth. Loss of the ozone layer may be a major risk factor in increasing the incidence of skin cancer.

Other Pollutants. Certain workplaces, including some mines, manufacturing plants, and old buildings, may expose workers to asbestos (see Asbestosis, page 942) and other particulate matter that can produce lung damage and tumors.

INDOOR POLLUTION

The inside of your home also is a potentially polluted place. Especially in homes that are superinsulated (tightly sealed to prevent the loss of heat or cooling), indoor environments can become contaminated with hazardous levels of pollutants.

Prolonged exposure to indoor pollutants can result in symptoms of allergies (including rashes, eye irritation, cough, sore throat, and other cold symptoms). There is also evidence of increased risk of cancer from exposure to certain indoor pollutants.

Among the most common indoor pollutants are the following.

Cigarette Smoke. High in carbon monoxide and particulates such as tar and nicotine, cigarette smoke is a health hazard, even for the nonsmoker who merely shares an interior space with a smoker (see Second-Hand Smoke, page 412, and Carbon Monoxide Poisoning, page 333).

Formaldehyde. Various construction products (including particle board and urea-formaldehyde foam insulation), some synthetic carpet and curtain material, fabric softeners, and many cosmetics can release formaldehyde in your home. Although the level of formaldehyde usually is negligible if materials are installed or used properly, an accumulation of high concentrations of formaldehyde may result in chest and lung discomfort. The risk generally is higher in mobile homes because materials that contain formaldehyde sometimes are used in building and decorating these structures.

Other Pollutants. Gas cookers produce nitrous oxide. Carbon monoxide may come from various indoor heating and cooking devices (see Carbon Monoxide Poisoning, page 333). Asbestos, most often from deteriorating insulation on heating pipes, is an especially dangerous risk (see Asbestosis, page 942). We discuss radon, another indoor pollutant, on page 335.

WHAT TO DO

Monitoring the quality of the air outside your home and enforcing the regulations regarding it are the responsibility of the federal Environmental Protection Agency (EPA) and other such agencies on the state and local level. In the workplace, the Occupational

---

TWENTIETH-CENTURY ALLERGY: FACT OR FICTION?

In recent years, a concept of illness variously named 20th-century syndrome (see page 455), total allergy syndrome, or multiple chemical sensitivities has been developed by "clinical ecologists," a group of physicians at the fringe of orthodox medicine.

The working hypothesis is that the health of some people is harmed by "unnatural elements" in the environment. Unnatural elements can range from exposure to synthetic materials to certain foods. People sometimes are told that their immune systems have been damaged. This damage supposedly renders them excessively sensitive to a wide range of naturally occurring and synthetic substances.

Various symptoms have been attributed to the supposed disorder, but the symptoms are not those that ordinarily result from an allergy. Symptoms commonly include fatigue, headache, depression, dizziness, anxiety, and mood swings. Furthermore, laboratory tests are never conclusive as to a po-tential cause for the discomforts these people describe.

There is no clear definition of the disorder. Its potential existence has attracted supporters because of widespread concern about the environment.

This supposed ailment has been examined in depth by the American College of Physicians. The conclusion of this group is that there is no convincing evidence to support the concept of a 20th-century allergy.

Persons for whom this diagnosis has been proposed may indeed have a disorder. Depression is one possible explanation. The physical discomforts commonly described by depressed people are numerous and vague and comparable to the symptoms people with 20th-century allergy complain of.

The practice of clinical ecology lacks scientific validation. In many situations, the lives of "patients" have been severely constrained because of recommendations made without validation. In addition, enormous costs are sometimes incurred for ineffective treatment while less costly methods that are potentially helpful are shunned.

Safety and Health Administration (OSHA) is charged with monitoring conditions. If you are aware of a source of air pollution in your neighborhood, town, or workplace, report your concerns to one of these agencies.

Make sure that pollution control devices on your car are functioning properly. Your state may require an emissions test as a part of the schedule of inspections.

In your home, be alert to potential airborne poisons. If your house often seems to accumulate smoke, fumes, or other indoor pollution, poor ventilation may be a problem. Have your ventilation checked by a heating/air conditioning specialist. If you live in a house with limited air exchange (a house tightly insulated to hold heat or cool air in), a duct system of air exchangers may be in order.

Make sure that your furnace is installed, maintained, and vented correctly. The same holds true for any other open-flame device you may have in your home (such as a fireplace or cook stove).

CARBON MONOXIDE POISONING

Carbon monoxide is tasteless, odorless, colorless—and deadly. Often referred to by its chemical formula, CO, this gas is produced by the incomplete combustion of carbon-based fuel. Many cooking stoves, lamps, space heaters, furnaces, hot water heaters, and engines produce it.

If the CO level is too high, it takes the place of oxygen in the hemoglobin in your red blood cells, preventing the vital function of this oxygen-carrying molecule.

CO CONTAMINATION IN THE HOME AND ON THE ROAD

The risk of CO poisoning is greatest during cold weather. We seal and weather-strip our homes as tightly as possible to conserve heat, but in so doing we also decrease ventilation and increase the accumulation of indoor pollutants such as CO (see also Indoor Pollution, page 332). CO buildup is most likely to occur as a result of defective control valves or pilot lights on cooking or heating units such as portable kerosene space heaters or of inadequately ventilated flame-burning heaters or cookers.

Many recreational vehicles, trailers, and pickup campers have been found to have engine exhaust fumes leaking into them. Such vehicles may have unvented ovens, stoves, and flame-burning lamps that also produce CO.

The signs and symptoms of CO poisoning are vague. Headache, nausea, vomiting, fatigue, and dizziness may occur but are easily confused with flu-like illnesses that are common in winter months. When the concentration of CO is very high, muscle paralysis and loss of consciousness may occur.

If you suspect CO poisoning, get away from the source immediately. Consult your physician, who will conduct a blood test to identify the amount of CO being carried by your hemoglobin.

Prevention Make sure your wood stoves, space heaters, fireplaces, and flame-burning appliances are properly installed, adjusted, operated, and ventilated. Never use ovens or gas ranges for heating purposes.

Do not operate gas-powered vehicles in confined spaces (such as your garage or basement).

Never burn charcoal inside your home, recreational vehicle, or tent.

RADIATION AND YOUR HEALTH

When necessary, your physician may schedule you for an x-ray examination (radiographic examination) to obtain information that will help assist him or her in diagnosing your problem. The examination itself will be performed by a radiologist or a radiology technician. The results will be interpreted by the radiologist.

WHAT ARE X-RAYS AND WHAT DO THEY DO?

X-rays are a form of radiation (energy that moves from one place to another). Most radiation is nonpenetrating—it cannot pass through structures. One example of nonpenetrating radiation is visible light. X-rays are one of the few types of radiation (called ionizing radiation) that can penetrate your body.

Because x-rays are able to penetrate your body, they can create a picture of internal body structures on film. This allows your physician to see inside your body without a surgical procedure.

Are X-Rays Safe? For most x-ray examinations, the amount of radiation you receive is small and the risk of harm is very low. This risk is outweighed by benefits of the examination. In addition, great care is taken to use the lowest dose possible to produce an image for your radiologist to evaluate. No radiation remains in your body after an x-ray examination.

Note: Neither magnetic resonance imaging (MRI) nor ultrasound examination involves the use of x-rays; thus, there is no ionizing radiation exposure with these procedures.

Are There Limits on the Number of X-Ray Examinations You Receive? Because the benefits from these examinations far outweigh the very low risk associated with this type of radiation exposure, limits have not been placed on x-ray examinations that are considered medically necessary.

How Is Radiation Measured? The amount of radiation to which you are exposed is measured in a unit called a roentgen, named after the man who discovered x-rays in 1895, Professor Wilhelm Konrad Roentgen. Other units, the rad and the rem, have technical differences from the roentgen but, for practical purposes, 1 roentgen equals 1 rad or rem. A smaller unit of measurement, the mrad (1/1,000 of a rad), is more useful for measuring exposures to radiation.

What Are the Sources of Radiation Exposure? Every year, the average person is exposed to approximately 360 mrad of ionizing radiation. This radiation comes from many sources. Natural sources of radiation, which include outer space, rocks, and soil, vary throughout the country. X-rays are a man-made source of radiation. They account for 11 percent of our average yearly exposure to radiation. In recent years, radon has become, in some situations, a significant source of radiation (see page 335).

Should I Have an X-Ray Examination When I Am Pregnant? The risk of ill effects from exposure of an unborn child to diagnostic x-rays or radiopharmaceuticals is very low. Nevertheless, because fetal tissues are growing rapidly, they are more sensitive to radiation than the tissues of an adult. Therefore, if you think you might be pregnant, tell your physician. If it is important for you to have an x-ray examination even though you are pregnant, special precautions can be taken to minimize the radiation exposure to your unborn child. For example, in the case of a chest x-ray, a CT scan of your head, or a mammogram, your unborn

Sources of radiation exposure of United States population. Total is 360 mrad per year. Courtesy: National Council on Radiation Protection and Measurements.

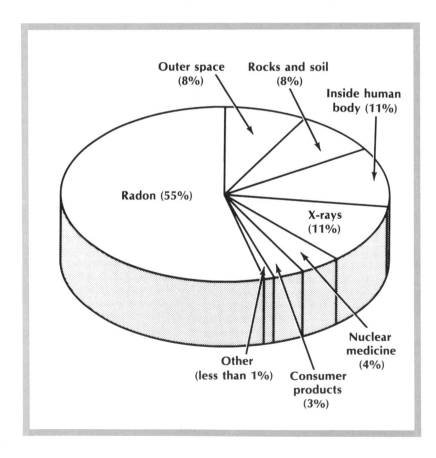

Outer space (8%)
Rocks and soil (8%)
Inside human body (11%)
Radon (55%)
X-rays (11%)
Nuclear medicine (4%)
Consumer products (3%)
Other (less than 1%)

THE RADON RISK

The element uranium is found in soil and in rocks that contain granite, shale, or phosphate (which means it is also found in masonry building materials such as bricks and concrete). As it decays, the uranium releases a gas called radon in such small quantities usually as to be harmless.

In some instances, however, especially in the interior of some homes, radon can accumulate and the level can become relatively high. Radon decays to radioactive atoms that may attach themselves to dust particles and, when inhaled, may release small bursts of energy that can damage lung tissue and may increase the risk of lung cancer after many years of exposure.

Measuring the Radon

A commonly used measure of radioactivity in the United States is the curie. The Environmental Protection Agency urges you to take action if the average annual radon level in your home is 4 picocuries per liter of air or more (a picocurie is one-trillionth of a curie). One recent survey found that nearly one in three basements tested contained higher levels.

The Testing Process

Several tests are available; we recommend use of an alpha tract detector in the fall and winter months. Available in hardware stores and supermarkets, this detector measures radon over several months to a year.

Use at least two detectors in your home. Place one in the lowest part used as a living area (such as a family room) and one in an upper area (such as a bedroom).

Follow the directions you receive with the testing device, and return the device to the manufacturer as soon as the testing period ends. The manufacturer will send you the test results, usually within 2 weeks.

Making Changes

If tests conducted over a period of years indicate that average radon levels in your home are greater than 4 picocuries per liter of air, minor adjustments to your home may be recommended. Rarely is expensive remodeling required.

Try the following approaches. In the cellar or crawl space, cover large openings to the soil; cover sump pumps and vent them to the outside. Use a high-quality caulk that adheres to concrete to seal cracks and other openings in your basement floors and walls. Insulate the floor above any crawl space and keep vents open on all sides of your home to ventilate the basement or crawl space.

If the radon reading is very high, you might consider installing a small fan that brings in fresh air. Another option is the installation of an air-to-air heat exchanger.

Retest your home after making the changes to determine whether you have decreased the amount of radon in the air.

Here, in descending order of frequency, are the six most common routes by which radon can enter your home: (1) open sump pump, (2) gaps between wall-to-wall joints, (3) cracks in foundation floors and mortar joints, (4) pores in concrete block, (5) building materials, and (6) water supply.

child can be shielded so there is virtually no exposure.

What About Radioactive Iodine? Occasionally, persons with thyroid problems are given a dose of radioactive iodine to help cure their disease (see Hyperthyroidism, page 727). When this happens, it is important to follow your physician's instructions in order to minimize radiation exposure to members of your family during the first few days after the radioactive iodine treatment. Because radiation exposure decreases rapidly with distance, these instructions usually consist of simple steps such as not holding children in your lap, not sharing eating utensils, and sleeping alone for several days. Such steps decrease radiation exposure of family members to nearly zero.

What About Other Radiation? There is little you can do about most natural radiation exposure. Radiation is in the air around us and we cannot avoid it. However, if your occupation or geographical location exposes you to greater than normal amounts of radiation, you might consider life-style changes to decrease your exposure. If levels of radon in your home are high, make adjustments to decrease them (see The Radon Risk, page 335).

CHAPTER 12
TRAVEL

CHAPTER CONTENTS

Traveling outside the United States brings you into contact with new sights, sounds, and foods—and perhaps with new bacteria and viruses that your body is not accustomed to. The result can be serious disorders or nagging, irritating discomforts such as traveler's diarrhea.

This chapter describes some of the illnesses that can affect you when you travel abroad and how to prevent them. There also is a discussion of the inconvenient discomfort often referred to as jet lag, with suggestions for minimizing its effects.

IMMUNIZATIONS

Before you leave on a trip out of the country, and especially if you are going to a less-developed country, make sure that you and your children are adequately immunized against any infectious diseases you might encounter.

Every adult and child should have up-to-date immunity against tetanus and polio, whether traveling or not. The other immunizations you need depend on the country you are going to and perhaps the region of that country. Generally, you are more likely to be exposed to an infectious disease in a rural area than in an urban one (particularly in less-developed countries) because water supply systems and sanitary conditions may not be as up-to-date in rural areas.

Each country has immunization requirements that travelers must fulfill before entering. These are listed in the booklet *Health Information for International Travel* which is written by the Centers for Disease Control (CDC) and published yearly by the US Government Printing Office. For more up-to-date information, you can call the CDC in Atlanta, Georgia. You can also ask your physician, local or state health department, or the consulate or embassy of the country you plan to visit. The Public Health Service recommends that you have only those vaccinations that are required.

If you are going to an area where diseases are prevalent, check with your physician about immunization at least a month before you plan to depart because some vaccines must be given several weeks before exposure to the infection.

Take vaccination records with you when you travel out of the United States. Some countries require certificates of vaccination against diseases such as cholera and yellow fever (see Your Medical Traveling Packet, page 340).

Some trip-related illnesses do not become evident until after you return home. If you are reporting symptoms to your physician, be sure to mention any trips you have recently taken.

Here are some suggestions for basic vaccination schedules.

TETANUS

Tetanus vaccination usually is given to children as a series of shots and is completed by the time the child enters school. A tetanus/diphtheria booster is given to adults and children over 12 every 7 to 10 years thereafter. Every child and adult should have up-to-date immunity at all times.

DIPHTHERIA

A killed vaccine is used. It usually is given to children. The vaccine is combined with tetanus and pertussis vaccines (DTP shot). It is given as a series of four shots. Children over 12 and adults should receive a tetanus-diphtheria toxoid, adult type, booster shot every 7 to 10 years. Make sure your immunization schedule is up-to-date.

POLIO

Poliomyelitis vaccination generally is performed by giving a live vaccine orally at ages 2, 4, and 18 months of age (and 6 months if polio is prevalent in the area) at the same time as the DTP vaccine. All adults and children should be immunized, whether they are traveling or not.

INFLUENZA

Immunization is not recommended for the general population, but certain persons who are at high risk of serious illness should be vaccinated (see page 854) before leaving the country. Elderly people in particular should be vaccinated.

PNEUMOCOCCAL PNEUMONIA

Elderly people who have not received this vaccine previously should be vaccinated once before traveling, several weeks before departure. Once a person has received this vaccine, however, no further doses should be given.

HEPATITIS B

There are two vaccines available for people who do not test positive for antibodies to the hepatitis B virus but are at risk of getting it. If you plan to travel to a country where hepatitis is prevalent or if you are at risk of acquiring the disease (see page 650), you should be vaccinated.

HEPATITIS A

A vaccine against hepatitis A is not available, but temporary immunity (1 to 2 months) can be acquired by receiving an injection of human gamma globulin. We recommend an injection of gamma globulin 1 or 2 days before departure if you are going to an area where sanitation is poor and you are at high risk of contracting hepatitis A from contaminated food or water or from contact with someone who is infected.

MENINGOCOCCAL MENINGITIS

If you are traveling to regions of Africa or South America where meningitis is prevalent, you should receive types A, C, W-135, and Y vaccines against this disease.

RABIES

If you plan to stay or live in areas where rabies is common in domestic animals, such as India and parts of South America, you may want to develop immunity to the virus before leaving by obtaining injections of

human diploid cell vaccine. It usually is given as three injections at intervals of 1 week with a booster 3 weeks later. Mild adverse reactions are quite common.

MALARIA

There is no vaccine, as yet, against malaria, but effective preventive medications are available. Consider taking chloroquine phosphate once a week, beginning a week before you arrive in a country where malaria is present. Continue taking the drug for 6 weeks after you leave the area. If you are traveling to countries where there is malaria that is resistant to chloroquine, consider an additional medication (Fansidar). Consult your physician about these prescription drugs and ask about possible adverse reactions to them.

CHOLERA

If you are traveling to certain areas of the Middle East or Asia or to other areas where cholera is present, you should be immunized against this disease. The vaccination is given as two injections, 2 to 6 weeks apart, with booster shots every 6 months while you are at risk of exposure.

TYPHOID

If you are traveling to a country where typhoid is prevalent, consider receiving the killed vaccine which is given in two doses at least 1 month apart. If you live in that country for an extended period of time, have a booster shot every 3 years while you are at risk of exposure.

PLAGUE

Vaccination consists of three injections a month or more apart and is given to people traveling to areas where the disease is still prevalent.

YELLOW FEVER

A live virus vaccine, available only at certain medical centers, should be given to those

YOUR MEDICAL TRAVELING PACKET

When we travel, most of us think to take our wallets, passports (if necessary), and suitcases. But also remember to take a range of items to fill any of your or your family's health needs during the trip. Here are our suggestions.

Medications

If you need a medication at home, you probably need it while traveling, too. Make sure that you have an ample supply of medications you take regularly. Prescriptions should be up-to-date; an extra supply is a good idea, too. You may stay longer than you anticipated. If you are traveling to third-world countries where you may encounter gastrointestinal distress, ask your physician to prescribe an appropriate medication.

Other Pharmaceutical Products

If you will need sunscreens, contact lens solution, insect repellant, or other familiar products, take them with you. A motion-sickness medication also may be a sensible precaution if you tend to feel nauseated during bumpy travels.

If you have allergies or other acute medical problems that you routinely treat with medications, take the medications along. A familiar remedy may not be readily available in a foreign land.

First Aid Kit

Taking a simple first aid kit is a sensible precaution. Antiseptic cream, aspirin or acetaminophen, adhesive and gauze bandages, a thermometer, and an elastic wrap (for sprains).

Medical Records

In case of emergency or illness, the physician you consult on your trip will need to know something of your medical history. Be prepared to inform him or her of the following:

• Any chronic diseases you have—in particular, diabetes, glaucoma, heart disorder, or hypertension.

• The prescription medications you are taking for either chronic or acute ailments; make sure you know the generic and brand names (if any) as well as the dosage and frequency at which you take them.

• Whether your physician has observed abnormalities on an x-ray or electrocardiogram; if so, have those test results with you.

• Your immunization record, because some countries require certificates of vaccination against diseases such as cholera and yellow fever.

• Any allergies you have, especially to drugs, foods, or insect stings.

Keep all this material together. Make sure other members of your family know where it is kept so they can quickly and easily provide relevant information to any medical professional who may need it. The package should also contain the names, addresses, and telephone numbers of your primary-care physician and your traveling companions' physicians.

---

traveling to certain areas of Africa and South America where the disease is widespread. Vaccination must be repeated at least every 10 years.

SMALLPOX

Smallpox has been eradicated as of 1980; therefore vaccination is unnecessary.

PREVENTION OF TRAVELER'S DIARRHEA

"Traveler's diarrhea," "turista," "Montezuma's revenge" are familiar names for a common ailment of travelers. A trip to a foreign country by no means guarantees a bout with gastrointestinal discomfort but, if you travel to a land whose climate, social conditions, or sanitary standards and practices are significantly different from yours at home, the risk may be high.

Traveler's diarrhea may be attributed to a number of causes, including unaccustomed food and drink, change in the bacteria that naturally live in the bowel, change in living habits, and, sometimes, viral infections.

PREVENTION

Taking antibiotics or other medications as a preventive measure before and during your trip is not generally recommended, but follow your physician's advice. Taking bismuth subsalicylate (Pepto-Bismol) tablets throughout your trip as a preventive measure can decrease your risk of diarrhea but the large amount necessary makes this an impractical approach.

Proper Water Sources.   The first rule for avoiding diarrhea while traveling: Do not drink the water—whether it comes from a stream, a well, or a tap—unless it has been sterilized. Bottled water may be safe, so long as it indeed is factory bottled. In addition, you can purchase water filter pumps from camping stores that remove many microorganisms.

Iodine tablets or crystals, which also can be purchased at camping stores, will kill most microbes. However, be sure to follow the directions and allow the treatment to continue long enough before drinking the water. (Drinking large amounts of water containing iodine is not always a good idea either.) Water that has been chlorinated or boiled is safe.

At some of the newer resort hotels you may be able to drink the tap water if the water system is up-to-date, but do not rely on it.

Often, tourists will conscientiously avoid drinking water from the tap, only to come down with traveler's diarrhea from drinking beverages that contain ice. If the water used to make ice is not free of bacteria, when the ice melts into your drink you will be exposed to foreign bacteria.

Be careful as well of fruit juices because they often are diluted with tap water. Bottled wine, beer, and carbonated sodas (without ice) are safe. Using tap water to brush your teeth is all right; however, do not swallow the water.

What Foods Can Travelers Eat Safely?
Cooked foods are usually safe, but do not

A DRINK TO REPLACE LOST FLUIDS

If you experience severe weakness after a bout of traveler's diarrhea, your body may have lost an excessive amount of vital fluids and salts. To help correct the problem if professional help is unavailable, prepare this replacement solution.

Mix one-half teaspoon of table salt (sodium chloride), one-half teaspoon of baking soda (sodium bicarbonate), and four tablespoons of table sugar (sucrose) in one quart of carbonated water. If carbonated water is not available, tap water boiled for 15 minutes is a suitable substitute.

You can prepare this solution in your hotel room. Drink it over the course of the day as a supplement to a clear liquid diet. Also drink orange, apple, or other fruit juices to replace lost potassium (but avoid juices that are diluted with tap water). Although generally not included in a clear liquid diet, bananas are a good source of potassium.

---

eat raw foods—especially do not eat salads that contain lettuce or raw vegetables. Fruits and vegetables that can be peeled immediately before you eat them are safe. Oranges, pineapples, melons, apples, and other fruits with a rind or skin that can be peeled off usually are safe. Eat in restaurants that have a reputation for safety. Do not eat foods from street vendors, and consume only foods (especially meat products) that are thoroughly cooked. If you cook your own food, keep cold those items that can spoil.

If all else fails and you do come down with a case of traveler's diarrhea, drink plenty of safe liquids. Broths, sweetened tea, and soda are good for keeping up your strength. As soon as you feel like eating again, start with bland, nonfatty foods in order to avoid irritating your intestinal system. Bland cereals, rice, gelatin, jellied consommé, simple puddings, and soft-cooked eggs and bland foods are possibilities (see also Infections of the Gastrointestinal Tract, page 617).

PREVENTION OF JET LAG

Perhaps you are familiar with that dragged-out, out-of-sync feeling referred to as jet lag. It occurs when the body is suddenly delivered to an unfamiliar time zone so that the patterns of eating, working, relaxing, and sleeping are abruptly changed. The symptoms may include fatigue, drowsiness, difficulty in sleeping, loss of mental acuity, minor coordination problems, and irritability.

The precipitating event that produces jet lag is clear: it is the sudden readjustment you demand of your body when traveling across time zones. But not all jet lag is the same.

Flying eastward (and therefore resetting your body clock forward) is often more difficult than flying westward and adding hours to your day (flying north or south does not produce jet lag). Most people's bodies adjust at the rate of about 1 hour a day. Thus, after a 4-time-zone change, your body will require about 4 days to resynchronize its usual rhythms.

PREVENTION STRATEGIES

You might try to schedule your arrival at your destination at roughly your usual bedtime according to the clocks in the time zone to which you are flying. Or try sleeping on the plane and planning to arrive at the hour you usually start your day. In this way, you immediately begin to orient your body systems to the new time schedule, a valuable psychological and physiological advantage. Getting added sleep before departure may help to ease the symptoms of jet lag.

Another strategy is to begin resetting your body's clock several days in advance of your departure by adopting a sleep-wake pattern similar to the day-night cycle at your destination. Or try setting your watch to the time of your destination when you are halfway through the trip so that you start thinking in terms of the new time.

If you have an important event or meeting at your destination, get there 2 or 3 days in advance. That way, you will not be disadvantaged by a fresh case of jet lag.

Limit food and alcohol intake during your flight. Eat a high-protein, low-calorie diet just before, during, and just after your flight. Drink lots of beverages, but avoid, or at least minimize, drinking beverages containing caffeine or alcohol. Bring or order fruit on the plane; avoid fatty foods.

Note that, if you are on a regimen of medications, you may have to make adjustments as to when you take them. Check with your physician before leaving. If you are diabetic and are taking long-acting insulin, you may have to switch to regular insulin until you adjust to the new time, food, and activities.

PART III

KEEPING FIT

The chapters that follow concern prevention. Whether it's a matter of what to eat, which exercise program to adopt, or how to amend certain destructive behaviors, you will find in these pages concrete advice on achieving, regaining, or improving your health and conditioning.

CONTENTS

CHAPTER 13

NUTRITION AND HEALTH

CHAPTER CONTENTS

WHAT IS A HEALTHFUL DIET?

Not many subjects are of consuming interest to virtually all of us—but food is certainly one of them. It is a principal pleasure of life and also a life-giving essential.

Without the continual replacement of nutrients in our bodies, we would die. Food is so important that from time immemorial it has formed the basis for rituals in every society. Much of the way we evaluate one another is based on how we look—and this is a link, albeit an indirect one, to food. The success of a society itself has traditionally been measured by the abundance and quality (or lack thereof) of its food.

As American society has evolved, we have made a national goal of having a rich and varied quantity of food. We have made it a point of national pride to be able to feed others the world over. We have become a rich nation, as is evidenced in part by our collective waistline.

As recently as 50 years ago, the focus of nutrition research was to fight malnutrition and diseases caused by a lack of basic nutrients. Today, the pendulum has swung, and overconsumption has replaced deficiency as America's leading nutrition problem.

In response, Dr. C. Everett Koop, Surgeon General under President Ronald Reagan, released a report on the nation's health. The report placed nutrition high on the nation's health agenda, along with reducing the spread of AIDS and eliminating smoking.

The report presented solid evidence based on years of research. It argued that for the two of every three of us who do not smoke or drink excessively, the choices we make that will most influence our long-term health prospects are dietary. The report gave recommendations on how Americans must change their diets to ensure better health.

These recommendations are covered in this chapter, along with basic information on how our bodies use food. The pages that follow also discuss weight control and how to eat well when faced with disease.

If you need specific advice about a nutrition question beyond what is offered in these pages, talk to a registered dietician. The letters R.D. (for Registered Dietician) after a person's name show that he or she is registered with the American Dietetic Association. To obtain this title, a person must earn an undergraduate degree in a 4-year program in food science and nutrition at an accredited college or university, complete 6 to 12 months of accredited or approved training in practical aspects of dietetics, and pass a national examination. In addition, Registered Dieticians must complete 75 hours of professional education every 5 years.

Some states have licensing procedures, and a dietician may also be a Licensed Dietician (L.D.) under the regulations of the state health department. Your local health department or physician can refer you to a competent dietician.

Other people may also be helpful in examining or improving your nutritional status. Some physicians have a particular interest in nutrition. Home economists are often a good source of information on meal planning, food preservation, and food preparation, but they are less qualified than an R.D. in advising about the nutritional needs of a specific person.

The term nutritionist is not specifically defined and, unfortunately, it is sometimes used by people who have no real nutritional training and who seek to sell dietary supplements or weight-loss schemes. Some may even display a diploma or certificate that may mean very little.

You can verify whether a school listed on a diploma is a bona fide educational institution by asking your local librarian to check whether the school is accredited by an agency recognized by the US Department of Education or the Council on Post-Secondary Accreditation. The nutritional staff at your local hospital may also be a help for evaluating qualifications.

IS THERE AN IDEAL DIET?

In this day of intense interest in diet and health, many people yearn and often search for the perfect diet—one that will produce super health, above-normal vigor, strength, and resistance to disease, one that will delay aging, and one that will keep them slim. So pervasive is this interest that thousands of people spend vast quantities of time and money searching for the perfect answer.

Does or can such a diet exist? In all likelihood, the answer is no. Our nutritional needs differ at each stage of our lives from infancy through childhood, maturity, pregnancy, and old age and in states of disease. We also vary in our genetic tendencies toward diseases, including hypertension, some cancers, and heart and other vascular diseases, so food elements such as salts or fats pose different risks to different people.

The human body needs various substances from the environment in order to grow, reproduce, and survive. We breathe air to acquire the oxygen our cells need to survive; we drink water to replenish vital supplies of liquid. And we eat to provide us with all-important energy sources since energy is provided by the body's use of ingested protein, fat, and carbohydrate. Other elements are also needed, although in much smaller amounts. These include essential amino acids, fatty acids, minerals, trace minerals, and vitamins.

All the foods we eat provide some level of nutrition. There may be no one perfect diet for all of us or even for one of us at all times. But a sound knowledge of nutrition is the best way to attain the best diet possible.

The Basic Components of Food. Our food is made up of many components that, when combined in appropriate proportions, provide a complete diet. The major groupings are carbohydrates, proteins, and fats. Other groups are trace nutrients, known as vitamins and minerals, needed in smaller amounts. Each category has a different function in the regulation, growth, and repair of the body.

Carbohydrates. Carbohydrates are starches or sugars and are found primarily in breads and cereals and in fruits and vegetables, including leafy greens such as broccoli and lettuce. The starches are referred to as complex carbohydrates, and sugars (found in fruits as well as in refined sugars) are called simple carbohydrates. Cane or beet sugar, known technically as sucrose, and corn syrup, which contains the sugar known as fructose, make up a considerable portion of the average American diet.

Proteins. Proteins are composed of building blocks called amino acids. Some of these amino acids can be produced by your body; others cannot. Those that must be obtained from the diet are called essential amino acids.

The essential amino acids in meat, eggs, milk, and cheese are very efficiently used. Such proteins have high biological quality. Proteins found in vegetables, cereals (such as wheat, rice, or corn), peas, and beans do not provide an optimal ratio of essential amino acids. Thus, a greater amount of protein of plant origin is needed to meet your body's requirements than of protein of animal origin. Protein of plant origin has a low biological quality.

Fats. Fats are found in various foods and in various forms. Fats are found in foods of animal origin, such as meat, poultry, and fish, and in foods of vegetable origin. Meats often contain a considerable proportion of fat, even after all visible fat has been removed. In general, the more tender and expensive a cut of meat, the more fat it will contain. Some fats, such as cooking oils and salad oils, are liquid; others, such as butter, margarine, vegetable shortening, and trimmed meat fat, are solid.

Chemists classify fats according to the structure of their building blocks, the fatty acids. Fatty acids are saturated or unsaturated. Unsaturated fats are further classified as mono-unsaturated (mono means one) and polyunsaturated (poly means many).

The chemical structure of saturated fatty acids is different from that of unsaturated ones, and this structure determines the characteristics of each type of fat. Saturated fats usually are solid at room temperature, and unsaturated fats are liquid at room temperature. Saturated fats are less likely to turn rancid, which is why they are used in many processed foods that must withstand long storage times.

Unsaturated fats can be made into saturated fats through a process called hydrogenation. This makes them more solid. Usually only a small proportion of the unsaturated fat in a product is converted to saturated fat during hydrogenation. Fats that contain a generous proportion of saturated fats are common ingredients in commercial baked goods and other processed foods.

No food contains just one type of fatty acid. All foods contain a mixture of fats in various proportions. For example, olive oil is termed a mono-unsaturated fat, but it contains small proportions of saturated and polyunsaturated fatty acids.

Various fatty acids have different effects on blood cholesterol levels, which have been shown to have a relationship to heart disease. Saturated fats tend to raise your total blood cholesterol level. Mono-unsaturated fats tend to raise the concentration of high density lipoprotein (HDL), the "good" part of blood cholesterol, without significantly raising the total blood cholesterol level. Polyunsaturated fats tend to reduce your total blood cholesterol level, but at the expense of the protective HDLs. (For more about fats and your health, see What Do Measurements of Blood Fats Mean?, page 789.)

Vitamins. Vitamins are substances that are essential in certain chemical transformations in your body and need to be present in your diet only in very small amounts. They help the body process proteins, carbohydrates, and fats. Certain vitamins also contribute to the production of blood cells, hormones, genetic material, and chemicals of your nervous system. Our bodies are unable to synthesize adequate amounts of most vitamins, so we must get them from the foods we eat.

The essential vitamins (there are 13 in all) are divided into two categories: fat-soluble and water-soluble.

The fat-soluble vitamins are A, D, E, and K. Vitamins A and D are stored in the liver, and reserve supplies there may be sufficient for as much as 6 months. Reserves of vitamin K, however, may be sufficient for only a few days, and the supply of vitamin E is somewhere in between.

Both vitamins A and D can produce toxic effects when taken in excessive amounts. Toxic effects from taking large amounts of vitamin E have not been clearly demonstrated, but it does accumulate in the body's fatty tissues. Vitamin K is scarcely stored at all, and toxic effects from taking large amounts have been found only rarely.

The water-soluble vitamins include vitamin C (ascorbic acid) and the B vitamins. They are stored to a lesser extent than fat-soluble vitamins. Although it is popularly believed that the water-soluble vitamins are harmless when taken in large amounts, this is not always true.

Some of the water-soluble vitamins may have strong medicinal effects—good and bad—when taken in large amounts. Large amounts of niacin, for instance, are sometimes used to reduce high levels of fats in the blood; on the other hand, they also can cause abnormal liver function and increase blood sugar levels. Ascorbic acid in high amounts can increase oxalate excretion in the urine. Thus, if you have oxalate kidney stones, avoid large amounts of ascorbic acid. In large doses, pyridoxine (a B vitamin) can cause nerve damage. In short, taking megadoses of vitamins is rarely warranted—and often is potentially hazardous.

Minerals. Minerals such as calcium, magnesium, phosphorus, potassium, sodium, and sulfur are also essential parts of the diet. Known as macrominerals, they are needed in relatively large amounts in the diet (those we need less of, termed microminerals, are discussed below). Calcium, phosphorus, and magnesium all are important in the development and health of bones and teeth. Potassium is a major component of our muscles. Sodium helps regulate the fluids of the body, and sulfur is a constituent of protein tissues.

The microminerals (trace minerals) are found in much smaller amounts in our food. Essential trace elements are minerals that, like vitamins, are needed in only small amounts. They include iron, iodine, zinc, copper, fluoride, selenium, and manganese, among others. They are all necessary for normal growth and health.

Calories. A calorie is a measure of energy rather than a discrete part of food. When carbohydrates, proteins, or fats are metabolized (burned) in the body, they produce energy, energy that is measured in a unit known as the kilocalorie. One kilocalorie—which consists of 1,000 calories—is defined as the amount of energy or heat required to raise 1 kilogram (2.2 pounds) of water 1° centigrade (1.8° Fahrenheit).

We all need energy, but our calorie needs vary considerably. A small, elderly, sedentary woman may need only about 1,000 calories (1 kilocalorie) per day, but a large, young, physically active man may need as many as 4,000 calories (4 kilocalories) daily.

Dieticians use tables to calculate the nutrient content of various diets; these tables give the calorie, protein, carbohydrate, and fat content of various foods. When such tables are used, the portion of food must be measured accurately, preferably by weighing it.

The term "empty calories" applies to sugars and to alcohol. These foods contribute energy (calories) but no other essential food elements such as vitamins or trace elements. Sugars include cane and beet sugar, fructose syrups, glucose, and lactose. Some of these sugars, such as fructose and lactose, are an inherent part of some of the foods we eat (fruit and milk, respectively). Consuming sugar and even alcohol in moderation should not affect your health adversely, as long as you eat a variety of other foods to provide a good pattern of essential nutrients.

However, if you derive too many of your daily calories from sugars and alcohol, you can develop nutritional deficiencies through simple dilution.

Your Body Composition. Understanding the principles of nutrition involves more than a basic understanding of the various kinds of food we eat. The next step requires some comprehension of the makeup of our bodies. The fact is that protein, fat, and carbohydrate are the largest "ingredients" of the human body.

Protein structures make up about 50 to 60 percent of body weight. These tissues (muscle and vital organs such as the liver) function as the machinery of your body.

Your body does not store extra protein. If you eat more protein than your body needs, your muscle mass will not increase, nor will you have protein on reserve should you need it. Rather, extra protein is converted to fat. In a state approaching starvation, your body will tear down protein tissues in order to use the amino acids as fuel for energy processes. Death by starvation occurs when the body uses up between a quarter and a third of its protein structures.

Carbohydrate exists in the liver and muscles of the body as glycogen stores. Carbohydrate in the form of glycogen makes up about 1 to 5 percent of your body weight.

If your diet is high in carbohydrates and you are eating your full complement of needed calories each day, your glycogen stores, found largely in the liver, will be maximized. This store of fuel can be quickly called upon. For example, marathon runners may eat a diet rich in carbohydrates before a race. Glycogen, after conversion to glucose, is used as a fuel for the brain during brief fasts—such as during an overnight sleep (see Special Athletic Diets, page 361).

Conversely, if you eat a diet low in carbohydrates or if you are on a restricted-calorie diet, your glycogen stores will be rapidly depleted. If you switch from a normal diet to a very low-calorie or a very low-carbohydrate diet, you may lose 3 or 4 pounds within a day or two of the change. Such weight loss, however, will be in the form of glycogen and not fat.

Another "ingredient" of your body is fat. Fat is unlike protein and carbohydrates in that it is an extremely concentrated form of reserve energy and is associated with very little water. Body fat represents nearly 10 times as much energy for its weight as protein or carbohydrate tissues, about 3,500 calories per pound. In a normal person, 15 to 20 percent of body weight is from fat, although extremely obese people may have as much as 50 percent of their body weight in the form of fat.

These discrepancies in stored fats are the result of the way our bodies work. If you eat larger amounts of food than your body can burn, whether in the form of protein, fat, or carbohydrate, your body will store the extra energy as fatty tissue. However, because fat in our diet is so high in calories, indiscretion in fat intake can supply more calories than if protein or carbohydrates were eaten. Conversely, if we eat less food than our bodies need, our fuel reserves are mobilized to meet the daily energy deficit, and fatty tissues diminish—but relatively slowly because of the caloric richness of the fatty tissue.

The primary function of body fat seems to be as a reserve of fuel, but it also constitutes a form of mechanical padding and insulation. Have you ever noticed how overweight people can sit longer and more comfortably on an unpadded bench or chair than can lean people? And how lean people become chilled more easily in cold surroundings?

Body fat also contributes to the regulation of certain hormones in women. Women whose body fat stores become very scant tend not to have menstrual periods. This is often the case with young women suffering from anorexia nervosa or some other form of starvation, and it can be a problem among lean women athletes.

Calibrating degrees of personal fatness is difficult. Skin-fold measuring is one method, but it requires special calipers and considerable skill and practice.

There are methods for reaching rough estimates for groups of people. Perhaps the easiest to use are weight and height tables (see Metropolitan Weight and Height Ta-

METROPOLITAN WEIGHT AND HEIGHT TABLES

Height and weight tables can help in estimating normal weight for average people. Many of these tables were developed by the insurance industry to predict optimal weight for longevity.

The tables of the Metropolitan Life Insurance Company are considered the standard. They are periodically adjusted to reflect new understandings of the relationship between weight and health.

These tables are meant to be used only as a guide and with an understanding of their limitations. You must take into account your particular skeletal structure and muscle mass, as well as your weight and age. If you are a muscular athlete and have an average amount of body fat, you will weigh more than the average given on the chart for your sex, height, and frame size because of your greater amount of muscle. Or, if your bones are small and you are not particularly muscular, your ideal weight might be on the low end of the range.

These tables also do not account for key individual factors such as the amount of body fat and its location on the body. These factors, more than weight alone, influence health.

Weights on most tables are not adjusted for age. The older we get, the more our weight tends to be in the form of fat rather than muscle. Also, we tend to weigh less in youth than in middle age.

bles, this page). Keep in mind, however, that the weight assigned to your sex and height does not take into account your individual makeup and such factors as skeletal structure (are you big-boned?) and the amount of muscle (are you unusually muscular?). These are useful averages, but they are not to be taken as the final word in establishing your place on the slimness-to-heaviness scale.

One final word on the subject of fat. Physicians and scientists often debate whether having a very small amount of body fat is a hedge against some degenerative diseases, such as coronary artery disease (see Atherosclerosis: What Is It?, page 786). In fact, one statistical study concludes that the greatest life expectancy occurs at weights at least 10 percent above the average in the United States.

Alternatively, having only a small reserve of calories in the form of minimal body fat may lessen your chances of survival in the event of serious injury, infection, or disease with prolonged stress and convalescence. Obesity can under no circumstances be termed healthy, but being underweight may offer other health risks.

Changing Body Composition. The composition of the adult body changes during the course of a lifetime. Muscle mass tends to decrease slowly after the age of 30 or 35 and more rapidly after the age of 55. Translated into what your scale tells you, that means that if at age 65 you weigh 10 pounds more than you did at 30, you may actually be 15 to 20 pounds "fatter."

If you have a disorder such as diabetes or hypertension that is aggravated by excess fat tissue in the later years of life, you can use your weight at age 25 or 30 as a desirable goal, as long as you were of fairly average weight at that time. Individuals and their health problems vary considerably, however, and your physician may have reasons to set a different weight as a goal.

We seem to be equipped genetically for a certain distribution of fat. Women tend to carry more of their fat around the hips and thighs. Men often carry excess weight around their abdomens.

The distribution of fat is also related to age. As we get older, our subcutaneous fat tends to shift from the periphery (face, arms, legs, and neck) to the center of our bodies (trunk and abdomen). Furthermore, as we age, fat seems to shift from the subcutaneous

Metropolitan Weight* and Height† Tables

Women (Weight in Pounds)		Height	Men (Weight in Pounds)	
Average	Range		Average	Range
117	102–131	4'9"	. . .	. . .
119	103–134	4'10"	. . .	. . .
121	104–137	4'11"	. . .	. . .
123	106–140	5'0"	. . .	. . .
126	108–143	5'1"	139	128–150
129	111–147	5'2"	142	130–153
133	114–151	5'3"	144	132–156
136	117–155	5'4"	147	134–160
140	120–159	5'5"	150	136–164
143	123–163	5'6"	153	138–168
147	126–167	5'7"	156	140–172
150	129–170	5'8"	159	142–176
153	132–173	5'9"	162	144–180
156	135–176	5'10"	165	146–184
159	138–179	5'11"	169	149–188
. . .	. . .	6'0"	172	152–192
. . .	. . .	6'1"	176	155–197
. . .	. . .	6'2"	180	158–202
. . .	. . .	6'3"	185	162–207

*Weights are at ages 25 to 59 years based on lowest mortality. Weight is in pounds (in indoor clothing weighing 3 pounds for women and 5 pounds for men).

†The table is adjusted to reflect subject without shoes for height measurement.

From *Mayo Clinic Diet Manual*, sixth edition. By permission of Mayo Foundation.

depots to accumulations within the body cavity and around the kidneys. This is one reason why older people often have thin faces and extremities. At the same time, they may have protruding stomachs but little "pinchable" subcutaneous fat over the abdomen.

Metabolism. The processing undergone by the carbohydrates, proteins, fats, and other food substances we eat is termed metabolism. It is the extremely complex process by which the food we eat is converted into energy and structure. The process produces heat, carbon dioxide, water, and waste products. The energy created is used to carry out essential chemical transformations in the body and for muscular activity, and the heat helps maintain body temperature.

The rate of metabolism can be determined by measuring how much oxygen is used and how much carbon dioxide is given off. This rate, measured shortly after waking and before eating, is called the basal metabolic rate (BMR). Physicians have formulas to calculate average BMR or resting caloric expenditure based on metabolic rate standards, but you can get a very rough idea of your daily calorie expenditure with normal activity by multiplying your weight in pounds by 12.

The rate of metabolism, and therefore production of body heat, increases for an hour or two after meals. The rate of metabolism also increases with physical exertion. When you exert yourself, fat and glycogen (stored starch) are used up at an increased rate (see Exercise and Fitness, page 377).

We now have discussed the basic components of food: fat, protein, carbohydrate, vitamins, and minerals. We have reviewed the process by which your body metabolizes fuel to keep you healthy and active. Now it is time to translate that knowledge into action and to identify what, for you, is a prudent, healthful diet.

THE SENSIBLE DIET

Except for people who are in need of a therapeutic diet to deal with a specific health problem, the best overall dietary plan can be stated simply: eat a wide variety of foods including plenty of carbohydrates from fruits, vegetables, and grains and foods including protein such as meats, fish, eggs, and dairy products. Vitamins and minerals exist in almost all of the foods we eat.

Dietary Guidelines for Americans. In recent years, the United States government has been actively encouraging healthful eating habits.

In 1989, the National Academy of Sciences released a report on diet and health. This report offers sound dietary guidelines, which are summarized below:

- *Reduce the amount of fat of all kinds in your diet.* It is estimated that the average American gets almost 40 percent of his or her daily calories from fat. A goal of reducing one's total fat intake to 30 percent of the day's caloric intake is sensible. The intake of saturated fat should be reduced to 10 percent of daily calories, and intake of cholesterol should be less than 300 milligrams per day.

  For many people, a diet high in fats leads to obesity, which in itself has various health implications. People who have a family background of certain forms of heart disease and hypertension can be at particular risk if they follow a diet high in fats (see Avoiding Heart Disease, page 367, and Salt and Hypertension, page 372).

- *Achieve and maintain a desirable body weight through diet and exercise.* Obesity is a major complicating factor of several diseases, including diabetes mellitus (see page 707), hypertension (see page 796), and coronary artery disease (see page 801).

- *Increase the amount of complex carbohydrates and fiber in your diet.* Americans tend to obtain too few of their calories in complex carbohydrates. By eating 50 to 55 percent of our daily calories in carbohydrates (fruits, vegetables, and grains), we can reduce fat intake while increasing consumption of certain vitamins, minerals, and fiber. Try to eat five or more servings (about ½ cup each) of fruits and vegetables daily—especially leafy green and yellow vegetables and citrus fruits. Eat six or more servings of complex carbohydrates, including breads, legumes, and cereals. Dietary fiber plays an important role in the digestion and absorption of nutrients.

- *Eat only moderate amounts of protein.* The American diet contains far too much protein, particularly from animals. Eating no more than twice the recommended dietary allowance (RDA) for protein is a good goal. You may also find that if you reduce the amount of protein that you eat, your intake of fat will decrease because much of our fat intake, particularly cholesterol, is found in animal products. However, don't give up meats; just eat less of them.
- *Select foods relatively low in sodium, and limit the amount of salt you add to your food in cooking and at the table.* Most Americans consume much more salt than they need. For most people, sodium levels may never be part of a health problem, but it still is a good idea to reduce excess salt in your diet. If you have a family background of hypertension or if you have a sensitivity to sodium, it is even more important to restrict salt in your diet.
- *If you drink, reduce your alcohol intake to one or two drinks per day.* If you are pregnant, do not drink at all (see page 429).
- *Adolescent girls and women need more calcium and iron in their diets.* Most women and girls consume about half the amount of calcium necessary for healthy growth and lifelong maintenance of bones. During childbearing years, many women and girls consume much less iron than is needed to maintain health.
- *Make sure your diet and your children's diets contain fluoride to help prevent tooth decay.* Fluoridated water can reduce significantly the development of tooth decay in children and adults. If your water supply is not fluoridated, consult your dentist regarding dietary fluoride supplements.
- *Do not take daily vitamin and mineral supplements in excess of the RDA unless your physician tells you to.* The theory that more is better does not necessarily hold true for vitamins and minerals. The best way to obtain the vitamins and minerals your body needs is to eat a diverse diet. A daily multiple vitamin and mineral supplement containing 100 percent of the RDA is not harmful and may be beneficial if your diet is lacking in certain areas, but anything more can harm your health.

These guidelines are for healthy people, not for those who need special diets because of disease and conditions that interfere with normal nutrition.

THE FOUR BASIC FOOD GROUPS

In the 1950s, the US Department of Agriculture developed the concept of four basic food groups. The goal was to help people choose appropriate kinds and amounts of foods to form the basis of a balanced, healthful diet. The groups include the following:

- Milk and dairy products
- Meat, fish, and poultry
- Fruits and vegetables
- Grains (such as breads and cereals)

There is also a fifth group for people who want to increase their caloric intake. It is comprised of fats, sugars, and alcohol.

If you select foods from these basic groups and then consume the recommended daily dietary allowances (amounts), you will achieve a balanced, healthful diet.

Milk and Dairy Products.   The milk group is composed of dairy products of all kinds. Dairy products such as milk, all forms of cheese, yogurt, ice cream, and ice milk provide protein, carbohydrates, fats, vitamins, and minerals. Dairy products, other than butter, are excellent sources of calcium, an important nutrient for the growth and maintenance of bones. Milk—whether whole, skim, or partially defatted (2% and 1%)—is fortified with vitamin D. The average adult requires two servings each day. Milk is also our major food source of calcium. Women, especially pregnant and lactating women, and growing children require more than two servings each day. Margarine is fortified with vitamin A.

Meats.   The meat group includes all meats, poultry, and fish, as well as some foods of vegetable origin. This group of foods is high in protein of good biological quality, which is important in the building and maintenance of body tissues. Foods in this group are also high in some vitamins and minerals. Eat a minimum of 4 to 6 ounces of meat each day or its equivalent (see The Daily Food Guide, page 353).

Fruits and Vegetables. Vegetables and fruits provide fiber as well as necessary vitamins, minerals, and carbohydrates. Much of the fiber found in apples and citrus fruits, unrefined oat products, dried beans, peas, and lentils is soluble. Soluble fiber acts like a sponge, absorbing water as it moves through your digestive system and producing larger and softer stools. Insoluble fiber passes through your body quickly and helps you maintain regulation in such body functions as elimination of stool. Insoluble fiber is found in whole wheat products and many vegetables.

Recently, soluble fiber has gotten much publicity for its possible effectiveness in helping to regulate or balance the production of cholesterol. Good sources of soluble fiber include oat products, dried beans, peas, lentils, apples, and citrus fruits (see Diet and Disease, page 366).

Vegetables such as peas and beans contain high amounts of protein. This form of protein is of somewhat lower biological quality than that in eggs or meat and should be combined at the same meal with certain grains such as corn, wheat, or rice to form a complete protein. We recommend four or more servings of fruits and vegetables each day.

Grains. Grain products such as breads and cereals are composed largely of complex carbohydrates. They also provide healthy doses of vitamins, minerals, and fiber. "Enriched" flour has had some of the vitamins that are lost in the milling of grain restored. Such foods include all forms of bread—wheat, corn, rice, oats—and grains such as rice, barley, and corn. Each day, eat four or more servings of grain products.

Water. Water often goes unmentioned in discussions of diet because it has almost no food value. Our bodies can exist for weeks without food, but if we stop replacing water we die within days.

Your body is able to store only a limited amount of water because water is continuously used in the workings of every cell. Thirst and mechanisms that regulate the amount of urine formed all act to keep the amount of water in tissues of your body within narrow limits. Nutrients, waste products, antibodies, hormones, and other elements are carried to and from body cells in

---

THE DAILY FOOD GUIDE

The following serving and food selection recommendations form the basis of a sound dietary regimen.

Group	Minimum Number of Servings	Examples of Serving Sizes and Food Selections
Milk		
Children < 9 yr	2–3	1 cup milk, 1 cup yogurt (plain),
Children 9–12 yr	3	1½ oz cheese, 2 cups cottage
Teenagers	4	cheese, 1¾ cup ice cream or
Adults	2	ice milk, or 4 Tbsp cheese
Pregnant women	3	spread or Parmesan cheese
Nursing mothers	4	
Meat		
Children	2	2–3 oz cooked lean meat,
Teenagers	2	poultry, or fish, 2 eggs, 1–1½
Adults	2	cup dried peas or beans, ½–1
Pregnant women	3	cup nuts and seeds, or 4 Tbsp
Nursing mothers	2	peanut butter
Fruits and vegetables		
Children	4	½ cup juice, ½ cup fruit or
Teenagers	4	vegetable (canned, cooked), 1
Adults	4	cup fruit or vegetable (raw),
Pregnant women	4	medium-size fresh fruit, or ½
Nursing mothers	4	grapefruit or cantaloupe
Grains		
Children	4	1 slice bread, 1 cup ready-to-eat
Teenagers	4	cereal, ½ cup cooked cereal
Adults	4	or grits, ½ cup rice, or ½ cup
Pregnant women	4	pasta
Nursing mothers	4	
Fats, sweets, alcohol*		
		1 tsp margarine or butter, 1 tsp sugar, 1 Tbsp mayonnaise, salad dressing, 1 Tbsp jelly, 1 cup soft drink, or 3½ oz wine

*Select these if you need additional calories after you eat the recommended number of servings from the food groups above.

From *Mayo Clinic Diet Manual*, sixth edition. By permission of Mayo Foundation.

---

water. Water is also a necessary part of the digestive process, it helps regulate your body temperature, and it carries away waste.

Water is in everything you drink and, to some degree, in the food you eat. Knowing when you are drinking enough is not usually too difficult to determine: thirst is a reasonable guide to the amount of water you need. Keep your thirst satisfied.

Generous water consumption can help prevent constipation (see Chronic Constipation, page 633) and keeps your mouth moist with a free flow of saliva, thus facilitating oral hygiene and lessening the risk of halitosis (see Bad Breath, page 579).

CALCIUM AND OSTEOPOROSIS

If you are a woman, you have one chance in four of developing osteoporosis after

DIETETIC FOOD LABELING

Today, grocery stores feature an increasing number of prepared foods marketed for people interested in modifying their diets. Such foods are intended to meet the desires of people interested in reducing calories, sugar, sodium, and fat in their diets.

Often, the labels on these foods speak directly to the concerns of the consumer. Yet the terms used are not always clear and sometimes can be misleading.

The Food and Drug Administration has labeling regulations for food manufacturers that, when fully understood, can be useful. But definitions for terms commonly used are not always immediately apparent. Some examples follow.

Low-calorie: A product bearing this claim can contain no more than 40 calories per serving, with no more than 0.4 calorie per gram as eaten. Foods naturally low in calories may not be labeled low-calorie.

Reduced-calorie: To earn this label, the food must be at least one-third lower in calorie content than the food to which it is being compared. The label must describe the comparison on which the claim for reduced calories is based.

Artificially sweetened, diet, dietetic: These terms may be used if a food product qualifies as a low-calorie or reduced-calorie food.

Sugar-free, sugarless, no sugar: Foods bearing these labels contain no table sugar (sucrose). However, they may contain calories from other sweeteners, including corn syrup, fructose, or honey. (The presence of these ingredients must be stated on the label.) Products containing saccharin, aspartame, sorbitol, or mannitol may also bear these labels.

Light and lite: If a product is labeled "lite" and claims are made for its value in reducing calories, the product must meet the same standards as for "low-calorie" or "reduced-calorie" labeling (that is, the product must have reduced calorie content from comparable products). There are no labeling regulations for "light." Often it is used to describe appearance (color) as well as content.

Nutritive and non-nutritive alternative sweeteners: The presence of sweeteners must be indicated on the label.

Sodium restrictions: Sodium-free means 5 milligrams or less of sodium per serving; very low sodium means 35 milligrams or less

of sodium per serving; low sodium means 140 milligrams or less of sodium per serving. Reduced sodium means that the sodium content is at least 75 percent less than the usual amount found in the food. Unsalted means no salt was added during processing to a food normally processed with salt. Note: Unsalted foods can still contain sodium. Check with your registered dietician if this is a concern.

Extra-lean: Products bearing this label are required to have a fat content of 5 percent or less by weight than a comparable product.

Lean or low-fat: Products with these labels have a fat content 10 percent or less by weight than a comparable product.

Light, lite, leaner, and lower fat: Foods with these labels contain at least 25 percent less fat than a similar product.

You may also see the following labels.

Cholesterol-free: Each serving of the food contains no more than 2 milligrams of cholesterol.

Low-cholesterol: Each serving of the food contains no more than 20 milligrams of cholesterol.

Reduced-cholesterol: Each serving of the food contains at least 75 percent less cholesterol than the food it replaces.

menopause. In osteoporosis, bones become thin, fragile, and prone to fracture. A stooped posture and fractures of the spine, wrist, and hip are common. For some older people, complications arising from such fractures can prove fatal (see Osteoporosis, page 982).

The cause of osteoporosis remains unclear. We do know that one factor seems to be the amount of dietary calcium you consume during your lifetime. That is why your diet should include adequate amounts of calcium.

The recommended dietary allowance (RDA) of calcium for men and women from ages 11 to 24 years is 1,200 milligrams per day, and from age 25 years on it is 800 milligrams per day. However, many women consume barely half the RDA for calcium. Dairy products, such as milk, cheese, and yogurt, are particularly rich in calcium. Many women avoid dairy products on the assumption that they are fattening. If this is your concern, consider this—dairy products made from skim milk supply as much or slightly more calcium than do higher-calorie products made with whole milk.

Other sources of calcium include canned salmon and sardines (with the bones), dark green vegetables such as broccoli, kale, spinach, and bok choy, and beans such as kidney, navy, pinto, soy, and black-eyed peas. Because of differences in absorption, the calcium in fiber-rich vegetables is probably less available to your body. Thus, if you consume a high-fiber diet, be careful to include other food sources that are high in calcium. (Note: If you take a bulk-forming agent containing psyllium, take it at times other than mealtime.)

Some brands of yogurt, orange juice, and milk are calcium-enhanced. They usually command a premium price, and may be worth it if your intake of calcium from other sources is low.

What about supplements? In general, it is better to get as much calcium as you can from your diet. However, if you cannot attain your RDA of calcium from food, supplements can help make up the difference. The most common recommended dosage for a supplement to prevent osteoporosis is 1,000 to 1,200 milligrams per day, which is slightly above the RDA for people who are 25 years and older. Discuss taking a dietary supplement with your physician, particularly if you are already through menopause.

Foods Rich in Calcium

Food	Amount	Calcium, milligrams
Dairy products		
Whole milk	1 cup	290
2% milk	1 cup	297
Skim milk	1 cup	302
Buttermilk	1 cup	285
Yogurt, plain low-fat	8 oz	415
Cheddar cheese	1 oz	206
Swiss cheese	1 oz	272
Processed American cheese	1 oz	174
Cottage cheese, creamed	½ cup	62
Vanilla ice cream	½ cup	88
Sherbet	½ cup	48
Grain products		
Bread, white	1 slice	30
Biscuit, homemade	1	34
Biscuit, from mix	1	58
Frozen waffle	1	85
Cereal, refined	½ cup, cooked	49
Vegetables		
Broccoli	½ cup, cooked	88
Brussels sprouts	½ cup, cooked	32
Cabbage	½ cup, cooked	44
Cress	½ cup, cooked	61
Beet greens	½ cup, cooked	99
Collards	½ cup, cooked	152
Dandelion greens	½ cup, cooked	140
Kale	¾ cup, cooked	134
Mustard greens	½ cup, cooked	138
Spinach	½ cup, cooked	83
Swiss chard	½ cup, cooked	73
Turnip greens	⅔ cup, cooked	184
Leeks	3–4 medium	52
Lima beans	⅝ cup, cooked	47
Okra	8–9 pods	92
Parsnips	½ cup, cooked	45
Rutabaga	½ cup, cooked	59
Fruit		
Orange, Valencia	1 medium	48
Rhubarb	½ cup, cooked	174

From *Mayo Clinic Diet Manual*, sixth edition. By permission of Mayo Foundation.

FOOD SAFETY IN YOUR HOME

Our food and water supplies generally are remarkably safe. However, the food you eat and the water you drink can make you sick. In the following pages, we review these risks and offer tips on how you can avoid trouble. The risks include food poisoning from bacteria or other organisms, natural toxins, and possible contamination from pesticides.

Federal and local health departments monitor our food supply, but their resources are not unlimited. There has been, and probably will continue to be, controversy regarding how much funding should be provided to these agencies and how their resources should be allocated. Should monitoring be done widely or should more intense scrutiny be given to certain target areas where the probability of difficulties is greater? How valid are assumptions based on observations made on test animals given large amounts of a substance that humans consume in very small amounts? These and other food safety issues may be better understood in the next several years so that our food supply perhaps can be made even safer.

Infectious Food Poisoning.   Food poisoning is a gastrointestinal infection caused by eating contaminated food. The most common symptoms are loss of appetite, nausea, vomiting, diarrhea, and stomachache. In most people, the discomforts of food poisoning pass within a few hours (see Infections of the Gastrointestinal Tract, page 617).

Bacterial contamination of food can occur if food is handled improperly. Thus, cleanliness in the kitchen is of paramount importance. Wash your hands before you handle food. Wash dishes in hot water. Cook foods at temperatures that minimize the number of bacteria. Cool and refrigerate foods adequately and rapidly (see Proper Handling of Food, page 358.)

The recent rise in popularity of salad bars in restaurants and grocery stores poses a potential new risk. Observe how well the items are chilled and how well they are protected from the inevitable sneezes and coughs of the public before buying from them.

Many of our common foods carry large numbers of bacteria. Raw vegetables, salads, and milk products, in particular, contain or carry bacteria. Ordinarily, these bacteria pose no risk because the body is capable of destroying them. However, people with suppressed immune function, such as those receiving chemotherapy or organ transplants, may become vulnerable to infections from uncooked everyday foods.

Staphylococcus aureus.   The most common bacterium that causes food poisoning is *Staphylococcus aureus.* Referred to as staph infections, such outbreaks can occur among large numbers of people. Sometimes these infections are traced to an open wound on the hand of a food preparer. Bacteria from the wound are passed to the food, where they can multiply rapidly if the food is left at room temperature.

Foods with mayonnaise or cream bases make particularly good environments for growth of bacteria. Within 3 to 6 hours after eating, people experience nausea, vomiting, and diarrhea, which persist for about 12 hours.

Clostridium perfringens.   A form of infectious diarrhea is caused by *Clostridium perfringens.* This can result from allowing cooked meat to cool slowly to room temperature over a period of 12 to 24 hours. Symptoms of abdominal pain and diarrhea begin within 6 to 12 hours after eating the contaminated meat and last about 24 hours.

Salmonella.   These bacteria are responsible for another common and potentially fatal form of food poisoning. The bacteria are found most commonly in poultry, eggs, and meat. Symptoms (which may last less than a day) usually appear 12 to 48 hours after you eat contaminated foods. In addition to gastrointestinal discomforts, you may run a fever. Infants or older people are especially at risk from this infection.

Botulism.   This is a particularly dangerous form of food poisoning. Fortunately, it is rare because of modern canning techniques. Unlike most other bacteria that cause food poisoning, *Clostridium botulinum* grows in the absence of oxygen. Botulism can occur when sealed foods are not processed at high enough temperatures to kill the organism. Also, cooking this canned food after you remove it from the container will not destroy the toxin. If you are about to open a canned food, be sure that the can is not swollen or that the safety button in the center of the lid has not popped up. If you see either, throw the food away.

Botulism can be fatal. It requires prompt treatment with a substance called antiserum (see Botulism, page 534). Symptoms include muscle weakness in addition to nausea, vomiting, cramps, headache, and double vision.

Traveler's Diarrhea. Another common bacterial food hazard is traveler's diarrhea. This form of poisoning results from eating strains of the common intestinal bacterium *Escherichia coli* (known as *E. coli*), which produces toxins. These toxins can cause a severe diarrhea that lasts several days. You are most likely to find strains of this bacterium, to which you have little immunity, when you travel abroad. In many countries it is common in the water supply and on foods prepared in a less-than-hygienic manner. Outbreaks of this form of food poisoning can occur among large groups of people.

When traveling in developing countries, shun untreated water and ice, salads, raw fruits and vegetables that you cannot peel, and uncooked milk products (see Prevention of Traveler's Diarrhea, page 340).

Contamination from *E. coli* bacteria also can occur from eating meat that has been handled, such as ground meat, and then not thoroughly cooked. Regardless of where you are in the world, avoid hamburgers that are pink in the middle.

Hepatitis A. Hepatitis A can be caused by eating raw shellfish harvested from sewage-contaminated waters. Even though federal regulations and posting of contaminated waters offer some protection, there is a risk to eating raw shellfish. The wisest course is to consume them in the cooked state (see Acute Viral Hepatitis, page 650).

Contaminated Fish. Other forms of food poisoning can occur from eating fish that have ingested certain one-cell organisms. Such infections occur occasionally from eating fish such as snapper, sea bass, barracuda, and amberjack caught off Florida or the West Indies, or puffer fish from the Pacific Ocean. In addition to the gastrointestinal symptoms common to food poisoning, symptoms include a rash, numbness in the hands and feet, headache, muscle ache, tingling of the lips and tongue, and face pain. In some cases, the debilitating symptoms can last for months.

Another form of food poisoning results from eating certain kinds of fish that are not fresh. Bacterial decomposition of tuna, mackerel, bonito, mahimahi, bluefish, or albacore can cause immediate gastrointestinal distress as well as a rash and pain around the abdomen. Symptoms usually last only a day or so.

One final note on food poisoning from seafoods: sushi, the popular Japanese dish made of raw fish, can be responsible for a form of gastrointestinal distress characterized by abdominal pain in addition to nausea and vomiting. Its cause is not a bacterium but a parasitic worm, anisakiasis, which infests small crustaceans upon which many kinds of fish feed.

Naturally Occurring Food Intoxicants. Certain foods contain toxins that can cause serious or even fatal gastrointestinal ailments. For example, certain forms of mushrooms, most commonly those of the amanita family, can produce poisons that cause severe intestinal distress as well as tearing of the eyes, salivation, sweating, dizziness, mental confusion, and coma. If not treated within a few hours you can die.

Amanita mushrooms are not cultivated, so they can be gathered only in the wild. To be safe, never eat mushrooms you find outdoors unless you are positive of their identity (see Poisonous Plants, page 302).

We all know the benefits of the potato. Not everyone knows, however, that potatoes can develop a toxin. This toxin can produce intestinal distress. Do not eat potato sprouts or potato eyes. If you prepare green potatoes, be sure to peel away all portions that have any tint of green.

Peanuts, another ordinarily healthful food, can develop an unhealthful mold when not stored properly. Do not eat moldy or shriveled peanuts.

Other Intoxicants. The possibility of contamination of foods with pesticides and other man-made substances is a continuing cause for concern. Always wash fruits and vegetables carefully. Pesticides and most other contaminants are likely to be on the surface.

One of the problems presented by such food intoxicants is largely psychological. Today's techniques for measuring such substances allow detection of exceedingly small amounts. Even if the quantities are thought to be harmless, our anxieties may be sustained simply by the knowledge that the intoxicants are present. Unless they reach a level determined to be harmful, these substances in our food supply do not seem to pose a significant risk. Still, alertness and monitoring programs conducted by our public health departments continue to be important.

Food Processing   Many people are concerned about the effects of food processing. "Processing" covers anything done to a food to prepare it for market. Processing efforts may range from simple washing to creation of a nearly new synthetic food.

For instance, soybean proteins can be prepared in a highly purified form and then used as a constituent in foods meant to resemble meats of various sorts. Such foods may contain substances for preservation, flavoring, and texture.

Some people focus their concerns on food preservatives. Chemical preservatives and antioxidants are present in many of the foods and beverages most of us consume each day. For several decades, sulfur dioxide and similar compounds have been used to preserve flavor and color. Commonly known as sulfites, these chemicals generally are useful and appropriate for human consumption. Sulfites are used by stores and wholesalers on fresh fruits and vegetables and by restaurants to keep certain foods fresh. Many processed foods also contain sulfites. By preventing spoilage, they help to keep food wholesome, palatable, and safe from molds and other decay.

Some people, however, have a sensitivity to sulfites and experience unpleasant symptoms shortly after eating or drinking foods or beverages containing sulfites. If you have this problem, avoid foods containing sulfites (see Food Allergies, page 469).

One concern about processed foods is whether the nutritional value is lost during processing. In commercial canning and freezing operations, losses of vitamins and minerals may occur. Ingredients such as sugar, salt, and fat—which sometimes are added in considerable quantities—can make these processed foods less nutritionally sound than those you prepare yourself.

PROPER HANDLING OF FOOD

Foods that present the greatest risk for contamination during storage, preparation, cooking, and serving are meat, poultry, and eggs. The principles of proper handling are as follows.

Wash Your Hands.   To avoid contamination by *Salmonella* bacteria or other organisms when preparing any food—especially poultry and meat—wash your hands thoroughly with soap and water before and after handling the food. Then, wash your utensils (or cutting board) with hot soapy water before allowing them to come into contact with any other food.

You can wash an acrylic board in your dishwasher, where high temperatures kill organisms. After use, disinfect a wooden cutting board with a solution of 2 teaspoons of household bleach mixed with 1 quart of water. Flush the board thoroughly after applying the bleach. To minimize contact with other foods, reserve a separate cutting board for poultry and meat.

Do Not Thaw Meat at Room Temperature.   Thaw meat or poultry in a microwave oven or in your refrigerator, then cook the meat immediately.

Do Not Consume Uncooked Marinades. If you marinate meat or poultry, do not serve the marinade unless it has been cooked at a rolling boil for several minutes. (Also, serve poultry and meat on a clean plate, with a clean utensil, so as not to contaminate the cooked food with its raw juices.)

Cook Poultry and Pork Thoroughly. Use a meat thermometer. Place it in the thickest portion of the pork or the poultry thigh (*not* in contact with a bone). Before the meat is done cooking, the thermometer should register 180° to 185° Fahrenheit for poultry and 137° Fahrenheit for pork. Juices should run clear when the meat is pierced.

FOOD SCARES

Our food and water supplies are the safest they have ever been and are among the safest in the world. Although continuing vigilance over the safety of the foods we eat and the water we drink is important to our individual and collective health, perhaps it is our overconcern that sometimes allows unnecessary food scares to develop.

We should not ignore possible risks to health from chemical agents in our food and water. However, we do need to keep the focus on more important, ongoing risks (such as smoking, use of alcohol, and lack of use of auto seat belts) and not be swept away by momentary panics. We need to be careful—but we have to realize that we can never make our lives absolutely free of risk.

Do not cook poultry such as turkey at low temperature over a long time.

Refrigerate Leftovers Promptly. Cool poultry and meat quickly when refrigerating it. In particular, do not let stuffed fowl stand for long periods before refrigerating it. Better yet, remove the stuffing promptly after cooking and before refrigerating.

Never Use Cracked Eggs. *Salmonella* bacteria can enter cracked eggs and contaminate them; therefore, it's safest to check eggs for cracks before you use them—and discard any questionable eggs.

Cook Eggs Thoroughly. Even an uncracked egg may contain bacteria, but *Salmonella* bacteria are destroyed by heat, so cook eggs thoroughly. Avoid dishes that use raw eggs such as Caesar salad dressing, hollandaise sauce, homemade eggnog, and high-energy drinks that use raw eggs. To keep eggs fresh longer, refrigerate them in their original cartons.

Do Not Eat Moldy Foods. Generally, it is best to throw out foods that are moldy, such as leftovers. Cheese is an exception—just trim off the mold before serving the cheese.

CAFFEINE AND YOUR HEALTH

You hear a great deal these days about caffeine. Can it harm you? How much is too much? We cannot know because the research is incomplete.

Most of us tend to associate caffeine exclusively with coffee. Coffee certainly is a large source of caffeine. Half the world's coffee supply is consumed within the United States. But coffee is not the only source of caffeine. Tea, carbonated beverages such as colas, cocoa, and chocolate all contain caffeine.

Certain medications, particularly nonprescription drugs for colds and allergies, use caffeine to counteract the sleep-inducing effects of antihistamines. Nonprescription stimulants such as NoDoz and Vivarin rely on caffeine as their main component—usually about twice the amount of caffeine per dose as a cup of coffee.

The Benefits. For all its recent bad press, caffeine does have benefits. Its most obvious effect is its ability to stimulate.

Caffeine has certain medical applications. It constricts blood vessels in the brain; thus, it is used to treat certain types of migraine headaches and to counteract certain drugs that depress the central nervous system. It is used to treat hyperactive children, upon whom it seems to have a calming effect.

The Drawbacks. Caffeine's disadvantages include potentially undesirable effects on health. People who drink large quantities of coffee run the risk of developing irregular or rapid heartbeats, insomnia, upset stomach, increased blood pressure, anxiety reactions, and increased body temperature. Caffeine also can interfere with fine muscle coordination and timing.

The Food and Drug Administration (FDA) warns pregnant women not to consume caffeine because it may harm the health of their fetuses. Some researchers believe there is a link between consumption of caffeine and stillbirth, miscarriage, and birth defects. Although such associations remain unproven, why take a chance? We endorse the FDA recommendation.

What Should You Do? As with many decisions regarding your diet, moderation is the best approach. For the average person, one or two 6-ounce cups of regular, caffeine-containing coffee or 20 ounces of a caffeinated soft drink per day are considered safe. If you have ulcers, avoid even decaffeinated coffee because of its acid-producing qualities. If you have hypertension, use caffeine with caution. It can raise your blood pressure. If regular coffee keeps you awake at night, switch to decaffeinated.

Cutting Down. To cut down on caffeine, do so gradually to avoid possible ill effects of sudden withdrawal. (People often report headaches, drowsiness, nausea, and reduced attention span when they stop abruptly.) There are several methods.

- Mix decaffeinated coffee in with your regular coffee when it is brewing.
- Substitute regular instant coffee because it contains less caffeine per cup than brewed coffee.
- Cut your consumption by 1 cup a day over the course of a week or two.

You can, of course, do the same with tea or other beverages that contain caffeine. Be

Approximate Caffeine Content of Foods	
6-ounce cup brewed coffee	100 milligrams
6-ounce cup instant coffee (1 rounded teaspoon)	55–60 milligrams
6-ounce cup decaffeinated coffee	2 milligrams
6-ounce cup tea	35–40 milligrams
6-ounce cup cocoa	5 milligrams
12 ounces cola	40–50 milligrams
1 ounce bittersweet chocolate	20 milligrams
1 ounce baking chocolate	25 milligrams

careful when switching to herb teas, however. Some types, particularly homemade varieties, can have the same or worse effects as coffee.

SPECIALIZED DIETS FOR THE HEALTHY

For various reasons, people sometimes follow special dietary strategies. For example, some vegetarians regard avoiding meats as a moral imperative. Athletes may select a diet in the hope of improving strength or endurance. For healthy, active people, there are alternatives to the rules of a conventional diet.

Normal Athletic Eating. Many people have a mental image of athletes at the "training table." The vision may be of a team of muscular football players devouring huge slabs of steak before a game or of runners swallowing mounds of spaghetti before a marathon. In fact, there is no one diet that produces optimal vigor or athletic performance—and there are as many misconceptions about so-called training diets as there are diets.

One misapprehension is that high-protein diets increase strength. Many athletes consume commercially prepared "protein supplements" in an effort to increase their muscle bulk and strength.

If you are an athlete and you eat a nutritionally balanced diet, you have no need for extra protein. The protein requirements of athletes are only a little higher than those of non-athletes. However, most athletes already receive this additional protein in their normal diets. The typical American diet is between 50 and 75 percent above the recommended dietary allowance for protein.

If increased muscle mass is your goal, weight-lifting and increased calorie intake can help (but select complex carbohydrates instead of, for example, meat or dietary supplements).

Similarly, exercise does not increase your body's vitamin needs. Thus, taking vitamin supplements cannot improve athletic performance.

All of us need fat in our diets. Although our bodies can make most fats from carbohydrates or protein, there are some fatty acids, known as essential fatty acids, which the body must have, that can be obtained only by eating foods containing fat. However, athletes, who burn a great many calories in exercise, need more than an average amount of fat if they are to maintain body weight. Alternatively, athletes who need to lose weight can begin by eliminating some of the fat they eat.

For the athlete and non-athlete alike, the need for carbohydrates is far greater than the need for protein or fat. In fact, the recommended distribution of dietary calories for athletes is the same as for healthy adults: 55 to 65 percent of your food should be complex carbohydrates, 25 to 30 percent fat, and only 12 to 15 percent protein. (This recommended nutrient distribution is the same for those wanting to lose, maintain, or gain weight.)

Drink Enough Water. Adequate fluid is vital for the athlete. Proper hydration is the most frequently overlooked aid to athletic performance. For most of us, thirst is a good sign of our need for water; however, it is not a reliable indicator during physical activity. If you are going to engage in vigorous exercise in which you perspire, drink an extra pint of water 2 hours before the competition or workout, and 3 to 6 ounces every 10 to 20 minutes during exercise.

To determine how much liquid you lose during a workout, weigh yourself before and after it. Then, over the course of a few hours afterward, drink about a pint of fluid for every pound you have lost.

Drinks containing a high percentage of sugar may delay stomach emptying; thus, avoid them. Instead, select a drink that contains less than 10 percent sugar. (The rate of stomach emptying is similar to that when water is consumed.) Orange juice is 11 percent sugar, and you can mix water with the orange juice in equal amounts to lower the sugar content.

Commercially prepared drinks are available. They contain sugars and electrolytes such as sodium and potassium. These drinks are designed with the intent of preventing undue depletion of body water and electrolytes during exercise. Such drinks ordinarily are unnecessary but may be useful if exercise is unusually intense and prolonged and is performed under hot, humid conditions that cause profuse perspiration.

If you train in a hot environment for several weeks, acclimatization will take place and the loss of electrolytes in your sweat will be reduced. Generally, the sodium and potassium you lose in your sweat are small enough that they can be replaced by eating ordinary food lightly salted. Also, you do not need salt tablets. They can irritate your stomach and cause nausea.

Iron-Deficiency Anemia. Certain kinds of athletic training can have an effect on your body and on its use of and need for certain nutrients. Blood hemoglobin concentrations tend to decrease in the highly trained athlete and may appear to be evidence of anemia (lacking in iron). This decrease in blood hemoglobin level appears to result from a dilution due to an increased amount of fluid in your blood vessels. (Runners who exercise several hours each day actually may lose small amounts of blood in the intestinal tract.)

As an athlete, eat foods rich in iron, such as meats, and also consume citrus fruits. Citrus fruits eaten or taken as juice help facilitate your body's absorption of the iron in vegetables, cereals, and other non-meat sources. These foods can help prevent potential iron-deficiency anemia. But consult your physician before taking iron supplements. Excess iron consumption over a period of time can pose a significant health threat.

Osteoporosis. Women athletes can be vulnerable to osteoporosis (the weakening of bones due to loss of calcium). When a woman's body fat content falls below a certain amount, her hormones react so that menstruation ceases. Because many women athletes are involved in sports in which lean-

ness is required for maximal performance, the diminished amount of female hormones in association with the cessation of menses may be a factor that contributes to future development of osteoporosis.

A lack of calcium in the diet does not seem to be the major factor, as it seems to be in other women, but if you are an athlete, be particularly careful to eat foods rich in calcium to achieve the recommended dietary allowance of this important mineral (see Calcium and Osteoporosis, page 354). You may need to take supplemental calcium carbonate tablets to reach the goal of about 1,000 to 1,200 milligrams per day (see Osteoporosis, page 982).

Special Athletic Diets. Carbohydrate seems to be the preferred fuel for working muscles. In general, like everyone else, athletes should rely on bread, cereals, vegetables, and fruits for at least 55 to 60 percent of their daily calorie needs. However, there are specific strategies you can use in advance of a particular event.

Carbohydrate Loading. Carbohydrate loading is a practice sometimes used by long-distance runners. It can only benefit athletes participating in endurance events (90 minutes or more), and it should be done no more frequently than three or four times per year. Two or 3 days before a competition, you eat a diet high in carbohydrates. You do this after consuming a low-carbohydrate, high-fat, high-protein diet in combination with continued exercise for up to a week before the competition.

Carbohydrate loading supplies your muscles with a large amount of glycogen, which is the most readily available fuel during competition. It also tends to increase your body weight by 2 or 3 pounds. The glycogen is stored in your muscles (and your liver), and this contributes to your body weight. The practice of carbohydrate loading will increase your endurance, especially if your diet is not normally high in carbohydrates.

We believe athletes who participate in endurance events such as long-distance running should follow a high-carbohydrate diet *throughout* training. From the seventh to the fourth day before competition, reduce your consumption of carbohydrates. At this time you should receive approximately 50 percent of your calories from carbohydrates. (Training activity remains intense on these days.) On the third to the second day before competition, you decrease training and increase carbohydrate intake to approximately 70 percent of daily calories. This modified sequence results in muscle glycogen levels equal to those provided by carbohydrate loading. In addition, most athletes find this new routine easier to follow.

High-Protein Diets.   A low-carbohydrate, high-protein diet tends to reduce glycogen stored in your muscles and liver and to impair endurance. Still, this diet often appeals to wrestlers, whose weight is crucial in qualifying to compete in a given weight class. If a wrestler wants to compete in a lower-weight category, a low-carbohydrate diet in the days immediately preceding the event can help keep weight down by several pounds while not greatly impairing strength. It will, however, affect endurance.

Water-Weight Diets.   Some wrestlers use sodium-restricted diets and diuretics in an effort to reduce body weight from water. Such practices can encourage faintness and weakness and may cause the loss of potassium, an essential nutrient. Avoid these diets.

The Pregame Meal.   In the past, much attention was given to the meal eaten before a competition. Often it consisted of meat and other high-protein foods.

Today we know that it is better to eat a meal primarily of carbohydrates, with a moderate amount of protein and a low amount of fat. Such a meal provides glycogen, the most readily available fuel during competition. Eat this meal 3 or 4 hours in advance of competition to ensure that the food has left your stomach (you should not feel full or heavy). Remember, as a general rule, carbohydrates empty from your stomach faster than proteins, and proteins empty faster than fats.

Vegetarian Diets.   Vegetarian diets appeal to people for various reasons. For some people, religious and philosophical teachings prompt adherence to a vegetarian regimen. Other people seek possible health benefits, because evidence suggests that vegetarianism may be a hedge against heart attacks, stroke, and possibly some cancers.

At the same time, a poorly planned vegetarian diet can put you at risk for disorders such as vitamin B_{12} deficiency, iron-deficiency anemia, growth retardation (in persons who have not yet achieved their full adult growth), and osteoporosis, to name a few. Avoiding these risks means devising a healthy vegetarian diet—that is, one in which all of your body's nutrient needs are met.

Careful planning is the key to such a diet. Because many of the nutrients a human body needs are found most readily in animal products, finding substitutes requires effort.

There are various degrees of food restrictions in vegetarian diets. Total vegetarians, known as vegans, restrict their foods to those of plant origin only. Fruitarians further restrict their foods to only raw or dried fruits and nuts, honey, and olive oil. Lacto-vegetarians eat foods of plant origin plus milk and other dairy products. Lacto-ovovegetarians eat plant foods, milk and dairy products, and eggs. Semivegetarians (partial vegetarians) eat certain animal foods such as poultry or fish but usually exclude beef, pork, and game.

Obviously, the question of the nutritional adequacy of a particular vegetarian regimen depends on the extent of food restrictions. Also, vegetarian children and teenagers, pregnant and lactating women, and people recovering from a serious illness or injury need to take precautions to ensure that all of their body's needs are met. Such people should follow a vegetarian regimen only with the careful supervision of an experienced, registered dietician.

Protein is the nutrient of primary concern when planning a vegetarian diet. Protein found in foods of plant origin tends to have only small amounts of one or more essential amino acids. (Essential amino acids are those that your body cannot manufacture—you must obtain them from your diet.) Protein from animal sources contains essential amino acids in an optimal proportion, and they are of high biological quality. (You need to eat relatively less of protein foods with high biological quality to meet daily needs.)

In adhering to a strict vegetarian diet, you must eat specific amounts and combinations of plant proteins if you are to get the complete protein your body needs. Grains and cereals with ingredients including wheat, corn, oats, and rice provide some essential amino acids, and legumes such as peas, peanuts, and beans provide others. When you combine a grain and a legume (such as rice) with peas, or cornmeal with beans, you have a more nearly complete set of essential amino acids.

Another important nutrient in the vegetarian diet is vitamin B_{12}. Vegetarians who consume milk or eggs will get enough of this vitamin. Those who do not can eat foods artificially enriched with vitamin B_{12}. Some commercial foods made from soybeans and other plant proteins are fortified with vitamin B_{12}. A deficiency of this vitamin is a serious medical disorder (see Pernicious Anemia, page 479).

Vegetarians who eat eggs and dairy products also usually receive enough calcium and riboflavin, but the pure vegetarian has to devise special dietary strategies. Many foods of plant origin contain calcium, but they may not be as easily used by the body because of the presence of fiber and oxalic acid in the foods. Oxalic acid and fiber may interfere with the body's ability to use the calcium present in the foods. Thus if you are a strict vegetarian, you may need calcium supplements.

Vitamin D, iron, and zinc are other nutritional elements needing special attention in the vegetarian diet. Most of us obtain vita-

RECOMMENDED DIETARY ALLOWANCES (RDAs)

You have heard advertisements touting foods containing "100 percent of the recommended dietary allowance" for this or that nutrient. Have you ever wondered what the term "recommended dietary allowance" means, and who devised all the numbers? Wonder no more.

RDAs are estimates of the amounts of essential nutrients you need to prevent nutritional deficiency, assuming you are healthy. RDAs currently show recommended amounts of nutrients based on age, sex, height, and weight. They are formulated by the Food and Nutrition Board of the National Research Council (part of the National Academy of Sciences).

These recommendations are meant to serve as guides rather than specific targets; thus, they have a substantial safety margin built in. This allows for variations in specific needs. A diet providing even substantially less of a given nutrient than specified by the standards will not necessarily cause a nutritional deficiency.

The United States Recommended Dietary Allowances (USRDAs) constitute simplified standards that are carried on vitamin bottles and boxes of packaged foods such as cereal. The USRDAs are based on the RDAs and recommend the highest RDA of each nutrient.

USRDAs for Children Age 4 and Older and for Adults

Shown here are the amounts of vitamins and minerals that equal 100 percent of the USRDAs. A daily allowance has been established for *only* these nutrients.

Look for the USRDAs on the labels of multivitamin/ mineral supplements and some packaged foods.

The label *must show* these seven essential vitamins and minerals:

Vitamins and Minerals	100 Percent USRDAs
Vitamin A	1,000 retinol equivalents (RE) or 5,000 International Units (IU)
Vitamin C (ascorbic acid)	60 milligrams (mg)
Thiamine (vitamin B_1)	1.5 milligrams (mg)
Riboflavin (vitamin B_2)	1.7 milligrams (mg)
Niacin	20 milligrams (mg)
Calcium	1 gram or 1,000 milligrams (mg)
Iron	18 milligrams (mg)

The manufacturer *may choose* to list the percentage of the USRDAs for these essential nutrients:

Vitamins and Minerals	100 Percent USRDAs
Vitamin D	400 International Units (IU)
Vitamin E	30 International Units (IU)
Vitamin B_6	2 milligrams (mg)
Folic acid (folacin)	0.4 milligram (mg)
Vitamin B_{12}	6 micrograms (μg)
Biotin	0.3 milligram (mg)
Pantothenic acid	10 milligrams (mg)
Phosphorus	1 gram or 1,000 milligrams (mg)
Iodine	150 micrograms (μg)
Magnesium	400 milligrams (mg)
Zinc	15 milligrams (mg)
Copper	2 milligrams (mg)

min D through fortified milk and exposure of our skin to sunlight. If you do not drink milk you must rely on sunlight or on a vitamin supplement. Only brief exposures to sunlight are usually sufficient for the manufacture of this vitamin by the body. However, vegetarian children and pregnant and lactating women should not rely solely on sunlight but should take a supplement.

The high fiber content of most vegetarian diets tends to impair absorption of iron and zinc. Good sources of iron include enriched cereals and grains, legumes, dates, prunes, raisins, and leafy green vegetables. You can enhance absorption of the iron in vegetables by drinking citrus juice with your meals. Good sources of zinc include legumes, nuts, and spinach.

In general, vegetarians are not healthier or less healthy than people who consume diets in which animal proteins are present. However, if you are a vegetarian, make a special effort to ensure that you get all the required nutrients in forms your body can effectively use.

SETTING THE PACE FOR WEIGHT CONTROL

Anyone who has struggled with a weight problem yearns for the ability to become thin immediately. Indeed, each year the market is flooded with the latest in instant weight-reduction plans.

Just remember this: most claims are greatly exaggerated.

Consider this, too: anything that makes you lose weight at a sustained overall rate of more than 2 pounds per week is a possible risk to your health.

The good news is that you need not master complicated formulas or scientific theories to learn about real, healthful weight loss. The concept is simple: your excessive stores of fat can be used up by expending more energy (calories) than you consume.

The Daily Calorie Deficit.   Let's take a more detailed look. The first step is to reduce your food consumption so that you eat less food than your body needs to perform the physical, mental, and other tasks that you demand of it. The difference between your daily calorie expenditure and calorie intake is called the *daily calorie deficit.*

The daily calorie expenditure can be calculated approximately by multiplying your weight in pounds by 12. This may underestimate your expenditure somewhat if you are younger or male—and overestimate it if you are older or female. The calorie intake of a diet can be estimated from food tables, although you must carefully measure amounts and sizes of portions. There may be substantial error in estimating both intake and expenditure of calories. A dietician can help with such a calculation.

The second step involves the way your body fills the daily calorie deficit. Ideally, to lose weight, your body would use only body fat to provide extra calories. In fact, however, body protein also is used (more is used if the deficit is large and if the dietary protein intake is small and of poor biological quality). Loss of this body protein increases the rate of weight loss because approximately the same number of calories is contained in a pound of body protein tissues as found in one-eighth to one-tenth of a pound of body fat.

The Rate of Weight Loss.   If you are considerably overweight and begin a weight-loss program by eating less food, you may notice a rapid loss during the first week or two. This initial weight loss can help give you confidence in your plan. However, be aware that such loss may not be limited to a loss of fat alone. Your weight loss also may be due in part to a loss of fluid and a depletion of glycogen stores in your muscles and liver. Thus, the 2 to 5 pounds you may lose those first few days can make you feel good about the plan, but permanent weight loss (fat loss) is a slower process.

To lose a pound of fat a day requires a deficit of 3,500 calories, a nearly impossible goal—although many quick-weight-loss schemes imply that this is possible. A more reasonable goal is to plan for a deficit of about 500 to 1,000 calories per day. Such a limitation will generally result in a weight loss of body fat of about 1 or 2 pounds per week.

The advantage of the smaller calorie deficit (500 calories) is somewhat greater confidence that the protein tissues of your body are not being lost in the process of weight reduction. The advantage of the greater calorie deficit (1,000 calories) is that a faster rate of weight loss results. Also, minor errors in measuring quantities of food are less likely to negate results of your dietary efforts.

Remember this: Any program that promises you more than 2 pounds of weight loss per week is unhealthful in that the additional weight loss will be in the form of water, protein, and glycogen—not just body fat.

You can calculate your approximate weight loss per week over a long term by multiplying your daily calorie deficit by 0.002. For example, if you expend 2,000 calories per day in energy and eat 1,500 calories worth of energy, your deficit will be 500 calories per day. Five hundred calories multiplied by 0.002 yields an expected weight loss of 1 pound per week.

The Setbacks. If you binge in the form of a single big dessert generous in calories and carbohydrates, you may well find your weight up 2 or 3 pounds the next day, mainly because of the increase in glycogen stores. This might lead you to the disheartening conclusion that a single meal or dessert can wipe out a week of dieting. Not so.

If you return to your dietary program promptly, most, but not quite all, of that increase in weight will disappear during the next day or two. The weight loss will be behind schedule by the amount of calories in the big dessert, but it usually amounts to the wiping out of no more than a day or two of previous dieting.

Half the process of dieting is controlling your intake of calories. The second half involves increasing the number of calories you burn.

THE ROLE OF EXERCISE IN WEIGHT CONTROL

Losing weight and keeping it off are much easier if you combine a food plan with an exercise plan.

Exercising increases your calorie expenditure. When it is combined with a reduction in calorie intake, exercise is a great asset to a weight loss program, *and* it can help strengthen and tone muscles and increase your vigor and feeling of well-being. Lack of vigor is a common complaint among people who are reducing (see also Exercise and Fitness, page 377).

The benefits of exercise are great, but do not expect a rapid loss of weight due simply to a vigorous exercise plan. Loss of weight should be steady and is best achieved by combining good eating habits with regular exercise. Keep in mind, however, that even a little exercise will help burn off fat. It may be too small to be apparent in the day-to-day fluctuation of weight, but every little bit does help. Remember also that with exercise, protein needs may increase.

Before embarking on an exercise and diet plan, visit your physician. If you have a physical disability that prevents even moderate exercise such as slow walking, don't despair. You can lose weight successfully solely by reducing your calorie intake. It just takes longer.

Motivation. One of the problems with exercising is keeping motivated. Many people find that once they reach their weight goals they gradually lose interest in their exercise programs as well as in their careful eating patterns. First they skip a workout or two, then several in a row. After a time they find themselves back in their old sedentary habits.

The only way to keep fit long-term is to incorporate your exercise into your normal routine—like managing your money and keeping in touch with family and friends. The following are some suggestions for creating an exercise plan that becomes part of your normal routine, one that you can use while you lose weight and, just as importantly, one you will maintain *after* you reach your goal.

Be realistic. Few of us will ever have the perfectly shaped bodies that exercise videos and some publications show. Do not be intimidated by them. Do not compare yourself with them.

Instead of trying to carve out the perfect physique, concentrate on toning your muscles and strengthening your heart and lungs. In this way you will be focusing your exercise toward the most important aspect of your program, your increased good health.

Choose your activities carefully. What you do should match your personality. Select an individual sport such as tennis or racquetball if you like to compete on a one-to-one basis. If you like to socialize, choose a team sport or one in an organized group, such as dancing or aerobic exercise classes. If you enjoy solitude, try walking (highly recommended for all ages and many stages of fitness), jogging, bike riding, or cross-country skiing. Whatever you choose, make sure it is something you can do regularly, at least three times each week for 20 minutes or more. Try to schedule the activity for a regular time. This helps you get into a habit of exercise (see also What Exercise Is Right for You?, page 382).

Set priorities. Lack of time is the most common excuse for dropping an exercise program. However, studies show that people who exercise have the same amount as or even less leisure time than sedentary people—it is just that they *find the time* for exercise.

Take charge of your time. If your schedule is in disarray, exercise becomes just one more nuisance. If you make a commitment, 30 minutes or an hour of exercise three to five times each week can be easy to maintain.

Vary your routine. If you get bored with a constant pattern of exercise, mix it up. Varying your activities is also a good way to prevent wear and tear on your body. Ride your bike one day, jog the next, dance another—they are all good aerobic exercises. Weight-lifting, calisthenics, and swimming all firm muscles.

Do not overdo. Some people who finally make a commitment to exercise over-train. They become so enthusiastic about exercise that they set unrealistic goals for themselves. This can lead to injury or frustration when the body does not respond as quickly as desired.

To get started on the right track without overexerting, use a trainer or fitness advisor for the sport you choose. Start your exercise program by investigating local community programs or membership in a health club. Adopt a moderate pace and be sure to get enough rest. If you develop problems, contact a trainer, physician, or specialist in sports medicine promptly.

Make an investment. Many people feel more committed to an activity if they put money into it. Some people also find that the peer pressure of a class helps keep them involved. Look on such spending as an investment in your health.

But spend wisely. You do not have to sign up for the deluxe membership if all you plan to do is take a few classes. You do not need the very best athletic equipment to pursue an activity. Buying a pair of jogging shoes may help motivate you to start your program, but buying the most expensive pair will not make your body tone up any faster.

Do not worry about how you may appear to others. The class is for your benefit. Forget about how you look in a leotard. Remember that most people in these classes are most concerned about their own appearance—not yours.

Reward yourself. Just as you may occasionally indulge yourself in a treat while on your eating plan, you may find that moderate self-indulgence in your exercise program helps keep you motivated. Treat yourself occasionally to a new tape to listen to while you walk, or to a new sweatshirt.

Have fun. "No pain, no gain." "Feel the burn." Unfortunately, such attitudes can make working out such serious business that you really do not look forward to it. And if it seems like a never-ending unpleasant chore, you may well look forward to stopping it. Try to look at exercise as a way to release tension or frustrations, a time for quiet reflection, or something that makes you feel good. That is why it is important to choose an activity that gives you some kind of pleasure.

DIET AND DISEASE

There are many theories regarding preventive nutrition. Claims seem always to be made that preventing or curing countless disorders, ranging from the minor and inconvenient to the debilitating and fatal, is merely a matter of using this or that food or food additive.

Not all diseases and disorders have a nutritional component. However, several ailments do, including diabetes, heart disease, hypertension, and various chronic gastrointestinal disorders.

In the following pages, we consider the diet-and-disease link for each of these ailments as well as some of the often ineffective therapies associated with various food fads and vitamin and mineral supplementation programs.

AVOIDING HEART DISEASE

Some factors that put you at high risk for heart disease are beyond your control (for example, your heredity). But one risk factor, a high blood cholesterol concentration, may be affected by what you eat.

In short, reduce the amount of fat and cholesterol you consume, particularly if you are susceptible to having a high cholesterol value. For most people, this need not involve a revolution in eating patterns. Moderation is the key. Small changes, consistently followed, can have a significant impact.

For a detailed discussion of preventing heart and blood disease, see Controllable Risk Factors, page 787.

FOOD FADS

Food can be symbolic. From ancient times, humankind has endowed particular foods with various attributes. In some of the early Near East civilizations, for example, foods were designated as having either hot or cold qualities, and one was advised not to mix these at the same meal. Certain primitive societies believed that eating a tiger's heart enhanced a man's courage.

Even now, the rhinoceros is being hunted to near extinction because of the belief that eating powdered rhinoceros horn will aid sexual potency. The simplistic expectation that the properties of foods are assumed by or passed into the eater with little alteration is exemplified in the modern Western world by the practice of athletes who eat large amounts of protein foods and take protein supplements for the purpose of building muscle.

Adoption of unusual eating habits can be a vehicle for expressing one's political views or a means of protest. Views on nutrition can even have a religious aspect.

There are certainly plenty of unqualified people ready to make nutritional claims. The fads they spawn come and go and are generally characterized by a brief but intense enthusiasm and then a fading away of interest, often to be supplanted by another similarly strong and then dwindling interest or hope. The "Beverly Hills diet" is one such fad. It requires that the person eat only fruit for the first 2 weeks to achieve weight loss and increase vigor. The "Scarsdale diet" is a low-carbohydrate, high-protein (ketogenic) diet for weight loss, as is the "Cambridge diet." All these diets are presented with appealing but incorrect theories on how you can achieve a shortcut to fat loss. Most of these have been published in book form and apparently have enjoyed commercial success.

Scientific exploration of various foods we eat and their relationship to health sometimes unwittingly spawns some of the fads we see each year. A few scientific reports about the properties of a specific food are published, sometimes in reputable publications, and soon the machinery of faddism is under way. Before long, newspapers and magazines across the country discuss the magical benefits or serious toxicity of certain foods.

An example is the current fad about oat bran. There are undoubted nutritional benefits from the use of fiber in the diet, soluble fiber in particular; but the manner in which oat bran has been promoted and the way in which it has been received by the public justify categorizing the current use of oat bran as a fad. Although there is research to support the idea that eating a serving or two of oat bran each day can help reduce cholesterol, such findings have led to an immense commercial tide. Despite the fact that you would need 6 or more cups of oat cereal to equal the recommended amounts of 35 to 40 grams of oat bran per day, many cereal companies have suddenly begun to tout the benefits of their oat bran products. There is also a spinoff effect, with other fiber sources such as psyllium seed. Even corn-cob flour is being incorporated into cereal or baking ingredients.

People consume oat bran believing that this is all they need to do to lower their cholesterol levels. They fail to recognize that other dietary changes are needed for proper control of blood fats. In addition, oat bran and other fibers may combine with calcium in the gut to form a compound your body cannot absorb. Thus, the calcium and the fiber are eliminated from the body before potentially beneficial effects occur. Thus, if your diet is high in fiber, you may need more calcium than usual.

Some of the preparations used to make oat bran palatable are extremely high in fat and sugar. Increasing your intake of fiber, in general, is a good idea, but focusing too closely on one specific food is not—especially if eating one muffin for its bran also means consuming quantities of butter, sugar, and other ingredients whose potential for increasing blood cholesterol far outweighs the potential benefits of the oat bran.

A similar fad several years ago involved a largely mythical disease. Hypoglycemia is a legitimate condition characterized by an abnormally low blood glucose level. It occurs in diabetics taking insulin or oral hypoglycemic drugs (see Diabetes Mellitus, page 707) and as a result of certain rare tumors (see page 723). At some point, however, a fad started. The fad suggests that people who are hungry, cranky, or nervous a few hours after eating are suffering from "hypoglycemia." The "treatment" is to eat something sweet or high in carbohydrates. There is nothing wrong, of course, with eating when you are hungry. Often it does make you feel better. But to self-diagnose your hunger as a "disease" is unwise.

Other common misconceptions about foods include the extraordinary powers sometimes attributed to vitamins and minerals. Vitamin E seems to be one target for commercial exploitation. One theory holds that large doses of vitamin E will increase sexual performance. Another claims that vitamin E can prevent heart disease. Vitamin C also has been touted as helpful in preventing colds. Controlled studies have not proved this to be true.

Claims often are made that honey has unique nutritional benefits. Not true. Honey has essentially the same nutritional properties as ordinary sugar. Your body does not seem to differentiate the way it processes and uses them.

Much has been made of supposed higher-quality nutrition in foods grown in "organic" conditions. Promoters claim that foods produced by using inorganic (chemically produced and processed) fertilizers are of poorer nutritional quality. However, when studied in a laboratory, foods grown using "organic" manure and those grown using commercial fertilizers show few or no such differences. Organic gardening and farming practices may be desirable from a conservation standpoint, but the food produced is not nutritionally superior to conventionally produced food.

For any person who eats a well-balanced diet containing the necessary proteins, fats, carbohydrates, vitamins, and minerals, fad diets promising healthy people improved health are less than useless. Because they are misleading, they are potentially harmful. The harsh reality is that additives or special foods cannot cure or prevent disease. The best way to avoid disease by dietary means is to eat a balanced diet (see The Sensible Diet, page 351).

NUTRITION AND THE CANCER PATIENT

Good nutrition is important for everyone. However, it is particularly important for people undergoing treatment for cancer; and proper eating can be especially difficult at this time. Treatments such as chemotherapy and radiation often disrupt eating patterns. You may feel nauseated. You may have no appetite, or find that medications change your ability to taste accurately. Foods may lose their taste.

You may find that you are so tired or ill that the last thing you feel able to cope with is eating. Some cancer patients lose their appetite even when they are not undergoing treatment.

Proper eating is vitally important to the success of cancer treatment. People who eat well during treatment maintain their stamina better and thus are more able to withstand potential side effects of chemotherapy and radiation therapy. They also tend to have fewer infections and remain more active during treatment.

What constitutes eating well? A healthful diet during cancer treatment is virtually the same as at any other time. You need to eat a variety of foods each day. You need servings from each of the four basic food groups (fruits and vegetables, meat and other proteins, grain products, and dairy products). Ideally, each day eat four or more servings of fruits and vegetables, four or more servings of grains (such as breads, cereals, pastas, and rice), two to three servings of proteins (such as poultry, fish, meat, and vegetable proteins such as beans, peas or nuts combined with grain), and two or more servings of dairy products that are high in protein, calcium, and vitamins (these include milk, cheese, yogurt, and ice cream).

DIET AND CANCER PROTECTION

These days there is a great interest in the effect of diet on cancer risk. Much research is under way to evaluate and clarify the role that diet and nutrition play in development of cancer. Although no direct cause-and-effect relationship has been proved, statistics do show that some foods may increase or decrease the risk for certain types of cancer.

The American Cancer Society and the National Cancer Institute have developed dietary guidelines to help people reduce the risk of developing certain kinds of cancer. These dietary recommendations are consistent with dietary guidelines for Americans put forth by the United States Department of Agriculture and the Department of Health and Human Services. They include general recommendations for an overall healthy diet, and are as follows:

- *Keep a normal body weight.* Obesity is linked to increased death rates from some cancers in humans, particularly those of the prostate, pancreas, breast, ovary, colon, gallbladder, and uterus.
- *Avoid too much fat in your diet, both saturated and unsaturated.* Evidence from epidemiologic studies suggests a relationship between dietary fat levels and the occurrence of prostate, colorectal, and other cancers. At present, the reasons for such correlations are unclear.

    Recent reports suggest that dietary fat intake may be unrelated to the incidence of breast cancer. No guideline for fat intake has been established, but it seems clear that in general the lower the fat intake, the less the risk of cancer. A prudent guideline for fat intake is 30 percent of your total calorie intake. (Do not try to eliminate fat from your diet; it is neither healthful nor possible.)
- *Eat foods rich in fiber.* The National Cancer Institute recommends a fiber intake of 25 to 35 grams each day. Dietary fiber appears to protect the body against some forms of cancer, particularly colorectal. The manner in which specific types of fiber work is unclear. Therefore, eat fiber daily from various dietary sources such as fresh fruits, vegetables, and whole-grain products.
- *Eat foods rich in vitamins A and C daily.* (Some examples include dark green and deep yellow fresh vegetables and fruits, such as carrots, spinach, sweet potatoes, peaches and apricots, as sources of vitamin A; and oranges, grapefruit, strawberries, and green and red peppers for vitamin C.) Vitamin A may help decrease the incidence of several cancers, including those of the oral cavity, pharynx, larynx, and lung. Also, animal studies have shown that ascorbic acid, commonly known as vitamin C, can inhibit the formation of some carcinogenic compounds that are produced when nitrates are eaten. Still, there is no suggestion that you should consume more of these vitamins than listed in the USRDAs (see page 363).
- *Include, as part of your regular diet, such vegetables as broccoli, cabbage, Brussels sprouts, kale, cauliflower, kohlrabi, mustard greens, and Swiss chard.* Research shows that these foods seem to offer protection from the development of colorectal, stomach, and lung cancers.
- *Eat only moderate amounts of salt-cured, smoked, and nitrate-cured foods.* This group of foods includes smoked and cured meats such as bacon, sausage, ham, and others. The incidence of cancers of the esophagus and of the stomach is higher among populations in which large quantities of these foods are eaten.

    Some cooking methods, such as barbecuing or smoking, can produce substances that might cause cancer—thus be moderate in using these methods.

    Limit the amount of salt you use in cooking to one-quarter teaspoon of salt per pound of meat and to one-eighth teaspoon of salt per serving of cooked vegetables or cereals. Bypass or eat infrequently and in small quantities high-sodium foods such as ham, bacon, soy sauce, or pickles.
- *If you drink alcohol, do so in moderation.* Drinking large quantities of alcohol over a long period of time increases your risk of liver cancer. Combining alcohol consumption with smoking or chewing tobacco increases your risk of cancer of the mouth, larynx, throat, and esophagus. A limit of two or fewer drinks per day is recommended.

These suggestions are reasonable. You can follow them with little alteration in your daily dietary regimen. Still, the degree of protection from cancer that such actions may confer remains uncertain.

Pay special attention to eating protein-rich foods. They are particularly useful in helping to repair and build body tissues. In general, you need to eat enough food so that your body does not need to call on its stores of protein for energy, thus leaving it less able to repair itself.

Tips for Eating Well During Treatment. How do you go about eating well when you feel ill? Choose foods that are most palatable, then time your eating to take advantage of the times when you feel up to it.

Many people find that some of their favorite foods have scant appeal during therapy. Thus they end up eating a very limited diet. As more foods seem unappetizing, their dietary choices shrink. Don't let this happen.

Keep an open mind about the foods you might eat. Something that is unpalatable today might taste better tomorrow or next week.

When you do feel well, make the most of it. Eat as much as you can of various foods. If you are cooking for yourself, prepare meals you can freeze and easily reheat if you feel ill. (This is the time to use time savers.) Frozen dinners and prepared foods can be a unique help if cooking requires special effort. To make cooking easier, combine canned soups and sauces with fresh foods.

Even if you do not feel like it, give meals a pleasant atmosphere. Surroundings can do a great deal to help you forget how poorly you feel. A meal eaten on your lap may not be nearly as appealing, especially if you have no appetite, as one eaten at the table— from attractive china, with flowers on the table.

Perhaps the biggest problem to overcome during treatment is finding foods that are both appealing and nutritious. Many people find that meats do not appeal to them. If this is a problem for you, try poultry, mild-flavored fish, or cheeses. Mild-tasting dairy products such as cottage cheese and tangy yogurt also are good sources of protein. Even ice cream contains some protein. Also, try eating a peanut butter sandwich or peanut butter spread on fruit such as apple slices. Legumes such as kidney beans, chickpeas, and black-eyed peas are good sources of protein, especially when combined with grains such as rice, corn, or bread.

Pack as many calories as possible into the foods you eat. Warm your bread, and spread it with butter, margarine, jam, or honey. Sprinkle foods with chopped nuts. Enrich foods with nonfat dried milk.

Many people report losing interest in foods that are not particularly healthful. Fried foods, candy, potato chips, and alcoholic drinks are often unappealing, as are coffee, tea, or red meat. Some vegetables, such as those that have a tendency to cause gas or bloating (broccoli, cauliflower, corn, and beans), also often are disliked.

Foods that seem to cause fewer problems include fresh fruits and many vegetables and foods that, in general, are easy to eat and digest. Lightly seasoned dishes made with milk products, eggs, poultry, fish, and pasta often are well tolerated.

If you have trouble eating an adequate amount of food at a single sitting, eat smaller amounts more frequently. Chew your food slowly. Drink liquids at other times. Also, make sure that liquids you drink have nutritional value, such as juices, milk shakes, or milk. If carbonated drinks help calm your stomach, mix fruit juice with sparkling water rather than relying on soda alone. Keep snacks handy so that when you do feel a little hungry you can eat easily. Also, avoid greasy foods and rich buttery sauces. They may make you feel satiated much faster than other foods.

If the aroma of food being prepared makes you feel ill, avoid these smells. Heat foods in a microwave oven, or choose foods that require little cooking or can be warmed at a low temperature.

Many people report problems of elimination, either constipation or diarrhea, during the course of treatment. These conditions may be due to various factors, including medication that irritates the intestine and causes diarrhea or that slows down action of the bowel and promotes constipation. Radiation to the abdomen also can cause diarrhea. A decrease in activity and in variety of foods eaten also can cause constipation and bloating from gas. Some people develop an inability to break down the lactose in milk products during treatment and have to refrain from eating them until treatments are complete.

In the case of constipation, eating foods rich in fiber often can help prevent or combat the problem. Such foods include fresh fruits and vegetables, dried fruits, whole grain cereals and breads, and nuts. Drinking plenty of fluids also helps (see Chronic Constipation, page 633).

Diarrhea can result in a loss of important minerals and fluids. Sometimes a high-fiber diet is effective in treating diarrhea because fiber tends to absorb liquid in the stool and solidify it. Your physician may prescribe an antidiarrheal medication. You may want to avoid dairy products until the diarrhea clears up. If you have cramps, avoid foods that

VITAMIN AND MINERAL SUPPLEMENTS

Many American adults take vitamin supplements regularly. Some people regard them as essential food replacements; others see them as harmless "insurance."

The recommended dietary allowances (RDAs) are amounts of vitamins and minerals estimated to meet or exceed the requirements of most healthy people. They are neither minimal nor required amounts (see Recommended Dietary Allowances, page 363).

A daily multivitamin and mineral supplement that supplies close to 100 percent of the RDAs is not harmful, and it could be beneficial if you eat a very limited diet—one that does not contain foods from the basic four food groups (fruits and vegetables, grain products, meats and other proteins, and dairy products). However, true vitamin or mineral deficiencies in the United States are rare, and few people need to take supplements of any kind.

There is also a danger: those who decide on their own to take megadoses (more than 10 times the RDA) of vitamins or minerals are taking significant health risks.

Food Is Better
The unglamorous but tried-and-true recommendation of eating at least four servings of fruits and vegetables, four or more servings of breads and cereals, two or more servings of low-fat milk and dairy products, and two servings of lean meat or meat substitutes a day is still the best way to ensure adequate nutrition. Food contains many components that work to-gether to maximize your absorption of nutrients.

Although a nutritionally balanced diet is ideal, it may be unrealistic for some people. If you routinely eat less than 1,200 calories a day, a balanced diet will be difficult to achieve. Regardless of how many calories you eat, if your diet regularly falls short in one or more of the four food groups, a daily multivitamin and mineral supplement may be a reasonable precaution.

Here is what to look for when choosing a supplement.

Avoid Gimmicks
Disregard labels that suggest the product is specially formulated for certain groups of people—such as women, the elderly, or the athlete—or for a specific purpose—such as "stress formula."

Maintain Balance
Read the label for the amount of vitamins and minerals or the percentage of the USRDAs (simplified RDAs) per dose. Choose a supplement that supplies close to 100 percent of all the vitamins and minerals instead of one that supplies, for instance, 500 percent of one vitamin and only 20 percent of another.

The exception to this is calcium. Multivitamin and mineral supplements do not contain 100 percent of the RDA for calcium because the tablets would be too large to swallow. Therefore, you take calcium supplements several times per day.

Organic Versus Synthetic
There is no advantage to taking "organic" or "natural" vitamins instead of synthetic ones. Your body does not know the difference and uses them in the same way.

Brand Name Versus Generic Name
Nationally advertised brands are not necessarily better than generic or store brands. Compare the list of ingredients and the percentages of the RDAs. The nationally advertised brands may cost more without offering any real advantage.

Special Needs
Physicians often prescribe specific supplements for persons with special needs. For example, women with heavy menstrual flow may need iron supplements. Women who are pregnant or breast-feeding need additional amounts of iron, folic acid, and calcium. Some vegetarians, especially those who eat no animal products, may not receive enough vitamin B_{12}, vitamin D, calcium, and iron in their diets; thus, a vitamin supplement may be essential.

Before taking any supplement other than a standard multivitamin and mineral supplement, check with your physician or a registered dietician. As little as 5 to 10 times the RDA for vitamin A, for example, taken over an extended period can harm your health.

Again, as is so often the case in matters of nutrition, moderation is the best strategy. Aside from supplements your physician prescribes (perhaps because of the action of a drug you are taking), we do not recommend mineral or vitamin supplementation that goes beyond 100 percent of the USRDA, and then only if your diet is significantly limited in one way or another.

cause gas, such as carbonated drinks of all kinds, cabbage, broccoli, cauliflower, highly spiced foods, and even some forms of chewing gum (those that contain sorbitol). Also, drink liquids between meals (see also Nutrition and Cancer, page 1249).

SALT AND HYPERTENSION

Too much salt (sodium) in the American diet has been the focus of much study and has been given much attention by the media in recent years.

Findings indicate that people in certain population groups that habitually consume large amounts of salt develop hypertension (high blood pressure) more frequently than do individuals who use less salt. Also, research shows that people with hypertension generally can lower their blood pressure if they follow a low-sodium diet.

Blood pressure refers to the force exerted by the bloodstream on the walls of arteries. When there is more fluid in the bloodstream or when the blood vessels are narrowed, the pressure is greater. Roughly 20 percent of people in the United States are sensitive to the effects of sodium.

The American diet tends to be high in salt. We all should be aware of the amount of salt we eat, but a major effort to restrict salt is necessary only if you have hypertension (or if you are prone to developing hypertension). Even then, reducing the amount of salt in your diet is but one important step in lowering your blood pressure.

Sodium is present in nearly all plants and animals we consume. Indeed, our bodies need a small amount of sodium to function properly (approximately half a gram daily, the equivalent of about a quarter teaspoon). The average American consumes 6 to 8 grams (2 or 3 teaspoons) per day. However, with current publicity about salt in the diet, this amount is decreasing.

If you need to limit your salt intake, begin with the food you prepare. Do not use salt when you cook, or use it only in very small amounts. Remove the salt shaker from your dinner table. If food tastes bland without salt, use herbs instead. Avoid salty foods such as chips and pickled foods. Switch from salted butter and margarine to unsalted. (You may be surprised by the good flavor of products now available.)

Be aware that many processed foods contain large amounts of salt. Get in the habit of scrutinizing food labels. These labels list ingredients in order of quantity. Avoid foods in which sodium is high on the list. Look for the terms monosodium glutamate (MSG), sodium chloride (table salt), and even baking soda (it contains sodium). Condiments such as ketchup, prepared mustard, and soy sauce are all high in sodium. Prepared foods such as canned soups, stews, and broths and cured foods such as ham, bacon, cold cuts, and hot dogs also are high in salt content.

For a detailed discussion of High Blood Pressure, see page 796.

THE DIABETIC'S DIET

It is increasingly clear that your weight is an important factor in your overall health. The link is especially strong when it comes to diabetes. *For a detailed discussion of the types of diabetes and its treatment, see Diabetes Mellitus, page 707.*

Obesity is associated with the most common form of diabetes (non-insulin-dependent diabetes mellitus—NIDDM). Evidently, obesity acts as a "trigger," causing genetically vulnerable people to develop NIDDM.

Although the supply of insulin produced by the pancreas might be adequate for a person of normal weight, the demand for insulin is greater in the overweight person. In the obese person with NIDDM the pancreas is not able to keep up with the demand.

Thus, weight control is a crucial element in prevention and treatment of non-insulin-dependent diabetes. About 10 million Americans have this form of the disease; 80 percent of them are overweight. Half of these people are unaware of their condition.

The American Diabetes Association has issued a series of recommendations. These revised guidelines are similar to those from the American Heart Association and American Cancer Society. The focus is on a moderate restriction of fats, with emphasis on complex carbohydrates (see page 347).

If you have NIDDM and you need to lose weight, you may only have to follow some rather general dietary rules, although you may also benefit from specific instructions from a dietician regarding the precautions appropriate to your particular needs. Diabetics and non-diabetics alike can lose weight by adhering to the following dietary guidelines.

Calories. A nutritionally balanced diet is essential to a successful weight-loss plan. Moderate calorie reduction, about 500 calories below daily requirements, seems to be best for ongoing permanent weight loss (see Setting the Pace for Weight Control, page 364). Once you achieve your desired weight, you can increase the amount of calories slightly, but be sure to maintain the lower weight.

Fats and Carbohydrates. Reduce your fat intake to less than 30 percent of your daily intake of calories. Limit saturated fat (fat from animal products) to 10 percent of your total calories. Approximately 50 percent of what you eat should be rich in complex carbohydrates such as whole-grain bread, cereals and other grains, potatoes, rice, and pasta.

Fiber. Some studies indicate that certain forms of fiber can help control glucose and cholesterol in the blood, especially when carbohydrates make up 50 percent of calorie intake. However, the results are not conclusive.

A diet rich in complex carbohydrates, including fresh fruits and vegetables, grains, and cereals, is relatively low in calories and high in fiber.

Reduce your consumption of foods that are high in simple carbohydrates and sugar (including desserts and baked goods such as doughnuts, pie, cake, and cookies). Many of these foods also contain large amounts of fat.

Protein. The standard recommendation that protein should provide 12 to 20 percent of your calories is valid for people who have diabetes and for those who do not. (Exception: if you have kidney or liver problems you may not be able to eliminate waste products produced by metabolism of protein. Therefore, you should consume less protein. See your physician for a recommendation.)

Other Lifestyle Factors. Learn to control your diabetes; don't let it control you. In addition to weight control, two other elements of diabetes management are important, as follows.

Medication. The use of oral medications or insulin injections may be necessary if diet alone cannot control your diabetes. Consistency in the timing and amount of what you eat is especially important if you take medications for diabetes.

Exercise. In addition to helping you control your weight, exercise can help lower your blood sugar concentrations. The key is a consistent pattern of moderate exercise. Get a medical checkup, begin slowly, and follow your physician's instructions carefully. Diabetics have special problems. Some have poor circulation or impaired nerves in the legs. Your physician can help you tailor an exercise program suited to your personal needs.

SPECIALIZED DIETS FOR CHRONIC DISEASES

Some chronic diseases require use of specialized diets. Such diseases include a sensitivity to gluten in foods (known as celiac sprue), liver failure, kidney failure, and kidney stones. When used with proper medical programs, appropriate diets can be important in controlling these conditions.

Celiac Sprue and the Gluten-Free Diet. Celiac sprue (also called non-tropical sprue) can cause improper absorption of nutrients (see page 621). The disease is caused by the body's intolerance of gluten, a protein found in wheat, rye, oats, and barley. The sensitivity to gluten causes the lining of the intestine to lose its many tiny folds (villi) through which nutrients are absorbed. In addition, necessary digestive enzymes cease to be produced in large enough quantities. Symptoms include foul-smelling diarrhea, weight loss, a bloated abdomen, and anemia. Children, who are among the most common sufferers, fail to grow and may develop rickets; adults may develop a bone disease called osteomalacia (see Osteomalacia and Rickets, page 985).

Strict adherence to a gluten-free diet is the main course of therapy. Such abstinence seems, at first glance, to be fairly easy. However, it is actually quite difficult. You must avoid all foods containing wheat, barley, oats, and rye. Products made from gluten-containing grains are staples of American and European diets.

For example, many processed foods contain emulsifiers, thickeners, and other additives derived from such grains. These foods include commercial beverages such as chocolate milk, dietary supplements, cold cuts and prepared meats, breaded prepared foods, cheese foods and spreads, commercial soufflés, omelets, fondue, and soy protein meat substitutes. Also included are commercial salad dressings and gravies, seasoned rice and potato mixes, vegetable mixes, canned baked beans, commercial soups and broths, and commercial ice creams and sherbets. Wheat breads of all kinds contain gluten, as do most baked goods. Commercially prepared condiments such as ketchup, mustard, soy sauce, meat sauces, vinegar, pickles, and syrups all may contain gluten unless the manufacturer specifically states the product is free of gluten.

Rice (which does not contain gluten) may become the mainstay of your diet insofar as grains are concerned. Breads and pastries made with rice flour, corn flour, or potato starch are acceptable. Plain meats, fish, fowl, eggs, dairy products, vegetables, and fruits contain no gluten. Beverages including coffee, tea, carbonated drinks, chocolate drinks made with pure cocoa powder, wine, and distilled liquor contain no gluten. If you are on a gluten-free diet, you can also eat such things as soups and desserts thickened with tapioca, cornstarch, arrowroot, or eggs (see Celiac or Nontropical Sprue, page 621).

Kidney Stones.   Renal lithiasis, the technical term for kidney stones, is a relatively common disorder. An estimated 5 percent of women and 10 percent of men will have at least one stone by the time they reach age 70 years. For most people it is a very painful experience.

A kidney stone is a hard mineralized deposit that occurs within the urinary passage. There are many kinds of kidney stones (see page 898). If you have kidney stones, your physician will determine the particular kind of stones you have and may make some dietary recommendations. In general, you will be advised to drink plenty of fluids each day—up to 3 or 4 quarts—to keep your urine diluted, particularly at night.

If you have calcium stones (the most common form), you will probably be advised to limit your intake of calcium to no more than 600 milligrams per day, to limit your salt intake to 2 grams per day, to avoid excessive protein, and to eat whole-grain foods.

If you have stones containing calcium oxalate, your physician may recommend first that you limit oxalate-containing foods (such as tea, chocolate, berries, and rhubarb) and second that you avoid supplements of vitamin C.

Kidney Failure.   Kidney failure occurs when the kidneys are unable to remove waste products from the blood. It may result from infection, injury, exposure to toxins, or disease.

The two types of kidney failure are acute and chronic; both have nutritional implications. If you have acute kidney failure you will probably be placed on a diet high in carbohydrates and low in protein. If you are on dialysis, you may need more protein and your sodium and potassium intakes may be restricted. (Your physician or dietician will monitor this carefully.)

Chronic kidney failure has many nutritional implications. Nausea, vomiting, and lack of appetite may be helped by eating a diet low in protein. A diet low in protein may also help preserve kidney function. You may also have to govern the amount of water you drink. If you have hypertension associated with the disease, you may need to restrict the amount of liquids you drink as well as the amount of salt you eat. Your physician may limit the amounts of phosphate and potassium you consume (for more information about kidney failure, see page 906).

Liver Disease.   Another problem that has nutritional implications is advanced liver disease. If this occurs, it may result in an increased amount of ammonia in your blood. Protein tends to be broken down into ammonia, so your physician may suggest a diet low in protein. Because vegetable and dairy proteins produce less ammonia than animal protein, your physician may also recommend these foods. People with liver ailments often retain fluids. To minimize this, you may need to restrict salt in your diet.

THE DIETARY RISKS OF ALCOHOLISM

Problems caused by alcoholism are many. They touch virtually every aspect of an alcoholic's life. Not least among them are the nutritional deficiencies and abnormalities that prolonged heavy drinking often will cause.

Alcohol contains only "empty calories"— those that have no nutritional value beyond their energy value. Alcoholics commonly substitute alcohol for food—thus their diets are lacking in essential nutrients.

Eating improperly, of course, is not the only problem they have. Many important nutrients, particularly thiamine and folic acid, are poorly absorbed. In addition, fat accumulates and is stored in the liver in only partially processed forms. Soon the liver swells, producing a condition called "fatty liver," and its function is impaired.

Excessive use of alcohol may result in a condition known as cirrhosis of the liver (see page 653). Some of the protein metabolized by the damaged (cirrhotic) liver is broken down into ammonia and substances called amines. These substances can build up in the body and can impair consciousness, resulting in a condition called hepatic encephalopathy (see page 657).

Consumption of large quantities of alcohol also may cause gastric bleeding or it can damage the pancreas, resulting in pancreatitis, both of which can be fatal (see page 668).

For a detailed discussion of Alcohol Abuse, see page 417.

CHAPTER 14

EXERCISE AND FITNESS

CHAPTER CONTENTS

THE BENEFITS OF EXERCISE

A century ago, most Americans lived and worked on farms. Just staying warm and well fed involved countless daily tasks, all of which required actual physical labor.

For many of us today, the daily routine involves little or no compulsory exercise. Our service economy and innumerable labor-saving devices have made our lives more pleasurable in many ways but have robbed us of the natural, regular exercise we need to achieve optimal levels of health, performance, and appearance.

Physical inactivity and the aging process can result in a steady decline in your capacity to do physical work. If you withdraw from a physically active existence, activities that require strength and stamina become more difficult, the chances of injury become greater, and your risks of heart disease and other ailments increase.

On the other hand, there has been a healthy trend in recent years to "work out." More and more men and women are working out regularly because they like the way it makes them feel as well as its long-term benefits. In some social circles, the after-work cocktail has been replaced by a workout at the club.

It is not hard to understand why so many are turning to a healthier lifestyle that includes regular exercise. After the "pain" of a vigorous exercise session has gone away and the sweat has been showered off, they like the healthy glow of the skin, the toned muscles, and the extra energy that comes from exercise.

The outward signs of a good exercise program are readily apparent. You can tell when your physical fitness improves: your ability to perform physical and even mental work increases. There may be an accompanying reduction in fatigue, tension, and anxiety.

Your muscles and joints will feel more flexible and seem to function better. You may be able to shed extra pounds, especially if a moderate reduction in food intake accompanies your exercise program. But perhaps the most important benefits cannot be seen.

When you exercise vigorously, your muscles require more oxygen. Thus, you must breathe more deeply to fill your lungs with air. Your body's most important muscle—your heart—must beat harder and faster to pump blood to your muscles. In time, your heart becomes stronger and more resilient.

In addition to a stronger heart, blood fat and sugar levels also may be decreased by exercise.

Women who exercise have a better chance of avoiding osteoporosis, a degenerative bone disease that afflicts many older women, provided that they do not become so thin that menstruation stops (see page 1064). An exercise program may even be a factor in helping you quit smoking. Exercise also relieves stress, gives you an overall feeling of well-being, helps you sleep better, and improves concentration.

Just as exercise is important to your health—setting aside time for three 20-minute workouts a week is a sound practice—it is also essential that you match the exercise to your age, physical condition, and temperament.

In the following pages, you will learn about exercise programs. If you can understand the goals, adopt or devise a suitable variety of exercise that fits into your lifestyle, and stay at it, your health will benefit. An important warning to remember, however, is that you should consult your physician before starting a new exercise regimen if you are obese, lead a largely sedentary life, or are over age 40; if you have diabetes, a kidney disorder, or other serious health problem or had a relative who died of a heart attack before age 50; or if you smoke or suffer from high blood pressure. Your physician may conduct an exercise tolerance test (see page 804) to help you establish safe limits for your exercise program.

WHAT IS A GOOD EXERCISE PROGRAM?

A key distinction between kinds of exercise is whether they are aerobic or anaerobic.

Aerobic exercise involves continuous motion. An aerobic activity is one that requires your heart and lungs to function at an increased rate to supply your cells with more oxygen (literally, aerobic means "exercise with oxygen"). The increased respiration and heartbeat improve the condition of those vital organs and thus improve your overall conditioning and endurance, words that often are used interchangeably with aerobic health (see Cardiovascular Fitness, page 793).

Walking, bicycling, jogging, aerobic dancing, and swimming are familiar aerobic exercises. They involve continuous activity and will help condition your cardiovascular system. They increase the rate and depth of breathing. Your body becomes warm and, if the exercise is sufficiently long and vigorous, you will also perspire.

Anaerobic exercise can be healthy, too, but does little for the health of your heart. Weight-lifting is a classic example: strong muscles may be the end result of a weight-lifting program, but lifting heavy barbells a few times offers little challenge to your heart and lungs to deliver oxygen in a sustained fashion to your body's tissues. A workout with light weights that is of sufficient duration may be aerobic, as evidenced by increased breathing and perspiration.

A personal exercise program is a logical way to incorporate physical activity into your daily routine. It need not be very strenuous exercise to improve your fitness. In fact, a moderate amount of exercise is sufficient and will be more enjoyable for most people.

An exercise program should also be gradual: do not try to whip yourself into shape overnight, or even in a week or two. By gradually increasing the amount of exercise performed and by allowing your body to adapt to the change in activity level, you can improve your fitness in 8 to 12 weeks.

Tailor your fitness program to your needs, abilities, schedule, and other personal factors. Develop a regimen that works for you and your lifestyle because you must do it consistently to benefit. If you make your program so difficult that you rarely find the desire to do it or if the length of your workout is such that you cannot seem to fit your workout into your schedule more than once or twice a week, rethink your fitness program. You need a minimum of three 20- to 30-minute periods of conditioning exercise each week.

For maximum gain and to avoid injury, any exercise program should consist of three distinct elements: the warm-up, the primary exercise or activity itself, and the cool-down.

THE ELEMENTS OF EXERCISE

THE WARM-UP

The purpose of the warm-up is to attain and enhance flexibility. Muscles that have been inactive are "cool"; stretching and other low-intensity exercise gradually increase heart rate (pulse), body temperature, and blood flow to your muscles. Your warm-up regimen can ease you into the principal exercise. It will help you to avoid muscle stiffness, soreness, and even injury.

Stretches. In performing stretching exercises, remember to *hold* each stretching position for 30 seconds—do not bounce rhythmically. You should experience a definite pulling sensation in the muscles you are stretching but it should not be painful.

We recommend at least 5 to 10 minutes of stretching at the start (and the end) of every workout. Your selection of stretches should depend on the kind of exercise that is to follow. For example, if you are a runner, emphasize your legs and lower back. Among good candidates for stretches are the following.

Calf Stretch. Stand an arm's length away from the wall. Lean forward, rest your forearms on the wall, and put your forehead on the back of your hands. Bend one leg at the knee and bring it toward the wall. Keep the other leg stiff with the heel on the floor.

Move your hips toward the wall, keeping your back straight. You will feel a stretch in the calf muscles. Hold this position for 30 seconds. Repeat with the other leg.

Thigh Stretch. Place your left hand on the wall for balance. Reach behind you and

Calf stretch

Thigh stretch

Hamstring stretch

hold onto your right foot or ankle with your right hand. Pull the foot toward your buttocks. Again, you will feel your muscles stretching, this time in the front of the thigh. Hold this position for 30 seconds and then repeat with the other leg.

Hamstring Stretch.   Sit on the floor and extend your left leg straight ahead of you. Bend your right leg so that the bottom of your right foot touches the inner thigh of your left leg. Bend forward from your waist and slowly move both hands down your left leg—you will feel a stretch in the back thigh muscles (hamstrings). Hold this position for 30 seconds, then repeat with the other leg.

THE EXERCISE

Your principal exercise should be a conditioning (aerobic) exercise. This is any activity that requires continuous rhythmic muscle contraction of the legs and possibly the arms and that increases the rate and depth of breathing. Common endurance activities include walking, cycling, jogging, swimming, cross-country skiing, rowing, rope skipping, dancing, and racket sports. The key is to find an activity that you enjoy.

Your selection of exercise should be made with three characteristics in mind: intensity, duration, and frequency.

Intensity.   The right intensity for your exercise will improve your fitness; on the other hand, your workout should not be too strenuous. In general, proper exercise intensity requires you to reach 50 to 80 percent of your "maximal endurance exercise capacity." For most people, the ideal is about 70 percent.

By measuring your heart rate (pulse) you can determine the intensity of a given workout: the more intense your aerobic exercise, the greater your heart rate. When you exercise as hard as you can (your "maximal endurance exercise capacity"), your heart will be beating at its maximum rate. This rate decreases as you age and is affected by heart disease and some heart medications.

Additional benefits from going full-tilt in your workouts are small. That is where your "target heart rate" comes in. You can measure the efficiency of your exercise by determining your target rate (a calculation that factors your age into the equation; see Finding Your Target Heart Rate, page 383). During the conditioning portion of your workout, your heart rate should reach the target rate and remain there for perhaps 20 minutes or more. Exceeding your target rate puts you at increased risk of muscle or joint soreness or injury.

To use your target heart rate as a guide, you need to take your pulse. With the tips of your index and third fingers, locate the pulsing artery (radial artery) between your wrist bone and tendon on the thumb side of either wrist. Do not press too hard on the blood vessel; you could temporarily obstruct the flow of blood. Count your pulse for 10 seconds timed by the sweep hand of a watch or clock. Multiply this count by six to obtain your pulse (see page 796).

At rest, the pulse is likely to be about 70 for men and about 80 for women. When you exercise your rate may more than double (depending on your age and the intensity of your workout).

Frequency.   Exercise three times each week on non-consecutive days. Exercising more often will increase conditioning and speed weight loss if you are overweight.

Duration.   The duration of your conditioning exercise should be at least 20 to 30 minutes; 45 to 60 minutes of exercise will produce faster progress in conditioning and weight loss. These times do not include warm-up and cool-down periods.

You may find lower intensity exercise more enjoyable; if so, then increase the duration of your exercise (from 20 to 40 minutes) and you will continue to reap the desired fitness benefits.

Getting Started.   Change your habits gradually. If you have not been physically active

---

GETTING STARTED: FIVE LITTLE RULES

First, visit your physician before you begin an exercise program. If you smoke, are overweight, are over 45 and have never exercised, or have a chronic condition such as heart disease, diabetes, high blood pressure, or kidney disease, it is particularly important that you check with your physician.

Second, begin gradually. Rome wasn't built in a day, and one doesn't go from strolls around the block to being a decathlete overnight. Do not overdo it. If you have trouble talking to a companion during your workout, you are probably pushing too hard. Slow down a bit.

A body not accustomed to vigorous exercise can be easily injured. Thus, in the beginning, your joints, ligaments, and muscles are vulnerable. Your body is less likely to be injured after it has been conditioned. Use your target heart rate (see Finding Your Target Heart Rate, page 383) to help you establish a suitable pace.

Third, select the exercise that is right for you. It should be something you enjoy—or at least find tolerable. Otherwise, in time you will avoid doing it. Vigorous walking, running, swimming, biking, racket sports, dancing, skiing, and aerobics are a few good forms of exercise.

Fourth, do it regularly. For real benefit, it is important that you have at least three exercise sessions of at least 20 minutes every week. When you exercise, it should be vigorous enough to make you breathless and sweaty. You should feel your heart pounding in your chest. However, never exercise to the point of nausea or dizziness.

Fifth, stay with your program. Do not get discouraged. You do not have to be a natural athlete to have a regular exercise program. Nor should you have unrealistic expectations. If you have short, thick legs, do not expect exercise to give you a ballet dancer's body. What you can expect is a better-toned body and more energy.

for the previous 2 months or more, start conservatively. If you are over 40, sedentary, obese, diabetic, or a smoker; if you suffer from hypertension, a kidney disorder, or other serious health problem; or if a relative died of a heart attack before age 50, consult your physician before starting any new exercise regimen. Your physician may conduct an exercise tolerance test (see page 804).

For the first several weeks of an exercise program, keep your target heart rate at the lower end of your target zone (perhaps 50 percent of your maximal endurance exercise capacity). Limit your weekly conditioning exercise program to three 10- or 15-minute workouts. Increase the duration by 1 to 5 minutes every other session. Increase intensity only after you have reached the desired duration. A month-long, graduated program should help you adapt to your individual exercise prescription.

If at any time during a workout you experience chest discomfort or pressure, faintness, shortness of breath, bursts of very rapid or slow heart rate, irregular heartbeat, excessive fatigue, or severe joint or muscle pain, stop your workout and consult your physician.

THE COOL-DOWN

Immediately after your conditioning exercise, allow your heart rate to return to normal. It also is important to stretch the muscles used during the endurance activity and prevent blood from pooling in your legs (which can cause dizziness).

Three to 5 minutes of low-level activity will help achieve these ends. Slow walking, for example, will allow you to cool down and your heart and respiration to return to normal levels. Then do stretching exercises to prevent soreness and stiffness as well as to maintain flexibility. Exercises like those described for the warm-up are suitable for the cool-down as well. Devote a total of 5 to 10 minutes to cooling down.

WHAT EXERCISE IS RIGHT FOR YOU?

The perfect workout for an Olympic high-jumper is very different from an appropriate fitness program for a pregnant woman or an elderly man. Yet, for each of these people, a good exercise program is equally important.

Two factors must be calculated into the fitness equation: your goals, and your physical status.

IDENTIFYING YOUR GOALS

If you are looking to increase your strength or quickness or some other athletic characteristic, your exercise program should be quite different from that of the person who is simply looking to maintain his or her basic good health.

Any exercise program should involve a mix of activities but, for practical purposes, there are three kinds of exercise. They are distinguished by the goals they are intended to help attain.

Strengthening Exercise. To increase strength, an exercise must involve weights (resistance). The exercise is usually done to the point, called momentary muscular failure, at which you can no longer complete the exercise in proper form. Strengthening exercises are not essential for a maintenance exercise program in which the goals involve weight control, cardiovascular health, or simply staying in shape.

Endurance Exercise. In contrast to strengthening exercise which involves working your muscles until they are too tired to move, endurance exercise involves conditioning your body so that it does not get too tired to move.

Endurance exercise involves less resistance and more repetitions. In working with weights, this means using less weight for a longer period. Many other kinds of exercise can build endurance, too. In particular, aerobic activities like running and swimming build the endurance of the heart and lungs (cardiovascular benefit).

Aerobic (cardiovascular) exercise requires continuous motion. It is a form of exercise that demands of your heart and lungs an increase in their ability to provide oxygen for your cells. Three 20-minute aerobic workouts a week should be a part of any basic conditioning program (see Cardiovascular Fitness, page 793).

Flexibility Exercise. Flexibility exercises also are basic. They are less about conditioning and more about avoiding injury and discomfort. Stretching and warm-up exercises get the blood flowing, literally warming up your muscles and getting them ready to work out. At the close of a period of activity, flexibility exercises are also essential to help your muscles cool down and to help prevent muscle tightness.

RECOGNIZING YOUR CONDITION

Your physical status is the other key factor—are you overweight, of a certain age, or pregnant? You and the members of your family each will be in one of the following categories.

Child. For many parents, the idea of having to encourage their children to be more active is absurd. Kids never stop running around. How could they possibly need more exercise?

For some children, however, particularly those who are overweight, an increase in physical activity may be important. Weight control at any age is largely a matter of balancing the intake of calories with the amount of energy burned in everyday activities—when more calories are burned than are consumed, the excess pounds will begin to disappear.

Scheduling regular workouts is a suitable approach for an adult, but it probably is not for a school-age or even teenage child. A better approach is to encourage sports or physical fitness activities at times of the child's choosing. These activities burn calories and may have a beneficial effect on self-esteem and self-image as well.

Healthy Adult. The aging process often makes us realize how important exercise is: our bodies grow less forgiving of our minor excesses and sedentary ways as we grow older. Muscles that are rarely used lose strength, tone, and definition. In particular, if your heart and lungs are unchallenged, you increase your risk of heart attack, atherosclerosis, and other disorders.

The good news is that there are a wide variety of exercise options for a healthy adult. You might consider jogging (see A Sample Regimen: The Starter Jogging Program, page 386), bicycling (see Bicycling for Fitness, page 386), swimming, rowing, or any number of other options.

The key considerations are: start slowly and work up gradually; eventually work out a minimum of three times a week; and determine your target heartbeat and work to maintain it for no less than 20 minutes at each workout (see Finding Your Target Heart Rate, below).

If you are over 35, overweight, or a smoker, or if you have had a heart attack or have diabetes, consult your physician first. An exercise stress test may be necessary to assess the risks and limitations (see The Exercise Tolerance Test, page 804).

Pregnant Woman. Reasonable exercise programs probably have little or no impact on your unborn child—but they can affect you in numerous ways, including your stamina (perhaps making labor shorter and

---

FINDING YOUR TARGET HEART RATE

Whenever you run, swim, or cycle, your heart beats faster—this is the point of a conditioning exercise. But is your increased heart rate fast enough that you are getting maximum benefit but not so fast that there is an unnecessary strain on your heart?

In selecting the right exercise for you and in creating your exercise program, look for the right pace: this means identifying your "target heart rate." To do this, subtract your age from 220, and then take 70 percent of this number. For example, if you are 40 years old, 220 minus 40 is 180; 70 percent of 180 is 126, so your target heart rate is about 125 beats per minute. That means that you should aim to reach and maintain that level or slightly above it for the duration of your workout.

However, if you have been inactive for several months or more, have a chronic health problem, or are recovering from an injury, consult your physician before starting a workout regimen. If you have high blood pressure, high cholesterol level, diabetes, or a family history of heart disease or if you are a smoker, your physician may recommend an exercise stress test to help determine the best approach for you (see The Exercise Tolerance Test, page 804).

Your physician may recommend that, rather than the 70 percent factor, a lower value, perhaps 50 percent, is appropriate, at least to start with.

easier) and even your overall attitude. However, during pregnancy you may be more vulnerable to injury, so take appropriate precautions when planning a program (see Exercise in Pregnancy, page 186).

Obese Adult.   Any complete weight-loss program should involve an exercise component: reducing your intake of calories is a key element, but exercise burns calories, tones muscles, and can help you firm up and feel better. However, if you are overweight and have been largely inactive for several months or more, consult your physician before embarking on an exercise regimen. He or she may give you an exercise stress test to determine the response of your heart to the stresses of exercise (see The Exercise Tolerance Test, page 804). When you begin to exercise, start slowly, perhaps with a walking program.

Heart-Attack Survivor.   Having had a heart attack *does not* mean no more exercise. On the contrary, appropriate workouts are an important part of your recuperation. Your physician can help you plan an exercise program. A local civic organization may even have group workouts for post-cardiac care patients (see also Cardiac Rehabilitation, page 815).

Elderly Person.   If you have led a sedentary life, consult your physician before starting a conditioning program. Your physician may conduct an exercise stress test to help you plan the pace of your exercise (see The Exercise Tolerance Test, page 804).

In general, walking is an excellent exercise for older people. It delivers cardiovascular benefit yet does not stress the bones and joints, in contrast to some more vigorous forms of exercise. In particular, women beyond menopause are at increased risk of fractures because of bone demineralization (see Osteoporosis, page 982) so avoiding unnecessary stresses is sensible.

If you experience chest pressure or pain, dizziness, shortness of breath, bursts of very rapid or slow heart rate, irregular heartbeat, excessive fatigue, or severe joint or muscle pain, stop your workout and consult your physician.

Disabled Person.   Exercise is as important to the disabled as to those without physical limitations. The health of the heart and lungs is equally crucial to the disabled person, and cardiovascular conditioning exercise should be sought.

COMMON FORMS OF EXERCISE

WALKING FOR EXERCISE

We take walking for granted. We do it every day, taking dozens or even hundreds of little trips to the kitchen, car, bathroom—going just about anywhere involves taking at least a few steps.

Yet, taking a brisk walk can be a safe, effective means of improving your physical fitness. Especially if you lead an inactive life and are a bit out of shape, a program of walking could be just the challenge you need, not too taxing yet providing fitness benefits.

An appropriate regimen of walking can help you increase the efficiency of your heart and lungs, improve the ability of your body to use oxygen during exertion, and decrease your resting heart rate. It also may decrease your blood pressure.

Walking burns calories—a 150-pound person burns 240 calories by walking 2 miles in an hour, 320 calories at 3 miles in an hour, and 440 calories at 4½ miles in an hour. Walking can improve muscle tone, which helps to shape and tone muscles in your legs, hips, buttocks, and abdomen. Walking also can be a valuable part of a weight-loss program.

Walking can be a tonic for the mind as well as the body. Walking can relieve stress, helping you unwind at the end of the day or after a difficult task.

Regular walking also can help you prevent age-related diseases. Walking increases bone density and, according to recent research, may lower the risk of osteoporosis developing (see page 982). For some people, regular exercise can lessen the pain of osteoarthritis.

About 30 million Americans today walk for fitness—in fact, fitness walking is the fastest-growing participant sport in the country. It requires no special skills or instruction. You can vary your route to keep it interesting. Walking is a convenient, inexpensive, and even social workout, if you can get a spouse or a friend to join you. Walkers also are less prone to injury than participants in most other kinds of physical activity.

ESTABLISHING THE ROUTINE

Decide *before* you begin what your goals are. For aerobic benefit, plan on a minimum of three workouts a week, on alternating days, of 20 minutes or more each.

Get yourself a pair of good walking shoes. Such shoes should be lightweight, fit comfortably, and have a slightly elevated heel. They should also provide substantial arch support, plenty of width in the toe area, a firm heel counter (the curved support at the rear of the shoe) to guide your foot through its roll forward, a well-cushioned heel and midsole to absorb shock, and a durable outsole with good traction. The rest of your attire is important, too, especially in an excessively warm or cold condition (see Exercise in the Heat and Cold, page 391).

Do stretching exercises before and after you work out. In fact, a safe, effective workout consists of the same basic components: a warm-up with flexibility and stretching exercises, the conditioning exercise itself (in this case walking), and a post-exercise cool-down period with more stretching and flexibility exercise.

Stretch for at least 5 minutes before the walking exercise. This gradually increases your heart rate, loosens joints, and stretches key muscles. After each walking session, cool down by walking slowly, and then conclude with 5 minutes of stretches.

Start slowly. If you are just beginning, increase the duration and rate of your workout slowly over a period of 4 to 6 weeks. By monitoring your pulse rate, you can slowly increase your levels of exercise.

Establish a routine and do it at least three times each week. Take your walk at the

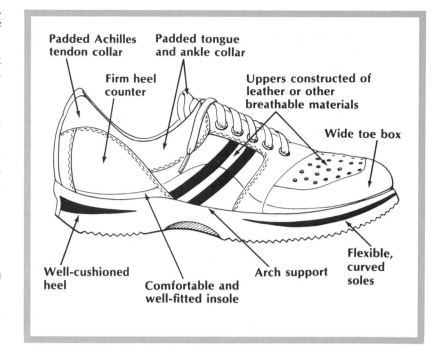

Padded Achilles tendon collar
Padded tongue and ankle collar
Firm heel counter
Uppers constructed of leather or other breathable materials
Wide toe box
Well-cushioned heel
Comfortable and well-fitted insole
Arch support
Flexible, curved soles

A good walking shoe should offer a variety of features.

same time each day; before breakfast or dinner is a good time.

The following chart outlines a walking regimen you might follow:

Week of Program	Distance, miles	Time, minutes per mile
1–2	1–2	15
3–4	2–2.5	12–15
5–6	2.5–3	12
7–8	3–4	12
9–10	4–5	12

Keep your water consumption high. When you exercise, you need the extra water to maintain your normal body temperature and to cool working muscles. Drink water before *and* after your workout.

And listen to your body. It will send warning signals—pain, nausea, dizziness—if something is amiss. Stop and rest. If symptoms persist, consult your physician.

Especially if you have been inactive for several months or more, have a chronic health problem, or are recovering from an injury, consult your physician before beginning walking workouts. If you have high blood pressure, high cholesterol level, diabetes, or a family history of heart disease or are a smoker, your physician may recommend an exercise stress test to help determine the best approach for you (see The Exercise Tolerance Test, page 804).

A SAMPLE REGIMEN: THE STARTER JOGGING PROGRAM

Jogging is not for everybody (if you have a heart or lung ailment, discuss jogging or any proposed exercise program with your physician *before* beginning it). But many people find that a regular program of jogging suits their exercise needs and can fit into busy schedules.

If you have not been active for several months, do not start with a multi-mile run. Begin by walking. When you are able to walk 2 miles in 30 minutes comfortably, you are ready to try alternating jogging and walking.

Follow the guidelines in the chart. Move from one step to the next every 2 to 7 days—your body will tell you when you have gone too far too fast. To minimize the risk of injury and of muscle and joint discomfort, do not jog more than three or four times a week and do it on alternate days.

Jog at a comfortable pace, aim-ing at the lower end of your target heart rate (perhaps 50 percent; see Finding Your Target Heart Rate, page 383). After step 12, you can then gradually increase the intensity of your workout.

Remember the warm-up and cool-down. Do not forget to allow 5 to 10 minutes before *and* after your jogging for stretching and ac-climating your body to the change in pace (see The Warm-Up and The Cool-Down, pages 379 and 382).

To begin, give your body a break. Do not try to accomplish too much. Step 1: Jog for 1 minute, and then walk for 1 minute. Repeat this sequence 12 times for a 24-minute workout. Exercise three times a week on alternate days. Each week, move up one step in your Starter Jogging Program.

Starter Jogging Program

| Step | Exercise Time, minutes | | Repetitions | | Total Time, minutes |
	Jog	Walk	Jog	Walk	
1	1	1	12	12	24
2	2	1	8	8	24
3	3	1	6	6	24
4	4	1	5	5	25
5	5	1	4	4	24
6	7	1	3	2	23
7	10	1	2	2	22
8	12	1	2	1	25
9	15	1	2	1	31
10	20	—	1	—	20
11	25	—	1	—	25
12	30	—	1	—	30

BICYCLING FOR FITNESS

As the old cliché has it, "You never forget how to ride a bicycle." This is more or less true, and a good thing to remember if you are looking for a conditioning exercise.

Cycling is not just for kids. Increasingly, fitness-minded adults are returning to cycling. About 20 million adults get on their bicycles at least once a week; many of them use their bicycles regularly in a pattern of three or more workouts a week for maximum aerobic benefit. However, there are some important considerations in planning for a true workout.

Selecting the Right Bicycle. Some bicycles are designed for smooth surfaces and high speeds; others are suitable for rougher terrain. Consider your needs: do you need a racing, mountain, or touring bicycle?

Racing bicycles are lightweight with narrow tires, low-slung handlebars, and many gear settings, usually between 10 and 18. When riding a racing bicycle, the upper part of your body is parallel to the ground.

Mountain bicycles have sturdier frames and wider tires that have more tread. They are designed for off-the-road riding and often have many gear settings, too. The handlebars are more upright. The riding posture is more erect.

Touring bicycles are between mountain and racing bicycles. The posture is more upright. Older models typically had gears for 3 to 5 speeds, but today's touring bicycles often have 10 or 12.

In selecting a bicycle, keep in mind that, when you are seated and have your foot on the pedal lowest to the ground, your leg

HOW MANY CALORIES DOES IT USE UP?

Even when you are asleep, you require energy (calories) to fuel your heartbeat, breathing, and other body functions. When you move about slowly, you burn more calories. When you exercise, your calorie consumption may increase dramatically.

In the chart below you will find the range of energy expended while performing various activities for 1 hour.

Remember that you will expend 50 to 100 calories, depending on body size, while sitting quietly for 1 hour.

From the numbers in the table it is obvious that calorie expenditure varies widely with different forms of exercise. You can indulge in an activity with a great intensity or with a low degree of intensity or any degree between. In addition, the trained athlete can carry out a given activity with greater economy of motion and less expenditure of energy.

Walking at ordinary speeds is the exception. The amount of energy you use for walking depends only on body weight and distance covered. The heavier the person, the greater the calorie expenditure; the greater the distance covered, the greater the calorie expenditure. The athlete has no advantage over the rest of us.

It also is apparent that all forms of activity cost a lean person fewer calories than they cost a heavy person. This is the reason that middle- and long-distance runners strive to be as lean as possible. With lesser body weight they need less oxygen and less fuel (calories) to cover the same distance.

Activity	Average Calories Expended per Hour	
	120–130 lb Person	170–180 lb Person
Aerobic dancing	290–575	400–800
Backpacking	290–630	400–880
Badminton	230–515	320–720
Basketball		
Game	400–690	560–960
Nongame	170–515	240–720
Bicycling		
Outdoor	170–800	240–1,120
Stationary	85–800	120–1,120
Bowling	115–170	160–240
Canoeing	170–460	240–640
Chopping wood	170–575	240–800
Dancing	115–400	160–560
Gardening	115–400	160–560
Golfing (walking, carrying or pulling bag)	115–400	160–560
Handball	460–690	640–960
Hiking	170–690	240–960
Jogging		
5.0 mph (12 min/mile)	460	640
6.0 mph (10 min/mile)	575	800
Racquetball	345–690	480–960
Rope skipping	345–690	480–960
Rowing	170–800	240–1,120
Running		
7.0 mph (9 min/mile)	690	960
8.0 mph (7.5 min/mile)	745	1,040
10.0 mph (6 min/mile)	860	1,200
Scuba diving	290–690	400–800
Skating, ice or roller	230–460	320–640
Skiing		
Cross-country	290–800	400–1,120
Downhill	170–460	240–640
Soccer	290–690	400–960
Squash	345–690	480–960
Stair climbing	230–460	320–640
Swimming	230–690	320–900
Table tennis	170–290	240–400
Tennis	230–515	320–720
Volleyball	170–400	240–560
Walking		
2.0 mph (30 min/mile)	115	160
3.0 mph (20 min/mile)	170	240
4.0 mph (15 min/mile)	260	360

should be not quite fully extended. You should be able to reach the handlebars and to work the brakes and shift mechanism while keeping your eyes on the road. When straddling a racing bicycle with your feet on the ground, there should be 1 to 3 inches of clearance above the crossbar; a mountain or touring bicycle should have 3 to 6 inches of clearance.

Designing Your Exercise Program. As with any form of conditioning exercise, schedule regular workouts. We recommend three rides a week (at least) of 30 minutes' duration or more. Stretch your muscles before and after you cycle.

Intensity is also a factor: you need to move your legs at least twice as fast as you would during a brisk walk in order to gain aerobic benefit. As you get comfortable with your bicycle and workout schedule, determine what your target heart rate should be and work up to maintaining it for the duration of your workout (see Finding Your Target Heart Rate, page 383).

If you have been inactive for several months or more, have a chronic health problem, or are recovering from an injury, consult your physician before starting a workout regimen. If you have high blood pressure, high cholesterol, diabetes, or a family history of heart disease or are a smoker, your physician may recommend an exercise stress test to help determine the

---

AVOIDING INJURY

Most injuries that occur during an athletic activity result from unusual demands on bones, muscles, or other tissues. The novice runner who struggles to complete 5 miles the first day on the track will experience aches and pains; the over-40 ex-jock who comes out of retirement for the company softball game is an excellent candidate for a sprain or some other painful injury.

An injury-free life is an unrealistic goal. But there are a few sensible rules to follow that will help you avoid inconvenient, painful, expensive, and, at times, disabling injuries.

Consult Your Physician

If you are over 40, obese, or a heavy smoker or have had unexplained chest pains, heart problems such as a previous heart attack, irregular heart rhythms, or other serious health problem, or lead a largely sedentary life, consult your physician before starting a vigorous exercise regimen. Your physician may suggest a stress test (see The Exercise Tolerance Test, page 804) to evaluate the condition of your heart and lungs and

will offer valuable do's and do not's specific to your physical condition.

Warm Up Before Exercising

To avoid injury, invest at least 5 to 10 minutes in stretching and loosening the muscles that will be used in your activity. The increased blood flow of such a warm-up will decrease tension in your muscles, improve their range of motion, and even may improve your performance. Simultaneously, you are significantly decreasing the chance of muscle pulls, strains, and other injuries.

Cool Down After Exercising

After your workout, allow your muscles to cool down. Muscles that have carried you through a workout have contracted, and a session of stretching is critical. Muscles that are not treated by this staged return to normal are more likely to sustain pulls, strains, and spasms.

Pace Yourself

Sudden and unfamiliar exertions are most likely to cause injuries. If you are bent on improving your performance, do so, but at a sensible pace. Do not double your distance or your duration overnight.

Develop a program that allows your body to become conditioned to the activity so that it adjusts over time to the challenges you offer it.

Select the Right Sport for You

If you have a bad back or perpetually sore knees, the pounding of jogging is not for you; perhaps a daily swim or riding on a stationary bicycle more nearly suits your needs.

Make It a Habit

Working out only once a week, no matter how vigorous the activity, puts you at risk of injury (and fails to provide you with maximum aerobic and conditioning benefits; see The Benefits of Exercise, page 378). Try to establish a schedule of a minimum of three 20-minute workouts a week.

Take Care of That Injury

If you sprain an ankle or twist a knee, make sure you get medical advice and then follow it. A key element is almost sure to be what physicians commonly refer to as "the tincture of time." Allow the injury to heal before testing it too vigorously (see Principles of Sports Rehabilitation, page 969).

best approach for you (see The Exercise Tolerance Test, page 804).

Select a time of day for your cycling that works for you. For example, if managing stress is a goal, perhaps your ride is best scheduled when you need a safety valve from pressure—a ride after work may relax you for your evening at home.

Do not be tempted to challenge yourself by setting the gears to make pedaling hard, producing a strain resembling that of a hard run. This does not work your heart and lungs effectively, except when you are ascending a hill. Pedaling more rapidly at all times— even while going downhill—will help you make your ride an aerobic activity.

Is the workout challenging enough? According to the "talk test," you should be able to carry on a conversation during your workout but have to time your words with your breathing pattern. If you can not talk, then slow down a bit. On the other hand, if you do not need a shower after your ride, you have not challenged yourself enough. (See also Basic Bicycling Safety, page 327.)

AT HIGH ALTITUDES

If you travel to an altitude much higher than that to which you are accustomed, you may experience a decrease in performance during endurance exercise. There is less oxygen in the air at higher altitudes (barometric pressure is lower), but do not allow that to deter you from exercise unless you experience symptoms of acute mountain sickness.

Acute mountain sickness is caused by a shortage of oxygen in the blood (hypoxia), and usually has symptoms such as headache, breathlessness on mild exertion, fatigue, nausea, vomiting, and disturbed sleep. It is much more likely to occur at high elevations (8,000 feet or more) and to people who have ascended rapidly.

WEIGHT-TRAINING

Weight-lifting is about more than big biceps. Lifting weights can increase muscle size but it also can tone and tighten muscles and enhance overall conditioning. However, weight-lifting is of limited aerobic value,

even if you move rapidly from one exercise to another.

Types of Weight-Training. Power-lifting is what the Olympian muscle-men do, powering hundreds of pounds of barbells toward the sky. Body-building is another category in which participants use weights for conditioning, but the emphasis is on shaping or "sculpting" the musculature for visual effect.

Today, more people are likely to incorporate resistance training into their exercise programs. At its simplest, resistance training is an overall weight-training approach for the purpose of conditioning muscles for other sports.

Resistance training works on the principle of overload. You exercise certain groups of muscles, such as in the arms, legs, or chest, to the point of fatigue. Then, after a recovery phase, you exercise them again, gradually increasing the amount of weight used (progressive resistance).

Designing Your Program. How much and how often should you lift? Get advice from a qualified instructor—many gyms and schools have qualified strength-and-conditioning professionals. Such an advisor can help you design a program that meets your needs and is varied enough to keep you interested.

The design of a weight-lifting program depends on your goals. To build strength, lifting a weight that will exhaust you after 6 lifts is appropriate; to enhance the size and contour of your muscles, weight that exhausts you after 8 to 12 lifts is best; for endurance (such as for swimming or running), lifting a weight that creates muscle exhaustion after 15 to 20 times is best.

Types of Weights. There are several varieties of weights that can be used for weight training.

Free Weights. These are what most people think of as traditional weight-lifting equipment. Free weights consist of dumbbells (weights held in one hand) and barbells (requiring a two-handed grip). You lift the weight and control its direction. These are inexpensive, suitable for home use, and effective, but their potential for injury should

TAKING CARE OF YOUR BACK

Many athletic activities put your back at risk for injury. If a sneeze can produce a twinge of back pain in some people, then lifting weights surely can, too. Reportedly, four of five Americans complain of back pain at least once in their lives.

As you go about your daily activities and, in particular, if you start a new exercise regimen, it is an excellent idea to keep some commonsense strategies in mind to avoid back discomfort.

Maintain Good Posture
Whether you are walking to the bathroom to brush your teeth or running a marathon, good posture is important. Keep your backbone straight. Hold your shoulders back. Pull in your stomach and buttocks. Trim your profile. Pull in your chin (see also The Importance of Posture, page 989).

Lifting
Whether the object to be picked up is a newspaper or a 100-pound barbell, squat down with your back straight and let your legs do the lifting. Bring tension on your muscles gradually: never jerk or lunge to lift the load.

Exercise
If you have had back problems, remember that sports involving sudden jerking motions (stops and starts, twists and turns) put your back at increased risk of stress and strain. Falls and collisions also can endanger the health of your back. Perhaps you should retire from the Saturday afternoon touch football game and take up swimming, bicycling, walking, or jogging instead.

If the muscles of your back are poorly toned, your chance of injury also is increased. Exercises can be done to stretch and strengthen your back muscles (see your physiatrist or physical therapist for instructions) (see Treatment for Your Backache, page 993).

Sleeping
Lying down provides relief for backache and also an opportunity for backache prevention. Do not sleep on your stomach unless your abdomen is cushioned by a pillow; sleep on your side with your legs drawn up slightly toward your chest. Pick a firm mattress, one that provides your back with proper support. If the mattress is too soft or sags, use a bed board of ½-inch plywood.

Avoid Stiffness
If you find yourself seated at a desk, standing in one position, or behind the wheel of a car for hours every day, you are at risk of stiffness and muscle fatigue. Make it a point to break the routine at frequent intervals. When standing, shift your weight from one foot to the other periodically; when sitting, get up, even for a few seconds, as often as possible. Take frequent breaks when driving and get out and stretch. A small pillow at the base of your back also can help to support your spine.

Weight Loss
One frequent cause of backache in the United States is being overweight. The extra pounds at your waistline put important strains and stresses on your back. An appropriate program of weight loss and exercise may help you avoid back pain.

When lifting any object, let your legs do the work. Bend your knees rather than your back. Hold the object close to your body and lift gently. Avoid jerking or lunging upward.

not be ignored. For safety, work with a training partner.

Machines. Machines can isolate a particular muscle or group of muscles and provide variable resistance. Some of these machines look very high-tech and intimidating, but in general they are easier and safer to use than free weights. Machines typically are found in health clubs, but they can be purchased for home use as well. Given the expense, however, it makes sense to try weight-lifting at a public gym and buy the machine later, after you know weight-training is for you.

Establishing Your Routine. An investment of time and energy is required to benefit from weight-training. Typically, strength increases are noticeable after 6 weeks of programmed lifting; improvement in muscle shape and size takes longer, perhaps 8 to 16 weeks.

Do not try to do it all at once: using too much weight too soon can result in injury.

For the same reasons, incorporate proper warm-up and cool-down periods into every workout.

Listen to what your body tells you: muscular aches are common after workouts, but lingering aches or burning sensations should not be. Take a day or two off; if the discomfort does not go away, consult your physician.

Some Cautions. If you have high blood pressure or heart disease, consult your physician before beginning a weight-training regimen. Lifting can cause your blood pressure to soar.

Be sure to use proper technique. Do not bounce the weight or bend and shift your body while lifting. Breathing correctly is important, too—inflate your chest to support your spine during exertion. (A support belt also can be helpful.) Set a regular rhythm, breathing in before the lift, exhaling after. Never hold your breath.

EXERCISE IN THE HEAT AND COLD

The environment in which you work out has a significant effect on your exercise. Extremes of heat or cold and high altitude may require that you adjust not only your attire but also the duration and intensity of your exercise. Listen to what your body advises you about extremes of temperature and climate: maintain your schedule of workouts if you can, but adjust to the conditions when necessary.

HOT WEATHER

On warm, humid days, more blood is directed to your skin to dissipate heat. This means that less blood is available for your muscles than on cool days, so your heart rate must increase. To compensate, decrease the intensity of your exercise to keep your target heart rate within sensible limits (see Finding Your Target Heart Rate, page 383).

Another strategy for hot days concerns scheduling: try exercising indoors or work out during a cooler time of day (morning or evening). Make sure you drink water before and after exercise in warm, humid weather.

If you exercise for a period in excess of 30 minutes, stop and drink water every 15 to 20 minutes during the exercise.

Proper attire also is important: wear lightweight, loose-fitting clothing made of fabrics that breathe. Wear reflective material on your jogging clothes and try to run in well-lit areas where traffic is limited.

COLD WEATHER

In extremely cold, windy weather, exposed skin may freeze (see Frostbite, page 279). Protect exposed skin as much as possible if you elect to exercise outdoors in such conditions; using an indoor facility is an alternative. Walking or jogging in snowy or icy conditions also puts you at risk of falling.

Breathing extremely cold air does not injure your lungs because the air is warmed to body temperature before it arrives in the air sacs (alveoli) of your lungs. However, if you have asthma or angina (heart pain), exercise in cold weather may worsen these symptoms. Try wearing a soft scarf or a cold-air mask over your mouth and nose in extremely cold or windy conditions. You can purchase a cold-air mask at your local drug-store or pharmacy. Also, breathe through your nose because your nose warms, filters, and humidifies the air before it enters your lungs.

When you exercise outdoors, dress for the conditions. Dressing in layers is the best strategy in the cold. This provides added insulation, and you can add or shed layers as appropriate to warm up and cool down. Thick, absorbent socks are important, especially for runners and walkers. A wind-breaker will help protect you against excessive heat loss in a strong wind.

CHAPTER 15
TOOTH CARE

CHAPTER CONTENTS

THE CARE OF YOUR TEETH

Your teeth are among your most important assets. Attached to jaws driven by powerful muscles, your teeth enable you to chew your food into a form that helps facilitate digestion.

Teeth, of course, also have a cosmetic dimension. Frequently, the first thing we notice about another person is his or her smile.

Clean, healthy-looking teeth seem to be a sign to the world of general good health. In the past, a healthy smile belonged only to the young because, until recently, most people lost their teeth by middle age. Now, however, dental care, improved nutrition, and good home hygiene make it possible for most of us to keep our teeth for our entire lives.

Essential to maintaining a set of healthy teeth is a lifelong program of good dental hygiene—one that you begin early and practice consistently through the years. This includes modifying your diet to lessen the effects of sugar and carbohydrates.

In most children and adults, tooth decay (cavities or, more formally, caries) is the primary problem. Tooth decay is mainly caused by bacteria and carbohydrates. Bacteria are present in a thin, almost invisible film on your teeth. Enzymes in your saliva change starches into sugar in your mouth. Bacteria convert the sugar to an acid that decays your teeth.

Start your child early on a program of regular brushing and flossing. Decay can begin as soon as your child's primary (baby) teeth begin to erupt.

Never allow your infant to sleep with a bottle of fruit juice or milk. The sugar content of these beverages encourages decay. If your baby seems to require the soothing presence of a bottle at bedtime, fill it with water.

Teach your toddler to brush his or her teeth at least twice a day. Reinforce the habit by setting a good example. Make sure that all of your children brush with fluoride toothpaste and have regular dental checkups, beginning no later than at age 3.

In adults, the principal cause of tooth loss is caries. In addition, advanced periodontal disease can lead to tooth loss (see Dental and Oral Disorders, page 561).

Periodontal disease is an infection of the gums and other tissues that support the teeth. The incidence of gingivitis (a mild form of periodontal disease) is high in all age groups—reportedly over 80 percent in adults age 45 and older. The incidence of periodontitis (a more serious form) increases with age. Close to 50 percent of those age 45 or older are thought to be affected.

Advanced periodontitis can lead to loosening and eventual loss of teeth. However, you can prevent gum disease with proper daily care of your teeth.

The most frequent sign of gum disease is swollen gums that bleed easily, especially during brushing and flossing. Other symptoms include bad breath, soft or tender gums, pus from the gum line (where the gum forms a collar around the tooth), shrinkage of the gum away from the tooth, loose tooth, and changes in the tooth in alignment and bite.

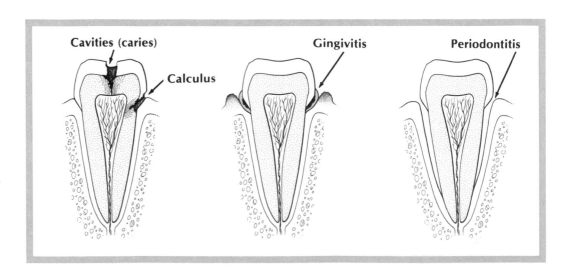

Three principal causes of tooth loss are dental cavities (caries), gingivitis, and periodontitis; the last two are disorders of the gums and other tissues that support your teeth.

Like tooth decay, the cause of periodontal disease is plaque. Plaque consists of an accumulation of bacteria and sugars on the surface of the teeth. Plaque forms constantly in your mouth and collects on the surfaces of your teeth. As plaque accumulates along the gum line, it irritates your gums, making them tender and likely to bleed. This condition is called gingivitis (see Gingivitis, page 570). If you do not remove the plaque daily by brushing and flossing, it continues to accumulate and reacts with minerals in your saliva to form a calcified deposit known as calculus (tartar).

As plaque builds up on top of the calculus, the gums slowly separate from the teeth, leaving pockets that fill with bacteria and sometimes pus. When the disease goes untreated, it attacks and destroys bone that supports the teeth. As a result, otherwise healthy, undecayed teeth loosen and can be lost.

The best method for controlling plaque and tartar is to brush thoroughly and regularly (at least twice each day) and to floss at least once a day. As with tooth decay, limit the amount of sugar you eat, particularly between meals (see Prevention of Periodontal Disease, page 573).

HOW TO CHOOSE A TOOTHBRUSH

A toothbrush with soft, end-rounded or polished bristles is best for cleaning your teeth and gums. Stiff or hard brushes are more likely to injure gum tissues.

The size and shape of the brush should allow you to reach every tooth. There are brush sizes for children and for adults as well as various configurations of bristles. Remember that only the tips of the bristles do the cleaning, so there's no need to exert a great deal of pressure.

Replace your toothbrush *every 3 to 4 months,* or sooner if the bristles become bent. In this way you always will be using bristles that are effective in brushing plaque (bacteria and sugars) from the surface of your teeth and gums. Splayed bristles are a sign that it is past time to replace your toothbrush.

If you have doubts about the proper brushes for you and your family, ask your dentist for a recommendation.

PROPER FLOSSING AND BRUSHING TECHNIQUES

Total mouth care depends more on brushing and flossing techniques than on use of any product. Rather than paying a premium price for a so-called antiplaque or antitartar toothpaste, your best aid is an investment of old-fashioned "elbow grease."

Brushing and flossing are the best ways to remove bacteria and food particles before dental problems begin. Start by flossing your teeth once each day and brushing them at least twice a day (in the morning and before going to bed). Better yet, brush after each meal or snack. A complete cleaning with a fluoride toothpaste, toothbrush, and dental floss (thread that you draw between your teeth) should take 3 to 5 minutes. The proper order is floss first, brush second. This way you can brush away food particles and bacteria loosened by the flossing.

FLOSSING

Take at least 18 inches of dental floss—unwaxed or waxed, whichever is more comfortable for you—and wind most of it around the middle finger of one hand. Wind a turn or two around the middle finger of the other hand so that there is 2 to 3 inches of floss between these fingers.

For your upper teeth, position the floss over the thumb of one hand and forefinger of the other hand. Use your thumb to hold back your cheek for better accessibility. Guide about an inch of floss into each gap between your teeth. Use a gentle up-and-down motion, holding the floss tightly, to rub the sides of each tooth.

When the floss reaches your gum line, curve it into a "C" shape around your tooth and move the floss up and down, gently scraping the wall of the tooth. Wind the used floss around your middle finger, exposing a fresh section, and repeat the procedure for each tooth.

For the lower teeth, wrap the dental floss around your forefingers and insert it between your teeth. Use the same motion as described for the upper teeth and repeat the procedure for each tooth.

Do not be alarmed if your gums bleed the first few times you floss. If the bleeding con-

To prevent dental problems, brush and floss your teeth regularly. Begin with the outer surfaces of all teeth and the inner surfaces of your back teeth. Position your toothbrush horizontally and brush back and forth vigorously (A). Next, to clean inner surfaces of upper and lower front teeth, brush vertically (B), moving your toothbrush over both teeth and gums. To clean the junction between your teeth and gums, brush at a 45-degree angle (see inset). To floss, wrap waxed or unwaxed dental floss around the middle fingers of both hands. For lower teeth (C), position floss between your index fingers, then insert it between your teeth and gently move it back and forth from the bottom to the top of your teeth. For upper teeth (D), a thumb and index finger technique works best.

tinues each time you floss, consult your dentist. The problem may be improper flossing. Your dentist can demonstrate the proper method for you.

BRUSHING

When you brush your teeth, position your toothbrush horizontally on your teeth. To effectively clean the top and bottom surfaces of all teeth, move the brush back and forth vertically in a series of short, scrubbing strokes.

For surfaces adjacent to your gums, move the brush in short back-and-forth strokes or in a rotary motion over both teeth and gums. Positioning your toothbrush at an angle will help clean the junction between your teeth and gums more effectively.

FLUORIDE AND TOOTH DECAY

Several decades ago, scientists found that adding fluoride to drinking water deficient in fluoride greatly decreased the number of cavities in children and adolescents who drank that water. Today, the scientific evidence is conclusive: the addition of fluoride to drinking water and toothpaste helps to prevent cavities, particularly among children.

Ingestion of fluoride is especially helpful during early childhood, when the teeth are developing. Fluoride is incorporated into the enamel structure and provides continuing protection.

You and your family should always brush with a fluoride toothpaste. Many fluoride toothpastes are available, including flavors specially formulated to appeal to children (see also Prevention of Tooth Decay, page 568).

The results of fluoride use are so impressive that now not only toothpastes but also some public water supplies contain fluoride. Fluoride is inexpensive, safe, and effective.

Still, only half of our population drinks fluoridated water. If you have children and your municipal water supply is not treated, ask about fluoridation for drinking water in your schools. In addition, persons of all ages who do not have access to fluoridated water will benefit from use of supplemental fluoride drops or tablets which are available by prescription from your dentist or physician.

Older children, adolescents, and senior citizens are most susceptible to tooth decay. For them, fluoride mouth rinses can be useful, as can topical fluoride treatments applied by a dentist.

DENTAL X-RAYS

Almost all of us have had dental x-rays taken. As in other medical fields, these x-rays are used to aid in diagnosing disease or injury. They often are useful in diagnosing the presence and extent of dental cavities, bone damage from periodontal disease, tooth abscesses, impacted teeth, fractures of the jawbone and teeth, and other abnormalities of the teeth and jawbone.

When it comes to cavities, x-rays can show the presence of decay in a tooth even when the enamel looks intact, particularly when the decay is hidden between teeth or under the gum line. If your dentist suspects that something may be wrong, an x-ray of the tooth may be taken.

The amount of radiation used to make dental x-rays is extremely small, and the pro-

Dental x-rays are useful in diagnosing the presence and extent of cavities and other abnormalities of the tooth and supporting structures. Shown below: full-mouth set of x-rays.

cess is simple. For the detection of cavities, most dentists use the x-ray procedure referred to as a bite-wing. A small piece of film is placed in your mouth, next to the teeth. You hold the film in place by biting down on the paper that covers the film. The x-ray machine is then aimed at the tooth, and the exposure is made. After the film is developed, which takes a few minutes, your dentist can determine an appropriate course of action.

X-rays, particularly a complete set of all the teeth, should not be taken as part of a routine examination but only as a diagnostic tool. No one should have more radiation exposure than absolutely necessary. A set of full-mouth x-rays should not be made more than once every 5 years, unless necessary for a specific purpose. Your dentist will advise you on the proper set of x-rays to obtain.

As a precautionary measure against excess radiation, your dentist may fit you with a lead apron that covers you from chest to lower abdomen. Everyone should wear the apron, but it is particularly important for pregnant women and women of childbearing age.

CONTROLLING TARTAR

Called calculus by your dentist, tartar is a product of minerals in your saliva and plaque. Tartar is a primary cause of gum diseases such as gingivitis and periodontitis. Tartar is most troublesome when it forms below the gum line.

Tartar is chalky, hard, and difficult to remove. Part of a regular dental checkup involves cleaning your teeth and removing tartar. This is often done by scraping the teeth, particularly below the gum line, with instruments known as scalers and curettes. The procedure can be uncomfortable and make your gums bleed. Another method uses a vibrating device that helps remove tartar.

Much advertising is being done these days for tartar-control toothpastes. These toothpastes have been found to decrease the accumulation of tartar on the teeth above the gums but have little or no effect on tartar below the gum line. Unfortunately, it is the tartar that forms below the gum line that can lead to periodontitis, the gum disease that can result in loss of teeth. Tartar-control toothpastes may have a cosmetic effect and make your teeth easier to clean when you see the dentist, but they are of little use in keeping the really harmful tartar from building up.

Special toothpastes designed to remove stains caused by cigarette smoking also are available. We do not recommend them. People whose gums have already recessed, exposing the softer layers beneath the gum line, may be at risk of further damage from toothpastes such as these. These toothpastes also can cause your teeth to become more sensitive to hot or cold foods.

The American Dental Association endorsement found on some brands of tartar-control toothpaste refers not to anti-tartar qualities but to the fluoride the toothpastes contain.

Tartar (calculus)

Tartar (your dentist may call it calculus) is an accumulation of minerals and plaque on the surfaces of your teeth. When cleaning your teeth, your dentist or oral hygienist will remove the tartar, especially at or below the gum line, because it is a primary cause of gum disease.

CHAPTER 16

CONTROLLING STRESS

CHAPTER CONTENTS

KEEPING YOUR STRESS UNDER CONTROL

Most of us know something about stress—the term has become common in our society. In addition, nearly everyone experiences stress on a day-to-day basis.

Stress is an individualized, personal response to situations and circumstances that create pressures. It is a normal and perhaps necessary part of our lives.

Stress is not an outside force; rather, it is our physiological response to specific stimuli or "stressors." These responses mobilize bodily systems so that they can help us adapt to the constant demands and changes of our lives. For example, athletes frequently perform best in competition rather than in practice. Many people find that goals and deadlines are stimulating and necessary for accomplishment.

Sometimes stress responses may be so mild that they go virtually unnoticed. At other times, they can seem to be an overwhelming burden. One of the greatest current stressors may be the feeling that we should not have the discomfort associated with increased stress. When this discomfort happens, some of us may assume that we are not coping well or that this is a sign of illness. The assumption that we should feel good all the time, no matter what changes or problems we are facing, can add to the pressures we already feel.

There are two basic types of stressful events: one is intense, an alarm reaction that readies your body for an emergency; the other is less intense and alerts your body to meet a long-term problem that calls for endurance.

In instances when the stimulus is intense, as in a perceived threat, a phenomenon referred to as "fight or flight" occurs. The physical signs of this stress response are almost always conspicuous and may include an increased heart rate, muscle tension, or perspiration.

The effects of stress are not always fleeting. In many people the impact can be deferred for weeks or months. As a result, many illnesses are thought to be affected by accumulated stress, whether the illness has been either brought on or worsened by stress. Simply stated, stress produces or worsens symptoms when demands outweigh personal resources to cope with them.

THE "FIGHT-OR-FLIGHT" RESPONSE

Since the phenomenon we refer to as "fight or flight" was first described nearly 50 years ago, we have learned much about how the body produces chemicals in preparation for a fight-or-flight response.

Your pituitary, a gland attached to the base of your brain, secretes hormones that regulate many body processes. When you perceive a danger, your pituitary secretes a hormone called adrenocorticotropic hormone (ACTH) which causes your adrenal gland to release other hormones. These hormones—adrenaline (epinephrine) and cortisol—immediately cause your pulse to quicken, your muscles to tense, and your blood pressure to increase. Your body is made ready to fight or to flee (see also The Endocrine System at Work, page 706).

The change in blood flow is produced by adrenaline (epinephrine). During an emergency, you need more blood in your large muscles, so your heart beats faster and the blood pressure increases abruptly. Also, blood is directed away from your stomach and skin. Your body also releases more fat into the bloodstream because fat is an excellent quick source of energy; your blood sugar concentration increases for the same reason. Your body even secretes certain chemicals that make it easier for your blood to clot in case of an injury.

Your nervous system also is brought into action so that the pupils of your eyes dilate (to permit better vision), your facial muscles become tense (possibly to look more menacing), perspiration increases (to keep your body cool), and respiration accelerates (to increase available oxygen in the blood). All of these changes prepare your body for an emergency, real or imagined.

RECOGNIZING STRESS

Many of us are not very good at recognizing the emotional reactions we have and so find that first we notice the physical responses.

Stress can produce such symptoms as headache, insomnia, upset stomach, or digestive changes. You may feel physical symptoms or emotional fatigue as the first clues of increased stress. An old nervous habit such as nail-biting may reappear. Because you may not recognize that you are under increased stress, you may interpret the symptoms as those of an illness rather than the manifestation of an adjustment or adaptation process.

The thought that you may have a new illness can be frightening and can add to the emotional burden you already have.

The stress experience also may become apparent through psychological changes. The most common change is increased irritability with people who are close to you. You also may feel more cynical, pessimistic, or resentful than usual. Many people report a sense of being victimized, misunderstood,

or unappreciated. You may find that things to which you normally look forward seem burdensome. Some people become anxious or reclusive or prone to crying or laughing or to inappropriate aggressive behavior. Occasionally, these changes are so gradual that you or others around you may not recognize them until your health or relationships change.

As with the physical symptoms described earlier, you may not recognize such emotional changes as what they may be, signals of increased stress. Many people find themselves perplexed by the changes and often feel guilty or prone to blame others. The term "burnout" often is used to describe a combination of physical and psychological responses to stress.

DEALING WITH STRESS

In the course of daily events, we develop various ways of dealing with stressors. We work hard to decrease the newness of the changes we face, we talk about the experience, and we use things that we can count on already in our lives as "safe havens" from the new or adaptive change.

Much of this we do without really thinking about it. However, some of these changes are monumental, such as switching jobs or moving to another home. Others are routine, such as turning in a report, taking a test, meeting a new client, interviewing a babysitter, meeting a new teacher, or dealing with a child's temper tantrum. Mostly, we do pretty well in getting through fairly major as well as minor crises. Sometimes, we could do better.

The first step in learning to manage our stress-related reactions better is to become more aware of the things that may be particularly stressful for us individually. Not everyone responds to the same life event with the same amount of distress. For instance, a so-called workaholic may be thought by others to be working into an early grave but he or she may have found that taking on extra challenges in a work-related environment helps him or her to feel more under control. For this person, the work itself may be a form of stress management, but the unstructured time of a holiday without goals or "relaxation" at home may be a much greater stress.

We must learn to recognize in ourselves those things that cause the most trouble. We may not be able to avoid them, but, when we encounter them, it may reassure us to know they are the source of our extra discomfort. Just recognizing such elements helps to make us feel more in control. Understanding the real cause of discomfort also can minimize anxiety about the manifestations of stress we experience.

As a part of our overall strategy to manage stress in our lives, most of us must become more self-tolerant. We need to understand and accept that we constantly have to adapt to changes, losses, and things over which we have no or, at best, only partial control in our lives.

Most of us tend to be a great deal more understanding of other people's distress than we are of our own. We tend to think that we should always feel all right. As long as we believe this, we are sure to be disappointed. Accepting the fact that we may experience stress-related discomforts and that they are normal is helpful in managing stress.

Another important step involves actually dealing with the stress. Most of us want to do *something* when we are distressed so that we can feel as if we are making an active choice to reassume control in our lives—the very thing we feel we have lost to some degree in facing life's challenges. What we do is largely determined by a method most easily called "trial and success."

Over the years, most of us have found techniques that help us feel more comfortable. These vary from person to person and from personality to personality, so there is no way to provide a list of things everyone should do.

Each person needs several tools, or techniques, at his or her disposal. Some of the tools may include learning and using specific relaxation techniques—meditation, exercise, hobbies, and such. Other tools may require interaction with others and may decrease the sense of social isolation that we may feel. They may include group sports or hobbies, attending social events, meeting with a group of friends, or talking with a particularly valued friend, among many things. Finally, more-specific treatment by a skilled professional may be necessary. Discuss this with your physician.

Be particularly careful about using drugs, either prescribed or recreational, as a management technique. The so-called happy hour, which many people use as a way to release tensions from their work, functions as a stress reliever not because of the alcohol consumed but rather because of the social setting. The happy hour works because the person has made a choice to be in a setting with friends with few work expectations.

Drugs, whether tranquilizers or alcohol, may increase symptoms of loss of control, depression, and emotional or behavioral impulsiveness. Conscious or regular use of drugs to manage stress can be a manifestation of problems with the substances (for more information about alcohol and substance abuse, see pages 417 and 431).

In summary, experiencing stress is an ongoing and normal part of living. We are constantly called on to adapt to changes within ourselves (such as aging or health problems), or in our surroundings (such as a new job, family structure, or social relationships). The reactions to these stressors may be physical or psychological and usually are unpleasant. The fact that they may be unpleasant does not mean that they are abnormal or that they constitute illness.

You can minimize the effects of stress by learning to recognize when you are experiencing it, by acknowledging and accepting it, and by choosing or learning to use methods for managing it. Some of these tools for managing stress include individual and interpersonal skills and techniques and include both physical and psychological approaches.

A caution. Physical or psychological symptoms that affect a person's ability to work, to play, or to find pleasure in life or hope for the future are unlikely to be merely due to stress. Consult your family physician immediately for further evaluation. Stress-management techniques alone are unlikely to provide relief.

TECHNIQUES FOR ACCEPTING STRESS

Events that cause stress will always be with us. We can do many things to lessen the effects of stress and to relieve the discomfort it causes, but some stress is inevitable. Accept situations that cannot be changed. But remember—you can make acceptance easier. Here are suggestions.

KEEP THINGS IN PERSPECTIVE

Most of us tend to worry about things over which we have no control. For instance, how many times have you worried about whether the weather will be pleasant for a special event, such as a wedding? Clearly, there is nothing you can do about it except to prepare for the possibility of inclement weather.

When faced with worries and fears, try to look beyond the specific event. Ask yourself a few questions, such as:

What is the worst thing that can happen?
How likely is it that the worst will happen?
Have I done everything I realistically can to influence the outcome of the situation?
Will the outcome change my life substantially, and will I even remember it several years from now?
How would I counsel a friend in a similar situation?

Try giving yourself a little pep talk of reassurance. Do not let feelings of defeat, fear, or disappointment overtake you. The more positively you can approach the situation, the more likely it is that you will be able to face and influence the outcome.

INTERPERSONAL CONFLICTS

Difficulties in coping are not always a matter of the individual and his or her circumstances. Often, life's hurdles include dealing with personality conflicts with others. Typically, such conflicts are of three kinds: family, marital, or job-related.

Family Conflicts

All families are a complex network of relationships. Each member has a different relationship with each of the others in the family. These differences may be a reflection of age, birth order, sex, or personality type, or a combination of several factors. Each of these relationships, in turn, affects the rest of the family.

Physicians often recommend family therapy—in which the client is the entire family unit and the sessions include the whole family—when more than one member seems to have serious emotional problems, when a pattern of blame has become entrenched, or when an adolescent is particularly rebellious.

Often, problems within the family as a whole may be brought to the attention of a professional therapist when one member of the family is showing signs of a problem—for example, trouble in school, substance abuse, or inappropriate sexual behavior. Through family therapy, each member can discover his or her role in the problem.

There may be a pattern of behavior that everyone is contributing to and that everyone needs to help change. Rather than focusing on the gripes of individual family members, the therapist will identify specific problems in communication that can be worked on by all. The therapist does not solve problems for the family but shows families how to understand their problems and how to cope with them more effectively.

Marital Conflicts

Marriage counselors frequently observe that one of the greatest problems in the marriages they observe is that partners often enter into the relationship with unrealistic expectations. Our culture's romantic view of marriage fosters this tendency. Instead of realizing that they are marrying ordinary human beings with strengths and weaknesses, people tend to idealize their mates and expect nothing short of perfection.

Over the life of a marriage, couples typically face a predictable series of transitions. Consequently, researchers often speak of "different marriages" within a single marriage. Adjustments to the first child and subsequent children, changes in jobs, loss of a spouse's parents, and changing sexual needs all present challenges. If the marriage is to survive, the couple must communicate and resolve inevitable conflicts effectively.

At a time of conflict in a marriage, a marriage counselor often can help bring such issues to light so that the couple can begin to deal with current problems in a more mature way.

Job-Related Conflicts

Interpersonal conflicts in the workplace can represent a multitude of issues. Competition between co-workers may reflect a genuine lack of the potential for upward mobility; there may simply be too many candidates for promotion. Conflict also can stem from an individual's desire for power and control. Problems result from a lack of proper communication between co-workers and between management and employees.

If conflicts prove to be a continuing problem, seek counseling.

SEEK HELP IF YOU CANNOT COPE

You do not need to handle all of your problems alone. Sometimes the help of a counselor, psychiatrist, psychologist, clergyman, or friend may be just what you need to help you handle stress. Many people believe that seeking outside help is a sign of weakness, which adds to their sense of despair, hopelessness, or anger. Nothing could be further from the truth. It takes strength to realize that you need help. Ask your physician, local community health organization, or employer for recommendations if you need help in finding appropriate assistance.

METHODS OF COPING WITH STRESS

Even if you cannot always identify causes of stress, you can relieve some of the discomfort. Just feeling that you *can* do something often is a help in itself.

RELAXATION TECHNIQUES

Many of us think of relaxation as simply not working. We tend to think that watching television with our feet up or reading a book or the newspaper is relaxing. Such activities may or may not be. If our teeth are clenched or our muscles tense as we follow the action or if we relive the irritations and problems of the day while paying only partial attention, we are anything but relaxed. Relaxing involves skills you can learn.

Relaxation techniques can help lessen the discomfort and duration of symptoms of stress such as headaches, anxiety, high blood pressure, trouble falling asleep, Raynaud's syndrome (see page 840) or other causes of cool or cold hands, hyperventilation, and clenching or grinding of teeth, to name a few.

One simple method of relaxation is to remove yourself from the stressful situation: block the world out and concentrate on your body. Here is how:

1. Sit or lie in a comfortable position and close your eyes. Allow your jaw to drop and your eyelids to be relaxed and heavy but not tightly closed.
2. Mentally scan your body, starting with your toes and working slowly up through your legs, buttocks, torso, arms, hands, fingers, neck, and head. Focus on each part individually; where you feel tension, imagine it melting away.
3. Tighten the muscles in one area of your body and hold them for a count of 5 or more before relaxing and moving on to the next area. This is a good method for releasing tension. Tighten the muscles of your face, shoulders, arms, legs, and buttocks.
4. Allow thoughts to flow through your mind but do not focus on any of them. Many people find using autosuggestion to be a great help: suggest to yourself that you are relaxed and calm, that your hands are warm (or cool if you are hot) and heavy, that your heart is beating calmly, or that you feel perfectly at peace.
5. Breathe slowly, regularly, and deeply during the procedure.
6. Once you are relaxed, imagine you are in a favorite place or in a spot of great beauty and stillness.
7. After 5 or 10 minutes, rouse yourself from the state gradually.

RELAXED BREATHING

Make relaxed breathing a part of your total relaxation program. This type of breathing can be helpful because of its quick, calming effect.

Different methods of breathing involve movement of different regions of your torso. Most adults breathe by expanding and contracting their chests (chest breathing). Some lift their shoulders in an attempt to fill their lungs (shoulder breathing). Infants and children, on the other hand, usually breathe from the diaphragm, the dome-shaped muscle that separates the chest cavity from the abdominal cavity. This diaphragmatic breathing provides a more efficient exchange of oxygen and carbon dioxide than chest or especially shoulder breathing. Diaphragmatic breathing also takes less effort.

Proper relaxed breathing is an important part of good physical and mental health. With relaxed diaphragmatic breathing, your shoulders do not move up and your chest does not move out noticeably. Air flows smoothly into and out of your lungs rather than being drawn in and blown out forcefully. Your abdomen rises with each inhalation and lowers with each exhalation. The overall effect is relaxing to your entire body.

With practice you can breathe in a deep and relaxing manner as a matter of course. At first, practice lying on your back while wearing clothing that is loose around your waist and abdomen. Once you can breathe easily in this position, practice while sitting and then while standing. After a while you will be able to breathe from your diaphragm whenever and wherever you wish.

1. Lie down on your back on a bed, a well-padded floor, or a recliner chair.
2. Place your feet slightly apart. Rest one hand comfortably on your abdomen near your navel. Place the other hand on your chest.
3. Inhale through your nose because this allows the air to be filtered and warmed. Exhale through your mouth. If you have trouble breathing through your nose, inhale through your mouth.
4. Concentrate on your breathing for a few minutes and become aware of which

hand is rising and falling with each breath.

5. Gently exhale most of the air in your lungs.

6. Inhale while slowly counting to 4, about 1 second per count. As you inhale gently, slightly extend your abdomen, causing it to rise about 1 inch. (You should be able to feel the movement with your hand.) Remember, do not pull your shoulders up or move your chest.

7. As you breathe in, imagine the warmed air flowing in. Imagine this warmth flowing to all parts of your body.

8. Pause 1 second after inhaling.

9. Slowly exhale to the count of 4. While you are exhaling, your abdomen will slowly fall as your diaphragm relaxes upward against your lungs.

10. As air flows out, imagine that tension is also flowing out.

11. Pause 1 second after exhaling.

12. If it is difficult to inhale and exhale to a count of 4, shorten the count slightly and later work up to 4. If you experience light-headedness, alter the length or depth of your breathing.

13. Repeat the slow inhaling, pausing, slow exhaling, and pausing 5 to 10 times. Exhale. Inhale slowly: 1, 2, 3, 4. Pause. Exhale slowly: 1, 2, 3, 4. Pause. Inhale: 1, 2, 3, 4. Pause. Exhale: 1, 2, 3, 4. Pause. Continue on your own.

As you practice you may notice that initially not every breath will reach the lower parts of your lungs. This will improve with practice. The idea is to concentrate on slow, even, easy breathing.

If it seems difficult to make your breathing regular, take a slightly deeper breath, hold it for a second or two, and then let it out slowly through pursed lips for about 10 seconds. Repeat this once or twice and return to the other procedure.

PHYSICAL FITNESS

Another method for coping with stress is physical activity. If you are physically fit, your body can handle stress better, both physically and emotionally.

Exercise also has a calming effect that lasts well after you finish your workout. Activities such as running and swimming which require repetitive movements can produce a mental state similar to that of meditation. Aerobic exercise that increases your heart rate for at least 20 minutes is good for cardiovascular fitness (see page 793) and also may decrease feelings of stress. Yoga and other nonaerobic stretching exercises are calming and produce a meditation-like state.

Almost any exercise can be good for you. Jogging, swimming, aerobic exercises, and brisk walking all may help to relieve symptoms of stress. Stretching can relieve tension in certain muscles or all over, and it can be done at almost any time.

Tension is common in the shoulders and neck. To relieve it, roll your shoulders, raising them toward your ears. Then relax your shoulders.

To reduce neck tension, move your head gently in a circle going clockwise and then counterclockwise.

Relieve tension in your torso by reaching toward the ceiling and doing side bends.

To help relieve foot and leg tension, draw circles in the air with your feet while flexing your toes.

To help ease muscular tension throughout your body, stand up and stretch all over.

CHAPTER 17
TOBACCO

CHAPTER CONTENTS

WHY SMOKERS SMOKE

The health-care costs of tobacco use in this country are staggering. Annually, we spend 23 billion dollars in medical costs and we lose 30 billion dollars because of loss of working time and decreased productivity from the effects of smoking. *Each year smoking kills more Americans than died in battle in World War II and Vietnam combined.*

The indirect costs of smoking are equally astonishing. Each year, fires started by cigarettes cause more than 400 million dollars in property damage. Higher insurance premiums and taxes needed to fund disability benefits for people made sick from cigarette smoking are part of the cost picture as well.

Warnings about the hazards of smoking have had an effect on smokers. Today, about 40 million Americans identify themselves as former smokers. The number of men who smoke has declined substantially, from one-half of the adult men in 1965 to about one-third today; among women, it has declined slightly to just under one-third.

Yet, in the face of the well-known dangers of cigarette smoking, an estimated 14 million of the more than 50 million people over the age of 20 who smoke are still unaware of or do not accept the health risks of their smoking. More than half of all Americans do not realize that cigarette smoking is addictive.

Very few people restrict their smoking to a few cigarettes a day or week. Fifty million American smokers consume 80 million packs of cigarettes each day.

Because tobacco use is legal and for the most part is still socially acceptable in this country, education about the perils of smoking may be the most effective way of providing reasons either to stop or to never start smoking. The following pages explain many of the health hazards of smoking and some of the methods for quitting.

The medical evidence is quite clear: smoking cigarettes, pipes, or cigars (or chewing tobacco) endangers your health. Even the infrequent use of tobacco is unhealthy.

The reasons people start smoking or refuse to quit are rarely clear. Some smokers report that their cigarettes offer them a surge of energy, especially to wake them up in the morning or keep them awake at other times (for example, while driving). Nicotine acts as a stimulant with an adrenaline-like effect. For example, it increases your heart rate and blood pressure while you are smoking.

Some smokers report that, when they are under tension, their cigarettes act to calm them. As a prop, the cigarette gives them something to do with their hands if they are nervous and provides a mild form of distraction or even a feeling of security.

The nicotine in tobacco is an addictive drug. Nicotine can provoke an addictive response in regular smokers that can be relieved only by smoking another cigarette. The degree of addiction depends to some degree on how much and how long the smoker has smoked.

The addiction most smokers experience may be both psychological and physical. For some, the regular use of cigarettes in many life situations may have persuaded them that they could not cope with life without smoking.

Advertising also affects smoking behavior. Cigarettes are the most heavily marketed consumer product in America, with the tobacco industry spending more than 2 billion dollars a year on advertising and promotion.

Many advertisements show smoking as part of physical, outdoor activities such as backpacking, jogging, and boating. Tobacco companies also sponsor events of high visibility with major crowds of young people, such as rock concerts, automobile and horse racing, and athletic events. In a far more aggressive form of promotion, tobacco companies continue to provide free sample packages of cigarettes to the public, many of which fall into the hands of youngsters.

To counteract the educational efforts of the medical community in this country, the tobacco industry through their public relations efforts, opinion surveys, and lobbyists persistently challenges the relationship between cigarettes and disease. Even though the tobacco manufacturers claim that their advertising is meant only to establish brand loyalty among existing smokers, the extravagantly expensive advertising, promotional, and political campaigns of the industry must be considered a significant influence on the many young people who start and continue to smoke.

HOW HAZARDOUS IS SMOKING?

Smoking is the single largest preventable cause of premature death and disability in this country. One in six deaths in the United States each year is associated with cigarette smoking. The American Lung Association states that smoking kills more Americans each year than cocaine, heroin, alcohol abuse, auto accidents, homicide, and suicide combined.

Each year almost 400,000 Americans die prematurely from the effects of smoking. Millions more live with damaged lungs and hearts. Cigarette smoking accounts for the vast majority of deaths from lung cancer and from chronic obstructive pulmonary disease (see Emphysema, page 929, and Chronic Bronchitis, page 927). For years, lung cancer has been the number 1 cause of cancer death in men; lung cancer has now surpassed breast cancer as the leading cancer killer of women, too.

Smoking contributes substantially to the development of atherosclerosis which affects the heart and peripheral blood vessels (see Atherosclerosis: What Is It?, page 786). Smoking is also implicated as a cause or is associated with other diseases and types of cancer (such as cancer of the larynx, oral cavity, esophagus, urinary bladder, kidney, pancreas, stomach, and uterine cervix).

COMMON HEALTH EFFECTS

Cigarette smoke contains about 4,000 chemicals including trace amounts of such known poisons such as DDT, arsenic, and formaldehyde. Carbon monoxide in cigarette smoke displaces oxygen from your red blood cells, thereby robbing your tissues of oxygen.

THE LOW-YIELD CIGARETTE

The low-yield cigarette is not a magic answer to the problems caused by smoking.

During the last 30 years, the average tar and nicotine yield of American cigarettes has declined substantially. On the face of it, the decrease in these substances is good news, and the implication from advertisers has been that the low-yield cigarettes may be safer than the older conventional cigarettes.

How Different Are Low-Yield Cigarettes?
The addition of a filter-tip that selectively removes tar and nicotine was an important first step in decreasing the levels of these substances in the smoke. Further refinements to decrease tar and nicotine have included expanded or puffed tobacco (so that there is less tobacco per cigarette), faster burning times, more porous paper, and ventilated filters that allow dilution of the tobacco smoke with air.

The fact is, however, that the low-yield cigarette contains the same tobacco and nicotine as the other cigarettes—it has simply been engineered to make less smoke available to the smoker. In addition, filters do not remove carbon monoxide or other gaseous components from the tobacco smoke.

Don't Be Misled
Most smokers smoke because they are addicted to nicotine. When using low-yield cigarettes, smokers tend to change their smoking behavior. They take more frequent puffs, inhale more deeply, and often smoke more cigarettes. After switching to low-yield cigarettes, you may still take in as much, or more, tar, nicotine, and carbon monoxide as with your old brand.

Use of low-yield cigarettes probably does not decrease the risk of cancer, emphysema, or other diseases—even if you do not increase the number of cigarettes you smoke per day.

In addition, there appears to be no difference in the risk of a heart attack between high-yield and low-yield cigarette smokers. However, the risk of a heart attack diminishes within a year after you stop smoking, no matter which type of cigarette you smoked.

The Bottom Line
Thus, even if you switched to a low-yield cigarette, the chance of decreasing your risks for lung cancer, emphysema, heart attack, or other diseases is probably very small. To decrease these risks significantly, there is only one clear message: stop smoking. Do not be confused; low-yield cigarettes are not safe cigarettes.

The delicate tissues of the mouth, throat (pharynx), and voice box (larynx) are exposed repetitively to the effects of cigarette smoke. The cancer-causing agents of tobacco smoke are directly responsible for most cancers of the mouth, pharynx, and larynx seen in this country. The profile of someone with oral cancer is a man over age 50 who has been a heavy cigarette smoker most of his life. Pipe and cigar smokers run the same risks of oral and laryngeal cancer; use of chewing tobacco is linked primarily to cancers of the lip and mouth.

After the smoke passes through your mouth, your lungs retain 70 to 90 percent of the compounds you inhale. A few puffs on a cigarette reduces the effectiveness of the cilia inside your bronchial tubes. These tiny hair-like bodies normally work like brooms to sweep foreign particles out from your lungs. Smoking just one cigarette can slow the sweeping action of the cilia. Regular smoking virtually paralyzes the cilia, leaving your lungs exposed to billions of tiny particles from cigarette smoke. With the cilia largely inactive, tar from the cigarette smoke begins to build up and damage delicate lung tissues. When cooled inside your lungs, the tar forms a brown, sticky layer on the lining of breathing passages. This layer contains chemicals that can produce cancer (see Lung Cancer, page 937).

The link between smoking and lung cancer is inescapable. At the turn of the century, lung cancer was relatively rare. But with the widespread practice of cigarette smoking among men after World War I, and then among women 30 years later, lung cancer has become the most common cause of cancer death in this country. The risk of having lung cancer is approximately 10 times greater for cigarette smokers than for non-smokers. Pipe and cigar smokers as a group have a somewhat smaller risk for developing lung and bladder cancer, probably because they generally do not inhale the smoke as deeply.

Various studies and reports issued by the Surgeon General of the United States clearly document that cigarette smoking is also the major cause of chronic lung diseases such as chronic bronchitis (see page 927) and emphysema (see page 929). In addition to paralyzing or destroying the cilia in your lungs, the smoke irrevocably damages or destroys the alveoli, the tiny air sacs in your lungs in

THE RISKS OF CHEWING TOBACCO

At the turn of the century, smokeless tobacco was the most popular form of tobacco used in this country. Chewing tobacco and snuff remained commonplace until the discovery that tuberculosis was transmitted through spitting, and it became both illegal and socially unacceptable to spit in public places.

Since the early 1970s, there has been an upswing in the use of so-called smokeless tobacco, especially among male adolescents. Surveys have found that in some areas up to one-third of all male high school and college students regularly use smokeless tobacco. Of the 10 million users in this country, an estimated 3 million are under age 21. Studies have also revealed that children as young as 8 and 9 years old use smokeless tobacco regularly.

Smokeless tobacco is sold in two forms. One is a cured, ground tobacco called snuff which may be dry, moist, or finely cut. The other form is chewing tobacco which is sold in loose-leaf, plug, or twisted forms. When you chew tobacco or place a small amount of it between your gum and cheek, the tobacco mixes with your saliva and nicotine is absorbed through the lining of your mouth into your bloodstream.

The use of smokeless tobacco is linked to an increased chance of oral cancer developing (see Oral Cancer, page 580). The cheek and gum are the locations most often affected. Leukoplakia—white spots or patches on the tongue, lip, or cheek which can become ma-

lignant—has been found in a high percentage of people who use smokeless tobacco. Smokeless tobacco has also been associated with cancers of the esophagus, larynx, and pancreas.

Another health problem associated with this use of tobacco is periodontal disease. Smokeless tobacco can cause the gums to become so inflamed that they swell and bleed (see Gingivitis, page 570). In addition, chewing tobacco extract can increase the growth of two types of oral bacteria that are associated with dental cavities.

Despite marketing claims or conventional wisdom, smokeless tobacco is *not* a safe alternative to smoking. On the contrary, it is clear that smokeless tobacco poses a serious threat to the health of anyone who uses it.

TEENAGE SMOKING

Most cigarette smokers start early in life. Among smokers born since 1935, more than 80 percent started smoking before age 21 and more than half started before age 18. Today, a million teenagers take up smoking each year.

A growing number of them are female. While smoking has generally declined since the mid-1960s, an increasing number of teenage girls smoke. This group continues to be a major target for advertising by the tobacco industry.

It has been well documented that a high percentage of teenagers who smoke are from families in which one or both parents smoke. An explanation of this may be that, because more mothers now smoke than in past generations, more of their daughters mimic their mothers' smoking behavior.

Cigarette smoking among teenagers also seems to be connected with peer pressure. In a survey of 3,000 junior high school students, the most likely predictor of whether a boy or girl smoked was having friends who smoked.

Education does not appear to be an effective deterrent to smoking among teenagers. Nine of every 10 teenagers recently surveyed believed that smoking was harmful to their health and 85 percent of those who smoked said that they did not plan to be smokers for more than 5 years. It is interesting to note that most of the teenagers who took up smoking had been adamantly against smoking in their younger years. But the power of example, good or bad, is often persuasive: children whose parents continue to smoke with no visible ill effects often tend to change their own attitudes. The teenagers' concerns about smoking diminish, and many take up smoking.

It has been found that young women smokers find it harder to quit than men do. One of their fears is that they will gain weight if they quit smoking. Yet the facts do not support a direct link between weight gain and quitting smoking. If you stop smoking, your senses of taste and smell tend to return and with this a greater enjoyment of food. Simply being on guard against the temptation to exploit the newly returned enjoyment of the taste of food may prevent undue weight gain. In a national survey, one of four exsmokers had actually lost weight.

Young people are not exempt from the health risks of smoking. Lung damage can begin at an early age, and atherosclerosis, which can lead to heart attacks and strokes, can have its start early in life, especially among smokers.

---

which carbon dioxide is exchanged for oxygen. When these air sacs are injured to a critical extent, your body is unable to transport adequate levels of oxygen to your vital organs and, eventually, the chronic bronchitis or emphysema becomes fatal.

LESSER-KNOWN HEALTH EFFECTS

It is well known that smoking is the leading cause of lung cancer and chronic lung diseases. Yet, the single most important health effect of smoking may be in the development of heart attacks: cigarette smoking is the suspected cause of approximately one-fourth of deaths from coronary artery disease. There are many different chemicals and substances in tobacco smoke that injure the cardiovascular system.

The nicotine in tobacco smoke acts on your adrenal glands, causing them to secrete hormones that temporarily increase your blood pressure and your heart rate, which makes your heart work harder. Tobacco smoke also contains carbon monoxide. When inhaled, the carbon monoxide binds to the hemoglobin, taking the place of valuable oxygen. Thus, smoking decreases the amount of oxygen available to your heart.

The result is that every cigarette places a small but unnecessary load on your heart and blood vessels. In addition, the carbon monoxide may have a direct effect on the heart muscle itself, on your blood vessels, and perhaps even on the clotting of your blood.

Smoking probably increases the clumping ability of certain blood cells (platelets). The mechanism is complex, but the result is that smoking is a contributing factor to the deposition of cholesterol in the arteries (see Atherosclerosis: What Is It?, page 786). This may be why smoking is also associated with stroke, the nation's third leading cause of death. Smokers may be at a 2 or 3 times greater risk of having a stroke.

Smoking contributes to peripheral obstructive arterial disease (see Circulatory Problems, page 834). This can result in leg or

SECOND-HAND SMOKE

The health threat to the non-smoker from exposure to tobacco smoke is well documented. As a result of the effects of this second-hand (passive) smoking, more than 30 states have enacted laws limiting smoking in public places.

The inhaling of second-hand smoke causes your heart to beat faster, your blood pressure to increase, and the level of carbon monoxide in your blood to increase. Sidestream smoke from a burning cigarette contains twice as much tar and nicotine as does the inhaled smoke, 3 times as much of a compound called 3,4-benz-pyrene (a cancer-causing agent), 5 times as much carbon monoxide, and possibly 50 times as much ammonia. Clearly, people with respira-tory or heart conditions, and the elderly in general, are at special health risk when exposed to second-hand smoke.

Children under 1 year of age who are exposed to smoke have a higher frequency of admissions to hospitals for respiratory illness compared with children of nonsmoking parents. Second-hand (passive) smoke increases a child's risk of getting pneumonia, bronchitis, or tonsillitis. Furthermore, children of parents who smoke are at increased health risk because their parents are more apt to have respiratory infections that they pass on to their children.

In conclusion, the health issues in regard to environmental smoke are so grave that all smoking parents should consider quitting if for no other reason than the health of their children.

thigh pain with exercise and, ultimately, in gangrene of the foot.

Women who use oral contraceptives and smoke, especially after age 35, are at risk of serious problems with their heart and blood vessels. The risk is so serious, in fact, that the Food and Drug Administration requires a warning on oral contraceptive packages.

Smoking decreases the senses of smell and taste which makes eating food less enjoyable. Smoking also can impair the healing of peptic ulcers (see Peptic Ulcer, page 603) and may increase the likelihood of a recurrence.

SMOKING AND PREGNANCY

Many women who smoke during their pregnancy fail to understand that there are unique health hazards both to themselves and to their developing fetuses. The primary risks associated with cigarette smoking during pregnancy or at the time of delivery include an increased chance of miscarriage, a low-birth-weight baby, and increased incidence of fetal or infant death (see Smoking and Use of Alcohol and Illegal Drugs During Pregnancy, page 188).

HOW TO STOP SMOKING

Most smokers understand that tobacco use, and smoking specifically, is a behavior that is hazardous to their health. What many beginning smokers fail to understand, however, is that smoking is also an addiction that involves chemicals that affect emotions and behavior.

The cigarette user smokes to maintain a certain level of nicotine in his or her blood. After the smoker has not had a cigarette for several hours, this level decreases and the smoker becomes irritable and edgy—he or she "needs a smoke." Smoking a cigarette may then relieve these symptoms of withdrawal. Smoking a cigarette will not relieve nervousness in a nonsmoker. The only kind of nervousness that smoking will relieve is the nervousness that comes from nicotine withdrawal.

Because nicotine is an addictive drug, quitting smoking can be difficult—in fact, most people fail in their first attempt. As difficult as it may be to stop, however, it is not impossible. Each year, 3 million Americans are successful, although many of them failed on previous attempts. The reasons many people initially fail vary, depending on how long and how much they smoked, their sensitivity to the drug, and how well they prepared for their attempt to stop.

Remember, there is no reason to give up trying to quit even after a failed attempt or two or more. If you failed in past efforts to stop smoking, do not be discouraged. Instead, learn from your experiences and set another stop date. Making a commitment to stop and then following through with an attempt to stop can be a most rewarding accomplishment and of incalculable importance to your continued good health and the health of others.

METHODS OF STOPPING

There is no one perfect plan or technique for quitting smoking. What most successful quitting approaches have in common, however, is a commitment on the part of participants to quit coupled with a realistic expectation that quitting probably will not be easy.

You may experience physical withdrawal symptoms for 3 to 10 days. When these symptoms begin to lessen, you may still have an impulse to smoke at those times you habitually would "light up" in the past (after a meal or when getting behind the wheel of your car).

For some exsmokers, periodic urges to smoke may come and go for months to years. However, the intensity and duration of these urges invariably grow smaller with the passage of time.

Most relapses occur within the first week after a person stops. The reason for a relapse depends on many factors, including the strength of the addiction. Occasionally, relapses occur because of a weakness in the smoke-ending program. A smoke-ending program should include various changes in your routine because it is thought that people revert to smoking during the first 3 months most often because of a lack of new nonsmoking behaviors.

Consider the following strategies in designing your personal stop-smoking regimen.

Set a Stop Date. Pick a date to quit, and make it reasonably soon. Then list on paper the reasons you want to stop. Review the points on your list both before you begin your attempt and periodically during the program.

Involve Other People. Do not make your plans to quit a secret merely to avoid talking about a potential failed effort. Tell your family, friends, and colleagues. Give them specifics of when and why you want to stop and ask for their support. Ask your spouse or a friend to quit with you.

Before You Reach Your Stop Day. You can switch to a brand whose taste, packaging, or some other aspect is less appealing. Decrease your nicotine dose by changing to a milder brand; smoke only half of each cigarette. Beware, however: if you switch to a milder brand there is a tendency to smoke a larger number of cigarettes because you tend to smoke enough to maintain the nicotine level to which you have become addicted (see The Low-Yield Cigarette, page 409). Taper off by beginning a gradual reduction in the number of times you smoke and in the number of cigarettes you smoke each day.

Use matches instead of a lighter, or vice versa. Make changes in your normal routine that are mildly disruptive. Get rid of favorite lighters and ashtrays, and clean your clothes to rid them of the cigarette smell. Throw out all but one ashtray, and clean it after each cigarette. Buy cigarettes by the pack instead of by the carton. Make cigarettes inconvenient by keeping them in another room. Delay smoking when you feel the urge.

Invent your own methods of making yourself conscious of every cigarette you are tempted to smoke. Remember, you are breaking a behavior, one that is likely to be a ritualized part of your life.

Take It One Day at a Time. On your stop day, quit completely. Make it your commitment to not smoke today. Focus all of your attention on achieving that goal. Tomorrow can be taken care of tomorrow.

Change Your Routine. Avoid or change situations in which you previously smoked. Drink your morning coffee in a different location. Leave the table immediately after meals if they formerly ended with a cigarette. Take a walk instead of lighting up. If you smoked while using the telephone, avoid prolonged conversations or change the location of the telephone you use. If you have a chair you favor for smoking, avoid it temporarily.

Alter Your Surroundings. Before the urge to smoke strikes, start activities that make smoking physically difficult to perform, such as washing the car, weeding the garden, or taking a shower. Almost any kind of physical exercise may help. Your smoking behavior may be very ingrained and seem automatic.

Anticipate this automatic behavior and plan alternatives.

Time the Urge. Check your watch whenever an urge hits. Most are short-lived. Once this is apparent, you will be better able to resist the urge.

Practice Positive Thinking. Reverse the negative "I can't do it" thinking. Take a positive approach. "I can make it another few minutes and then the urge will pass and I will be okay."

If you do light one up, you do not have to smoke it. If you start it, you do not have to finish it. And if you do finish it, you are not a failure. This is nothing more than a temporary setback. Experts in the field suggest that it is important to retain a vision of the day when you no longer smoke and to refer to it when the urge to smoke comes on: no more messy ashtrays, stained yellow teeth, cigarette breath, or burn marks on your furniture, rugs, or clothes. No more breathlessness and lack of stamina.

Another positive step is to reward yourself. With the money you save by not buying tobacco, buy or treat yourself to something.

Aids for Nonsmoking. A nicotine resin (nicotine polacrilex), popularly known by its tradename Nicorette, may help as an adjunct to a treatment program. This product, often called nicotine gum, gradually releases nicotine when it is chewed. Chewing too rapidly will release too much nicotine and cause nausea.

The goal is to use just enough nicotine polacrilex to maintain your nicotine level, thus holding in check any withdrawal symptoms. Nicotine polacrilex is designed to be "parked" between your cheek and gum in order to maximize its absorption. Meanwhile, the smell of cigarette smoke begins to disappear from your home and your clothing—and the habit of reaching for a cigarette is slowly being broken.

Once you feel comfortable in your smoke-free behaviors, it is time to begin gradually decreasing the amount of nicotine polacrilex you use. You can taper off any time within 3 to 6 months after you stop smoking. By the end of 6 months, however, discontinue the nicotine polacrilex.

We emphasize that the nicotine gum is only an aid and may not be appropriate for everyone. Some heart patients, people with peptic ulcers, and pregnant women should not chew the gum. In addition, it does not mimic other effects of smoking. Although it is lightly spiced to mask the nicotine's bitterness, most smokers find that it takes several days to become accustomed to the unusual taste. There may be side effects such as indigestion or stomachache, but these discomforts usually are mild and short-lived. Nicotine gum is available only by prescription from a physician. Other prescription medications are being studied for their potential in assisting smokers to stop.

Do Your Homework First. In organizing your plan for quitting, your physician can be helpful or you can seek a smoking cessation program in your community. Before you start your program, examine the wide range of self-help materials available from the local chapters of your American Lung Association, American Cancer Society, and American Heart Association.

Many chapters of the American Lung Association have programs that can help you identify the situations or moods that trigger your urge to smoke. The assistance of a trained facilitator can help you develop a personalized plan of coping strategies for quitting. Some offer weight control and stress management skills as well.

PROBLEMS OF STOPPING

Immediately after quitting, you may feel edgy and more hungry, tired, irritable, and short-tempered than usual. You may have strong cravings for a cigarette. You also may have trouble sleeping and may notice an increase in coughing.

Nicotine withdrawal symptoms are the result of your body's clearing itself of the nicotine. Most of the nicotine will be gone in 2 or 3 days but your body's desire for it may continue for several weeks.

You may experience an increased hunger or an improvement in your senses of taste and smell. Indirectly, this can result in weight gain. Quitting does not mean that you automatically will gain weight; besides, a modest, temporary weight gain is a small price to pay for eliminating what may be your single greatest overall health risk and, specifically, for significantly decreasing your chances of having cancer or heart or lung disease. Some tips for guarding against a major weight gain are as follows:

- Drink a glass of water before every meal.
- Plan well-balanced menus carefully and literally count the calories.
- Arrange beforehand that you will eat only low-fat, low-calorie snacks, including low-calorie beverages.
- If oral gratification becomes a problem, chew sugarless gum or snack on foods such as carrots, pickles, sunflower seeds, or celery.
- Weigh yourself weekly and exercise regularly.

If you become constipated during your recovery, add some roughage to your diet, such as raw vegetables and whole-grain cereals.

Tension and irritability are common withdrawal symptoms. Become familiar with suitable relaxation techniques. Take a walk or a shower or soak in the bathtub. Breathe deeply and slowly, as though you are inhaling a cigarette, and repeat this procedure several times.

Remember: if unsuccessful, try again.

BENEFITS OF STOPPING

Within a few days, you will begin to notice some remarkable changes in your body. Your senses of smell and taste may improve. You may breathe easier, and your smoker's cough will begin to disappear, although you may still cough and bring up mucus for a while. You may also notice an improvement in your stamina.

The more lasting and serious benefits of quitting smoking begin almost immediately. Within 24 hours the levels of carbon monoxide and nicotine in your system will decrease rapidly. The effects of smoking on bronchitis will begin to be reversed from the very first day you quit. Although the effects of emphysema are irreversible, breathing is made easier and the progress of the disease is slowed.

By the end of the first nonsmoking year, your risk of a heart attack begins to decrease; by the 10th year it is almost the same as for lifetime nonsmokers. The American Cancer Society believes that quitting smoking immediately decreases the chances of esophageal or pancreatic cancer; within 7 years your risk of bladder cancer will drop to that of a nonsmoker, and after 10 to 15 years of not smoking the statistical risk of the exsmoker getting cancer of the lung, larynx, or mouth approaches that of people who have never smoked.

CHAPTER 18

ALCOHOL ABUSE

CHAPTER CONTENTS

UNDERSTANDING ALCOHOL

Alcohols are a group of compounds, many of which are ingredients in perfumes, extracts, tinctures, paints, and other products. Alcohols are also essential to many manufacturing processes.

The form of alcohol in the beverages we drink is ethyl alcohol (ethanol), a colorless liquid that in its pure, undiluted form has a biting or burning taste. It is produced by the fermentation of sugars that occurs naturally in cereals and fruits, such as barley and grapes.

Historically, alcohol has enjoyed a reputation as the "elixir of life." Because of its many reported medicinal properties, alcohol was once thought to improve life, perhaps even prolong it. Over the years, however, virtually all of the magical claims have proved to be untrue.

Alcohol depresses the central nervous system, acting as a sedative or tranquilizer. It is also a consciousness-altering drug. Taken in large enough quantities, alcohol is a lethal poison. Technically, alcohol is also a food because it provides calories (slightly less than the number of calories per gram found in fat).

Unfortunately, millions of people use alcohol excessively. According to the National Institute on Alcohol Abuse and Alcoholism, two-thirds of all Americans over the age of 14 use alcohol—approximately 10 million of them can be classified as alcoholics, and another 7 million are alcohol abusers. Equally tragic is the fact that no more than about 15 percent of these people receive treatment for their condition.

Alcoholism has become a major social, economic, and public health problem. In the United States alone, the annual cost of lost productivity and health expenses related to alcoholism is estimated to be well over 100 billion dollars. Alcohol is involved in more than half of all accidental deaths, suicides, and homicides and in only slightly less than half of all traffic fatalities.

An additional expense is the cost of treating the approximately 1.5 million Americans who enter substance abuse centers each year. Indirect costs of alcohol include alcohol-related work accidents and days lost from work as a result of alcohol-related injury or illness.

HOW ALCOHOL WORKS IN YOUR BODY

Ethyl alcohol (ethanol) is a central nervous system depressant that relaxes you and reduces your inhibitions because it depresses the controlling centers of your brain. The more you drink, the more you are sedated. In sufficient amounts, alcohol can impair your speech and muscle coordination. Large quantities can produce sleep and in some cases life-threatening coma by severely depressing the vital centers of your brain.

The principal site for alcohol absorption is your small intestine, although very small amounts are absorbed in the mouth and esophagus and only slightly more is absorbed in your stomach. The rate at which the alcohol is absorbed in the small intestine depends on several factors.

If your stomach is empty, most of the alcohol is usually quickly absorbed. Food in the stomach or small intestine, especially solid and fatty foods, slows the emptying of the stomach and therefore the absorption of alcohol.

Once the alcohol has been absorbed into the bloodstream, it is quickly transported throughout your body. In fact, the alcohol is moved to wherever there is water in your body, including inside individual cells. This distribution accounts for the intoxicating effects of the alcohol. In pregnant women, alcohol eventually reaches the fetus, and in lactating women, alcohol passes into breast milk.

Nearly all of the alcohol is burned as fuel for your body, although small amounts are lost in your urine and from the lungs. It is the alcohol in the air we exhale that is measured in breath tests to determine the amount of alcohol in our bodies. The level of alcohol in the exhalations closely parallels the concentration of alcohol in the blood.

The smell of alcohol on your breath is usually the result of both the metabolism of other parts of the drink and the nearly odorless but slightly astringent smell of the alcohol itself. Beer, for example, will produce a breath odor different from that produced by whiskey. Gin and vodka are less likely to produce the readily identifiable drinker's breath.

Like an anesthetic, alcohol gradually and progressively depresses brain function. As you consume alcohol, areas of thought, emotion, and judgment are affected initially. As you continue to drink, motor control areas of your brain also are affected, resulting in slurred speech, unsteady balance, and slower reactions.

Alcohol also dilates the peripheral blood vessels (those nearest your skin) to produce an initial feeling of warmth. Your pulse rate rises and more urine is produced because of the increased fluid intake and the diuretic action of the drug on your kidneys. Alcohol also stimulates your stomach to secrete acid.

Your body uses alcohol just as it uses other food—by burning (metabolizing) it in the liver to gain heat and energy. For each gram of alcohol burned, 7 calories are produced. A 4-ounce drink of 12 percent wine, 12 ounces of beer, or 1 ounce of 100 proof liquor all may produce about 80 calories from their alcohol content alone. Beer or sweet wine will have additional calories from their sugar or carbohydrate content.

The food value of alcohol is limited, however, because its calories are "empty," providing no vitamins, minerals, or proteins.

Chronic alcoholics often have deficiencies in nutrients. Common deficiencies include thiamine (vitamin B_1), riboflavin (vitamin B_2), niacin, folic acid, pyridoxine (vitamin B_6), magnesium, potassium, and zinc.

Physicians once thought that the effect of alcohol on nutritional status was the only cause of long-term liver damage so commonly found in chronic alcohol users (conditions called fatty liver and cirrhosis; see Enlarged Liver, page 659, and Cirrhosis, page 653). Today it is known that the toxic effect of alcohol can harm the liver directly.

ALCOHOLISM

Alcoholism is a chronic and often progressive disease characterized by periods of preoccupation with the drug alcohol, impaired control over alcohol intake, and repetitive use of alcohol despite the presence of adverse consequences related to drinking. In this context, alcoholism is equated with al-

---

HOW MANY CALORIES ARE THERE IN MY DRINK?

Are you counting calories? Don't forget to include any alcoholic beverages you may consume.

You burn most of the calories in alcohol as fuel for your body, or it is transformed into body fat.

To determine the calorie content of an alcoholic beverage, read the label first. If the beverage is a distilled liquor such as whiskey or vodka, what is the proof? If it is a wine, what is the percentage of alcohol?

A distilled liquor identified as 100 proof is 50 percent alcohol by volume. "Proof" is twice the percentage of alcohol contained. Thus, a liquor that is 80 proof contains 40 percent alcohol; and if a wine label states that the alcohol concentration is 10 percent by volume, then it is 20 proof (although wine is not traditionally referred to by its proof).

Although the label on beer only rarely indicates its alcohol content, beer is usually 4 to 5 percent alcohol and is, therefore, about 8 to 10 proof.

The amount of calories contributed by the alcohol portion of various forms of alcohol drinks can be calculated by the following formula: Number of ounces $\times$ proof $\times$ 0.8 = number of calories. For example, a 2-ounce drink of 80 proof gin: $2 \times 80 \times 0.8 = 128$ calories.

Because dry wines and distilled liquors contain essentially no calories beyond those found in the alcohol, this formula can reveal the calorie content with good accuracy. Remember, though, that sugar in a sweet wine contributes additional calories; likewise, the carbohydrates in beer may furnish perhaps a fourth or half again as many calories as the alcohol itself. "Light" beers have smaller amounts of carbohydrates and often lesser amounts of alcohol.

---

cohol dependence. In other words, this is a type of drug dependence.

To be dependent on alcohol implies that you have a psychological need for its effects. It also suggests that you continue drinking despite the harmful effects it may cause you, your family, friends, and your work. To be dependent also suggests that you have a physical dependence on the drug.

In addition, a hereditary predisposition to alcoholism has been demonstrated, particularly in the sons of men who became alcoholic at an early age. These genetic factors also may influence the tendency for some alcoholics to have neurological complications (see Short- and Long-Term Effects of Excessive Alcohol Use, page 421).

The telltale symptoms of a physical dependence on alcohol are tolerance to the effects of alcohol or withdrawal symptoms that develop when you abstain from its use. These symptoms are relieved when the alcoholic takes another drink. Signs of withdrawal may range from a protracted headache, anxiety, insomnia, and nausea to tremors, delirium, and seizures (see Alcohol Withdrawal and the Dreaded DTs, page 422).

Tolerance may be an early sign of alcohol dependence. Tolerance occurs when, after a period of alcohol use, the drug effects that are usually seen are not as readily apparent. Thus, the alcoholic may appear sober even if he or she has a blood alcohol concentration that would normally indicate intoxication. A long-time user of alcohol may also metabolize (break down) the alcohol slightly more rapidly than someone whose body is not accustomed to chronic alcohol consumption.

Beware. No matter how much tolerance someone seems to develop, his or her liver is still unable to metabolize pure alcohol at a rate faster than approximately 1 ounce of 80 proof liquor every hour. After heavy drinkers develop a high tolerance, they may discover that their tolerance gradually declines and that they become drunk on progressively smaller amounts of alcohol. This decrease in tolerance probably occurs because their damaged livers metabolize or break down the alcohol more slowly. In addition, the effects of aging and the involvement of your nervous system may play a role. High tolerance is a sign of probable alcohol dependence.

What are the signs of abuse or dependence other than tolerance and withdrawal symptoms? Your physician can conduct tests to reveal clinical signs of serious physical damage caused by alcohol abuse, such as cirrhosis of the liver (see Cirrhosis, page 653), alcoholic hepatitis (see page 651), or cardiomyopathy (see page 831). However, the diagnosis of alcoholism should be made long before these complications develop.

Early signs of the problem are behavioral. An example would be someone who continues to ignore repeated warning signs that alcohol is causing problems in his or her marriage. Rather than admit the problem, the alcoholic becomes separated or divorced and continues to drink. Other warnings are alcohol-related problems on the job that result in the drinker missing many days of work or being fired or laid off, more than

one arrest for an alcohol-related incident such as driving while intoxicated, or signs of impaired health due to alcohol use.

Learning how to drink safely is important. Using tolerance as the sole measure of how much someone should drink is unsafe because it may permit someone to believe he or she does not have a drinking problem when, in fact, that problem is very real indeed. Remember: the earliest signs of alcohol abuse are simply the harmful effects of drinking that are ignored by the drinker, who continues to drink in the same manner (see Recognizing the Alcoholic, page 422).

ALCOHOL INTOXICATION

The effect of a given amount of alcohol on a particular person varies significantly because of several factors. The ingestion of equal amounts of alcohol is likely to achieve a higher blood alcohol concentration and, therefore, have a greater effect on the average woman than on the average man. This is because, in general, women's bodies are smaller and have a higher percentage of fat tissue than do men's bodies.

The effects of alcohol also depend on how much food has been consumed and how recently. The more food in the stomach, the slower the absorption of alcohol into the blood. Taking a drink on a full stomach spreads the metabolism of that drink over a longer period so the concentration of alcohol attained in the blood will be lower.

Intoxicating effects of alcohol correlate roughly with the concentration of alcohol, which, in turn, reflects levels present in the brain. In persons who are not alcoholics, a blood alcohol concentration above 25 mg/dL is associated with mild intoxication, including symptoms of altered mood, impaired thinking, and incoordination. At blood alcohol concentrations of more than 100 mg/dL, the person without alcoholism may experience double vision, difficulty in speaking, and pronounced incoordination. As the concentration increases, mild confusion may give way to stupor and, ultimately, coma.

Legal intoxication in most states is defined as a blood alcohol concentration of at least 80 to 100 mg of alcohol per deciliter of blood (mg/dL, or 0.1 percent).

Even at concentrations much lower than the legal limit, most people will have lost some coordination and reaction time. (Reaction time is the speed with which you can react to a situation—for example, how rapidly you can apply the brakes while driving a car when something unexpected happens.)

SHORT- AND LONG-TERM EFFECTS OF EXCESSIVE ALCOHOL USE

Alcohol abuse is a major social and medical problem. Very moderate drinking is acceptable in many social circles. However, excessive alcohol use can damage your liver, pancreas, brain, nerves, and cardiovascular system.

Brain and Nervous System. Excessive drinking of alcohol can produce several harmful effects on your brain and the nervous system. Alcohol can cause a temporary memory loss (blackout). It is not uncommon for heavy drinkers, and many first-time drinkers as well, to forget all or part of what occurred during the time they were drinking. Some heavy drinkers can have problems with their short-term memory that may persist for several weeks after stopping drinking. However, the memory is usually restored with abstinence.

Excessive alcohol use can cause insomnia and also can leave the user tired and exhausted in the morning, even after a full night's sleep. Guided by the activity of the brain, we move from periods of light or moderate sleep to intervals of dreaming sleep. These dreaming periods are called rapid-eye-movement (REM) sleep, and our physical and mental health are dependent on them (see Sleep Disorders, page 1028). Unfortunately, the anesthetic effect of alcohol interferes with the brain's ability to produce an adequate amount of REM sleep, which partially accounts for the morning fatigue many heavy drinkers experience.

A neurological disorder called Wernicke-Korsakoff's syndrome is found in some chronic alcoholics. This disorder primarily occurs in alcoholics with a poor nutritional intake, particularly of thiamine (vitamin B_1). This syndrome consists of two separate disorders that often occur together in the alcoholic.

The first symptom of Wernicke's syndrome is often a sudden weakness and paralysis of the eye muscles, which may result in double vision. Over time, the alcoholic with Wernicke's syndrome cannot stand or walk without aid. Korsakoff's syndrome results in severe amnesia, particularly involving recent memory. People with Wernicke-Korsakoff's syndrome exhibit symptoms of profound and deteriorating memory loss, including episodes in which the person may forget his or her identity. Furthermore, the person may mutter to himself or herself, become disoriented or delirious, and suffer hallucinations.

Treatment for Wernicke-Korsakoff's syndrome is very straightforward: abstinence from alcohol with thiamine supplements to relieve symptoms of the vitamin deficiency. However, the symptoms of this disorder are usually not completely reversible.

Gastrointestinal System. Alcohol can irritate the mucous lining of your stomach and produce gastritis (see page 608). This also may cause vomiting, which, in turn, can cause small tears in the upper stomach and lower esophagus. These tears, called Mallory-Weiss tears, can bleed. Persistent drinking can interfere with the absorption of some of the B vitamins, particularly folic acid and thiamine, and other nutrients. Most of these problems will disappear if you stop drinking. However, problems such as a fatty or enlarged liver, alcohol-induced hepatitis (see page 651), or esophageal varices (see page 601) may require immediate medical attention. The damage caused by cirrhosis of the liver (see Cirrhosis, page 653) tends to be progressive.

As the circulating alcohol moves through your liver, it is broken down (metabolized) by enzymes. A healthy liver can process alcohol at a rate of about 50 calories per hour. This is equivalent to about 1 ounce of 80 proof whiskey in about an hour. If your liver becomes overwhelmed by large amounts of alcohol, the alcohol will circulate in your body until it can be processed by your liver.

The cause of the common hangover (typically, the symptoms include headaches and dry mouth) is not entirely clear. One possibility is that alcohol is a diuretic, causing loss of water through the urine. This can lead to dehydration. The treatment for hangover symptoms is rest, plenty of liquids, and aspirin or other simple analgesics.

Alcoholics also may develop both acute and chronic pancreatitis (see pages 667 and 668).

Cardiovascular System. A drink of alcohol may temporarily reduce blood pressure but, taken regularly, alcoholic beverages can elevate blood pressure.

Chronic heavy drinkers frequently develop a condition called cardiomyopathy, a disease that destroys the heart muscle and produces symptoms that range from arrhythmias (irregular heartbeat) to heart failure (see Cardiomyopathy, page 831). In some people, a daily practice of only moderate alcohol intake may increase the possibility of heart disease.

Sexual Functioning. Alcohol abuse can cause impotence in men. In women it can interrupt menstruation. Pregnant women are routinely cautioned against using alcohol because it can pose a threat to the health and development of the fetus (see Pregnancy and Alcohol, page 429).

Cancer. After cardiovascular disease, cancer is the next leading cause of death among alcoholics. Alcoholics have a rate of cancer higher than that of the general population, especially cancer of the larynx, esophagus, stomach, and pancreas.

RECOGNIZING THE ALCOHOLIC

No longer do we accept the stereotypical view of alcoholics as limited to derelicts or people easily recognized by an unkempt appearance or public drunkenness.

Experience reveals that alcoholism knows no social or economic bounds. It strikes the young and old, men and women, rich and poor, and people of all races. Seemingly happy and successful people are just as likely to suffer from this disease as are those whose lives are filled with disappointments and failures. Many alcoholics are highly regarded people in society and pass for years among their friends and associates as healthy and normally functioning people. The problems that are brought on by their alcoholism, such as a broken marriage or lost job, are seen by them as the consequence of bad luck, something caused by others, or simply a character flaw.

For centuries alcoholics were viewed as people who suffered because they were weak-willed, and only personal resolve and willpower were considered ways to correct their drinking behavior. Since they lacked this strength of character, there was little or nothing one could do to help them.

These views have changed. Since the 1950s, the American Medical Association has characterized alcoholism as a disease. Other organizations, such as the National Council on Alcoholism, have worked to improve our understanding of alcoholism. Acceptance of alcoholism as a disease in this country has been slow, and many people still believe that the alcoholic is someone who has disgraced himself or herself because of personal weakness.

The truth is that alcoholics are sick people. Because of the social stigma placed on the disease of alcoholism, many alcoholics also view themselves as weak and bad peo-

---

ALCOHOL WITHDRAWAL AND THE DREADED DTs

The alcoholic who suddenly stops drinking is likely to experience physical and psychological withdrawal symptoms. In most people, the symptoms are minor: perhaps the "shakes" are evident in the hands; there may be a mild increase in pulse, blood pressure, and body temperature; nausea, diarrhea, and other gastrointestinal discomfort may occur; insomnia also may result. These symptoms generally run a course of 3 to 5 days; minor discomforts may last for weeks.

However, delirium tremens (DTs) make alcohol withdrawal a fearsome and dangerous prospect for some alcoholics. In most people, bad dreams, anxiety, and minor panic attacks are the worst effects of withdrawal; in a few others, more severe withdrawal symptoms occur. Often beginning with periods of confusion, the DTs also may involve vivid hallucinations, severe tremulousness, paranoid ideas, and even seizures. These symptoms often last for 3 to 5 days, sometimes longer.

The cause of both the minor and the more serious symptoms is the withdrawal of alcohol: the brain and other organs have become accustomed to tolerating elevated levels of ethanol, and when it is withdrawn the abstinence symptoms result.

If you are a chronic drinker seeking to stop drinking, anticipate a period of withdrawal symptoms. Sometimes admission to a hospital detoxification program is appropriate. Consult your physician: he or she can help you deal with withdrawal symptoms by addressing issues of safety, nutrition, and rest and by taking appropriate measures to deal with any underlying health problems (see The Treatment of Alcoholism, page 425).

ple. This burden of shame and blame is one of the stumbling blocks to the alcoholic's recovery.

How can you tell whether a friend or loved one is alcoholic? In most cases, it is not difficult. Early abuse, however, often goes undetected.

Anyone with a pattern of abusive drinking is someone with a drinking problem and may be an alcoholic. At a minimum, it can be said that an alcoholic is someone whose drinking causes problems. The following drinking patterns are indications of alcohol abuse or alcoholism.

Preoccupation. People who are alcohol-dependent tend to look forward to the next time they will be able to drink. They may select social activities on the basis of whether alcohol is available, talk a lot about drinking, and feel more comfortable if the liquor cabinet is well stocked. Feeling the need to be prepared for any emergency, they may store liquor in the car or at work.

Symptomatic Use of Alcohol. A common behavior of an alcohol-dependent person is to use alcohol as a medicine to relieve aches and pains, to relax, or to induce sleep.

Increased Tolerance. The alcoholic may be able to tolerate more alcohol than the occasional drinker. This increased tolerance is due to the brain's ability to adapt to the presence of higher concentrations of alcohol (see Alcoholism, page 419).

Loss of Control. The alcohol-dependent person cannot always predict how much he or she is going to drink. This person will often drink more than planned; he or she may stop for a "quick one" on the way home and stay an entire evening. This person may become intoxicated without intending to.

Solitary Drinking. Company is not important to an alcohol-dependent person—but the alcohol is. Drinking alone is a part of the dependency pattern.

Drinking Excessively and Often. Gulping drinks, ordering doubles, becoming intoxicated intentionally to feel good, or drinking to feel normal are indications of alcohol dependency.

Making Excuses for Drinking. Alcoholics may rationalize their drinking behaviors by making excuses for drinking. Any event is a sufficient reason for drinking.

Blackouts. Alcoholics may suffer temporary lapses of memory for periods of time when they have been drinking. These lapses may be followed by feelings of anxiety, concern, and guilt over what may have taken place.

SELF-ADMINISTERED ALCOHOLISM SCREENING TEST (SAAST)

Some disorders have symptoms that make a diagnosis easy. Alcoholism, however, defies easy classification: the symptoms vary greatly from one problem drinker to the next.

To cope with this difficulty, Mayo Clinic has developed the Self-Administered Alcoholism Screening Test (SAAST). Based in part on the Michigan Alcoholism Screening Test, the SAAST consists of 37 questions. In use since 1972, the test has been found to identify 95 percent of alcoholics ill enough to be hospitalized.

The test is non-threatening: it attempts not to accuse but to identify behavior patterns, medical symptoms, and consequences of drinking in the alcoholic.

Here is a sample of questions from the test.

1. Do you have a drink now and then?
2. Do you feel you are a normal drinker (that is, drink no more than average)?
3. Have you ever awakened the morning after drinking the night before and found that you could not remember a part of the evening?
4. Do close relatives ever worry or complain about your drinking?
5. Can you stop drinking without a struggle after one or two drinks?
6. Do you ever feel guilty about your drinking?
7. Do friends or relatives think you are a normal drinker?
8. Are you always able to stop drinking when you want to?
9. Have you ever attended a meeting of Alcoholics Anonymous (AA) because of your drinking?
10. Have you gotten into physical fights when drinking?

These responses suggest you are at risk of alcoholism: 1. Yes; 2. No; 3. Yes; 4. Yes; 5. No; 6. Yes; 7. No; 8. No; 9. Yes; 10. Yes.

Responses to the SAAST questions are best put into perspective by a psychiatrist, psychologist, or your physician. If your answers to the above-listed questions suggest you might have a drinking problem, use the results as a point for discussion of your alcohol use with your physician.

Denial.   Denial is a psychological mechanism often used by alcoholics to protect themselves from the truth about their drinking. Denial acts as a powerful barrier to recovery and is one of the reasons why so many alcoholics continue their abusive drinking for years without seeking help. Initially, they are unable to see the damage that their drinking is causing them and their families. Even if the consequences are plainly evident, they may persist in the belief that the ruin of their lives is caused by factors other than their drinking. Alcoholics continue to believe they are acting freely and that the alcohol is not controlling their lives.

An excellent source for helpful literature on recognizing all the possible symptoms of alcoholism and details about recovery is Alcoholics Anonymous. Their materials are written by alcoholics and people who treat alcoholics (see Alcoholics Anonymous and Al-Anon, page 428).

HELPING THE ALCOHOLIC

Most alcoholics who enter treatment do so reluctantly, usually under pressure from their family, employer, friends, or the legal system. This pressure often is necessary because of the denial used by the alcoholic, allowing him or her to believe there is no need for treatment.

Penetrating the Protective Shell.   The alcoholic often builds a protective shell by developing strategies, both conscious and unconscious, to avoid being found out.

The subconscious denial may be so profound that the alcoholic may genuinely not recognize the extent of the problem. One of the first goals of treatment is the penetration of the personal defenses that have developed over the years and that have allowed the alcoholic to continue the destructive drinking.

Alcoholism Is a Disease, Not a Character Flaw.   It is important to understand that alcoholism is a disease and that the alcoholic is someone who has been made ill by the disease. Blaming the alcoholic for the illness only feeds the alcoholic's feeling that no one understands him or her. The monumental damage some alcoholics continue to inflict on themselves and others is evidence of lives that are out of control.

Intervention.   As painful as it may be, you must confront the alcoholic with the complete truth about his or her drinking. Do not allow the alcoholic to deny alcoholism.

In a kind but candid way, tell the alcoholic to either get help or be prepared to suffer the consequences—such as being fired, divorced, or expelled from the family. This is not the time for the alcoholic to be bailed out of trouble or given another chance. An escape from the consequences of drinking usually is interpreted as permission to drink once again. Responsibility for the alcoholic is simple and unambiguous: stop drinking and faithfully follow a program of recovery.

There is no ideal time or place for a confrontation. However, do not confront an alcoholic when the person is drunk or even while drinking. Do pick a time when the alcoholic is sober.

There is no ideal person or persons to confront the alcoholic. An employer or an authority figure that the alcoholic respects is sometimes appropriate. Sometimes the best person to intervene is a recovering alcoholic. At other times, the initial confrontation should be by a group of people aware of the problem.

Family Members.   Family members are usually the first people to confront the alcoholic; they are also the people most injured by the disease. Often angry and hurt, they blame the alcoholic for the ruin the disease has caused in their lives.

As understandable as these feelings are, they are counterproductive when trying to help an alcoholic. To direct anger at the sick person who has alcoholism will only drive the alcoholic further away and perhaps deeper into the grip of the disease.

Many alcoholics might stop drinking earlier if they were confronted sooner. One reason why alcoholics are left alone for so many years is because their families fall prey to the same denial that holds the alcoholic. Family members may be unable to believe that the problem is as bad as it really is. Consequently, they make excuses for the alcoholic's drinking and forgive the alcoholic's bad behavior. They continue to rescue the alcoholic from trouble, pay the bills, and nurse him or her back to health. In effect, they enable the alcoholic to continue drinking.

Alcoholism creates victims out of the people closest to the alcoholic. Treatment for the disease should involve the non-alcoholic members of the family. In some cases all members of the family are affected, spouses and children alike.

Especially important in treating an alcoholic and his or her family is addressing the needs of the children. The resentments and the fear of trust and intimacy are some of the crucial problems that children of alcoholics may need help with.

THE TREATMENT OF ALCOHOLISM

Virtually every treatment and recovery program dealing with alcoholism has certain basic elements. If you are an alcoholic, here is what you might expect from a treatment program.

DETOXIFICATION AND WITHDRAWAL

Your treatment may begin with a program of detoxification. In a detoxification unit, you will receive medical care and you will be carefully monitored as you move through the withdrawal process. This usually takes about 4 to 7 days and often requires administration of tranquilizers or sedatives.

A physician's guidance may be required if you have withdrawal symptoms. Some alcoholics need treatment for depression during the withdrawal period. Alcoholics in severe withdrawal may become highly agitated, aggressive, or delirious or even have seizures.

Administration of medications (benzodiazepines) under the supervision of a physician may be necessary to prevent delirium tremens (DTs) or withdrawal seizures (see Alcohol Withdrawal and the Dreaded DTs, page 422).

MEDICAL TREATMENTS

If you have medical problems associated with your alcoholism, they will be treated. Common medical problems include such conditions as high blood pressure, increased blood sugar level, liver disease, and heart disease. In addition, nutritional problems associated with your disease can be diagnosed and treated. Your physician can instruct you about proper dietary regimens that can correct any long-term nutritional deficiencies you may have. Usually, this amounts to nothing more than resumption of a balanced diet (see Nutrition and Health, page 345) once you cease drinking.

RECOVERY PROGRAMS

What follows detoxification for most residential recovery programs is a period of rehabilitation. For 3 to 4 weeks, you probably will be counseled about the nature of your disease, the damage alcohol does to your body, problems caused by drinking, and what you may experience while recovering. During this phase of recovery, you may receive psychological support, counseling, and, if needed, additional nursing and medical care. Most of these programs include daily lectures or films, group therapy, counseling, activity therapy, and an introduction to the principles of Alcoholics Anonymous.

Many of the trained professional staff involved in recovery programs are recovering alcoholics themselves, which means they are able to offer insiders' knowledge of alcoholism and recovery. They also serve as role models. Seeing other recovering alcoholics working and leading healthy lives can encourage you to press on in your treatment program.

COMPLETE ABSTINENCE

Remember this: If you continue to drink you will have little or no control over your disease. Therefore, treatment programs for alcoholics involve complete abstinence.

ACCEPTANCE OF THE DISEASE

You must also be willing to acknowledge the fact that you have a disease. Specifically, you must readily admit to being addicted to alcohol and being unable to control your disease. Many alcoholics struggle to escape the shame and guilt. If you refuse to see yourself as someone with the disease of alcoholism, your denial may hamper treatment or even render it useless.

This admission of powerlessness over alcohol is a form of surrender (letting go) of the lies that once supported you. *It is the first and most important step to recovery.* It is not another form of compliance, nor is it only a matter of obeying conditions of your recovery program. Perhaps for the first time you will be acknowledging the power of the disease.

PSYCHIATRIC TREATMENT AND PSYCHOLOGICAL SUPPORT

Often, emotional symptoms alcoholics experience mimic psychiatric disorders; thus a psychiatrist may need to help differentiate alcoholic symptoms from a primary psychiatric illness. If the psychological aspects of your disease are not dealt with, you will not recover. These needs can be provided for in several ways, including group and individual therapies. Occasionally, alcoholics have other psychiatric disorders, such as a major depression (see page 1038). If you have a psychiatric disorder, it will require specific treatment apart from your alcoholism.

DRUG TREATMENTS

If you are engaged in a long-term recovery program, don't expect to receive tranquilizers or sedatives. These too are drugs. Like alcohol, they are subject to abuse. (An exception is use of medications to treat symptoms during a period of acute withdrawal.) Appropriate medications are sometimes needed if a psychiatric illness is present in addition to alcoholism.

If you have trouble abstaining from alcohol, a drug called disulfiram (Antabuse) may be useful. Taken orally, this drug disrupts the metabolism of alcohol in the liver. If alcohol is consumed, the drug produces a severe physical reaction that includes flushing, nausea, vomiting, headaches, and abdominal pain. In those using the drug, mild reactions can also be triggered by skin creams, mouthwashes, or anything else that contains alcohol.

This drug will not cure your alcoholism, nor can it remove your compulsion to drink. But it can be a strong deterrent. Other medications such as metronidazole and chlorpropamide will cause the same symptoms as Antabuse when taken with alcohol.

REFOCUSING YOUR LIFE

Recovery focuses on living for the present and on confronting guilt of the past and fear of the future. Therefore, sobriety is far more than just not drinking.

For many alcoholics, drinking furnishes illusions, usually of power and freedom. While under the influence of alcohol, they feel freed of whatever inhibition was present when they were sober. Don't be fooled. In truth, you grow less able to escape from darker aspects of your life that fuel your drinking. Many alcoholics become consumed with resentment and anger. Remember that successful recovery centers on facing and mastering emotions that otherwise will disable you.

Alcoholism can cause an impairment of relationships. The family is one of the first places where dysfunctional relationships begin to develop; the workplace is another. The National Council on Alcoholism estimates that 1 employee in 20 has an alcohol or drug abuse problem that affects work performance, whether it is an abuse problem of his or her own or one of a close family member. Treatment and recovery must concentrate on learning to acquire healthy, truthful relationships built on the strength of self-understanding and personal growth rather than on bad faith, denial, and lies.

CONTINUING SUPPORT

What happens after treatment ends will be critical to the success of your recovery program. The chronic nature of your disease calls for constant use of support systems and other resources. Aftercare programs are designed to help recovering alcoholics continue lives of abstinence from alcohol and other addictive drugs and to identify actions to take if a relapse occurs.

A major part of aftercare focuses on helping the alcoholic person and his or her fam-

MYTHS ABOUT ALCOHOLISM

Although the facts about alcoholism are only now emerging, there never has been a shortage of myths. Here are examples of some of the more common untruths.

Alcoholics Lack Willpower

During the past 20 years, the medical profession and much of the general public have come to view alcoholism as an addictive illness over which the alcoholic has little control. Still, many people continue to believe that the alcoholic suffers only from a weakness of character.

People who have the most difficulty admitting that willpower has little or nothing to do with alcoholism are the alcoholics themselves. Most active alcoholics believe they can, although not without some struggle perhaps, stop drinking at any time. It is this self-deceit that remains one of the most formidable barriers to recovery for any alcoholic. Ironically, some of the strongest-willed people in history have been alcoholics.

The Elderly Do Not Become Alcoholics

Alcoholism can strike at any age, although statistics demonstrate that the older the person, the less likely he or she is to become an active alcoholic. Alcoholism is a problem for many men and women after retirement. The stresses of retirement, forced changes, and the feeling of being useless may contribute to alcoholism at this age.

If You Admit To Being an Alcoholic, You Can Never Get Another Decent Job

It is illegal to discriminate in hiring on the basis of any medical disability, including alcoholism. Often, recovered alcoholics are admired by potential employers for the strength of character that is necessary to overcome the problem.

If you are an alcoholic who already is employed, remember this. Employers are learning that it often is less expensive to support an employee in treatment, usually through a health insurance policy, than it is to replace him or her. Don't allow recovery to hold you hostage to the fear of losing your job.

A Drink Can Warm You Up

Alcohol dilates your blood vessels. As a result, alcohol may give you the sensation of temporary warmth by sending more blood rushing to your skin's surface. This increased blood flow to the capillaries draws blood from vital inner organs and brings heat nearer the surface of your body, where it is lost through your skin; thus, the temperature of your body is lowered. Consequently, the risk of serious or even fatal low temperature (hypothermia) is increased if you drink alcohol. For example, if you fall into cold water or are exposed to cold temperatures while wearing thin or wet clothing after ingesting a quantity of alcohol, hypothermia is a distinct possibility.

When Drunk, You Reveal Your True Personality

Although alcohol may permit traits to surface that are denied when you are sober, excessive drinking can distort your personality. A person's true personality is revealed when he or she is sober.

Recovered Alcoholics Can Become Responsible Social Drinkers

This may be the most common illusion that active alcoholics carry with them before they begin recovery. The truth is that most can never safely resume drinking once they are addicted to the drug. The best policy is total abstinence.

Alcohol Is a Stimulant

The initial reaction to alcohol may be stimulation in some people. However, sedative effects occur as drinking continues.

Strong Black Coffee Can Help You Sober Up

Black coffee contains the stimulant caffeine, which will counteract the depressant effect of alcohol. If you are intoxicated or otherwise physically affected by alcohol consumption, caffeine may improve your level of awareness or reduce feelings of lethargy.

Coffee can neither increase the rate at which alcohol is processed by your liver nor change your blood alcohol levels. Unfortunately, the initial lift that coffee provides may lead you to believe that you are reasonably alert and sober when, in fact, you are not.

The consequences are self-evident when viewed in light of the many thousands of alcohol-related traffic deaths and injuries that occur annually in the United States.

ily make the decisions that will assist in adjustments they all must make to home life. One of the support systems we recommend is attendance and participation in Alcoholics Anonymous and in Al-Anon for your spouse, if you have a spouse.

ALCOHOLICS ANONYMOUS AND AL-ANON

The Fellowship of Alcoholics Anonymous was formed in 1935. As a self-help group of recovering alcoholics, Alcoholics Anonymous (AA) offers a sober peer group as an effective model of how you can achieve total abstinence.

The AA program is built around Twelve Steps, which are a dozen straightforward suggestions for men and women who choose to lead sober lives. The Twelve Steps are not requirements for membership but rather are guides for people who choose to live their lives sober.

As guides to recovery, the Twelve Steps help alcoholics accept their powerlessness over alcohol. Among other concerns, they also stress the necessity for honesty about the past and present. Recovery in AA is based on accepting the unique experience of each alcoholic. Through listening and sharing stories, alcoholics learn that they are not alone.

There are no fees for membership, only a willingness to remain sober. No matter what type of rehabilitation program you choose, consider joining Alcoholics Anonymous.

Initially, Alcoholics Anonymous was a family affair. Parents, spouses, and children all attended meetings. But as spouses and other members of the alcoholic's family shared their stories, these family members came to realize that many of the difficult family problems remain after the alcoholic was sober. It became apparent that family members also are deeply affected by the disease and need to change as well. In the middle 1950s, family members of recovering alcoholics formed a complementary self-help group called Al-Anon.

Al-Anon is designed for people who are affected by someone else's alcoholism. In sharing their stories they gain a greater understanding of how the disease affects the entire family, not just the alcoholic. Al-Anon also accepts the Twelve Steps of AA as the principles by which they are to conduct their lives. It also emphasizes how members need to learn detachment and forgiveness if they too are to be free of the disease.

Anyone with an alcohol-related problem is welcome in AA or Al-Anon. Simply look for a listing in your telephone directory and make the call.

In many communities, Alateen groups provide support for teenage children of alcoholics.

HOW TO CUT DOWN ON YOUR DRINKING

To reduce your drinking, work toward understanding situations that led you to drink in the past. Ask yourself, for example, what your mood was on those occasions. Did you feel anxious? Were you angry or lonely? Were you drinking because you were tired, or depressed, or hungry? Did you drink because your host urged you to?

Of course, none of these are good reasons to use alcohol. Learn to cope with life without using alcohol.

Ask yourself what drinking habits have caused problems in the past. Do you gulp your drinks? Are your drinks too strong? The faster you drink and the more you drink, the more likely it is that you will have problems.

Decide in advance how much you intend to drink and when. Never drink beyond this limit. A reasonable limit is two drinks a day; even that may be excessive if it is a regular practice. In fact, if you believe you must have two drinks each day, it suggests that you may have developed a dependence on alcohol.

Keep in mind that alcohol is a drug. Treat it as a drug. Always drink slowly. Never drink an alcoholic beverage (even beer) to quench your thirst. A glass of water or fruit juice is a far better choice.

TEENAGE DRINKING

Every year in the United States, more than 10,000 young people between the ages of 16 and 24 are killed in alcohol-related automobile accidents. Nearly 40,000 are injured. But the high cost of alcohol abuse extends beyond what these statistics reveal. Alcohol often is implicated in other deaths—drownings, suicides, fires.

Consumption often increases dramatically in high school years, especially among boys during the 10th and 11th grades. Also, although drinking continues to be statistically a male problem, the gap between teenage boys and girls is decreasing as more adolescent girls take up drinking.

An obvious danger of teenage drinking is that it can lead to addiction. More than half of the nearly 20 million adults who abuse alcohol in this country started heavy drinking as teenagers. But alcohol addiction is not reserved for adulthood. Although it often takes years for an adult to develop an addiction, teenagers can become addicted in months.

The reasons anyone, much less an adolescent, becomes an alcoholic are complex. For young people, however, the likelihood of addiction probably depends, in part, on factors such as their susceptibility to advertising campaigns, the influences of role models (peers and parents, for example), how early in life they begin to use alcohol, their psychological need for alcohol, and perhaps genetic factors that might predispose them to addiction.

Alcohol abuse among teenagers is a problem that affects families, schools, communities, and nations. There are no simple answers. Still, two of the most important elements in any effort to prevent the abuse of alcohol or cope with it are understanding and education.

Your Role as a Parent. Schools are growing increasingly aware of the need for alcohol and drug education. An equally important area for education is the family, which is where children should first learn how and why they must resist alcohol. Parents need to learn more about how alcohol and other drugs work, about the appeal alcohol holds for young people, about telltale signs of abuse, about short-term and long-term effects of abuse, about how to handle a child they suspect is abusing alcohol or other drugs, and about what type of help to seek.

Self-esteem and communication also play vital roles in alcohol abuse. Many young alcoholics report that their parents had little understanding of their personal sense of inadequacy and that it was impossible to communicate with their parents meaningfully on a wide range of sensitive matters. Trusting communication must be established early in your child's life and maintained (by both of you) as your child grows to maturity. Early communication is necessary because, in the school-age child, peer pressure becomes the source of many value judgments, especially those regarding use of alcohol.

Children learn by what they see and hear. Many child psychologists believe that before the fifth grade the attitudes children form toward use of alcohol are drawn primarily from their home life and television. Parents: It's up to you to set a good example, and do it early. By adolescence, when peer pressure becomes a dominating influence, a history of a good example in the home is crucial. If you abuse alcohol, there is greater likelihood that your child will too. If your children see you treating alcohol as a drug, whose abuse is dangerous, they are far more likely to adopt a healthy respect for its use.

We live in a culture that poorly educates young people about alcohol abuse. It is foolish and irresponsible for parents to permit young people to be guided solely by their peers on such matters as the use of alcohol. Many young people feel invulnerable to developing any physiological or psychological problems as a result of occasional alcohol abuse. If you fail to lovingly and wisely guide them through this period, you risk tragedy.

PREGNANCY AND ALCOHOL

If you are pregnant, use of alcohol presents much the same hazards to you as you would experience if you were not pregnant. To your unborn child, however, your alcohol consumption poses major risks.

In the past 15 to 20 years, there has been increasing recognition that many infants born to mothers who consumed excessive amounts of alcohol during pregnancy were smaller than normal. In addition, a pattern of birth defects has been observed, consisting of unusually small heads, heart defects, a shortening of the eyelids, and various other abnormalities. This has come to be called fetal-alcohol syndrome (see page 188). As these children have grown older, many have been found to be mentally retarded.

The means by which alcohol does this damage is not clearly understood. Most heavy drinkers are also heavy smokers, and it is known that smoking results in low birth weights (although birth defects have not been so clearly linked to smoking). Deficiencies of vitamins that may occur in heavy drinkers do not appear to contribute to this problem.

It is not known how much alcohol must be consumed in order to cause an abnormal infant; nor is it certain that drinking will cause abnormalities in every case. Good sense, however, suggests that women who think they might become pregnant should abstain completely from use of alcohol.

Remember that a certain proportion of infants are born with defects even under the best of circumstances. Thus, the occasional use of alcohol during pregnancy cannot always be blamed for a child's birth defects.

CHAPTER 19

MEDICATIONS AND DRUG ABUSE

CHAPTER CONTENTS

USE VERSUS ABUSE

Drug use is part of modern life in the United States. Annually, American physicians write countless prescriptions and consumers purchase hundreds of millions of dollars worth of nonprescription (over-the-counter) medications.

When taken as directed, prescription or nonprescription drugs are effective treatments of many illnesses. However, if they are not used as directed or are intentionally abused, health problems can result. In the following pages, we discuss the misuse and abuse of legal and illegal drugs.

WHAT IS DRUG ABUSE?

The abuse or misuse of addicting drugs is an increasing public health issue in this country. Drug abuse and dependence is one of the most frequently reported psychiatric disorders for men ages 18 to 65 years and for young women ages 18 to 24.

Abused drugs are not just those substances that are considered illegal or used illegally (that is, without a prescription). Drug abuse occurs if you take any drug for purposes other than for what it was intended or in a manner or in quantities other than directed.

Drug abuse also applies to the excessive consumption of drugs that are socially acceptable, such as nicotine (see Tobacco, page 407) and alcohol (see Alcohol Abuse, page 417). Both nicotine and alcohol have properties that categorize them as addictive drugs. They also may cause dangerous medical problems.

Through the Controlled Substances Act, the federal government has classified all potential drugs of abuse under five separate categories (schedules). The higher the classification of a drug, the greater the likelihood of abuse and the more exacting the federal regulations are for its use.

In Schedule I are drugs that are highly addictive, have no accepted medical use, and have no accepted level of safe use, such as heroin. These drugs are not legally available for medical use, although they may be used for research purposes.

Schedule II includes drugs that have a high potential for dependence or addiction but also have some accepted medical uses. Examples are cocaine, phencyclidine (PCP), and the opium derivatives codeine and morphine. Telephone prescriptions and refills are not allowed for Schedule II drugs.

Schedule III includes certain drugs that are combinations of narcotics such as codeine with other nonnarcotic drugs, certain appetite suppressants, and some hypnotic drugs. Schedule IV drugs include the benzodiazepines (tranquilizers such as diazepam, sold under the trade name Valium) and certain hypnotics (sleeping pills such as pentobarbital, sold under the trade name Nembutal). Telephone prescriptions are permitted for both Schedule III and IV drugs, but no more than five refills are permitted. Schedule V drugs are those with the least potential for abuse and dependence.

People abuse drugs for various reasons: mind-altering psychedelics produce effects that alter the way we see or hear, stimulants such as amphetamines increase energy and lift spirits, analgesics reduce the sensation of pain and induce drowsiness, and antianxiety and antidepressant drugs create a feeling of relaxation. To get "high" or intoxicated deliberately is a frequent motivation.

RECOGNIZING SIDE EFFECTS

Along with the intended effects, most drugs can produce unwanted effects. Some side effects will disappear as your body becomes accustomed to the presence of the drug. Other side effects are more serious and will require medical attention.

Learn what side effects are common with the drug you are taking. Know whether the potential side effects may require medical attention. When a drug is prescribed for your use, your physician will brief you on the usual side effects. He or she will also tell you about signs and symptoms that may alert you that a serious or even dangerous side effect may be occurring.

Be aware of effects that indicate that you should stop taking the drug and see your physician. Some of the symptoms may be related to an overdose. These symptoms may occur when you take a larger dose or take the drug more frequently than was prescribed. If upon taking a new medication you experience worrisome symptoms, consult your physician immediately.

Most of the millions of people who take drugs do not abuse them. However, many misuse them, sometimes out of ignorance and carelessness. Others, particularly the elderly, underuse prescription drugs, often in an attempt to reduce the cost of their medical care. It is important to your health that you follow your physician's instructions as to proper drug use, that you not use someone else's medication, and that you report any persistent side effects to your physician. At no time should you use drugs for any means other than what they were prescribed for.

HOW TO RECOGNIZE DRUG ABUSE AND ADDICTION

Drug abuse occurs if you take any drug for purposes other than for what it was intended or in any manner or in quantities other than directed. The abuse of drugs may lead to an addiction, now often referred to as drug dependence.

An addiction may be considered to be the compulsive and continued use of a drug, or the loss of control over its use, despite adverse consequences produced by the drug. Drug dependence has both psychological and physical characteristics. If unable to obtain the drug, the addicted person may experience symptoms of distress or withdrawal and a need to take the drug again.

Recognizing the signs of addiction (to legal or illegal drugs) in someone else can be difficult. These signs vary from drug to drug and person to person. However, people who are addicted to one or more drugs often will exhibit changes in their behavior that may gradually affect personal relationships and work performance.

Their behavior may be erratic and their moods unpredictable, alternating between periods of exhilaration or agitation and exhaustion or lethargy. Some addicted persons find that they no longer sleep well, and others will "crash" and sleep for long periods. They may lose their interest in eating or experience an unexplained loss of weight.

Eyes that are bloodshot or that have a dazed or expressionless appearance can be clues to drug abuse. Persons abusing hallucinogens may appear to be daydreaming and may have to be spoken to several times before responding, or they may gaze at or examine an object without explanation for long periods.

Other drugs may produce excessive sweating or flushed skin. An unexplained rash or an irritated nostril or running nose may be a sign that someone has been using an opiate (for more signs, see Teenagers and Drugs, page 437). Alternatively, many drug-dependent persons appear normal to their friends.

If someone close to you has several of these signs or symptoms, he or she is not necessarily a drug addict. But you may know the person well enough to recognize whether genuine changes in personality have taken place. If changes include spending increasing amounts of time away from home, a shift in classroom behavior or missed classes, or a constant demand or need for money, you may have grounds for concern. However, as with all medical conditions, proper evaluation must be done to assess the true nature of the problem or to rule out disorders that might cause similar behavior.

ABUSE AND MISUSE OF LEGAL DRUGS

Drug abuse and drug dependence in this country involve more than just the better-known illegal (street) drugs. Millions of Americans abuse legal prescription and nonprescription drugs, sometimes with tragic results.

In fact, these drugs dominate the statistics on drug-related deaths and emergencies. They are associated with most of the deaths attributed to drugs. Hospital emergency rooms report that approximately the same percentage of drug emergencies are due to misuse of legal drugs as compared with misuse of illegal drugs.

The abuse of prescription or nonprescription drugs, especially painkillers (see Dependence on Analgesics, page 436) and tranquilizers (see Dependence on Tranquilizers, page 436), is widespread. Also, many other drugs, including numerous drugs that are available without a prescription (over-the-counter drugs), can be misused.

The misuse of drugs such as laxatives, for example, can have long-term effects. This

DEFINITIONS RELATED TO DRUG ABUSE

Drug abuse or drug dependence can cause health problems that range from physical to psychological, mild to severe, and reversible to permanent. For purposes of discussing and describing some of the conditions associated with addiction, the following general categories may be useful.

Psychological dependence: This describes the state in which a drug is required for the abuser to feel better.

Tolerance: Tolerance occurs when progressively more and more of the drug is required to get the same effect.

Addiction: An addiction is the compulsive use of a drug, loss of control over its use, and continued use despite adverse consequences. The state of addiction may include psychological dependence (when the desire or need grows to a desperate craving for the drug) and physical dependence (when distinctive withdrawal symptoms appear shortly after the drug abuser stops taking the drug). There is a need to take the drug again.

Withdrawal symptoms: Symptoms that develop after discontinuing use of the drug are termed withdrawal symptoms. These may become severe and possibly life-threatening, sometimes requiring immediate medical attention. Examples of these symptoms include agitation, tremulousness, anxiety, insomnia, depression, convulsions, and hallucinations.

---

form of drug misuse is common among people who have chronic constipation or irregularity. The habitual use of certain kinds of laxatives can, over time, damage the muscular action of the large intestine (colon). The result may be a worsening of chronic constipation that is the reason for taking the medication in the first place (see Chronic Constipation, page 633).

Nasal sprays are another example of an over-the-counter drug that can produce a dependence. People who have used a nasal spray for an extended period often find that when they stop using the spray their noses become stuffy sooner and they feel even worse (see Beware: Nose-Drop Addiction, page 695).

Aspirin, cough medicines, laxatives, diet pills, nasal sprays, and numerous other medications can be abused or misused, especially if taken in higher dosages or more frequently than recommended. Read the instructions on the package and follow them. If you find your condition fails to improve or if you are concerned that you are misusing the drug, consult your physician.

DRUGS IN THE ELDERLY

Pharmacokinetics is the study of how drugs work in the body. This relatively new medical discipline examines the time required for drugs to be absorbed, how they are distributed in your body, how long they remain effective, and how they are eliminated.

Through the study of pharmacokinetics, we are coming to understand more about the interactions that determine specific drug effects and the individual diversity of different drug responses. Depending on several factors, including body weight, health, and age, we all respond to drugs differently.

One age group that is particularly sensitive to the actions of many drugs is the elderly. With age come changes in how your body responds to drugs. For example, there are changes in your digestive system that may alter absorption of drugs; in the functioning of your liver that can make it harder for your body to break down (metabolize) and eliminate certain drugs; in your kidneys that slow the rate at which drugs are eliminated from your body; in your circulatory and nervous systems that affect responsiveness to many drugs; and in mental functioning such that taking medicines according to instructions is more difficult.

Establishing Dosages and Monitoring Side Effects. Because physical changes make older people more sensitive to drugs, the elderly generally require lower doses to achieve the desired effects and to avoid toxic overdoses. Unfortunately, the side effects of drugs, and the misuse and abuse of drugs, are distinctly more serious problems in the elderly: adverse reactions to medication occur frequently in our older population, and it is often more difficult for the elderly to eliminate their effects. It has been estimated that as many as one in four drugs administered to the elderly in institutions may be ineffective or unneeded. Compounding the problem, many elderly people use nonprescription drugs without the knowledge of their physician. In addition, many elderly people misuse drugs by taking less than the prescribed dosage in a misguided attempt to reduce costs.

Beware of Specific Drug Problems. Some drugs widely used by elderly people may present special concerns.

Diuretic drugs are commonly used because they reduce the amount of water in the body, an effect that ultimately reduces the workload of the heart and arteries. These "water pills" increase the flow of urine and are used to treat hypertension, heart failure, and other ailments common to older people, but they can also cause a loss of potassium and other minerals from the body. A potassium deficiency will produce symptoms that range from weakness, listlessness, and a loss of appetite to an irregular heartbeat. A potassium deficiency can be resolved by reducing the dosage, changing the diuretic, or taking a potassium supplement. Many foods contain potassium, but it is difficult to increase the amount of dietary potassium by selecting certain foods. Generally, problems of potassium depletion will require taking a potassium supplement to prevent or resolve the problem if you continue to take the same diuretic.

Many older people receive other antihypertension medications that may make them feel depressed, drowsy, or suddenly faint, especially when they try to stand up. The elderly are also more likely to experience adverse effects from sedatives and tranquilizers. Barbiturates are particularly risky because they can cause severe mental confusion or even psychosis if taken to excess. Benzodiazepine tranquilizers, taken to ease the nervousness and stress of everyday life, also may cause drowsiness, shakiness, and confusion in older people. If it is necessary for you as an older person to take a tranquilizer, your physician will choose the drug carefully and probably will prescribe a dosage that is lower than what is normally indicated for a younger person.

Digitalis medicines, prescribed to improve the strength and efficiency of the heart, also can be a serious problem for older people. Older people sometimes develop symptoms of toxicity from these drugs, including excessive fatigue, loss of appetite, vision problems, and psychological disturbances. These symptoms occur in the elderly because they are commonly given digitalis for longer periods and they do not eliminate the drug as readily as younger persons. Older people sometimes will receive lower doses of digitalis medications because, over time, the medicine can accumulate to toxic levels.

Beware of Mixing Drugs and Alcohol. In an effort to alleviate some of the age-related problems of loneliness and boredom that many elderly people face, some older people use drugs, such as alcohol, prescription drugs, and illegal (street) drugs. A National Institute of Drug Abuse survey indicated that two-thirds of all persons over the age of 65 use prescription drugs and, except for cardiovascular medications, the most commonly used drugs were sedatives and tranquilizers. More than half of all the persons using tranquilizers and sedatives said they could not perform their daily activities without these drugs. If you use sedatives or tranquilizers, take special care not to abuse them (see also Dependence on Tranquilizers, page 436). The use of many drugs along with alcohol can cause harmful interactions.

Multiple Drug Use. Perhaps the most common form of drug misuse in the elderly is multiple drug use. This involves taking too many drugs or inappropriately taking drugs that interact with each other.

Elderly persons often have numerous symptoms or illnesses. Sometimes there is a tendency for each new symptom to result in a visit to the physician and a new prescription, all too frequently without sufficient regard to the schedule of medicine already being taken. This pattern can lead one to take a surprising number of medicines, some of which may interact harmfully with each other.

Do not expect a medicine for every new symptom. Sometimes a symptom can be resolved by reducing the dose of another medicine or reorganizing the schedule of medicine. Also, review the schedule of all your medicines with your physician on every visit (particularly if a medicine is added) to determine whether the schedule can be simplified.

With multiple drug use, it is hardly surprising that in many instances a person can get confused and take too little or too much of one or more drugs or experience unwanted side effects from drug interactions.

Older people often need assistance in following drug therapies, especially if they have multiple diseases that require the correct use of several medicines each day. When the drugs are not taken as prescribed, they may be ineffective; with the mixing of certain medications, negative drug interactions are far more likely and more severe (see Problems Related To Too Many Medications, page 244).

DEPENDENCE ON TRANQUILIZERS

Addiction to tranquilizers is a major drug problem in this country. There are no reliable figures for the number of people thought to be addicted, but as many as 10,000 emergency room visits a year result from this particular addiction; every year thousands of people enter drug treatment centers for the same reason. Many of the more than 1.5 million people who each year take tranquilizers continuously for 4 months or more may be addicted.

Part of the problem appears to be that strong tranquilizers, such as diazepam (Valium), alprazolam (Xanax), triazolam (Halcion), and chlordiazepoxide (Librium), all part of a family of drugs named benzodiazepines, are initially prescribed or used to treat the nervousness or tension caused by the stress of everyday life or for psychosomatic symptoms (physical symptoms that may be secondary to a mental or emotional source). They are often used for an inappropriate duration or at too high a dose. As a general rule, physicians do not treat minor stress and tension with drugs; at most, use of drugs for this purpose is limited to a short period of time.

Are Tranquilizers Addicting?   Another issue related to the abuse of benzodiazepines is the mistaken belief that they are not addicting. When first available, they were widely adopted because barbiturates, another family of tranquilizing drugs, were known to have a high risk of overdosage and toxicity. Subsequently, benzodiazepines have been found to have strong addictive potential. In fact, virtually all of the drugs in the benzodiazepine group can cause physical and psychological addiction if used in high doses or over a prolonged time. Even relatively low doses may result in an addiction if taken over a sufficient period. People who have taken only the prescribed doses for several months have developed signs of dependence.

What are the signs of addiction? The most serious signs are withdrawal symptoms that appear when someone abruptly stops taking a drug and that quickly disappear when use of the drug is resumed. These symptoms may start anytime from the first day to several days after you stop taking the drug. They can persist, although probably not with the same intensity, for as long as 7 to 10 days. The symptoms usually include anxiety, restlessness, nausea, loss of appetite, sleeping difficulty, blurred vision, tremors, and twitching or muscle pains. In severe cases, delirium or convulsions may occur.

People withdrawing from tranquilizers may also suffer changes in the senses, especially of taste and smell, and become nauseated and vomit. They frequently lose weight and generally feel listless and depressed. Far more dangerous withdrawal symptoms are possible, including seizures, paranoia, hallucinations, and loss of touch with reality (psychosis).

Mixing Medications.   It is never a good idea to take several drugs together without your physician's knowledge. In combination with tranquilizers, some otherwise safe drugs may cause adverse symptoms. For example, the action of some medications may slow the elimination of the tranquilizer from your body, thereby increasing the risk of a toxic buildup. Let your physician know you are taking tranquilizers before other medications are prescribed.

Alcohol Interactions.   Avoid alcohol when taking tranquilizers. In fact, mixing alcohol with almost any drug is ill-advised. With tranquilizers it can cause drowsiness, intoxication, impaired memory, or even death. Taken together, these two depressant drugs are the cause of hundreds of fatal drug overdoses each year.

Benzodiazepines are more likely to have side effects in older persons. The drugs remain in the body for a much longer time in the elderly and can accumulate to hazardous levels. If you are an older person using one of these drugs, your physician may decrease the dosage.

DEPENDENCE ON ANALGESICS

The ideal analgesic (painkiller) would be one that furnishes sufficient pain relief, produces a minimum of unwanted side effects, acts promptly and over time with a minimal amount of sedation, prevents any tolerance from developing, and is nonaddicting. Unfortunately, there is no one ideal painkiller.

Individual needs determine the suitability and choice of the most appropriate drug, each of which has advantages and disadvantages. Analgesics can be divided into addictive and nonaddictive types. The first group includes the opiates (and opioids) such as morphine (and methadone); the second group includes non-opioids such as aspirin and acetaminophen.

The strongest painkillers, although not always the most effective, are opiates and opioids. Opiates are narcotic drugs derived from opium, and opioids are synthetic narcotic substances with the same properties. Morphine, a frequently used opiate for the treatment of severe pain, is prescribed for only short periods because it is addictive. In the case of terminally ill persons who are in severe pain, there is no reason, other than the possibility of causing confusion or excessive sedation, to be concerned about the addictive property of morphine or other narcotics. The opiate codeine often is used in combination with other nonnarcotic drugs as a pain reliever and cough suppressant.

People most likely to develop an addiction (see Definitions Related To Drug Abuse, page 434) with the use of narcotic analgesics are those with chronic pain. To avoid developing a drug dependency or addiction, the treatment of chronic pain usually includes other therapies (see Chronic Pain Centers, page 1052).

Symptoms of withdrawal from opiate abuse include diarrhea, depressed respiratory rate and blood pressure, dizziness, nausea, sweating, uncoordinated muscle movements, general weakness, body pain, insomnia, and intense drug craving. The withdrawal symptoms begin within 8 to 16 hours after the last dose, which explains why some addicts wake every morning in mild withdrawal.

TEENAGERS AND DRUGS

The best time to prevent drug abuse is before it begins. For parents, however, it may be very difficult to learn much about the potential for drug use among their children. It is critical that parents learn to talk to their children and develop good listening skills.

What is not being said, however, may be even more revealing than what is reported. Teenagers who use drugs are often unhappy, especially lonely and anxious, although they are not eager to talk about their problems. Yet, many of them want their parents' understanding.

Pay attention to what evidence you are offered. Do you know your children's newest friends? The pressure of peers cannot be exaggerated during adolescence. Studies generally indicate that the approval of peers is often decisive in a teenager's decision to use drugs.

How can you know definitely whether your youngster is using drugs? In lieu of an admission or direct evidence of drug use (such as a "high"), there are signs that may indicate abuse. Keep in mind, however, that these clues are not definitive signs but only possible indications that something is troubling your youngster.

School. Many children may grow to dislike school at some point, but the child who suddenly shows an active dislike of school and looks for excuses to stay home may be in trouble. Contact school authorities and especially the child's teachers: does your son's or daughter's official attendance record match what you know about his or her sick days? What about missed classes? An unexplained pattern of tardiness at school is also telling.

Another change that is a matter of concern is a student whose grades are generally A or B who suddenly begins to fail courses or receives only minimal passing grades and expresses general indifference toward school performance. Again, it is a sudden change that is most likely to be a significant sign.

Other causes for concern include temper tantrums, unexpected displays of anger over relatively small matters, or the onset of discipline problems, both in and out of school.

Physical Health. Most healthy youngsters have sufficient stamina to see them through their busy lives. Many sleep long hours during weekends and vacations. However, listlessness and apathy are not common characteristics of teenagers.

Clothing. Despite the varied and changing dress codes of young people, appearance is important to adolescents. Thus, it can be a significant warning sign if your youngster suddenly shows little interest in his or her clothing.

Personal Behavior.   Teenagers enjoy their privacy and often will go to great lengths to protect it. However, exaggerated efforts to bar parents from going into their bedrooms or knowing where they go with their friends can be a signal. Unexplained and lengthy stays in the bathroom for the sake of privacy cannot be ignored if other behavioral changes are observed.

If your teenage child suddenly makes requests for more money without a reasonable explanation for its use, it may be for the purchase of drugs. Other sudden and unexplained changes may also be signs: one example is a school athlete who stops participating in his or her favorite sport for no apparent reason.

Adolescents need to feel that there is an open line of communication with their parents in which they can risk sensitive disclosure without the fear of being censured. During adolescence, children find it difficult to share their concerns with their parents. Many young people choose peers as their only confidants. Even in the face of your child's reluctance to share, continue to express an interest in listening to the experiences of your children.

Most children want their family relationships to be marked by understanding and forgiveness. In these circumstances, even if drug abuse has begun, your child must believe that help and understanding will always be available (see also The Teenage Years, page 141).

DRUGS AND SPORTS

When you exercise, your nervous system is naturally aroused. Your stimulated nervous system boosts production of hormones, including adrenaline (epinephrine). These hormones increase the amount of blood your heart pumps, resulting in more blood for muscles and a release of sugar (glucose) from the liver and of fatty acids from body fat to serve as fuel for the muscles.

These effects are important to anyone who is exercising. The increased blood flow ensures that the muscles receive a constant supply of oxygen and nutrients, and potentially toxic waste products produced by the accelerated metabolism are more quickly removed.

At times, athletes have used drugs or other substances in abnormal quantities with the sole intention of improving performance in an artificial, unfair manner. Such risky practices are called "doping." In some cases, a medical disorder is treated with banned drugs that may also boost an athlete's performance in competition in an artificial or unfair manner. These practices not only give the athlete an unfair advantage but also can threaten his or her health.

Sympathomimetic Amines.   Some professional and world-class athletes have admitted using sympathomimetic amines, a class of stimulant drugs that mimic the natural effects of a stimulated sympathetic nervous system. These include ephedrine and its derivatives (pseudoephedrine and phenylpropanolamine), which are often present in cold and hay fever preparations as decongestants. Ephedrine is also a common ingredient of asthma medications. The use of ephedrine has been the reason for disqualification of athletes who have asthma and who have used this drug to prevent asthma during competition.

These drugs can increase alertness and physical endurance as well as postpone the onset of fatigue; they have been banned by most athletic organizations including the International Olympic Committee.

Psychomotor Stimulant Drugs.   Athletes also have been disqualified for using psychomotor stimulant drugs. The drugs in this category that are most often abused are amphetamines (namely, amphetamine, dextroamphetamine, and methamphetamine) and methylphenidate hydrochloride (Ritalin). The most common street name for these drugs is *speed.* Other slang names include *bennies, dexies, greenies,* and *pep pills.* Amphetamines are usually taken orally, but chronic abusers often prefer to inject the drug because it produces a more immediate and stronger effect.

The effects of psychomotor stimulants are not unlike those of sympathomimetic amines. They increase heart rate, respiration, and blood pressure and generally heighten the activity of the sympathetic nervous system. These drugs also affect the brain so that the athlete feels more alert, confident, and perhaps even euphoric. Consequently, psychomotor stimulants may lead to an improved athletic performance, more through their psychological than their physical effects; however, apart from increasing endurance, the benefits of these stimulants on athletic performance are limited.

Amphetamines have a role in medicine, especially in the treatment of hyperactive children (see Hyperactivity, page 136) and of narcolepsy (see page 1030). But amphetamines have no place in sports, and their unprescribed use is illegal. In addition to the dangers of a physical and psychological addiction, they generate many adverse physical and psychological reactions such as insomnia, dizziness, tremors, heart palpitations, irregular heartbeat, sexual impotence, and possibly amphetamine psychosis. Deaths have resulted even when normal doses have been used under conditions of maximal physical activity.

Beta$_2$-Agonists. These medications often are used in the treatment of asthma and other respiratory ailments. Like ephedrine, they can have stimulant properties. Currently they are banned when taken orally, but their use is permitted in aerosol or inhalant forms. Examples of these medications include metaproterenol (brand names, Alupent and Metaprel), salbutamol or albuterol (brand names, Ventolin and Proventil), and terbutaline (brand name, Brethaire).

Narcotic Analgesics. Narcotic analgesics (painkillers) may produce a sensation of euphoria or psychological stimulation. They also may increase the pain threshold so that an athlete may fail to recognize injury, leading to more serious injury. These drugs have been banned by the International Olympic Committee.

Note that the nonnarcotic analgesics such as aspirin or the nonsteroidal anti-inflammatory drugs have good analgesic and anti-inflammatory actions and have been useful in treating minor injuries. These drugs are not banned. But if you are an athlete, be careful that a narcotic such as codeine is not included in combination with another medicine such as aspirin.

Anabolic Steroids. Another group of drugs illegally used by athletes are androgenic-anabolic steroids. These drugs gain their name from the two Greek words *andro*

and *gennan,* meaning male-producing, and from another Greek word, *anabold,* which means to build up. Because these drugs are closely related chemically to the natural hormones of the male, anabolic steroids mimic the effects of the male sex hormone testosterone. Athletes have used these drugs illegally because they stimulate the buildup of body tissue.

Anabolic steroids have several legitimate medical uses. They are used to treat skeletal and growth disorders and certain types of anemia and to offset the negative effect of irradiation and chemotherapy.

Whether you take them in large or moderate doses over a prolonged period, anabolic steroids have many potentially serious side effects, especially on the liver, cardiovascular system, and reproductive system.

Liver. An overload of anabolic steroids can cause liver damage to the point that jaundice and even liver failure occur. Another potential liver problem from anabolic steroid use is peliosis hepatis. In this instance the liver develops blood-filled cysts that can rupture. Liver failure can result. There is also the potential for liver tumors forming as a result of anabolic steroid use. Most liver function problems associated with anabolic steroid use are not fatal, and most are reversible after use of the steroid is discontinued.

Cardiovascular System. Use of anabolic steroids has been linked to an increase in several risk factors leading to the development of cardiovascular disease. These include decreased blood concentrations of HDL (the "good" cholesterol; see also Atherosclerosis: What Is It?, page 786) and an increase in blood pressure. Animal research has shown that use of anabolic steroids also can lead to damage of the heart.

Reproductive System. Anabolic steroids can reduce sperm production, decrease the size of the testes, and reduce the amount of sex hormones produced, resulting in a diminished sex drive. Among female athletes, these drugs have reduced the production of female sex hormones (both estrogen and progesterone), inhibited development of eggs and ovulation, and disrupted the menstrual cycle. All of these changes are reversible when use of anabolic steroids is discontinued. Female athletes, however, sometimes find that male secondary sex characteristics, such as an increase in facial hair or a deepening of the voice, remain after they stop using anabolic steroids.

Other undesirable effects associated with abuse of anabolic steroids include a reduction of breast size and changes in overall hair growth patterns in women, an increased thinning of hair or hair that falls out, and acne. Another concern is the effect the drug has on behavior, which may result in increased aggressiveness.

Beta Blockers. These are drugs commonly used in cardiovascular disease to lower blood pressure and decrease heart rate. Beta blockers also block stimulatory responses. Thus, they have been used in sports such as shooting to steady the trigger finger and to relax the nerves. This use is considered doping, and therefore these drugs have been banned.

Growth Hormone. Use of this hormone is considered doping by the US Olympic Committee and is therefore prohibited.

Diuretics. Diuretics increase the elimination of fluid from the body as urine. They sometimes are misused by athletes to reduce weight quickly in sports such as wrestling in which strict weight classifications are involved; diuretics have also been used illegally to reduce the concentration of drugs in the urine so that other illegal drugs are not detected. The use of diuretics can affect the balance of such minerals as potassium and sodium in the body and can result, among other things, in heart arrhythmias and even death.

Blood Doping. Blood doping is the intravenous administration of red blood cells or related blood products for reasons other than a medical need. Some athletes have had blood withdrawn weeks or months before an event and then reinfused into their system just before an event in which they are competing. The risk of receiving blood from another donor includes the development of allergic reactions, viral hepatitis (see page 650), and AIDS (see page 848). The practice of blood doping also is banned by the International Olympic Committee.

Corticosteroids. The use of corticosteroids is banned by the International Olympic Committee if the drugs are taken by mouth or injected into a muscle or a vein. Corticosteroids can be used topically (in the ear, eye, or skin), in local or intra-articular injections such as for bursitis, or in inhalation therapy for disorders such as asthma (see also Corticosteroid Drugs, page 1005).

Dangers and Risks. The abuse of anabolic steroids and other drugs is often front-page news. The problem is international in scope, involving professional and amateur athletes who participate in a wide range of sports.

This elevated level of consciousness of the problem has led to more drug testing. The result is that today there are two important reasons for an athlete not to get his or her "competitive edge" from anabolic steroids or other medications. First, these drugs can put your future as an athlete at risk because of the bans and penalties now meted out for offenders. Second, and even more important, these drugs might put your health at risk.

MARIJUANA ABUSE AND DEPENDENCE

The most popular illegal drug in America is marijuana. It is estimated to be a 10 billion dollar a year crop in the United States, which would make it our third largest agricultural crop. A significant percentage of high school seniors have smoked marijuana, and studies indicate that at least a few of these students smoke it every day.

The hemp plant *(Cannabis sativa)* from which marijuana is derived contains more than 400 chemicals including tetrahydrocannabinol (THC). The THC in marijuana is what gets someone "stoned" and is probably responsible for the hunger many people experience after using marijuana.

Marijuana cigarettes are made from the leaves and tops of the plant. The amount of THC varies from plant to plant and from cigarette to cigarette. Hashish, a more powerful derivative drug prepared from the resin of the hemp plant, contains far greater concentrations of the psychoactive THC.

If you smoke marijuana, THC is quickly absorbed from your lungs into your bloodstream and rapidly distributed to most tissues and organs of your body. To eliminate THC, your liver converts the substance into waste products (metabolites). Most of these metabolites are excreted through the feces and urine. The rate at which they are cleared from your body is slower than that of many other psychoactive drugs. If you smoke marijuana regularly and then stop, THC can be found in your urine for more than 4 weeks after use.

The effects of marijuana are almost immediate, especially if you smoke it. Your pulse quickens by as much as 50 percent, depending on the potency of the marijuana. People with a poor blood supply to the heart may have chest pains.

Most people experience a feeling of relaxation and mild euphoria. Some first-time users undergo an acute panic reaction in which they feel they are losing control. This panic usually subsides within a few hours. Depending on the level of intoxication, some people have trouble remembering events that happened while "high" and experience difficulty in performing functions that require concentration, rapid reactions, and physical coordination. High doses of marijuana may produce many of the same behavioral effects as severe alcohol intoxication. Although the high may subside, many of the negative effects may linger for up to 6 hours after you smoke marijuana.

Chronic marijuana smokers show evidence of decreased lung capacity and chronic bronchial irritation. Marijuana also may contain the fungus *Aspergillus*. Studies suggest that serious lung infections may result from inhaling this organism. Because chronic marijuana smoking may impair your body's immune system, your lungs may be more susceptible to this and other infections.

Regular daily marijuana smokers often inhale the smoke deeply and retain it in their lungs as long as possible to increase their "high." This practice also increases the risk of damage to the lungs.

Marijuana is occasionally contaminated by animal droppings containing *Salmonella* bacteria either at the time of drying or during storage. This organism, which is not destroyed by drying, can cause diarrhea, abdominal pain, and fever (see page 619). A herbicide called paraquat, widely used by the government to destroy marijuana plants, poses another kind of health hazard. If plants sprayed with paraquat are harvested before exposure to sunlight, unaltered paraquat remains on the leaves. This herbicide is highly toxic to humans and can cause irreversible damage to the lungs.

Clinical testing suggests that marijuana may have a negative effect on the human reproductive system, possibly causing irregular menstrual cycles in women and a temporary loss of fertility in both men and women. Some studies have suggested that there may be a significant relationship between heavy use of marijuana during pregnancy and premature birth.

Depending on the length of use and the potency of the marijuana you use, you may experience withdrawal symptoms when use is discontinued. Some of the mild or moderate symptoms are tremors, sweating, nausea, vomiting, diarrhea, irritability, and sleep disturbances. However, these withdrawal symptoms are usually mild compared with those of heavy opiate or alcohol use, and they rarely require medical attention.

Although often misunderstood and misrepresented to the public, marijuana clearly is a drug of dependence. Regular use often results in the same type of drug dependence described for other substances (see also page 1048).

STREET DRUGS

Street drugs is another term for drugs sold illegally—often, these drugs are sold in the street.

The popularity of different drugs changes with the times. Twenty-five years ago, psychedelics were some of the more commonly used street drugs; in the 1980s, LSD was far less common than cocaine or cocaine derivatives such as crack. However, marijuana remains the most common street drug (see Marijuana Abuse and Dependence, page 440).

Cocaine. Cocaine was once referred to as the champagne of drugs, in part because it was an expensive drug preferred by the well-to-do. Unfortunately, today it is one of the most widely used illegal drugs in this country. Cocaine is eagerly sought by drug users because it sharply increases alertness and creates a sense of euphoria. These effects are the basis of the profound psychological dependence associated with the drug.

Cocaine dilates your pupils and accelerates your heart and respiratory rates. It also causes a slight rise in body temperature.

These effects are mostly short-term. They reach their peak about 15 to 20 minutes after you inhale the drug (snort it) through your nose in the form of a powder, and they dissipate in approximately an hour. Unwanted effects of chronic use of cocaine are a persistent restlessness, anxiety, and sleeplessness.

Another problem associated with inhaling cocaine is a mildly stuffy or running nose; long-term use can cause ulcers on the mucous membrane of your nose and even cause a hole (perforation) in your nasal septum. In addition, people who chronically abuse cocaine may develop paranoid hallucinations, called cocaine psychosis, that may involve the sense of touch, sight, taste, or smell.

Smoking (free-basing) cocaine creates a faster and more intense high. In this form the drug can cause confusion, slurred speech, and anxiety. Crack cocaine is smoked and has essentially the same effect as free-base cocaine; both forms are smoked and are highly addictive.

Crack is aptly named because it produces an intense high in a matter of seconds. Within a few minutes a profound low follows that usually leaves the chronic abuser despondent and desperate for more.

Short-term physical effects of crack are increased heart rate and increased blood pressure. Smoking this form of cocaine (as well as using the free-base) poses additional health problems because it increases the risk of emphysema (see page 929) and the risk of a heart attack due to the intensity of the high. In some instances, people who were using the free-base have set themselves on fire because this requires the use of flammable solvents that can explode. Injecting cocaine by means of shared needles increases the risk of exposure to AIDS and other communicable diseases that are passed by sharing nonsterile needles or solutions that are contaminated (see Central Nervous System Stimulants, page 1047).

Hallucinogens. Hallucinogenic drugs were widely used in the 1960s and early 1970s. The popularity of such drugs diminished during the next 20 years. Some observers report that there may be a renewed interest today in the use of hallucinogens, especially lysergic acid diethylamide (LSD).

Hallucinogens were popular because they produced vivid changes in sensation, depth perception, passage of time, and body image. Some experimenters reported experiencing a mixing of the senses—under the influence of LSD, one could seemingly "hear" colors or "see" sounds.

LSD also can cause powerful negative experiences, referred to as "bad trips," in which there is an overwhelming sense of fear, perhaps of being abandoned, going insane, or dying. In some instances, abusers have had no comprehension of their limitations and have died because they tried to fly out windows or walk on water.

An effect of hallucinogenic drugs is the production of sustained altered mental states that last for 8 hours or more. Flashbacks also may occur days or weeks after the conclusion of the initial trip, in which previous effects are reexperienced even though no more of the drug has been ingested.

LSD and other psychedelics, such as mescaline, increase heart rate and blood pressure, dilate pupils, and cause loss of appetite, sleeplessness, and tremors. Death from overdose is also possible.

It is not yet known whether all of the symptoms dissipate after LSD is no longer ingested. Heavy long-term use of hallucinogens, however, is known to cause impaired memory, abbreviated attention span, and a difficulty with abstract thinking (see also Hallucinogens, page 1049).

Phencyclidine (PCP). This powerful hallucinogen, referred to as "angel dust," was used by veterinarians to sedate large animals. From this use came other street names for the drug, such as "hog" and "horse tranquilizer." But the drug so disturbed and bewildered the animals before it put them to sleep that its use was abandoned.

Taken in very small doses by humans, however, the drug causes a loss of inhibition and induces a state of general euphoria. Other physical symptoms are increased heart rate and blood pressure, sweating, flushing of the skin, and an increase in body temperature. It also may cause some unsteadiness and muscle numbness. But what makes the drug so dangerous is its unpredictability.

Almost any increase in dosage may result in destructive, violent behavior. When users have turned violent or acted in bizarre ways, they have been known to lose all control.

Other symptoms are muscle rigidity, loss of concentration, vision disturbances, speech impairment, convulsions and delirium, fear of isolation, and paranoia. PCP also can lead to heart and lung failure or a stroke. It has been known to induce a toxic psychosis that resembles schizophrenia (see also Hallucinogens, page 1049).

Inhalants. Some people inhale a prescription drug called amyl nitrite. This drug is a vasodilator that relaxes smooth muscle in small blood vessels, causing them to expand and so lower the blood pressure. It is usually prescribed for the treatment of angina pectoris (see page 803). But people inhale amyl nitrite, or "poppers" as they are sometimes called, because it produces an intense and immediate high and seems to intensify orgasm during sex. The effects are short-lived, lasting only minutes.

Amyl nitrite is not physically addictive, but it is not free of side effects. Users suffer headaches, dizziness, accelerated heart rate, nasal irritation, and cough. The headaches seem to be the one side effect that can persist long after use.

People inhale various other substances that can give them a high, many of which do not require a prescription. One category of volatile inhalants, sold as room deodorizers, contain butyl and isobutyl nitrite. Butyl nitrite is also thought to intensify a sexual experience. Other inhalants that some young people use are solvents such as Freon (trichlorofluoromethane), halogenated hydrocarbons (for example, trichloroethylene), esters (for example, ethyl, amyl, and butyl acetates), and aromatic hydrocarbons (for example, benzene). The physical risks from inhaling these solvents range from cardiac arrhythmia from Freon and trichloroethylene to liver and kidney impairment from aromatic hydrocarbons and ethyl acetate.

Opiates. Heroin, methadone, morphine, and opium all are considered opiates because they all are derived from opium. Generally, opiates are prescribed to relieve severe pain. Given in low doses over short time periods, they are not addictive, but in large doses given over time, these drugs are highly addictive. Side effects include respiratory and circulatory system depression (in high dosages), dizziness, nausea, sweating, uncoordinated muscle movement, general weakness, and euphoria. Heavy use also will depress the sex drive.

When the drug is injected using a shared needle, users sometimes develop diseases or disorders such as AIDS, hepatitis, blood poisoning, congested lungs, and pneumonia. When the drug is taken with other sedatives, death can result (see also Opioids, page 1048).

Drugs and Pregnancy. Many drugs pass through the placenta and reach the fetus or enter the breast milk. During the first trimester of pregnancy, the fetus may be the most sensitive to drugs in the mother's body. Therefore, inform your physician if you have been taking any drugs just before becoming pregnant.

Some drugs are known to cause problems with pregnancy and the reproductive system. Marijuana, for example, causes irregular menstrual cycles in women and can cause a temporary loss of fertility in both men and women. Women who have smoked marijuana during their pregnancy have given birth to low-birth-weight and premature babies.

Among other drugs to avoid, especially during pregnancy, are tranquilizers and amphetamines, which may cause congenital malformations, and barbiturates, opiates, and cocaine, which can cause addiction in babies (see Smoking and Use of Alcohol and Illegal Drugs During Pregnancy, page 188).

PART IV

HUMAN DISEASE AND DISORDERS

The focus of the following chapters is on what ails you. You will find detailed discussions of a multitude of medical problems, ranging from the minor to the serious.

CONTENTS

CHAPTER 20

ALLERGIES

CHAPTER CONTENTS

UNDERSTANDING ALLERGY

Allergies are the result of a response by the body's immune system to agents perceived as possibly dangerous to the body. These agents are usually benign (in the case of foods) or even beneficial, but somehow the body reacts against them, by producing quantities of antibodies to defend itself. To understand allergies, it is important to have some idea about how the immune system works.

The job of the immune system is to protect the body from invaders that can harm it. An invader that prompts the body to produce antibodies is called an antigen (a term derived from the fact that these substances *gen*erate *anti*bodies). Antigens include harmful germs, viruses, and other foreign agents that can attack the body, and the immune system is vigilant in its search, recognition, and destruction of them. When the immune system recognizes a harmful invader and produces antibodies, these molecules circulate in the blood or reside in certain cells where they specifically counteract the invader.

The key actors in the defense system are white blood cells known as lymphocytes which are manufactured in enormous quantities in the bone marrow, lymph nodes, and spleen. Lymphocytes can produce plasma cells which in turn produce the antibodies that react with specific antigens. The reaction with antibodies circulating in the bloodstream neutralizes antigens by blocking them from entering cells or by making them susceptible to attack by roaming scavenger cells (known as macrophages).

There are two major kinds of lymphocytes, the B cells and the T cells, and these are responsible for two kinds of responses.

B cells produce antibodies that circulate in the bloodstream and act against invaders that also are circulating. The immunity these cells provide is known as humoral, meaning it is located in the body's fluids.

T cells are activated in the thymus gland. They attack antigens directly rather than by producing antibodies, and they also can act in concert with B cells to destroy antigens. The immunity the T cells provide is known as cell-mediated because the reaction between the antigen and the immune mechanism takes place on or within the cell. These

Your immune system reacts to foreign invaders, including harmful bacteria, viruses, and other perceived enemies (antigens). The response may produce one or both of two kinds of "fighters." One kind involves antibodies that circulate in the bloodstream; the second type stimulates specific cells to take on the unwanted invaders.

Invaders — Immune system — Fighters

Bacteria
Viruses
Other invaders
(Antigens)

Two kinds

B cells produce antibodies that circulate in the bloodstream

T cells do not produce antibodies but do produce lymphokines that stimulate specific cells (macrophages)

Counteract invaders

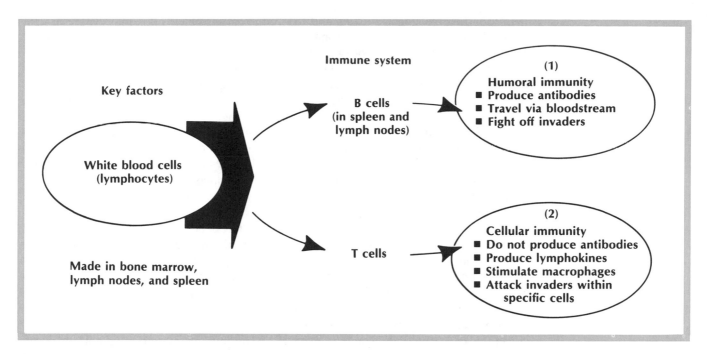

White blood cells, known as lymphocytes, are divisible into two major kinds: B cells and T cells. Both act in the short and long term to provide you with immune protection. In the short term, the B cells are responsible for humoral immunity and are activated in the lymph nodes and spleen to produce antibodies to fight off invaders in the blood stream. The T cells from the thymus gland produce lymphokines, which stimulate macrophages to attack the invaders within specific cells.

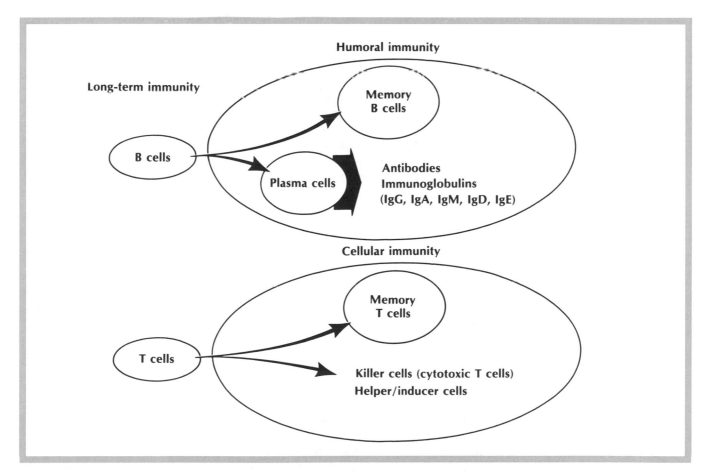

In the long term, the B cells and T cells "remember" (memory cells) the antigens they have done battle with, and are prepared to act if the same invader (antigen) reappears.

cells respond to malignant growths and to some viral and bacterial infections. They are important in the rejection of foreign tissue such as transplants. T cells make substances, called lymphokines, that can stimulate cells called macrophages to engulf (phagocytize) bacteria.

The antibodies produced by B cells are made of a special kind of protein known as immunoglobulin. There are five kinds of immunoglobulins (Igs) known as IgA, IgD, IgE, IgG, and IgM. Of these, IgE is the one that is most involved in allergic responses.

One of the things that makes the immune system efficient is its memory capacity. When lymphocytes are called into action to protect the body, some of the cells "remember" the chemical identity of the invader cells from a previous encounter. Thus, they already are programmed to destroy those cells. In this case, the body is able to react to invasion by these antigens immediately upon their reappearance.

It is largely due to this memory part of immunity that we stay well. Humans are born with natural immunity as a result of antibodies acquired from their mothers, but this immunity lasts only a few months before disappearing, to be replaced gradually by each infant's own immunity. The new immunity is acquired after the infant's own immune system has been exposed to a foreign agent. An example of such a developed immunity to a disease is the situation in chickenpox. Once you have had chickenpox, your body's immune system will prevent another bout of the disease, even though the virus that causes chickenpox may persist in your body for years (herpes zoster; see Shingles, page 1176).

Immune responses also develop when a very small amount of an antigen is intentionally introduced into the system in the form of a vaccine, such as for polio, diphtheria, tetanus, or measles. These antigens have been altered so that they cannot produce a full-scale infection of the disease but they can produce an immune response. This is why you may have mild muscle cramps and a low-grade fever for a few days after a vaccine has been injected. The most important result of the injection of this antigen is that it prepares the memory in certain lymphocytes which then are ready to block a full-scale invasion, should one occur. The memory for many antigens generally is lifelong.

The immune system does not attack everything foreign that enters the body. Most of the foods, drinks, and drugs that we ingest do not trigger an immune response. However, the immune system does respond to agents such as germs, viruses, and other invaders that cause harm such as infection. Occasionally, the immune system does react to a harmless invader, and this reaction is known as an allergy.

Many problems related to allergies can be handled by your primary-care physician. Occasionally, however, you may be referred to an allergist, a specialist who deals with allergies. If your allergic problems are skin-related, consultation with a dermatologist may be necessary (see page 457).

HOW ALLERGIC REACTIONS OCCUR

In most people, and for the vast majority of the time, the immune system works efficiently in protecting the body. In some people, however, it occasionally misreads the signals and responds to substances that actually are benign but are perceived as harmful antigens. Such reactions involve an interaction between a specific foreign substance, known as an allergen (an antigen that can stimulate antibody production), and a specific antibody (usually a protein).

When an allergen enters the system, it reacts with antibodies (IgE type) on the surface of basophils (a type of circulating white blood cell) or mast cells (a type of cell that lines respiratory and gastrointestinal tracts and the skin). The basophils and mast cells then release histamine (a body chemical that can act as an irritating stimulant) and other harmful chemicals into the tissue to combat the allergen, which they perceive as dangerous.

The eosinophil, another circulating white blood cell, also is involved in the allergic reaction by increasing its numbers in the blood and in the nasal and bronchial secretions of the allergic person.

The result is a host of symptoms that vary in severity.

When histamine is released in the lungs, it

causes secretion of mucus and narrowing and swelling of the lining of the airways. This leads to wheezing, coughing, and, sometimes, shortness of breath. When histamine is released in the nose and, rarely, the sinuses, it produces a running nose, tearing eyes, and itching of the nose, throat, roof of the mouth, and eyes. In the skin, histamine produces hives and other rashes. When the digestive system is the site, stomach cramps and diarrhea may result. Occasionally, the entire system will be affected in a response known as anaphylactic shock in which blood vessels dilate and air passages narrow, causing a slowing of the pulse, breathing difficulty, and other symptoms. Unconsciousness and occasionally death may result (see Anaphylaxis, page 474).

Each allergen produces its own specific set of IgE antibodies. For this reason, a person may be sensitive to ragweed but not to mold allergens. It is possible for a person to have many different specific IgE antibodies, making him or her sensitive to many allergens. Indeed, it is not unusual for a person who is allergic to one substance to be allergic to one or two others.

The intensity of the allergic reaction varies widely. Some people have only mild sniffles during ragweed season; others react violently with an attack of asthma. The number of IgE antibodies present in the system controls the severity of symptoms: the more antibodies present, the stronger the reaction.

TYPES OF ALLERGENS

A surprising number of different things can cause allergic reactions. These include substances found outdoors, indoors, and in the foods we eat. Allergens may be present in certain medications, in parts of plants (such as pollen), in house dust, in animal dander, in molds, in fungi, in foods, and in insect venom. In these cases, it is a specific allergen that causes the body to overreact. However, some people can be sensitive to the chemical changes caused by exposure to heat or cold and by exercise.

USUAL KINDS OF EXPOSURE

Those who are sensitive to certain allergens may be at risk of exposure daily because these allergens are common. Different allergens have different routes of entry into the body.

Exposure to the allergens of plants such as poison ivy, poison oak, and poison sumac occurs when a person merely brushes against the leaves. The allergic reaction usually occurs at the body site where the contact was made. For instance, one commonly gets poison ivy as a result of brushing up against it accidentally while walking in a wooded area or handling it while gardening. The plant resin that causes the reaction is thus transferred to the skin, and a reaction subsequently occurs. The same reaction also may develop if the resin is deposited on clothing that then rubs against your skin.

Other contact reactions can be caused by prolonged exposure to certain metals such as nickel (used in costume jewelry) and chromium. People who are sensitive to certain cosmetics can develop rashes after exposure to nail polish, hair dyes, eye makeup, or lipstick.

Perhaps the most common exposure is by inhaling an offending allergen. Millions of people experience the effects of sensitivity to pollen as hay fever (although neither hay nor fever is involved). The medical term is allergic rhinitis. The respiratory system is affected when wind-borne pollen is inhaled. Exposure is inevitable during spring, summer, and autumn, the pollen-producing seasons.

Molds release particles during their reproductive cycle and these are borne in the air. When inhaled, they also can trigger a reaction in the respiratory system. A similar reaction can occur when a sensitive person inhales animal dander or house dust. These allergens tend to affect people more during the winter months, when more time is spent indoors.

In addition to these inhaled allergens, other materials in the air such as smoke, fumes, mists, and baby powder may cause allergic reactions in sensitive persons. Some hypersensitive people may react to the formaldehyde present in household products such as insulation, pressed board, permanent-press clothing, new furniture, and polishes.

For most people, the reaction to an inhaled allergen is characterized by cold-like symptoms—running nose, cough, and itchy, teary eyes. An asthma reaction can occur but is more rare. In this case, the airways in the lungs become swollen so that a wheezing and a feeling of tightness in the chest are produced; often there also is production of thick mucus and a cough. During such a reaction, the affected person sometimes has difficulty breathing, and severe cases can be life-threatening.

Certain foods can cause an IgE response in very sensitive people. The foods found to be the cause in most reactions include milk, eggs, nuts, shellfish, fish, wheat, corn, berries, and legumes. In addition, certain materials used in the processing of foods cause allergic reactions; these include salicylates (found in all foods processed with cider or wine vinegar), tartrazine or Yellow Food Dye no. 5 (found in processed foods treated to enhance their color), sulfites (used to preserve fruits, vegetables, meats, and beverages such as wine), and gum arabic (used as a thickener in processed foods) (see Food Allergies, page 469).

People can be allergic to certain drugs taken orally, intramuscularly, or intravenously. The most common offender by far is penicillin and its relatives, followed by other antibiotics, insulin, local anesthetics, and the contrast agents used in certain x-ray tests. Many people are sensitive to aspirin, even though the reaction it causes is not truly an allergic reaction. Rarely, an individual will react to aspirin by having a rash, hives, and aggravation of asthma. Almost any medicine has the potential to cause a reaction (see Drug Allergies, page 471).

The bite or sting of insects can be responsible for exposure to an allergen for extremely sensitive people. In most people, the sting of a bee, wasp, or yellow jacket is uncomfortable for a couple of hours. However, in highly sensitive people, such a sting can trigger a systemic reaction (see Insect Bite Allergies, page 472 and Anaphylaxis, page 474).

In rare cases, people are sensitive (not allergic) to heat, cold, pressure, or light and sun rays and they have responses such as skin rashes, but these are not true allergic reactions (see Skin Allergies, page 457). Just as rare is sensitivity to changes in the body that are caused by exercise. The responses usually are wheals and tiny hives. In some people, vigorous exercise may provoke the symptoms of asthma.

DISCOVERING CAUSES

No one knows why some people become sensitive to certain substances such as plant resins, pollens, molds, house dust mites, foods, and drugs. Your physician will ask you a series of questions about your symptoms, your family's medical history, past medical problems, past and current emotional and social conditions, lifestyle including work, eating, and recreation habits, and possible exposure to certain allergens. This interview is one of the most important sources of information useful in making a diagnosis.

One important clue in the medical history will be the answer to the question "Does either of your parents have allergies?" It is known that the tendency to develop allergies is inherited. People who have allergies frequently have a close relative who also has allergies or a hypersensitivity. However, they do not necessarily have to be sensitive to the same allergens. You are less likely to inherit the sensitivity to a specific agent than you are to inherit the general tendency to develop sensitivities.

Other questions your physician asks will try to determine how various factors may cause an increased sensitivity to certain substances. Repeated or prolonged exposure to a specific substance might be responsible for a reaction—for example a person who works outside as a gardener in the spring and summer may experience an increase in hay fever symptoms when leaving the house. Such an observation is important because it suggests that the cause of the symptoms may be pollen or outdoor mold. As another example, the physician might ask for a list of all the foods eaten within the last five days to 2 weeks to determine if consumption of a certain food can be linked with the occurrence of the symptoms. The list of questions can be quite extensive.

TESTING FOR ALLERGENS

After the full medical history has been taken and affected areas of the lungs, skin, eyes, nose, and ears have been examined, the physician will select a testing method. The type of test to be used depends on the cause that is suspected.

Skin Test. The most commonly used test is the skin test, and several methods can be used. In the most common, a small amount of a suspected allergen is placed on the skin of either the forearm or the upper arm. Occasionally, skin on the back is used. The area is then pricked or scratched to introduce the allergen beneath the skin surface. Another common method is known as the intradermal method. It involves injecting a tiny amount of an allergen directly into the skin. With either method, the results are checked after 15 or 20 minutes.

If there is swelling and redness of the skin at the test site, the test is considered to be positive for that allergen. In skin tests, several allergens are tested at the same time, both to eliminate possible allergens and because people often are sensitive to several agents.

When a skin test is positive, the person being tested may experience symptoms of allergy when exposed to the allergen in its usual form. However, these tests are not foolproof: a person may test positive and yet not respond to the allergen in the course of everyday life. Also, a negative result does not rule out the possibility that the person is sensitive to that allergy. Skin tests must be interpreted cautiously. Tests with food allergens have the widest margin of error. This possibility of error on all tests is one reason why diagnosing allergies can be very difficult.

Skin tests are conducted for many forms of allergies. They are particularly useful for respiratory allergies, penicillin allergy, and insect bite allergy. They may not be as useful for diagnosing food allergies. Drug allergies other than penicillin and closely related drugs cannot be diagnosed with a skin test.

Skin tests must be conducted carefully. If too much allergen is placed on the skin, a positive reaction will be produced even in persons who are not allergic. Also, in rare instances, an extremely sensitive person can have a full-scale anaphylactic reaction, requiring immediate treatment with an injection of adrenaline (see page 474). The skin tests for airborne substances such as dust mites, animal dander, and pollens are the most reliable.

Skin test shows typical wheal and flare (see arrow) allergic reaction to allergen introduced beneath the skin surface.

INAPPROPRIATE TESTS

If you think you may have food allergies, be wary of certain tests and procedures that have not been proven to be valid. Do not accept cytotoxic testing, provocation and neutralization testing, or yeast hypersensitivity treatment.

Cytotoxic testing involves mixing extracts of foods in vials with samples of the patient's white blood cells. If the cells change shape in any way, the individual is said to be allergic to that food. There is no proven correlation between this shape change and a food allergy.

In provocation and neutralization testing, the person is injected with a small amount of food extract to provoke symptoms. When symptons occur, he or she is given "neutralizing" injections of the food on the theory that this will neutralize the effects of the first dose. This is an unproven test method.

There is one treatment to be aware of. Yeast hypersensitivity treatment is based on the theory that a yeast-like fungus called *Candida* is the cause of all allergies. People are told to remove from their diet all foods containing yeast and mold, including fruits, milk, refined carbohydrates (such as breads), and processed foods. Supposedly, this enables the body to correct the condition. There is no evidence to support the notion that *Candida* has any relation to food allergies.

Double-Blind Food Allergy Test. This test is used with care for diagnosing food allergies. Because the symptoms of food sensitivities are often affected by what a person believes he or she is allergic to, it can be useful to use a test in which neither the patient nor the physician knows what is being administered. In this test, the physician administers a series of foods and placebos in disguised form. The test substances are labeled in code, and neither the physician nor the patient knows what the test substances are (a third party in the office knows the code). After the test is finished, the identities of the substances are revealed. Because emotions and attitudes can easily affect the outcome of a test, such double-blind tests can be useful. These tests should not be done in people who report a history of severe food reactions.

RAST. A new laboratory test—the radioallergosorbent test (RAST)—has been found to be useful in discovering the causes of some allergies to inhaled substances.

The RAST measures the amounts of specific IgE antibodies in the patient's blood. In this test, all testing is done on a blood sample, which is an advantage over skin tests because it is more convenient and does not have even the slight risks of skin tests. Also, the test is not affected by the antihistamine drugs the person may be taking to lessen the allergic symptoms.

The disadvantages of the RAST are that the results are not available immediately but must come from a specialized laboratory, the test is not as sensitive as skin tests, and fewer allergens can be tested. It also may be considerably more expensive than skin tests.

WHAT YOUR DOCTOR CAN DO

IS THE CONDITION A TRUE ALLERGY?

Because allergies often seem to have no explanation, a wide range of complaints are often blamed on them. However, allergic responses are fairly specific, even if the causes are often hard to pinpoint. A true allergy usually involves IgE antibodies of the immune system. During the allergic reaction, histamine is released into various tissues, which causes such symptoms as skin rashes and hives, respiratory discomfort including nasal congestion and asthma, and internal problems such as nausea and diarrhea.

Plants such as poison ivy, poison oak, and poison sumac react with the immune system's T lymphocytes. An itchy rash with blisters develops in sensitive people after contact with the resin of such plants.

Occasionally, people have reactions that may closely resemble an allergy but in fact are due to something other than an IgE immune response. Such reactions are particularly common in response to food. A food reaction can be caused by many factors other than an allergen. For instance, the food may be contaminated with toxin-producing bacteria, or the person may experience the effects of irritable bowel syndrome (see page 632), stress, or a food intolerance (such as lactose intolerance; see page 470). The resulting symptoms, such as diarrhea and vomiting, may be confused with an allergy because they seem to happen whenever a person eats a particular food. The only way to assess the cause fully is to see a physician who can diagnose the problem and prescribe a suitable course of action.

Certain drug reactions commonly mimic allergic responses although they do not involve the immune system. Aspirin produces non-allergic reactions as well as idiosyncratic reactions that resemble allergic reactions. The antibiotic ampicillin also produces a non-allergic skin rash.

GENERAL PRINCIPLES OF TREATMENT

Effective methods of treatment for allergies involve several strategies. First, a proper diagnostic effort must be made to discover the true cause of your allergies. Your physician then must determine the best course of action to eliminate the problem or to alleviate the symptoms. The proper diagnostic effort includes evaluating your history and con-

20TH CENTURY SYNDROME: CAN YOU BE ALLERGIC TO MODERN TIMES?

In most people, allergic reactions are the result of sensitivities to specific agents such as pollen, mold, insect venom, and others. Strong flower odors, exhaust fumes, ozone, cigarette smoke, and even temperature changes can affect sensitive people. However, some insist that they are allergic to all of these agents and more, almost everything in the modern lifestyle and environment. These people, more often women than men, experience dizziness, impaired concentration, headaches, and joint pain. Known as 20th century syndrome in America and Total Allergy Syndrome in Europe and Australia, this disorder is difficult to treat because it seems to be the result of emotional upheaval. The symptoms are real, but the allergy is not.

20th century syndrome does not come on suddenly. It usually emerges gradually, often after a traumatic event such as the death of a child or the loss of a job. As the symptoms increase, the person often becomes preoccupied with the problem. Frustrated that physicians can find no physical cause for the symptoms, the individual often sees dozens of physicians and other health practitioners before someone diagnoses the problem as allergy.

Unfortunately for the people who suffer from the syndrome, there are physicians, known as clinical ecologists, who are at the fringe of orthodox medicine and who prescribe treatments that are expensive, that are disruptive to patients' lives, and that occasionally can be physically debilitating. Such treatments often require the person to avoid all "unnatural elements." This may require drastic measures such as quitting one's job to move to the mountains to live in a rustic home in which there are no man-made materials. Only organic foods may be eaten and often on a strict regimen. The prescription may require the consumption of several quarts of water a day and bathing with coconut oil rather than with soap. Despite all of these accommodations to a "natural" lifestyle, rarely are the symptoms relieved permanently.

There is effective treatment for 20th century syndrome. After a thorough examination to rule out any physical illness, a program of psychiatric therapy to treat emotional stress provides the best long-term treatment. Unfortunately, it is one that people who suffer from the syndrome usually shun, preferring instead unscientific and potentially harmful "allergy therapies."

---

ducting tests such as skin tests, RAST, or an elimination trial for food allergies.

Avoidance.   The best therapy for allergies is avoidance of the allergen. Avoiding a known allergen is fairly simple in the case of allergy to something like poison ivy, penicillin, or strawberries. However, it is not so simple for hay fever because these allergens are constantly in the air during certain months of the year or for allergy to house dust which is present year round even in the best-kept homes.

Medication.   The basic drug treatment for most allergies is the administration of antihistamines. These drugs block the action of histamine, the substance that is largely responsible for the symptoms.

Many antihistamines are available in nonprescription preparations intended for relieving symptoms of colds. For many people who have respiratory allergies such as hay fever or mold and house dust mite sensitivity, these drugs can control the nasal conges-tion, running nose, itchy eyes, throat, and mouth, and cough. In more severe cases and for hives, swelling of mucous membranes, or food allergies, antihistamines obtained by prescription are required.

The corticosteroid drugs (such as cortisone) are used for severe symptoms. These powerful anti-inflammatory drugs come in various forms for administration by injection, by swallowing a pill, by nasal spray, and by topical application of a cream (see Corticosteroid Drugs, page 1005). Available only by prescription, except for mild topical creams, these drugs can be very useful in the treatment of allergies, but they have side effects that may need to be weighed against the seriousness of the symptoms. Generally, the side effects of nasal sprays are minimal. The corticosteroid-containing creams often used in the treatment of contact dermatitis can cause skin problems in sensitive people and therefore should be used with care.

Cromolyn sodium is a non-corticosteroid drug that is prescribed in the treatment of some forms of allergies, particularly respiratory allergies. Use of this drug, in the form of a nasal spray and eye drops, usually is begun in advance of the allergy season because the drug must be used for several weeks before its benefits become apparent. It helps to prevent severe symptoms in the nose and eyes when used daily.

The most severe allergic reaction is life-threatening anaphylaxis. In this situation, blood vessels are dilated and air passages in the lungs are constricted (sometimes causing wheezing, low blood pressure, unconsciousness, and, occasionally, death). Treatment is injections of adrenaline (also known as epinephrine). This drug is used as an emergency medication most commonly for insect stings, drug allergies, and food allergies (see Anaphylaxis, page 474).

Allergy Shots. Certain allergies, including those to pollens, molds, and insect poisons, often can be treated by immunotherapy (known as allergy shots). This form of therapy involves injecting very small amounts of known allergens to stimulate the body to produce a neutralizing antibody. Some allergists believe that neutralizing antibody blocks the interaction of IgE antibodies with the allergen. Other mechanisms also are probably involved. The treatment requires regular injections, often on a weekly basis, of increasing doses of the allergen until a maintenance dose is established. Then, injections of the maintenance dose are given monthly for up to several years.

MYTHS ABOUT ALLERGY

The causes of an allergy are not always readily apparent. Allergies often appear to be vague in origin and unpredictable in response. They are difficult to treat successfully. Therefore, it is not surprising that a host of misconceptions and myths has arisen about them.

Few people affected by allergies have escaped without hearing someone's notion of sage advice about what causes his or her allergies and how to cure them. Here are our comments on the most common myths about allergies.

Allergies Are Psychosomatic. Although some allergies affect the nose and sinuses, they are not "all in your head." Allergies are real; they are the result of a response by the immune system to specific allergens. The symptoms may be affected by stress or emotions—science does not fully understand the relationship between body chemistry and emotions—but emotions do not cause the allergy.

Moving to Arizona Will Cure Allergies. For years, people who were bothered by seasonal allergies to pollens and molds thought that if they moved to the Southwest, where the foliage and climate are different from other regions, their allergies would disappear. Many enjoyed relief for a time but, although the desert is lacking in maple trees and ragweed, it does have other pollen-producing plants such as sagebrush, cottonwood, ash, and olive trees. People sensitive to some pollens and molds may develop allergies to the pollens and molds found in

ANTIHISTAMINES

When the immune system identifies an invader and produces IgE antibodies in response to it, one of the chemicals that is released is histamine. Histamine is partly responsible for most allergic responses, including running nose, itchy eyes, throat, and mouth, skin rashes and hives, asthma, anaphylactic shock, nausea, and diarrhea.

The drugs most widely used to combat the effects of histamines are known as antihistamines. This is a broad class of drugs that, as the name suggests, work to block the actions of histamine.

Antihistamines also have been found useful in the treatment of motion sickness, dizziness, and itching and as tranquilizers and local anesthetics. They are found in many non-prescription cold and allergy remedies, lotions, and creams as well as in prescription medications.

Although very useful in treating the symptoms of various allergies, antihistamines do have side effects. They can cause drowsiness, dryness of the nose and mouth, and blurred vision. Some antihistamine preparations contain decongestants, and some have fewer side effects than others. Recently introduced prescription antihistamines such as terfenadine (Seldane) and astemizole (Hismanal) have virtually no side effects. Because of the sleepiness that most antihistamines cause, avoid driving a car or operating heavy machinery when you are taking these drugs. Alcohol speeds the absorption of some antihistamines and also intensifies the drowsiness. Check with your physician before taking antihistamines. Antihistamines prescribed by a physician may be stronger than those available over-the-counter, and therefore instructions should be followed carefully. Sometimes the side effects can outweigh the benefit of antihistamines.

new environments. For example, people sensitive to ragweed may become sensitive to sagebrush pollen.

Allergies Are All Sniffles and Scratches, But No One Ever Dies From Them.   Most allergic reactions do indeed mimic some of the symptoms of a head and chest cold. However, some allergic reactions can be very serious indeed. Highly sensitive people can enter a state of life-threatening shock as a result of being stung by a bee, wasp, hornet, or yellow jacket or the injection of penicillin. A person highly sensitive to certain foods can experience severe abdominal distress or shock after eating those foods. A rare form of hereditary angioedema can cause swelling of the throat that can block breathing. Although it is true that many allergies are merely an inconvenience, severe reactions must be taken seriously and treated promptly and properly.

Short-Haired Pets Do Not Cause the Allergies.   The length of an animal's fur does not determine whether or not the fur can be responsible for an allergy. In fact, the fur itself is not the culprit. The cause is the dander, the scales of skin that are constantly shed by all animals with hair or feathers. In addition, saliva and urine may cause a sensitivity. If you have allergies to furry pets, the only really safe pets are fish and reptiles.

You Can Catch Poison Ivy by Just Standing Near the Plant.   The resin responsible for the sensitivity to poison ivy, poison oak, and poison sumac must actually touch the skin or clothing of a person to cause a reaction. The resin can be transferred from clothing to skin quite easily, which may explain why people who think they haven't touched the plants do have reactions. The irritating resins even can be carried in the smoke if the plant is burned.

SKIN ALLERGIES

Most Americans are susceptible to skin allergies or reactions at some time during their lives. The most common such sensitivity is to plants such as poison ivy, poison oak, or poison sumac. In susceptible individuals, contact with one of these plants produces an itchy, blistering rash. The swelling and itchy wheals of hives sometimes are caused by allergies. Another type of allergy causes swelling of tissues beneath the skin or in the throat (a condition called angioedema) for no apparent reason.

All of these discomforts are caused by histamines and other chemicals released into the skin or under the lining of the throat or bronchial passages as a result of an allergic response (see Understanding Allergy, page 448). In the following pages, each of the common skin allergies, including dermatitis, hives, and angioedema, will be described.

CONTACT DERMATITIS

Signs and Symptoms
- Itchy rash consisting of small bumps, blisters, and general swelling;
- Burning sensation of the eyes and mucous membranes.

Each year, millions of people have a contact dermatitis, an irritation of the skin caused by direct contact with certain plants, cosmetics, chemicals, metals, or drugs. Contact dermatitis is a hypersensitivity produced by T cells, not by the more common IgE antibodies (see Understanding Allergy, page 448). The most common irritants include the resins of poison ivy, poison oak, and poison sumac; the chemical *para*-phenylenediamine, which is used in hair and fur dyes, leather, and rubber and in printing; nickel compounds often used in jewelry; rubber compounds; ethylenediamine, a preservative used in creams and ophthalmic solutions; and dichromates used in textile ink, paints, and leather processing.

"Leaves of three, let them be," is a familiar phrase for many people, and with good reason. Certain three-leaved plants, particularly poison ivy and poison oak, are probably the most common causes of contact dermatitis. Poison sumac, which has multiple leaves, is a common offender as well. Four of every five Americans become sensitive to these in some degree. Although the plants are different, the problem-causing substance is the same, an oily resin called urushiol.

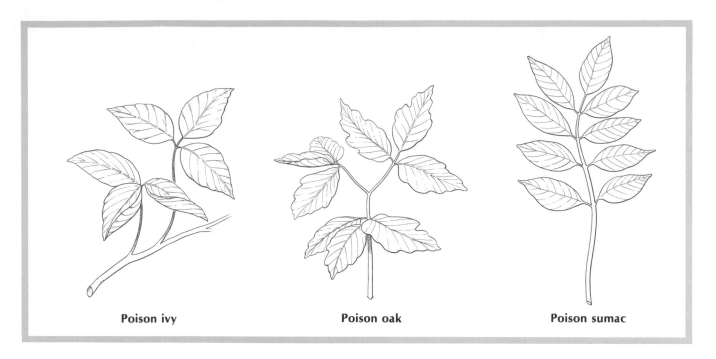

Poison ivy   Poison oak   Poison sumac

A reaction occurs when a sensitive person comes in contact with a resin-containing plant (by brushing against the plant itself or against something, such as clothing or pet fur, that has brushed against it). It takes only a tiny amount of the resin to cause a reaction, but direct contact is essential. For this reason, poison ivy and other such rashes do not develop as a result of a person's being merely near the plant. Nor does the rash spread as a result of washing or scratching open rash blisters, because the resin is not present in blister fluid. However, it can be spread by accidentally rubbing the resin on other areas of the skin before all the resin is washed off. For example, the eyelids often become inflamed as a result of touching or rubbing the eyes with fingers or hands that have resin on them. Thorough bathing with soap after an exposure to one of these plants may prevent a reaction or lessen its severity.

Other plants also can cause contact dermatitis. These include: heliotrope, found in the deserts of the Southwest; ragweed, both the leaves and the pollen; daisies; chrysanthemums; sagebrush; wormwood; celery; oranges; limes; and potatoes.

Certain chemicals and metals can cause rashes similar to poison ivy among persons who are particularly sensitive. Often, such sensitivities develop over a period of years of low-level exposure. These agents include the chemicals formaldehyde, chlorine, phenol (carbolic acid), and alcohols and metals such as nickel, chromium, mercury, and be-

ryllium. Perhaps the most common reaction to metal occurs when costume jewelry containing nickel (watchbands, earrings, bracelets) comes into contact with sensitive skin over a prolonged period. An itchy, flaky, red patch develops over a period of weeks or months. (See color photograph, page B-3.)

We most often think of exposure to chemicals as primarily an occupational hazard but many such substances, particularly formaldehyde, are found in household products ranging from permanent-press clothing to dyes, polishes, plaster, paper, rugs, foam insulation, and the particle board used in home construction and furniture. Formaldehyde causes a burning sensation in the eyes and mucous membranes.

Some people are sensitive to allergens in eye makeup, hair dye, lipstick, and nail polish. Occasionally, perfumes, colognes, and antiperspirants also can cause skin reactions.

The Diagnosis. A rash develops within 2 days after exposure. In very sensitive people it can develop as soon as a few hours. The affected area reddens and swells, and small itchy blisters and bumps form. The blisters first fill with clear fluid and then burst, revealing raw skin susceptible to bacteria and infection. The itching can range from minor to severe. The rash usually reaches its peak after about 5 days and is usually gone within 1 to 2 weeks.

Reactions to plants rarely develop on the soles, palms, and scalp. In the case of formaldehyde, a burning sensation of the eyes and linings of the nose, mouth, throat, or eyes (mucous membranes) develops.

How Serious Is Contact Dermatitis?

Contact dermatitis is an irritating condition that causes pain and discomfort, and the blisters can become infected. It can be temporarily debilitating, but it has no lasting effects.

Treatment.   The itching of the contact dermatitis rash can be relieved by applying a paste made of baking soda or Epsom salts and water or using calamine lotion or nonprescription hydrocortisone creams. (Some people are sensitive to the agents in certain creams and lotions, which can aggravate the condition.) Do not apply alcohol because this tends to make the itching worse. Cover open blisters with sterile gauze to prevent infection. Creams and lotions do not help much when the blisters open, but they can be used again when the blisters close. Try not to scratch.

Severe cases or those in sensitive areas such as face, eyes, and the genital region should be treated by a physician who may prescribe application of a cortisone ointment, use of an antihistamine, or taking a cortisone drug orally.

Prevention.   Avoidance is the best way to prevent contact dermatitis. Allergens in household agents are not always easy to detect, but harmful plants are. Poison ivy is found in woodlands almost everywhere in the United States except California, where poison oak is found.

Learn to recognize offending plants, and avoid them or wear protective clothing when exposure seems likely. Poison ivy may be a low-growing plant, a bush, or a vine. Its leaves usually are glossy green in the summer and turn an attractive red, pink, or yellow in the autumn. They generally are elliptical in shape and grow in groups of three on a stem. Poison oak can grow as low plants or bushes. Its leaves also grow three to a stem, and they resemble oak leaves. Poison sumac may be a bush or a tree. It has two rows of leaflets, opposite each other, per stem and a leaflet at the tip. It can be distinguished from its harmless relative by the smooth edges of its leaves. Poison sumac tends to grow in marshy areas such as swamps and bogs.

If one of these poisonous plants grows in your yard, you can kill it with a herbicide. Pulling it out alone will not necessarily cure the problem because new growth can develop from the roots. These plants should not be burned because the resin can be carried in the smoke and cause internal as well as external reactions. They should not be composted but rather should be disposed of in a plastic bag.

Washing the harmful resin off the skin with soap within 5 or 10 minutes after exposure can avert an episode of contact dermatitis. Washing after this brief period will not always prevent a reaction but may help to contain it within a smaller area. Clothes that have brushed against such resinous plants should be removed carefully and washed.

If your reactions are to household chemicals, you can take steps to decrease your exposure. Wash all new permanent-press clothing several times before wearing it, avoid insulating a home with formaldehyde foam, and apply a varnish to all particle board in the household to seal it. In the case of metal sensitivity, wear solid (not plated) gold and sterling silver jewelry.

Cosmetics free of problem-causing ingredients are available.

ATOPIC DERMATITIS

Signs and Symptoms

- Extreme, persistent itching and thickening of the skin in patches.

Atopic dermatitis, also known as eczema, generally occurs in babies and children, although it can occur at any time of life. There is a strong genetic component. About 70 percent of affected people have a family history of atopic dermatitis. Although atopic dermatitis itself is not an allergy, in about a third of individuals who have it respiratory allergies such as hay fever and asthma do develop (see also Atopic Dermatitis, page 1157, and color photograph of eczema, page B-2).

The Diagnosis.   Atopic dermatitis consists of patches of dry, extremely itchy, thickened skin. Characteristically, it affects the skin behind the knees and in the folds of the elbow. The itching is persistent, and it often drives the sufferers to frantic scratching. Babies and children who have it sweat more than normal, and they have a dry skin and a greater than normal tendency to itch. Abrasion, heat, or stress can start these children scratching. (See color photograph, page B-2.)

Most infants with atopic dermatitis (about 3 percent of the population) are from families in which other members have allergy-related diseases such as hay fever or asthma. Children usually outgrow their atopic dermatitis by about age 6, although in some the improvement does not occur until puberty and in some it lasts into adulthood.

How Serious Is Atopic Dermatitis? This form of eczema is irritating but for most people it is a passing problem.

Treatment. Treatment for atopic dermatitis is primarily a matter of using creams, lotions, and antihistamines. The objective is to stop the intense itching because it causes scratching and thus more itching.

Keep the skin moist with creams and lotions. If the itching and scratching continue, your physician may prescribe antihistamines. Coal-tar ointments are often used when the condition has been present for months or years and the skin has become thickened and leather-like, a process known as lichenification. Corticosteroid creams and ointments are very useful in reducing the inflammation and itching.

Children should be bathed no more than three times a week, and these baths should be done rapidly with a mild neutral soap. Use of bath oil sometimes keeps the skin from drying too much. The fingernails should be kept short to decrease the damage caused by scratching.

HIVES AND ANGIOEDEMA

Signs and Symptoms

Hives
- Raised red, often itchy, welts of various sizes that appear and disappear at random on the surface of the skin;
- New welts develop where the skin is scratched (dermatographia).

Angioedema
- Large welts below the surface of the skin, particularly around the eyes and lips but also on the hands and feet, and in the throat.

About one in five people experience hives at one time or another. The condition also is called urticaria (from the Latin *urtica,* for nettle). The lesions usually occur in batches rather than singly, and they may last a few minutes or for several days. Hives occur on the surface of the skin. Angioedema is a similar swelling that occurs beneath the skin (see color photograph, page B-9).

Hives and angioedema may result from the release of histamine and other chemicals into the bloodstream. The cause of the reaction often is unknown, although all sorts of things have been found to cause hives, including foods, pollen, animal dander, drugs, insect bites, infections, illness, cold, heat, light, and emotional distress. As with many allergies, there is a hereditary component to the development of hives and angioedema.

Foods that may cause problems in some sensitive people include berries, shellfish, fish, nuts, eggs, and milk. Penicillin and aspirin are known culprits. Pollen and animal dander are common inhalant agents.

The Diagnosis. The primary symptom of hives and angioedema is a swelling of the skin into red welts. In the case of hives the swellings, which are often intensely itchy, appear on the surface of the skin. In angioedema, the swellings are deeper and appear primarily around the eyes and mouth, making them appear swollen. They also occur on the hands and feet, although less frequently.

In treating hives, your physician will begin by asking about your medical history. This may include asking you to create a detailed diary of exposure to possible irritants over a period of 2 weeks to a month. Because hives and angioedema can be caused by many different things and can be exacerbated by emotional conditions, it sometimes is impossible to determine the cause. (See color photograph, page B-9.)

How Serious Are Hives and Angioedema? Hives and angioedema generally are harmless. They leave no lasting marks and sometimes are not even uncomfortable. However, there is one rare form, hereditary angioedema, that is more troublesome and can be dangerous. It is a disorder of a blood protein that is part of the immune system and may require special treatment. This reaction includes non-itchy swelling, possibly with painful abdominal cramping and diarrhea. When angioedema affects the throat or tongue, it causes the air passage to be blocked and can be life-threatening.

Treatment. Sometimes treatment is not needed. The standard treatment for hives and angioedema is antihistamines, but other drugs may be used, including adrenaline (epinephrine), terbutaline, and cimetidine. Occasionally, physicians prescribe a corticosteroid drug for oral use (see page 1005). People who are allergic should avoid substances that they know cause attacks in them.

ALLERGIC REACTIONS TO HEAT OR COLD

Signs and Symptoms
- A rash or swollen welts such as hives appear as a result of exposure to heat, cold, sun, or rubbing.

Emergency Symptoms
- Muscle cramping, vomiting, and fainting as a result of immersion in cold water.

One of the most puzzling of allergy-like reactions is that to physical stimuli such as pressure, heat, cold, light, and sunlight. Hives are the most common symptom. People who have this sort of response often have very sensitive skin. Sometimes, just the rubbing of a blunt object on the skin produces a swelling within a few minutes. In the condition called dermographia, when the skin is stroked lightly, as with a fingernail, it reddens almost immediately and a wheal develops where the skin is touched. (See color photograph, page B-9.)

The Diagnosis. Physical allergy-like symptoms include: tiny hives in response to vigorous exercise, a hot shower, or emotional stress; swelling of the hands and feet in response to pressure; and hives in response to rewarming of body parts that had been exposed to cold air. In testing for heat and cold reactions, your physician will take a complete history and conduct a test in which cold and hot objects are applied to the skin to see if a reaction occurs.

Treatment. The best method for treating hypersensitivity to heat and cold is to avoid them as much as possible. Wear warm clothing during cold weather. Take warm showers and baths rather than hot or cold ones. Avoid swimming or bathing in cold water if hives develop where your body is exposed to cold. Your physician may prescribe a strong antihistamine drug.

Sun-induced hives is best treated by avoiding the sun (or using sunscreens), perfumes, and drugs such as antibiotics, antihistamines, diuretics, antifungal agents, tranquilizers, and hypoglycemics that have been known to cause such reactions.

RESPIRATORY ALLERGIES

Allergies of the respiratory tract often produce symptoms that are similar to those of a cold: congested head and chest, stuffy or running nose, cough, and sneezes. Occasionally, wheezing also occurs with a respiratory allergy. In fact, allergies and colds are sometimes confused until one realizes that the symptoms of the allergic response last far longer than those of a cold, or they seem to appear (and disappear) with a suddenness uncharacteristic of the common cold.

For some people, such symptoms appear during a pollen season—spring, summer, or autumn. For others, the symptoms are manifested primarily in the winter when their home is closed to ventilation and house dust mites, and molds are common. Still others experience symptoms when they enter a room in which a furred animal lives.

All respiratory allergies represent responses of the immune system to airborne allergies (see Understanding Allergy, page 448). The following pages will discuss the common kinds of allergies to pollen, molds, dusts, and dander as well as asthma and nasal polyps.

HAY FEVER (ALLERGIC RHINITIS)

Signs and Symptoms
- Stuffy or running nose;
- Frequent sneezing;

- Itchy eyes, nose, roof of mouth, or throat;
- Cough.

It's springtime. The air is sweet with the smell of fresh new flowers but you can't enjoy it because your head is stuffed up, your nose is sore, and your throat itches. Or it's autumn and the ragweed and other autumn plants are blooming and spreading their wind-blown pollen everywhere, including into your respiratory system—making your eyes teary, your head and nose congested, and the roof of your mouth itchy.

The sum of these symptoms is known as hay fever (technically, it is allergic rhinitis), although things other than hay usually cause the problem and no fever is present.

No one knows why some people are more susceptible than others to the tiny airborne pollens of certain seasonal plants. In all likelihood a person's sensitivity is partly an inherited trait that affects the ability of the immune system to deal with potential invaders. Many believe that hay fever is a childhood disorder, something you grow out of by the time you reach adulthood. However, hay fever can develop at any time during life, and you can recover from it at any time. A person who has other allergies such as dermatitis or asthma or who has relatives with allergies is more likely to have hay fever.

People with hay fever react to specific allergens. Some are sensitive to only one or two substances; others are sensitive to many. When an allergic person inhales the pollen to which he or she is allergic, antibodies react with the pollen and this causes histamine to be released. This histamine causes the lining of the nose, sinuses, eyelids, and eyes to become inflamed. The sinuses may become congested, the nose runs, and the eyes, nose, throat, and roof of the mouth often itch. You may sneeze, sometimes violently and repeatedly—as many as 10 to 20 times in a row. Usually, attacks of the symptoms last about 15 to 20 minutes and happen several times a day. Many people find that their hay fever doesn't interfere with their lives in any substantial way. Every year at a certain time their noses are congested and they sneeze frequently for a couple of weeks.

The Diagnosis. For many people, hay fever is a minor inconvenience at certain times of the year. If it is a significant interference in your life, a visit to an allergist is in order.

Your physician will begin by asking a series of questions to determine what sort of allergens cause congestion and how much they interfere with your normal habits. You may be asked to keep a diary to determine when reactions occur most frequently, in order to determine the frequency accurately. For instance, if your symptoms come on only in the spring, then you probably are allergic to pollens found only in the spring. If you have allergy attacks throughout the growing season, you may be allergic to several pollens.

Sometimes a series of skin tests may be used to determine which pollens you are most sensitive to. These include prick tests and occasionally a radioallergosorbent test (RAST) (see Testing for Allergens, page 452).

Treatment. The most effective method for controlling the symptoms of hay fever is to avoid the allergens. During pollen season, this means staying indoors a good deal, especially on dry windy days when pollen counts are high. Keeping doors and windows closed is useful. Air conditioning, particularly a filtered central system, also is helpful.

In mild cases of hay fever, relief often is provided by non-prescription antihistamines and decongestant tablets. However, antihistamines can produce drowsiness and a dryness of the throat and mouth that can cause as much discomfort as that of the hay fever. Newer antihistamines such as terfenadine or astemizole have very few side effects.

Avoid chronic use of over-the-counter nasal sprays and drops. Although they relieve symptoms at first, they can be addicting. After a number of weeks or months of daily use of these agents, the nose becomes increasingly congested and more frequent doses of the spray or drops are needed to clear it. The only way of resolving nose drop addiction is to stop the use of the spray or drops and wait for the rebound congestion to subside. This usually takes a month or two.

If you are particularly bothered by hay fever, consult an allergist who can determine what pollens you are allergic to and the best course of treatment. The allergist may prescribe an antihistamine that works well for you. Over-the-counter antihistamine tablets and eye drops may give comfort. Your physician may prescribe a corticosteroid nasal spray in addition to other measures. Another useful drug is cromolyn; it is available both as nasal spray and as eye drops. It must be used for several weeks before you can expect to experience benefits.

The closest thing to a cure for hay fever is a series of immunizing injections (immunotherapy) which desensitize the system to allergens. In this series, increasing amounts of the offending allergen are given over time. Many people who undergo this therapy lose their sensitivity, usually within 2 years. However, the procedure is long and expensive and is not effective for 20 to 30 percent of patients.

NASAL POLYPS

Signs and Symptoms
• Chronically blocked nasal passages.

When the mucous membrane that lines the inside of the nose swells and protrudes into the nasal passage, the swelling is known as a polyp. A polyp may appear singly or in clusters so that it is difficult for the person who has them to breathe or to smell odors. Nasal polyps are caused by an overproduction of fluid in the mucous membrane, sometimes as a result of hay fever or some other nasal allergy. Often, no specific cause can be identified.

The Diagnosis. If you notice that your nose never seems to clear, making it difficult to breathe through it or to smell odors, you may have nasal polyps. Headaches are a sign that a polyp may be blocking the opening between the nasal cavity and one of the sinuses.

Occasionally, you may be able to determine if you have polyps yourself. When you shine a light up your nostrils and examine them with a mirror, you may see pearl-like lumps. However, because polyps often are at the back of the nose, they are not seen easily.

Nasal polyps must be treated by a physician. To determine if polyps are present, your physician will use a nasal speculum, which looks like a pair of sugar tongs, to examine the inside of your nose.

How Serious Are Nasal Polyps? Nasal polyps are an inconvenience but generally are not a serious threat to health. Sometimes they obstruct the drainage of the sinuses enough to cause recurring sinus infections and significant difficulty in breathing through the nose. Occasionally, there may be an association between use of aspirin and nasal polyps or between cystic fibrosis and nasal polyps (see page 934).

Treatment. Nasal polyps are removed surgically in an operation usually performed under local anesthesia. Polyps can reappear and may need to be removed as they develop.

ALLERGIES TO MOLD, DANDER, AND DUST

Signs and Symptoms
• Stuffy, runny nose;
• Frequent sneezing;
• Itchy eyes, nose, roof of mouth, or throat;
• Cough;
• Wheezing.

Pearl-like lumps in the lining of the nasal passage are called nasal polyps. If they cause breathing difficulty or recurrent sinus infections, these polyps can be removed in a simple surgical procedure.

POLLEN

The pollens that are carried by bees from plant to plant are relatively harmless to humans because they are relatively large grains and have a waxy texture. However, those that are carried by the wind are lighter and smaller and do cause hay fever.

Where there are plants, there is pollen at some time of the year. Trees, both deciduous and evergreen, produce pollen in the spring. Grasses and most flowers produce their pollen during June and July. Late-blooming plants such as ragweed produce pollen in the early autumn. In warm climates with long growing seasons, pollen may be present in the air for 8 or 9 months of the year, whereas in climates with shorter growing seasons the pollen is present for less time.

Certain plants are more likely to cause reactions than others. The roadside plant ragweed heads the list of hay-fever-causing plants east of the Rocky Mountains. Other pollens that produce allergy but much less commonly include sagebrush, tumbleweed, redroot pigweed, spiny amaranth, burning bush, and English plantain.

Grasses also provide their share of allergy-causing pollens. Grass varieties that cause trouble include rye, timothy, redtop, Bermuda, orchard, sweet vernal, and bluegrasses. Most trees produce pollens that can cause problems; these include maple, oak, ash, birch, poplar, elm, pecan, juniper, and cottonwood.

The amount of pollen in the air depends on the weather. Hot, dry, breezy days stir up more pollen than do damp, rainy ones when the pollen is washed to the ground. Most pollen particles are so small that they can be carried, by the air, into the house through open windows as well as through doors and screens. If kept well maintained, the filters in central air-conditioning systems may help remove pollen.

It does not take much pollen to produce a reaction, as little as 20 particles per cubic yard. Considering that the particles are often invisible and that many plants can produce up to a million such particles, it's not surprising that sneezing and runny nose are common during the pollen season.

Not all hay fever (allergic rhinitis) (see page 461) is caused by pollen. Identical reactions may occur from sensitivity to other inhaled allergens such as molds, animal dander, and the microscopic mites that live in house dust.

Some people experience an allergy attack when they enter an empty room. Others find they have the symptoms of nasal allergy at random times all year long. Still others have the symptoms seasonally. All of these people may be reacting to airborne allergens other than common pollen.

The Diagnosis. For most people, allergy to molds, dust, or animals is primarily an inconvenience. When it lasts only a few weeks each year it can be ignored or treated as the symptoms of a cold. Indeed, the symptoms are similar to those of a cold except that they last longer and the mucus discharge usually is clear. When the symptoms interfere with normal activities, a visit to an allergist is in order to determine the exact causes and a method of treatment.

When diagnosing inhalant allergies such as those to molds or dust, your allergist will ask a series of questions designed to determine how severe the reaction is, how often it occurs, whether it is year-round or seasonal, and the situations in which it occurs most frequently. You may be asked to keep a detailed diary for up to a month to determine frequency and possible causes. A series of skin tests may be used to identify the allergens to which you are most sensitive. The prick test is a common one. Occasionally, the radioallergosorbent test (RAST) also is used (see Testing for Allergens, page 452).

Some people may be sensitive to more than one allergen; some or all of these may be responsible for their symptoms. Therefore it is difficult to pinpoint which allergens cause the most trouble.

How Serious Are These Allergies? The cold-like symptoms of allergies are inconvenient and annoying but are not serious problems to general health.

Treatment. The most effective treatment for allergy to molds, dust, and animals is avoidance. This may be easier said than done because some allergens, particularly mold spores, are borne on the wind just like pollen. In those cases, staying indoors in an air-conditioned atmosphere is often the most useful preventive measure. When the allergen is dust, animal dander, or feathers, you can take steps to avoid some sources of irritation (see page 463).

The medical treatment for allergies to molds, dust, and animals is often identical to that for allergic rhinitis. Non-prescription antihistamine tablets (see Antihistamines, page 456) and decongestants relieve the symptoms for many people. When the reactions are severe or interfere with a person's life, a physician's care may be needed to provide a course of treatment. An allergist may prescribe antihistamine tablets, cromolyn eye drops, and steroid nasal sprays to reduce the swelling of the mucous membrane of the nose. Oral doses of steroids may be prescribed when reactions are severe (see Corticosteroid Drugs, page 1005).

Drugs used to control allergic rhinitis have drawbacks. Many antihistamines cause drowsiness in most people, although they occasionally can have the reverse effect in others, causing them to be wakeful and nervous. When taken over a prolonged period the powerful anti-inflammatory steroids given orally can induce a number of side effects.

As in allergic rhinitis, in the other respiratory allergies the closest thing to a cure is a course of desensitization. The allergens that cause the most trouble are diagnosed with skin tests and the patient is periodically injected with small doses of the offending allergens. The doses are increased gradually as the body produces protective mechanisms to limit the release of histamine and other chemicals. Such therapy often is given on a weekly basis, and the course can run anywhere from 3 months to several years. After the main course is concluded, a course of maintenance shots begins, given every 2 to 6 weeks. This may last for several years.

Immunotherapy works well for many people, but it is not without a few problems. It is expensive and inconvenient, carries risks of reactions, and it doesn't work for everyone. Discuss the pros and cons with your primary-care physician and your allergist.

Molds. Many allergy sufferers are sensitive to the spores of common molds that are carried by the air. Outdoor molds produce spores mostly in the summer and early autumn and these are carried by the wind, although in warm climates they can be present all year. Indoor molds shed spores all year long, producing constant problems for sensitive people.

Molds thrive indoors in damp locations such as basements and bathrooms and in upholstered furniture and beds, rugs, stuffed animals, wood, books, and wallpaper. Outdoors they live in the soil and on compost or damp vegetation. Susceptible people react most noticeably when mowing grass, harvesting crops, or walking through tall grass and plants. Common offending molds include the indoor molds *Penicillium, Aspergillus, Mucor,* and *Rhizopus* and the outdoor molds *Alternaria* and *Hormodendrum.*

Mold spores are everywhere, so they cannot be eliminated. However, you can minimize the exposure. During the summer and autumn you can stay inside in air-conditioned surroundings as much as possible. You can dry out a damp basement by using a dehumidifier. Discard moldy or mildewed articles such as books, old shoes, and bedding. Wash wooden furniture with a weak solution of bleach and air it in the sun. Use synthetic fabrics for upholstery and bedding. Clean bathroom and basement walls with disinfectants. Instead of using wallpaper, paint walls with mold-proof paint.

Dust. Common house dust is a major cause of year-round suffering for sensitive people. House dust harbors all kinds of substances, including pollen, mold spores, fabric fibers, and detergents, but the primary cause of allergic reaction is mites which are microscopic insects. Mites thrive during the summer, but most people's reactions are worse in the winter. This is probably due to the fact that the disintegrated fragments of the spider-like insects are more easily inhaled than the live animals. Disintegrated fibers from stuffing materials, mattresses, toys, furniture, blankets, carpets, and draperies also can be irritants.

The best way to deal with dust is to keep the house as clean as possible. This means not only vacuuming up visible dust frequently but also damp-mopping and dusting often. Wash scatter rugs and furniture covers weekly if possible. Pay particular attention to the bedroom, the most-used room in the house. Keep furniture simple and avoid dust trappers such as bed ruffles, canopy beds, bunk beds, rugs, curtains, upholstered furniture, and Venetian blinds. Enclose pillows, mattresses, and box springs in allergen-proof coverings.

A central heating and air-conditioning system that filters and humidifies the air is a help. You can attach special air filters to the system. Individual room air cleaners can be of limited help as well.

Animals. Another household substance to which some people are allergic is the dander shed from the skin, fur, and feathers of animals and birds. The fur and feathers themselves are not the cause of year-round irritation. It is the scales shed from the skin that cause the allergy, along with the pet's saliva and urine. People allergic to pollens or molds may become allergic to animal dander as well. The only way to eliminate the problem is to avoid the source. This means not keeping pets. If you are sensitive to the tiny amounts of dander found in wool, avoid products made mostly with wool.

Miscellaneous Irritants.   Dozens of other substances can cause reactions among a very small percentage of people. These factors include smoke and fumes from industrial activities; tobacco smoke from cigarettes, cigars, and pipes; face and baby powder; and powdered laundry detergents. People sensitive to respiratory allergens are more likely to be sensitive to other irritants.

Avoid irritating substances as much as possible. Avoid smoking and avoid smoke-filled environments when possible. Use liquid laundry detergents. Do not use body or facial powders.

ASTHMA

Signs and Symptoms
- Wheezing;
- Difficulty in breathing;
- Painless tightness in the chest;
- Coughing up of excess mucus.

Emergency Symptoms
- Extreme difficulty in breathing;

- Bluish cast to the face and lips;
- Severe anxiety;
- Increased pulse rate;
- Sweating.

Asthma, characterized by periodic tightness in the chest, cough, wheezing, and difficulty in breathing, may be caused or aggravated by allergy to pollen, mold spores, animal dander, or house dust mites. However, its cause often is unknown. Respiratory infections, exercise, and anti-inflammatory drugs, including aspirin, can cause or aggravate asthma. Emotional distress once was thought to be a major contributing factor in asthma attacks, but research has shown that it is less significant than previously thought.

As in other allergies, IgE antibodies react with allergens, which produces histamine and other chemicals. The result is a tightening of the muscles and swelling of the lining of lung airways and increased production of mucus. Air flow through the swollen bronchial tubes is restricted, producing a wheezing sound that is loudest during exhaling of the breath.

Asthma affects almost 10 million Americans. It is seen most often in children and usually is an inherited condition. Asthma is not contagious and may remain chronic throughout childhood. It is the leading cause of chronic illness in children. Up to 10 percent of children have asthma, being twice as common in boys as in girls. About half of the cases develop before age 10; another third develop by age 40. Some children outgrow it because no more than 3 to 5 percent of the adult population have it.

ASTHMA AND EXERCISE

In some people, asthma attacks are induced by exercise. This does not mean, however, that you need to eliminate exercise from your life. Although it may make breathing uncomfortable, regular exercise does not harm your lungs and it keeps your muscles in tone, which is important to your overall health.

The cause of the asthma attack after exercise is not known. Vigorous exercise is more likely to cause an asthma attack than is mild exercise. During cold weather, it is generally a good idea to exercise indoors because cold, dry air worsens the symptoms.

When you go out in cold weather, be sure to wear a soft scarf or a cold-air mask over your mouth and nose, even if you are just walking a short distance. You can purchase a cold-air mask at your local drugstore. Also, breathe through your nose so that your nose can warm, filter, and humidify the air that enters your lungs.

Taking medications to prevent asthma immediately before exercising also may help. Some of the medications that are effective are albuterol aerosol (Ventolin or Proventil) and, for some people, cromolyn aerosol or powder (Intal). If you have asthma, be sure to talk to your physician about how to incorporate exercise into your lifestyle.

AVOID THOSE ALLERGENS AND IRRITANTS

Avoiding the things to which you are allergic or sensitive is one way to help prevent asthma attacks. Among the strategies you can use are the following.

Avoid Smoke, Smoking, and Smokers

Do not smoke, and avoid exposure to smoke of all types. Smoke from cigarettes, wood fires, burning leaves or rubbish, or other sources irritates your bronchial tubes, eyes, and nose. Ask relatives and friends who smoke to avoid smoking around you.

Avoid Using Analgesics if You Are Sensitive to Them

Some people with asthma experience severe attacks after they take aspirin. Often, these people also have nasal polyps. If you are sensitive to aspirin, do not use it and make sure that any over-the-counter cold or pain medications you take do not contain aspirin (also called acetylsalicylic acid). Ibuprofen, available in over-the-counter form (Advil and Nuprin) and by prescription (Motrin or Rufen), also should be avoided because it may cause reactions in as-pirin-sensitive people. The same goes for the other nonsteroidal anti-inflammatory drugs taken for pain and arthritis, including indomethacin (Indocin), naproxen (Naproxyn), mefenamic acid (Ponstel), sulindac (Clinoril), and piroxicam (Feldene).

Keep the Dust Down

Avoid dusty jobs, if possible; if not possible, wear a dust mask. Avoid paint and paint remover fumes, sawdust, and similar irritants. Remodeling a room often makes asthma worse temporarily. If you are allergic to dust, minimize use of carpets, overstuffed furniture, and draperies which attract and hold dust.

Condition Your Air

If you are allergic to airborne pollens and molds, use air conditioning in your home, car, and office, particularly during the seasons when these allergens are more prevalent. If your asthma attacks are precipitated by changes in temperature, you may not be able to do this, but keeping doors and windows closed also helps keep out allergens.

If you live in a house with a forced-air furnace and are allergic to dust, put a filter for dust control into your furnace. For limited areas, portable air purifiers are somewhat effective, but obtain one that does not produce ozone because it is a respiratory irritant.

If you have a humidifier, be sure to clean it regularly; otherwise molds and other growths can develop and may aggravate your asthma.

Animal Trouble

Many people are allergic to animal dander. If you are, do not have dogs, cats, or other animals in your home. Also, do not buy furniture or rugs made with animal hair.

Food Allergies

If you are allergic to certain foods, eliminate those foods from your diet. About 4 to 8 percent of people with asthma are sensitive to sulfites which are often used in restaurants and markets to keep lettuce and fruits looking fresh. They are also used in wine, beer, dehydrated fruits, potatoes, and some seafoods. Dehydrated soups often contain sulfites, as do maraschino cherries and some soft drinks and avocado mixtures. If you are sensitive to sulfites, you will probably experience a reaction in a few minutes after ingesting them.

The Diagnosis. Difficulty in breathing is the primary symptom of asthma. This usually is accompanied by wheezing as the air is forced through narrowed bronchial tubes. A cough, often in bunches and sometimes producing mucus, also is very characteristic. The symptoms of an asthma attack can occur within minutes after exposure to an offending allergen but they also may occur for no apparent reason.

Physicians use various tests to help diagnose asthma. A chest x-ray, complete physical examination, and special lung (pulmonary) tests may be called for. Your physician may also ask you to keep a diary to determine if there is a pattern to the attacks and thus narrow the list of possible causes.

How Serious Is Asthma? Asthma attacks are irritating more often than dangerous, especially when breathing is only partially restricted. The attacks last minutes to hours and sometimes even days. Often, a cold is the trigger for an asthmatic attack and the symptoms of asthma may last as long as the cold. Asthma attacks can be dangerous when air flow is severely obstructed. A person with asthma should be under the care of a physician. With help, the attacks can be

PROPER USE OF THE METERED-DOSE INHALER

One very useful aid in the treatment of asthma is the metered-dose inhaler (MDI). These devices allow administration of medication into the lungs in specific amounts and are used for asthma medicines such as bronchodilators, cortisone, and cromolyn.

To take full advantage of the inhaler, you must use it properly. It takes a little practice to coordinate squeezing the device and inhaling through it. You may find that having a friend or family member observe as you practice the following steps will help you perfect your technique. The idea is to mix the medication with incoming air and pull this mixture into the lungs slowly.

1. Shake the inhaler well, perhaps five or six times.
2. Attach a spacer to the nozzle end of the inhaler. A spacer is a 6- to 8-inch-long tube that helps to distribute the medication evenly in the bronchial tubes. Many expensive commercial spacers are available, but any tube of similar size may be used effectively as a spacer.
3. Breathe in and out normally once, then stop for a moment. Do not try to push all the air from your lungs.
4. Close your mouth around the end of the spacer.
5. Squeeze the inhaler once, as you breathe in slowly. Keep inhaling even after finishing the squeeze. Continue inhaling for 5 to 7 seconds.
6. After inhaling, remove the spacer from your mouth and press your lips together for 10 seconds. Then, exhale through your nose.
7. If you need a second dose, breathe normally four or five times and then repeat the sequence from step 1. You usually should not take more than four to eight doses in any 24-hour period.

controlled so that they seldom become disabling or life-threatening.

Treatment.   Asthma is a disease of the airways, and allergies may be the trigger for an attack. Therefore, the treatments for asthma are similar to those for other forms of allergy. Avoiding the offending allergens as much as possible is the first step, if the allergen can be identified. For example, if the allergy is to pollen, it may be helpful to spend a good deal of the worst of the season indoors in an environment with filtered air.

If dust is the problem, your house should be kept as dust-free as possible. If the problem is animal dander, you should not keep any pet that produces allergens. Often, no cause can be found (see page 467).

An allergist may prescribe a drug called cromolyn that helps prevent attacks. This medication is often prescribed as a maintenance drug for children and young adults. In addition, theophylline, inhaled bronchodilators, and oral doses of steroids are used for immediate relief (see The Lungs and the Respiratory System, page 913).

ALLERGIES TO FOODS, DRUGS, AND INSECT BITES

Allergies to food, drugs, and insect bites may be the result of antibody responses to allergens that have come into contact with the internal systems of the body (see Understanding Allergy, page 448). The symptoms may range from a simple skin rash to a systemic reaction involving the gastrointestinal tract and the respiratory and cardiovascular systems.

The symptoms may appear immediately after a specific food is eaten, a drug is administered, or a bee sting occurs. With some allergens it may take several days, or even several weeks, for the reaction to develop.

FOOD ALLERGIES

Signs and Symptoms

- Abdominal pain, diarrhea, nausea, or vomiting;
- Fainting;
- Hives, swelling beneath the skin (see Angioedema, page 460), or eczema;
- Swelling of the lips, eyes, face, tongue, and throat;
- Nasal congestion;
- Asthma.

Emergency Symptoms

- Severe symptoms of the above reactions;
- Anaphylaxis (see page 474).

Few things are more distressing than a reaction to food because food represents something that nourishes and comforts. If you have experienced severe symptoms after eating, you may fear a recurrence. Perhaps this is why food allergies are the subject of widespread apprehension and misinformation.

Food allergies are specific responses of the immune system to a particular food or food component. The immune system produces vast numbers of antibodies to attack the food or food component, an occurrence that in turn releases histamine which causes the symptoms.

Food allergies may be the most misunderstood of the allergies. Two out of five Americans believe they are allergic to specific foods. However, fewer than 1 percent have true food allergies. Most other discomforts do not involve release of histamine and should be termed food intolerances. Children have a higher percentage of food allergies than adults, but many of them grow out of these, often by around age 6. About 70 percent of the food allergies develop in persons less than age 30.

Ninety percent of the food allergies are caused by certain proteins in cow's milk, egg whites, peanuts, wheat, or soybeans. Other foods that can cause problems include berries, shellfish, corn, beans, and gum arabic (a thickener found in processed foods). Yellow Food Dye no. 5 is known to produce an allergic response. Chocolate, long thought to be allergenic (particularly among children), has been found to seldom be a cause of allergy.

The Diagnosis. Suppose you ate strawberries 2 days ago and now you have hives on your feet and hands. Yet you ate them a week ago and had no reaction. How could you be allergic to strawberries?

Most foods provoke an almost immediate reaction. For instance, if you eat something and within a few minutes your tongue and lips are swollen, it is easy to determine the cause. It is unusual for a food to cause a reaction that occurs more than 2 hours after eating.

To determine the cause of the problem, you may begin with a self-conducted elimination diet. Eliminate suspected foods from the diet for a week or two, then add them back to your diet one at a time. Such a method is not foolproof because psychological factors as well as physiological factors come into play. If a person thinks he or she is sensitive to a food, this conviction well may play a part in triggering a response that may resemble but is probably not a true allergic reaction.

Your physician will ask a series of detailed questions to determine your eating habits,

FOOD ALLERGY FACTS AND FICTIONS

Some people are intolerant to certain foods, in some instances because they lack the enzymes needed to digest them fully. Many just believe that they are allergic—actually, they may have other problems such as irritable bowel syndrome or recurring stress or may have eaten food contaminated by a toxin that produces a reaction. Emotional and physical stresses are important factors when it comes to properly digesting food because they can trigger adverse reactions.

For a person with a true food allergy, an offending food will cause antibodies to form to protect the body from what it deems a foreign invader. Tracking food allergies and responses can be tricky. Sometimes, no cause for particular problems is ever found. This leaves a wide open field for businesses that are less than scientific and sound to develop.

People claiming cures find a ready market. Unsound and untested theories abound, partly fueled by faddish self-help diet and nutrition books that label some foods as allergenic for conditions such as menstrual cramps, fatigue, nervousness, and hyperactivity and bed-wetting in children. Food plays no part in these. Tests such as the cytotoxic test, provocation and neutralization, and yeast hypersensitivity therapy are unproven and should be avoided (see page 453).

FOOD ALLERGY VS. FOOD INTOLERANCE

Food allergy and food intolerance are frequently lumped together as a single condition. There is a difference, however. When a person allergic to a specific food has a response, it is a true allergic reaction in that the body produces histamine and other substances to combat what it perceives as bacterial invaders. The histamine irritates the body tissues, producing the gastrointestinal, respiratory, and skin symptoms that we associate with food allergies.

Food intolerance can produce somewhat similar symptoms, but the chemistry is quite different. No histamine is released. One cause for a food intolerance is absence of an enzyme that is needed to digest a specific food fully. Thus, the symptoms are not responses to antibodies.

Lactose Intolerance

Probably the most common item to which people are intolerant is lactose, a sugar found in milk. Most people are able to tolerate less lactose as they grow older. About 70 percent of the world's population—virtually everyone except Western Europeans and their descendants—are unable to process lactose efficiently after age 6. Even in infancy, 1 to 3 percent of all babies are lactose intolerant (see also the discussion on lactose intolerance on page 623).

Many people who are lactose intolerant can eat dairy products in which much of the lactose is already digested. These products include hard cheeses and cultured milk products such as yogurt and sour cream.

Wheat and Vegetable Intolerances

Other common intolerances include the intolerance to gluten, found primarily in wheat products. Young children are most commonly affected, and they may or may not grow out of their sensitivity. Other common foods that people are intolerant to include some vegetables (particularly broccoli and peas, which produce intestinal gas), mushrooms, and wines (which produce indigestion and diarrhea).

Chinese Restaurant Syndrome

Monosodium glutamate (MSG), a commonly used flavor-enhancer, is thought to cause flushing, headache, and numbness about the mouth in susceptible people. Because many Chinese restaurants use MSG, these symptoms may occur after a susceptible person eats Chinese food; the reaction has come to be known as Chinese restaurant syndrome. MSG is also found in some seasoning mixtures and prepared foods.

Sulfite Sensitivity

Sulfites are present in various products, particularly wine, and they cause problems for sensitive people. However, few people are sensitive to sulfites, and for the most part these people have asthma. Sulfites have been used to sanitize and preserve foods, particularly in salad bars. For most people, sulfites have no perceptible effect, but for those who are sensitive care is needed when eating salads, fresh fruits, potatoes, shellfish, and wine. Ask whether sulfites have been used. Check labels, too, looking for the terms sodium bisulfite, potassium bisulfite, sodium sulfite, sulfur dioxide, and potassium metabisulfite.

Food Dye Sensitivity

Tartrazine, also known as Yellow Dye no. 5, is a food coloring used in foods, drugs, and cosmetics, and it may produce allergic responses in some people who have asthma. Recent investigations question the role of tartrazine in these reactions. Foods colored yellow, orange, or yellow-green may contain tartrazine. Read the labels; many show the complete contents. If a label does not, you can write to the Consumer Service Department of the manufacturer for a complete listing.

Food Ingredient Sensitivity

One of the tricky aspects of diagnosing a food sensitivity is that some people are allergic not to the food itself, such as peanuts, but to a substance used in the preparation of the food. This is particularly true of foods containing salicylates, sulfites, and possibly tartrazine. Salicylates appear in nature and frequently are used in the preparation of processed foods.

Very few people are sensitive to salicylates, which is a good thing, because they appear in various foods, especially fruits. For instance, salicylates are found in apples and grapes and in their derivatives—cider, wine, and vinegar. If you are sensitive to salicylates avoid any food prepared with them, including pickles, vinegar-based dressings, mayonnaise, tartar sauce, and catsup.

Salicylates are also present in many other foods in all categories. These include beverages such as tea, root beer, fermented and distilled alcoholic beverages (except vodka), meats such as corned beef and those processed with vinegar, sauces such as mayonnaise and salad dressings made with vinegar, vegetables including avocado, corn, cucumbers, peppers, white potatoes, olives, and peppers, fruits such as apples and their products, apricots, berries, cherries, currants, grapes and raisins, and melons, peaches, nectarines, plums, and prunes. In addition, avoid mint- and wintergreen-flavored foods.

your diet, and their relationship to the symptoms. You may be asked to keep a detailed diary of everything you eat for several weeks. Your physician also may conduct a series of skin tests to determine possible causes. Positive skin tests are not particularly reliable in the case of food allergies because a test often can be positive for a substance that causes no reaction when it is eaten. Negative skin tests for food, however, are usually reliable. A special approach is the double-blind challenge test. In this test, the person is given doses of suspected foods in disguised form so that neither the individual nor the physician knows what food is being administered. These results seem to be more conclusive, but this test is difficult and time-consuming.

How Serious Are Food Allergies? For most people, food allergies are uncomfortable, and often extremely so. Responses vary from minor sniffles and a cough to severe abdominal cramps, vomiting, and even anaphylactic shock. When a person reacts severely with an anaphylactic response—narrowed air passageways, rapid pulse, decrease in blood pressure, cardiovascular collapse, and shock—food allergies can be life-threatening.

Treatment. The only significant treatment for food allergy is avoidance of the food that causes the problem. For some people, eliminating certain foods from the diet is no hardship; for others who are allergic to foods common in the average diet it means living on a severely restricted diet that may make social eating difficult. People on restricted diets must replace those nutrients lost because they are in the forbidden foods with substitutes. Thus, these people should be careful to avoid only those foods clearly shown to cause symptoms.

Emergency treatment is necessary when anaphylaxis develops. This includes an immediate injection of adrenaline (epinephrine) and a visit to the emergency room.

Sometimes it is not practical to avoid a food, particularly when that food is widely used. Occasionally, a reaction-causing food will not be detected. Also, some reactions may be irritating but not particularly dangerous or uncomfortable. If reaction to certain foods is a nuisance but not life-threatening, symptomatic relief may be considered. Your physician may prescribe antihistamines to relieve some symptoms. Skin reactions can be relieved with creams.

There are no ideal methods of treatment for food allergy, but people are not necessarily saddled with them for life. Children frequently grow out of their food allergies, often by age 6. Even adults may lose their sensitivities. Individuals of all ages lose sensitivities to milk, eggs, and soy products more quickly than to peanuts, walnuts, fish, and shellfish.

DRUG ALLERGIES

Signs and Symptoms
- Wheezing and difficulty in breathing;
- Hives;
- Generalized itching;
- Skin rash;
- Shock.

Emergency Symptoms
- Anaphylaxis with: severe swelling of eyes, lips, or tongue; swelling of the throat that causes difficulty in breathing; coughing or wheezing; hives; slurred speech; mental confusion; cramps; nausea and vomiting; anxiety; severe decrease in blood pressure resulting in unconsciousness (see page 474);
- Severe asthma;
- Obstruction of the throat by swelling.

Almost any drug can cause an adverse reaction in someone. Reactions to most drugs are not common, but they can range from merely irritating to life-threatening. Some reactions are true allergic responses (IgE antibodies are mobilized against the invading substance and histamine is released). Others are side effects of a particular drug. Some are toxic effects of the drugs. Still others are reactions that are poorly understood or not understood at all. Your physician will determine the nature of the reactions you experience and what to do about them.

Penicillin and its relatives are responsible for many drug allergy reactions ranging from mild rashes to hives to immediate anaphylaxis. Most reactions are minor rashes. Only those who are extremely sensitive have the severe reaction of anaphylaxis. Many who are treated with another antibiotic, ampicillin, have a rash that is not an allergy.

Drugs that cause reactions include sulfas, barbiturates, anticonvulsants, insulin, and local anesthetics. In addition, contrast dyes that are injected into blood vessels to help outline major organs in x-ray studies contain iodine and so may be allergens.

Almost a million Americans, primarily adults, have reactions to a common drug, aspirin. The response, hives, mimics the symptoms of a true allergy but has no immunological basis. Almost a quarter of those who have chronic hives experience a worsening in their condition after they take aspirin. About 10 percent of those with asthma are sensitive to aspirin, too; in these persons, it can cause acute spasms of the bronchial tubes.

The Diagnosis.   Skin rash is the most common allergic reaction to drugs. Penicillins cause both a skin rash and hives and can be responsible for another reaction known as serum sickness. This reaction, which can take up to 3 weeks to develop, is characterized by fever, aching joints, swelling of the lymph glands, and skin rash. In very rare cases, penicillins, as well as streptomycin, insulin, and tetracycline, can cause anaphylactic shock.

Sensitivity to penicillin drugs can be diagnosed with a skin test. However, sensitivities to other drugs are not so easy to detect because for these the skin testing is ineffective or dangerous. That means that the physician must rely on the patient's memory about when and how certain drugs were taken, how much was taken, whether it was in combination with other drugs, how long after the dose the symptoms developed, and what other medications were being used at the time, including non-prescription items such as vitamins, laxatives, nose drops, cold remedies, and aspirin.

How Serious Is a Drug Allergy?   Severe reactions such as anaphylaxis or acute asthma are very serious because they can be life-threatening. Such reactions are rare. Most reactions are limited to rashes and hives. However, this does not mean that they can be ignored.

Treatment.   The most common drug allergy reactions—rash, itching, and hives—are treated with antihistamines or, occasionally, steroid drugs (see Corticosteroid Drugs, page 1005). Asthma reactions are treated with bronchodilators (see page 466) and steroids. Anaphylaxis is treated with adrenaline injections (see page 474).

Most drug allergies cannot be cured. The allergy to penicillin is an exception. In some cases, this sensitivity can be reduced enough so that the person can tolerate the drug. Small amounts of the drug are given in slowly increasing amounts. Sometimes antihistamines and steroids are given before and along with the penicillin doses to lessen the allergic reaction.

People who know they are allergic to certain drugs should avoid them. This means alerting their physicians of the sensitivity before treatment. It also may involve avoiding foods that may contain certain drugs. People sensitive to aspirin should avoid all aspirin-containing drugs.

Wear at all times an alert necklace or bracelet to indicate your allergy.

If you have a drug allergy, carry appropriate identification at all times.

INSECT BITE ALLERGIES

Signs and Symptoms
- Hives;
- Itchy eyes;
- Constricted feeling of the throat and chest.

Emergency Symptoms

- Anaphylaxis with: severe swelling of eyes, lips, or tongue; swelling of the throat that causes difficulty in breathing; coughing or wheezing; hives; slurred speech; mental confusion; cramps; nausea and vomiting; anxiety; severe drop in blood pressure resulting in unconsciousness (see page 474).

Most people consider the bite of a mosquito or the sting of a bee or wasp to be an irritation. The area may swell and itch or sting for several hours and then it returns to normal. However, perhaps as many as 10 to 15 percent of the population are extremely sensitive to insect venom, particularly that of insects such as bees, wasps, hornets, yellow jackets, and fire ants. Of these, yellow jackets are responsible for most of the reactions. Milder reactions that are not the allergy type can be caused by mosquitoes, ticks, biting flies, and some spiders.

The venom of most insects is composed of a number of chemicals. The toxic effects of the venom bother everyone by causing the redness, swelling, and itching at the site of the sting. In addition, in a sensitive person, an IgE antibody response occurs, thus releasing histamine into the system.

There is no one type of person likely to be allergic to insect stings. With some allergies, being sensitive to pollen or dust may dispose a person to being sensitive to other allergens. Such is not the case with insect bite allergies. People who work with bees often develop sensitivity as a result of multiple stings, but others can develop it at any time, after one or two stings or with the first one.

The Diagnosis. Symptoms of insect bite allergy usually appear within a few minutes after the sting occurs. In people mildly sensitive to the venom, hives may develop, and, in addition to the pain and intense itch around the site of the sting, the eyes may itch. Extremely sensitive people may have more serious symptoms such as severe hives and anaphylaxis with constriction of the throat causing difficulty in breathing, abdominal and uterine cramps, nausea, vomiting, dizziness, severe drop in blood pressure, disorientation, and severe anxiety. They may also lapse into unconsciousness.

Severe reactions to insect stings can happen within 10 to 20 minutes, or they may not appear for several hours or even days. Generally, the sooner the reaction begins, the more severe it will be. If a person exhibits any of the symptoms of a severe reaction, he or she should be treated immediately with adrenaline (epinephrine).

When the reaction is delayed, it often is in the form of serum sickness. The symptoms are fever, painful joints, hives, and swollen lymph glands. A person can experience both an immediate reaction and a delayed one from the same sting.

Diagnosis of the exact cause may not be possible immediately, but at some point your physician will ask questions about where the insect stung you; what it looked like; how it moved; what the sting looked like; and at what time of day and where the incident occurred. To confirm a diagnosis, your doctor may perform skin tests several weeks after the incident.

How Serious Are Insect Bite Allergies?
Insect bite allergies are not to be taken lightly. The reactions can range from mild to life-threatening. A person who knows he or she is sensitive to stings should be under the care of a physician for any sting. Many people do not know they are highly sensitive, however, and their past experience is not always dependable because sensitivity can develop at any time.

Treatment. In the case of severe reactions, a physician or emergency medical team may perform cardiopulmonary resuscitation. Occasionally, if the throat is constricted enough to block passage of air, a tracheostomy will be performed and a tube will be inserted. An injection of adrenaline (epinephrine) will be administered. A strong dose of antihistamine can help decrease the severity of the reaction.

Corticosteroids, which act over a longer period of time than the emergency treatment with adrenaline, are often prescribed to reduce hives and other swelling (see Corticosteroid Drugs, page 1005).

When the reaction is less severe, the person can help minimize the effects by keeping the venom as localized as possible. Remove the stinger. Place a cold pack on the wound to keep swelling and itching down.

Once the diagnosis of insect bite allergy is made, there are a number of things you can do. For one, immunotherapy can be used to build your tolerance to the offending venom. Injections of small amounts of the venom will be administered every week until you can tolerate the amount of venom in a sting or bite. From then on, you will receive maintenance injections every 4 to 6 weeks, indefinitely.

There are other things you can do, too. Begin by avoiding these kinds of insects as much as possible. Beekeepers should give up their hives. Avoid the things that attract these insects, too. Black and brown clothing are attractive to certain insects, as are sweet perfumes, scented soaps, suntan lotions, and other cosmetics. White clothing does not interest bees and the insects related to them. Wear shoes and long-sleeved shirts when you are outside. Wear close-fitting clothes that will not allow insects to fly inside them.

Avoid places where bees and other stinging insects are found. Orchards attract bees, as do flower gardens and fields or lawns containing clover. The food at picnics and outdoor concessions attracts wasps and bees.

If you feel in danger of being stung, act calm. Move away from the insect slowly and without sudden movement. Panicky flailing only agitates insects.

Extremely sensitive people can safeguard themselves by keeping an emergency kit containing antihistamine tablets and a syringe filled with adrenaline (epinephrine). Your physician can prescribe such a kit, to be used until you can reach a hospital. Wearing an alert bracelet or necklace or carrying an identification card will provide helpful information if an emergency team is summoned in the case of a severe reaction.

ANAPHYLAXIS

Signs and Symptoms
- Constriction of airways, including swollen throat, resulting in breathing difficulty;
- Shock associated with severe decrease in blood pressure;
- Rapid pulse;
- Cardiovascular collapse;
- Hives and angioedema;
- Nausea, vomiting, or diarrhea;
- Dizziness, mental confusion, slurred speech, or extreme anxiety.

Anaphylaxis is the most severe and frightening allergic response. Luckily, it is also the most infrequent, although each year several hundred Americans die from the reaction.

Anaphylaxis is an IgE antibody response to a large number of different antigens. The anaphylactic reaction is systemic, meaning that it is not limited to the site of the irritation. A mild reaction may cause only generalized hives and intense itching. A severe reaction is life-threatening because its most characteristic symptom is constriction of the air passageways in the bronchial tract or in the throat, or in both. It is often accompanied by shock—a situation in which there can be sudden decrease of blood pressure that causes rapid pulse as well as weakness, paleness, mental confusion, unconsciousness, and cardiovascular collapse. These can cause death if not treated immediately.

Almost any allergen can cause the response, including insect venoms, pollens, the horse serum used in a few vaccines, certain foods, drugs such as penicillin, aspirin, insulin, and the contrast agents injected as part of some x-ray procedures. Some persons have anaphylactic reactions of unknown cause.

The anaphylactic response is quick, beginning seconds or minutes after an allergen is encountered. Anaphylaxis occurs more commonly after certain insect stings and bites and intravenous injection of certain drugs. Only rarely do pollens cause the anaphylactic response. Certain foods such as peanuts, true nuts, and shellfish also can cause fatal reactions.

A person who experiences a mild reaction may have a severe reaction upon a subsequent exposure. A person also may become hypersensitive at any time, whether previously sensitized or not.

Treatment. The standard treatment for anaphylaxis is injection of adrenaline (epinephrine) which opens the airways and blood vessels. Cardiovascular resuscitation and emergency tracheostomy sometimes have to be performed as life-saving measures.

CHAPTER 21
THE BLOOD

CHAPTER CONTENTS

UNDERSTANDING YOUR BLOOD

The blood that circulates through your body carries out a number of crucial functions. In the tissues of your lungs, inhaled oxygen is picked up by your blood and delivered, by your arteries, to tissues throughout your body. At the same time, the blood removes carbon dioxide from these tissues and, through the veins, returns it to your lungs where it passes into the exhaled air.

The blood also carries life-sustaining nutrients from your intestines to cells throughout your body. When waste products from these cells need to be removed, the blood transports them to the kidneys where they are excreted (see The Kidneys and Urinary Tract, page 881).

By serving as the vehicle for long-distance messengers such as hormones, the blood helps the various parts of your body to communicate with each other and to coordinate their functions. The blood acts as a medium for your immune system by carrying antibodies (proteins that help protect your body against foreign substances) and cells that fight infections (see also page 844). And it even helps to regulate your body temperature by dissipating the heat produced in the muscles.

These different functions are performed by blood cells and the liquid part of the blood, called plasma. Most of the cells are red blood cells (erythrocytes). These are the cells that contain the hemoglobin, a red, iron-rich, complex substance. Hemoglobin binds to oxygen in the lungs in order to carry it through the bloodstream to tiny blood vessels (capillaries) where the hemoglobin releases the oxygen so that it can move out of the bloodstream to the cells that need it.

White blood cells (leukocytes) defend your body against foreign matter, including infection-causing bacteria, viruses, and fungi. There are three main types of white blood cells. One type, the granulocytes (grainy cells), includes neutrophils, eosinophils, and basophils. These and the second type, the monocytes, respond to many different types of infection and also defend by engulfing foreign substances. The third type of white blood cells, known as lymphocytes, react specifically to specific infecting agents. The lymphocytes include B cells and T cells. B cells produce antibodies, and T cells attack foreign and virus-infected cells. (For more on the immune system, see The Workings of the Immune System, page 844.)

Platelets (thrombocytes) are colorless blood cells that repair injured blood vessels. They stop loss of blood from the bloodstream by forming plugs in vessel holes. When any of your blood vessels is damaged, platelets gather to plug the site of injury. This is the first step in clot formation (coagulation), a process that is completed by proteins, called clotting factors, that travel in the plasma.

The plasma, a yellowish liquid, carries other proteins as well as the clotting factors. Plasma can be defined as what is left after the cells are removed from your blood. Serum is plasma from which the clotting factors also have been removed.

There is another circulatory system in your body, the lymph system which carries a fluid called lymph. The lymph helps to return water and proteins from the tissues to the blood.

Most of the blood cells are produced in the bone marrow, a material in cavities inside many of your bones. Most of these cells continue to mature and develop further into specific types of blood cells within the bone marrow. However, for some blood cells this maturation process occurs in the spleen or lymph nodes.

When your physician suspects that you might have a blood disorder, he or she will have blood tests performed. Samples for these tests can be collected by drawing blood from a vein in an arm or from capillaries in a fingertip. Blood tests generally are part of the routine physical examination.

The most common blood test is the complete blood count (abbreviated as CBC). This involves counting the number of each type of blood cell in a given volume of your blood and examining the cells under a microscope to check for any abnormalities in their size or shape. Part of the complete blood count is determining the hematocrit value, the percentage of your total blood volume that the red blood cells occupy. The hematocrit value normally is about 42 percent in women and 47 percent in men. Another part of the complete blood count is assessing the hemoglobin status (hemoglobin is the iron-rich molecule in the red blood cell that binds oxygen and delivers it to the cells of your body).

If your physician thinks you may have a disorder that involves a specific type of white blood cell, he or she will do a differential count. This determines the relative amounts of each kind of white blood cell. Other blood tests measure the number of platelets and the bleeding time (a useful indication of how well your platelets are functioning).

To study how well your body is making new blood cells, your physician may examine a sample of your bone marrow under a microscope. This marrow usually is taken from the back of the large pelvic bone (see page 1284).

Many problems with your blood can be treated by your family physician. Occasionally, you may be referred to a specialist in disorders of the blood, a hematologist.

Some blood disorders are a type of cancer. Examples include leukemia, lymphoma, and multiple myeloma. Hematologists traditionally treat these types of cancer. Another specialist, the oncologist, deals with the treatment of various cancers with drugs called chemotherapeutic agents. Hematologists and oncologists cooperate closely with radiation specialists who treat cancers with x-rays. Sometimes, a physician will specialize in both oncology and hematology.

In the following pages, we will discuss various blood disorders. These are divided according to the part of the circulatory system in which they arise. The anemias are problems caused by too few red blood cells. Symptoms of anemia may include paleness as well as breathlessness and lack of endurance. Decreased numbers of white blood cells impair your body's resistance to infection. The leukemias are usually accompanied by too many white blood cells. The lymphomas involve the lymph nodes, spleen, and bone marrow. The clotting disorders result from defects in platelets or in clotting factors.

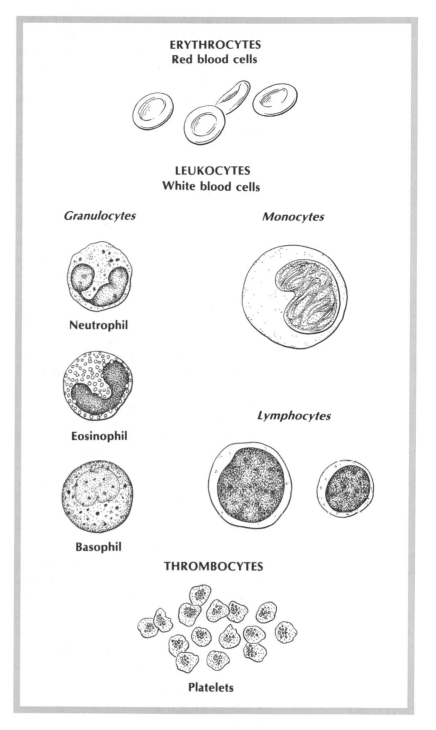

Erythrocytes (red blood cells) are the cells that contain hemoglobin. Leukocytes (there are three types: granulocytes, monocytes, and lymphocytes) are white blood cells that defend your body against foreign matter. Thrombocytes (platelets) repair injured blood vessels.

ANEMIAS

Anemia is a state in which hemoglobin is diminished. In addition, the number of red blood cells (erythrocytes) usually is decreased. There are many anemias that have various causes. As a group, the anemias are the most common blood disorders.

When anemia starts, the signs and symptoms tend to be so mild that they often go unnoticed, but their severity increases as the condition progresses. At first, you may be more tired and paler than usual. The best places to check for pallor are your nail beds, the undersides of your eyelids and lips, and your palms. Anemia often causes the creases in your palm to be as pale as the surrounding skin. When you exercise, you may feel more out of breath than is usual. You also may be aware that your heartbeat is faster than normal.

Iron deficiency is the most common cause of anemia. Without enough iron, your body cannot produce adequate amounts of hemoglobin. When you have a shortage of vitamin B_{12} (as in pernicious anemia) or of folic acid (folic acid deficiency), you cannot make sufficient numbers of red blood cells. If you inherit a disorder such as sickle cell disease, thalassemia, or a rare hemoglobin disease, your body produces a defective form of hemoglobin.

In the hemolytic anemias, the red blood cells are broken down (hemolyzed) faster than the bone marrow can produce new red blood cells to replace them. Inherited defects of enzymes such as glucose-6-phosphate dehydrogenase (G6PD) can cause hemolytic anemia. Many infections and chronic diseases, including some cancers, can interfere with the production of red blood cells and thus result in anemia.

Despite the many similarities among the signs and symptoms of the following anemias, each of these disorders has a different cause.

IRON-DEFICIENCY ANEMIA

Signs and Symptoms
- None are apparent early in this disorder;
- Pallor;
- Fatigue.

Iron-deficiency anemia occurs when the amount of iron in the body is not enough to permit manufacture of the amount of hemoglobin needed. There are several main causes of the deficiency, including insufficient consumption of iron-containing foods, poor absorption of iron by the body, and loss of blood.

Worldwide, iron deficiency is the most common cause of anemia. It is estimated that 20 percent of the women in this country have iron-deficiency anemia. It occurs particularly frequently among women of childbearing age. In nonpregnant women, the cause is the monthly menstrual loss of blood. Without iron supplementation, iron-deficiency anemia occurs in virtually all pregnant women because their iron stores have to serve the increased blood volume of the mother as well as be a source of hemoglobin for the growing fetus.

The condition occasionally is seen in infants, children, and adolescents. All three age groups go through spurts of rapid growth that require a great deal of iron for the manufacture of new muscle and hemoglobin. In addition, lead poisoning can contribute to iron-deficiency anemia in children (see Lead Poisoning, page 76). In men, the most common cause of the condition is blood loss from the digestive tract, which can occur with long-term daily use of aspirin, peptic ulcers, or cancer of the colon.

The Diagnosis.   The symptoms of iron-deficiency anemia tend to appear so gradually that they are often hard to notice. As with other anemias, you may feel tired and less tolerant of exercise. Your skin, gums, nail beds, and eyelid linings become pale. Eventually, the anemia may become severe enough that your heartbeat seems more rapid and noticeable.

Rarely, people with this condition develop a craving for substances that are not foods. This craving is called pica. They may eat ice, clay, or soil. Some of these substances will interfere with absorption of iron in the intestinal tract and thus may worsen the iron deficiency.

Your physician can use various blood tests to diagnose iron-deficiency anemia. The size of the individual red blood cells is diminished but the number of them may be nearly normal. The amount of hemoglobin in the cells is low and, under a microscope, individual red blood cells will appear pale.

When there is a question of blood loss from the digestive tract, special tests (such as a HemoQuant study of the stool) (see page 641) can precisely measure the amount of blood in the stool.

How Serious Is Iron-Deficiency Anemia?
This is a chronic condition. When iron-deficiency anemia is severe enough, it may interfere with work performance. However,

this and other effects usually can be reversed quickly by iron replacement therapy. When iron-deficiency anemia is found, the cause of the deficiency must be uncovered. It may be the first symptom of a serious disorder such as cancer of the colon. It may be the result of other serious disorders. Do not be satisfied until the definite cause is found and treated.

Treatment. The key to prevention of iron-deficiency anemia not due to disease is adequate nutrition.

Nutrition. Foods rich in iron that your body can readily absorb include meats (especially liver), fish, poultry, eggs, legumes (peas and beans), potatoes, and rice. Many wheat products receive added iron when they are processed, but this iron is not in a form that your body can easily use. The iron in many vegetables is poorly absorbed. You can enhance your body's absorption of iron by drinking citrus juice when you take a supplement or eat an iron-containing food. In contrast, milk and tea decrease iron absorption.

Eating plenty of iron-containing foods is particularly important for people who have high iron requirements, such as children and pregnant or menstruating women. It is also crucial for those whose diets are low in iron, including strict vegetarians, people on weight-reduction diets, and infants.

Breast milk contains iron in a form that is particularly easy for the body to use. However, it does not contain enough iron to allow the maximal growth of an infant who is more than 4 months old. So breast-fed infants should start receiving supplemental iron drops or iron-fortified cereal at that age. Iron-fortified formula is available for formula-fed infants.

Iron supplements can be helpful during times of great need, such as growth spurts in children and pregnancy. However, be careful not to overdo it (see The Dangers of Too Much Iron, above).

Medication. To treat iron deficiency, your physician will give you supplemental iron salts (ferrous sulfate). These are usually taken orally, and only rarely is it necessary to give iron by intramuscular injection.

Surgery. If the underlying reason for the iron deficiency is loss of blood from the di-

---

THE DANGERS OF TOO MUCH IRON

Too much of a good thing may be dangerous—so don't take too much supplemental iron.

Iron supplements are appropriate only when you need more iron than a balanced diet can provide. If you think you need an iron supplement, check with your physician before taking any. The reason is that overloading your body with iron can be even more serious than iron-deficiency anemia.

You are especially likely to collect too much iron in your body if you have inherited one or two genes for a relatively common condition called hemochromatosis (see page 656). This disorder is caused by excessive absorption of iron by the digestive tract, and the consumption of iron supplements could greatly accel erate the course of the disease.

Excess iron accumulation can damage your liver and cause cirrhosis. You can get a type of diabetes called bronze diabetes in which your skin may turn a bronze-like color. Your heart may fail, or its rhythm may be disturbed if overloaded with iron. Iron deposits in your joints can cause arthritis. Injury to the testes by iron accumulation can cause impotence and sterility. Hemochromatosis is treated by phlebotomy, the removal of 1 unit of blood (approximately a pint) once or twice a week.

If you are losing blood because of some serious condition such as colon cancer, taking an iron supplement may delay the diagnosis. Iron-deficiency anemia is an important diagnostic clue that should be pursued by your physician.

---

gestive tract, such as in colon cancer, an operation will be required.

Other Therapies. Your physician may consider giving you a transfusion of packed red blood cells (see also page 500), but only if you have extremely severe anemia is immediate correction needed.

PERNICIOUS ANEMIA

Signs and Symptoms
- Usually, none are apparent early in the disease;
- Reduced exercise endurance and rapid, noticeable heartbeat;
- Sore tongue;
- Low appetite and loss of weight;
- Disturbed walking gait and balance;
- Mental changes, including memory loss, depression, and dementia;
- Numbness in hands and feet.

Pernicious anemia is caused by a deficiency of vitamin B_{12} which is needed for normal production of red blood cells. It is often hereditary. The term pernicious was adopted when no effective treatment was known and the condition was inevitably fatal.

The foods that contain vitamin B_{12} are meat and dairy products. However, except in strict vegetarians, this disorder is not a result of not eating enough of these foods. Rather, pernicious anemia results from the failure of the digestive tract to absorb vitamin B_{12}. This impaired absorption is thought to be a complex process.

The cells that line a part of the stomach produce a substance called intrinsic factor (IF) which is necessary for absorption of vitamin B_{12} in the small intestine. Intrinsic factor attaches itself to vitamin B_{12}, and it is this combination that is absorbed in the lowest portion of the small bowel (ileum), just before the small bowel enters the colon. A vitamin B_{12} deficiency also can result when the ileum is diseased or removed in the course of surgery because then the intrinsic factor-vitamin B_{12} combination is not absorbed.

The condition is unusual. It occurs most often in older people. Men and women are affected in similar numbers. It is most common among people of northern European descent. Those with the disorder tend to be fair-haired.

The Diagnosis.   To check for pernicious anemia, your physician can perform various blood tests. One test measures the amount of vitamin B_{12} in your blood. Also, your blood is examined under a microscope to assess the size and shape of red blood cells. If you have pernicious anemia, your red blood cells will be enlarged and there will be fewer of them.

It may be necessary to study a sample of your bone marrow, where the red blood cells are produced (see page 1284). Your physician may order a test to determine whether antibodies to intrinsic factor are present, an indirect way of telling whether intrinsic factor itself is present or absent. He or she also may order a Schilling test to determine whether you have a vitamin B_{12} deficiency due to a lack of intrinsic factor (and therefore pernicious anemia) or there is a failure to absorb the vitamin for some other reason.

How Serious Is Pernicious Anemia?   This chronic disease progresses slowly but steadily if not treated. In the past, before proper treatment was developed, it eventually caused death after many years. Now, replacement therapy with adequate amounts of vitamin B_{12} corrects the deficiency and allows a normal life. However, if the condition progresses for a long time before detection, it may cause some damage to certain parts of the body, primarily the nervous and digestive systems.

Treatment.   Recognition of the disorder's hereditary nature makes it possible to prevent the development of symptoms. If you have a relative who has pernicious anemia, inform your physician so that he or she can test your blood every few years, before any symptoms appear. If your physician decides that you do have pernicious anemia, he or she can treat you for it.

Medication.   To treat pernicious anemia, vitamin B_{12} is injected beneath the skin with a hypodermic needle. At first the injections may be done once daily, but after several days the injection can be once a month. These injections must be given indefinitely. Neither oral supplements nor dietary changes are useful treatments because the underlying problem is the inability of the digestive tract to absorb the vitamin.

FOLIC ACID ANEMIA

Signs and Symptoms

- Usually none are apparent early in the disease;
- Low exercise endurance and rapid, noticeable heartbeat;
- Weight loss;
- Diarrhea.

As in pernicious anemia (see page 479), folic acid deficiency interferes with the production of red blood cells. Folic acid, which is also known as folate, is a member of the vitamin B group. Lack of it causes an anemia characterized by red blood cells that are large but few in number. Deficiency can result if you do not get enough folic acid in your diet to meet your body's demands or if your intestines cannot absorb it.

The disorder is not uncommon. Alcoholics often develop it if they become malnourished when drinking becomes their principal source of calories and their digestive tract does not absorb as well as it used to. The ailment sometimes develops in pregnant women and during the growth spurts of infancy and adolescence. At these times, the body's demand for folic acid may outrun its supply. Folic acid anemia is often present in malabsorption problems (see page 621). Certain anticonvulsant medications may induce folic acid anemia.

The Diagnosis. The symptoms of folic acid deficiency are similar to those of pernicious anemia, so your physician will perform various blood tests to distinguish between the two disorders. These include counting the cells in your blood, examining the cells under a microscope, and measuring the amount of folic acid in the blood. If folic acid anemia is present, your physician may perform more tests to look for an underlying cause.

Treatment. Depending on its underlying cause, folic acid deficiency may be chronic or acute. Proper treatment will let you lead a normal life.

Prevention. Most people can prevent folic acid deficiency by eating a balanced diet, controlling their consumption of alcohol, and taking prescribed supplements during pregnancy. If you have folic acid deficiency, it is important to eliminate the condition that was its underlying cause. For instance, if alcoholism was the reason folic acid deficiency developed, you must stop drinking.

Nutrition. In some cases, adequate nutrition is the remedy. The main food sources of this vitamin are raw fruits and vegetables, liver, and kidney. Folic acid is found in a wide variety of foods but it can be destroyed by extensive cooking.

Medication. In most cases, supplemental folic acid is given orally every day. It is injected only if the underlying problem is a disorder of the intestinal tract that severely interferes with absorption.

SICKLE CELL DISEASE

Signs and Symptoms
- Fatigue, breathlessness, and rapid heartbeat (as in other anemias);
- Delayed growth and development;
- Susceptibility to infections;
- Skin ulcers on the lower legs;
- Vision problems when the retina is affected.

Emergency Symptoms
- Attacks of pain caused by blocked blood vessels and damaged organs;
- Aplastic crises, in which the number of red blood cells decreases drastically;
- Symptoms of anemia—severe shortness of breath, fatigue, light-headedness, particularly on standing.

In sickle cell disease, the red blood cells become rigid and shaped like crescents or sickles rather than being flexible and round. These changes in the red blood cells may precipitate attacks of pain. The disorder gets its name from this change of shape (sickling), which results from the presence of an abnormal type of hemoglobin known as hemoglobin S. These cells are fragile and tend to undergo hemolysis—that is, the red blood cell breaks up and its hemoglobin is released into the plasma, resulting in anemia. The disease is also called sickle cell anemia.

This is an inherited disorder and is relatively common in black people. If you have sickle cell disease, you received one gene for hemoglobin S from each of your parents. This gene is recessive, so if you have only one copy of it, you are a carrier of sickle cell trait.

If you are a carrier, your red blood cells may be deformed but no symptoms occur unless you are at high altitude. Some carriers of sickle cell disease will experience symptoms during an unpressurized plane flight or while traveling in a car at high altitudes. The lack of oxygen at higher levels renders the red blood cells more fragile and deformed, thus increasing their tendency to sickle and break up (hemolysis).

The Diagnosis. To detect sickle cell disease, your physician will perform various blood tests. The test that confirms the diagnosis is hemoglobin electrophoresis, a laboratory procedure that isolates and identifies the telltale hemoglobin S.

How Serious Is Sickle Cell Disease?   It is a chronic disease that makes your body vulnerable to infection. You can limit its progression by avoiding infections or by getting

Normal and sickled red blood cells. The sickled cells assume a crescent shape.

them treated early. For the disease itself, no effective therapy is available. New treatments continue to be tested.

Two types of acute, severe episodes can occur, spontaneously or when triggered by infection or other stress. These are the crises produced by acute sickling and may be associated with obstruction of small blood vessels, pain, and the breakdown of red blood cells. At times, there also may be a temporary failure of red blood cell development in the bone marrow that can result in exceptionally severe, life-threatening anemia. Repeated crises can produce increasing damage to the kidneys, lungs, liver, and central nervous system, at times resulting in death.

In contrast, the sickle cell trait is harmless and is of concern only when you are considering marriage and children.

If you know that sickle cell disease runs in your family, genetic counseling may help you prevent passing it on to your children. If both you and your spouse carry the trait, the risk is 1 out of 4 that your child will have sickle cell disease. The disease can be detected before birth, and some couples choose to abort an affected fetus.

Treatment. *Medication.* Your physician may prescribe a daily oral supplement of folic acid, because the disease increases your body's need for this vitamin. Your physician will also be on the lookout for infections. Antibiotics are given to treat infections and sometimes to prevent them. During crises, you will receive medications to relieve the pain and to prevent dehydration. Oxygen is given if there is not enough oxygen in your bloodstream. Antisickling drugs are being tested.

Other Therapies.   Blood transfusions are occasionally used to prevent crises.

HEMOLYTIC ANEMIAS

Signs and Symptoms
- Fatigue;
- Paleness;
- Breathlessness;
- Heartbeat faster and more noticeable, particularly on exertion;
- Yellow-tinged skin;
- Dark urine;
- Enlarged spleen.

RARE HEMOGLOBIN DISEASES

Rare hemoglobin diseases, also called hemoglobinopathies, are caused by the presence of variant forms of hemoglobin. Over 400 variants have been identified. These abnormal hemoglobins tend to be less efficient than the normal form at carrying oxygen to the cells of the body.

One example is hemoglobin S-C. In this case, the affected person inherits the sickle cell trait (hemoglobin S) from one parent and another variant (hemoglobin C) from the other parent. With this condition, life span is almost normal, but with mild to moderate anemia. However, these people occasionally can suffer attacks of pain as in sickle cell disease (see page 481).

An even more rare hemoglobin disease is hemoglobin E which tends to occur in people of Southeast Asian origin. It also causes mild to moderate anemia.

Emergency Symptoms

• Sudden onset of pain in the upper abdomen.

The hemolytic anemias are conditions in which red blood cells are destroyed and the hemoglobin is liberated from these cells. In these disorders, old red blood cells are broken down faster than the bone marrow can produce new red blood cells. The word hemolytic comes from Greek roots meaning destruction of blood.

There are inherited and acquired forms of hemolytic anemias. In one hereditary type, called spherocytosis, the red blood cells are small, round, and fragile. Other inherited hemolytic anemia disorders include sickle cell disease (see page 481) and thalassemia (see below).

Hemolytic anemias can be caused by certain medications and infections. Sometimes they result from an immune response against your own red blood cells (autoimmunity). Some types of hemolytic anemia are hard to treat, but they seldom are fatal.

The Diagnosis. If your physician thinks you may have a hemolytic anemia, he or she will have a sample of your blood examined to count the number of young red blood cells (called reticulocytes) and to see if the red blood cells are deformed. The number of young red cells is increased in hemolytic anemia. Your physician also will examine your upper abdomen to see whether your spleen or liver is enlarged.

Treatment. *Medication.* If your hemolytic anemia was caused by a drug, your physician will have you stop taking that drug. If your condition resulted from autoimmunity, your physician can prescribe medications to treat this problem. Corticosteroid medications such as prednisone are often helpful in preventing the destruction (hemolysis) of red blood cells.

Surgery. Some cases, especially those involving hereditary spherocytosis, are treated by surgical removal of the spleen (splenectomy).

OTHER ANEMIAS

In addition to the usual types of anemias discussed above, rarer forms may occur as the result of genetic factors or as a consequence of certain diseases or the use of certain drugs. Among these types of anemias are the following.

Glucose-6-Phosphate Dehydrogenase Deficiency

This is the result of an inherited defect in an enzyme, glucose-6-phosphate dehydrogenase, in the red blood cell. Like hemolytic anemia (see page 482), this disorder causes the untimely breakdown of red blood cells. It occurs commonly in people of Mediterranean ancestry and in black people.

The symptoms range from mild to severe, depending on which type of defective gene for the enzyme is present. In blacks the symptoms tend to be milder; in people of Mediterranean ancestry the symptoms tend to be more severe.

The gene for the enzyme is sex-linked (carried on the X chromosome). Therefore, like hemophilia (see page 496), this disease almost always affects boys and men (who have only one X chromosome) rather than girls and women (who have two such chromosomes).

Thalassemia

There are two types of this unusual disease. Both are based on inherited defects in hemoglobin. In alpha-thalassemia, not enough of the part of hemoglobin called alpha-globin is produced. In beta-thalassemia, beta-globin is lacking.

Alpha-thalassemia occurs most often in people of southeast Asian descent. Beta-thalassemia is also known as Cooley's anemia after the American physician who described it and as Mediterranean anemia because it is common in that region. The name thalassemia comes from Greek roots for sea and blood.

The genes for both thalassemias are recessive, so you have to inherit them from both parents to get the disease. If you have only one gene, you are said to carry the trait but you will have no symptoms. When inherited from both parents, thalassemia frequently causes severe chronic anemia with poor growth, enlarged spleen, and, sometimes, heart failure.

Without treatment, death occurs in early childhood. There is no cure, but therapy can prolong life into the 20s or 30s. The treatment is repeated transfusions of packed red blood cells. These cells carry a great deal of iron which can overload the body's vital organs. To lessen this effect, a medication may be given to cause the iron to be excreted in the urine. A treatment that still is experimental is bone marrow transplantation (see page 488). Genetic counseling may help you to avoid passing the disorder on to your children.

A milder form of thalassemia, thalassemia minor (or thalassemia trait), is quite common. This disorder produces blood cells that look like those present in iron-deficient blood, but there are no symptoms. Iron therapy may be harmful because it causes iron overload. This disorder by itself does not cause problems.

Anemia of Chronic Disease

Occasionally, an anemia can develop as the result of a chronic disease. There are four groups of chronic diseases most often associated with anemia: chronic inflammation, such as rheumatoid arthritis (see page 997); uremia (uric acid in the blood), as in kidney failure (see page 906); endocrine failure, in which a hormone is deficient (for instance, hypothyroidism, see page 730); and chronic liver disease (see page 649).

Anemia of chronic disease is curable only if the underlying disorder can be cured or made less severe.

Aplastic Anemia

Aplastic means a failure in development, and aplastic anemia is an anemia caused by a drastic decrease in the bone marrow's production of all types of blood cells. This unusual and serious disease can occur spontaneously or it can be triggered by certain medications or toxic substances.

The disorder may be acute or chronic. It always is progressive. The symptoms of the anemia, if severe enough, resemble the response of a normal person to high altitude. Because the platelet count also is low, easy bruising and bleeding may occur. The low number of white blood cells leaves you vulnerable to bacterial infection. Infection and hemorrhage are emergency symptoms.

To diagnose aplastic anemia, your physician will use the complete count of the cells in your blood and an examination of a sample of your bone marrow. Treatment starts with elimination of the cause, if it is known. Your physician will try to protect you from infections and will treat any that do occur aggressively with antibiotics. Transfusion of red blood cells, white blood cells, and platelets may be necessary. Corticosteroid drugs may be tried. You may be a candidate for bone marrow transplantation (see page 488) if your case is severe and a suitable donor is available.

Prevention may be aided by avoiding exposure to organic solvents, volatile chemicals, cleaners, and paint removers, particularly in a confined space. Certain medications and diseases can also be responsible.

Sideroblastic Anemia

Sideroblasts are young red blood cells that contain excess iron. The name is derived from the Greek roots for iron and germ. Sideroblastic anemias are rare disorders in which the red blood cells are overloaded with iron, the blood contains a high concentration of iron, and hemoglobin production is defective.

The treatment depends on the cause. You can acquire this anemia as a result of exposure to drugs or toxins such as alcohol and lead. When the offending agent is removed, the anemia may disappear entirely. It is also associated with certain cancers such as leukemia (see page 484), lymphoma (see page 489), and myeloma (see page 493) and with inflammatory diseases such as rheumatoid arthritis (see page 997). In such cases, the underlying condition should be treated. There is also an inherited form of sideroblastic anemia.

In some cases, no cause can be identified. In these cases, blood transfusions may be needed, along with a drug to remove the iron, via the urine, that accumulates from the transfused red blood cells.

LEUKEMIAS

Leukemias are cancers of the body's blood-forming tissues including the bone marrow and lymph system. These cancers cause the formation of large amounts of abnormal white blood cells. These abnormal white blood cells reach high concentrations in the bone marrow, lymph system, and bloodstream, and their accumulation can interfere with the functions of the vital organs. Eventually, they overwhelm the production of healthy blood cells, including white and red blood cells and platelets.

In addition to the overabundance of abnormal white blood cells, there is an insufficient number of healthy ones. Therefore, the body's ability to fight infections is decreased. The abnormal white blood cells interfere with the production of red blood cells and platelets in the bone marrow. The deficiency in red blood cells means that the body's organs do not receive enough oxygen; the shortage of platelets makes the blood clotting process less effective, leaving the body more vulnerable to bleeding and bruising. Because of all these effects, leukemia is fatal without successful treatment.

The causes of leukemia are not known. Researchers have proposed that certain chemicals and viruses might play a role. Susceptibility to leukemia may be inherited. The ailment runs in some families, and people with certain congenital disorders, including Down's syndrome (see page 57), are at higher risk of developing it.

Leukemias are classified as lymphocytic, myelogenous, or monocytic, depending on which type of white blood cell is affected. Myelogenous leukemia is a cancer of the granulocytes, a type of white blood cell that is formed in the bone marrow. Lymphocytic leukemia involves the lymphocytes, a type of white blood cell produced in the lymph system and marrow. Monocytic leukemia involves the monocytes, white blood cells of the bone marrow.

Types of leukemia are further divided according to how quickly they progress and the maturity of the cells affected. Acute leukemia progresses quickly with proliferation of immature cells. These cells, called blasts, are precursors of more mature white blood cells. Chronic leukemia progresses slowly and is characterized by overproduction of mature white blood cells as well as blasts. Both acute and chronic forms occur somewhat more frequently in men than in women.

CHRONIC MYELOGENOUS LEUKEMIA

Signs and Symptoms
- Symptoms of anemia (see page 477);
- Bone pain;
- Fever and infections;
- Weight loss;
- Swollen lymph nodes;
- Pressure under the left ribs from an enlarged spleen;
- Bleeding and bruising;
- In some cases, none.

Emergency Symptoms
- Severe bleeding;

- Sudden appearance of small red marks on the skin.

Chronic myelogenous leukemia is characterized by an overproduction of cancerous versions of granulocytes, a type of white blood cell formed in the bone marrow. This type of leukemia also may be called myeloid, myelocytic, or granulocytic. The disorder tends to occur in middle-aged persons.

The Diagnosis. The disease can develop insidiously. In about a third of the cases, there are no symptoms at the time of diagnosis. These cases are detected when routine blood tests give abnormal results.

To determine whether you have chronic myelogenous leukemia, your physician will perform certain blood tests. These include a complete blood count (see page 476), a differential count of the various types of white blood cells, and measurement of an enzyme called leukocyte alkaline phosphatase. Your physician will also determine whether you have an abnormal chromosome known as the Philadelphia chromosome; this abnormality is found in 90 percent of those with chronic myelogenous leukemia. A small sample of the bone marrow may be examined (see page 1284).

How Serious Is Chronic Myelogenous Leukemia? Chronic myelogenous leukemia is a progressive disease that cannot be cured except by bone marrow transplantation (see page 488). In most people with this disorder, an acute phase, called a blast crisis, develops within 5 years. The blast crisis is characterized by a high concentration of blasts (immature white blood cells) in the blood and by red pinpoints (petechiae) on the skin that result from bleeding as a consequence of a lack of platelets. Death ensues because the blast crisis is a form of acute leukemia that is particularly resistant to treatment. So far, the only treatment that has been found to alter the course of this disease is high-dose chemotherapy with total-body irradiation followed by bone marrow transplantation.

Treatment. *Medication.* Treatment of the chronic phase generally is simple chemotherapy given by mouth. High-dose chemotherapy with bone marrow transplantation sometimes is used. Other drugs, such as interferon, are being tried experimentally.

Surgery. If your spleen is extremely enlarged, it may be removed surgically (splenectomy). This has not been found to increase the duration of survival and usually is done only to relieve pain and bleeding if the spleen ruptures.

ACUTE NONLYMPHOCYTIC LEUKEMIA

Signs and Symptoms
- Fatigue and lack of feeling of well-being, due mainly to anemia;
- Fevers;
- Bruising, small red marks on the skin, or a rash;
- Weight loss;
- Overgrowth of the gums;
- Blurred vision or loss of vision;
- Headaches or seizures;
- Swollen lymph nodes;
- In some cases, none.

Emergency Symptoms
- Bleeding from the digestive tract; altered state of consciousness or inability to talk or move an extremity;
- Fever, with bacterial infection in the blood.

Acute nonlymphocytic leukemia is a cancer that causes overproduction of immature white blood cells known as blasts; ordinarily, these cells would have gone on to become granulocytes. The word nonlymphocytic distinguishes it from leukemias that affect the lymphocytes or their precursors. This form of acute leukemia is also called myelogenous, monocytic, myelogenic, or myelocytic in reference to the bone marrow, the site of origin of the affected cells. It is the most common type of leukemia in adults.

The Diagnosis. Diagnosis of acute nonlymphocytic leukemia is based on a complete blood count (see page 476), a differential count of the various types of white blood cells, and examination of a sample of bone marrow. Your physician also will look for certain chromosome abnormalities which can help establish the diagnosis or predict how your body will respond to the disease. In some cases, your physician also may have a sample of your spinal fluid analyzed.

How Serious Is Acute Nonlymphocytic Leukemia? The onset of acute nonlymphocytic leukemia can be extremely rapid. Without treatment, death can occur within weeks. Treatment with combinations of certain drugs (chemotherapy) frequently produces remission, a condition in which the body is rid of all evidence of the disease. However, recurrences occur in more than 80 percent of the patients who enter remission, and death ensues in an average of 1½ years. If the remission lasts for 5 years after treatment, there is a high chance of cure. However, it is also possible for the disease to relapse even then.

Treatment. ***Medication.*** Combinations of different chemotherapeutic drugs are given under the direction of your physician. Therapy with antibiotics can help to prevent or can treat the bacterial infections that are frequent complications. Your physician will choose an appropriate antibiotic based on the results of cultures of the blood, sputum, or urine specimens.

Other Therapies. Bone marrow transplantation may be performed in remission, in relapse, or in second remission, if an appropriate donor can be found.

CHRONIC LYMPHOCYTIC LEUKEMIA

Signs and Symptoms
- Swollen lymph nodes;
- Fatigue and lack of feeling of well-being, mainly due to anemia;
- Infection;
- Weight loss;
- Bleeding;
- Night sweats;
- Pressure under the left ribs from enlargement of the spleen;
- In some cases, none.

Chronic lymphocytic leukemia is a cancerous proliferation of the white blood cells known as lymphocytes. It is most common among older adults; 90 percent of the cases are in people more than 50 years old. It occurs 2 to 3 times more often among men than among women. This difference in frequency between the sexes is more marked in this leukemia than in the other leukemias.

The Diagnosis. The onset of chronic lymphocytic leukemia tends to be insidious, with symptoms developing gradually. Most cases are detected by routine blood tests performed in people who have no symptoms. These tests include complete blood count (see page 476) with a differential count showing a high proportion of lymphocytes.

If your physician finds that you have the disease, he or she may conduct further tests to establish what subtypes of lymphocytes have been affected. The results of these tests will help predict how rapidly or slowly the disorder will advance and how you should be treated.

How Serious Is Chronic Lymphocytic Leukemia? The course of chronic lymphocytic leukemia varies widely. Because it is an overproduction of mature, functional lymphocytes, persons with this disorder may survive for many years, even without treatment.

In contrast, in some the disorder progresses more rapidly, and earlier treatment may be required and usually is very helpful.

Treatment. If your disease is not advanced, your physician may choose not to start any form of treatment but instead just keep track of your condition with periodic complete blood counts.

Medication. Treatment for advanced disease includes appropriate chemotherapy. Corticosteroid drugs such as prednisone also may be used.

Surgery. Rarely, removal of the spleen (splenectomy) may be performed if it has become massive or if immune complications have arisen and are resistant to treatment with drugs.

ACUTE LYMPHOCYTIC LEUKEMIA

Signs and Symptoms
- Abnormal bruising, including small hemorrhages into the skin;
- Bleeding from mucous membranes;
- Fatigue and lack of feeling of well-being;
- Fever;
- Paleness;
- Enlarged liver, spleen, or lymph nodes;
- Bone pain.

Emergency Symptoms
- Fever;
- Bleeding.

Acute lymphocytic leukemia is a cancer that produces overproduction of immature blood cells known as blasts (these cells would otherwise have become lymphocytes). This particular type of blast is also called a lymphoblast, so the disorder is also known as acute lymphoblastic leukemia. It has been called childhood leukemia because it most frequently affects children.

The Diagnosis. The symptoms of acute lymphocytic leukemia may appear suddenly or may be present weeks or months before the diagnosis is made. If the disease is suspected, your physician will perform blood tests including a complete blood count (see page 476) with a differential count of the various types of white blood cells. If the results of these tests suggest acute lymphocytic leukemia, a sample of your bone marrow will be examined to see whether it contains a high concentration of blasts (see page 1284).

In most medical centers, further tests are performed to determine what subtypes of lymphoblasts are present. These and other tests on the leukemic cells can help your physician characterize the disease and choose the most appropriate treatment.

How Serious Is Acute Lymphocytic Leukemia? Without treatment, bleeding and infection lead to death within months. Before current treatments were developed, this was the inevitable course of the disease. Today, however, one of the great success stories of cancer treatment is the treatment of this leukemia.

The younger you are and the lower your white blood cell count at the time of diagnosis, the higher your chances are of being cured. With proper combination chemotherapy, up to 70 percent of children are in complete remission at 5 years after detection of the disease and most are probably

BONE MARROW TRANSPLANTATION

Bone marrow transplantation, a new technique, offers hope to seriously ill people. Bone marrow transplantation permits use of higher doses of chemotherapeutic agents and thus an enhanced anti-cancer action.

Types of Transplants

Syngeneic

The donor of a syngeneic transplant is the identical twin of the recipient. Identical twins have the same genetic makeup so the recipient is not at risk for a severe reaction to the transplant, called graft-versus-host disease, or rejection of the transplant. However, few patients have identical twins.

Allogeneic

The donor is a brother, sister, or parent of the recipient. In order to establish the compatibility of the potential donor's bone marrow, a test for human lymphocyte antigens (HLA test) is done to determine whether there is an HLA match. This test examines six proteins, the HLAs, found on the surface of the white blood cells and most other cells of the body. The odds of an HLA donor/recipient match are about 25 percent if two siblings in a family are tested but increase to about 75 percent if there are six.

Autologous

In autologous bone marrow transplantation, bone marrow is taken from the person with the cancer. Then this person is subjected to high doses of chemotherapy and perhaps irradiation. After this treatment has been completed, the bone marrow is returned to the person. There is no risk of graft-versus-host disease in autol-ogous bone marrow transplantation.

Unrelated Donors

This type of bone marrow transplantation uses unrelated donors for allogeneic bone marrow transplantation. These donors are selected on the basis of their HLA system being identical or nearly identical to that of the recipient. A National Bone Marrow Registry has been set up to help locate HLA-matched bone marrow donors.

The Transplantation Process

Bone marrow donation is more complicated than blood donation. Bone marrow is removed from the donor's hipbone, under general anesthesia in the hospital. This bone marrow is then injected into one of the recipient's veins. From there it travels in the bloodstream and eventually occupies the bone marrow space and produces new cells.

Throughout the transplantation process, the recipient stays in a special hospital room that is ventilated with filtered air to minimize the risk of infection; intravenous treatment with antibiotics also is used. If there are no major complications, the recipient can leave the hospital within 4 to 6 weeks.

In allogeneic and syngeneic bone marrow transplantation, the bone marrow generally is removed from the donor and injected into the recipient the same day. In autologous transplantation, the bone marrow is stored frozen (these cells can remain frozen for months to years) until the person has completed the high-dose chemotherapy, with or without radiation therapy. Then, the stored marrow is thawed and injected back into the body.

Bone marrow transplantation is a unique process of donation because the marrow that has been donated replaces itself, and the loss of bone marrow is not significant. Therefore, there is no long-term concern about having only one organ, such as there is in kidney transplantation.

When Is Bone Marrow Transplantation Appropriate?

The best results after allogeneic and syngeneic bone marrow transplantation have been obtained in cases of severe aplastic anemia (see page 484), chronic granulocytic leukemia (see page 485), and relapses of acute non-lymphocytic leukemia (see page 486). There have been clinical trials to evaluate bone marrow transplantation for treating acute nonlymphocytic leukemia in remission (see page 486), acute lymphocytic leukemia in remission (see page 487), lymphoma in remission (see page 489), and neuroblastoma in remission (see page 538). People with these diseases have a very high risk of dying in a relatively short time unless they receive some form of treatment such as transplantation.

In autologous transplantation, the best results have been obtained in treating Hodgkin's lymphoma (see page 489) and non-Hodgkin's lymphoma (see page 491). At the present time, it appears that individuals whose disease is responsive to chemotherapy or who again achieve complete remission after relapsing after chemotherapy are the best candidates for this procedure. Pilot programs are evaluating the use of bone marrow transplantation for other tumors such as breast cancer.

What Are the Risks?

The major cause of disease and death in bone marrow transplantation is graft-versus-host disease, not graft rejection. This complication can affect the skin, liver, gastrointestinal tract, and lungs. This is the major complication in allogeneic transplantation but is not a problem in syngeneic or autologous transplantation.

The mortality is 25 percent in the first 10 days after an allogeneic bone marrow transplantation, from infection or graft-versus-host disease. The second major problem is a type of pneumonia which can be caused by infection or other complications.

The Future
Additional techniques are being developed for treating leukemia and lymphoma. One is the use of specific antibodies (monoclonal antibodies) that are directed against the disease cells. After the marrow is removed, it is treated with the monoclonal antibodies, and possibly other chemotherapeutic agents, prior to being given to the patient. This has been utilized in autologous transplantation.

---

cured. However, the prognosis is not as good for older children and adults; only about 20 percent achieve long-term survival. The outcome also depends on the particular type of lymphoblast that is present.

Treatment. *Medication.* Treatment of acute lymphocytic leukemia has three or four phases.

First, an attempt is made to achieve remission, usually by administering anticancer drugs in combination. Using combinations of drugs maximizes the effect on the leukemic cells. Your physician also may inject a chemotherapeutic drug such as methotrexate into your spinal fluid. Unfortunately, however, adverse effects still can create problems because some of these drugs can interfere with the normal functions of the bone marrow, the immune system, and other organs. In addition, some chemotherapeutic drugs temporarily slow the growth of children, but these children usually catch up after treatment is finished.

Second, once remission has been achieved, your methotrexate may be continued and radiation therapy to your central nervous system also may be recommended. These treatments are designed to kill the cancer cells that may linger in your central nervous system beyond the reach of medications given orally or intravenously. If not destroyed, such cells could cause a relapse later on.

For some individuals, additional courses of chemotherapy, at times with different drugs, are given during remission in the hopes of eliminating the last surviving leukemic cells.

Last, maintenance treatment may be used to ensure that the remission continues. This involves relatively low-dose chemotherapy over the course of several years.

Other Therapies. Bone marrow transplantation may be performed after a relapse or in persons deemed to be at high risk of relapse.

LYMPHOMAS

Lymphomas are cancers of the lymph system. The lymph system includes the lymph nodes, or lymph glands, which are located throughout the body and are connected by small vessels called lymphatics. The spleen is also part of the lymph system. Often, the first symptom of lymphoma is enlargement of lymph nodes with no other obvious symptoms.

Swelling of the lymph nodes, which are normally the size of a bean, is not necessarily a sign of lymphoma; many other conditions can cause nodes to enlarge. However, if your glands stay swollen for more than 3 weeks, consult your physician.

Lymphomas are a diverse group of diseases. They include Hodgkin's disease and non-Hodgkin's disease which are described below.

HODGKIN'S DISEASE

Signs and Symptoms
- Painless swelling of lymph nodes in the neck, armpits, or groin;

- Persistent fatigue;
- Fever and chills;
- Night sweats;
- Weight loss and loss of appetite;
- Severe itching.

Emergency Symptoms
- Sudden onset of high fever from any cause;
- Loss of bladder or bowel control;
- Numbness or loss of strength in the arms and legs.

Hodgkin's disease is named after Thomas Hodgkin, a 19th-century English physician. Four major types can be identified on the basis of the appearance of the tissue under the microscope (histologic subtypes). There is no major difference in outcome despite differences in cell types if the extent of disease is similar.

Your lymphatic system consists of lymph nodes found throughout your body. The nodes are connected by vessels called lymphatics. Your spleen is part of the system.

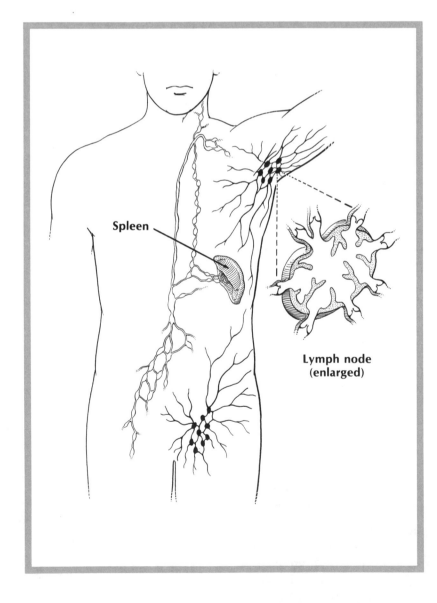

Spleen

Lymph node
(enlarged)

Hodgkin's disease usually affects people between 15 and 35 years old, but it can occur in those over 50. The presence of Hodgkin's disease often is suspected when an enlarged lymph node is detected.

The Diagnosis. To determine whether or not you have Hodgkin's disease, your physician will ask about previous medical problems, conduct a thorough physical examination, take a chest x-ray, and obtain tests of your blood and urine. Most important will be a lymph node biopsy in which lymph node tissue is removed and studied for the presence of the patterns typical of Hodgkin's disease. Occasionally, only a portion of the node is removed for examination under a microscope. The remainder of the node, still in place, is then used as a marker to evaluate your response to treatment.

If your physician finds that you have Hodgkin's disease, he or she will conduct more tests to find out how advanced the tumor is and to decide how best to treat it. This testing process is called staging the tumor and may involve a bilateral bone marrow biopsy (see page 1284), a computed tomographic scan of your abdomen and chest (see page 1286), or an operation to explore the abdomen (a laparotomy).

How Serious Is Hodgkin's Disease?
When Hodgkin's disease is detected early and treated properly, as many as 90 percent of the cases can be completely cured. Years ago, before current treatment was developed, the disease was almost always fatal. Of patients with the most advanced stages of the disease, 50 to 80 percent have no disease 10 years after chemotherapy and are considered cured.

Treatment. *Radiation Therapy.* Radiation therapy is the main treatment when the spread of the disease is limited. Radiation therapy is sometimes used in combination with chemotherapy. When one lymph node region is involved, 90 percent of affected persons are disease-free after 10 years. For those who have two lymph node regions involved, either above or below the diaphragm, 70 percent are alive and disease-free after 10 years.

Medication. For advanced Hodgkin's disease, chemotherapy is the primary treatment. If there is a relapse after chemotherapy, the treatment can be repeated at higher doses, with or without radiation therapy, followed by autologous bone marrow transplantation (see Bone Marrow Transplantation, page 488). In this process, bone marrow is removed before chemotherapy and replaced afterward, allowing the use of larger doses of anticancer drugs.

Surgery. Occasionally, an operation will be performed to explore the abdomen (laparotomy) in order to determine the stage of the disease.

NON-HODGKIN'S LYMPHOMA

Signs and Symptoms
- Painless enlargement of lymph nodes, with or without swelling of the abdomen;
- Persistent fatigue;
- Fever or chills;
- Night sweats;
- Loss of appetite.

Emergency Symptoms
- Sudden onset of high fever, from any cause;
- Severe constipation or profuse urination;
- Mental confusion, drowsiness;
- Involuntary loss of urine or stool;
- Numbness or loss of strength in the arms and legs.

Non-Hodgkin's lymphomas are a group of tumors that arise from the lymphocytes (white blood cells). These tumors are classified according to their cell size as seen under the microscope. They are also grouped into three broad categories by level of activity of the malignant cells: low grade, intermediate grade, and high grade.

These tumors are seen more commonly than Hodgkin's disease. They occur more frequently among people who have received organ transplants and whose immune mechanisms are inhibited by immunosuppressive therapy. The disease typically is detected in persons in their mid-40s but, unlike Hodgkin's disease, it often occurs in older persons.

The Diagnosis. If your physician suspects that you have non-Hodgkin's lymphoma, he or she will do a physical examination and obtain laboratory tests on your blood and urine, a computed tomography scan of your abdomen (see page 1286), and a bone marrow study by aspiration and biopsy (see page 1284). Your physician will also perform a lymph node biopsy for classifying the disease.

How Serious Is Non-Hodgkin's Lymphoma? Low-grade non-Hodgkin's lymphoma is not curable *but* the survival rate is good and it is very responsive to initial therapy. The 5-year survival rate is greater than 80 percent, and the 10-year survival rate is approximately 75 percent. If you have this disease but have no symptoms, your physician may recommend observation only.

In contrast, some of the intermediate- and high-grade non-Hodgkin's lymphomas are curable with aggressive treatments, but survival is usually less than 1½ years if treatment does not produce a complete remission.

Treatment. *Medication.* Chemotherapy with a combination of anticancer drugs is usually used.

Surgery. An operation to decrease the size of the tumor (debulking) has been used when the lymphoma involves the stomach or in cases of other unusual appearances of the disease, but it is not used in treating most people.

Other Therapies. Radiation therapy is used in some instances of low-grade and intermediate-grade non-Hodgkin's lymphoma.

Nutrition. To maintain your quality of life, it is important that you follow guidelines for proper nutrition. However, this has not been proved to increase the chances of survival.

GROWTH DISORDERS OF THE BONE MARROW

The marrow lies in spaces within your bones and normally produces all of your red blood cells and platelets and most of your white blood cells. When something goes wrong with your bone marrow, the consequences are serious. Production of cells is no longer

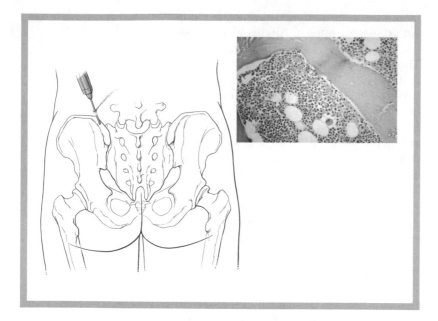

In a bone marrow biopsy, a sample of bone marrow is removed for examination under a microscope (see inset).

Emergency Symptoms
- Blood in the vomit or stool;
- Stroke.

Polycythemia vera occurs when the bone marrow produces too many blood cells. The word polycythemia refers to many cells in the blood; vera means true.

In this disorder there is a high concentration of red blood cells in the circulating blood, but white blood cell and platelet counts also are increased. The condition is unusual, and its cause is not known.

Polycythemia vera generally appears in late middle age; it is extremely rare in children. It is slightly more common among men than women.

orderly and deficiencies may occur, leading to anemia, bleeding disorders, and vulnerability to infections.

In a young child, all of the bones contain active marrow that forms blood cells. As the body matures, active blood-forming marrow is found only in the bones of the spine, skull, ribs, and pelvis. However, if for some reason the body requires extra blood cells, the bone marrow in the arms and legs may be stimulated to revert to active production.

If your physician thinks that you may have a bone marrow disorder, a sample of your bone marrow will be removed for study under a microscope. In a process called aspiration, a special needle is inserted into your hipbone or breastbone and a small amount of the marrow is withdrawn through it. Often a biopsy of the bone marrow is obtained at the same time. The site of the biopsy is infiltrated with an anesthetic, a needle is inserted into the bone, and a small piece of bone marrow is removed for examination under the microscope (see page 1284).

POLYCYTHEMIA VERA

Signs and Symptoms
- Weakness;
- Itching, especially in a warm bath;
- Dizziness;
- Sense of fullness in the head and redness of the face and hands;
- Fullness in the left upper abdomen.

The Diagnosis.   The symptoms of polycythemia vera appear gradually. If your physician thinks that you may have it, he or she will order various blood tests including a complete blood count (see page 476) and possibly measurement of the vitamin B_{12} and certain other substances, such as leukocyte alkaline phosphatase, in your blood. The values often are unusually high in this disorder. Uric acid levels are also increased, which may cause attacks of gouty arthritis (see Gout, page 1003).

Another sign is an increase in the volume of blood without much of an increase in its plasma component. Your physician can measure the increase with special blood tests.

Additional tests are used to differentiate polycythemia vera from secondary polycythemia which has other causes such as heavy cigarette smoking, severe lung disease, abnormal hemoglobin, or living at high altitudes.

In secondary polycythemia, the blood's high content of red blood cells is a response to the low oxygen concentration in the air and therefore in the blood. Because there is less oxygen in the blood, the body attempts to overcome the deficiency by making more red blood cells until there are too many.

How Serious Is Polycythemia Vera?
Without treatment, the symptoms of polycythemia vera worsen and the risk of death from stroke (see page 508) or heart attack (see page 809) increases. The reason for this is that the high concentration of blood cells makes the blood thicker (more viscous) and

so it has greater difficulty flowing through the blood vessels.

With proper treatment, you generally feel normal and the risk of stroke or heart attack lessens. Although there is no cure, most people live for more than 10 years with the disease. In a small percentage of those with polycythemia vera, acute leukemia develops after a period of years.

Treatment. To decrease the volume of the circulating blood, blood is withdrawn from a vein (phlebotomy). This is effective in decreasing the viscosity of the blood and lessening the danger of stroke. Generally this is the first treatment used. The schedule of withdrawal is about a pint of blood at intervals of a few days initially to weeks or months. The goal is to maintain the blood hemoglobin level within the range of low to normal values. Often, blood withdrawal can be stopped for months at a time if the hemoglobin level remains in the required range.

Medication. If your blood has quite high white blood cell and platelet counts, in addition to a high content of red blood cells, your physician may prescribe a drug that cuts down blood cell production by the bone marrow, such as radioactive phosphorus. A disadvantage of radioactive phosphorus therapy is that it has been associated with transformation of normal white cells to leukemia cells in some cases over a period of years. One advantage of it is that one treatment a year may be enough. Other medicines may be used on a daily basis.

Surgery. If your spleen becomes extremely enlarged, which happens in rare cases, your physician may consider surgical removal of it (splenectomy).

AGNOGENIC MYELOID METAPLASIA

Signs and Symptoms
- Breathlessness on exertion;
- Rapid heartbeat;
- Paleness;
- Enlarged spleen;
- Night sweats;
- Weight loss;
- Stuffed feeling after eating.

In agnogenic myeloid metaplasia, the bone marrow gradually becomes scarred and less able to manufacture blood cells. Then, blood cells are also produced outside of the marrow, in the spleen and liver, and both of these organs can become enlarged. The name of the disorder means bone marrow transformation of unknown origin. It is also called idiopathic myelofibrosis.

Treatment. Medications are available, but there is no cure. Most affected persons become dependent on blood transfusions.

Enlargement of the spleen may cause pain or reduce the number of platelets in the blood (by trapping them in the spleen), and your physician may consider surgical removal of the spleen (splenectomy).

MULTIPLE MYELOMA

Signs and Symptoms
- Fatigue, as a result of anemia;
- Back pain that progresses insidiously;
- Unexplained bone fractures, especially in the vertebrae or ribs;
- Vulnerability to infection;
- Bleeding problems, such as nosebleeds and bleeding gums;
- Bone fracture.

Emergency Symptoms
- Severe constipation and profuse urination;
- Excessive sleepiness or fluctuating level of consciousness;
- Significant decrease in urine flow;
- Incontinence of stool or urine;
- Numbness or loss of strength in extremities.

Multiple myeloma is a cancer that produces uncontrolled multiplication of a type of white blood cell in the marrow called a plasma cell. As these cells grow and take up more space in the marrow, the bones may weaken, causing pain, particularly in the back and ribs. As the bones become more fragile, they break more easily.

Eventually, the growth of plasma cells interferes with the production of normal red blood cells, white blood cells, and platelets by the bone marrow. Anemia, susceptibility to infection, and bleeding problems can result.

MONOCLONAL GAMMOPATHY OF UNDETERMINED SIGNIFICANCE

The finding of a monoclonal protein in the blood in older people is not uncommon. This protein is an abnormal antibody-like protein that comes from a single line (or clone) of plasma cells. Plasma cells are a type of white blood cell in the bone marrow that produce the antibodies needed for normal immunity.

Monoclonal gammopathies are usually detected in the course of routine physical examinations. They occur in 1 percent of healthy persons over age 50 and in 3 percent over age 70.

In 80 percent of cases, they never cause a problem. However, in the remaining 20 percent, the amount of the abnormal protein in the blood eventually increases, indicating the presence of a disorder that will probably require treatment. Such conditions include such disorders as lymphoma (see page 489), multiple myeloma (see page 493), and amyloidosis (see page 495). Therefore, if you have a monoclonal gammopathy, your physician will want to check your blood to identify the protein and recheck you at intervals, perhaps yearly.

The name of this unusual disorder means a bone marrow tumor that occurs in many sites. The disease primarily affects persons past the age of 50 with the average age being 63 years at the time of diagnosis. It occurs slightly more often in men than women, and it is almost twice as common among blacks as whites. This disease is not inherited.

The Diagnosis.   A common symptom of multiple myeloma is back pain that is slowly progressive. The pain eases with rest and increases with movement. It eventually may also be felt in the ribs, neck, and hips.

If your physician suspects that you have multiple myeloma, he or she will have a sample of your bone marrow examined for myeloma cells. X-rays of your skeleton will show whether or not your bones have any of the thinned-out areas that characterize the disease. Your physician also will have various blood tests performed including a complete blood count (see page 476) and measurements of calcium, uric acid, creatinine, and blood proteins.

Ordinarily, the plasma cells produce antibody proteins to fight infections. In this disorder, mutation of one such cell gives rise to a new line of abnormal cells. When this happens, another small molecule, called Bence Jones protein after the 19th century English physician who discovered the substance, may be produced. Therefore, your physician will check samples of your blood and urine for the presence of these proteins.

Increased amounts of protein from these abnormal cells are common in the blood of older people, and the discovery of one increased protein does not necessarily signify multiple myeloma. Such a state may be referred to as monoclonal gammopathy of undetermined significance (see this page). When such an abnormal protein is found, your physician will carry out examinations to exclude multiple myeloma. Occasional checkups thereafter may be advised.

How Serious Is Multiple Myeloma?

There is no cure. However, treatment can prolong your life for years and can relieve the symptoms. Your physician will watch your progress to judge your response to treatment and to avoid complications.

Treatment.   If you have multiple myeloma, remain active, drink plenty of fluids, and eat a balanced diet. Staying active helps to retain the calcium in your bones (not the blood), which keeps your bones strong. Some restrictions, such as avoiding heavy lifting, may be necessary. If pain is disabling, a back brace, cane, or other orthopedic support device may help you remain active. Drinking fluids prevents dehydration. The amount of protein you eat does not need to be restricted.

Medication.   If your multiple myeloma is detected in its early stages, you may not need treatment. If treatment is required, however, your physician will prescribe appropriate medication, either by pills or by intravenous delivery. Corticosteroids such as prednisone also can help. Analgesics can alleviate bone pain.

Surgery.   If your bones become unstable, surgical repairs may be necessary to strengthen them.

Other Therapies.   Radiation directed at specific sites, usually on the back and neck, can control severe pain and disease in that area.

AMYLOIDOSIS

Signs and Symptoms
- Fatigue or weakness;
- Numbness of hands or feet;
- Weight loss;
- Shortness of breath;
- Swelling of the legs.

In amyloidosis, a protein called amyloid is deposited in sites throughout the body. The term amyloidosis is something of a misnomer because it suggests a condition involving a starch-like substance, but the material in question is a protein, not a starch. The disorder is rare.

The Diagnosis.   The diagnosis of amyloidosis hinges on the detection, by biopsy, of amyloid deposits in tissues in your body. The biopsy sites frequently used include the gums, rectum, abdominal fat, and kidney. Biopsies of the heart, nerves, and bone marrow occasionally are performed to establish the diagnosis.

As in multiple myeloma (see page 493), the plasma cells may produce abnormal proteins. Your physician may check your urine for the presence of these proteins.

How Serious Is Amyloidosis?   No effective treatment has been found. The condition is chronic, progressing slowly and usually leading to death after a number of years.

The severity of the disorder depends on which organs are affected by the amyloid deposits. Potentially life-threatening situations, including kidney failure (see page 906) and congestive heart failure (see page 807), may occur. If the accumulations of amyloid are limited to less crucial sites, there may be no symptoms. Most cases are somewhere between these two extremes.

Treatment.   *Medication.*   There is no specific medication that is effective against this disorder. However, your physician may prescribe certain medications that still are undergoing experimental trials to see if they may be effective. In addition, your physician may prescribe diuretics and other medicines if your heart is affected and analgesics, if necessary, for pain. It is wise to avoid direct exposure to people with known infections.

Nutrition.   Changing the amount of protein you eat will not affect the disease, but other special diets may be necessary, depending on which organs are affected. Your physician will discuss with you any dietary restrictions or nutritional supplements that may be necessary.

GRANULOCYTOPENIA AND AGRANULOCYTOSIS

When your physician conducts tests of your blood, a wide variety of findings may emerge. Among the more unusual disorders may be granulocytopenia or agranulocytosis.

These uncommon problems are usually caused by other disorders, possibly leukemia (see page 484) or aplastic anemia (see page 484). They also may be side effects of certain medications or exposure to poisons.

Granulocytopenia
When the blood contains less than the normal number of a grainy type of white blood cell called 'granulocytes,' the condition is called granulocytopenia. Either the bone marrow does not produce enough of these cells or they are being destroyed at a rate that is higher than usual.

The condition is also known as neutropenia because the granulocytes that most often are affected are the neutrophils. The name neutrophil, or neutral loving, comes from the fact that it is stained about equally by acidic and basic dyes. This subtype of cell is considered to be the body's first line of defense against bacterial or fungal (but not viral) infection. Therefore, granulocytopenia increases the body's susceptibility to infections. Antibiotic treatment can help ward these off.

Granulocytopenia can be the first sign of leukemia (see page 484) or aplastic anemia (see page 484). Granulocytopenia that is secondary to another problem or medication, such as chemotherapy, is more common than spontaneous occurrence of the ailment.

Agranulocytosis
This rare condition is a drastic decrease in the blood's content of granulocytes. Almost all of the neutrophils are destroyed, leaving the body particularly prone to infection. Therefore, people with this ailment must be watched carefully for the development of infections and must be treated with antibiotics.

Most often, the disorder occurs as a rare, acute response to exposure to certain chemicals, solvents, or hydrocarbons or to certain medications including penicillins, phenothiazines, and anti-inflammatory agents.

The usual treatment is to remove the affected person from additional exposure and to protect him or her against serious infection until the bone marrow can recover.

BLEEDING DISORDERS

Bleeding disorders result from disruption of the body's elaborate process by which blood clots form. This coagulation process, which involves platelets as well as plasma proteins called clotting factors, begins when platelets stick to the site of injury to a blood vessel. An intricate cascade of enzyme reactions occurs to produce a web-like protein network that encircles the platelets and holds them in place (platelet phase) to form the clot (coagulation phase). In this cascade, each clotting factor is transformed, in turn, from an inactive to an active form.

Specialized laboratories can study the coagulation mechanism in an affected person's blood to pinpoint the place in the cascade at which the fault lies.

Problems with clotting factors cause bleeding disorders such as hemophilia, von Willebrand's disease, and disseminated intravascular coagulation. Bleeding disorders based on clotting factor problems generally tend to cause bleeding deep in the tissues and joints, although excessive bruising, severe nosebleeds, and other types of bleeding can occur as well.

When platelets are too few (thrombocytopenia) or fail to function, one result is red pinpoint hemorrhages known as petechiae, seen in the skin.

HEMOPHILIA

Signs and Symptoms
- Many large or deep bruises;
- Pain and swelling of joints, caused by internal bleeding;
- Blood in the urine or stool;
- Prolonged bleeding from cuts or injuries or after surgery or tooth extraction.

Emergency Symptoms
- Bleeding into the head, neck, or digestive tract;
- Sudden pain, swelling, and warmth of large joints such as the knees, elbows, hips, and shoulders and of the muscles of the arms and legs;
- Bleeding from any injury (especially if you have a severe form of hemophilia).

Hemophilia, named from Greek roots meaning fond of blood, includes several inherited disorders of specific clotting factors (the proteins in the plasma that cause the blood to clot). The most common is hemophilia A, also called classic hemophilia, in which there is not enough of clotting factor VIII. Hemophilia B (or Christmas disease), in which factor IX is lacking, makes up most of the remaining cases.

Both the A and B forms of the disorder have also been called the royal disease, because hemophilia was inherited by descendants of England's Queen Victoria and introduced into the royal houses of Spain, Germany, and Russia. Although hemophilia is one of the most commonly inherited bleeding disorders, it is still a rather unusual ailment.

Hemophilia A and hemophilia B are caused by genes that are recessive and sex-linked (carried on the X chromosome), so the disorder almost always occurs in boys, not girls (see also page 45). Girls who inherit a hemophilia gene usually are symptomless carriers (they are said to have hemophilia trait) because they are protected by the normal gene on their other X chromosome. Most often, hemophilia occurs in families who have a history of the disease which passes from grandfather to grandson through a mother who is a carrier. However, new cases sometimes occur in families in which the disease has not previously been apparent.

The Diagnosis. The major problem for people with hemophilia is not the superficial external cuts which can be easily treated with pressure and a bandage but is uncontrolled internal bleeding. The severity of bleeding varies from person to person. The more severe forms become apparent early in life. Newborns often show no signs of hemophilia unless they are circumcised, but marked bruising may develop beneath the skin as the child starts to crawl or walk. In more severe forms of hemophilia, excessive bleeding happens often and even spontaneously without any apparent cause. However, in its mild forms, hemophilia may not become apparent until later in life; and troublesome bleeding episodes may happen only after surgery, tooth extraction, or major injury.

Your physician can establish the diagnosis by using specialized laboratory tests that measure the clotting activity of factors VIII and IX (or other factors) and determine the presence or absence of an inhibitor of these factors.

How Serious Is Hemophilia? With current medical treatment, people with hemophilia can have close to an average life expectancy. Although the disease is lifelong, it can be controlled with medication or by the administration of clotting factors, allowing a relatively normal life. Depending on the severity of the hemophilia, it may be necessary to take extra care to minimize bleeding as a result of physical activity or surgical or dental procedures. Sometimes the disorder becomes more difficult to control because antibodies develop to the clotting factor that has been used in the treatment.

Without treatment, recurrent bleeding into the joints can cause chronic pain and weakness and even can destroy the joint (through osteoarthritis, see page 995). Bleeding into muscles and soft tissue may put pressure on nerves, producing pain, stiffness, and numbness. Without adequate control, permanent nerve damage and muscle wasting eventually may occur. When blood collects in the head, neck, or digestive system, the condition is considered to be extremely serious. So it is important to stop these episodes promptly. To prevent joint destruction, all bleeding episodes should be treated promptly by infusion of a clotting factor replacement or, for mild hemophilia A, a medicine called desmopressin (see below). If you have hemophilia or think you may carry the trait, prenatal testing and genetic counseling can help you learn whether you could pass the disorder on to your children (see also page 45).

Treatment. Despite having hemophilia, you may lead a relatively normal life.

Exercise. Physical therapy can help damaged joints to function better. Swimming, bicycle riding, and walking can build up your muscles, thus helping to protect your joints. Do not engage in contact sports.

Medication. If you have mild hemophilia A, your bleeding episodes may be treated with infusion (slow injection into a vein) of

desmopressin (also known as DDAVP). This drug helps stop bleeding by stimulating the release of factor VIII and making blood vessels contract.

If you have hemophilia B or more severe hemophilia A, bleeding episodes may stop only after the missing clotting factor is replaced by infusion. These clotting factors are derived from donated human blood and are supplied as purified concentrates, as fresh frozen plasma, or as cryoprecipitate (a clotting factor concentrate derived from donated human blood). The clotting factor concentrates are now heat-treated to prevent transmission of the AIDS virus (see AIDS, page 848). With special training (available through your physician or a regional hemophilia center), you can learn to infuse DDAVP or some of these blood products yourself as soon as you show signs of bleeding. Do not use medications that might worsen bleeding, such as aspirin.

Surgery. If recurrent internal bleeding has destroyed any of your joints, you may choose to have that joint replaced surgically with an artificial joint (see Joint Replacement, page 998).

VON WILLEBRAND'S DISEASE

Signs and Symptoms
- Nosebleeds or excessive menstrual bleeding;
- Easy bruising;
- Blood in the stool, characterized by a black or tarry appearance.

This chronic bleeding disorder is caused by a defect in a clotting factor called von Willebrand factor. In many cases, there also is a deficiency of factor VIII. Ordinarily, these two factors combine to form the active complex that is needed to cause platelets to gather at the site of blood vessel injury. In von Willebrand's disease, the platelet aggregation and clot formation are impaired.

The disease is named after the early 20th-century Finnish physician who described it. It has also been called pseudohemophilia or vascular hemophilia. It is the most common hereditary bleeding disorder.

The severity of symptoms varies from person to person. The most severe form of the disease is rare, but milder forms are now recognized as being much more common. It affects both sexes in equal numbers. Before adolescence, a key symptom is nosebleeds that may be severe enough to require a visit to your physician or emergency room. In women, the menstrual flow is heavy. Other symptoms are marked bruising, blood in the urine or stool, and bleeding during and after surgery or tooth extraction.

The Diagnosis.   To diagnose the disease, your physician will arrange for specialized blood tests. He or she will look for prolonged bleeding time, impaired platelet function, and a shortage of active von Willebrand factor and, in some cases, of factor VIII as well.

Treatment.   If you have von Willebrand's disease, the treatment to prevent or to stop the bleeding may be infusion of the drug desmopressin which stimulates release of von Willebrand factor and factor VIII from blood vessel walls. Transfusion of plasma or cryoprecipitate also may be used (cryoprecipitate is a clotting factor concentrate derived from donated human blood). Avoid medications that might worsen bleeding, such as aspirin. There is no prevention for this inherited disorder aside from genetic counseling of prospective parents who have it. If you are found to have von Willebrand's disease, it is possible that your brothers, sisters, or children also might have it. Therefore, they may wish to seek appropriate testing and counseling (see also page 45).

DISSEMINATED INTRAVASCULAR COAGULATION

Signs and Symptoms
- Severe bleeding from many sites in the body;
- None may be apparent.

Emergency Symptoms
- Severe bleeding, especially with trauma or at surgical incision sites.

This is a nonhereditary bleeding disorder that actually results from excessive coagulation. It occurs when activated clotting factors are present throughout the bloodstream instead of being limited to sites of injury. These factors cause circulating platelets to clot (coagulate) in small blood vessels all over the body, hence the name disseminated intravascular coagulation.

So much of the body's supply of clotting factors and platelets is used up by this unnecessary coagulation that not enough is available for the formation of clots at injury sites. The body also reacts by stepping up the system that dissolves clots, and this promotes generalized bleeding.

The disorder is also known by the acronym DIC, as intravascular coagulation and fibrinolysis, and also as defibrination syndrome. It occurs only occasionally, almost always as a complication of one of a large variety of serious underlying diseases.

The Diagnosis.   If your physician suspects that you have disseminated intravascular coagulation, he or she will perform various blood tests. These include platelet count, measuring the fibrinogen concentration in your blood, and determining the time required for your blood to clot in a standardized procedure.

How Serious Is Disseminated Intravascular Coagulation?   The diseases that cause the disorder tend to be life-threatening but, if they are treated successfully, the disseminated intravascular coagulation will stop. These diseases include various obstetrical emergencies, widespread cancer, massive trauma, shock, and bacterial sepsis (blood infection).

The severity of the disorder itself varies. When disseminated intravascular coagulation occurs with cancer or some other disorder it can be chronic, being detected only in blood tests but not causing any spontaneous bleeding. More often, it is acute, causing severe bleeding from multiple sites such as surgical incisions. Rarely, it is serious enough to cause gangrene in the fingers, genitals, or nose.

Treatment.   The only really effective approach is to treat the underlying condition that caused the disseminated intravascular coagulation. However, transfusion of various blood products also may be necessary to replace the clotting factors depleted by the widespread coagulation. Rarely, treatment with heparin (a drug that is given through a vein and prevents clotting) may be needed.

THROMBOCYTOPENIA

Signs and Symptoms
- Easy or excessive bruising;
- Measles-like rash, usually on the lower legs;
- Nosebleeds;
- Blood in vomit or stools;
- Heavy menstrual flow;
- Bleeding during surgery.

Emergency Symptoms
- Serious or widespread bleeding, including bleeding in the brain and digestive system.

Thrombocytopenia, a common bleeding disorder, results from a shortage of platelets in the blood, hence its name which is derived from Greek roots meaning a poverty of clotting cells. The disorder is divided into two types: idiopathic and secondary. Most often it is an acquired condition rather than a hereditary one.

Idiopathic thrombocytopenia is also known as idiopathic thrombocytopenic purpura (ITP). Purpura (derived from the Greek word for purple) is a rash made up of small red marks (petechiae) caused by bleeding into the lower layers of the skin. Although idiopathic means of unknown cause, most cases of idiopathic thrombocytopenia are a result of production by spleen and lymph tissue of antibodies against the body's own healthy platelets. These antibodies destroy the platelets prematurely. Because of this process of immunity against oneself (autoimmunity), the disorder is also called autoimmune thrombocytopenic purpura (AITP or ATP). It occurs most often in children and young adults but can occur at any age. It affects more women than men, but this condition is equally likely to occur in boys as in girls.

In secondary thrombocytopenia, there is some other cause of the ailment. The underlying disorders include viral infections, systemic lupus erythematosus (see page 1006), and blood diseases such as aplastic anemia (see page 484), leukemia (see page 484), and lymphoma (see page 489). Secondary thrombocytopenia also can occur as a side effect of therapy with radiation, transfusions, and many medicines including anticancer drugs.

The Diagnosis. To detect thrombocytopenia, your physician will obtain a platelet count and an examination of a stained smear of your blood under a microscope. If it appears that you have thrombocytopenia, your physician may proceed to special blood tests and a bone marrow examination to determine what is causing the concentration of platelets in your blood to be low (see page 501).

How Serious Is Thrombocytopenia?
Particularly in children, idiopathic thrombocytopenia can sometimes go away without any treatment. In these cases, the bone marrow may make up for the shortening of the life span of the platelets by producing large numbers of new ones while the initiating cause appears to subside. The young platelets are especially active in clotting, so even though the total concentration of platelets is low, bleeding problems may not occur. Thus, your physician may decide that no special treatment is necessary.

In adults, acute thrombocytopenia often becomes a chronic ailment. It may vary in severity over time, and it can even recur after an apparently complete remission. The most serious complications, bleeding into the brain and digestive tract, occur only rarely.

Treatment. If you have secondary thrombocytopenia, your physician will treat the underlying condition or will stop the treatment that caused it.

Medication. Various medications that suppress or otherwise alter the immune system, including prednisone (a corticosteroid drug), are used to treat idiopathic thrombocytopenia. Do not use medications such as aspirin that impair the function of platelets.

Surgery. Surgical removal of the spleen (splenectomy) is sometimes undertaken to relieve symptoms or to help cure chronic idiopathic thrombocytopenia that does not respond to medication.

Other Therapies. With severe bleeding, lost blood is replaced with transfusions of packed red blood cells, whole blood, or, occasionally, platelet concentrates (see page 501). The infusion of plasma is sometimes used when there is an urgent need to increase the platelet count in a person with idiopathic thrombocytopenia.

Sometimes, treatment is not needed. In such cases, despite the low concentration of platelets, no bleeding complications result and the condition simply may go away.

BLOOD TRANSFUSIONS

Blood transfusions often are necessary to save the life of a person who has a blood disorder, some other disease, an accident, or surgery. Blood donations are always needed, so consider giving blood if you possibly can. Only about 5 percent of the people in the United States who are eligible to donate blood actually do so.

BLOOD GROUPS

Blood groups were discovered around 1900 when it was observed that blood collected for transfusions was compatible in some recipients but not in others. It was found that each person spontaneously forms antibodies against antigens that his or her own red blood cells lack. If you receive blood that contains blood group antigens different from your own, then your antibodies attack the cells in the transfused blood that carry these antigens—that is, foreign cells. The blood groups are based on which antigens (proteins) are carried on your red blood cells. Like other physical characteristics, which antigens you have is controlled through pairs of genes inherited from your parents.

There are four major blood groups: A, B, AB, and O. Each of these groups is divided into two Rh types, positive and negative. The most common blood group in the United States is O positive, followed by A positive, B positive, O negative, A negative, AB positive, B negative, and AB negative. The four major blood groups are inherited in a consistent manner. They can be used to exclude paternity.

Today, the blood groups of donors and recipients are matched to make transfusions safe. If your blood group is A, your red blood cells are coated with A antigens, and your plasma carries antibodies against B. If your blood group is B, you have B antigens and antibodies against A.

If your blood is Rh-negative, your red blood cells do not carry an antigen called the "rhesus factor (Rh factor)." You do not spontaneously produce antibodies against this factor. However, Rh typing is particularly important if you are a woman because you may start developing anti-Rh antibodies after exposure to Rh-positive blood at the time of your first pregnancy. Then, if you are exposed again to Rh-positive blood, serious complications and even death could result. (For information on pregnancy in Rh-negative women, see Health Problems of Women, page 1053.)

Many other minor blood subgroups also occur that become important only in special circumstances such as organ transplantation.

THE DONATION PROCEDURE

If you are more than 17 years old and weigh at least 110 pounds, you may be a suitable blood donor. However, you must not donate if you have had certain diseases, such as hepatitis, or if you are a member of a risk group for AIDS (acquired immune deficiency syndrome). (For more on these diseases, see pages 650 and 848.)

To give blood, go to a blood donation center or a hospital. There, trained staff members will take a small sample of your blood to check whether you have enough hemoglobin; they also will ask some questions about your health. If your health is good and your hemoglobin concentration is normal, they will draw a pint of blood from a vein in your arm.

Giving blood is quick and painless. It also is completely safe, because a new, sterile, disposable syringe is used for each donor. Therefore, there is no risk of getting any disease by donating blood.

The average volume of blood in the body is 10 to 12 pints in men and 8 to 9 pints in women. The usual amount of blood taken during donation is 1 pint. If you are a healthy adult, you can spare this amount without affecting your own well-being. Within a few hours, your body will have replaced the fluid you have lost. Your red blood cells will have returned to their usual numbers well before you are eligible to give blood again (in 8 weeks).

TRANSFUSION TYPES

When donated blood that has been stored as collected is infused, this is known as whole blood transfusion. More often, however, donated blood is separated into its various components—packed red blood cells, fresh-frozen plasma, cryoprecipitate, coagulation factor concentrate, granulocytes (a type of white blood cell), and platelets—and these components are given as needed.

Whole Blood. You may need a transfusion of whole blood if you have lost a large amount of your own blood through recent bleeding from your digestive tract, major surgery, or trauma. Whole blood can be stored for a maximum of 5 weeks and then can no longer be used.

Red Blood Cells. If you are deficient in red blood cells but not in the other components of blood, a transfusion of red blood cells, rather than whole blood, is best. This provides only the red blood cells you need, without any extra volume from the other blood cells and plasma. Thus, the risk of increasing the circulating blood volume too high above normal is minimized.

Transfusions of red blood cells are often used to treat various types of anemia such as disorders that involve depression of the bone marrow's production of these cells. Red blood cells are also transfused during the acute crisis of such inherited anemias as sickle cell disease (see page 481), thalassemia (see page 483), or glucose-6-phosphate dehydrogenase deficiency (see page 483).

Red blood cells can be kept in storage for a maximum of 7 weeks.

Fresh-Frozen Plasma. Fresh-frozen plasma can be used to treat clotting disorders, including mild forms of hemophilia and von Willebrand's disease, as well as serious burns. This blood product can be stored frozen for 1 year.

Cryoprecipitate. Cryoprecipitate is prepared from fresh plasma and stored frozen. It is enriched for three clotting factors: factors I and VIII and von Willebrand factor. Cryoprecipitate is used to treat clotting disorders including hemophilia (see page 496) and von Willebrand's disease (see page 497).

Coagulation Factor Concentrate. Coagulation factor concentrates are freeze-dried preparations of specific clotting factors from plasma. Before being transfused, the concentrate must be reconstituted. It is used to treat clotting disorders such as hemophilia.

Granulocytes. Transfusions of granulocytes can be used to treat severe granulocytopenia or agranulocytosis (see page 495). These cells can be stored for only about 12 hours. These transfusions are rarely needed today because of the availability of modern antibiotics.

Platelets. Platelet transfusions can control bleeding in people who have lost blood by a process called massive blood replacement or from prolonged surgery or other reasons.

The production of platelets can be suppressed in leukemia (see page 484), lymphoma (see page 489), or thrombocytopenia (see page 499) that has been caused by treatment with chemotherapy or radiation therapy. Therefore, such patients often receive transfusions of platelets. However, platelet transfusions tend not to be useful for those with idiopathic thrombocytopenia because they induce destructive antibodies against these cells (see below).

Platelets can be stored for only about 5 days before they become useless.

ADVERSE REACTIONS TO TRANSFUSIONS

When you receive a blood transfusion, you are given donor blood that has been matched with your own blood group (see Blood Groups, page 500). Before the actual transfusion starts, the blood bank mixes a sample of your blood with some of the donor's blood to double-check that they are compatible.

Antibody Reactions. Despite the precautions, sometimes a transfusion recipient will be carrying antibodies against the donor's red blood cells, white blood cells, or platelets. An immune reaction results. If you receive incompatible blood, you may experience fever, shaking, chills, chest pain, low back pain, pain along the vein that received the transfusion, shortness of breath, pink urine, hives, and nausea. Shock, kidney failure, or intravascular coagulation can ensue and, rarely, even death may occur.

Your risk of having this kind of immunological reaction is increased if you have received multiple blood transfusions in the past. As you are exposed to blood antigens from more and more different donors, you may develop antibodies against obscure blood groups.

Communicable Diseases. Blood transfusions can spread diseases such as hepatitis, cytomegalovirus infection, syphilis, malaria, toxoplasmosis, and AIDS. Various tests are performed on donated blood to minimize the risk of infection.

For AIDS, testing starts with the enzyme-linked immunosorbent assay (ELISA). If this test is positive, a more specific assay, a Western blot or immunoblot assay, is performed to confirm the result. If a blood bank determines that you have this virus, it will discard your blood and notify you. However, never donate blood if you think you may have the virus. Instead, see your physician.

Symptoms of hepatitis include fatigue, jaundice, dark urine, nausea, and vomiting (see page 652). Symptoms of AIDS include unexplained weight loss, diarrhea, swollen lymph nodes, and unusual skin cancers (see page 1172).

Other Reactions. There are other possible adverse reactions to transfusions. For instance, if you have heart trouble, you may have difficulty handling an increase in blood volume. In addition, if you receive repeated transfusions of red blood cells (200 transfusions or more), you may experience iron overload.

It is important to realize that the vast majority of persons who receive a transfusion have no adverse reactions or infections as a result. If you truly need a transfusion, you should not let unfounded or exaggerated fears prevent you from accepting it.

TRANSFUSION WITH YOUR OWN BLOOD

The safest blood for you to receive is your own. Your immune system will not react to your blood as foreign, and you cannot give yourself any infections that you do not already have. Giving one's own blood, also known as autologous transfusion, is becoming more popular.

In an emergency, you may have to rely on transfusions from random donors unless you are at a medical center that can salvage your own blood during surgery (see below). However, if your physician is planning to do elective surgery for you, ask him or her if you can donate your own blood ahead of time. Usually, you give it over a period of a few weeks in advance of when your operation is scheduled. Your blood will be stored and used, if necessary, to replace blood that you lose during the operation.

It costs more to receive your own blood than to get a random donor transfusion. The reason is the extra work involved in specially labeling your own blood, storing it separately, and delivering it to you at the right time. However, many people consider the added expense to be well worth it.

You might assume that if, for some reason, you cannot donate your own blood, the next-best thing is to receive blood from a designated donor. This person is a friend or relative who has the same blood group that you do. However, a blood bank is much better than you are at selecting donors whose blood will not cause an adverse reaction. Blood from designated donors chosen by you may not be as safe as you think.

There will always be situations in which using your own blood is impossible. So, the growth of this approach will not abolish the need for blood donors.

The Future: Synthetic Substitutes. Researchers at many centers are working on the development of synthetic substitutes for blood. There are several reasons for this effort. Having such materials could help to prevent transfusion complications such as infection and immunologic reaction as well as to overcome shortages of donated blood. However, these synthetic blood substances are still experimental. In addition, although they are designed to carry oxygen, they cannot perform any of the myriad other functions of the blood. Therefore, the best way to prevent adverse reactions to transfusions is to donate your own blood beforehand for your own use.

USING YOUR OWN BLOOD DURING SURGERY

It is possible to recover the blood a patient loses during an operation for return to that patient. In this procedure, known as intraoperative autologous transfusion, surgeons salvage blood cells from the wound while they are operating. The cells are washed free of debris from the wound and then returned to the patient.

CHAPTER 22
THE BRAIN AND NERVOUS SYSTEM

CHAPTER CONTENTS

THE WORKING OF THE SYSTEM

The brain and nervous system are your means of receiving input from various body parts and the outside world and also your means of transmitting messages throughout your body. These messages affect functions such as coordination, learning, memory, emotion, and thought.

The basic unit in the system is the nerve cell (neuron). A neuron consists of a cell body, one major branching fiber (axon), and numerous smaller branching fibers (dendrites). Each neuron is connected to other neurons by contacts (synapses) on the axons and dendrites. A neuron receives chemical signals from other neurons through the synapses. All of these incoming signals are combined as an electrical signal within the neuron, and it may or may not send an outgoing chemical signal through its synapses.

Your brain is composed of approximately 100 billion neurons and their connections and supporting cells, which add up to roughly 3 pounds of tissue. This dense network of interconnected, transmitting neurons is organized to convey all the control signals necessary for your activities. The components of this system are the cerebrum, the brainstem, the cerebellum, and the spinal cord.

Your spinal cord is connected to your brain by the brainstem, which is composed of the medulla, the pons, and the midbrain.

Your brainstem controls many of your vital functions, such as breathing and circulation of blood. Cranial nerves (nerves connected to your brain) exit from the brainstem to control muscles in your face, eyes, tongue, ears, and throat; they also convey sensations from these parts back to the brain.

In addition to the brainstem, your brain has two other major parts: the cerebrum and the cerebellum. The cerebrum consists of thick, convoluted masses of nerve tissue. It is divided into two sides (cerebral hemispheres), which are connected in the middle by the corpus callosum. Conscious functions such as speech, memory, and vision are controlled in the cerebral hemispheres. Specific areas within these hemispheres are known to be responsible for certain functions, such as speech and the control of muscles in particular parts of the body. In general, control of the muscles of the right side of the body resides in the left hemisphere of the brain, and muscles of the left side of the body are controlled by the right hemisphere of the brain. Other functions, such as memory, recognition, and personality, are not localized to any specific cerebral area. The linking of higher brain functions with cerebral areas is a very active field of research. The other major portion of the brain, the cerebellum, is tucked beneath the cerebral hemispheres. It helps control your coordination, balance, and other functions that you are not usually conscious of.

At the core of your brain, atop the brainstem, are the hypothalamus and the thalamus. The hypothalamus is an endocrine regulatory center that affects sleep, appetite, and sexual desire. (See The Endocrine System, page 705.) The thalamus is a collection of nerves whose function is the integration and transmission of many of your sensations.

Your brain and spinal cord, collectively called the central nervous system, are encased in bone. The brain is protected by the skull, and the spinal cord is protected by the vertebrae. The brain and spinal cord are sheathed in three layers of membranes (meninges): dura mater (outermost), arachnoid (middle), and pia mater (innermost). These layers provide cushioning for the brain and spinal cord; in addition, a liquid,

The nerve cell (neuron) is the basic unit of the brain and nervous system. It consists of the cell body, a major branching fiber (the axon), and numerous smaller branching fibers (dendrites). Each neuron is linked to adjacent nerve cells at contact points called synapses.

Nerve cell

Synapse

Axon

Dendrite

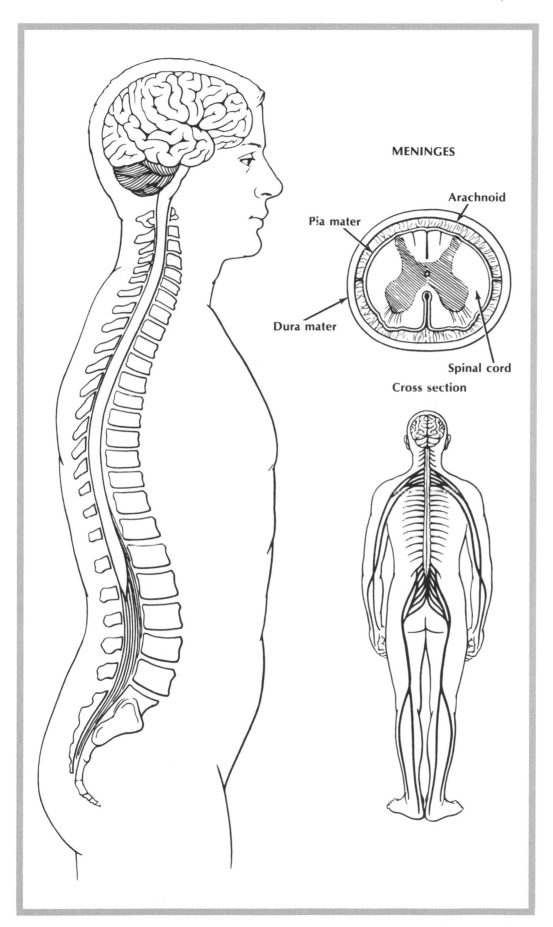

MENINGES

Pia mater

Arachnoid

Dura mater

Spinal cord

Cross section

Your central nervous system (brain and spinal cord) is protected by your skull and vertebrae and by three layers of membranes: dura mater, arachnoid, and pia mater (collectively known as meninges). Your peripheral nervous system (lower right) extends from your brain and spinal cord to all other parts of your body.

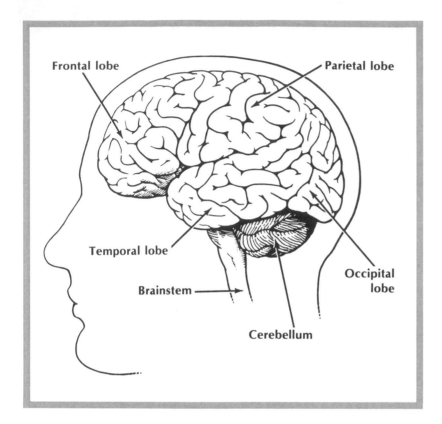

Frontal lobe

Parietal lobe

Temporal lobe

Brainstem

Occipital lobe

Cerebellum

The cerebrum is composed of the frontal, parietal, occipital, and temporal lobes. Other major areas of your brain include the brainstem and the cerebellum.

Like other organs in your body, your brain depends on a constant supply of blood to provide oxygen and nutrients for normal function. Blood is supplied through several key arteries.

called cerebrospinal fluid, between the arachnoid and pia mater further protects your brain and spinal cord from injury by the surrounding bones.

Peripheral nerves run from the brain and spinal cord to all other parts of your body. The parts of this system are named for the four spinal regions from which they branch: neck (cervical), chest (thoracic), lower back

(lumbar), and pelvis (sacral). The spinal cord acts as a central communication network to transmit signals back and forth between your brain and the farthest reaches of your peripheral nervous system.

Your autonomic nervous system is the nerve distribution to smooth muscles in blood vessels (vascular) and internal organs (visceral), to exocrine and endocrine glands, and to functional cells of internal organs. This system controls unconscious but vital activities, such as distribution of blood flow, regulation of blood pressure, heartbeat, sweating, and body temperature. Connections between autonomic and other brain functions occur at the brainstem.

The arterial blood supply, carrying oxygen and nutrients, is critical to the functioning of your brain. Despite its small size and weight, your brain uses 20 percent of the heart's output of blood and 20 percent of the oxygen consumed by your body at rest. Blood is brought to the brain by the vertebral-basilar and carotid arteries, which extend up through your neck from your heart. These large arteries then divide into smaller ones to distribute blood to various regions of your brain.

This complicated system is vulnerable. Disturbances in the blood supply to the brain cause strokes. Degeneration of nerve cells causes illnesses such as Alzheimer's disease, amyotrophic lateral sclerosis, and Parkinson's disease. Inflammatory reaction of the brain to infection causes meningitis and encephalitis. Polio is a viral infection in parts of the spinal cord and brain. Head injury or a tumor of the brain may cause

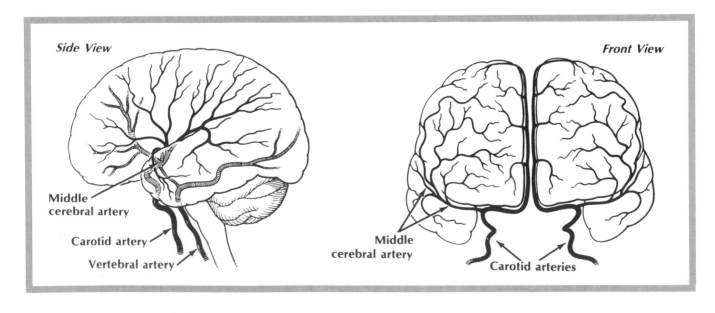

Side View

Front View

Middle cerebral artery

Carotid artery

Vertebral artery

Middle cerebral artery

Carotid arteries

THE NEUROLOGICAL EXAMINATION

The most important element in the diagnosis of a nervous system disorder is a description of your symptoms and how they developed. Headaches, blurred vision, or tingling sensations, for example, can be caused by many disorders. To determine what disorder you might have, your physician may need to ask questions about your family history and then conduct a neurological examination.

The examination systematically tests how well the various parts of your nervous system are functioning. Abnormalities that you may not notice can be detected with simple tests done in your physician's office. The tests are not painful, and no surgical procedure or injections are required. Some of the routine tests for nervous system functions are described below.

Tendon Reflexes
Your tendon reflexes are tested to evaluate motor nerve functions, spinal cord connections, and peripheral nerve conditions. For example, your physician will stimulate your reflexes by tapping your knee or ankle lightly with a special rubber-tipped hammer.

Babinski Reflex
Light stroking of the underside of your foot may produce an involuntary movement of your big toe, which can suggest an abnormality in the nerve tracts that originate in the brain.

Muscle Strength
Weakness of a muscle or group of muscles can be a manifestation of a neurological disorder. Therefore, your physician will test your muscle strength as part of your examination.

Muscle Tone
To test your muscle tone, your physician moves your arm or leg to assess the muscle strength and also the ease and range of movement. For example, both legs may be tested to check for differences between the two sides of your body. Spasticity, rigidity, or flaccidity can indicate particular problems in the nerves that stimulate different muscle groups.

Sensory Function
Sensory tests are important in a neurological examination because sensations such as pain, heat, touch, and vibration travel through your peripheral nerves to your central nervous system. Your physician evaluates these functions by asking what you feel when your skin is touched lightly by a pinprick, a hot or cold object, a cotton ball, or a tuning fork.

Nervous system disorders also can affect your eyes and senses of taste, smell, and hearing. Eye testing is particularly useful. The size of your pupils, difference between them in size, range of eye movement, gaze, and field of vision are often useful for diagnosing disturbances in the nerves that control your vision.

Your physician also will evaluate your gait, posture, coordination, and sense of balance. You may be asked to stand, walk, or move your body in a particular way to reveal possible abnormalities.

Mental Status
Your physician also may ask you questions that help determine whether your thinking, judgment, or memory is disturbed.

structural damage. Problems in mental processing, called cognitive disorders, such as focusing attention or interpreting written words, can interfere with learning. Seizures are caused by abnormal firing of nerve cells. Neuralgias are problems that affect nerves. The following sections describe these and other common nervous system disorders in detail.

Neurologists and neurosurgeons are the medical specialists who treat nervous system disorders. Diagnosis can be difficult because the symptoms and signs are numerous and diverse. Difficulties also may be encountered in distinguishing between neurological and psychiatric disease. A careful assessment of the character and pattern of symptoms over time, in addition to laboratory tests, may be required to decide among several possible diagnoses.

STROKE AND VASCULAR DISORDERS

Your brain requires 20 percent of your heart's output of fresh blood and 20 percent of the blood's oxygen and glucose contents. Two major artery systems extend through your neck to distribute this blood supply throughout your brain.

Any disturbance in blood flow—even for a few seconds—usually produces a dramatic effect on your brain's functions. Depending on what areas of your brain are affected, you can have vision or speech difficulties, paralysis in part of your body, or loss of consciousness.

If this disturbance continues for more than a few minutes, brain cells in the affected area may be destroyed, causing permanent impairment or death. Two important types of blood supply disturbance are described in this section: reduced blood flow (ischemia) and bleeding (hemorrhage).

STROKE

Signs and Symptoms
- Deterioration in vision, speech, or sensation over minutes to hours;
- Sudden weakness or loss of sensation in one limb or in an arm and leg (usually on the same side), with or without involvement of the face;
- Acute onset of double vision, slurred speech, vertigo, incoordination, or swallowing difficulty.

Emergency Symptoms
- Abrupt loss of consciousness (not due to injury);

- Sudden onset of partial or complete paralysis or numbness of face, arm, or leg;
- Sudden disturbance in or loss of vision;
- Rapid onset of a speech disorder;
- Sudden onset of severe headache.

Stroke is the common name for several disorders that occur within seconds or minutes after the blood supply to the brain is disturbed. Symptoms may progress or fluctuate during the first day or two after onset; this is called stroke in evolution. When no further deterioration occurs, the condition is considered to be a completed stroke. The only warning signal that suggests you may be prone to a stroke is a transient ischemic attack (TIA) (see page 510).

The medical term for stroke is cerebrovascular disease, which indicates that it originates in the blood vessels (from the Latin *vasa* for vessels) of your brain (*cerebrum* is Latin for brain). Strokes are characterized by the location and type of disturbance. The most common disturbance is a deficient supply of blood through an artery (ischemia). When this happens, the nerve tissue served by that artery rapidly loses its ability to function and may die. The dead tissue is called an infarct.

The most common arterial disease leading to ischemia is atherosclerosis, a condition in which a fatty deposit forms in the inner layer of an artery and results in the formation of plaque (see page 786). A blood clot (thrombus) may then develop at the site in the ar-

If circulation to the brain is blocked, brain tissue may die. If the middle cerebral artery becomes obstructed, the portion of the brain shaded here (illustration on right) will be affected, producing an ischemic attack or stroke.

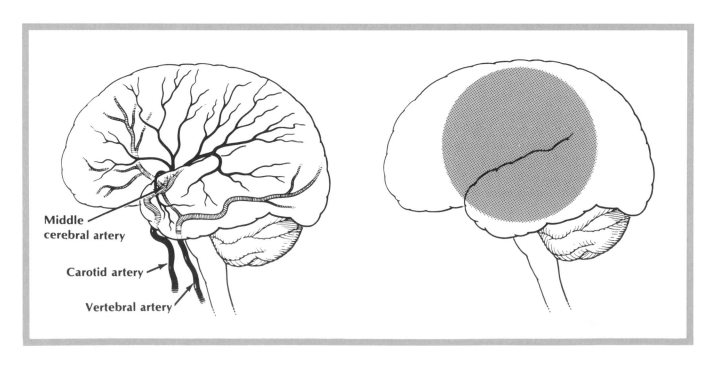

Middle cerebral artery

Carotid artery

Vertebral artery

tery narrowed by the plaque and block the flow. This type of ischemic stroke is a cerebral thrombosis. Another type of ischemic stroke, cerebral embolism, may occur when either a plaque fragment or a blood clot (the embolus) that is formed elsewhere is carried by the blood until it lodges in one location and blocks the flow. Emboli may arise from another vessel or from the heart.

A less common type of stroke (cerebral hemorrhage) occurs when an artery leaks blood into the brain, causing compression, displacement, and death of nerve tissue. The initial effect of a hemorrhagic stroke is often more severe than that of an ischemic stroke; the long-term effects, however, are similar in both cases. A severe headache followed by the other signs and symptoms described above is more typical of hemorrhagic than ischemic stroke.

A subarachnoid hemorrhage occurs when there is bleeding between the arachnoid membrane and the surface of the brain. Spontaneous subarachnoid hemorrhage most commonly occurs after the rupture of a saccular aneurysm. A saccular aneurysm is a balloon-like bulge with a narrowed neck that develops in the artery wall. Aneurysmal bleeding sometimes produces an intracerebral hemorrhage.

An arteriovenous malformation develops as a tangle of abnormal blood vessels between the arteries and veins where there should be small capillaries. These large, thin-walled vessels usually present with bleeding into the subarachnoid space. At times they may present with seizures. Occasionally, arteriovenous malformations run in families.

Stroke is the third leading cause of death in developed countries. Approximately 300,000 Americans suffer a stroke each year; one-fourth of them die, and half the survivors have long-term disabilities. Stroke is more likely to occur as you get older, and the risk doubles each decade after age 35 years. Five percent of the population older than 65 years has had a stroke.

Several risk factors are associated with stroke. It is estimated that 70 percent of all strokes occur in persons with high blood pressure (see page 796). Some forms of heart disease such as valvular heart disease or recent heart attack (see pages 822 and 809) increase the chance of stroke because blood clots from the heart may travel up the major arteries to the brain. Smoking, diabetes, and high blood cholesterol concentra-tion also are thought to be liabilities (see pages 787, 788, and 789). Although young women have a very low risk, their chances may be slightly increased by the use of birth control pills. For women who smoke, chances are greatly increased. Men have a higher risk than women.

The Diagnosis. The diagnosis of stroke does not depend on any single symptom, but a rapid development of symptoms is significant. A large blockage such as a clot or a fragment from a cholesterol plaque deposit that is carried in the blood until it blocks flow (embolism) tends to cause a completed stroke within a few minutes. A blockage that develops in place (thrombus) often occurs more slowly. The presence of symptoms that correspond to specific arterial areas within the brain is further evidence of stroke.

In order to select a treatment, your physician must decide what type of stroke occurred and its location. In addition, other

Arrow reveals area of brain tissue affected by stroke as shown in magnetic resonance imaging (MRI) scan.

possible causes of your symptoms, such as tumor, need to be excluded. One or more of the following diagnostic tests may be used to study your blood vessels: arteriography (see page 513), computed tomography (CT, see page 539), and magnetic resonance imaging (MRI, see page 539).

How Serious Is Stroke?   Stroke is a very serious illness. A physician's attention is required immediately.

After any kind of stroke, an area of dead nerve tissue (infarct) may remain after the stroke is complete. Recovery depends on whether other nerve tissue can assume the function of that area. A series of strokes can lead to multi-infarct dementia (see page 518).

Stroke is an acute (immediate) illness that most frequently stems from chronic conditions such as high blood pressure, atherosclerosis, or heart disease. If you suffer from one or more of these chronic disorders, you need close medical supervision.

Treatment.   Intensive care for a comatose stroke victim includes life-support equipment to supply oxygen, nutrients, and medications and catheterization for bladder functions. If the ability to swallow is lost, it may return within 1 to 2 weeks or may never return. In the interim, food and water can be supplied intravenously or directly to the stomach after a procedure called a gastrostomy (see page 612). Sometimes a stroke results in much less neurological damage and requires less care.

Medication.   No medication can cure a stroke once it has occurred, and the medication used for one stroke victim can cause further damage in another. For example, medications called anticoagulants (such as heparin or sodium warfarin) may be used to prevent damage to brain tissue, but these drugs are potentially dangerous in persons with high blood pressure and extensive damage to brain tissue because they increase the possibility of hemorrhage. (The term blood thinners is used commonly to describe these medications, which decrease the tendency of the blood to clot but do not actually thin the blood.)

For hemorrhagic stroke, pain relievers may be needed to relieve headache. If nausea and vomiting are present, intravenous administration of nutrients and fluid may be required for a few days.

Surgery.   Surgical procedures sometimes are used to remove blood that has leaked into the tissues from a cerebral hemorrhage. The decision depends on where the hemorrhage occurred and how far it has progressed. If a subarachnoid hemorrhage has occurred, surgical treatment of the underlying aneurysm or arteriovenous malformation is often needed. Although surgery is used rarely during ischemic stroke, an operation called carotid endarterectomy (see page 514), which removes arterial plaque deposits, may be used as a preventive measure in some cases.

TRANSIENT ISCHEMIC ATTACK

Signs and Symptoms

- Sudden onset of weakness, tingling, or numbness typically involving one side of the body;
- Vision loss;
- Speech difficulty, vertigo, double vision, imbalance, or incoordination of the limbs.

A transient ischemic attack (TIA) is caused by a temporary deficiency in the blood supply to the brain. Most episodes last only a few minutes. It has the same origins as ischemic stroke (see page 508).

A TIA most frequently is due to a disease called atherosclerosis, which develops when plaque deposits form inside arteries (see page 786). Plaque forms after the inner lining of an artery is injured. This, then, allows platelets to clump at the area of injury. This, along with the formation of cholesterol at the same site, forms a mass that protrudes into the artery. With further injury, other changes such as ulceration of the plaque and the local formation of a clot (thrombosis) can occur. A plaque fragment can break off and be carried by the blood and lodge at a distant site in the brain. This may cause a TIA.

The major risk factors contributing to TIAs are high blood pressure, some types of heart disease, smoking, diabetes, and advanced age.

The Diagnosis.   The most significant symptom of TIA is the speed at which it comes and goes: rapid onset, brief duration, and then a return to normal is the usual sequence. Recurrence of the same or similar symptoms is also significant. You may be aware of the physical symptoms as a mild loss of function or sensation.

A complete description of your symptoms is helpful for diagnosing TIA. Weakness in only one arm or leg, for example, may point to a disturbance in a branch of the internal carotid artery, whereas weakness in both arms or legs suggests disturbances in the vertebral-basilar artery. Other information that assists in diagnosis includes your eye and arm blood pressure and the noise (bruit) heard with a stethoscope when there is impairment of blood flow in various arteries. Tests might be required to gather complete information. These could include CT or MRI (see page 539) or arteriography (see page 513) to provide images of the arteries for evaluation.

How Serious Is Transient Ischemic Attack?   The signs and symptoms of TIA are similar to those of ischemic stroke, with an important difference—the symptoms disappear completely within 24 hours. A TIA may be repeated in the same day or sometime later, and each episode typically lasts only a few minutes. You should regard it as a warning that a stroke may follow. Approximately a third of persons with TIAs will later have a stroke, a third will have more TIAs, and a third will have no further cerebrovascular symptoms.

Arterial plaque deposits are very common, but they do not necessarily cause a TIA. The separate arterial networks in the brain have a built-in safety factor through extensive, small interconnections between them. When blood flow is gradually impeded in one network, these interconnections tend to enlarge so another arterial network can take over the blood supply to that region, a phenomenon called collateral circulation. As a result, a completely blocked artery may be harmless if collateral circulation is sufficient.

An additional safety factor is that the arteries to the brain are large enough to provide an adequate blood supply even when they are narrowed up to 75 percent by a plaque deposit. A TIA, therefore, is a warning that your safety factors are being overwhelmed.

Treatment.   The purpose of treatment of TIA is prevention: to improve the arterial blood supply to the brain and avoid stroke.

Medication.   If you have high blood pressure and TIAs, your high blood pressure generally is treated first (see page 796). In the absence of high blood pressure, medication may be prescribed to reduce the tendency of the blood to clot. The most common medication used for this purpose is aspirin. (In addition to its pain-relieving ability, aspirin also inhibits the way platelets clump together; the presence of too many platelets at a narrowed site may further compromise the flow of blood to the brain.) Your physician may prescribe it first as trial therapy. Anticoagulants (such as heparin or sodium warfarin) may be recommended in some situations. Anticoagulants reduce the tendency of the blood to clot. They are sometimes referred to as "blood thinners," although they do not actually thin the blood. Pharmaceutical firms are testing new drugs that reduce or eliminate plaque deposits, and some of these may be available in the 1990s.

Surgery.   In carefully selected cases, a surgical procedure, called carotid endarterectomy (see page 514), to remove arterial plaque may prevent further TIAs. The ideal candidate for this operation has had a TIA caused by plaque deposits in the neck arteries to the brain, has no further symptoms of stroke, and is thought to be a good surgical candidate.

SUBDURAL HEMORRHAGE

Signs and Symptoms
- Steady or fluctuating headache, drowsiness, seizures, or confusion after a head injury;
- Partial paralysis on one side of the body;
- Slowed thinking or changes in personality.

Emergency Symptoms
- Convulsions, stupor, or loss of consciousness after a head injury;
- Enlarged pupil(s).

Subdural hemorrhage is caused by an injury to the head. It may be the result of a car accident or a seemingly trivial event such as bumping your head. The hemorrhage occurs when blood vessels (usually veins) rupture between the brain and the dura mater, the

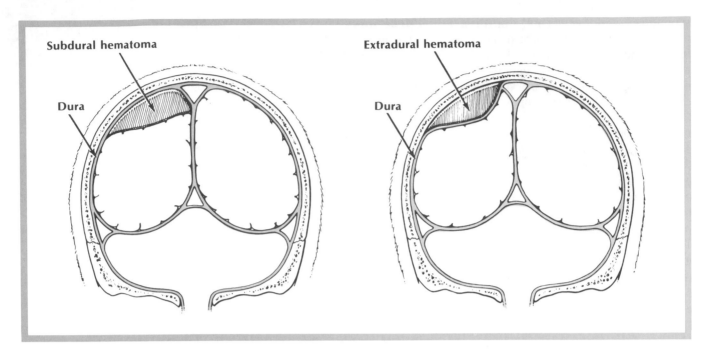

Subdural hematoma   Extradural hematoma

Dura   Dura

When an injury results in bleeding between the brain and the dura mater (left drawing), blood may accumulate, producing a mass called a subdural hematoma. When bleeding occurs between the dura mater and the skull (right drawing), the accumulation is termed an extradural hematoma. Both of these conditions can put pressure on the brain, may produce unconsciousness, and may require immediate treatment.

outermost of three membrane layers that cover the brain. The leaking blood forms a mass (hematoma) that compresses the brain tissue. If the hematoma keeps growing, there is a progressive decline in consciousness that can culminate in death.

The interval between injury and the onset of significant symptoms, such as headache, confusion, paralysis, and loss of consciousness, can vary. The hematoma is considered acute if the interval is less than 48 hours, subacute if it is between 48 hours and 2 weeks, and chronic if it is more than 2 weeks. Infants and elderly people are most likely to suffer chronic subdural hematoma, and the injury that caused it may not be remembered.

The Diagnosis. Chronic subdural hematoma is hard to diagnose. The progressive loss of consciousness after a head injury, however, generally is presumed to be caused by a hemorrhage inside the head (intracranial) until proved otherwise. The best method to define the position and size of the hematoma is CT (see page 539), if there is time to perform it. In some cases, arteriography may be used instead (see page 513). When there is no time to do these tests, immediate surgery may be required.

How Serious Is Subdural Hemorrhage?
Acute subdural hematoma is often fatal with or without immediate surgery, and

death may occur despite prompt medical attention.

The subacute and chronic forms have less risk, but they also require medical attention as soon as symptoms are apparent or permanent brain damage may result. The risk is greater for persons who use aspirin and anticoagulants on a daily basis.

Treatment. *Medication.* Intensive care includes various procedures and medications such as corticosteroids and diuretics to control the brain swelling (edema) due to other fluids accumulating after a head injury. After surgery, anticonvulsant drugs, such as phenytoin, may be prescribed to control or prevent posttraumatic seizures. Seizures can begin as late as 24 months after the trauma.

Surgery. Removal of the hematoma usually requires an operation. If the blood is localized and liquid, the only procedure required may be a perforation (creation of a hole through the skull) and evacuation by suction. Large hematomas or clotted blood may require that a section of skull be opened (craniotomy) to remove the blood. Some subdural hematomas are small, do not cause symptoms, and do not need to be removed.

Convalescence. Amnesia, giddiness, attention difficulties, anxiety, and headache may occur and continue for some time. In

CEREBRAL ARTERIOGRAPHY

Cerebral arteriography, also called angiography, is a form of x-ray imaging that permits a physician to see the blood circulating through the brain. This diagnostic procedure is used to locate the specific source of a blood vessel abnormality in the brain or neck so treatment can be prescribed. Cerebral arteriography also is useful to evaluate mass abnormalities such as tumors, especially if surgery is contemplated.

In preparation for the procedure, you will be hospitalized and not given food for several hours before the test. You will receive a mild sedative, but you will remain awake during the procedure because your cooperation is necessary in monitoring your neurological status.

The test may last 1 to 3 hours.

As a precaution, a device will be inserted in a vein in case some form of medication is needed during testing. A long, thin, flexible tube (a catheter) is then inserted through a small incision, usually in your groin. A local anesthetic generally is applied at the point of insertion. The catheter is manipulated up through the major arteries of the trunk and into the carotid or vertebral artery. Once the catheter is in place, dye (contrast medium) is injected through it. The dye outlines arteries not normally seen in x-ray imaging and helps to reveal abnormalities or obstructions.

Cerebral arteriography is a tiring procedure. You may have to lie in awkward positions for short periods, and you will normally be kept in the hospital for 24 hours after the test. The dye sometimes causes a brief burning sensation in the head.

Although arteriography is a wonderful diagnostic tool, it has its drawbacks. The procedure may cause a stroke if the catheter dislodges a blood clot or plaque deposit in an artery. Other risks involve possible allergic reaction to the dye. If you previously have shown a sensitivity to dye, special preparations are required, or this test may be avoided. Much of the risk depends on the training and experience of the team that performs the test. Statistics show that when the procedure is performed in a hospital that does fewer than 100 of these tests a year, the risks are 8 times greater than in a hospital that does at least 400 procedures a year.

As with many medical decisions, you must weigh the risks against the benefits. The risk of a complication with this test is about 0.5 percent.

With the advent of effective CT and MRI (see page 539), cerebral arteriography increasingly has become a supplementary technique in brain imaging. Cerebral arteriography nevertheless continues to be useful, especially for identifying the site and nature of problems in the brain's blood vessels. These problems include plaque deposits in the arteries, the source of hemorrhages, aneurysms, and blood vessel malformations.

This test almost always precedes the decision for or against a surgical procedure to be done on a blood vessel, such as carotid endarterectomy (see page 514). Arteriography also may be used to establish the location of brain tumors and abscesses. To date, there is no substitute for arteriography if you are suspected to have had a stroke or series of TIAs and need immediate diagnosis and therapy to avoid further and more serious damage.

Cerebral arteriography allows your physician to view how blood circulates within vessels leading to and through your brain.

adults, most recovery occurs within the first 6 months, and smaller improvements occur over 2 years. Incomplete recovery is due to brain damage. Children fare better; they have superior immediate recovery and small improvements spread over a longer period.

CAROTID ENDARTERECTOMY

Endarterectomy is a surgical procedure that removes the plaque from inside a blood vessel. This plaque can reduce the flow of blood or be the source of particles that break off and flow to the brain. Plaque formation is a common disease; it is also called atherosclerosis (see page 786). It frequently occurs in the neck arteries to the brain, particularly where the two branches of the carotid artery meet.

Plaque at this juncture is a common cause for transient ischemic attack (see page 510) or ischemic stroke (see page 508). Carotid endarterectomy usually is done after one or more transient ischemic attacks in order to prevent their recurrence and subsequent stroke. Occasionally, it will be done during the first few hours of an evolving ischemic stroke.

Although it has a high success rate, the procedure has its risks, and your physician will have to weigh several factors when deciding its benefits in your case. If you have symptoms, such as transient ischemic attack, that may be due to plaque in the carotid artery, your physician will check several indicators, including the sound (bruit) made by your blood flowing through a narrowed segment of the carotid artery and the blood pressure in your arms and in your eyes. If these indications are positive, you may need arteriography (see page 513) to locate and evaluate the blockage.

Your physician also will assess other factors before recommending this operation, including the possibility of high blood pressure and other cardiovascular disease. Active coronary artery disease may make the risk of this operation too great. Chronic high blood pressure generally must be corrected preoperatively. Another condition that requires special consideration is complete blockage of the artery.

In some persons, the combined risk of diagnostic arteriography and this surgical procedure may be greater than nonsurgical therapy, such as medication to control clotting of the blood. The risk is highest for persons with acute stroke or stroke in evolution (see Stroke, page 508) and lowest for those with no stroke symptoms at the time of surgery. For those without stroke symptoms, the rate of mortality and major neurological complications ranges from 1 to 4 percent at medical centers that have special expertise in the treatment of this condition.

The procedure begins with an incision in the neck to expose the carotid junction. Clamps are inserted to stop blood flow. The artery is opened to remove the plaque. Closure of the artery may require a patch of synthetic material. Restoring the blood flow must be done carefully to prevent clots from entering the flow.

Complications can arise during this operation. When one happens, inoperable stroke can occur. The electrical activity of your brain will be monitored by electroencephalography (see page 1294), which will warn your surgeon that steps are required to improve your circulation.

As with any surgical procedure, the success rate of carotid endarterectomy depends on the expertise of your physician and surgical team. Blockage may recur after surgery, but this is uncommon. In properly selected persons, the operation is usually successful because it eliminates further transient ischemic attacks and reduces the chance of a stroke.

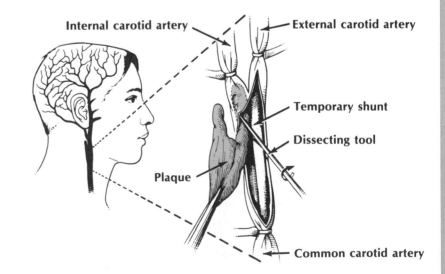

Internal carotid artery
External carotid artery
Temporary shunt
Dissecting tool
Plaque
Common carotid artery

If blood flow to the brain is blocked by an obstruction in the carotid artery, a surgical procedure called an endarterectomy may be done. This involves temporarily rerouting blood flow around the affected artery while plaque deposits are removed.

REHABILITATION AFTER A STROKE

Some 500,000 Americans survive strokes each year. Half of them live 5 years, and 10 to 15 percent live for 10 years.

An estimated 2.5 million disabled stroke survivors are alive in the United States.

Some persons live with only minor disabilities despite having had additional strokes. Four out of five long-term survivors will walk again without help, and two out of three will be able to care for themselves. One-third can return to work. But 2 out of 10 stroke survivors require extended care, some because of the mental or physical disabilities that result and others because they lack a family member or helper at home.

After a stroke, rehabilitation is crucial for morale and a return to maximal function. Those who return to work are usually white-collar workers younger than 65 years who were not totally disabled at the time they started rehabilitation.

A healthy home environment has a beneficial effect on rehabilitation. Regardless of age, stroke survivors who can go home to a healthy spouse or other companion are more likely to become independent and productive. Encouragement and early treatment are important. Various adaptive devices and architectural modifications such as ramps, hand bars on the tub and toilet, and walking frames facilitate independence

and safety. Contact your physician, local rehabilitation professionals, or independent living center for information and assistance.

Recovery and rehabilitation depend on the area of the brain involved and the amount of tissue damaged. Harm to the right side of the brain may impair sensation and movement on the left side of the body. Damage to brain tissue on the left side may affect movement on the right side and, in right-handed people, may also cause speech and language disorders. Speech disorders may include difficulty in understanding or in expressing words and can be very frustrating for the stroke survivor. Some loss of vision may occur regardless of the area of the brain that is affected. A stroke that occurs in the brainstem can cause disturbances in breathing, swallowing, balance, hearing, and eye and tongue movements. There may be a loss of sensation also. Bladder and bowel function are disturbed in many people.

In addition to the various physical side effects, depression is a common response to stroke. Affected individuals may feel helpless, frustrated, and uninterested in activities they once enjoyed. Diminished sex drive, mood changes, and thoughts of suicide are not unusual. The way in which a person thinks, interacts with others, or interprets everyday events may be affected. These side effects may be due in part to changes in the production of chemical transmitters within the

synapses, and antidepressant drugs may be prescribed.

The professional rehabilitation team normally includes a rehabilitation physician, a nurse, a dietician, a physical therapist, an occupational therapist, a recreational therapist, a speech therapist, a social worker, a psychologist, and a chaplain. The makeup of the team varies with the needs of the individual. Therapy is focused on maximizing the individual's capabilities. Early and repeated appraisals of status are needed to design the remedial program. This program will emphasize the use of the remaining function for self-care, mobility in the home and community, and reestablishing recreational and vocational pursuits tailored for the individual. Many survivors regain partial use of affected limbs, especially with the help of rehabilitation professionals. Rehabilitation returns $10 for every $1 invested by reducing costs of long-term care, and it improves quality of life.

Some persons recover satisfactorily without specific rehabilitation therapy; in others, damage is so severe that intensive rehabilitation is impractical. Prevention of complicating contractures, skin ulcers, pneumonia, malnutrition, bowel and bladder dysfunction, social isolation, and depression is a minimal objective and should be provided in any living setting. The most important and effective help over the long term may come from family and friends, and it must be given with patience and persistence.

EXTRADURAL HEMORRHAGE

Signs and Symptoms

- Headache, drowsiness, or confusion after a head injury;
- Nausea, vomiting, or dizziness;
- Enlarged pupil.

Extradural (also called epidural) hemorrhage occurs when a blood vessel (usually an artery) ruptures between the outer surface of the dura mater (the outermost of three membrane layers that cover the brain) and the skull. The blood vessel usually is damaged by a skull fracture. Blood then leaks between the dura mater and the skull to form a mass (hematoma) that compresses the brain tissue.

Extradural hemorrhage is caused by injury to the head. It occurs most frequently as a result of automobile or motorcycle accidents. There may be no visible signs, such as an open wound or bruise.

In extradural hematoma, pressure on the brain increases as more and more blood flows into the narrow space between the brain and skull. The signs and symptoms described above may lead to unconsciousness, permanent brain damage, and even death. Immediate diagnosis and treatment are important.

The Diagnosis. Symptoms are likely to occur within minutes to hours after injury. Several tests may be required to locate and assess extradural hemorrhaging, such as a skull x-ray and CT scan (see page 539). When there is no time to do these tests, immediate operation may be required.

How Serious Is Extradural Hemorrhage? Head injuries are common, but only approximately 10 percent require hospitalization. Although only a small percentage of head injuries result in acute extradural hemorrhage, the risk of dying is substantial unless prompt treatment is obtained. Up to a third of victims may remain conscious, but most are drowsy or comatose from the moment of trauma.

Treatment. *Surgery.* If diagnostic tests indicate the presence of extradural hemorrhage, operation will be necessary to stop the bleeding. The surgical procedure will involve drilling perforations or holes in the skull (craniotomy) or excising a portion of the skull to remove the blood clot and stop the bleeding. Prompt surgery usually results in complete recovery.

Convalescence. A period of convalescence may be required after a significant injury to the head. Amnesia, giddiness, attention difficulties, anxiety, and headache may occur and continue for some time. Personality changes and memory deficits may go unnoticed unless tested for. Speech disorders and paralysis usually disappear. In adults, most recovery occurs within the first 6 months, and smaller adjustments are made over 2 years. Incomplete recovery is due to brain damage. Children fare better; they have superior immediate recovery and small improvements spread over a longer period.

DEGENERATIVE DISORDERS

Your brain, spinal cord, and peripheral nerves form an intricate organization consisting of billions of nerve cells. Each of these cells is a complex electrical and chemical transmitter that carries signals to make your muscles move and to relay information throughout your nervous system.

If a few scattered cells die or malfunction, you will not notice any change because surrounding cells then carry the transmissions. When there is progressive deterioration in any part of your nervous system, however, you gradually will lose some ability to function. This loss can involve mental ability (dementia), muscular movement (paralysis), muscular control (tremor), or impaired coordination.

Compared with many other diseases, the degenerative disorders described in this section are less well understood and their prognosis is often less hopeful. These disorders may be disabling and, in most cases, there is no known cure.

ALZHEIMER'S DISEASE

Signs and Symptoms
- Gradual loss of memory for recent events and inability to learn new information;
- Growing tendency to repeat oneself, misplace objects, become confused, and get lost;
- Slow disintegration of personality, judgment, and social graces;
- Increasing irritability, anxiety, depression, confusion, and restlessness.

Dementia is a syndrome (collection of symptoms) characterized by a decline in intellectual and social abilities to a sufficient degree to affect daily activities. Alzheimer's disease is the most common form of dementia. It is due to a degeneration of brain cells. Some forms of dementia are caused by specific neurological or medical diseases and may be treatable. The cause of Alzheimer's disease, however, is unknown, and no effective treatment exists. The symptoms of Alzheimer's disease are progressive, but the rate of degeneration varies greatly from person to person.

Alzheimer's disease gradually produces abnormalities in certain areas of the brain. The particular behavioral characteristics of the disease depend on which area of the brain is most affected by the disease process. The brain cells of persons with Alzheimer's disease have characteristic features that were first described in 1906 by Alois Alzheimer, a German neurologist. The brain also has chemical abnormalities related to the substances that allow the brain cells to communicate with one another.

Research on the cause and treatment of Alzheimer's disease is progressing. Among the several possible causes that are being explored are genetic factors, toxic exposures, abnormal protein production, viruses, abnormalities in the barrier between the blood and the brain, and neurochemical abnormalities. No particular hypothesis has turned out to be the entire answer thus far, but aging and genetic factors seem to contribute to the disease.

Alzheimer's disease accounts for approximately 50 to 60 percent of all cases of dementia. About 2.5 to 2.8 million persons in the United States have Alzheimer's disease. The disease occurs in approximately 4 percent of persons 65 to 74 years old, 10 percent of those 75 to 84 years, and 17 percent of those 85 years or older. Alzheimer's disease is extremely rare in young people and is uncommon in middle age.

The Diagnosis.   No single test can be used to diagnose Alzheimer's disease, with the exception of a brain biopsy or an autopsy. Many of the signs and symptoms of Alzheimer's disease, such as memory loss, occur as a normal part of aging or as a part of other diseases such as vitamin B_{12} deficiency, hypothyroidism, depression, an adverse reaction to prescribed medications, or a chronic subdural hematoma (see pages 479, 730, 243, 244, and 511). Many of these disorders can be treated, and thus it is important for an individual with mental status abnormalities to have a thorough medical and neurological evaluation.

A person with dementia may lack insight into his or her disability. Consequently, if you know someone who shows signs of changes in mental ability, encourage him or her to be evaluated. The person's family and friends are essential in helping diagnose dementia or Alzheimer's disease and also are needed for ongoing support.

Alzheimer's disease is diagnosed by eliminating other possible causes for the changes in mental status. Initially, the person's history is reviewed in detail, and additional information from family or friends is obtained. The person then has a thorough physical examination and a neurological examination (see page 507) to determine whether some other disease is present. Hearing is often evaluated. A series of laboratory tests then are used to assess other possible causes for the changes in mental status.

A neuropsychologist may be asked to evaluate the person's cognitive function. In particular, performance on various memory and intelligence tests will be compared with performance by normal persons of the same age. Laboratory tests to rule out other causes of the changes in mental status may include chest x-ray, electrocardiography, blood tests, CT or MRI of the head, electroencephalography, and lumbar puncture. The tests for dementia are described in greater detail on page 519.

How Serious Is Alzheimer's Disease?
Alzheimer's disease is generally not an acute condition and often does not require emergency treatment. Abrupt changes in mental status may be due to other diseases, and they warrant medical attention. Alzheimer's disease, however, is ultimately fatal. Affected persons eventually may become bedridden and unable to care for themselves. They eventually may die of malnutrition or an infection because of this disability. The course of Alzheimer's disease can run from a few years to as many as 10 to 15 or more years. In the final stages, persons with Alzheimer's disease may be unable to communicate or feed themselves and may have bowel and bladder incontinence.

Treatment. During the early stages of the disorder, you can provide care at home for a friend or member of your family who has Alzheimer's disease. It is necessary, however, to care for the person under the direction of a physician. Providing care for an individual with Alzheimer's disease can be difficult and may be stressful to the spouse and family members. Often, those providing care need assistance from support organizations and a network of family and friends. Caring for someone with Alzheimer's disease requires patience and compassion to deal with the frequent repetition of stories and questions and the occasionally offensive behavior. Eventually, the person's condition deteriorates such that additional full-time nursing care is required, and often placement in a nursing home is necessary.

Medication. Several experimental drugs are being evaluated for the treatment of Alzheimer's disease. Thus far, none have proved successful for reversing the course of the disease. However, medications can be prescribed to deal with some of the behavior problems that may accompany Alzheimer's disease. Occasionally, mild sedatives, antidepressants, or antipsychotic medications may be necessary to control behavior. These drugs, often used in low doses, can improve the person's quality of life and assist the family in caring for the patient.

Other Therapies. A person with Alzheimer's disease should be encouraged to continue his or her daily routines, physical activities, and social interactions as much as possible. General health maintenance, including proper nutrition and fluid intake, is critical, but generally special diets and supplements are unnecessary. Exercise is important, and your physician may recommend specific physical therapies. The person should not be restricted from trying new activities, and travel with a supportive companion may be possible if arrangements are not overly complicated.

Avoid dramatic changes in routine, such as moving to a new location, reorganizing furniture, and disrupting daily habits. Avoid dangerous equipment or materials in the living environment, and monitor carefully the person's ability to drive.

Provide practical assistance by using notes as reminders of activities. The living situation can be modified to provide calendars, lists of routine tasks, and directions for daily activities. A medical bracelet may be helpful in case the person becomes disoriented and wanders into unfamiliar settings.

Alzheimer's disease can be a difficult disorder to deal with, but concern and compassion on the part of the persons providing care can make a difference. The assistance of a physician and the services provided by Alzheimer's disease support groups should be sought.

MULTI-INFARCT DEMENTIA

Signs and Symptoms
- Step-by-step loss of memory, marked by clouding of consciousness at each step;
- Disintegration of personality with increasing depression;
- Sudden, involuntary laughing and crying;
- Partial paralysis on one side of the body.

Emergency Symptoms
- Abrupt change in mental state.

Multi-infarct dementia is caused by a series of strokes (see page 508) that leave areas of dead brain cells (infarcts). The disorder produces a step-by-step degeneration in mental ability, with each step corresponding to a stroke. Memory, particularly of recent events, usually is affected first.

Approximately 10 percent of all cases of dementia are classified as multi-infarct, and 10 percent are attributable to a combination of Alzheimer's disease (see page 516) and multiple infarctions. More than 4 million Americans have moderate to severe mental impairment due to dementia.

In the early stages, before too much damage has occurred, the affected person often is aware of impaired ability, and frustration tends to increase the characteristic depression.

Strokes and the resulting multi-infarct dementia are typically the consequences of one or more underlying disorders, including high blood pressure and resultant artery damage (see High Blood Pressure and Atherosclerosis, pages 796 and 786). Tests for this and other forms of dementia are described on page 519.

Treatment. Prevention of stroke is the only potentially effective treatment for this

TESTS FOR DEMENTIA

Dementia is a syndrome characterized by a decline in intellectual and social abilities that affects a person's daily functioning. The symptoms of dementia are a progressive loss of memory and other mental abilities, often accompanied by increasing behavior abnormalities and personality changes. These symptoms are not specific for dementia and may be caused by various other disorders, such as depression, adverse reactions to medication, vitamin B_{12} deficiency, thyroid function abnormalities, alcoholism, drug abuse, or diseases affecting other organs in the body. The purpose of testing an individual for dementia is to identify a possible treatable cause of the changes in mental status. Therefore, an accurate diagnosis is important.

The evaluation of a person with dementia begins with a detailed history of the symptoms and physical and neurological evaluations (see page 507). The laboratory tests that are then ordered are selected to identify a specific cause of the abnormality in mental status. A mental status examination is often part of the neurological evaluation. This test is not an evaluation for sanity; rather, it assesses various mental functions such as memory, attention, language, and perception skills. Your physician or a clinical psychologist may ask questions to assess several mental processes. These questions may include an evaluation of insight into the problem (What is your difficulty?), orientation (What is the date, month, and year? Where are you now?), memory (learning a list of words and repeating them

later), recall (remembering information learned at a previous time), abstract reasoning (explanation of a proverb), attention (recite the months of the year forward and backward), language (name objects and demonstrate an ability to read, write, and comprehend the spoken word), general information (Who is the President? How many weeks are there in a year?), and thought content (What are your fears and concerns?).

Memory function may be tested in more detail because impairment of memory is a prominent finding in dementia. Various tests of a person's ability to learn both verbal and nonverbal information and to recall items from the remote past may be used. The ability to construct objects by drawing also may be assessed, and the person may be asked to recall these drawings at a later time.

Cognitive function also may be assessed in more detail by formal neuropsychological testing. This uses standardized tests of intelligence (such as the Wechsler Adult Intelligence Scale—Revised), memory (such as the Wechsler Memory Scale—Revised), language (such as the Boston Diagnostic Aphasia Examination), and prior academic achievements (such as the Wide Range Achievement Test). These tests have been standardized using large groups of people. Typically, an individual's performance score is compared with scores obtained from other persons of the same age. These tests will help to determine whether any changes in mental status performance are within the normal range of aging or whether they may be due to other disease processes. For example, depression may interfere

with some attention and memory tasks in a manner somewhat similar to that found in Alzheimer's disease.

After the clinical examinations, several laboratory tests may be done to identify a specific disease that may be causing the symptoms. These diseases include certain brain disorders, such as strokes, tumors, abscesses, or fluid accumulations, and other general medical disorders that may affect mental status, such as heart and lung disease, liver disease, kidney disease, and infections such as AIDS or syphilis. Because some of these disorders are treatable, a thorough evaluation is essential in newly diagnosed cases of dementia.

Tests that may be ordered to assess the presence of these disorders include CT or MRI of the head (see page 539), electrocardiography (see page 1293), chest x-ray (see page 1210), blood chemistry and urine tests, and drug screening. Additional neurological tests that may help in the diagnosis include electroencephalography (see page 1294), lumbar puncture (see page 530), and radioisotope studies (see page 1287).

If no specific cause for the decline in mental status is identified after a thorough medical, neurological, neuropsychological, and laboratory evaluation, the person may be suffering from Alzheimer's disease. As indicated on page 517, in the absence of a brain biopsy or an autopsy, the diagnosis of Alzheimer's disease is based on exclusion of other causes of the symptoms. The diagnosis of Alzheimer's disease must not be assigned before a thorough evaluation of all other treatable causes has been completed.

dementia. If you have high blood pressure (see page 796) or transient ischemic attacks (page 510) or have had a stroke, you will

need continuing treatment for these diseases to minimize their recurrence and avoid multi-infarct dementia. Affected persons require care similar to that needed for those with Alzheimer's disease (see page 516).

PARKINSON'S DISEASE

Signs and Symptoms
- Shaking at rest (rest tremor);
- Masking or reduction of facial expression;
- Slowness of movements;
- Shuffling gait;
- Stiffness or rigidity of limbs;
- Slow, low-pitched, monotone voice;
- Difficulty in maintaining balance;
- Stooped posture;
- Small, illegible handwriting;
- Difficulties in speech, swallowing, and chewing.

Parkinson's disease, also called shaking palsy or paralysis agitans, was first described by Englishman James Parkinson in 1817. It is a progressive degeneration of nerve cells in part of the brain that controls muscle movements.

This particular group of nerve cells makes a chemical called dopamine. Dopamine is important for transporting signals from one cell to another within your brain. In Parkinson's disease, the dopamine is lost, resulting in impairment of walking, arm movement, and facial expression.

Although much research has been done on Parkinson's disease, the cause remains unknown.

Parkinson's disease manifests itself in various manners. These may include 1) only one side of the body, 2) both sides, 3) both sides with mild postural imbalance, 4) both sides with critical postural instability, and 5) severe and fully developed disease so that you may be restricted to a bed or chair.

If the disease becomes severe, your facial expression becomes fixed, your eyes are unblinking, and your mouth may open slightly with an excess of saliva at the corners. Your posture is typically stooped. Your limbs or trunk may be rigid. Some people find it hard to start walking, beginning with hesitant, small steps, but then they have to break into a run to avoid falling forward. Some patients stop their movement in a "frozen" position and are unable to resume movement.

If your symptoms include tremor, it may be aggravated by tension or fatigue. Tremor of the hand may take the form of a continuous rubbing of thumb and forefinger (called pill-rolling tremor). The tremor disappears during sleep.

Parkinson's disease ordinarily starts in middle or late life and develops very slowly. More than 1 million Americans have the disorder.

The Diagnosis. Similar symptoms are caused by other disorders, including adverse reactions to prescribed medication, carbon monoxide poisoning, stroke, head injury, and brain tumors. Tremors, although commonly associated with Parkinson's disease, may have many other causes, such as essential tremor, which is described on page 521. Many persons with Parkinson's disease have little or no symptomatic tremor.

The onset is not readily apparent, and you may not recognize the early symptoms as a medical problem for some time. The first symptoms you experience may be a slight dragging of one foot while walking, a sense of stiffness in a limb, or a mild tremor in the fingers of one hand.

Symptoms beyond these early indications become so clear-cut, however, that your physician may be able to diagnose the disorder by a simple examination. Other possible disorders may have to be excluded by tests such as blood tests and CT or MRI (see page 539).

How Serious Is Parkinson's Disease? Parkinson's disease tends to be progressive. There currently are no medications that stop the progression. Thus, the symptoms worsen eventually. The time involved in this process varies greatly, and you may have years of productive living after developing this disease. During the later stages, however, you may need assistance. In its most severe form, you may become helplessly incapacitated by rigidity and tremor. Fortunately, this occurs only in a small minority.

Many individuals with Parkinson's disease suffer depression. In addition, some degree of mental deterioration occurs in about one-third of those persons with Parkinson's disease. In the later stages, auditory and visual hallucinations may develop; these may be activated by the medication prescribed to lessen other symptoms of the disease.

Treatment.   In early stages of the illness, you may not require therapy. Medication normally is introduced at a time when Parkinson's disease interferes with daily activities.

It is critical that you maintain good general health and continue to exercise. Your energy level may go up and down, and you will need to adjust your activities accordingly. Rest periods during the day are needed, and a contented frame of mind is important because fatigue, anxiety, and unhappiness may aggravate your symptoms considerably. You will need emotional support and encouragement to deal with the illness. There are support groups nationwide for this purpose. The National Parkinson's Foundation is a resource for information. Getting involved in physical and occupational therapy programs is stimulating both physically and emotionally. This can help you maintain a positive mental attitude and avoid depression.

Medication.   The main goal of treatment is to reverse the problems with walking, movement, and tremors by restoring your brain's supply of dopamine. A medicine called levodopa is used to increase the amount of dopamine in your brain. Levodopa can be dramatically effective for improving the deficits in movement and balance. Your physician may prescribe levodopa in combination with another medication (carbidopa) that is designed to reduce the side effects of levodopa and make levodopa more potent. Anticholinergic drugs also may be used to decrease tremor. Other drugs that might also be prescribed include amantadine, pergolide, or bromocriptine.

Close medical supervision is required during drug therapy. Dosage and the time at which you take the medication must be changed as your symptoms change. You may experience side effects such as involuntary movements, nausea, dizziness, and mental changes. Report these changes to your physician so that medication can be adjusted to your needs. Most people respond, in some degree, to drug therapy. Some are relieved of symptoms almost completely; however, over a period of years, control of symptoms may become less complete with a varying response to medication.

Surgery.   Various surgical procedures have been used to destroy tissue deep in the brain in an effort to decrease tremor. Because of computer-assisted technology now available, these procedures are being done much more precisely than in the past.

Currently, the transplantation of adrenal gland tissue to precise locations deep in the brain is under investigation. Although early reports on this form of treatment were encouraging, more recent experience with this type of transplantation is much less encouraging. Much more investigation needs to be done to determine its exact role in the treatment of conditions such as Parkinson's disease.

ESSENTIAL TREMOR

Signs and Symptoms
* Rhythmic, alternating movement of your hands, arm, head, tongue, or larynx;
* Arm and head symptoms worsen with use.

Essential tremor is not a serious condition. When there is a family history, it is called familial tremor. Although it is the most common form of tremor, its cause is unknown. The rhythmic tremor may range from a moderate to a rapid frequency (6 to 10 tremors per second).

Almost half the cases run in families, appearing at adolescence or later. It most commonly begins in middle to late life and develops slowly. Over time the tremor may affect your entire arm or both arms, your head, your voice, and even your eyelids. Your voluntary movements, such as holding a coffee cup or a fork, usually make the tremor worse. This is in contrast to Parkinson's disease (see page 520), in which the tremor tends to decrease with movement.

Stress also may increase the rhythmic shaking of essential tremor. You may notice that it usually appears while you are active. It disappears during sleep.

The diagnosis is usually made on the basis of a history and examination. Only limited laboratory tests are necessary.

Treatment.   Often, treatment is unnecessary. The usual medications include propranolol, which reduces the tremor (and also slows heart rate and reduces blood pressure), Mysoline (an antiseizure drug), or limited tranquilizers.

Avoid stimulants, such as caffeine, which may increase the tremor. Consumption of alcohol tends to decrease the tremor but can lead to alcohol abuse.

MULTIPLE SCLEROSIS

Signs and Symptoms
- Numbness, weakness, or paralysis in one or more limbs;
- Impaired vision with pain during movement in one eye;
- Tremor, lack of coordination, or unsteady gait;
- Rapid, involuntary eye movement.

Multiple sclerosis (MS) is a disease of your central nervous system. Its cause is unknown. It generally proceeds in episodes (attacks) that last weeks or months and can be separated by periods in which symptoms diminish or even disappear (remission). Attacks ordinarily recur (relapse), however, and disability may persist and the symptoms may increase in severity. MS is the chief cause of major disability in adults of working age.

Attacks are most frequent 3 to 4 years after they begin. The first attack, sometimes too mild to be remembered, most commonly happens between the ages of 20 and 40 years.

MS has a wide variety of symptoms because of the way it affects the central nervous system. Each attack is thought to be due to inflammation in an area of your nervous system. This may result in the destruction of the insulating sheath (myelin) that covers nerve fibers, leaving multiple areas of scarring (sclerosis). Muscle coordination, visual sensation, and other signals are slowed or blocked.

The most common general symptoms of MS are movement or coordination problems; sensory problems such as brief pain, tingling, or electric shock sensations; vision problems such as blurred or double vision; and problems with bladder control or mental functions. Lack of energy and easy fatigability are also common complaints of persons with MS.

Any of these symptoms may be caused by other disorders. One of the early indications that MS may be present is symptoms that appear briefly (usually lasting days to weeks) and then disappear completely or become less noticeable. This pattern corresponds to the attack-and-remission cycle of MS. Symptoms may become more prominent when your body temperature is raised by a hot bath, by being out in the sun, or by a stressful situation.

The cause of MS is not completely understood, but medical research is very active. Preceding the MS symptoms, the concentration of immune cells in your central nervous system is high. These cells are usually beneficial for fighting disease. When you have MS, however, they are thought to destroy the cells that produce the myelin sheath. The presence of a virus, in either immune cells or sheath-producing cells, is one suspected cause.

Your risk for MS is greater if a relative has the disease. An environmental source of the virus or an inherited factor in the immune system genes or a combination of the two may be involved. Your susceptibility to MS probably is acquired before you are 15 years old.

The chances for developing MS also vary with geography; the risk is greater in northern states than in southern states. More than 200,000 Americans have MS. Women have a slightly higher risk than men.

Your nerve fibers are protected by an insulating sheath (myelin). In multiple sclerosis, the sheath is damaged, producing symptoms of MS.

Normal myelin sheath

Nerve fiber (axon)

Damaged myelin sheath

The Diagnosis. The neurological symptoms of MS are varied and difficult to diagnose in the initial stages. However, the sequence of an attack, remission, and yet another attack strongly suggests MS. It is very important to get an accurate diagnosis because all subsequent symptoms may be attributed to MS, and the onset of another neurological disease may be overlooked. If MS is suspected, your physician probably will refer you to a neurologist for a detailed examination.

Criteria for diagnosing MS include a reliable history of at least two attacks and an observable abnormality of the central nervous system such as altered reflexes or sensation. Because the lesions tend to be distributed randomly in the brain and spinal cord, the symptoms can vary considerably.

Laboratory tests may be used to help establish the diagnosis. Recordings may be made of the electrical activity in the brain (electroencephalogram, see page 1294) when your senses are stimulated. You may be given a standard visual stimulus to determine how your brain's nerve cells process this input signal. Other tests may include magnetic resonance imaging (see page 539). Lumbar puncture (see page 530) also may be used to check the concentration of immune cells and proteins in your cerebrospinal fluid.

How Serious Is Multiple Sclerosis? The effect of MS is unpredictable. The average life expectancy is more than 35 years after onset of the disease, and it has increased 10 to 15 years in the past few decades as a result of better medical care, particularly in dealing with complications of the disease. Most persons with MS are ambulatory, and many are employed even after having MS for 20 years. An uncommon acute form of MS can be fatal within weeks or months.

Treatment. Currently, there is no cure for MS. Medication varies depending on the symptoms. Baclofen is sometimes useful for suppressing muscle spasticity. For severe attacks, corticosteroid drugs or the hormone ACTH may be prescribed to reduce inflammation and provide temporary relief. Several experimental drugs are being evaluated; most of them are designed to suppress the immune system.

Physical and occupational therapy are important for maintaining a positive mental attitude and avoiding depression. A planned exercise program may be needed.

AMYOTROPHIC LATERAL SCLEROSIS

Signs and Symptoms
* Slow loss of strength and coordination in one or more limbs;
* Muscle twitches or cramps;
* Increasingly stiff, clumsy gait;
* Swallowing, speaking, or breathing difficulty.

Amyotrophic lateral sclerosis (ALS) is a progressive degeneration of the nerve cells in the brain and spinal cord that control your voluntary muscles. It commonly is called Lou Gehrig's disease after the baseball player who died of ALS in 1939.

The cause of ALS is unknown. The affected nerve cells shrink and disappear with no other signs of abnormality. The muscle tissues then waste away because the nerves that stimulated them are gone.

ALS is not contagious. Occasionally other family members are affected. Nearly 5,000 Americans are affected each year, men more frequently than women.

The onset is gradual. Most often there is increasing weakness in one limb, especially a hand. Later, other limbs may be affected. This may be accompanied by twitching and cramping. Additional muscle areas become affected as ALS progresses, and complete paralysis may result. One in five patients lives longer than 5 years, but death generally occurs within 2 to 10 years after diagnosis.

The disease may be well advanced before you seek medical attention; if so, the diagnosis may be based on your symptoms and signs. Electromyography (see page 1294) to test for nerve damage may be required.

Treatment. There is no cure for ALS. Individually designed therapy is useful for maintaining your muscle function and general health during the early stages. The disease does not affect your mind, and several years of enjoyable life may be possible. A distressing feature is the difficulty in swallowing and the tendency for food and saliva to be inhaled into the windpipe. This complication can be avoided by insertion of a tube through the wall of the abdomen and into the stomach through which liquid feedings can be given (see Gastrostomy, page 612).

Emotional support from family and friends helps encourage positive attitudes. The ALS Society of America can provide information and help.

HUNTINGTON'S CHOREA

Signs and Symptoms
- Wide, prancing gait;
- Hesitant speech;
- Involuntary, jerky movements in arms, neck, trunk, and face;
- Personality changes;
- Intellectual deterioration.

Emergency Symptoms
- Abrupt change in mental state.

Huntington's chorea (Huntington's disease) is a progressive degenerative disease stemming from a disorder within the cerebrum that causes certain nerve cells to waste away. The severity of the symptoms is related to the degree of cell loss.

The disorder was first documented in 1872 by American physician George Huntington. Chorea comes from the Greek word for dance and refers to the characteristic incessant, quick, jerky, and involuntary movements.

Onset is usually between ages 35 and 50 years. Younger patients often have a more severe condition. Rare cases may occur in children. One or 2 in 20,000 people have the disease.

It is an inherited disease. If one parent has the single faulty gene, the chance that an offspring will have the defect, in some degree, is 50 percent. Because the onset is typically in middle age, it is difficult for young parents to know the chances for occurrence of the disorder in their children. If your family history includes this disease, it is important to get genetic counseling (see page 45).

The development of the disease is slow. Personality changes, from moodiness to paranoia, may occur first. Involuntary facial movements may begin mildly and develop into grimaces. Other symptoms, including severe chorea and mental impairment (de-

mentia), appear as the disease progresses. Death occurs after many years, by infection or, not uncommonly, suicide.

Treatment.   *Medication.*   No satisfactory treatment is available. Medication may be prescribed to lessen the chorea symptoms.

FRIEDREICH'S ATAXIA

Signs and Symptoms
- Difficulty in maintaining balance while walking or standing;
- Abnormal speech rhythm or articulation;
- Weakness in limbs;
- Tremor of hands or arms;
- Deformed spine or feet;
- Paralysis, particularly of the legs.

Friedreich's ataxia, named for German physician Nikolaus Friedreich in 1863, is a rare inherited disease. The symptoms, which begin in youth, are due to nerve fiber degeneration in areas of the spinal cord, peripheral nerves, or cerebellum. The diagnosis relies on a family history and on eliminating other diseases.

Survival beyond early adulthood is rare. Death is frequently caused by impairment of heart muscles (myocardia, see page 832).

Treatment.   No specific treatment is available. Continued physical activity is recommended for general health.

CEREBRAL PALSY

Signs and Symptoms
- Full or partial spastic paralysis or weakness in one or more limbs;
- Tremor or other involuntary movements;
- Vision, speech, or hearing disorders;
- Occasionally, mental retardation.

Emergency Symptoms
- Convulsive seizures.

Cerebral palsy refers to a group of disorders caused by injuries to the cerebral area of the brain that occur before or during birth or in the first few months after birth. Damage to the cerebrum may cause paralysis (palsy) in one or more parts of the body.

Cerebral palsy is the most common crippling childhood disorder. Although the damage sustained by your child continues throughout adult life, it usually does not get worse.

Cerebral injury occurs in several ways, including inadequate blood or oxygen supply to the fetus, premature birth, birth trauma, diseases in infancy (encephalitis, meningitis, or herpes simplex), subdural hemorrhage, or blood vessel damage.

Any resulting paralysis is classified clinically after the child is 2 years old. There are three main categories, and a fourth category is used to indicate mixed symptoms.

The first classification, spastic cerebral palsy, is the most common and the mildest form, occurring in 50 percent of cases. Your child may have varying degrees of paralysis in paired limbs (paraplegia), one side of the body (hemiplegia), or all four extremities (quadriplegia).

The second classification is dyskinetic or athetoid cerebral palsy; it occurs in 20 percent of cases. Your child may have abnormal involuntary movement, such as twisting, twitching, or writhing, or abrupt, jerky movements that may increase with tension and disappear during sleep.

The third classification is ataxic cerebral palsy. It is the least common form, occurring in 10 percent of cases. Your child may have tremor, unsteadiness, incoordination, and choreal movements (see Huntington's chorea, page 524).

The Diagnosis. It is difficult to diagnose cerebral palsy in early infancy, although some babies exhibit symptoms after age 6 months. Their symptoms can include a tendency to tuck their arms into their sides, to cross their legs in a scissors-like fashion, or to point their feet downward from the ankle.

Once the symptoms develop, laboratory tests may be required to exclude other disorders. If your child shows signs of mental retardation, blood tests may be needed to check for abnormalities in amino acid levels and other biochemical abnormalities.

How Serious Is Cerebral Palsy? Cerebral palsy is a chronic ailment that may require long-term care, but it is not life-threatening. The seriousness of the disorder depends on the amount of cerebral damage and can range from a speech disorder to mental retardation and a physical handicap. With special treatment, many children with cerebral palsy grow up to live long and productive lives.

Treatment. The goal of treatment is to develop your child's maximal level of independence. Regular attendance at school is recommended if the symptoms are not too severe. Physical and occupational therapy may be needed (see page 526). Some children may require an orthopedic operation. Guidelines for treatment should be determined by your child's learning capacity and physical limitations. You will need guidance and help in understanding your child's disorder and future potential.

Medication. Your child's physician may prescribe medications to alleviate some symptoms. These may include muscle relaxants to ease muscle stiffness and anticonvulsants to reduce the seizures that some children experience.

MYASTHENIA GRAVIS

Signs and Symptoms
- Facial muscle weakness (including drooping eyelids), double vision, and difficulty in breathing, talking, chewing, or swallowing;
- Muscle weakness in the arms or legs.

Emergency Symptoms
- Increasing difficulty in breathing or swallowing.

Myasthenia gravis is a chronic disorder characterized by weakness and rapid fatigue of your voluntary muscles. It is apparently caused by a problem relating to the immune system. Antibodies that are normally formed by your body's immune system to fight infection react instead against normal tissue. Most persons with myasthenia gravis also have abnormalities of the thymus gland, which is an organ that helps resist infection.

Muscle weakness develops gradually and may appear first in your face.

Myasthenia gravis is rare; in the United States it develops in 1 of 20,000 persons. Although the disease may strike any race, age, or group, it occurs most frequently in women between ages 20 and 40 years.

PHYSICAL THERAPY IN THE REHABILITATION OF CHRONIC NEUROLOGICAL PROBLEMS

Physical therapy, also called physiotherapy, is used to achieve maximal potential in persons with a disability resulting from stroke, cerebral palsy, muscular dystrophy, traumatic brain injury, multiple sclerosis, and many other disorders. Physical treatments can be valuable for helping to relieve pain, to improve your strength and mobility, and to train you to perform essential tasks so that you can regain as much independence as possible.

Before you begin a program of physical therapy, have a complete medical examination with diagnostic, functional, and psychological testing, as determined by your physician. Your physical therapist, usually at a local hospital or clinic, will consult closely with your physician. Testing and consultation are needed to plan a program that will work best for you and to reevaluate the therapy frequently as you make progress.

Physical testing will include a determination of your joint mobility, muscle strength (any weakness or paralysis), coordination, heart and lung response to exercise, posture, and ability to change position, walk, communicate, follow directions, and perform other essential daily activities.

Physical therapists are trained and licensed in the use of exercise, water, heat, cold, light, electricity, ultrasound, and other agents that may help relieve symptoms and signs of disease.

Exercise is the most varied and widely used of all physical therapy techniques. Your exercise routine will be designed to overcome the manifestations of your disorder as much as possible, whether it be to increase the degree of joint mobility, muscle strength, or endurance or to retrain your muscles to contract and relax in useful coordination with other muscles.

Exercises may be simple or complex. They are performed actively by you alone or with the help of your therapist or passively as your physical therapist moves your arm or leg through some prescribed motion. Active exercises are necessary to improve your muscle function, but passive exercises are helpful when you have muscle contractures or need to relearn certain movements. Exercises against resistance can improve your strength.

Various types of equipment may be used for this therapy, including an exercise table or mat, a stationary bicycle, walking aids, wheelchair, practice stairs, curbs, ramps, parallel bars, and pulleys and weights.

Heat generally is used to stimulate circulation, relax tense muscles, and relieve pain. It is applied with hot-water compresses, infrared lamps, shortwave radiation, high-frequency electrical current, ultrasound, hot paraffin wax, or warm baths. In some cases, cold treatment may be necessary. This is applied with ice packs or cold-water soaking. Alternating hot and cold water immersion of the hands or feet may be used in certain circumstances.

Whirlpool baths can ease the pain from muscle spasm and help guide or strengthen your movements because the water partially supports you and provides resistance to your motion.

Massage is used to aid circulation, help you relax, relieve local pain or muscle spasms, and reduce swelling. It can be done by trained therapists with special equipment or by family members trained in specific techniques.

Electrical currents of very low strength may be applied through your skin to stimulate superficial muscles and make them contract. This helps paralyzed or weakened muscles to respond again. For example, if you have amyotrophic lateral sclerosis, such therapy may be used to maintain your muscle function as long as possible. Electrical instruments also are used to test the condition of the nerves supplying your muscles and affecting sensation in your skin. Certain medications can even be supplied through your skin by means of a low-voltage electrical apparatus. Portable electrical current devices (TENS units) frequently are used to control chronic pain.

Your therapy may include learning how to use assistance devices for walking (cane, crutches, walker, braces, or others), mobility aids to substitute for walking (wheelchairs or motorized scooters), or transfer aids for changing position (boards, lifts, and bars). Special equipment that you may be trained to use ranges from simple aids, such as a cane or walker, to sophisticated devices that can make it easier to fasten buttons, hold a fork, dial a telephone, or drive a car.

Many persons are involved in the team approach to rehabilitation. In addition to your physician and physical therapist, other members of your rehabilitation team may include a corrective therapist who uses physical education techniques and an occupational therapist to help you regain the ability to perform routine daily tasks such as grooming and dressing or to help you develop an alternative to compensate for a lost function. Sometimes an orthotist may be needed to construct braces or other devices needed for mobility. Often, a rehabilitation counselor advises you on how, where, and from whom to get the necessary rehabilitation.

The Diagnosis.   The key symptom that will alert your physician to the possibility of myasthenia gravis is muscle weakness that improves with rest. Tests to confirm the diagnosis may include a neurological examination (see page 507), electromyography (see page 1294), and a blood analysis for the presence of certain antibodies. After the strength of various muscles is tested, you may be given a drug called edrophonium. Improved muscle strength after taking this drug is suggestive of myasthenia gravis.

How Serious Is Myasthenia Gravis?
There is no cure for myasthenia gravis, but treatment can often induce a remission. In a crisis phase of the illness, affected persons become so weak they need help breathing, but this effect rarely persists beyond a few weeks. With proper treatment and an accommodation in lifestyle, most can lead productive lives.

Pregnancy is possible for women with myasthenia gravis, although you should stay in close consultation with your physician. Your baby may need medication for the first few weeks of life but will be free of the disease.

Treatment.   Plan activities to take advantage of your energy peaks and schedule daily rest periods. Arrange to eat meals about 30 minutes after taking your medication to minimize chewing and swallowing difficulty. To relieve double vision, wear an eye patch. Stress also can worsen your condition, and you and your family will need to cooperate in minimizing your level of stress.

Medication.   Drugs may be prescribed to increase the amounts of nerve chemicals at the junctions of your nerves and muscles. Medications such as prednisone also may be prescribed to decrease your body's immune response.

Other Therapies.   Plasmapheresis is a treatment in which the plasma component in your blood is removed and discarded because it contains antibodies that may contribute to your disease. Your blood cells along with other fluids that replace your plasma are returned to your body. This treatment may reduce the immune response and improve muscle strength temporarily.

Surgery.   In some cases, removal of the thymus gland may be recommended. This can lead to permanent improvement in symptoms.

INFECTIONS

Infections can attack your central nervous system in several ways. They can be direct invasions by a virus or bacteria. They also can attack you indirectly when some minor condition, such as an ear infection or a case of measles, leads to a major infection of the nervous system. You also can be infected by bacterial toxins or certain tick bites.

These infections vary in seriousness. They may result in several days in bed, months of sickness with residual mental and physical impairment, or even death.

MENINGITIS

Signs and Symptoms
- Fever, severe headache, or vomiting;
- Confusion or drowsiness;
- Stiff neck.

Emergency Symptoms
- Stupor or coma;
- Convulsions.

Acute bacterial meningitis is an infection and inflammation of your central nervous system that attacks the membranes (meninges) and cerebrospinal fluid surrounding your brain and spinal cord. Bacteria usually invade through the bloodstream, but direct spread to the brain or spine can occur.

Bacteria generally enter the blood as a result of infections in other parts of your body. The infection often starts in the respiratory system. Infection of the heart valves, bones, or other areas of the body also can spread to the meninges via the bloodstream. Infection also can occur by direct invasion of bacteria already localized near your cen-

Like the brain, the spinal column is protected by several layers of membranes (meninges): dura mater, arachnoid, and pia mater. Cerebrospinal fluid (shown in blue) surrounds your brain and spinal cord. If you have meningitis, your meninges and cerebrospinal fluid are affected.

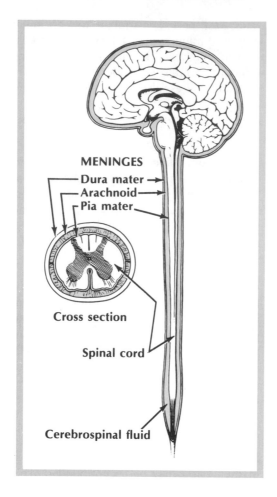

MENINGES
- Dura mater →
- Arachnoid →
- Pia mater →

Cross section

Spinal cord

Cerebrospinal fluid

tral nervous system—for example, from an infected ear, sinus, nose, or even tooth.

Other less frequent causes for acute bacterial meningitis include epidural abscess and medical procedures such as lumbar puncture. Alcoholism, diabetes mellitus, drugs used for organ transplantation, and AIDS may make you more vulnerable to meningitis. In Lyme disease, there can be an inflammation of the lining of the brain from the organism that causes the disease.

The incidence of meningitis is 5 to 10 cases per 100,000 persons annually. About 70 percent of all cases occur in children younger than 5 years, but the disease can strike at any age.

The Diagnosis.   Symptoms of meningitis include fever, headache, stiff neck, progressive lethargy, and sometimes confusion or even seizures. All these symptoms may not develop early in the course of the infection but, if meningitis is suspected, seek immediate medical consultation.

Your physician will examine your head, ears, and skin (especially along the spine) for sources of infection. Samples of pus from

the middle ear or sinuses may be obtained for study. You probably will have x-rays taken of your chest, skull, and sinuses. CT (see page 539) may be done to determine whether there is an abscess or deep swelling. The definitive diagnosis, however, will be made by analyzing your cerebrospinal fluid, which is extracted by lumbar puncture (see page 530). One of the signs of the disease is a low glucose level and increased white blood cell count in the fluid. Some of the fluid will be cultured to determine what type of bacteria may be present.

How Serious Is Meningitis?   Acute bacterial meningitis is a medical emergency. The longer you have the disease without diagnosis and treatment, the greater your risk of permanent neurological damage, such as hearing loss, brain damage, retardation, or loss of vision. Meningitis is most dangerous to infants and elderly persons.

Other, normally less acute, forms of the disease include aseptic, subacute, and recurrent meningitis. Aseptic meningitis is an inflammatory reaction of the meninges that is not caused by bacteria. This disease is most commonly caused by certain viruses but also can be a reaction to certain medications or cells that are not normally present in the cerebrospinal fluid. This form causes many of the same symptoms as a bacterial infection.

Subacute meningitis can be caused by fungal infections, the dissemination of malignant cells, or syphilis. Subacute symptoms evolve over a period of weeks.

Recurrent meningitis may be the result of a channel between the nose and the areas between the brain and one of its protective layers (subarachnoid space). This channel, usually the result of an injury, permits loss of fluid through the nose in certain positions; it also may allow bacteria to travel from the nose or sinuses to the subarachnoid space.

A certain bacterial strain (meningococcal meningitis) may cause local epidemics within relatively confined environments, such as boarding schools or military bases. It produces a purplish rash in 50 percent of cases. The disease may be rapidly fatal if not treated promptly with penicillin or another suitable antibiotic. In addition, other bacterial strains that cause sporadic cases of meningitis include *Haemophilus influenzae, Streptococcus,* and *Staphylococcus.*

Treatment. *Medication.* After diagnosis of acute bacterial meningitis, antibiotic drug therapy is instituted immediately and will vary depending on the type of bacteria causing the infection. In some cases, treatment for brain swelling, shock, convulsions, or dehydration may be needed.

Certain forms of bacterial meningitis can occur in family members. Your physician may prescribe an antibiotic to prevent this. In addition, a *Haemophilus* vaccine is available for children who are at least 18 months of age (see page 867).

Other Therapies. Drainage of infected sinuses or mastoids may be needed. If fluid has accumulated between your brain membrane layers, it may need to be drained or surgically removed.

ENCEPHALITIS

Signs and Symptoms
- Confusion, drowsiness, and disorientation;
- Sudden fever;
- Severe headache;
- Nausea and vomiting;
- Tremor;
- In infants, bulging in the soft spot of the skull;
- Occasionally, a stiff neck.

Emergency Symptoms
- Altered levels of consciousness.

Encephalitis is a rare and acute inflammatory disease of the brain caused by a viral infection. Encephalitis sometimes occurs in a primary form when the disease is due to a direct viral invasion of your central nervous system. Its most common form, however, is secondary (postinfectious) encephalitis, which follows or occurs with a viral infection in some other part of your body such as measles, chickenpox, rubella, or mumps. The cause in some of these secondary cases is believed to be a hypersensitivity reaction.

Secondary encephalitis arises from within your body, but the primary form results from the environment around you. The viruses can be sporadic or epidemic. The most common sporadic form, herpes simplex encephalitis, can be particularly deceptive when it starts as a minor illness with headache and fever. This is followed by neurological symptoms, which may include difficulty in talking, confusion, unconsciousness, repeated seizures, and the symptoms described above. Epidemic varieties may be due to arboviruses; these are mosquito-borne and infect you only in warm weather.

Some 1,500 to 2,000 cases of encephalitis are reported annually in the United States.

The Diagnosis. In infants, a bulging in the soft spot of the skull (the fontanelle) and a stiff neck are key symptoms. In older children, severe headache and sensitivity to light may be more significant. In adults, mental disturbances, from severe disorientation to coma, may be the most outstanding clinical feature.

After the initial signs, the onset of neurological symptoms can be variable. You may be severely ill within 24 hours, or a week may pass before the neurological symptoms are apparent. In the case of secondary viral encephalitis, the disease may develop 5 to 10 days after onset of the initiating viral infection.

Encephalitis usually is diagnosed by analyzing your cerebrospinal fluid, which is extracted by a lumbar puncture (see page 530). Analysis of the fluid reveals a normal glucose level, increased white blood cell count, and failure of culture of the fluid to show the presence of bacteria. Your physician will be able to rule out acute bacterial meningitis (see page 527). When hemorrhages are part of the illness, your cerebrospinal fluid may be slightly bloody. Electroencephalography, MRI, or CT (see pages 1294 and 539) can help to confirm the diagnosis of encephalitis.

Diagnosis of herpes simplex encephalitis is difficult and requires a biopsy of the brain. Because this biopsy involves some risk, treatment with an antiviral agent is initiated early and the response is observed. If no response occurs with antiviral treatment, a brain biopsy may be advised.

How Serious Is Encephalitis? The course of viral encephalitis is variable. It may be of short duration and benign, or it may strike with great severity and leave significant mental impairment. Such impairment can include loss of memory, the inability to speak coherently, lack of muscle coordination, paralysis, or hearing or vision defects.

The most acute phase of the illness can

LUMBAR PUNCTURE

Lumbar puncture (spinal tap) is the procedure used to measure pressure in your cerebrospinal fluid (CSF) and to extract small samples of CSF for laboratory analysis. It also is used to inject spinal anesthetics, some medications, and substances for diagnostic tests.

A local anesthetic is used at the puncture site. A thin, hollow needle then is inserted between two vertebrae in your lower back (lumbar region), through the spinal membrane, and into the spinal canal. The vertebrae must be spread apart slightly to provide access, so you will be asked to lie on your side with your knees drawn up to your chest and both arms clasped around your knees. This position flexes the back and spreads the vertebrae. Some conditions, such as a spinal fluid blockage in your middle back, require the puncture to be made between two cervical vertebrae in your neck rather than the lower back.

Once the needle is in place, the fluid pressure is measured, CSF is extracted, and then the pressure is measured again. If a drug or substance is being injected, its volume will equal the volume of CSF that is withdrawn. The substance is at body temperature and injections are made slowly to avoid any shock to the central nervous system. The procedure usually takes about 30 minutes when a CSF sample is being extracted, but more time may be required for an injection. After the procedure, the puncture site is bandaged to prevent infection.

You may have a feeling of pressure during the procedure. Afterward, you may have a headache because of a decrease in CSF pressure related to a persistent leak of CSF into the tissues. Lying down usually alleviates the headache, and it usually goes away as the pressure returns to normal in a few days.

A sample of your CSF may be required to diagnose various diseases. These include multiple sclerosis, Reye's syndrome, Guillain-Barré syndrome, infections of the central nervous system (meningitis, encephalitis, polio, or AIDS-related diseases), certain kinds of tumors, and subarachnoid hemorrhage that cannot be seen on a CT scan (see page 539). The CSF sample can be tested for protein, sugar, red and white blood cells, and malignant cells. The sample can be cultured to identify bacterial and viral infections.

Lumbar puncture also is used for injecting dye (contrast material) or radioactive substances when they are needed to make diagnostic images of CSF flow (see Myelography, page 555). Medications such as antibiotics and antitumor agents occasionally are injected with this procedure.

There are some risks with lumbar puncture, although they are fewer now than previously. Greater care is used to prevent infection, and the procedure is used more selectively. The availability of CT, for example, reduces the need to use lumbar puncture for diagnosing most types of intracranial hemorrhage when a lumbar puncture may be dangerous. The risks remain for persons with blood coagulation disorders, in which the procedure can cause bleeding where the needle penetrates the spinal membrane, and for persons with increased spinal fluid pressure, which can lead to movement of the brain in a small area when the CSF is removed.

Spinal cord

In a lumbar puncture (spinal tap) you lie on your side, knees pulled to your chest, while a needle is inserted between two vertebrae and a small amount of cerebrospinal fluid is extracted for laboratory testing.

last from a few days to a week. The duration of the characteristic fever may be 4 to 14 days. Resolution may be gradual or abrupt. Resultant neurological defects can continue to resolve over weeks or months. Even severely ill persons may experience complete recovery.

The mortality rate varies with the source of the virus. Insect-borne sources might cause low mortality one year but severe mortality in the next.

Treatment.   *Medication.*   In the case of herpes simplex encephalitis, an antiviral agent such as acyclovir has been used with success in the early stages. For some patients, anticonvulsant medication may be needed.

Other Therapies. Because viruses that cause encephalitis do not respond to antibiotics, basic treatment is supportive and consists of rest, nourishment, and sufficient fluid intake to let your natural defenses fight the virus. In early convalescence, irritability is common. For persons left with mental impairment, physical and speech therapies may be needed.

REYE'S SYNDROME

Signs and Symptoms
- Persistent nausea and vomiting after a viral infection.

Emergency Symptoms
- Drowsiness, stupor, loss of consciousness, or coma;
- Delirium, seizures, or convulsions.

Reye's syndrome is relatively rare. It was first identified as a distinct disease in 1963. This is a serious disturbance that follows a viral infection in children. It affects the blood, liver, and brain. Characteristics include high levels of ammonia and acid but a low level of sugar in the blood, fat formation and swelling in the liver, and brain swelling that produces the emergency symptoms listed above.

The specific cause for Reye's syndrome is unknown, although giving aspirin may trigger it in children. It occurs mostly in children between 2 and 16 years old, soon after a viral infection such as chickenpox or influenza or an ordinary upper respiratory infection. There is, however, almost never any evidence of a virus in the liver or brain, which are the two areas most affected by Reye's syndrome. Fever is usually not a symptom, although fever occurred with the prior illness.

The Diagnosis. Symptoms typically start almost a week after the viral infection. At first there is persistent nausea and vomiting for 1 to 3 days, followed by a progressive decline in your child's mental alertness as the brain swelling increases. This progression goes from lethargy and drowsiness to stupor and deepening stages of coma. Episodes of agitation, seizures, or convulsions may occur. These symptoms develop rapidly over a few days, and immediate medical attention is required.

After examining your child, your physician may require further tests to complete the diagnosis. A blood analysis may give evidence of Reye's syndrome, but a liver biopsy is the definitive test. Cerebrospinal fluid may be extracted by lumbar puncture (see page 530) to test for other diseases with similar symptoms, such as meningitis or encephalitis (see pages 527 and 529).

How Serious Is Reye's Syndrome? Although the severity varies greatly, Reye's syndrome is usually an acute, life-threatening disorder. Emergency treatment is required. The chance for your child's survival depends on how far the disease has progressed and how quickly the body chemistry is stabilized.

Previously, the fatality rate was more than 40 percent. Now, with earlier diagnosis and better treatment, this rate has decreased to about 10 percent. Most children recover completely in 2 to 3 months, but brain damage may persist in a few cases.

Treatment. *Prevention.* The occurrence of Reye's syndrome is reduced by avoiding the use of aspirin in children younger than 16 years who have a viral infection. Moreover, aspirin is not recommended for children younger than 12 years with any illness. Other, safer alternatives include acetaminophen or ibuprofen.

Medication. Your child may require hospitalization in an intensive-care unit while medications are given and vital signs are monitored. Medications usually are given intravenously. Your child's blood sugar level is raised by giving glucose, the blood chemistry values are corrected with electrolyte solutions containing sodium, potassium, and chloride, and acidity is treated with basic solutions. Small amounts of insulin may be given to increase glucose metabolism. Brain swelling is controlled with a corticosteroid (dexamethasone) to reduce inflammation, and a diuretic (mannitol) is given to increase fluid loss through urination. Other medications may include purgatives, vitamin K_1, and oral nonabsorbable antibiotics (neomycin).

Monitoring of the pressure inside your

child's skull may be used to guide the therapy. Arterial catheters commonly are used to monitor blood gases, acidity, and pressure. Other common procedures include the insertion of a tube into your child's throat to aid breathing.

POLIOMYELITIS

Signs and Symptoms (for the acute paralytic form)
- Fever and headache;
- Stiff neck and back;
- Muscle weakness;
- Difficulty in swallowing.

Emergency Symptoms
- Weakness or paralysis;
- Respiratory failure.

Poliomyelitis, also called polio or infantile paralysis, is the result of a viral infection. The virus gains entry through your mouth, invades your body through the throat and digestive system, and spreads throughout the lymphatic system and the bloodstream. The poliovirus is contagious and is passed by direct contact with contaminated feces or saliva.

The disease manifests as a minor illness (sore throat, mild upset stomach, and low-grade fever), as aseptic meningitis (see page 539), or as paralytic poliomyelitis. The paralytic form occurs when the virus goes from your bloodstream into your central nervous system and then infects nerve cells of your brainstem or spinal cord that control muscular activity.

The Diagnosis. Paralytic poliomyelitis sometimes is preceded by fever and a brief illness. The incubation period is usually 7 to 14 days and can be up to 35 days.

The key symptom is limb paralysis without loss of sensation. An analysis of your cerebrospinal fluid, extracted by lumbar puncture (see page 530), will show a normal cell count but increased protein level.

How Serious Is Polio? A minor illness with complete recovery in a few weeks occurs in 90 percent of cases, mostly in children. Paralytic poliomyelitis, however, is an acute disease that strikes adults most severely, and you will need prompt medical attention.

The paralysis varies depending on the area of your nervous system that is affected. Brainstem infections, for example, cause weakness in muscles used for swallowing, talking, facial expression, breathing, and blood circulation. Spinal cord infections cause paralysis of the legs, arms, or trunk.

Less than about one in four people with polio incur permanent disability.

About 2 to 5 percent of children and 15 to 30 percent of adults with paralytic forms of poliovirus die. For survivors, recovery from paralytic symptoms occurs gradually over 6 months. The paralysis that remains after 6 months is usually permanent and may be accompanied by severe pain.

Other possible complications include diseased heart muscles, high blood pressure, fluid in the lungs, shock, and urinary tract infection.

In some people, progressive weakness and atrophy of muscles occur many years after an acute episode of polio. The cause of this is uncertain but may be a reactivation of the virus.

Treatment. *Prevention.* The two forms of vaccine are the Salk vaccine, which is given in a series of intramuscular injections and boosters, and the Sabin vaccine, which is administered orally. The Sabin vaccine is favored in the United States for routine childhood immunization. The Salk vaccine is recommended if you have an immunodeficiency. The incidence of polio is low in the United States because of widespread vaccination. If you have never been immunized or are traveling to a developing country, consult your physician (see page 338).

Other Therapies. Mild illness requires bed rest for several days. Persons with paralysis need to be on a firm bed with a foot board to prevent the permanent inability to flex the foot (footdrop). Medications may include bethanechol for urine retention and antibiotics for urinary tract infections. Artificial respiration may be required if the paralysis affects the respiratory muscles. A surgical incision into your windpipe (tracheotomy) may be needed if swallowing is difficult. Physical therapy (see page 526) is important during convalescence.

EPIDURAL ABSCESS

Signs and Symptoms
- Ear or nose pain with pus discharge;
- Unrelenting headache;
- Fever, nausea, and vomiting;
- Back pain and tenderness.

Emergency Symptoms
- Increasing speech difficulty;
- Growing loss of sensation, weakness, or paralysis in one side of the body or both legs;
- Seizures or convulsions.

Epidural abscess is usually due to bacterial infection that causes pus to form between the outermost brain membrane (dura mater) and the bone of your spine or skull. Sometimes it invades the bone surface inside the skull or vertebrae. It also can penetrate the membrane layers to become a subdural abscess, a brain abscess, or meningitis (see page 527).

Epidural abscesses in your head may originate as infections in your sinuses, your ears, or the mastoid bones behind your ears. Head injuries also may allow the infection to penetrate the skull. Occasionally, bacteria will be carried by the blood to the epidural space from an infection elsewhere in the body. Abscesses in the spine can start from a boil on your skin, an infection in your lung or abdomen, or an infection associated with operation.

Epidural and similar abscesses are now relatively rare because the widespread use of antibiotics controls many infections in their early stages. The greatest risk is from chronic sinus or ear infections.

The Diagnosis. As with meningitis, epidural abscess can be caused by direct infection or by an infection that is carried to the epidural area by the blood. Progressive headache or back pain with fever and tenderness around the infection site may develop. As the abscess enlarges, it can cause direct pressure on the spinal cord or brain, resulting in pain and the loss of neurological function.

The diagnosis of epidural abscess is suggested by the presence of an infection and the subsequent development of symptoms. Your physician probably will require an x-ray or MRI or CT scan (see page 539) of your head or spine to complete the diagnosis.

How Serious Is Epidural Abscess? An epidural abscess can cause serious neurological damage or even death if it is not treated promptly. Prompt treatment generally results in complete recovery.

Treatment. *Medication.* You will be given intravenous antibiotic therapy immediately to start controlling the infection. Epidural abscess sometimes is not cured by antibiotics alone, however, and an operation may be needed to drain the infected area. After the operation, antibiotics are usually given for 1 to 2 months.

Surgery. Prompt operation is sometimes required to empty the abscess and remove the pressure (decompression) on your spinal cord or brain. A section of your skull or spine is opened to provide access to the abscess and to facilitate drainage. If the abscess has penetrated any area of your skull or vertebrae, some of the affected area may be removed. Sometimes it is difficult to find and remove all traces of the infection, and your recovery may be complicated by reinfection.

AIDS AND THE NERVOUS SYSTEM

Signs and Symptoms
- Headache, fever, nausea, vomiting, sore throat, or stiff neck;
- Speech difficulty or vision impairment;
- Loss of memory, concentration, or other mental abilities;
- Weakness, loss of sensation, or incoordination.

Emergency Symptoms
- Partial paralysis, seizure, or convulsions;
- Stupor, loss of consciousness, or coma.

Acquired immune deficiency syndrome (AIDS) may lead to various nervous system diseases. AIDS is caused by a virus called human immune deficiency virus (HIV). HIV may directly infect your central nervous system and cause progressive degeneration of nerve cells. The AIDS virus also suppresses your immune system. Thus, other microorganisms have an opportunity to infect you (opportunistic infection), and tumors may invade the nervous system. HIV can infect any level of the nervous system, including the meninges (outer covering of the brain), brain, spinal column, or peripheral nerves.

Most persons with AIDS develop pneumonia or a rare skin cancer (Kaposi's sarcoma). Approximately a third develop nervous system diseases which include viral, fungal, or bacterial infections that cause meningitis, encephalitis, or myelitis (inflammation of the spinal cord). Other diseases of the nervous system that occur in association with AIDS include parasitic cysts in the brain, abnormal growth in nervous system lymphoid tissues, and a progressive form of dementia. Peripheral nerve disease also has been associated with AIDS.

The occurrence and diagnosis of AIDS is described on page 848. If symptoms of secondary diseases appear, your physician may require a CT scan (see page 539), lumbar puncture (see page 530), or other laboratory tests for diagnosis.

Treatment.   Some AIDS-related diseases of the nervous system are treatable, but the effectiveness of standard treatments (such as antibiotic therapy for bacterial infections) is limited by the state of immunodeficiency. Research on treatment is very active, and new medications are being tested.

BOTULISM

Signs and Symptoms
- Weak, limp muscles within 12 to 36 hours after consuming the contaminated food;
- Double vision;
- Dry mouth;

- Speech and swallowing difficulty;
- Vomiting and cramps.

Emergency Symptoms
- Rapidly progressive weakness or paralysis;
- Breathing difficulty.

Botulism is acute poisoning from the toxin produced by a microorganism *(Clostridium botulinum)* commonly found in soil. The organism is similar in many ways to that causing tetanus (see page 857).

You can be poisoned from canned or home-preserved foods that were not cooked enough to destroy the organism's spores. Your infant may be poisoned by sources, such as raw honey, that do not affect adults. It also can occur from wounds that get contaminated by soil. Usually, but not always, cans of food contaminated by this organism will bulge.

The poison blocks nerve signals to the inner lining of the mouth and muscles; this effect begins 3 hours to 14 days after consuming the poison. The diagnosis is based on the signs and symptoms and is confirmed by identifying the toxin in blood, food, or feces. Respiratory failure because of weakness of the muscles that control breathing causes death in 10 percent of food botulism cases and in 2 percent of botulism cases in infants. The disorder is now very rare because of careful preparation of food. Heating to boiling for 10 minutes will destroy the toxin.

Treatment.   Avoid obviously contaminated or poorly prepared foods. Giving honey to infants is not recommended. Specific treatment consists of administration of antitoxins.

If the person affected with botulism survives the first few days, recovery is usually complete.

STRUCTURAL PROBLEMS

The nerve tissue in your brain is delicate and easily torn, bruised, or damaged by pressure. Under ordinary circumstances, your skull and spinal membranes (meninges) provide protection, but during automotive, industrial, and other accidents the skull and membranes may prove inadequate. Structural damage to your brain from an accident

can range from a mild concussion to permanent disability or death.

Other structural problems described in this section include tumors inside your head. Structural problems from bleeding inside your skull are described under subdural and extradural hemorrhage (see pages 511 and 515, respectively). Structural problems with your spinal cord are described under spinal trauma (see page 552) and spinal tumor (see page 554).

HYDROCEPHALUS

Signs and Symptoms
- Abnormal enlargement of the head in newborns;
- Mental decline, slow and restricted body and eye movements, and urinary incontinence in older children or adults.

Hydrocephalus is caused by interference with the normal circulation of the cerebrospinal fluid (CSF) in the brain. CSF filters through a membrane in your brain and later is reabsorbed from the subarachnoid spaces above your brain.

Congenital or postnatal hydrocephalus in infants can be due to a blockage in the brain's CSF circulation system or to an inability to reabsorb the fluid. The resulting pressure expands the loosely connected sutures in the skull so that in a newborn or young child the head is enlarged abnormally in all directions, especially in the frontal area.

Your infant's symptoms may be mild and the progression might stop but then reappear in later childhood. The skull becomes firmly closed by age 5 years, so subsequent symptoms do not include appreciable head enlargement.

Congenital or childhood hydrocephalus due to a blockage in the circulation of CSF in the brain may be caused by various congenital malformations of the brain, a fetal viral infection, birth injury, or tumor. Hydrocephalus due to problems of reabsorption can result from brain malformation, an infection such as bacterial meningitis (see page 527), subarachnoid hemorrhage (see page 511), or spinal cord defects such as syringomyelia (see page 558) and myelomeningocele (see page 559).

In adults, a variation of hydrocephalus may occur in which the CSF pressure is normal (normal-pressure hydrocephalus) but the reabsorption of CSF is defective. The symptoms arise slowly after meningitis, head injury, or subarachnoid hemorrhage, but they also may develop for no known reason.

Hydrocephalus in children is relatively uncommon—it occurs in approximately 1 of 1,000 children. In adults, normal-pressure hydrocephalus is also uncommon and occurs most frequently among elderly people.

The Diagnosis.   Your child's head may be measured at birth. If the circumference of the head exceeds a certain size, hydrocephalus may be suspected and the head will be measured frequently during the first weeks of life.

In later childhood and adulthood, symptoms will lead to further testing. In all cases, the diagnosis may require a skull x-ray or CT or MRI scan (see page 539) and an examination and culture of a CSF specimen (obtained by lumbar puncture, see page 530).

How Serious Is Hydrocephalus?   The severity depends on the time of onset and whether the disease is progressive. If the condition is well-advanced at birth, major brain damage and physical handicaps are inevitable. Death usually occurs early from an underlying infection. In less severe cases, with proper treatment, 40 percent of the affected persons have a nearly normal life span and intelligence.

Treatment.   The goal of treatment is to reestablish the balance between CSF production and reabsorption. In young children with a slowly progressive condition, the drug acetazolamide sometimes diminishes CSF production. When the imbalance is due to a reabsorption problem, treatment may consist of repeated lumbar punctures to relieve pressure.

Surgery.   An operation to implant a shunt is effective in many children and adults. The shunt, with tubing or valves (or both), is placed to circumvent the blockage or to divert excess CSF into the bloodstream or abdominal cavity where it is reabsorbed. A successful shunt procedure will allow an infant's head size to become normal and will relieve symptoms in older children and adults. Shunt tubes may require replacement as a child grows. Successful shunts usually are maintained for life, but shunt infections can be a serious complication.

CONCUSSION

Signs and Symptoms
- Brief loss of consciousness or memory after a head injury;

- Headache;
- Faintness, nausea, or vomiting;
- Slightly blurred vision or difficulty concentrating.

Emergency Symptoms
- Persistent confusion, drowsiness, or delirium;
- Speech difficulty or partial paralysis;
- Stupor or coma;
- Dilation of a pupil;
- Progressive lethargy.

Concussion is a brief loss of consciousness after a head injury. The impact creates a sudden movement of the brain within the skull. Such traumatic movement can produce a wide range of injuries, and concussion is the mildest form of these. No evident structural damage to your brain occurs with concussion, although there may be cuts or bruises on the skin outside your skull.

Head injuries usually are caused by traffic or industrial accidents, falls, and physical assaults. Accidents are the leading cause of death for males younger than 35 years, and head injuries are involved in more than 70 percent of these accidents.

The fatality rate due to head injury has been reduced in recent years through the use of motorcycle and sports helmets, hard hats, and seat belts and because of better ambulance services. Nevertheless, head injuries remain a serious problem.

The Diagnosis. Get prompt medical attention for any impairment of consciousness or dazed feeling after a head injury. Diagnosis is complicated by the possibility of serious bleeding within the skull, and this could require emergency surgery. Serious damage may include epidural or subdural hemorrhage (see pages 515 and 511, respectively) or other brain injuries (see this page).

Symptoms of serious damage may be immediately obvious or they may not appear until hours or days after injury. Your state of alertness and attentiveness provides the key information for how much damage has occurred.

Your physician will examine you for signs of skull fracture and brain damage. Skull x-rays or a CT scan (see page 539) may be required to determine whether serious damage has occurred and whether your injuries are limited to a concussion. An observation period of 24 to 48 hours is recommended, in a hospital or at home with your family or friends checking to see whether further symptoms develop.

How Serious Is Concussion? Concussion is a minor, temporary injury without permanent brain damage. Accidental head injuries, however, cause death or brain damage in one out of five cases, and any head injury is potentially serious.

The loss of memory (amnesia) associated with concussion usually involves only your experience just before and during the accident that caused the concussion. It may, however, encompass a few weeks (or rarely months) before the accident. Your recovery of memory commonly progresses from the more distant past to the recent experience.

About a third of all persons with concussion have a combination of symptoms, called postconcussive syndrome or posttraumatic syndrome, for some time after a head injury. In addition to headache and dizziness, these symptoms may include insomnia, irritability, restlessness, inability to concentrate, depression, or personality changes such as moodiness. Precisely why these symptoms occur in some people is unknown.

Treatment. Concussion is generally self-healing and little or no treatment is required. Your physician may prescribe acetaminophen or a stronger painkiller, such as codeine, to relieve your headache. Aspirin should be avoided because it can contribute to bleeding. Rest and relaxation with no activities requiring concentration or vigorous movement usually will facilitate recovery within a few days.

Athletes, such as football players or boxers, who have had a concussion should have a medical evaluation before returning to their sport.

OTHER BRAIN INJURY

Signs and Symptoms
- Headache after a head injury.

Emergency Symptoms
- Persistent confusion, drowsiness, or delirium;
- Speech or breathing difficulty;
- Difference in size of eye pupils;

- Partial paralysis;
- Seizures or convulsions;
- Stupor or coma.

Brain injury may result from a blow to the head or from an object that penetrates the head, such as a bullet or piece of industrial equipment. Traffic accidents, falls, industrial accidents, and physical assaults are the major causes of such injuries. Accidents, usually involving head injuries, are the leading cause of death in males younger than 35 years.

Concussion (see page 535) is the mildest form of head injury resulting in loss of consciousness without brain damage. Brain damage does occur, however, in about 20 percent of the 10 million head injuries reported each year.

Moderate to severe brain injuries can be associated with a fracture, torn membranes or nerve tissue, and bruises or hemorrhaging within your brain. There may be brain swelling or leaking of cerebrospinal fluid. Subdural or extradural hemorrhage is possible (see pages 511 and 515, respectively). Your symptoms may not appear for several days after the accident.

The Diagnosis. Get prompt medical evaluation for any head injury that causes even a brief loss of consciousness or persistent symptoms. After an examination, your physician probably will recommend hospitalization for observation, testing, and treatment if you show any indications of brain injury. A CT scan (see page 539) may be needed.

How Serious Is Brain Injury? Most persons with moderate head injuries recover in 1 to 6 weeks, although some disability may persist. Continuing convulsive episodes may occur in up to 50 percent of those who experience seizures after injury (see page 541). Severe injuries can be fatal or permanently disabling despite the best medical and surgical treatment.

Treatment. Emergency treatment is required for comatose patients with severe brain injuries. Medications, such as corticosteroids (see page 1005), and possibly an operation are sometimes needed to control brain swelling, which can cause death.

BRAIN TUMOR

Signs and Symptoms
- Headaches of recent onset;
- Vomiting;
- Weakness and lethargy;
- Personality change;
- Double vision;
- Recent incoordination or clumsiness of arm or leg;
- Intellectual deterioration.

Emergency Symptoms
- Vision, sight, or speech difficulty;
- Seizures;
- Stupor.

A tumor is any mass or growth of abnormal cells. Whether it forms in your brain or elsewhere, it can be benign or malignant. A malignant tumor is cancer. The disorders described here relate to the two major categories of brain tumor: primary and secondary.

Primary brain tumors develop directly in your brain. Their cause is unknown, and occasionally they are congenital or hereditary.

Secondary (metastatic) brain tumors originate elsewhere in your body and are more common than primary tumors. They occur in one-fourth of persons with a malignant condition in other parts of the body (systemic cancer). Secondary tumors most often originate in your lung or breast. Tumor cells in these areas move through the bloodstream (metastasize) to the brain, which is a common target of metastasis.

Both primary and secondary tumors may be located within your brain or in proximity to it, such as in the skull, brain membranes, supportive tissue, cranial nerves, or pituitary or pineal gland. Many types of tumors can develop in these locations, and each has its own symptoms, treatment, and prognosis.

Brain tumors can occur at any age. They may produce no symptoms (asymptomatic), or they can grow very slowly over many years and remain asymptomatic until they become large. Progressive problems then can develop rapidly.

The Diagnosis. The symptoms listed above are typical of any expanding tumor because they increase the pressure in your skull and compress brain tissue, cranial nerves, and blood vessels. Emergency symptoms indicate the onset of serious

Magnetic resonance imaging (MRI) scan shows tumor in mid brain (see arrow).

Treatment.   Your therapy may include surgery, x-ray radiation to kill tumor cells, or anticancer drugs (chemotherapy) to halt the progress of the disease. Corticosteroid drugs to diminish brain swelling, anticonvulsants for seizures, and analgesic painkillers for headaches also may be prescribed. Some benign and malignant tumors can be removed completely at operation. Others can be removed only partially or not at all, and radiation or chemotherapy may be recommended. Advances in computer-assisted surgery (stereotactic surgery) are making it possible to remove some tumors deep within the brain. If widespread cancer is present, the primary consideration is to provide comfort and preserve neurological function.

NEUROBLASTOMA

Signs and Symptoms
- Pallor;
- Hypertension;
- Diarrhea;
- Abdominal mass, perhaps accompanied by liver enlargement if the tumor has spread there;
- Bone pain if tumor has spread to bone;
- Respiratory distress if tumor has spread to chest.

neurological involvement. Headaches of recent onset may be the key symptom. Neurological problems then may be evident within days or weeks. Seek medical attention for any new or persistent headache.

A thorough physical examination might be required to establish the diagnosis of brain tumor. A CT or MRI scan of the head (see page 539) might be needed to confirm the diagnosis. A chest x-ray to check for possible metastasis from the lung or other tests to evaluate other areas of the body may be needed. Cerebral arteriography (see page 513) may be required if an operation is planned.

How Serious Is a Brain Tumor?   Once a brain tumor has caused neurological symptoms it is extremely important to proceed quickly with appropriate treatment. Benign tumors frequently are curable, although sometimes their location makes total removal impossible. If a tumor infiltrates the brain in an area where the tumor tissue cannot be totally excised, recurrence is likely after surgery. Both benign and malignant tumors can produce profound and irreversible neurological impairment.

A neuroblastoma is a malignant tumor that, in 70 percent of cases, occurs first in the abdomen, often around the adrenal gland. The disease then may spread to various parts of the body, including the liver, bone marrow, and bones.

Unlike most tumors, neuroblastoma has a high rate of spontaneous regression, although why this occurs is not clear.

Neuroblastoma is found in one out of 100,000 children under the age of 15; 75 percent of cases are diagnosed by the time a child is 5, with 24 months being the median age at time of discovery. The tumor occurs slightly more often in boys.

The Diagnosis.   If your physician suspects a neuroblastoma, the site of the suspected tumor and whether it is believed to have spread will determine what diagnostic studies will be done. If there is an abdominal mass, for example, a CT scan (see page 539) may be done. To determine whether it has

CT HEAD SCAN AND MRI SCAN

The computerized scanning equipment introduced during the past 15 years has virtually revolutionized diagnostic neurology and neurosurgery. The two types of procedures most commonly available are computed tomographic (CT) scanning and magnetic resonance imaging (MRI).

Although their computerized scanning techniques are similar, CT and MRI rely on two distinct methods for producing the diagnostic image. CT scanning uses an ultrathin x-ray beam and MRI uses a very strong magnetic field. Both procedures are noninvasive.

During CT scanning, an x-ray beam passes through your body. Various tissues, such as bone or fluid, absorb different amounts of the beam; the intensity of the beam that emerges from your body is then measured by an x-ray detector. Your tissues appear as different shades of gray on the scan. Bone is at one end of this spectrum and appears white on the image; air is at the opposite end of the spectrum and appears black.

When you are in a magnetic field during MRI testing, each hydrogen atom in your body responds to the magnetic field. The degree of hydrogen response depends on the type of tissue or its water content. A magnetic field detector measures the responses of the atoms. You receive no radiation. The magnetic field may affect metallic devices such as a heart pacemaker, inner ear implant, brain aneurysm clip, or embedded shrapnel.

Scanning with CT or MRI is done by taking detector measurements from thousands of angles all around your body while you lie on a special table. These measurements are made automatically by the equipment, and all the data are then processed by computer to create a composite, three-dimensional representation of your body. Any two-dimensional plane, or slice, can be selected electronically from this representation and displayed on a television-type screen for examination. Photographic images can also be produced from the screen for further analysis.

CT and MRI scanning has several advantages over other procedures. CT shows internal structures (soft tissues) much better than conventional x-rays do, and it often reduces the need for higher-risk invasive procedures, such as cerebral arteriography (see page 513) or exploratory surgery. It is particularly useful for clear images of brain disorders, including strokes, hemorrhages, injuries, tumors, abscesses, cysts, swelling, fluid accumulation, and areas of dead brain tissue. CT scanning sometimes can distinguish benign from malignant tumors because it is sensitive enough to show their different densities.

MRI applications still are undergoing rapid development. It is particularly useful for imaging areas of your head where soft and hard tissue meet, your spinal cord, and areas affected by stroke that cannot be seen well on CT scans. MRI often is used in the diagnosis of nerve fiber disorders, such as multiple sclerosis, because of its high-resolution images of the brain's white and gray matter.

CT and MRI also are finding significant applications in the diagnosis of disorders in other parts of the body, including the kidneys, urinary tract, pancreas, and liver.

CT and MRI are safe, painless, simple procedures often done on an outpatient basis. They allow prompt diagnosis and treatment and enable effective follow-up studies.

Computed tomography (CT) is a safe, painless way to obtain a detailed image of the brain.

spread to the bone, a bone scan and bone marrow biopsy may be done.

How Serious Is Neuroblastoma?   The prognosis of this disease depends on the age of the child and how advanced the disease is. The older the child and the more widespread the disease, the more likely that the cancer will not respond to treatment.

Treatment.   If the tumor has not spread and is small, surgery alone or with local radiation therapy may offer a cure. In more advanced disease, chemotherapy may be successful. In persons with the most advanced disease, the long-term survival is less than 10 percent. A bone marrow transplantation in these children may achieve a 25 percent survival rate.

BELL'S PALSY

Signs and Symptoms
- Sagging muscles and weakness on one side of the face;
- Inability to close one eye.

Bell's palsy (also known as facial palsy) is a paralysis of the muscles that control expression on one side of your face. Bell's palsy results from damage to the facial nerve, a nerve that runs beneath the ear to the muscles of the face of the same side. This

If you have Bell's palsy, one corner of your mouth may droop and you may have difficulty retaining saliva on that side of your mouth. Most often, this disorder is temporary.

damage results in weakness of these muscles because the electrical impulses directed to them are impaired by the damaged nerve.

The cause of the disorder is unknown, and its development is not well understood. The prevalent theory is that the facial nerve becomes swollen and injured, perhaps by a viral infection such as herpes zoster (see Shingles, page 1176). The nerve then has no room to expand within its bony channel. Bell's palsy is due to this restriction or compression.

Full paralysis on one side will leave you looking expressionless, and you will have virtually no movement of the muscles from the forehead to the mouth on the paralyzed side. The corner of your mouth may droop, and you may have difficulty retaining saliva on that side of your mouth. When you move the muscles of the unaffected side, facial distortions result. The eye on your affected side may close only partially, and tears may leak from that eye. Some persons complain of pain behind the ear, in the jaw, or on the entire side of the face. You may feel that the unaffected side is twisted or contracted, and you may experience changes in salivation and sense of taste, heightened sensitivity to sound, or difficulty in speaking or eating. Extra tearing from your eye on the affected side may result if the lid loses its normal function of moving tears into your tear ducts.

One-sided facial weakness is a common neurological sign, and Bell's palsy is the most common cause. It occurs at any age, but it is most common between 30 and 60 years. Sometimes it seems to be associated with an infection of the middle ear. Annually, about 40,000 Americans get the disorder (1 person in 60 or 70 during their lifetimes). If it involves both sides of the face, other disorders such as Lyme disease or sarcoidosis may be the cause (see pages 854 and 934, respectively).

The Diagnosis.   The onset is fairly abrupt, and you may notice it when you wake up. Pain behind your ear can precede the palsy by a day or two. Maximal weakness or paralysis may be apparent within 48 hours after onset.

Your physician may be able to make a preliminary diagnosis by looking at your face and asking you to attempt to move your facial muscles. Other conditions, such as a stroke (see page 508), can cause one-sided facial paralysis, and careful evaluation is needed to exclude these disorders. Abrupt onset with no prior symptoms, however, is indicative of Bell's palsy. After several days, your physician may arrange for you to be tested by electromyography (see page 1294) to determine the severity of your nerve damage.

How Serious Is Bell's Palsy?   Bell's palsy is usually a temporary problem. In 80 percent of cases, recovery begins in 2 to 3 weeks and is complete within a few months. A mild case may be noticeable only when you smile, and it normally disappears in 1 month. A partial resolution of the paralysis by the end of the first week suggests a favorable outcome.

Recovery after total paralysis is variable, and electromyography (see page 1294) may be helpful for determining the possibility of long-term or incomplete regeneration of nerve fibers. If the damage to the facial nerve is unusually severe, the fibers may become irreversibly damaged. Another

complication can arise from misdirected regrowth of nerve fibers, which can result in contraction of other muscles during facial movement or ''crocodile tears'' during salivation.

Treatment.   Treatment is controversial. Some physicians believe that recovery, to whatever extent, will occur without treatment. If you cannot close your eye, however, it will need to be protected. Excessive dryness in your eye may lead to a corneal ulcer. A temporary patch or ointment may be recommended for sleeping. Use of moisturizing eye drops, such as methylcellulose drops, during waking hours will help guard your eye from dust and dryness. Use of eyeglasses also may help.

Physicians sometimes prescribe a corticosteroid medication, such as prednisone, to reduce the suspected swelling of your facial nerve. Physical therapy and facial massage to prevent long-term contracture may be recommended.

SEIZURES AND TICS

During normal working and sleeping, the brain cells produce various electrical patterns that can be recorded and identified with a test called electroencephalography (EEG) (see page 1294). If the electrical discharges by the brain cells become disorganized, a convulsion or seizure occurs.

Seizures have many causes, and a single episode does not always mean you have a seizure disorder. When seizures recur, however, the condition is termed a seizure disorder. This designation is preferred to the older term epilepsy.

Nervous tension or pain can cause you to engage in habitual movements, known as tics, which are not seizures. These disorders are described on the following pages.

GRAND MAL SEIZURE

Signs and Symptoms
* Episode of loss of consciousness with convulsions.

A grand mal seizure starts with a loss of consciousness and falling down, followed

by a 15- to 20-second period with muscle rigidity (tonic phase) and then a 1- to 2-minute period of violent, rhythmic convulsions (clonic phase). The seizure ends with a few minutes of deep, relaxed sleep before consciousness returns with no memory of the seizure. You may experience a headache and drowsiness or confusion afterward. A grand mal seizure also is called a generalized tonic-clonic seizure in reference to its phases.

Generalized or total seizures such as grand mal seizures are due to abnormal electrical activity throughout the brain. In most cases seizures seem to occur randomly, but for some susceptible persons, they are associated with menstruation and, rarely, reactions to a specific stimulation by light, sound, touch, or reading. Sometimes the seizures will involve only a few muscles, such as one side of the face or one extremity. This is called a focal seizure, in contrast to the usual generalized seizure, or jacksonian seizure.

Research has shown that seizures can be produced in normal brains by various chemical and electrical stimulants. Sometimes seizures run in families. Other identified causes for recurring seizures include scar tissue from brain disease or injury; brain infection, tumor, abscess, or hemorrhage; alcohol or drug withdrawal; and metabolic disturbances from kidney or liver disease. Nevertheless, the cause frequently is unknown when the disorder starts before age 25 years. Seizures that start after age 25 years may be caused by slowly growing brain tumors.

Up to 2 percent of the population have a seizure disorder, and as many as 10 percent of the population have a single seizure episode. Of these, the vast majority are grand mal seizures, sometimes in combination with other types of seizure. Two other types of seizure disorders are discussed below.

The Diagnosis.   Grand mal seizure is recognized easily, but the cause may be difficult to diagnose. Your physician will need a detailed medical history. After physical and neurological examinations, you will need electroencephalography (see page 1294). Other diagnostic tests may include CT or MRI (see page 539), blood tests, or lumbar puncture (see page 530). Focal or jacksonian seizures are sometimes caused by scarring or tumor in a specific part of the brain. A CT or MRI scan may help confirm such a diagnosis.

How Serious Is Grand Mal Seizure?   A single seizure, with no other signs of abnormality, does not necessarily mean you have a seizure disorder. Recurrence, however, may indicate a serious underlying disorder.

A seizure that produces either loss of awareness or control can be dangerous if you are driving a car or operating other equipment. Therefore, many states have licensing restrictions that are related to how well your seizures are controlled. Seizures also can produce injuries associated with falling.

Treatment.   If your seizures are infrequent, you can lead a relatively normal life with the grand mal form. Medication may be very successful in controlling this type of seizure disorder. Discuss antiseizure medication side effects with your physician. Pregnancy may alter your need for medicine. Inform your physician if you are contemplating becoming pregnant. Avoid lack of sleep, forgetting medication, and excess alcohol. Reg-

ular and adequate rest is important. Wear a bracelet or necklace stating who should be contacted if a seizure occurs.

Children with a seizure disorder may attend school while taking medication.

Medication.   Medication controls or greatly reduces seizures for more than 75 percent of the affected persons. Drug selection and dosage requires close medical supervision and testing. You may have side effects such as drowsiness, restlessness, upset stomach, or a rash. In some cases, the medication can be discontinued after several years without seizures, but this must be done by a gradual decrease in dosage, not abruptly. If your seizures are due to an underlying condition such as an infection or endocrine disorder, they may be eliminated when the cause is treated.

Surgery.   Seizures caused by a brain tumor, abscess, or hemorrhage may stop after surgical removal of the lesion.

PETIT MAL SEIZURE

Signs and Symptoms
* Brief, sudden absence of conscious activity;
* Decline in a child's learning ability.

Petit mal seizure, also called absence seizure, is a form of seizure disorder. Each seizure lasts only seconds or minutes, but hundreds may occur each day. In typical seizures, there may be no movement at all, fluttering eyelids, or a twitching hand during the brief lapse of consciousness. Full recovery takes only seconds, and afterward you will have no confusion. You will not remember the incident.

Atypical petit mal seizures include more noticeable muscle movement such as rhythmic convulsions, rigidity, or falling down. After atypical seizures there may be a period of confusion and recovery takes longer than after typical petit mal seizures.

In either case, these seizures almost always begin in children age 6 to 12 years, and they rarely start after age 20 years. After onset, they may occur for weeks or months before any adult notices them because they usually occur when the child is sitting quietly and seldom during physical activity. Your child may begin to have learning problems before you or a teacher discovers the seizures.

Less than 10 percent of all persons with seizure disorders have petit mal seizures, sometimes in combination with other types of seizure. Usually, no identifiable cause is found for the typical seizures, and your child probably is neurologically normal otherwise. Atypical seizures often are associated with other neurological disorders that may or may not have identifiable causes, such as congenital malformations in the brain, chemical disturbances from kidney or liver disease, or brain tissue scarring from head or birth injuries.

The Diagnosis. No findings on physical or neurological examination will confirm the diagnosis of petit mal seizures. Your child will need electroencephalography (see page 1294) to test for signs of the distinctive brain electrical pattern associated with these seizures. Your physician also may order blood tests or a CT scan (see page 539) to check for other possible causes for the symptoms.

How Serious Is Petit Mal Seizure? About 90 percent of all children with petit mal seizures have significantly fewer or no seizures when they take medication. About a third outgrow the seizures, a third continue with only petit mal seizures, and a third continue with petit mal and have occasional grand mal seizures (see page 541).

Treatment. Most children with typical petit mal seizures can live fairly normal lives and should be encouraged to do so. Your physician probably will advise you that your child can participate in physical activities and school with few restrictions. There may be some restrictions with driving or operating dangerous equipment when your child gets older.

Medication. Petit mal seizures are very responsive to antiseizure medications. On these medications, most persons are seizure-free. Close medical supervision and testing are required to determine the best drug and dosage for your child. These drugs may cause side effects such as dizziness, upset stomach, or lethargy.

FEBRILE SEIZURE

Signs and Symptoms
• Brief episode of loss of consciousness and convulsions during fever.

Febrile seizure is a type of grand mal seizure (see page 541). It frequently occurs in young children between 3 months and 5 years old during an illness with fever. Susceptibility to fever-induced seizures often runs in families, and your child probably will outgrow this reaction to fever.

Approximately 2 to 5 percent of children have seizures when they get a fever. The cause is unknown, but seizures can occur easily and from many causes. Children also can have recurring seizures (epilepsy) that are not associated with fever.

The Diagnosis. If your child has a convulsion while a fever is present, seek medical attention immediately. Often the seizures occur when the temperature is either rising or falling rapidly. Other, more serious diseases such as meningitis (see page 527), encephalitis (see page 529), or poisoning also may first become apparent with this combination of symptoms, and emergency treatment may be required.

Your child's physician will ask about your family medical history and will perform physical and neurological examinations on your child. A lumbar puncture (see page 530) may be required at this time to help rule out the presence of serious infections that may have caused the seizures. If the fever is clearly due to a common childhood illness, only electroencephalography (see page 1294) will be required to test for abnormalities in the electrical activity of the brain. If there is no sign of abnormality, the diagnosis is usually febrile seizure.

When there is any sign of another cause for the fever or the seizure, however, a CT scan or MRI (see page 539), lumbar puncture (if not done earlier), blood tests, and further EEG testing may be required.

How Serious Is Febrile Seizure? Febrile seizure is not a chronic condition. It happens suddenly and only when your child has a fever. If the seizure causes a loss of consciousness that does not last more than 5 minutes, the chances of mental impairment or a convulsive disorder are minimal.

There is a significant risk of future seizures, however, if your child has a prolonged seizure, local rather than general convulsions, an abnormal electroencephalographic recording, or signs of any neurological abnormality. Most often, seizures can be controlled or reduced significantly with medication.

Treatment. Your child's febrile seizure should last only a few minutes. Place your child on the ground or lying flat and remove any nearby objects that could be a source of injury. Do not put anything into your child's mouth during a seizure. Roll the child onto his or her side to make sure the tongue does not block breathing, and then call your physician. Rapidly cooling the child does not prevent further seizures.

Medication.   After your child has a single episode of seizure during a fever, your physician may or may not prescribe medication. When susceptibility to febrile seizure is demonstrated by at least two episodes, your physician may recommend quick and vigorous control of fever during childhood illness as a way to avoid seizures. An alternative procedure is continuing treatment with anticonvulsant medication. In this event, extensive medical tests and supervision are required to select the best drug and dosage. Side effects, such as restlessness, may result from the medication.

If no seizures occur after a few years or less and results of electroencephalography and neurological examinations are normal, your physician will start reducing your child's medication dosage. Many children eventually can stop taking all medication and remain free of seizures.

TEMPORAL LOBE SEIZURE

Signs and Symptoms
- Sensory or mental aberrations preceding a seizure;
- Brief loss of awareness.

Temporal lobe seizures frequently are preceded by a peculiar sensation (aura) and are followed by physical movements. These seizures most often originate in the temporal lobe areas of your brain, the portion that extends from your temple to just past your ear. If the seizure is associated with loss of consciousness, it may be termed a complex partial seizure. Another name for this disorder is psychomotor seizure. The recurrence of this or any other type of seizure is called a seizure disorder.

Temporal lobe seizures frequently are characterized by 1- to 2-minute episodes of lost awareness or contact with your surroundings. The physical movement can be a simple repetitive act such as lip smacking or picking at your clothes. You may take seconds to hours to recover normal mental activity, and you will not remember the seizure.

Complex partial seizures are due to abnormal electrical activity in the temporal lobe or, less frequently, in another part of the brain. The aura, the first symptom, is caused by an electrical discharge in the area. This is followed by spread of the abnormal firing of the brain's nerve cells, which gives rise to other manifestations of the seizure such as loss of awareness.

The aura, which usually precedes the seizure by seconds or a few minutes, is variously described as hallucinations (sight, sound, or smell), visual illusions (rotating, shrinking, or magnifying), distorted understanding (déjà vu, or recurrent memory), and sudden, intense emotion (anxiety or fear).

Seizures sometimes are caused by a specific disorder in the temporal lobe, such as microscopic scars or a tumor, but often there is no identifiable cause. Of the 1 million to 5 million persons in the United States with a seizure disorder, about one-half have complex partial seizures.

The Diagnosis.   Your physician will need an extensive medical history for you and possibly your family. Diagnostic tests usually include electroencephalography (see page 1294), blood tests, and CT scan or MRI (see page 539).

How Serious Are Temporal Lobe Seizures?   Once they begin, these seizures may become a chronic condition and may not be controllable with medication. Sometimes the source of the abnormality can be removed surgically; the frequency of seizures is reduced significantly in three or four out of five persons who have such an operation. Associated congenital or personality disorders sometimes exist and may not change after operation.

A medical bracelet can be helpful. These bracelets state who should be contacted if a seizure occurs and what medications are to be used.

Treatment. *Medication.* You will require long-term use of medications to minimize seizures. Medication may not completely control these seizures. Selection of the drug and its dosage requires close medical supervision and testing. These medications may produce side effects such as restlessness or sedation. Complex partial seizures are harder to control with medication than are other seizures. New anticonvulsant drugs are being tested for this purpose.

Surgery. When the cause of temporal lobe seizures can be identified as a tumor or can be localized to an area within one lobe, operation may be recommended to remove the source.

FACIAL TICS

Signs and Symptoms
- Habitual, repetitive movements or twitches of the face.

Facial tics are semivoluntary mannerisms, usually starting in childhood and occurring without your awareness. Grimaces, eye or mouth twitches, and head turning may be chronic, benign disorders with no known cause except tension.

Multiple tics, such as in Gilles de la Tourette's syndrome, include facial tics, shoulder or arm movements, and vocalizations (sniffing, grunting, or compulsive swearing). This syndrome is 4 times more frequent in boys than girls and sometimes runs in families. An evaluation is needed to exclude other disorders.

Treatment. *Medication.* Sometimes no medication is needed. Small dosages of anticonvulsants can be used for mild tics. Other drugs (called neuroleptic drugs) control multiple tics in a significant number of persons.

HEADACHES

Almost everyone experiences a headache at one time or another. During a few hours of television viewing, you probably will see several advertisements for painkillers to ease this common complaint. Headaches have many causes, and the site, severity, and frequency with which they occur vary greatly.

Your brain tissue cannot ache. In fact, pain cannot occur in most of your skull and a large portion of your brain membranes. Observations made during surgery indicate that only certain structures in your head are pain-sensitive. On the outside of the skull, these structures include your skin and the tissues lying just beneath it: muscles, arteries, the skull coating, eyes, ears, and nasal and sinus cavities. The pain-sensitive structures inside your skull include arteries, venous sinuses and their tributary veins, parts of the brain's outer membrane at the base of the brain, and certain cranial and cervical nerves. Pain is practically the only sensation produced by stimulating these structures.

Cranial or cervical nerves send pain sensations from these parts of your head to your central nervous system. Dental and jaw pain, for example, is conveyed by the cranial nerves. Your cervical nerves convey messages about pain in your neck and the base of your head.

Outside your skull, pain is caused by inflammation or tension in muscles, inflammation of scalp arteries, and inflammation in your sinuses, ears, or gums. Inside your skull, enlargement or contraction of arteries, inflammation of brain membranes, and pressure from a tumor or hemorrhage can cause a headache.

Inflammation of your scalp arteries and subsequent stretching of pain-sensitive structures is associated with migraine and cluster headaches. Research suggests that migraine may be due to changes in your brain's blood vessels from disturbances in a chemical called serotonin, which is produced by nerve cells. Cluster headaches are more likely due to an interaction of the nerves and arteries of the head and release of a brain chemical transmitter. Tension headaches may be a combination of spastic contraction of muscles and enlargement of arteries in your scalp. Physicians usually refer to headaches in two major categories: muscle-contraction headaches and blood vessel (vascular) headaches.

Your physician's diagnosis will require a medical history and examination. If your headache is of recent onset, if it occurs in abrupt attacks, if it is triggered by exertion, if it is typically present in the morning and accompanied by vomiting, or if it is associated with other symptoms such as fever, weight loss, or neurological abnormalities, further testing may be required.

Testing may include a CT scan of your head (see page 539) to look for any structural abnormalities and to examine your sinuses, facial bones, and neck tissue and bones. X-rays of the upper spine may be needed if your headaches began after a head or neck injury. Your physician may require other tests such as MRI (see page 539), a lumbar puncture (see page 530), or cerebral arteriography (see page 513) and also may consult with medical specialists to complete your diagnosis.

Your headache might feel dull, throbbing, or sharp. Your description of the quality of your pain will be helpful in diagnosing what type of headache you have. A throbbing pain is usually a vascular headache. When accompanied by nausea or transient visual disturbances, it is probably a migraine. Sharp, stabbing pain is more likely to be neuralgia (see page 559). Steady, nonthrobbing pain that may feel like a tight band is usually a tension headache.

Unrelieved headache pain that continues for 6 months or more as a major and disabling condition is considered chronic. Approximately 42 million Americans have chronic headaches, of which migraine and tension headaches are some of the most common forms. These two types of headaches are described on pages 549 and 547, respectively.

Another common form is sinus infection headache. It usually is felt in your forehead, cheek, eye, or top of your skull. Headaches of this sort may also be caused by a vacuum or suction on the sinus wall. This occurs when air can enter the sinus because of congestion of the nose due to an infection or allergy. The vacuum effect also may be the source of the ear and sinus pain many people experience during the descent of an airplane, especially when they have a cold.

Premenstrual headaches, typically migraine or tension headaches, occur in some women during the premenstrual syndrome and usually disappear during the first day of vaginal bleeding. Headaches from high blood pressure tend to occur in the morning, are uncommon, and occur only with very severe hypertension. Vascular headaches are also common in the morning. Headache can result from an infection in your nasal cavity, and it can be particularly painful when you bend over. Eyestrain headaches may occur after long periods of reading or driving a car at night. Headaches may occur from overexertion and can last intermittently for weeks or months.

Head pain also can be an indication of many underlying diseases. An acute, severe headache with tingling sensations, nausea, and vision or speech difficulties, for example, may be a symptom of a very serious cerebral hemorrhage. Any persistent headache of recent onset is potentially serious because it may be a symptom of a tumor, hemorrhage, or an aneurysm and also of meningitis, encephalitis, polio, abscess in the brain, or hemorrhage within the head. You need not be concerned by the occasional headache, but if one appears with other less-usual symptoms or if you have one that you might call "the worst ever," seek medical help.

For the common, everyday headache that may be caused by fatigue, stress, or overuse of alcohol or tobacco, your physician may advise you to avoid the offending activity and take a non-narcotic analgesic painkiller such as aspirin or acetaminophen.

Chronic headaches are more of a problem; non-narcotic analgesics may relieve your pain but not get rid of it completely or prevent it from coming back. Antidepressant drugs may be prescribed; they are believed to work on certain brain chemicals to lessen pain and to modify your perception of it. Narcotic analgesics, such as codeine, may bring relief and can be particularly useful in combination with aspirin or acetaminophen. However, these should be used with caution because of the risk of addiction. The stronger the dose, the worse the side effects of nausea, constipation, and drowsiness. Ergot preparations or methysergide may be

ASSESSING YOUR HEADACHES

To help assess your pain, your physician may ask several questions about your headaches, such as the following.

- What is your age?
- What is the circumstance of a headache's onset?
- How frequently do they occur?

- Do they occur at regular intervals, and at what time of day or night do they occur?
- Where do you experience the first pain?
- What does the pain feel like? Is it intense?
- Do your headaches begin slowly or rapidly and how fast do your headaches go from beginning to peak?
- How long do your headaches typically last?

- Do other symptoms precede your headache?
- Do symptoms accompany your headache?
- What kinds of things make them go away?
- Is there a history of headaches in your family?
- What are your present and past responses to medication?
- What ideas do you have about your headaches?
- Why are you seeking help now?

---

used to treat severe vascular headaches. These two types of medication are unsafe if you are pregnant or breast-feeding or have high blood pressure or poor blood supply to your brain or legs.

Your physician will have two goals in helping control your chronic pain. First, he or she will try to simplify and minimize your medications to eliminate redundant and ineffective drugs. Dosages of your remaining medication will be decreased systematically until you are taking only those drugs that have the most benefit and the least side effects. Second, your physician will try to help you develop a better understanding of your pain and the factors that make it worse so that you can avoid them and increase your ability to function. Antidepressant medication may be useful for helping you do whatever is required to cut down your rate of headaches, from practiced relaxation techniques (see page 548) to a serious change in lifestyle.

TENSION HEADACHES

Signs and Symptoms
- A dull or pressure-like pain in the scalp, temples, or back of the neck.

A tension headache (also known as a muscle-contraction headache) is usually felt as diffuse and intense pain over the top of your head or back of your neck. It may feel like fullness or pressure, as if your head were surrounded by a constricting band or vise. The cause for this sensation is thought to be,

at least in some cases, a tight, spastic contraction of the cranial and cervical muscles on the outside of your skull. There is some evidence that enlargement of the blood vessels in your scalp also may contribute to the pain.

You may find it difficult to sleep. Some people complain of a superficial stinging or burning sensation on their skin. The headaches may be episodic. These headaches are very common in the general population. Because they respond well to over-the-counter analgesic painkillers, persons with episodic headache usually do not consult their physicians. Tension headaches that occur two or more times weekly for a period of months or longer are considered chronic. Some persons report such headaches over a period of years or even decades. The headache pain usually has a waxing and waning quality.

Tension headaches are probably the most common cause of head pain. Some of them may be caused by poor posture, working in awkward conditions, or a sudden strain. Stress, depression, and anxiety are the most common triggers.

These headaches may strike persons of any age or sex. The chronic form most frequently develops during middle age, and it can last for several years after onset.

The Diagnosis. To establish a diagnosis, your physician will exclude other possible sources for your pain. Tests may include a urinalysis, vision tests, sinus x-ray, skull x-ray, or a CT scan (see page 539).

MUSCLE RELAXATION TECHNIQUES

When physicians refer to a muscle-tension problem, primarily involving pain, they are speaking about a habit. People sometimes develop, over years, *habitual* muscle responses to stress (a tension habit). Muscle relaxation techniques have been developed to deal with pain from muscle tension. These techniques have been useful in disorders such as tension headaches, TMJ syndrome (see page 584), and backaches.

You may set yourself up for your symptoms. After a particularly trying day you may wonder just when your headache will begin. You need strategy and discipline to break this cycle of tension causing pain causing more tension. Relaxation classes, yoga, walking, and jogging are a few of the many ways people help themselves. Practiced relaxation techniques have been successful stress relievers for many individuals.

Techniques vary, and there are many cassettes, books, and videotapes to help you. The more you practice, the easier it will become to avoid your particular expression of stress.

If you feel anxious, sit in a comfortable chair or lie down. Close your eyes. Begin to breathe slowly and deeply. Keep breathing deeply and rhythmically throughout the session. As you breathe in, let your stomach and chest expand with air. Contract them as you breathe out. In between, hold your breath for a few seconds. After some practice, a few breaths taken this way can calm you down during stressful situations.

Now tense the muscles of your toes and press down your feet. Hold them taut. Feel the tension in your toes and feet. Notice where the tightness is. Keep the muscles tight and concentrate on the tension for about 20 seconds. Then relax your toes and feet. Feel the tension leave your muscles. Feel them grow more and more relaxed, more and more heavy. Feel the warmth circulate through them as the tension drains away. Let all the tension in your toes and feet go. Say the words "calm" and "relax" silently to yourself. Put away all other thoughts. Let yourself feel more and more relaxed, and let that feeling increase.

When your feet and toes feel limp, perhaps in 30 seconds or more, go through the same procedure with another set of nearby muscles, moving very slowly up your body with one group of muscles at a time: your ankles and lower legs, your thighs, your pelvis and buttocks, your stomach, your fists, your arms, and your shoulders. Do not rush. Press your head into the cushion or pillow and tense the muscles in your neck. Clench your jaws. Frown and squint your eyes. As you relax each section of your neck and head, keep telling yourself "calm" and "relax." Tell yourself how good it feels when you relax that part, and breathe deeply and fully.

When your entire body feels relaxed, keep your eyes closed and feel your heaviness. Press your heaviness into the surface you are on. As you breathe deeply, tell yourself several times that you are feeling very refreshed. Count to three and open your eyes (see Controlling Stress, page 399).

Your physician may want information about how you feel and will look for evidence of anxiety or depression and of whether you have any unusual fears about the state of your health. You may be asked whether there is any particular stress in your job or family situation that is associated with worsening of the headache.

How Serious Are Tension Headaches?
Tension headaches are not life-threatening and do not lead to more serious disorders. They may, however, be a sign that you are depressed and anxious or subject to stress. Some persons who have tension headache need treatment for depression.

Treatment. Tension headaches respond best to massage, hot and cold showers, practiced relaxation techniques (see Biofeedback, page 1036), and close attention to adequate rest and exercise. Physical therapy may be helpful. Keep a headache diary, as described in the section on migraine headaches (see page 549), to try to identify the source of your pain. Medication is not a cure. Moreover, the effectiveness of your painkillers or other drugs may eventually wear off. If tension headaches persist, your body may be telling you that serious changes are needed in your lifestyle.

Medication. Simple analgesics such as aspirin, acetaminophen, or ibuprofen are usually effective. Antidepressant drugs may be prescribed for a chronic problem. Avoid tranquilizers.

MIGRAINE HEADACHES

Signs and Symptoms
- Intense head pain, sometimes accompanied by nausea and vomiting;
- Sparkling, rainbow-like colors, blank spots in your field of vision, or other auras.

Migraines are also known as vascular headaches. The exact cause of migraines is unknown, although evidence suggests involvement of the blood vessels of your head.

A migraine headache usually begins in the early morning or during the day with intense, gripping pain on one side of your head that may gradually spread. The pain begins to throb on one side or over your entire head. It reaches the peak of severity in minutes to an hour or two and lasts for hours to 2 days unless it is treated. It is often terminated by sleep, but you may be listless after waking up. The frequency of attacks can range from daily to one in several months. These attacks can be associated with nausea and, at times, vomiting.

Migraine has several clinical patterns: classic migraine (migraine with typical aura), common migraine (migraine without aura), and complicated migraine.

In classic migraine, your headache is preceded by warning symptoms. Hours before the headache you may feel elated, full of energy, thirsty, hungry for sweets, drowsy, irritable, or depressed. About 20 minutes before the headache, neurological symptoms often appear, including sparkling flashes of light, dazzling zigzag lines, slowly spreading blind spots, dizziness, or a feeling of numbness on one side of your body. The symptoms preceding the headache are referred to as the aura.

Common migraine has no characteristic warning symptoms. The headache usually builds to full intensity over several minutes or longer.

Complicated migraine is associated with prolonged neurological symptoms that may outlast your head pain. These may include a slowly spreading weakness or numbness of your face, a hand, or a leg; a tingling and numbness in your lips; or difficulty with talking or writing. Rarely, these symptoms can be permanent, presumably because of a stroke (infarct).

Less common forms of migraine headache include familial hemiplegic migraine (migraine with aura and paralysis of one side of the body, and the affected person has at least one immediate relative who has identical attacks), migraine aura without headache (occurs mostly in elderly persons), ophthalmoplegic migraine (migraine with partial paralysis of the eyes), status migrainous (migraine persisting longer than 72 hours), and migrainous infarction (one or more aura symptoms that persist unabated for longer than 21 days).

Migraines may begin in childhood, adolescence, or early adulthood and tend to taper off in number and intensity as you grow older. It is a common disorder that strikes many persons. Women are 3 times more likely to have migraines than men. Migraine may be associated with premenstrual tension. Attacks tend to decrease during pregnancy. There is a family history of migraine in about half of all cases.

The biological causes of migraine are unknown, but many precipitating factors have been identified. A period of hard work followed by relaxation may lead to a "weekend migraine." Stress, premenstrual changes, alcohol consumption, hunger, or use of oral contraceptives causes migraines in some persons. Certain foods may produce attacks; these include red wine, chocolate, aged cheese, milk, chicken livers, meats preserved in nitrates, or anything prepared with monosodium glutamate. Some persons even report that exposure to sunlight or exercise triggers their attacks.

The Diagnosis.   If you have migraines with characteristic warning symptoms or a family history of these headaches, your physician probably will have little difficulty diagnosing the condition. If you do not have these traits or if the headaches are severe and of recent onset, you may need testing to rule out tumors, aneurysms, or other structural disorders that could cause your pain. You may need to have a lumbar puncture (see page 530) so that your cerebrospinal fluid can be analyzed, skull and sinus x-rays, vision tests, and CT scanning (see page 539).

How Serious Are Migraine Headaches?
Migraine is a chronic disorder without cure.

The headaches are not life-threatening, and there is no proof that they lead to other disorders. With treatment, you should be able to reduce the number and severity of attacks.

Treatment. *For Acute Attacks.* Mild analgesics such as aspirin, acetaminophen, ibuprofen, naproxen sodium, or other nonsteroidal anti-inflammatory drugs may provide relief for mild to moderate migraines.

A combination of analgesic and barbiturate agents (such as aspirin, caffeine, and butalbital) helps some patients. The regular use of barbiturate compounds, however, may trigger daily headaches, and therefore they should not be used more than 2 days a week.

Antinauseants, such as metoclopramide, may be prescribed if your headaches cause nausea or vomiting. Some antinauseants can be prescribed in suppository form.

A drug called ergotamine has been used effectively for acute migraine. Sometimes an analgesic painkiller is used in combination with it. Ergotamine can bring on headaches and other side effects such as nausea, vomiting, cramps, and tingling sensations. It should be used only a few times a week and not at all during pregnancy or breastfeeding.

Isometheptene is a drug related to ergotamine and provides relief for some patients when it is given in combination with an analgesic and a mild sedative (isometheptene, acetaminophen, and dichloralphenazone). Isometheptene may not be as effective as ergotamine, but it is better tolerated and produces fewer side effects.

After taking medication when the first symptoms appear, some persons respond well to rest in a darkened room and sleep, if possible, especially during a fully developed attack.

If your migraine is prolonged with continued attacks of vomiting, seek emergency medical treatment to replace lost fluids and to control the pain.

Prevention. If you know that certain foods trigger a migraine, avoid them. It also may help to avoid oversleeping on holidays and weekends. You might consider discontinuing the use of birth control pills if you take them; about 30 percent of women with migraine have increased attacks when they take oral contraceptives.

If you have frequent headaches, keep a diary to give yourself clues about what triggers your attacks. Note the time a headache began, what you ate during the preceding 24 hours, how you felt (and what you were doing) when the headache started, unusual stress, how long the headache lasted, and what made it stop. Relaxation techniques (see page 548) help some persons cut down the number of headaches.

If you have more than two migraines a month or your pain is especially prolonged, medications such as beta-adrenergic blockers, calcium entry blockers, nonsteroidal anti-inflammatory drugs, or methysergide maleate may be prescribed for daily use to prevent attacks.

CLUSTER HEADACHES

Signs and Symptoms

- Steady, boring pain in and around one eye, occurring in episodes that often begin at the same time of day or night;
- Watering and redness of an eye with nasal stuffiness on the same side of the face.

Cluster headaches are characterized by intense burning, boring pain frequently located in or around one eye and temple and occasionally in one cheek or jaw. Your affected eye is bloodshot and teary. The nostril on that side often becomes blocked and may run profusely. Other features can include reduced pupil size on the painful side, a drooping eyelid, and a flushed face.

The pain swiftly intensifies within 5 to 10 minutes to a peak that typically persists for 30 minutes to 2 hours. Affected persons usually do not lie down during an attack because this usually worsens the pain.

Cluster headaches have an abrupt onset and can happen at any time, but they most commonly occur 2 to 3 hours after you fall asleep, usually during the phase of deep sleep known as rapid eye movement (REM). Headaches can occur daily for days, weeks, or months before a remission period that lasts weeks or years (episodic attacks), or they can occur for a year or more without remission (chronic attacks). A chronic phase may begin after a period of episodic attacks.

Unlike migraine headaches, which more often affect women, cluster headaches predominantly affect men. The first attack most frequently strikes men during adolescence or their early 20s. Almost all affected persons are heavy smokers. There is usually no family history of similar headaches.

No specific cause has been found for cluster headaches. Some researchers believe these headaches are related to a chemical present in the brain and certain cranial nerves. This chemical causes blood vessels to enlarge and become painful. Consumption of alcohol can trigger cluster attacks if you are predisposed to them. Rarely, some foods may precipitate a cluster headache.

The Diagnosis.   If your symptoms are typical of cluster headaches, your physician might have little difficulty in diagnosing the condition. Nevertheless, you may need tests to exclude other ailments that can cause similar pain, including an aneurysm of the carotid artery in your head, a tumor made up of newly formed blood vessels, sinusitis, or glaucoma.

How Serious Are Cluster Headaches?
Cluster headaches are a chronic ailment. There is no known cure and little understanding of the periodic pattern of attacks. The headaches can be a lifelong disorder. The pain during an attack can be debilitating, but there is no permanent harm, and the condition does not lead to other disorders.

Treatment.   If you have cluster headache attacks, keep a diary of your personal patterns and try to identify a trigger (see Migraine Headaches, page 549).

Cluster headaches are resistant to analgesic painkillers because these drugs take effect too slowly. Inhalation of 100 percent oxygen often provides relief. This may be the most effective treatment for frequent cluster headaches that occur primarily at night.

Ergotamine tartrate in suppository, tablet, or aerosol form is an effective pain reliever for some people, but the dosage must be limited to avoid side effects, especially nausea. It also may be prescribed to prevent attacks.

Corticosteroid medications, such as prednisone, may be prescribed if your cluster headaches are of recent onset or you have a pattern of short attack episodes and long remissions. Side effects prohibit long-term use.

About 60 percent of persons with cluster headache respond to methysergide maleate, which acts to relieve and to prevent the attacks. It is used during periods of pain and is tapered off slowly during remission.

Lithium carbonate can be effective during a chronic phase of cluster headaches; then its dosage is tapered to avoid side effects.

Calcium channel blocking agents such as verapamil are effective for the prevention of cluster headaches in many persons. They often are continued for 3 to 4 weeks after the last headache and then gradually tapered and discontinued under the direction of your physician. Occasionally, if the headaches are chronic, long-term use is required.

Chronic cluster headaches may require a management program that includes two or more of these medications. Surgery on certain groups of nerve cells near the brain may be recommended if drug management has not worked for you. Operation provides relief for approximately 66 percent of persons with chronic cluster headaches, but residual muscle weakness or sensory loss in certain nerves of the face and head can be a permanent disability.

PROBLEMS OF THE SPINE AND PERIPHERAL NERVES

Your peripheral nervous system runs from your brain and spinal cord to all other parts of your body. It is the network of nerves that you use for all your movements and sensations. Damage to your spine or peripheral nerves can interfere with communication between your brain and other areas of your body.

Your symptoms can include pain in the affected area, impairment of your ability to move muscles, and numbness or abnormal sensations. The seriousness of damage may range from mild numbness that disappears in a short time to more chronic symptoms or even permanent injury such as paralysis. The following sections discuss many disorders that involve your spine and peripheral nerves.

SPINAL CORD TRAUMA

Emergency Symptoms
- Weakness, incoordination, or paralysis in a part of the body after an accident;
- Numbness or loss of sensation;
- Loss of bladder or bowel control.

Most spinal cord injuries are the result of traffic or industrial accidents, falls, gunshot wounds, and sports injuries such as from

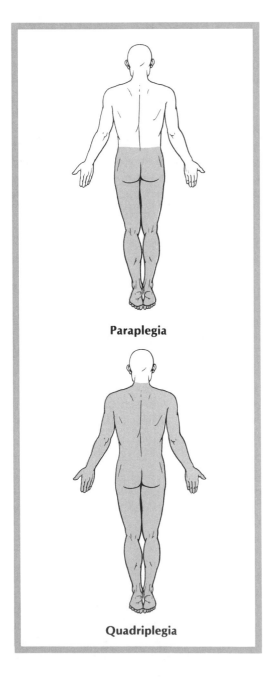

Paraplegia

Quadriplegia

diving or sledding. Sometimes a minor injury can produce severe trauma if you have a predisposing condition such as rheumatoid arthritis.

Various parts of your body can be affected by trauma at different places along your spinal cord because of the way its nerve fibers are organized. Your spinal cord is composed of long nerve fibers (tracts) leading from your brain.

The nerve tracts of the spinal cord feed into nerve roots that emerge between the vertebrae and organize into peripheral nerves that extend to your skin and muscles. If the spinal cord is injured, the nerve tracts passing through the injured region can be affected so that part or all of your corresponding muscles and sensations below that level may be impaired.

Spinal injuries occur most frequently in the lower back (lumbar) and neck (cervical) areas of the spine. A lumbar injury can affect leg and bowel and bladder control and sexual function in men. A neck injury may affect breathing and movements of the arms and hands. Trauma on one side of the spinal cord typically impairs the muscles on the same side and some sensations on the same and opposite sides of your body.

Injury may result from your spinal cord being pulled, compressed, pushed sideways, or cut. It also could result from bleeding or the accidental insertion of a fragment of bone or metal into your spinal cord. Striking your chin on the steering wheel during a traffic accident, for example, may stretch your spinal cord and cause a tear. A bullet or knife wound can cut the cord. Often, injury to the spinal cord in the neck area occurs from a sharp bending of the neck during contact while playing football, from a shallow-water dive, or from a motor vehicle accident. Injury to the lower spine may result in a compression injury of the spine. Again, car and motorcycle accidents are common causes.

Bleeding within the spinal cord can cause some permanent loss of sensation and muscle weakness. When bleeding occurs outside the spinal cord, however, the cord may be compressed; this compression results in weakness or loss of sensation of the limbs and trunk, depending on the site of the problem.

Compression also may occur from fluid accumulations and swelling in your spinal

REHABILITATION IN PARAPLEGIA AND QUADRIPLEGIA

In the first stages of paraplegia or quadriplegia, your physician will treat the injury or disease that caused the paralysis. Your physician also will watch for possible dangers such as stool or urine retention, respiratory or cardiovascular difficulty, stomach or intestinal ulcers, breakdown of skin, contractures, and phlebitis in the extremities.

After the initial injury or disease has become stable, care will focus on problems that may arise from immobilization, such as deconditioning, muscle contractures, bedsores, urinary infection, and blood clots. Early care will include changing your position frequently, range-of-motion exercises for paralyzed limbs, help with your bladder and bowel functions, applications of skin lotion, and use of soft bed coverings or flotation mattresses. Hospitalization will last from several weeks to several months, depending on the cause of the paralysis and the progress of your therapy.

During this time, a hospital social worker will begin assembling a rehabilitation team to work with your physician. Your team may include a physiatrist, a physical therapist, an occupational therapist, a rehabilitation nurse, a rehabilitation psychologist, a medical social worker, a recreation therapist, and any other professionals needed to design an appropriate therapy program for you. Their main goals will be to improve your remaining muscle strength and to give you the greatest possible mobility and independence for living a full and active life.

Physical therapy (see page 526) will include exercise and various therapeutic agents, such as whirlpool baths, to relieve your pain and relax your muscles. You will be given training on day-to-day tasks and on the devices you need to assist you, such as a wheelchair or equipment that can make it easier to fasten buttons or dial a telephone. This therapy may require several months in a rehabilitation facility.

The rehabilitation team will smooth your transition to living at home through short-term leaves from the hospital. They will acquaint you with support services in your community and share information and expertise for optimal care. The medical services in your community will be directed by your physician: he or she will monitor your health and help you, with the assistance of your family or friends, to adapt to a lifestyle that is healthy and as independent as possible.

Needed equipment and modifications in your home should be determined with your rehabilitation professionals: the goal is optimal independence and efficiency at minimal cost. Transportation needs also are best addressed in collaboration with the rehabilitation team.

Your mental state is extremely important. Sudden disability almost always is followed by devastating depression. Many handicapped persons learn to counter their depression by vigorous rehabilitative activity. It is essential for you to find or rediscover interesting things to do for yourself and for and with others. In addition, there are many support groups and peer counselors to help you.

---

cord. The resulting paralysis may continue for several days and then improve dramatically when the swelling subsides or the accumulated fluid is removed surgically, although some impairment may persist.

Most cuts and other severe forms of trauma to the spinal cord will cause permanent disability or paralysis because nerve fibers seldom regenerate. Paralysis below the neck can involve all four extremities (called quadriplegia) or only the legs and lower body (called paraplegia). Approximately 10,000 persons, mostly young and otherwise healthy, become paraplegics or quadriplegics each year in the United States because of spinal cord trauma. Currently, about 200,000 persons in the United States have quadriplegia.

The Diagnosis. Numbness or paralysis may occur immediately after the injury. These symptoms also might appear gradually as fluid accumulates in or around the spinal cord after an accident. Urgent medical attention is required to minimize the long-term effects of this trauma.

After a physical and neurological examination, diagnostic tests probably will be needed. These usually include x-rays, CT scanning or MRI (see page 539), or myelography (see page 555). Occasionally, lumbar puncture (see page 530) is also necessary.

How Serious Is Spinal Cord Trauma?
The immediate effect of a spinal cord injury is often paralysis or loss of sensation in part of

your body. This can be fatal if a neck injury has paralyzed breathing. The time between injury and treatment is a critical factor that can determine the extent of your recovery.

Recovery of movement or sensation within the first week usually means the eventual recovery of most or all functions. Any impairment remaining after 6 months probably will be permanent. If your bladder control remains paralyzed, as is often the case with quadriplegia or paraplegia, you become susceptible to recurring urinary tract infections. You also will be susceptible to injury of any part of your body that has impaired sensation.

Treatment. You will need emergency care, prolonged hospitalization while the injuries heal, and possibly months of specialized therapy for rehabilitation.

Medication. You may be given corticosteroids (dexamethasone or methylprednisolone) to reduce any swelling that compresses your spinal cord. Antibiotics may be required for urinary tract infections.

Surgery. Surgical procedures may be necessary to remove fragments of bone or foreign objects, to fix fractured vertebrae by fusing the bone or inserting metal pins, or to decompress the spinal cord by draining accumulated fluids.

Other Therapies. Traction may reduce some dislocations of your spine and immobilize the back for healing. Sometimes traction is accomplished by placing fixation tongs into the skull to hold it in place. Bed rest is the primary treatment. Further neurological assessment is used to check for signs that reflexes and sensations are returning.

Injuries will heal in 2 to 4 months, and then the physician can estimate how much disability will remain. At that time you may require the services of a special therapy team to obtain the best use from remaining muscle strength and to learn how to move with mechanical assistance.

SPINAL TUMOR

Signs and Symptoms
- Steadily increasing back pain;
- Numbness or cold sensations;
- Muscle weakness in one or more limbs.

Emergency Symptoms
- Loss of bowel or bladder control;
- Progressive loss of lower limb strength or sensation.

Spinal tumors are abnormal growths that can occur within your spinal cord, between its covering membranes, or outside the membranes in the spinal canal. These growths are malignant in 40 percent of cases, and the remainder are nonmalignant. Spinal cord tumors are similar to brain tumors (see page 537) but are only one-fourth as common.

Sometimes spinal tumors start elsewhere in your body (usually a lung or breast) and move through your bloodstream (metastasize) to the spinal area. More commonly, they originate in the spine itself. The cause is often unknown, although nonmalignant tumors can be congenital or hereditary.

Symptoms appear when the growing tumor presses against the spinal cord. Similar symptoms are caused by other spinal disorders that are not tumors.

If a spinal cord tumor is suspected after a physical and neurological examination, your physician may require x-rays, CT scanning or MRI (see page 539), and usually myelography (see page 555) to complete the diagnosis.

If you are diagnosed as having a spinal tumor, seek treatment as quickly as possible to minimize the risk of permanent impairment.

Treatment. Corticosteroids (such as dexamethasone) are used to reduce spinal cord swelling. Surgical removal is usually successful for isolated tumors outside the spinal cord. Other tumors may not be completely removable, and radiation therapy may be needed. Early diagnosis and treatment provide a higher success rate, although neurological symptoms often may continue after initial treatments. Physical therapy programs often are needed after completion of surgical or radiation therapy.

CERVICAL SPONDYLOSIS

Signs and Symptoms
- Pain or stiffness in the neck;

- Pain, numbness, or pins-and-needles sensation in the shoulder or arm;
- Numbness or weakness in the legs or arms;
- Bladder control problems;
- Imbalance or stiffness of the legs.

Cervical spondylosis (cervical osteoarthritis) is the growth of bone spurs on the vertebrae in your neck. This happens slowly, and your neck will become stiff gradually. The bone spurs eventually may press against the peripheral nerve roots leading to your shoulders and arms. This compression causes pain or other sensations in these areas. If the spurs also press against your spinal cord, your leg muscles and bladder and bowel muscles can be affected.

A neck injury can lead to spondylosis many years later. However, the bone spurs generally are caused by normal aging, and this disorder is common in older people. As the discs of your neck vertebrae become worn and thin, they can prolapse (see page 990) or allow the bone growths of spondylosis, or both. The symptoms are similar, but spondylosis is usually much less acute than a herniated disc.

MYELOGRAPHY

Myelography is a diagnostic examination that is performed while you are lying face down on a tiltable x-ray table. A local anesthetic is injected into the skin over the small of the back. A needle is inserted between two of your lower vertebrae, and a small amount of your cerebrospinal fluid is withdrawn.

Contrast medium then is injected slowly through the lumbar puncture needle. A series of x-rays are then made to show the configuration of the space around the spinal cord and whether it is distorted by the presence of a protruded disc or bony spur. After this injection, your diagnostic team can see the medium in your spinal area on x-rays. The table is tilted up and down to move the medium to the location of the suspected disorder in your spine.

Once the medium is appropriately located, x-rays are taken from different directions until the problem area can be seen clearly. Most contrast agents are absorbed by the bloodstream and excreted in the urine. Therefore, they generally do not have to be removed when myelography has been completed.

You may feel pressure or nausea during the injection, although your preparation beforehand should minimize these effects. Afterward, you may have a head-

In myelography, a liquid "dye" (contrast medium) is injected through a needle (see arrow) into the space around your spinal cord.

ache because of changes in the pressure of your cerebrospinal fluid. Lying down will help alleviate your headache, which is usually short-lived.

You probably will be hospitalized for the test, and no food or drink will be allowed for several hours before it. You may be given a sedative. The procedure generally requires 45 to 90 minutes.

There are risks associated with myelography. Some conditions, such as pressure on your spinal cord from a tumor or herniated disc, can be worsened from the change in cerebrospinal fluid pressure, and prompt operation may be required.

The risks involved with myelography are well understood, and significant complications are rare. Noninvasive diagnostic tests, such as CT or MRI, provide good resolution and often are used for a general diagnosis of spinal disorders. In many cases, however, myelography continues to be the preferred test because its resolution generally is sharper and fluid obtained from the puncture provides additional diagnostic information. With myelography, your physician can test your cerebrospinal fluid for evidence of infection, inflammation, and cancer cells.

The Diagnosis. A stiff neck is the key symptom, and it may not be very painful. If your symptoms become troublesome, your physician may require a neck x-ray or a CT or MRI scan (see page 539) to diagnose how much the spurs interfere with your nerve roots and spinal cord. When there is pressure on the spinal cord or nerve roots, your physician probably will need a myelogram (see page 555) to determine whether you need an operation.

How Serious Is Cervical Spondylosis?

The symptoms of cervical spondylosis are often mild, and you may never require medical treatment. Your discomfort may be chronic or occur only under certain circumstances, such as sleeping in the wrong position or turning your head suddenly.

Cervical spondylosis causes permanent disability in a few cases when there is pressure on the spinal cord or nerve roots.

Treatment. For a mild case of cervical spondylosis, your physician may recommend exercises, the use of a neck collar, or traction therapy at home. Traction involves using a head halter, carefully selected weights, and a pulley arrangement to stretch your neck for 15 to 30 minutes at a time.

For a more severe case, you may need 1 or 2 weeks of hospitalization, complete bed rest, and neck traction. You may need exercises and medication to loosen your neck muscles and to relieve symptoms.

Medication. Your physician may prescribe analgesic drugs (painkillers) or a muscle relaxant.

Surgery. Surgery may be required to remove the bone growths and to fuse your vertebrae. Fusion of two or more vertebrae may help by stiffening that part of the neck or back and thus preventing painful movement or neurological problems related to compression of the spinal cord or nerve roots by the unstable spine.

GUILLAIN-BARRÉ SYNDROME

Signs and Symptoms
- Spreading numbness and tingling in the fingers or toes;
- Muscle weakness.

Emergency Symptoms
- Widespread tingling and numbness;
- Difficulty breathing.

Guillain-Barré syndrome is acute and frequently causes severe damage to all or part of your peripheral nerves (see also Peripheral Neuropathies, page 557). The illness results from inflammation and destruction of the myelin sheath that covers your nerve fibers.

The cause of Guillain-Barré syndrome is unknown, but in two-thirds of the cases it occurs after a viral infection, either one you know about or one that is found by subsequent blood tests. The viral infection may be a form of herpes, such as Epstein-Barr virus, but it also can follow flu, a cold, or other minor infection. The syndrome also may develop with other conditions such as Hodgkin's disease (see page 489).

Guillain-Barré syndrome sometimes is associated with medical procedures. Five to 10 percent of all cases occur after an operation. For a brief period, a vaccine was thought to be a potential cause. Initial concern was raised after many cases of Guillain-Barré syndrome were reported after a major flu vaccination program in 1976 and 1977. Further study revealed that the number of cases was no greater than what would have occurred without the vaccination.

Your symptoms can appear a few days to a week or two after the causative infection or 1 to 4 weeks after operation. Tingling sensations in your fingers and toes may be followed by general muscle weakness. A sensation of weakness usually spreads from your legs to your arms and face. In severe cases, weakness becomes paralysis, and your respiratory muscles also are affected. The muscles responsible for eye movement, facial movements, speaking, chewing, and swallowing also may become weak or paralyzed.

The syndrome occurs at a rate of 3,500 cases annually in the United States and Canada. It can strike any race at any age.

The Diagnosis. The diagnosis will be based on your symptoms, a physical examination, tests such as electromyography (see page 1294), and analysis of cerebrospinal fluid extracted by lumbar puncture (see page 530).

How Serious Is Guillain-Barré Syndrome?

In its severe form, Guillain-Barré syndrome is a medical emergency and may require intensive-care hospitalization. A few persons with Guillain-Barré syndrome need respiratory assistance at some point during the illness.

Most often, recovery occurs over a period of months. If you are severely affected, you will need long-term rehabilitation to regain your independence. Some permanent impairment remains in about 10 percent of cases. The mortality rate is 3 or 4 percent.

Treatment.   Guillain-Barré syndrome generally is treated by supportive care. A procedure called plasmapheresis, which removes plasma and damaging antibodies from your blood, is used during the first few weeks of a severe attack. This may improve your chance for full recovery.

Once your condition is stabilized, rehabilitation therapy is initiated. Whirlpool hydrotherapy is used to relieve pain and facilitate retraining of movements. Physical therapy (see page 526) such as passive exercise can be done safely during the acute phase of the illness. After your symptoms subside, your rehabilitation team will prescribe an active exercise routine that will help you regain muscle strength and independence. Training with adaptive devices, such as a wheelchair or braces, may be needed to give you mobility and self-care skills during the protracted recovery period.

PERIPHERAL NEUROPATHIES

Signs and Symptoms

*   Tingling sensation in the hands or feet;
*   Numbness in the same areas;
*   Unsteadiness or lack of coordination;
*   Weakness and pain of the feet and hands.

Your peripheral nervous system is the network of nerves used for all of your movements (motor nerves) and sensations (sensory nerves). This network of nerves is connected to your central nervous system at your brainstem and at many points along your spinal cord. It reaches to the remote parts of your body.

Your peripheral nerves provide communication between your brain and your organs, blood vessels, muscles, and skin. Your brain's commands are conveyed by motor nerves, and information is delivered back to the brain by your sensory nerves.

Damage to a peripheral nerve can interfere with communication between the area it serves and your brain. This can impair your ability to move muscles or to feel normal sensations in an affected area. It can produce a painful sensation along the involved peripheral nerve.

Peripheral neuropathy is the term used to describe damage to your peripheral nerves that does not affect your brain and spinal cord. With minor damage, you may have acute burning pain, whereas major damage can result in imbalance or muscle weakness and even paralysis. You may have damage to a single nerve, as is the case in carpal tunnel syndrome (see page 974), or damage to many nerves at the same time, as in Guillain-Barré syndrome (see page 556).

The causes for peripheral neuropathy are numerous. A partial list includes immediate injury, continuing pressure on a nerve, and nerve destruction from disease or poisoning. The most common causes of peripheral neuropathies are diabetes mellitus, vitamin deficiency, alcoholism associated with poor nutrition, and inherited disorders.

Pressure on a nerve can be due to a tumor, abnormal bone growth, use of a cast or crutches, or prolonged periods in cramped postures. Rheumatoid arthritis, excessive vibration from power tools, bleeding into a nerve, herniated discs (see page 990), exposure to cold or radiation, and various forms of cancer also cause pressure on nerves. A common peripheral neuropathy, meralgia paresthetica, is characterized by burning sensations, numbness, and sensitivity of the front of the thighs.

Microorganisms can attack your nerves directly and result in peripheral nerve damage. The cause also can be toxic substances, including heavy metals (lead, mercury, arsenic), carbon monoxide, and solvents.

Your symptoms usually begin gradually over many months but, in certain cases, such as arsenic poisoning, the onset may be abrupt. A tingling sensation usually begins in your toes or the balls of your feet and spreads upward. Occasionally it begins in your hands and extends up your arms. Then numbness may proceed in the same way. Your skin can become sensitive, and even the lightest touch can be painful. In severe forms, a gradual weakness in the muscles may occur.

With diabetes mellitus (see page 707), symptoms of a peripheral neuropathy may not appear until you have had the disease for 15 or 20 years; if blood glucose levels are poorly controlled, the symptoms may occur much earlier. Specific symptoms, in addition to those described above, also can include intermittent episodes of sharp pain.

A severe form of vitamin B_{12} deficiency, known as pernicious anemia (see page 479), occurs when your body cannot absorb vitamin B_{12} as it should. Specific symptoms before the onset of peripheral neuropathy include paleness, weakness, fatigue, faintness, or breathlessness. Your skin may turn yellow, and your mouth and tongue may be sore.

Alcoholics may be the most prone to peripheral neuropathies. Their frequently inadequate diet (especially for the vitamin thiamine) contributes to the neuropathy. Pernicious anemia may occur and increase the chances for peripheral neuropathy.

The Diagnosis. Because peripheral neuropathies are a complex of symptoms rather than a single disease, the cause for your particular disorder may be difficult or impossible to diagnose. Your physician will conduct physical and neurological examinations and will probably ask you questions about which symptoms appeared first, recent viruses, new medications you may be taking, kinds of toxic exposure, similar symptoms in your family or co-workers, and your level of alcohol consumption. A detailed history of your known medical disorders will be needed.

Your physician may require further testing to verify whatever cause is indicated by your responses to the questions. These can include blood tests, urinalysis, a chest x-ray, electromyography (see page 1294), metabolic tests, nerve biopsy, thyroid function tests, and lumbar puncture (see page 530).

How Serious Are Peripheral Neuropathies? In contrast to the nerve fibers of your central nervous system, peripheral nerve fibers have a good ability to regenerate with proper care. In some disorders, recovery occurs, but the symptoms may recur if the cause is not eliminated.

Treatment. Specific therapy will be directed at the cause of your peripheral neu-

ropathy. This may mean closer control of your underlying disease, such as regular injections of vitamin B_{12} for pernicious anemia, returning your blood glucose level to normal if you have diabetes mellitus, or avoidance of alcohol. Multivitamin therapy may be appropriate.

In severe cases with permanent impairment, physical therapy (see page 526) will be needed to maintain as much muscle strength as possible and to avoid muscle cramping or spasms. Mechanical devices may be needed for mobility. Also, check your skin regularly and report any severe bruises or open sores to your physician.

CHARCOT-MARIE-TOOTH DISEASE

Signs and Symptoms
- Weakness in legs;
- Absence of stretch reflex;
- Foot deformity.

Charcot-Marie-Tooth disease is a relatively common hereditary disorder caused by degeneration of the insulating sheath (myelin sheath) covering nerve fibers, or of the nerve fibers themselves, in your legs. Onset is usually between mid-childhood and age 30 years. The disorder develops slowly and may stabilize spontaneously. Diagnosis may require biopsy of a leg muscle or nerve.

Treatment. Vocational counseling or leg braces may be needed, as may an orthopedic operation or corrective shoes to improve walking. The disorder does not necessarily affect your life span, and you may be active for years.

SYRINGOMYELIA

Signs and Symptoms
- Gradual loss of sensation in the nape of the neck, shoulders, and upper arms;
- Weakness of the arms or legs.

In syringomyelia, a fluid-filled cavity grows within your spinal cord, usually in the neck area. The cavity may expand gradually across or along your spinal cord, initially reducing your sense of heat or touch and then causing wasting of your muscles. Severe disability can develop. Frequently, the progression of symptoms is very slow.

Syringomyelia can be caused by spinal cord trauma, tumor, or a congenital defect that triggers syringomyelia in adolescence or early adulthood.

Treatment. Surgical therapy to drain the cavity and decompress the spinal cord frequently stops progression of the disorder. About half of the persons with syringomyelia improve significantly after an operation.

MYELOMENINGOCELE

Signs and Symptoms
- Sac protruding from the spinal cord on a newborn's back;
- Weakness of lower limbs.

Myelomeningocele is a congenital defect that leaves your baby's spinal canal open along several vertebrae in the lower or middle back. The spinal cord and membranes protrude shortly after birth. Neurological impairment below the defect, often including either partial or complete paralysis, is common.

Other congenital malformations often are associated with myelomeningocele, such as syringomyelia (see page 558), clubfoot, or hip dislocation. Meningitis (see page 527) can occur and should be treated surgically, especially if there is drainage from the spinal cord. If there are problems with neurological control of the bladder, urinary infections are likely to occur as your child gets older.

Treatment. Immediate surgical repair frequently is recommended. With proper care, a long life is possible in some cases, although problems, particularly impaired bladder and bowel function, may persist.

NEURALGIAS

Signs and Symptoms
- Attacks of extremely sharp, stabbing pain, or constant burning pain.

Neuralgias consist of severe spasms of pain that extend along the path of one of your nerves. They may be due to injury or irritation of the nerve, but in many cases the cause is unknown.

Your pain may have a background sensation of burning and aching with sharp, stabbing jabs superimposed on it. The pain comes in episodic attacks that might last for seconds or minutes, and the episodes may recur for days or weeks.

During an acute phase of your disorder, you may be hypersensitive to touch and to any slightly painful sensation, and you may even perceive that nonpainful sensations cause you pain.

Some neuralgias can occur as a result of a herpes infection, usually shingles (see page 1176) and occasionally infection by herpes simplex virus. Postherpetic neuralgia, for example, can be a most debilitating complication of herpes zoster virus. It typically produces a constant burning pain that is more prominent than the brief shooting or jabbing component. New attacks are provoked by contact or movement such as sneezing or eating. Your nerve pain can continue for weeks, months, or sometimes years after all signs of the herpes virus have disappeared.

Glossopharyngeal neuralgia is characterized by recurrent attacks of severe pain in the back of your pharynx, tonsils, middle ear, and the base of your tongue. The attacks may be precipitated by movements such as talking or swallowing, and the pain can be intense.

Occipital neuralgia causes pain in the back of your head. Intercostal neuralgia occurs between your ribs. Trigeminal neuralgia, the most common of all forms, is severe shooting spasms on one side of your face (see page 560).

Neuralgias usually strike after age 40 years and occur most commonly in elderly persons. Fortunately, postherpetic (that is, neuralgias that occur after shingles) and trigeminal neuralgia are the only neuralgias that occur commonly.

The Diagnosis. Your physician's diagnosis is determined by your symptoms and by exclusion of other disorders that may be causing your pain. You may need to see a neurologist for a thorough examination. Your dentist also may need to examine your teeth and gums when your face is affected. If you also have swelling as a sign, rheumatic diseases (see page 823), phlebitis (see page 838), and bone fractures will need to be ruled out.

How Serious Are Neuralgias? Although your pain may be incapacitating, it is not life-threatening. Your attacks may come and go variably, but the time between attacks can grow shorter as you get older.

Treatment. *Medication.* Treatment will depend on your symptoms, but analgesic drugs (painkillers) commonly are required. For mild neuralgias, your physician may prescribe non-narcotic analgesics such as aspirin, acetaminophen, or ibuprofen. In more severe cases, a narcotic analgesic such as codeine may be temporarily necessary. Carbamazepine is used for trigeminal neuralgia. Sometimes an antidepressant medication is prescribed to help control your pain. Physical therapy may be useful in the treatment of postherpetic neuralgia.

TRIGEMINAL NEURALGIA

Signs and Symptoms
* Brief flashes of excruciating pain in the

lips, gums, cheek, chin, or, rarely, forehead.

Trigeminal neuralgia, also called tic douloureux, is a condition of recurring pain on one side of your face emanating from one or more of the three branches of the fifth cranial (trigeminal) nerve. The pain may be a tearing, darting, or sharp cutting sensation that occurs in a portion of the face. An attack may last for seconds or a few minutes, and its intensity may make you contract your facial muscles, hence the term tic. Episodes may recur for days or weeks or months. The cause of the disorder usually is considered to be a blood vessel or sometimes even a tumor pressing on the nerve inside the skull.

Often there are trigger zones—spots on the face or certain movements—that precipitate the pain. These may include smiling, talking, chewing, brushing your teeth, or blowing your nose.

The disorder is found almost exclusively in persons older than 50 years and often in those older than 70 years. Women are 3 times more likely to have it than men.

Your physician usually can diagnose the disorder after excluding other disorders that may cause pain in your head, jaw, teeth, or sinuses. Multiple sclerosis (see page 522) can cause trigeminal neuralgia. Frequently, a delayed diagnosis results in multiple unnecessary dental procedures in an attempt to correct the pain.

Although the pain may be incapacitating, it is not life-threatening. Attacks come and go variably, but periods of remission may grow shorter as you age.

Treatment. In general, attempts to control the pain of trigeminal neuralgia begin with medications such as phenytoin or carbamazepine. If drug treatments fail to control the discomfort, nerve blocks or surgical procedures to reduce the sensitivity of the nerve are an option. An operation to free the nerve from the blood vessel or tumor compressing it also can eliminate the pain permanently. However, this is a major neurosurgical procedure with several potential complications.

If you have trigeminal neuralgia, pain may occur in areas supplied by one of the three branches of the trigeminal (fifth cranial) nerve.

Trigeminal nerve

CHAPTER 23

DENTAL AND ORAL DISORDERS

CHAPTER CONTENTS

YOUR HEALTHY TEETH

Few parts of your body play as many roles in everyday life as your mouth and teeth do. Many of the most important acts of self-expression—such as speaking, singing, and simply smiling—utilize the teeth to shape the sounds we make and to help form our appearance. Crucial to health, the mouth and teeth are responsible for the first phase in the process of digesting food.

Our teeth may seem only minor health concerns, but tooth and oral disorders can disrupt almost every aspect of our lives.

TOOTH DEVELOPMENT

We are born toothless—or so it appears. In actuality, tooth development is well advanced by the 3rd month of pregnancy, and by the 4th month there is evidence of enamel and dentin, the hard tissues of the primary or deciduous teeth (the baby teeth).

The first teeth appear in the mouth 6 to 7 months after the baby is born. The time these first teeth emerge varies greatly from child to child, but in most children the teeth have broken through the gums before the end of the first year.

In general, the first teeth to emerge are the incisors, the front teeth in the lower jaw, followed by the front teeth in the upper jaw.

THE ADULT MOUTH

Molars

Bicuspids

Canine

Incisors

Last to appear are the molars. Most children have a full set of primary teeth by age 3.

There are only 20 primary teeth. Each primary tooth is normally replaced by one permanent tooth, incisor-for-incisor, canine-for-canine, and bicuspid-for-molar. The permanent first molars erupt behind the primary molars.

For many children, the emergence of permanent teeth begins at about age 5 to 6. The lower front incisors tend to come in first, followed by the upper front incisors and first molars. Permanent bicuspids and cuspids emerge later.

The process of shedding primary teeth to be replaced by permanent teeth usually lasts through the elementary school years. By age 14, 28 permanent teeth should be in place. The last four molars, the wisdom teeth, usually emerge in early adulthood, around age 20, to complete the permanent set of 32 teeth.

We have several kinds of teeth. From the center of the mouth toward the back on the top and bottom jaws, there are 8 incisors (4 in each jaw), 4 canines (cuspids), 8 bicuspids, and 12 molars.

THE PARTS OF THE TOOTH

The basic structure of every tooth is essentially the same. The part of the tooth that is visible, the crown, is covered with enamel. The crown extends from just beneath the gum line to the top of the tooth. The hard enamel protects the structures of the tooth beneath. The enamel coating has no sensation and cannot heal after an injury.

Just beneath the crown lies the largest portion of the tooth, the dentin. The dentin is composed of millions of tiny cells arranged in tubules. It is a hard material (but not as hard as the enamel) and, unlike the outer layer, the dentin is sensitive to temperature and touch. Below the gum level, the dentin is covered by a layer called cementum. A connective tissue called the periodontal ligament connects the cementum to the bone that forms the socket.

Inside the dentin, at the center of the tooth, lies the pulp chamber and the pulp. The pulp includes the blood vessels that feed the tooth and the nerves of the tooth. The

PARTS OF THE TOOTH

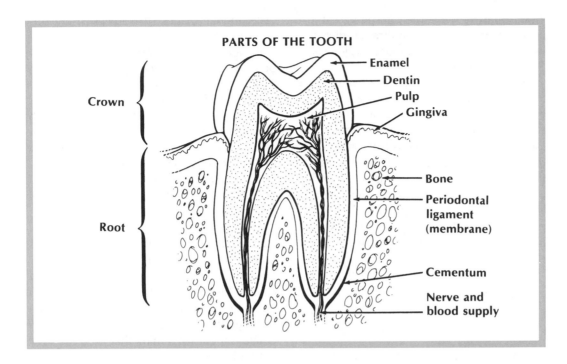

nerves and blood vessels enter the teeth from the end of the roots.

This chapter describes disorders and diseases of the teeth and mouth. Many people experience some of these problems during the course of their lives; in fact, one of the most common human diseases is dental caries (tooth decay). Another very common disorder is periodontal disease which contributes to the loss of teeth in adults.

Tooth decay and periodontal disease lead the list of oral disorders, but many others exist. These include other bacterial and fungal infections, oral cancers, salivary gland problems, problems of malformed and misaligned teeth, loss of teeth, and facial trauma.

DENTISTS AND THEIR SPECIALTIES

Just as there is no one type of physician who can handle all possible health problems, dentists also have specialties. Your general practitioner dentist may have special expertise in several areas, but for certain problems out of his or her training, you may elect to see or may be referred to a specialist. These include:

Periodontists who diagnose and treat disease of the tissues supporting and surrounding teeth (gums and bone);

Pediatric dentists who specialize in treating children from birth through adolescence;

Orthodontists who diagnose and correct malpositions of the teeth and jaws;

Endodontists who diagnose and treat diseases and injuries of the tooth pulp and surrounding tissues;

Oral and maxillofacial surgeons who extract teeth and who diagnose and treat injuries, diseases, and defects of the jaw, face, and mouth; and

Prosthodontists who create and fit artificial replacements for defective or missing teeth, including crowns, bridges (fixed partial dentures), and dentures.

TOOTH DECAY

Tooth decay is a bacterial disease of the teeth. After the common cold, tooth decay is one of the most common of all human disorders. Dental caries affects children and young adults most frequently, although it re-

mains a problem for many people throughout their lives.

Decay is the primary cause of tooth loss among people of all ages. Almost half of all American children have tooth decay by age

4, and many even earlier, despite great improvements in prevention through diet, the use of fluoride, and proper oral hygiene (see Tooth Care, page 393).

In the past, few people had their own teeth past middle age. Today, however, use of fluoride and better dental care, nutrition, and hygiene allow people to keep their teeth longer. This makes a relatively new problem, root caries, more common. Root caries is the decay of tooth roots and is an increasing problem among older people. A similar, lifelong program of appropriate dental care, preventive nutrition, and good oral hygiene are also the keys to combating this form of dental caries.

HOW TOOTH DECAY DEVELOPS

Tooth decay is the result of three interacting factors: bacteria, dietary sugar, and vulnerable tooth surface.

Your mouth, like other parts of your body, is host to bacteria. These bacteria convert some of the sugars and carbohydrates you eat into acid. The bacteria and the acids they form become part of the sticky deposit,

called dental plaque, that clings to the surfaces of your teeth.

In addition to bacteria, plaque is composed of mucus and food particles. You can feel the plaque when you pass your tongue over the surface of your teeth several hours after brushing. The texture is slightly rough and is particularly noticeable on the surfaces of back teeth. Plaque adheres most strongly in pits and fissures of the molars and premolars, in the areas just above the gum line and between teeth, and at the margins of dental restorations (fillings).

The decay-producing acid that forms in plaque attacks the mineral in the tooth's outer enamel surface. The erosion caused by the plaque leads to the formation of tiny cavities (openings) in the enamel, which you probably will not notice at first. Indeed, the first sign of decay may be a sensation of pain when you eat something that is sweet, very cold, or very hot.

Once the enamel has been penetrated, the softer dentin beneath becomes vulnerable. The dentin contains tiny canals leading to the pulp at the core of the tooth. Inflammation results if bacteria reach the sensitive pulp. Blood vessels within the pulp swell and, because there is no room within the rigid tooth to expand, you experience pain. In addition, your body sends white blood cells to counteract bacterial invasion from the tooth into the surrounding tissues.

This kind of bacterial infection is known as a tooth abscess. Blood vessels around the tooth enlarge. The enlarged vessels press on nerves in the area, causing even more pain. Often, despite the body's efforts to fight it off, the infection overwhelms the pulp, and the nerve and blood vessels die. The toothache will cease, but the tooth will become vulnerable to the formation of an abscess later, sometimes years later.

Tooth decay takes time to develop, often a year or two in permanent teeth but less in primary teeth. The initial formation of acid occurs within the first 20 minutes after you eat. Fortunately, you are not totally vulnerable to the effects of bacteria, acid, and the foods you eat. The chemistry and the mechanics of the mouth provide a certain amount of protection: your saliva and the actions of your tongue will wash away some of the destructive material. Today's dentistry also provides treatment and preventive measures to lessen the effects of dental caries (see Prevention of Tooth Decay, page 568).

Dental cavities (caries) are common causes of tooth loss.

THE CHECKUP

One of the important steps in preventing tooth decay is to visit your dentist regularly for a thorough checkup.

How Often Should I See My Dentist?

You and your children (beginning at age 3, or earlier if symptoms appear) should visit the dentist usually twice a year. You may need to see your dentist more frequently if certain conditions or problems exist.

People who have several cavities per year and who pay little attention to oral hygiene at home may need to see their dentist more often, perhaps every 3 months, for treatment and cleaning. Adults over 35 who are still getting cavities, take only moderate care of their teeth, and smoke and drink alcohol to excess also may need to visit the dentist frequently. Even people without natural teeth should see their dentist periodically.

On the other hand, adults who have few cavities, take very good care of their teeth, and do not smoke or drink may need to visit their dentist only once a year. Your dentist will determine your examination schedule according to your specific needs.

The Medical History

Before your dentist asks you to "Open wide, please," he or she probably will ask a few questions about your general health. The answers can have a direct bearing on your treatment.

For example, certain kinds of heart conditions make people susceptible to an infection of the heart valves when their gums are manipulated, such as in a thorough dental cleaning or when a tooth is filled or extracted. Therefore, these people usually take an antibiotic before dental treatment (see Infective Endocarditis: Protection and Prevention, page 824). People who are allergic to penicillin can have a reaction when it is prescribed for tooth infections. Diabetics whose disease is poorly controlled can become ill after the stress of dental treatment. People who have been ill with jaundice occasionally can carry the hepatitis virus without knowing it. Your dentist or dental assistant will probably also ask if you are on any medications, so that the dentist can avoid prescribing any that could cause harmful interactions.

The Examination

Once the preliminary questions are over, your dentist will begin examining your mouth and teeth. Your gums and the soft tissues of your mouth will be examined first for signs of gingivitis (see page 570), periodontitis (see page 571), and less common disorders such as leukoplakia, oral lichen planus, or oral cancer (see pages 578 and 580). If you have dentures, your gums will be examined for signs of pressure and uneven wear, indicated by patches of thickened skin, soreness, or reddened areas.

The next step is examination of each tooth by using a needle-shaped probe and a small mirror. Your dentist will be looking for signs of decay, including discolored areas and small fissures in the tooth enamel. Existing fillings will be checked for deterioration and for signs of new cavities around their edges. Your dentist will use a probe to check for periodontal disease around the base of your teeth.

Sometimes your dentist may suspect the presence of a cavity even when the enamel looks intact. He or she may then take x-rays of the area to check the teeth and surrounding tissue and bone. In addition, periodic x-rays are often necessary if you have periodontal disease or have had the root canals of a dead tooth filled or to determine the status of wisdom teeth or, in younger people, of other unerupted permanent teeth.

The Cleaning Process

Your dentist or dental hygienist also may clean your teeth (a process called dental prophylaxis). This is an essential step in maintaining the health of your teeth and gums. Plaque is a sticky substance that collects on teeth as a result of improper brushing or flossing. Calculus, often referred to as tartar, is plaque that has hardened and adheres tightly to the teeth.

Your dentist or dental hygienist can remove calculus in one of two ways. The traditional method involves scraping the deposits from your teeth with a sharp instrument known as a scaler. Some dentists also use an ultrasonic device that loosens the tartar through vibration. Whatever method is used, you may experience some bleeding of the gums. In some people, calculus develops quickly and must be removed every few months.

Once the calculus has been removed, the teeth are polished. Smooth teeth slow down the deposit of plaque. Polishing is done with a special toothpaste applied by a device with rotating rubber heads. With children, dentists often finish checkups with an application of fluoride to help prevent dental caries (see also Tooth Care, page 393).

TREATMENTS FOR TOOTH DECAY

Most cavities are discovered during a dental examination because the early stages of decay usually are painless. Detecting and treating tooth decay early can save pain, expense, and, most importantly, your teeth.

The sooner a cavity is detected, the less painful the situation is likely to be because the outer parts of the tooth, the enamel and dentin, are far less sensitive to pain than is the pulp. One way of ascertaining whether you have a cavity is with dental x-rays. Your dentist will determine, on the basis of your dental history and the current condition of your teeth, whether and how many x-ray examinations are appropriate.

Even if you have a seriously decayed tooth, modern dentistry is equipped to deaden the discomfort of the treatment process and often can save the tooth through such procedures as dental fillings (restorations) or root canals (in which the diseased portion of a tooth is removed, leaving the unaffected portions of the root and tooth in place, covered with a crown).

Fillings. Most often, you have not noticed symptoms but when you visit your dentist for a regular checkup he or she finds a cavity. In some cases, however, you may notice mild pain in one tooth when you eat something that is sweet, very hot, or very cold. This is likely to be the earliest symptom of tooth decay that you will experience. If you feel a sharp pain when eating sweet, hot, or cold foods, this may signal a more seriously decayed tooth. In each of these instances, the decay process usually can be halted by removing the decayed portion of the tooth (drilling) and replacing it with a restorative material (filling).

If the decay seems to be extensive or you are especially sensitive, you may be offered a local anesthetic (injected into the gums) to keep you from feeling pain. On occasion, some dentists will offer nitrous oxide gas to decrease discomfort and anxiety. If you are taking any medications, mention this to your dentist before accepting any anesthetic because certain medications and anesthetics taken together can produce adverse reactions.

Once the affected area has been cleared of decay, your dentist will prepare to restore the tooth. The kind of filling used depends on the location and function of the tooth. Molars, which do most of the work of chewing, experience the most stress and require more durable materials than do front (anterior) teeth. In addition, if possible, a filling in a front tooth should blend in color with the tooth itself.

Sometimes when decay is extensive, a temporary filling will be inserted to provide your dentist an opportunity to observe the tooth's response and sensitivity to treatment. After several weeks, if there are no adverse signs or symptoms, your dentist removes the filling and replaces it with a permanent one.

The most common restorative material is silver amalgam and is used in the back teeth. Such fillings are actually alloys of mercury, silver, and other metals. The recent addition of copper to the standard mixture makes today's "silver fillings" far more durable than those of even a few years ago.

Gold inlay, a more expensive restoration, is sometimes used in place of amalgam where more strength and support are necessary. Such a filling does not readily tarnish.

Fillings in front teeth need to be as invisible as possible. Silicate, a form of porcelain cement which resembles tooth enamel, was the standard choice until recently. Now, plastic resins are being used with increased frequency. Both forms can be tinted to match the color of the tooth that is filled. In the future, composite materials may be made strong enough to be used for the chewing surfaces of the molars and bicuspids.

Occasionally, gold foil is used as a restorative material for small cavities in front teeth. It is more expensive than porcelain or plastic composite materials but is more durable.

If your tooth is so decayed that it cannot support several fillings or a single large one without danger of breaking, your dentist may remove the decay, fill the site with cement or amalgam, and fit a porcelain jacket, a metal crown, or a combination metal and porcelain crown over the tooth to restore it. A model is usually made from an impression of your tooth and a crown is fabricated in the laboratory. This crown is then fitted, shaped, and finally cemented in place on what is left of the tooth.

Root Canal. If you have a tooth that is so severely decayed or infected that it is in danger of being lost, your dentist or an endodontist will perform a root canal. This procedure involves removal of the nerve and vascular tissue (pulp) from the root and pulp chamber as well as any associated decayed tooth structure. It allows for the root and base of the tooth itself to remain in place.

A root canal is performed as an office procedure and often requires local anesthesia. In this multistage procedure, the pulp is removed and the cavity that is created is then sterilized and filled with an inert material (gutta-percha) and cement. The remaining tooth structure will be more brittle than before and therefore will require permanent restoration, most often with a crown.

TOOTH ABSCESS

Signs and Symptoms
- Persistent aching or throbbing pain in a tooth;
- Sensitivity to hot or cold foods or liquids;
- Pain on chewing;
- Swollen lymph nodes in the neck;
- Fever and general malaise.

Some people do not view tooth decay as a potentially serious health problem but, if not dealt with promptly and properly, it can lead to a more troublesome ailment.

Decay can allow bacteria to infect the pulp of a tooth. The infection may spread to the root and into the surrounding bone. This is known as an abscess. If the infection reaches the bone, the tooth may loosen. The infected root and swollen tissue cause pain. If the root dies, the pain will go away, but the infection may remain, slowly destroying adjacent bone. The resulting breakdown material (pus) that forms as part of the infection can erode a channel through the jaw and form a swelling or boil on the gum.

The Diagnosis. If you have persistent throbbing pain in a tooth, find chewing painful, or are sensitive to hot or cold foods or liquids, you may have an abscessed tooth. You may have a slight fever and swollen lymph nodes in the neck and feel generally unwell.

A swelling that forms on the gum near the sore tooth may at some point burst, releasing into your mouth a quantity of thick liquid material with a foul taste and smell; simultaneously, the pain probably will be relieved.

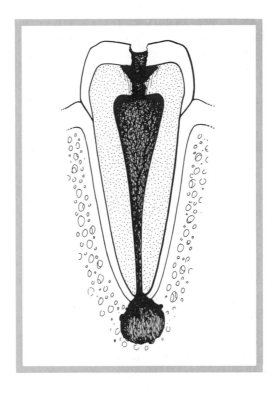

A tooth abscess occurs when bacteria enter through a decayed area and spread inward, infecting the pulp, root, and even bone surrounding the tooth.

If you experience any of these symptoms, see your dentist immediately. Your dentist will examine the tooth and decide on a proper course of action.

Treatment. Before you get to your dentist, you can help relieve the pain of an abscess by taking aspirin or another pain reliever. Do not apply aspirin directly to the tooth or surrounding tissue. Rinsing your mouth with warm, salted water every hour or so may be soothing but is not curative.

In the past, the only treatment for an abscessed tooth was extraction. Under certain conditions, extraction still is appropriate. However, dentists today often can save abscessed teeth.

As a first step, your dentist probably will prescribe an antibiotic to clear up the infection and keep it from spreading to other parts of your body. He or she can also prescribe pain relief medications to make you more comfortable.

To save the tooth, your dentist may anesthetize the area and then open a hole into the pulp chamber of the tooth. This will release the pressure. The pulp chamber can then be cleared out, disinfected, and filled with an inert material. If swelling persists after an abscessed tooth has been removed, your dentist may want to obtain special cultures to rule out a condition called actinomycosis.

Next, your dentist will place a temporary filling in your tooth. After the infection has cleared (usually within a few weeks), your tooth can receive a permanent filling.

Your dentist most likely will want to see you again in a few months, at which time x-rays will be taken of the tooth to determine whether bone and tissue are growing into the pocket left by the abscess. If the pocket appears to be healthy, the treatment is finished. If the infection persists, additional treatment is necessary and your dentist may refer you to a specialist who will perform a surgical procedure to remove the remaining diseased tissue, sometimes including a small portion of the root tip.

PREVENTION OF TOOTH DECAY

A successful plan of decay prevention involves three steps: taking good care of your teeth; proper diet; and, in the case of children, application of sealants to the chewing surfaces of back teeth and application of fluoride to all teeth. Such a plan involves thorough brushing and flossing on a daily basis, seeing your dentist regularly for checkups, controlling the intake of sugar and carbohydrates in your diet, and using fluoride and sealants to help prevent caries.

In an ideal world, everyone would brush their teeth after each meal and all snacks. A more realistic goal is to brush at least twice each day—in the morning and before retiring—and to floss once. Much decay-causing activity occurs at night when your mouth is dry from lack of saliva and your tongue is inactive in cleaning your mouth. Brushing and flossing before retiring thus are very important because they eliminate foods and bacteria that otherwise can cause decay.

Another strategy is to rinse your mouth with water after snacks (see also page 395 for a discussion of proper methods for brushing and flossing teeth).

A key to developing lifelong good habits is to start early. Teach your children the ritual of brushing even before they have a full set of teeth. Similarly, your child's dentist will demonstrate the proper methods of flossing.

Control Sugar and Carbohydrate Intake. The concept that sugar contributes to tooth decay is not new. But the evidence points to all fermentable carbohydrates, not just sugar, as foods that cause tooth decay. Fermentable carbohydrates include all sugars and most cooked starches.

Because carbohydrates are an important part of a healthy diet, do not cut down on them. Instead, the following tips may be helpful in discouraging tooth decay. This does not mean that you may never allow yourself or your child to have ice cream, cake, pie, or candy. The amount of sugar you eat is less important than how and when it is eaten. Sweets eaten between meals do more harm than those eaten with a meal.

Try to incorporate the following strategies into your eating habits and your children's:

1. Avoid chewy, sticky foods, particularly as snacks. Such foods as candy, candy-coated nuts, sticky dry cereal, doughy bread, raisins, and dry fruit cling to your teeth. Do not eliminate raisins and dried fruit; just brush within 20 minutes after eating them (acid production by the bacteria that promote tooth decay is most active after this time), or rinse your mouth with water.
2. Choose snacks carefully. Snacking on foods that promote tooth decay is worse than eating the same foods during meals. Nibbling on snacks throughout the day allows bacteria to produce a constant supply of acid on your teeth. Do not constantly sip sugar drinks or suck on hard candies, sugar-sweetened breath mints, cough drops, or chewing gum.

Even babies are at risk of tooth decay. Babies put to sleep with a bottle of milk (or juice) are at risk of damaging teeth. Both contain sugars. If your baby needs a bottle to settle down, fill it with water.

Recent research suggests that, when eaten along with carbohydrates, certain foods can neutralize the effects of sugar on teeth. You are more likely to eat combinations of foods at meals rather than as snacks. These combinations can alter the microbial effect and have the potential to decrease tooth decay.

The Value of Fluoride. Persons living in parts of the country where the public water supply naturally contains an optimal amount of fluoride have been found to have almost no dental caries. In a few communities, the natural fluoride content of drinking water is so high that brown stains appear on the teeth. Correct knowledge of the action of fluoride enables communities to avoid this cosmetic risk. There is no evidence that fluoride, whether added to water supplies or occurring naturally, constitutes any health risk.

Fluoride is especially helpful when it is ingested by children whose tooth development is in progress. The fluoride is incorporated into the enamel structure and offers continuing protection.

Many communities in the United States add small amounts of fluoride to their water systems because the water supply is deficient in fluoride. This approach is both cost-effective and safe. If your municipal water supply is not treated, ask about fluoridation for drinking water in your children's schools. Supplemental fluoride drops or tablets are available by prescription from your dentist or physician.

Children, adolescents, and elderly people are most susceptible to tooth decay. For them, topical application of fluoride, including fluoride toothpastes, is desirable. Fluoride mouthwashes can be useful as well. Many dentists also treat children's teeth with a fluoride solution as a part of regular checkups.

Fluoride is most effective in preventing caries on the smooth, nonchewing surfaces of your teeth. Consequently, most cavities occur on the chewing surfaces. The reason: these surfaces of your back teeth (premolars and molars) have depressions and grooves (pits and fissures) that are almost impossible to clean with a toothbrush.

Tooth Sealants. Besides good oral hygiene, the single best method to prevent decay of the chewing surfaces of back teeth is use of dental sealants. Sealants provide a thin plastic-like coating, usually clear or white. The application is painless and easy. First, your dentist cleans the chewing surface of your premolars and molars. Then, these surfaces are etched with a mild acid to improve adhesion. The teeth are thoroughly washed and dried. Then your dentist paints sealant onto each tooth in much the same way fingernail polish is applied. The sealant hardens into a shield that prevents accumulation of plaque in the pits and fissures.

Dental sealants can last up to 10 years, although various conditions may shorten their effectiveness. Regular visits to the dentist permit necessary touch-ups to extend the life of the sealant. If the sealant layer is lost, it can be replaced. If the sealant is damaged, the underlying tooth surface is at no greater risk for cavities than it would be if the sealant had never been applied.

Sealant protection is most appropriate for children. It should be applied when the first permanent molars erupt, at about age 6, and again when permanent second molars and premolars erupt, around age 11 to 13. Older people, the disabled, those who live in institutions, and people from groups with a high incidence of cavities also can benefit from sealants.

PERIODONTAL DISEASE

Tooth decay (dental caries) is the primary cause of tooth loss. After age 35, periodontal disease also becomes an important cause of tooth loss. Many people who have natural teeth experience periodontal disease in some form over the course of their lives, although they will not necessarily lose teeth.

The tissue in which the disease occurs is called the periodontium. This includes the gums (gingiva), the periodontal ligament, and the alveolar bone (tooth sockets). These structures support your teeth.

Periodontal disease is neither a disease that develops in 1 day nor an ailment that, with prompt attention, can be cured, never to appear again. Rather, periodontal disease results from a combination of factors involving bacterial plaque—the sticky substance found in everyone's mouth—and its long-term effects on the periodontium. It can take several forms, but the result is weakened tooth support.

The two most common forms of periodontal disease are gingivitis (inflammation of the gums) and periodontitis. Gingivitis is often a precursor of the more serious condition of periodontitis. Both of these diseases are discussed in the following pages, as is trench mouth and ways to prevent periodontal disease.

GINGIVITIS

Signs and Symptoms
- Swollen, soft, red gums;
- Gums that bleed easily.

The term gingivitis refers to inflammation of the gingiva or gums. It can be caused by deposits of plaque, the sticky film that forms on the exposed portion of teeth and irritates the gums.

Many people experience gingivitis first in their puberty and then at various degrees of severity throughout life. Mild forms of the disease are very common among adults. People with uncontrolled diabetes and pregnant women are particularly prone to the development of gum inflammation.

The Diagnosis. Healthy gums are firm and pale pink. If you notice that your gums are swollen, very tender, and bleed easily, you may have gingivitis. Often, people first detect a change in their gums when they notice that the bristles of their toothbrushes are pink after brushing, a sign that their gums are bleeding even with the gentle pressure of brush bristles. Further examination usually reveals red, inflamed gums. Gingivitis often causes no direct pain or discomfort and thus is frequently overlooked.

If your gums seem swollen and red, consult your dentist. He or she will examine your gums carefully, looking for inflammation and excess deposits of plaque at the base of your teeth. As the gum margin swells, more plaque can be trapped, thus irritating the gum further.

How Serious Is Gingivitis? Gingivitis often goes unnoticed because it usually is painless. If left unchecked, however, gingivitis can lead to periodontitis, a more serious disease that affects not only the gums but also the other supporting structures of the teeth, leading to tooth loss.

Treatment. Your dentist will treat your gingivitis by using several techniques. The first step is a thorough cleaning of the teeth to remove the plaque and calculus (a chalky material composed of mineralized plaque, often called tartar). This cleaning can be uncomfortable, particularly if your gums are sensitive or if your teeth are encrusted with plaque and calculus. The removal procedure, known as scaling, is designed to remove the deposits of bacteria, plaque, and calculus.

Sometimes the inflammation is enhanced by misaligned teeth, overhanging fillings, or poorly contoured restorations such as crowns and bridges that make plaque removal more difficult. Teeth can be straightened to minimize plaque accumulation, fillings can be replaced, and restorations can be recontoured.

If plaque accumulates on a normal tooth and is not removed promptly, it can harden into a mineral deposit called calculus (tartar). Gradually, the nearby gums become inflamed and swollen, a disorder known as gingivitis.

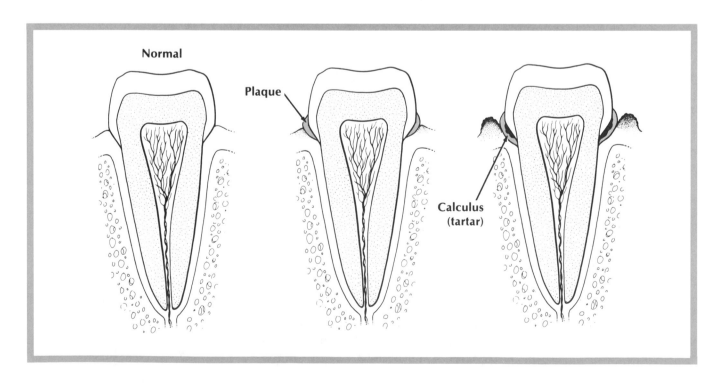

Normal

Plaque

Calculus (tartar)

Prevention.   Gingivitis most often is the result of poor dental hygiene. If you take good care of your teeth with thorough, daily brushing, regular flossing, and frequent professional cleaning, your chances of serious gingivitis developing are greatly decreased (see also Prevention of Periodontal Disease, page 573).

Once you have gingivitis, a strict program of oral hygiene is necessary to keep the disease from becoming worse. This includes flossing as well as brushing. Your dentist or dental hygienist will show you how to brush and floss properly (see Proper Flossing and Brushing Techniques, page 395).

At first your gums may bleed after brushing. This should last only a couple of weeks. Soon your gums should be pink and firm, a sign of their improved health. The program must be followed indefinitely, however, for your gums to remain healthy.

PERIODONTITIS

Signs and Symptoms

- Swollen gums or recessed gums;
- Unpleasant taste in mouth;
- Bad breath;
- Pain in a tooth when eating hot, cold, or sweet foods;
- Dull sound when a tooth is tapped;
- Loose tooth.

If gingivitis (see above) goes untreated or treatment is delayed, periodontitis may develop. Periodontitis gets its name from the Latin *peri* meaning around, *odont* meaning tooth, and *itis* for inflammation.

In this disease, which was formerly known as pyorrhea (Greek for flowing pus), not only are the gums affected but also there is inflammation of the periodontal ligament and alveolar bone (tooth sockets) which help hold the teeth in place.

In periodontitis, plaque-filled pockets are formed between the teeth and gum. The gums become inflamed, enlarging the pockets and trapping increasing amounts of plaque. The prolonged and increasing inflammation also damages the periodontal ligament of each affected tooth. Over time, the gums gradually detach from the teeth. Pus forms in response to infection from invading bacteria and may, in severe instances, ooze from around the teeth. The result of such long-term infection is an ero-

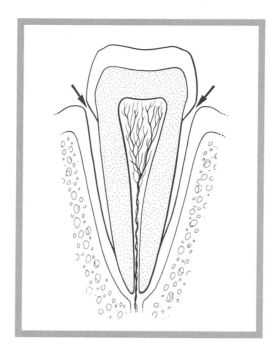

Untreated gingivitis can result in periodontitis, in which the inflamed gums gradually withdraw from the tooth (arrows); the tooth loosens and eventually may fall out.

sion of the bony socket housing the tooth. The tooth loosens and eventually may fall out.

Despite its long-term risks, periodontitis usually is painless. In some cases, however, an acute infection forms as an abscess in one or more of the pockets. This produces pain and eats away at bone even more quickly than the chronic condition does.

Generally speaking, the younger a person is when bone loss begins, the less the chances of saving the tooth. People who grind their teeth also may have more periodontal problems than those who do not.

The Diagnosis.   If your gums are swollen, if you have an unpleasant taste in your mouth and odor to your breath, if you experience pain on eating hot, cold, or sweet foods, or if you notice that a tooth is loose, see your dentist.

Your dentist will examine your teeth and gums for signs of periodontitis. Your gums will be examined for inflammation and deposits of plaque and calculus at and below the gum line and for erosion or withdrawal from the teeth. You may also be asked a series of questions to determine if a systemic disorder such as diabetes is present. If such indications are found, you may be referred to a physician for a thorough examination and treatment.

Treatment.   Conservative (nonsurgical) therapy is the first step in treating periodontal disease. This includes meticulous cleaning of the root surfaces of your teeth by your dentist or hygienist. A strict program of oral hygiene also is required. This includes flossing as well as brushing. Initially, your gums may bleed after brushing, but this unpleasant condition should disappear within 2 weeks.

Your dentist will evaluate the condition of your teeth and gums after several weeks. Generally, gums respond to the flossing and brushing by becoming pink and more firm. If you are able to maintain your gums and teeth in this condition, you may be able to avoid surgical treatment.

Orthodontic Treatment. If your teeth are malaligned and crowded, plaque accumulation may be increased and removal of it may be more difficult, but the arrangement of the teeth does not cause periodontitis. Orthodontic treatment can correct the positions of the teeth. Uneven biting and chewing surfaces can be recontoured to decrease pressure. If you grind your teeth during sleep (bruxism), you can be fitted with a device to protect your teeth from excessive pressure; however, bruxism may have other causes that may have to be identified.

Surgery. In more advanced cases, your dentist may perform a surgical procedure. For example, a flap procedure is sometimes done to clean calculus from teeth, remove infected tissue, and recontour bone. The gum tissue surrounding your teeth is lifted, the area around the teeth and bone is cleaned and recontoured, and the tissue is replaced and sutured in place.

Another technique, known as gingivectomy, may be performed under local anesthesia. In this procedure, the gums are trimmed to decrease the depth of the pockets. After the procedure, the gum line is covered with a protective putty-like packing to allow your gums to heal. The dressing should not interfere with normal eating and drinking. If it does, call your dentist or the specialist who performed the surgery.

A similar procedure, a gingivoplasty, sometimes is performed to remove excessive gum tissue and to reshape the gums to enable them to stay self-cleaning.

Sometimes an operation on the underlying bone may be performed to correct anatomic deformities or damage caused by periodontal disease. Grafting with bone or a bone substitute is often used to replace lost bone.

Prevention. In addition to techniques your dentist or periodontist can perform, you will be instructed in the proper care of your teeth. The goal is to prevent periodontitis from progressing or recurring. Good dental hygiene is paramount in the control of periodontal disease (see Prevention of Periodontal Disease, page 573).

TRENCH MOUTH

Signs and Symptoms
- Profuse bleeding from and pain in the gums after slight pressure;
- Grayish film on the gums.

Trench mouth, also known as necrotizing ulcerative gingivitis or Vincent's infection, is a painful form of gingivitis. It affects young adults most often; it can be mild or severe. This condition received the name trench mouth because during World War I it occurred in soldiers who were living in trenches under conditions of poor hygiene and poor nutrition.

Trench mouth is characterized by profuse bleeding at the slightest pressure or irritation. The condition is the result of an infection with bacteria that normally inhabit the mouth. It is not passed from one person to another.

The onset of this disease is often sudden. The points of gum between teeth (the papillae) are usually damaged, leaving craters that collect plaque and food debris. The area is covered with a grayish layer of decomposing gum tissue. The inflammation and infection also may involve other parts of the mouth.

The Diagnosis. If you experience the symptoms of gum pain and profuse bleeding after slight irritation or pressure on the gums, see your dentist immediately.

Treatment. Your dentist will begin by gently and thoroughly cleaning your gums. Irrigation of the mouth with salt or peroxide solution often helps to relieve symptoms. Your dentist may recommend taking a nonprescription pain reliever to lessen the discomfort. You will also be advised to get plenty of rest, eat a balanced diet, and avoid irritation from smoking or eating hot or spicy foods. Antibiotics may be prescribed if you have an accompanying high fever.

PREVENTION OF PERIODONTAL DISEASE

Periodontal disease (including gingivitis and periodontitis) is due in large part to poor dental hygiene. Inadequate care of your teeth will allow plaque to form and to become anchored to your teeth.

Some plaque is removed by the action of your tongue and saliva when you chew. However, in certain areas of the teeth, particularly near the gum line and between teeth, sticky plaque and hard calculus (calcified plaque, also known as tartar) collect and tend to adhere to your teeth. Thorough brushing and flossing of teeth are your best techniques for keeping plaque and calculus from forming.

Brush your teeth at least twice daily. Floss them once daily. Many dentists recommend brushing and flossing after every meal whenever possible. Be sure to brush at bedtime because the action of plaque is most damaging at night when the amount of saliva in your mouth decreases (see Proper Flossing and Brushing Techniques, page 395).

In some people, plaque develops in unusual quantities or especially quickly. If you have this problem, your dentist may recommend special toothpicks, stimulators, or toothbrushes. Devices that irrigate with water under pressure can be used to flush the toxic products found in plaque out from between the teeth. Such devices do not remove the plaque but they can help neutralize some of its effects.

Electric toothbrushes have not been found to be superior to regular toothbrushes in removing plaque. They are useful, however, for people whose dexterity is impaired.

Over-the-counter mouth rinses that are claimed to decrease plaque have yet to be proven more beneficial than brushing and flossing. The slick feel that some of these products impart to teeth is not due to the absence of tartar and plaque but rather to the glycerine manufacturers include in the rinse.

For people with chronic periodontal problems, one plaque-fighting rinse, chlorhexidine, is effective. It is available by prescription only. It is superior to over-the-counter rinses but has not cured gingivitis, even in Europe where it has been available for several decades. Side effects include an unpleasant taste, irritation of the soft tissues of the inner mouth, and staining of the teeth. For this reason, chlorhexidine may be undesirable for routine dental hygiene over a prolonged period of time.

Recently there has been promotion of and subsequent demand for toothpastes that claim to control calcified plaque (tartar). The effectiveness of these products in the prevention of periodontal disease has yet to be proven. Antitartar toothpastes may prevent the formation of tartar on the surfaces of teeth and make your teeth more cosmetically appealing. However, they do not help remove tartar below the gum line and between teeth where periodontal disease develops (see Controlling Tartar, page 398). One side effect of antitarter toothpastes is that they often cause teeth to become sensitive to cold.

No matter how careful you are, you are bound to have some plaque and calculus. The calculus must be removed by your dentist or dental hygienist with various instruments or an ultrasonic device that vibrates the deposits from your teeth. Consult your dentist every 6 to 12 months, depending on your dentist's recommendation, for such treatment. People with periodontitis and those who develop large amounts of calculus quickly find it necessary to visit their dentist more frequently.

DEVELOPMENTAL DISORDERS

In most people, the mouth and teeth develop in a fairly orderly and normal manner (see Tooth Development, page 562). However, problems may occur, often as a result of improper prenatal development or some-times environmental or genetic factors.

Modern dentistry and oral surgery often can minimize the effects of the developmental disorders discussed in the following pages.

IMPACTED TEETH

Signs and Symptoms
- Pain in the gums;
- Recurrent infection of partially buried tooth;
- Bad breath;
- Unpleasant taste.

Teeth emerge through the gums primarily at three times during life. The first time is when the baby or primary teeth emerge after the first year or so; the second is when permanent teeth emerge during early school years; and the third is when the last teeth, the so-called wisdom teeth or third molars, appear during the late teens or early twenties.

The wisdom teeth frequently have trouble emerging properly as a result of an inappropriate size of the jaw. Wisdom teeth often are too large for the jaw and thus become rotated, displaced, or tilted as they attempt to emerge. This can cause pain and occasionally infection when the tooth traps food debris in the soft gum tissue surrounding it. If the tooth comes in at an angle, it can push on the adjacent tooth, sometimes damaging it and sometimes causing pain and possibly some shifting of the bite.

The Diagnosis.   Impacted teeth do not always cause discomfort. When they do, the experience is unpleasant. The tissues overlying the third molars may enlarge. If you feel pain in your gums or have an unpleasant taste when you bite on or near where a wisdom or other unemerged adult tooth should be, you may have an impacted tooth. The

If a tooth does not emerge through the gum, it is said to be impacted. This most often occurs with the wisdom teeth at the back of the mouth.

tooth may be partly visible with the surrounding gums infected. The impacted tooth may press on other teeth, causing pain. Consult your dentist.

Treatment.   Before you see your dentist, you can help relieve the pain by taking an analgesic such as aspirin or by rinsing your mouth with warm salt water.

Your dentist will examine your mouth for signs of unemerged teeth and infection. X-rays will be taken to determine the exact location and position of the tooth. If you have an infection around the tooth, called pericoronitis, your dentist may prescribe an antibiotic.

The usual treatment for an impacted wisdom tooth is extraction. Wisdom teeth that emerge crooked can compromise your bite. Also, wisdom teeth are difficult to clean because they are so far back in the mouth and thus are prone to decay and periodontal disease.

Your dentist may remove the tooth or teeth in the office under local anesthesia. If your case is more complicated, your dentist may refer you to an oral surgeon for the removal. If the tooth lies at a difficult angle or you have several teeth impacted, the procedure may require general anesthesia and may need to be done in a hospital.

MISSHAPEN OR DISCOLORED TEETH

Signs and Symptoms
- Misshapen teeth;
- Discolored enamel on primary or secondary teeth.

In rare cases, a child's teeth may not be normal in shape or color. Such abnormalities can be caused by many factors including early illness or trauma, hereditary predisposition, or an environmental factor such as excessive fluoride in the drinking water or the mother's ingestion of tetracycline drugs during pregnancy and nursing. Most often, such abnormalities affect both primary and secondary teeth.

Misshapen teeth are caused most often by infection, high fever, or malnutrition during infancy or early childhood. The eight front teeth and the 6-year molars are the teeth most frequently affected because these develop first. The crowns of the teeth can be

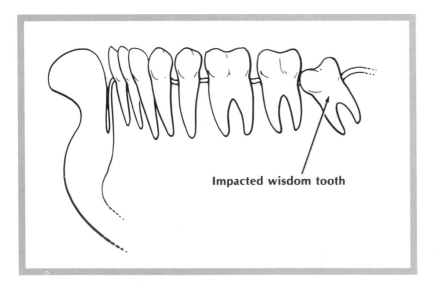

Impacted wisdom tooth

ORTHODONTICS AND SURGICAL CORRECTION

Few people have a perfect bite and pearly white, symmetrical teeth. For some of us, our teeth are slightly misaligned, perhaps where the uppers and lowers clamp together to form the bite or, in some cases, in the front where the teeth are most visible.

Some misalignment or crowding may be minor, requiring little or no attention. However, a significant number of children and adults have problems that do require treatment. Most of us are familiar with the term orthodontics, the branch of dentistry that deals with the correction of misaligned (maloccluded) teeth.

In general, orthodontists are concerned with producing an even bite, with the teeth aligned and balanced within the jaws and face. Such manipulation of the teeth usually requires the use of appliances (braces) that gradually move the teeth into the desired positions in the jaw.

Identifying the Problem

In the ideal bite, the teeth of the upper jaw slightly overlap those of the lower jaw. The points of the molars fit into the grooves of the opposing molars. In the ideal jaw there is room for all teeth to fit neatly, neither crowded nor spaced. There are no rotations of teeth or any teeth that twist or lean forward or backward.

When teeth do not fit together properly, they can cause chewing problems (and therefore eating and digestion difficulties). Increased tooth decay also can result. The abnormal forces on the improperly fitting teeth may be a contributing factor in periodontal disease. Misaligned or protruding teeth can cause emotional distress if they affect appearance. Jaw surgery sometimes is needed to correct serious problems when both the teeth and the jaws are misaligned.

Your child's regular dentist will monitor the development of the secondary teeth and recommend consultation with an orthodontist if problems seem imminent. Most problems of alignment become apparent once the secondary teeth begin to erupt, often as early as age 6. However, in some instances the problems can be appropriately treated earlier.

Your orthodontist will thoroughly examine your child's mouth. He or she may take a series of x-rays. Some of the x-rays are used to determine the position of teeth, both erupted and yet to erupt. Special x-rays of the head may help to determine the size, position, and relationship of the jaw and teeth.

If the lower jaw is significantly smaller than the upper jaw, the upper teeth may protrude excessively over the lower (a condition called overbite). Similarly, if the lower jaw is larger than the upper, the upper front teeth can bite behind the lower ones (underbite). When significant discrepancies exist between the upper and lower jaws, an operation (orthognathic surgery) may be desirable. However, most often these problems can be corrected with various appliances. Similarly, teeth that are rotated, overlapped, or spaced are candidates for correction.

Today, more and more adults are seeking orthodontic correction of problems that were not treated when they were younger. Although in adults the treatment time often is longer because tooth movement is slower, the results usually are pleasing. More corrective jaw surgery is performed on adults than on children.

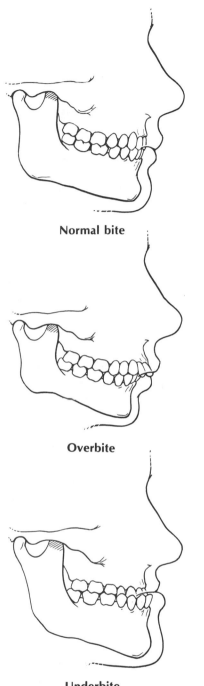

Normal bite

Overbite

Underbite

Other possible diagnostic studies include making impressions of your upper and lower teeth from which plaster models are constructed. Your dentist will ask you to bite down on a thin, wax-like material to make an impression that can be used to position plaster models accurately to represent the actual bite of your upper and lower teeth. Photographs of your teeth and face and other measurements and recordings also may be made.

Making Changes

If severe overcrowding is the main problem, certain permanent teeth, usually premolars, can be extracted to create room and the remaining teeth are realigned by fitting appliances (braces) to them.

Fixed braces, usually made of an alloy, are either ring-like bands that encircle the molar teeth or bonds that are attached only to the outside surfaces of the premolar and anterior teeth. Clear or tooth-colored ceramic or inside braces are other options for fixed braces.

Wires, springs, and other force-producing devices place a tension on the teeth that gradually shifts them into new positions. The jaw responds to the pressure by dissolving bone in front of the moving tooth and laying down new bone behind it. Occasionally, tension will be drawn from the opposite jaw, usually achieved with elastic bands placed on upper and lower teeth and connected to an opposite tooth.

Sometimes extra anchorage or support is needed outside the mouth. In these instances, special head or neck gear is designed for attachment to the appliances within the mouth. Such appliances are often worn only at night or for specific periods during the day.

There may be times, particularly in the growing child, when certain removable appliances may be appropriate. These appliances may be designed to move certain individual teeth or groups of teeth.

Routine treatment time with braces ranges from approximately 6 months to 2 years or more. The correction is made during this time, but this is not the end of treatment. The teeth then must be stabilized for months, years, or sometimes indefinitely to keep the moved teeth in place.

To accomplish this stabilization, the teeth are usually fitted with one or more of various devices called retainers. Examples of retainers include: positioners (rubber-like mouthpieces the person wears at night and bites into for a few hours during the day), removable retainers (with plastic material on the inside and wires on the outside of the teeth), removable, clear plastic retainers (completely cover the sides and biting surfaces of the teeth), and semi-rigid wires (most often are adapted to and bonded on the inside of the front teeth).

Oral Hygiene

Take special care to clean your teeth regularly during the course of orthodontic treatment. Food and plaque accumulate around orthodontic appliances. If you do not remove these deposits, de-

mineralization occurs and may leave permanent whitish marks (scars) on your teeth. Brush with a fluoride toothpaste and rinse with a fluoride mouthwash recommended by your dentist. Although somewhat more difficult, we also recommend flossing.

Corrective Surgery

In extreme cases when conventional orthodontic treatment is not enough to correct a problem, your dentist may recommend corrective surgery. This is more common in adults than in children.

Protrusion of the upper or lower jaw can be corrected by removing a section of bone and setting the remainder in its correct position. Conversely, short jaws can be lengthened; or the height of the lower face can be shortened or lengthened to provide better facial esthetics and function. Surgery can adjust other misaligned bites that may not respond fully to orthodontic treatment alone. Surgery also may shorten the overall time of orthodontic treatment.

Corrective surgery usually requires hospitalization for a few days, usually is performed under general anesthesia, and has a relatively short recuperation period. The jaws often are wired together for a few days to a few weeks during the initial healing. During healing, chewing and other activities involving the jaws must be curtailed to some extent.

pitted or grooved and may be discolored. In rare cases, misshapen teeth are related to serious disorders such as syphilis (see page 876) or Down's syndrome (see page 57). Occasionally, the enamel covering the teeth will be imperfect. Although this can be caused by several factors, most often it is the result of a genetic trait that recurs in families. The enamel may be discolored, thin, or even absent. Discoloration also can be caused by living in an area with fluoride content in

drinking water of more than 2 parts per million. This amount of fluoridation is not a result of added fluoride but rather occurs naturally in some areas.

Another cause of discolored teeth is the ingestion of tetracycline drugs. Enamel is completely formed on all but the wisdom teeth by about 8 years of age. Therefore, physicians do not prescribe a prolonged course of tetracycline treatment for pregnant women or children under age 8.

Treatment. Misshapen teeth can be treated by adding a restorative material or by covering them with crowns. Teeth without a complete covering of enamel and some very discolored teeth also may be treated in this manner. Sometimes this is done on primary teeth if the enamel is so malformed that serious cavities or wearing down of the teeth occurs. In these instances, the molar teeth often are fitted with stainless steel crowns.

INFECTIONS AND DISEASES OF THE MOUTH

Almost everyone occasionally experiences some sort of infection or disease of the mouth. Often we are not even aware of the problem, as in the case of gingivitis (see page 570), or it is so minor that it is merely a mild and passing irritation, as with the occasional canker sore or cold sore.

Other problems are more debilitating, as in the case of certain tongue, jaw, and salivary gland problems. Still others, such as oral cancer, can be life-threatening. We discuss each of these infections and diseases in the following pages.

CANKER SORES

Signs and Symptoms
• Small, painful, white ulcers in the mouth.

Canker sores, or aphthous ulcers, are common, annoying infections of the mouth. They occur singly or in clusters on the inside surface of the cheeks and lips, on the tongue, at the base of the gums, and on the soft palate (the movable flesh at the back of the roof of the mouth).

The cause of canker sores is unknown, although there seems to be an inherited disposition to them. Recurrent canker sores seem to occur in association with an injury to the mouth, such as that caused by a prick, puncture, or irritation as from orthodontic appliances. Physical and emotional stress also seem to trigger attacks of canker sores, as do dietary deficiencies in some people. People lacking iron, folic acid, vitamin B_{12}, or a combination of these nutrients often are susceptible. In some women, canker sores develop just before the onset of menses.

Treatment. Canker sores develop quickly and disappear quickly, usually within 7 to 10 days. They can be treated with soothing over-the-counter ointments. If they become infected, see your physician or dentist who may prescribe antibiotics to clear the infection. If a canker sore lasts more than 14 days, consult your dentist (see also Cold Sores and Canker Sores, page 1175).

(See page B-10 for color photograph of canker sores.)

GINGIVOSTOMATITIS

Signs and Symptoms
• Mouth and gum sores;
• Bad breath;
• Fever and a feeling of malaise.

Gingivostomatitis is a common infection of the mouth among children. The condition is a viral infection and often accompanies an upper respiratory infection such as a cold or the flu.

Gingivostomatitis infections range from mild to severe. Generally they last about 2 weeks.

The Diagnosis. If your child has sores on the gums or on the insides of the cheeks, has bad breath, runs a fever, and feels generally unwell, consult your dentist or physician. Your physician will examine your child's mouth and will check for any underlying infection, particularly of the chest or throat. A sample may be taken for culture.

Treatment. Treatment of any underlying infection or disorder will help clear the mouth infection. A medicated oral rinse may help relieve the pain and promote healing. Good oral hygiene and a nutritious diet of soft foods and plenty of fluids are important. Use of a mouthwash made of half a teaspoon of salt dissolved in 8 ounces of water, or an over-the-counter mouthwash, may be soothing.

ORAL THRUSH

Signs and Symptoms
- Creamy-white sore patches in the mouth or throat.

Your mouth houses many different kinds of microbes in very small numbers. One of them, the fungus *Candida albicans* (which is also found elsewhere in the body), on occasion can reproduce uncontrollably to produce an infection known as oral thrush. Thrush may extend downward into the esophagus (see also Other Causes of Esophageal Inflammation, page 595).

This fungus is the same microbe responsible for the vaginal yeast infections that many women experience. Oral thrush tends to occur most often when your natural resistance to disease has been weakened by illness or when your mouth's natural balance of microbes has been upset by medication such as antibiotics, immunosuppressive drugs, or corticosteroid drugs.

Many people experience an outbreak of oral thrush at some point in their lives. The infection is most common among babies and young children and the elderly, although it can occur at any time of life.

Oral thrush can be painful, but ordinarily it is not a serious disorder. However, it can interfere with eating and thereby impair your nutrition. It can be treated by your physician or dentist, but it tends to recur.

The Diagnosis.   If slightly raised, creamy-white sore patches develop in your mouth or on your tongue, you may have oral thrush. The patches may be brushed off when you clean your teeth or eat. Brushing may make them sore and they may bleed slightly. The infection can spread to the roof of your mouth, to your gums or tonsils, and into your throat. (See color photograph, page B-10.)

If you have any of these symptoms, see your dentist or physician who will examine your mouth and throat and will determine whether there may be an underlying cause for the condition.

Treatment.   Your dentist or physician will prescribe a course of oral antifungal medication, often to be taken for 7 to 10 days. Any underlying disorder must be treated as well.

LEUKOPLAKIA

Signs and Symptoms
- Thickened, hardened, white patch on a cheek or tongue.

The term leukoplakia comes from a Greek word meaning white plate, an apt description of the white patches that characterize this disorder. Ill-fitting dentures or a rough tooth rubbing against the cheek or gum is a common cause. (See color photograph, page B-10)

When white patches develop in the mouths of smokers as the body's natural protection against the heat of tobacco smoke, the condition is called smoker's keratosis. Patches of leukoplakia also occur if a cud of chewing tobacco or snuff is held within the mouth for extended periods.

You can have leukoplakia at any time during your life, but it is most common among the elderly.

The Diagnosis.   You may notice a white or grayish patch that develops on the inside of one cheek or on your tongue over the course of several weeks. At first it may not be noticeable. After a while it may become rough and sensitive to hot or spicy foods.

If you observe such a patch, see your dentist or physician. If the patch persists after treatment, your physician or dentist may take a biopsy specimen of the area for examination under a microscope. About 3 percent of such patches are early signs of mouth cancer.

Treatment.   Most treatment of leukoplakia involves removing the source of irritation. If a rough tooth or denture is the cause, the offending tooth will probably be filed down or replaced. If the patch is linked to smoking or chewing tobacco, you will be advised to quit the habit. Once the source of irritation has been removed, the patch may clear up, usually within weeks or months.

ORAL LICHEN PLANUS

Signs and Symptoms
- Small, pale pimples that form a lacy network on the tongue or cheeks;

- Shiny, slightly raised patches on the tongue or cheeks;
- Sore, dry mouth with a metallic taste.

Oral lichen planus may be limited to a network of pale pimples or shiny red raised patches. Both are found on the sides of the tongue or inside the cheeks, or it may advance into a painful erosive lesion. Your mouth may be sore and dry and have a metallic taste. Some people experience no symptoms other than the raised pimples or bumps. (See color photograph, page B-10.)

The cause of oral lichen planus is uncertain. Emotional stress seems to trigger the response in some people. At other times, oral lichen planus is a side effect of certain medications. Any adult can have this rare disorder, but it affects middle-aged women more frequently than any other group.

There seems to be a relationship between the oral form and the skin form of lichen planus (see Lichen Planus, page 1161) be-

BAD BREATH

Just about everyone would like to have breath that always is "kissing sweet." Because fresh breath is important to us, manufacturers of mints and mouthwashes harvest substantial profits from this multi-million dollar industry.

Advertisements for many of these products maintain that your breath can be made wonderfully fresh; the accompanying implication often is of an increased attractiveness to the opposite sex. Sad to say, these products do not always succeed in curing your bad breath (halitosis)—or have any effect on your social life.

At best, these products are only temporarily helpful in controlling breath odors. They actually may be less effective than simply rinsing your mouth with water, brushing and flossing your teeth, or just eating a meal.

What Causes Bad Breath?

There are many causes of bad breath. First, your mouth itself may be the source. Bacterial decomposition of food particles and other debris in and around your teeth can produce a foul odor. Pockets of infection, as in periodontitis (see page 571), are obvious causes of odor. A dry mouth, such as occurs during sleep or as the result of some drugs or of smoking, will enable dead cells to accumulate on your tongue (coated tongue), gums, and cheeks, and these will undergo bacterial decomposition.

Another cause of bad breath is eating foods containing volatile oils with a strong, distinctive odor. Onions and garlic are the best known examples, but there are other vegetables and spices that also may cause bad breath. After this food is digested in your stomach and small intestine and the volatile substances are absorbed into your bloodstream, they are carried to your lungs and are given off in your breath. (Alcohol behaves in the same fashion, thus allowing measurement of blood alcohol levels by tests of the breath. Alcohol itself has almost no odor, however. The characteristic smell on the breath is mainly the odor of other components of the beverage.)

Lung disease can cause bad breath. Chronic infections in the lungs, such as bronchiectasis (see page 921) or lung abscess (see page 923), can produce very foul-smelling breath. Usually, much sputum is produced in these cases. If you have impaired motility of your stomach you may have bad breath from fermentation of the stomach contents. Belching may produce the odor. Esophageal reflux also can be a cause of bad breath (see page 593).

There are several general health problems that can cause a distinctive odor to the breath. Kidney failure (see page 906) can cause a urine-like odor; liver failure (see page 653) may cause an odor sometimes described as "fishy." Acetone in the breath causes a fruity odor and may occur in diabetics who are developing ketoacidosis (see page 709) or commonly in children with childhood illnesses who have eaten poorly for several days.

Treating Your Halitosis

Odors coming from the mouth itself (these are the most common kinds) often can be eliminated by good oral hygiene: brush your teeth after every meal; floss to remove any food particles; have gum diseases treated and corrected; keep your mouth moist with frequent sips of water; and brush your tongue if it is coated (see Tooth Care, page 393).

Avoiding the foods that cause bad breath is another obvious precaution. However, no amount of toothbrushing or use of mouthwashes can do more than partially disguise any odors of garlic or onion that come from your lungs.

Causes such as lung disease, impaired emptying of the stomach, liver failure, and kidney failure must be corrected by treatment of the underlying conditions.

cause almost half of those with the oral version also have it on the skin.

If you notice any of the signs described above, see your dentist.

Treatment. Sometimes, treatment is unnecessary. If the cause is a certain medication, your dentist may advise you to discontinue its use. If you are experiencing discomfort, your dentist will prescribe appropriate medication.

TONGUE DISORDERS

Signs and Symptoms
- Tongue becomes smooth, dark red, and sometimes sore;
- Tongue becomes discolored black or dark brown;
- Tongue appears hairy or furry.

Glossitis is an inflammation of the tongue. Normally, the surface of your tongue is covered with small hair-like projections (papillae) of tissue. When glossitis occurs, the papillae are lost and a range of changes may occur, including discoloration. Specifically, the tongue loses its usual pink and velvety character. It may become sore.

Glossitis can be caused by various factors, including bacterial or fungal infection, iron deficiency anemia (see page 478), and pernicious anemia (see page 479). Most tongue problems are minor, but if the symptoms persist for more than 10 days, visit your physician or dentist for an examination.

Acute Glossitis. This condition can occur as the result of a local infection, burn, or trauma. It may develop quickly and produce swelling and tenderness; it may cause difficulty in chewing, swallowing, and speaking.

If your tongue swells a great deal, it can obstruct your air passages. If this happens, call an emergency medical team (see also Choking, Breathing Emergencies, and Resuscitation, page 268). Immediate corticosteroid treatment usually relieves the swelling.

Geographic Tongue. This disorder is characterized by absence of papillae in patches, which makes the tongue appear smooth and bright red within those patches. In some cases, soreness or burning is an ac-companying symptom. The cause is not completely understood.

Geographic tongue varies from day to day and may be persistent. There is no specific treatment. Avoiding hot or spicy foods, tobacco, and alcohol may help relieve the soreness of geographic tongue.

Hairy Tongue. Occasionally, hair-like papillae on the tongue grow profusely, producing a condition in which the tongue looks as though it is covered with hair. The tongue usually is not sore, but its appearance can be alarming.

Hairy tongue often is a result of antibiotic therapy, excessive use of certain mouthwashes, decreased saliva flow, or lack of adequate oral hygiene. The condition is not serious, and it usually clears after discontinuation of the antibiotic or the offending mouthwash or when the fever breaks. You can remove the hair-like growths by brushing gently with a toothbrush. (See color photograph; page B-10.)

Discolored Tongue. Bacteria normally live in the mouth and are part of your body's natural balance. Occasionally, however, these bacteria can grow excessively and accumulate on the papillae or in the fissures of the tongue. The tongue then appears black or dark brown. Bismuth-containing medications (Pepto-Bismol) also can cause black tongue.

The discoloration can be caused by antibiotic therapy, a fungal infection, smoking, or chewing tobacco. You can help remove the discoloration by brushing your tongue with a toothbrush gently twice each day. You may wish to dip the brush in an antiseptic mouthwash. If the condition persists, see your dentist or physician.

ORAL CANCER

Signs and Symptoms
- Small, pale lump or discolored thickening along the side or on the bottom of the tongue, on the floor of the mouth, inside the cheeks, or on gums, roof of the mouth, or palate.

Cancer of the mouth is common. As with most kinds of cancer, early detection is important to successful treatment.

Routine self-examination of your mouth and tongue may enable you to see or feel an oral cancer when it is small and treatment may be most effective.

The vast majority of oral cancers are of the squamous (scale-like) cell type. Sometimes the cause is unknown, but use of tobacco and excessive alcohol consumption are well-known risk factors (this includes chewing tobacco and snuff as well as smoking).

Oral cancer is less common in people who do not use either tobacco or alcohol. Chronic irritation from jagged tooth surfaces or poorly fitting dentures also may play a role.

The Diagnosis.   Most oral cancers occur along the side or on the bottom of the tongue or on the floor of the mouth. The tumors usually are painless at first and often are visible or can be felt with a finger.

Periodic examination of the soft tissues of the mouth is essential for early diagnosis. If you notice any persistent change from the usual appearance or feel of the soft tissues in your mouth, consult your dentist or physician. He or she will examine your mouth carefully. If an oral cancer is suspected, a local anesthetic will be applied to the area in question, and a small amount of tissue (biopsy) will be taken for laboratory study.

How Serious Is Oral Cancer?   If treated early, oral cancer often can be cured. Unfortunately, more than half of all mouth cancers are well advanced at the time of their detection. Often they spread into nearby lymph nodes of the neck. This requires treatment that is more extensive. The chance of a cure is diminished. Almost 25 percent of people with oral cancer die because of delayed discovery and treatment.

Treatment.   Early surgical removal of the tumor gives the best chance of cure with the fewest side effects. Radiation therapy is an alternative to surgery and is particularly useful for tumors too large for surgical removal.

After the operation, rehabilitation programs can help restore comfort, speech, chewing ability, and a more normal appearance. Again, early detection and treatment offer the best chance of complete recovery.

SALIVARY GLAND PROBLEMS

The saliva produced by your salivary glands serves several purposes. It aids in the mechanical cleaning of your mouth and teeth, it aids in swallowing, and it contains enzymes that help control infection.

There are three major sets of salivary glands as well as numerous smaller glands located throughout your mouth. The parotid glands are located on each side of your mouth. The submandibular glands are under your jaw at the front of your mouth, and the sublingual glands also are in the floor of your mouth. Secretions from these glands drain into the mouth.

Possible malfunctions of the salivary glands include excessive secretion (sialorrhea) and decreased salivation (xerostomia or dry mouth). An excess of saliva is characteristic in childhood, when certain oral infections are present, and often in mentally

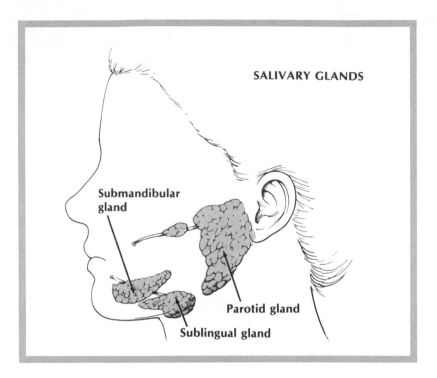

SALIVARY GLANDS

Submandibular gland

Parotid gland

Sublingual gland

retarded persons. Too little saliva may result from use of certain drugs, radiation treatment, certain systemic diseases, and the aging process.

SALIVARY GLAND INFECTIONS

Signs and Symptoms
- Swelling in the floor of the mouth, under the jaw, or in front of the ears;
- Decrease in saliva flow;
- Peculiar tastes in the mouth;
- Pain in the mouth.

Infections of the salivary glands are not uncommon. Viral infections, such as mumps (see page 865), may affect the salivary glands. Bacterial infections may occur after obstruction of a salivary gland or may be associated with poor oral hygiene.

The enlarged gland may be quite painful and may limit your ability to open your mouth wide. Also, pus may be evident at the opening of the duct.

Treatment. Your physician or dentist probably will prescribe a course of antibiotics to clear a bacterial infection. Warm salt water rinses often will aid in removal of the pus.

SALIVARY DUCT STONES

Signs and Symptoms
- Swelling under the chin or in front of the ear, particularly at mealtimes;
- Lack of saliva, particularly when eating;
- Pain in the mouth.

The submandibular glands on the floor of the mouth can become blocked. Such blockages are caused by the formation of a small hard particle, a stone, composed of chemicals from the saliva that harden into a solid material. When this stone partially blocks the duct, pain may be produced, particularly during mealtimes when large quantities of saliva are needed. The engorged gland also may become swollen.

The Diagnosis. If you notice a swelling under your chin or in front of your ear, especially at mealtimes, you may have a blocked salivary duct. You also may notice a lack of saliva and pain in the bottom of your mouth. See your dentist or physician who will probably order an x-ray of your mouth to identify a duct blockage.

Treatment.   A stone in a salivary duct can be removed by one of two methods: manipulation or excision. Your physician may be able to push the stone out of the salivary duct. If not, the stone can be removed by a surgical procedure.

In occasional instances, a gland that has had repeated infections and recurrent salivary duct stones may need to be surgically removed.

SALIVARY DUCT TUMORS

Signs and Symptoms
- Swelling under the chin or in front of your ears.

Rarely, the cells in one of the salivary glands, usually one of the parotid glands (in the cheeks) or submandibular glands (under the jaw), multiply to form a tumor. In most cases the growth is benign and self-contained. Such tumors develop over a period of years and cause the gland to swell gradually. This swelling usually is the only symptom.

Treatment. If one of your salivary glands seems swollen, see your dentist or physician who will examine it and possibly refer you to a radiologist for a special x-ray called a ptylogram or sialogram. This test helps determine the nature of the problem.

Treatment usually involves surgical removal of the gland. If the tumor is malignant, and thus likely to spread (metastasize), radiation therapy or additional surgery may be recommended as well.

FACIAL AND MANDIBULAR TRAUMA AND FRACTURES

When an accident happens, the most likely dental and oral injury is a dislocated or fractured jaw or having a tooth knocked out (tooth avulsion). Such traumas to the jaw are usually medical emergencies that should be attended to without delay.

BROKEN OR DISLOCATED JAW

Signs and Symptoms
- Teeth do not come together normally;
- Jaw cannot be closed or when moved causes intense pain.

Emergency Symptoms
- Obstructed airway;
- Profuse bleeding.

Most jaw trauma involves the mandible (lower jaw). If you sustain an injury to your mouth or face, seek help from your physician, an oral surgeon, or the nearest hospital emergency room immediately for a diagnosis of the extent of the problem and appropriate treatment.

The Diagnosis. Your physician will examine your jaw and take a series of x-rays to determine if the bone is fractured. A CT scan (see page 1286) may be performed to be sure that no other bones of the face have been fractured. If the blow has been strong enough to break other bones of your face, there also may be damage to your neck and back.

Emergency symptoms include an obstructed air passage and profuse bleeding or both.

A fracture is suspected if you are unable to close your mouth, if your teeth are misaligned when your mouth is closed, or if you experience tenderness or numbness around your jaw. An upper jaw that can be moved is a definite sign of fracture. If you are unable to close your jaw, it may be dislocated. Swelling and bruising are likely to accompany all jaw injuries.

Treatment. If you have any of the above symptoms after an accident involving your jaw, go to the nearest hospital without delay. If breathing is difficult or much blood is present, call for an ambulance. The emergency medical technicians may insert a tube to make breathing easier (see also Choking, Breathing Emergencies, and Resuscitation, page 268). If the lower jaw is hanging free, you may wish to cradle it very carefully in your hand until you reach the hospital.

Jaw Dislocation. If your jaw is dislocated, it may be treated by moving it back into place by manually manipulating it, sometimes after administration of an anesthetic.

Once the jaw is reseated, it may be stabilized with a bandage to keep your mouth from opening too wide and causing another dislocation. Avoid opening your mouth very wide for up to 6 weeks after the injury. When you feel a yawn coming on, place your fist under your chin to keep your mouth from opening wide.

If you have dislocated your jaw more than once, consult an oral and maxillofacial surgeon (a surgeon who specializes in problems of the jaw and the bones of the face) for possible treatment.

Jaw Fracture. The first step in treating a jaw fracture is to immobilize the jaw by using a bandage. Once you have been examined, a course of action will be chosen. In many cases this involves surgery to realign the bones and allow them to heal. Often the jaw will need to be immobilized for 6 to 8 weeks, perhaps by wiring it to the opposite jaw. During this time you will be able to eat only soft or liquid foods, and talking may be difficult.

LOSS OF A TOOTH (AVULSION)

When a permanent tooth is accidentally knocked out through accident (avulsion), appropriate emergency medical care is required, whether a child or an adult is involved (see Tooth Avulsion, page 316).

TEMPOROMANDIBULAR JOINT PROBLEMS

Signs and Symptoms

- Tenderness of your jaw muscles;
- Dull aching pain in front of your ear;
- A clicking sound or grating sensation on opening your mouth or chewing;
- Locking of the joint, making it difficult to open or close your mouth.

Your temporomandibular joint (TMJ) is a hinged joint situated on each side of your head where the lower jaw bone (mandible) connects with the temporal bone of your skull. Inflammation, injury, or dislocation of this joint can cause pain.

Your temporomandibular joints (TMJ) are the hinged joints that connect both sides of your lower jaw (mandible) to your skull. As with other joints, the bony surfaces are covered with cartilage and are separated by a small disc that prevents the bones from rubbing against one another. Muscles that enable you to open and close your mouth also serve to stabilize these joints which are located about one-half inch in front of each ear canal.

As with other joints, the TMJ is susceptible to a variety of disorders such as osteoarthritis, rheumatoid arthritis, and other forms of inflammation. In rare instances, tumors may arise in this area.

When you open your mouth, the mandible moves downward and forward. For normal jaw function, your left and right TMJs must work in synchrony. If the movement of both joints is not coordinated, the disc that separates the lower jaw from the skull can slip out of position, resulting in malfunction of the jaw. Should your mouth be forced open rapidly or too far, dislocation also can result.

Overuse of the joint by grinding your teeth (bruxism) or trauma to the side of your face also can cause TMJ pain. Extreme jaw clenching can lead to pain in your TMJ as well as over the temples. This occurs because the muscles that control jaw movement are also attached to a nearby bone of your skull.

In most cases, headaches or pain in the side of your face or jaw are not related to the abnormalities of the temporomandibular joint.

The Diagnosis.   Tenderness over the joint (with or without movement), a clicking or grating sensation when you open or close your mouth, and locking of the joints (making it difficult to open or close your mouth) when accompanied by pain may suggest a TMJ problem. See your dentist or physician.

He or she may order x-rays or a MRI scan (see page 1287); in most cases they are normal. Your dentist or physician will also examine your bite to see if there are abnormalities in the alignment of your teeth and in the movement of your jaw. Such conditions as a high filling, a tipped tooth, teeth displaced due to earlier loss of other teeth, or certain inherited characteristics may produce such misalignments.

Bruxism can exist without your being aware of it. Often, the grinding occurs during sleep. Your dentist can determine the presence of a tooth grinding habit by noting excessive wear on the biting surfaces of your teeth. Another result of excessive grinding and jaw clenching is a dull discomfort in your jaw and head areas on awakening in the morning. This is termed a musculoskeletal headache or tension headache (see page 547).

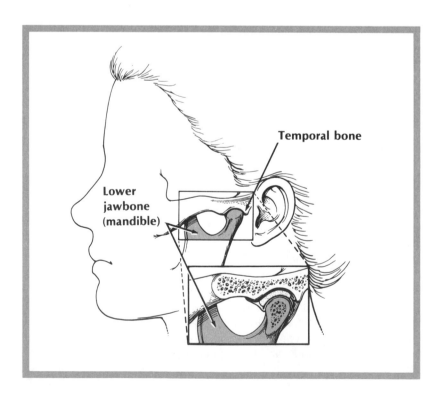

Temporal bone

Lower jawbone (mandible)

Treatment. Most cases of TMJ disorder are the result of inflammation within the joint. In these instances, physical therapy and medications (such as aspirin or other nonsteroidal anti-inflammatory drugs) used for treating similar symptoms in larger joints work effectively. Occasionally, a corticosteroid drug can be injected into the joint to reduce severe pain and inflammation.

If abnormalities in the alignment of your teeth are present, your dentist may correct this by balancing biting surfaces, replacing missing dentition, or replacing defective fillings or crowns.

If your TMJ is misaligned, your dentist may recommend a plastic bite plate (splint) to promote better alignment of jaw bones. This corrective device is worn over your teeth and helps to reestablish proper alignment. The device may need to be adjusted periodically by your dentist.

Splints typically provide relief from jaw locking, pain, and noise. In addition, your dentist may recommend modifications in your chewing habits. For example, he or she may discourage chewing of gum or of firm foods such as caramels, nontender meats,
raw carrots, and celery as well as excessive mouth opening during yawning.

If symptoms continue and the use of a splint is unsuccessful, a specialist in oral and maxillofacial surgery may need to repair or to remove the disc that separates the adjacent bony surfaces of the TMJ, or portions of the bones themselves, or both.

Bruxism can be a difficult habit to break, especially if it occurs while you sleep. However, your dentist may provide either a soft or a firm appliance that you can insert over your teeth at bedtime to offset the effects of the clenching or grinding and to protect your teeth from excessive wear. In addition to these "nightguard appliances," biofeedback/relaxation therapy, physical therapy, and other behavior modification efforts can be of great help.

When symptoms of TMJ disorder occur without evidence of a physical abnormality, psychological factors could be responsible for the pain. For example, chronic tension and anxiety might cause you to maintain a clenched jaw, leading to TMJ disorder. In these situations, biofeedback/relaxation therapy may provide relief (see page 1036).

PROSTHODONTICS

We have all seen the picture of George Washington with a slightly pained look on his face. And most of us have been told that his expression was due to a pair of ill-fitting wooden dentures.

Before modern dentistry, losing one's teeth was an inevitable part of aging. Rare was the person who by old age had any teeth left. In the 18th century, the very fact that Washington had dentures at all shows that he was one of the lucky few who were able to take advantage of the then latest advances in dentistry.

Today, however, the story is different. Fewer and fewer people need to have their teeth removed and replaced with dentures. If you lose an adult tooth, a prosthodontist can make a replacement tooth.

Partial dentures (bridges) may be placed permanently (fixed) in your mouth or may be removable, depending on conditions in your mouth. Partial dentures may be made when one or more teeth need replacement. Replacement of all teeth is achieved with complete dentures, removable sets of artificial teeth.

PARTIAL DENTURES

Once a permanent tooth has been lost, it should be replaced without delay. Your teeth are positioned such that every tooth holds its position and helps the adjacent teeth retain their proper positions, too. If you lose a tooth and do not replace it, the teeth on either side can gradually drift or tilt toward the open space. This can alter your bite, sometimes making it more difficult to chew.

Your dentist will determine what sort of partial denture, also called a bridge, is best suited to your needs. If you have healthy teeth on each side of the missing tooth or teeth, a fixed partial denture may be made. In this procedure, the healthy teeth are decreased in size to receive a retainer. The retainer and an artificial tooth are then joined together, and the retainer is cemented to the supporting teeth.

Another type of prosthetic device is known as a removable partial denture. This prosthesis has artificial teeth joined together with a metal or plastic base to which clips are attached at either end. The prosthesis then fits into the opening left by the missing tooth and attaches to surrounding teeth. Removable partial dentures are less costly than fixed partial dentures, and more teeth can be added to it if you lose neighboring teeth.

You must be very careful to keep all prosthetic appliances clean because they are all particularly prone to plaque buildup. If the partial denture is fixed, be sure to floss and brush it carefully. If it is removable, remove the prosthesis and brush it and surrounding teeth carefully after every meal. Also, remove partial dentures at bedtime.

PROPER CARE OF YOUR DENTURES

A set of dentures can last from 6 months to 5 years or more, depending on how well they fit, the condition of your jaw, their material, and how well they are maintained.

For dentures to be comfortable and durable, they must be cared for properly. Good maintenance is not difficult, particularly if you take these steps.

1. Make sure your dentures fit properly. If they seem uncomfortable after the initial adjustment period, see your dentist or prosthodontist.
2. Remove your dentures each night at bedtime. Your gums need a period of rest in order to remain healthy.
3. Store your removed dentures in water to which a denture cleaning agent may be added when needed. Dentures not stored in water can warp, making them uncomfortable to wear. Removable partial dentures with metal bases should not be left to soak in cleaning agents longer than 15 minutes.
4. Clean your dentures each day, according to your dentist's instructions. Food particles and plaque must be removed regularly.
5. Brush and floss your remaining natural teeth each day. It is imperative to keep the remaining teeth and gums as healthy as possible, particularly because they often are the support to which a partial denture is secured.
6. Clean and massage your mouth and gums each day using a brush, cloth, or your finger. It is as important to keep the gums and soft tissues of your mouth clean and stimulated as it is to keep your teeth clean.

DENTURES

If, as a consequence of serious periodontal disease or decay, you need to have all of your teeth removed—a decision to be made in concert by you and your dentist—your dentist or prosthodontist will make a set of artificial teeth (dentures).

Dentures can never replace the function and feeling of natural teeth but certainly are a better alternative to no teeth at all. You will lose some sensation in eating as your hard palate (roof of your mouth) is covered by the upper denture. Also, you may be limited in regard to what foods you can eat. Foods such as corn on the cob, whole apples, and hard candies may be difficult to eat because pressures exerted by biting or chewing such foods can cause dentures to loosen in your mouth.

Accustom yourself to different methods of food preparation such as cutting corn kernels from the cob and slicing apples.

The chewing pressure you can exert with dentures is much less than you can exert with your natural teeth (which are anchored in your jaw). Well-fitted dentures usually do not require use of denture adhesives.

Fitting Dentures.   There are two standard methods for fitting dentures. The teeth can be extracted and then the gums and jaw be allowed to heal before dentures are fitted. The other method is to prepare dentures in advance and insert them immediately after the extraction.

Not everyone is eligible for immediate dentures. Your dentist will be able to assess the conditions in your mouth and recommend the best approach for you.

Immediate dentures save you the inconvenience of being without teeth for a period of time. However, they often must be refitted once the jaw heals, and occasionally new ones must be made if the jaw changes shape significantly after extraction.

A full set of dentures usually consists of complete upper and lower bases that fit over the gums, but there is a variation known as an overdenture. When a few acceptable teeth remain in the jaw, the denture can be constructed to cover them. The covered teeth may need to have the nerve removed (root canal therapy) and be covered with a

OSSEOINTEGRATION OF TEETH

More than 40 percent of Americans age 65 or older and 4 percent of employed adults ages 18 to 64 have lost all of their natural teeth. Technology has come a long way since George Washington's legendary ill-fitting dentures, but dentures still can be troublesome.

The development of a new dental implant technique called osseointegration (osseo means bone; integration means to unite with something else) may help to diminish the problems of dentures in the future. The procedure was developed in Sweden in the 1960s and became available in this country in the early 1980s. In this procedure, titanium fittings are implanted in the bone of the jaw. Fixed or removable dentures or individual teeth can be attached to them. This procedure is often used for people who cannot tolerate standard dentures because of physical or emotional reasons.

In osseointegration, artificial teeth are attached to the bones of the lower or upper jaw. One tooth or all of the teeth in either jaw can be replaced. Conventional dentures rest upon a thin layer of gum tissue, which can become sore or infected. Osseointegration anchors the artificial teeth in the upper or lower jaw in much the same fashion as normal teeth are held in place. Chewing pressure, therefore, can be nearly normal whereas with conventional dentures the chewing pressure generally is much less. In this way, osseointegration helps to prevent deterioration of the jaw.

The Procedure
The procedure involves several steps over a period of months. It is expensive. The surgical phase may require a general anesthetic and 1 or 2 days in the hospital in complex cases. For routine cases, the surgery may be performed in the dental office.

Holes are drilled in your upper and lower jaw and hollow threaded cylinders made of titanium are placed in the holes. The bony tissue of your jaw grows around the implanted cylinders. Your old dentures can be adjusted for use during this period.

Several months after the operation, solid metal posts are screwed into the cylinders. One or 2 weeks later you return to have a cast made of your jaw with the posts in place. Then, artificial teeth are constructed and attached firmly to the posts by tiny gold screws.

The success rate for some implant procedures is more than 90 percent. Such high success rates are derived from the skill and painstaking care with which osseointegration is performed and the discipline of patients in caring for their mouths.

Osseointegration is a relatively new process whereby artificial teeth are permanently anchored into the mouth using tiny screws implanted in the jawbone.

restoration prior to construction of the overdenture.

An overdenture is especially useful in the lower gum because it sometimes is difficult to keep a denture in place there. The remaining teeth must be carefully and regularly maintained to keep them healthy. Your dentist or prosthodontist will advise you on the possibility of using an overdenture.

Whatever kind of removable denture you have, it will need periodic fitting to keep it comfortable and to help prevent bone loss and mouth sores.

DENTURE PROBLEMS

Signs and Symptoms
- Persistently loose lower denture;
- Pain in the mouth when dentures are in place;
- Inflamed gums;
- Sores in the mouth at denture pressure points.

Because dentures are foreign to your mouth, the chances are good that you will experience a problem with them. A lower denture may be loose-fitting, or sores may develop, or your gums may become inflamed. The lower denture usually does not remain in place by itself, and successful use may depend upon your ability to control a denture with the muscles surrounding it.

Many people in the United States suffer from ill-fitting lower dentures. Your natural teeth are supported by a specialized type of bone in your upper and lower jaws. When teeth are lost, the supporting bone begins to shrink. This bony shrinkage may be accelerated by the aging process and also by wearing ill-fitting dentures.

The result may be loose dentures. Loose dentures cause soreness during chewing and may become dislodged when you are talking or laughing. Changes in the bone make it difficult for your dentist to construct a properly fitting denture unless something

can be done to improve the foundation on which it rests.

A loose lower denture is only one of the problems you may encounter as a result of the pressure that your dentures place on your gums. The denture rests on soft tissues in your mouth. In some areas, this tissue is more vulnerable to injury than in other areas. Your denture may cause pressure over this less-resilient tissue. This pressure is uncomfortable and can lead to the formation of sores and mouth ulcers.

Partial dentures place pressure not only on the ridges but also on the natural teeth surrounding the denture. Partial dentures can trap food, particularly when they do not fit properly. Good oral hygiene is important because retained food particles lead to plaque, calculus, periodontal disease, and decay of the natural teeth.

The Diagnosis. If your dentures are uncomfortable for more than the initial few minutes after you put them in, if you experience pain when chewing, or if you notice that your gums are red and swollen or have sore white patches, see your dentist for an examination. Your dentist will study both the state of your jaw and the condition of your dentures and gums.

Treatment. Your dentist may be able to adjust your dentures to relieve the pressure on your gums or, if necessary, make a new set of dentures that conform to the current shape of your bones and gums. If your gums are red and swollen because of a fungal infection, your dentist can prescribe an antifungal medication.

If your jaw has shrunk and your prosthodontist has trouble making dentures that will fit well, several surgical techniques are now available that may provide a better foundation upon which a new denture can be constructed. These techniques include operations to build up the soft tissue of your gum or hard tissue of your jaw. Sometimes a metallic support can be implanted in the bone.

CHAPTER 24

THE DIGESTIVE SYSTEM

CHAPTER CONTENTS

THE DIGESTIVE SYSTEM AT WORK

The digestive system consists of many parts. Among them are the esophagus, stomach, and the small and large intestines, tubular structures through which food and waste products pass and in which digestion takes place. Two large glands, the liver and the pancreas, furnish some of the enzymes and other substances needed for digestion. The gallbladder, a hollow organ located just under the liver, stores the bile manufactured in the liver.

The food you eat is propelled through your digestive tract by muscular contractions that for the most part are automatic (involuntary). The process of digestion changes the components of food into a form that eventually can be absorbed into your bloodstream. After the nutrients are absorbed, your digestive tract eliminates unwanted material.

Digestion begins when you chew your food. The food is broken into smaller pieces by your teeth and, at the same time, is mixed with saliva secreted by your salivary glands. Your saliva contains an enzyme, called ptyalin, that begins to change starches (carbohydrates) into sugars. Chewing reduces the food to a mushy consistency. When you swallow, the food is propelled into the back part of your throat, past the opening of the voice box (larynx), and into the upper part of your esophagus. Food is prevented from entering your larynx by a flap of soft tissue (epiglottis) that closes as food passes into the esophagus. When the epiglottis fails to close completely, a minor coughing fit may result. Such an episode is said to be the result of the food "having gone down the wrong way."

ESOPHAGUS

Once you swallow your food, it moves down into the esophagus, a tube approximately 10 inches long that leads directly into your stomach. The food is moved into your esophagus by muscles in the back of your throat (pharynx). When it enters the main part of the esophagus, muscles there undergo a series of wave-like contractions, called peristalsis, to move the food into your stomach. Peristalsis is the mechanism by which the food is moved throughout the remainder of its trip through your digestive tract until the waste products reach the muscles of the anus.

A muscle that encircles the bottom portion of the esophagus (lower esophageal sphincter) is critical in the passage of food into your stomach. When this valve-like sphincter relaxes, it opens and permits food to enter your stomach. It then closes, which prevents any food from flowing back (regurgitating) into your esophagus. When this sphincter muscle fails to work properly, stomach contents regurgitate into the esophagus. Called esophageal reflux, this partial regurgitation may be damaging to the sensitive lining of your esophagus by allowing stomach acid to come into contact with it. If this occurs, you may experience the symptoms of heartburn and have a condition called esophagitis (see Esophageal Reflux, page 593, and Other Causes of Esophageal Inflammation, page 595).

STOMACH

The walls of your stomach consist of various layers of powerful muscles. These muscles serve an important mechanical function as they cause the stomach to churn, breaking the food into smaller and smaller pieces. In addition, gastric juices manufactured by the glands that line your stomach mix with the food particles. These juices contain pepsin, a digestive enzyme that begins to break down proteins in the mixture, and hydrochloric acid, which creates the proper environment for pepsin to work.

Although it serves a useful function, your stomach is not vital to the breakdown of food and its subsequent absorption. Only small amounts of such food as alcohol, simple sugars, and some medications are actually absorbed in the stomach.

There is a delicate balance in your stomach between the acid produced by its glands and the resistance of your stomach lining to that acid. If this balance is upset, the result may be damage to the stomach lining, such as a peptic ulcer (see page 603) or gastritis (see page 608).

Food leaves your stomach in two phases. The upper portion of your stomach contracts first, pushing the more liquid material into your small bowel. The more solid food leaves later, primarily by the action of the muscles in the lower part of your stomach. The partially processed food (called chyme) then travels through the pyloric canal into the first portion of your small intestine, the duodenum.

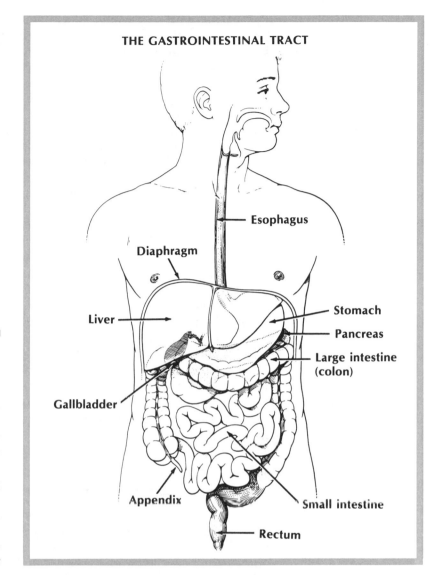

THE GASTROINTESTINAL TRACT

Esophagus

Diaphragm

Liver

Stomach

Pancreas

Large intestine (colon)

Gallbladder

Appendix

Small intestine

Rectum

SMALL INTESTINE

The small intestine (or small bowel) is an elongated tube whose length in adults varies from 12 to 22 feet, depending both on the tone of its muscular wall and on the way it is measured.

The small intestine is divided into three parts. The duodenum is the smallest part, and it is here that the absorption process truly begins. The jejunum, the largest portion of the small bowel, is where the majority of absorption takes place. The final section of the small bowel, the ileum, has some absorptive function (for vitamin B_{12}, for example) in addition to being responsible for the passage of food into the large intestine.

The duodenum contributes to the mixing of food material and also neutralizes acid coming from your stomach. Bile ducts from the liver and gallbladder and the pancreatic duct from the pancreas empty their digestive juices into the duodenum to aid in preparing the chyme for maximum absorption.

As the semi-solid food continues its movement downward through your small intestine, it undergoes further digestion by various enzymes. In this process, the food is broken into smaller particles that then can be readily absorbed through the lining of the small intestine into your bloodstream. The starches (carbohydrates) are broken down into simpler sugars, and proteins are broken down into amino acids. Fats are broken down by enzymes from the pancreas. Because of their detergent-like properties, bile acids from the liver render the fat molecules soluble in water so that they can then be absorbed into your bloodstream. In addition, minerals, vitamins, water, and electrolytes (such as sodium and calcium) are absorbed through the wall of the small intestine into your bloodstream.

By the time the food is ready to pass into your large intestine, almost all its nutrients have been absorbed.

LARGE INTESTINE

At this point, the role of your digestive system changes. Now its job is to remove the waste, consisting mainly of undigested and nonabsorbed food, fiber, and water.

The liquid (primarily water) from the small intestine is carried into the large intestine (colon) where most of it is reabsorbed. Your colon is extremely efficient in this process— of the 10 quarts of fluid that enter it every day, approximately 9.9 quarts are reabsorbed before reaching the anus.

The rest of the waste material moves through the three major segments of your colon—right, transverse, and left descending colon—then into the S-shaped sigmoid colon in the left lower abdomen, and finally into the rectum, the last 16 inches of the colon. It is here that the material collects until the voluntary muscles of the anus expel it.

LIVER

Your liver produces bile, a fluid containing cholesterol and bile acids. Bile flows from the liver through the cystic duct to your gall-

bladder where it is stored. It is eventually emptied into the duodenum, where it performs its major function of assisting in the absorption of fats through the lining of the small bowel into the bloodstream. The bile acids are then reabsorbed in the small intestine and cycled into the liver to be used again.

The liver has other functions also. One is the storage of glycogen, a complex carbohydrate that is converted to sugar for release into your bloodstream when your blood sugar level falls. Glycogen is deposited in the liver when the level of sugar in the blood increases. Many proteins also are synthesized in the liver.

The liver helps determine the amount of nutrients that are sent to the rest of your body. It also serves as a clearinghouse to eliminate some foods and substances that have served their purpose but are no longer useful. In addition, your liver breaks down some medications to enable them to be eliminated in the stool. Alcohol also is metabolized in the liver to supply energy or to be deposited as fat.

GALLBLADDER

The gallbladder is a pear-shaped organ that sits beneath the liver. It is a storage site for much of the bile that is produced in the liver. The bile passes into the gallbladder through a duct (cystic duct) and is stored until it is needed for the digestion of fats that have passed into the small intestine. It is discharged through the cystic duct into the lower portion of the bile duct and then into the duodenum.

Usually, the amounts of bile acids and cholesterol are balanced, but sometimes the concentration of cholesterol becomes too high. The result may be the formation of gallstones.

The gallbladder serves a useful function but is not vital to maintaining your normal body functions because bile can be delivered directly from the liver into the duodenum.

PANCREAS

Shaped somewhat like a banana, the pancreas stretches from your duodenum, to which its head is attached, to the spleen.

This vital organ produces two kinds of secretions. One is pancreatic juice which passes through the ducts of the pancreas into the duodenum where it aids in the digestion of fats and proteins. The other kind includes the hormones insulin and glucagon which pass directly into your bloodstream and help regulate the metabolism of glucose and protein in the liver and other tissues.

Given the numerous parts and the complexity of the gastrointestinal tract, it is hardly surprising that many types of disorders and diseases can occur. In discussing the normal functions and dysfunctions of the stomach, intestines, and the rest, this chapter will follow the same path as the food you eat. First, we will explore problems associated with the esophagus and stomach. We will then proceed to problems of the intestines and then to anorectal diseases. Finally, we will discuss diseases of the liver, pancreas, and gallbladder.

ESOPHAGEAL PROBLEMS

When you swallow food, muscles at the back of your mouth (soft palate) form the food into a soft mass called a bolus. The epiglottis, a leaf-shaped structure at the root of your tongue, folds over the top of the windpipe to protect your trachea and airway. The food is propelled from the back of your mouth into your esophagus.

Your esophagus is a muscular tube, approximately 10 inches long, that leads directly into your stomach. The food automatically travels through the esophagus as a result of wave-like muscular contractions called peristalsis.

At the lower end of the esophagus is an area of specialized muscle called the lower esophageal sphincter. This opens to allow the food to pass into the stomach. The lower esophageal sphincter then closes to prevent return (reflux) of food and stomach juices (including acids) from the stomach back into the esophagus.

This section will discuss problems of the esophagus. The most common problem is heartburn which, incidentally, has nothing to do with the heart but is the result of stomach acid returning (refluxing) back to the esophagus.

Other problems covered in this section include inflammation of the esophagus, swallowing problems, rupture, tumors, and constriction of the esophagus.

ESOPHAGEAL REFLUX

Signs and Symptoms
- Heartburn—a burning sensation in the chest that may start in the upper abdomen and radiate into the neck;
- Regurgitation of sour or bitter-tasting material into the throat and mouth, especially when you are lying down or sleeping.

Esophageal reflux, more commonly known as heartburn, is a frequent complaint. About 1 in 10 adults has heartburn at least once a week; 1 in 3 has the problem at least once a month. Moreover, due to hormonal changes and increased pressure within the abdomen, one in four pregnant women experiences heartburn daily.

Most infants are born with an incompetent lower esophageal sphincter. This allows stomach contents to reflux back up into the esophagus. By age 12 months, the lower esophageal sphincter has matured in most infants and reflux becomes a less common occurrence.

Heartburn occurs when acid-containing stomach contents are allowed to regurgitate back into the esophagus. Under normal circumstances, food passes into the stomach from the esophagus and is prevented from traveling back up the esophagus by the lower esophageal sphincter which remains tightly closed except when you swallow food. Sometimes, however, the sphincter muscle becomes lazy and relaxes (opens), allowing acidic stomach contents to move back up the esophagus, producing the symptoms of esophageal reflux.

The Diagnosis.   Usually a description of your symptoms will be all your physician needs to establish the diagnosis of heartburn.

However, if your symptoms are particularly severe or do not respond to treatment, tests such as a barium x-ray of the esophagus and stomach (see The Barium X-Ray of the Esophagus, Stomach, and Intestine, page 613) or an endoscopic examination (see Upper Gastrointestinal Endoscopy, page 611) may be necessary. In an infant with severe reflux, a barium x-ray of the esophagus may be done.

A hiatal hernia (a protrusion of part of the stomach through the diaphragm) often is found on barium x-ray in people with heartburn, but many hiatal hernias cause no symptoms and require no treatment (see Hiatal Hernia, this page).

How Serious Is Heartburn?   Occasional heartburn can be uncomfortable but is not a serious problem. However, if your heartburn occurs frequently, there is a chance of esophagitis, an irritation (inflammation) of the esophageal lining caused by stomach acid. If the esophagitis becomes severe, the result can be bleeding and difficulty in swallowing due to a constriction (stricture) of the esophagus. Some people with severe esophagitis develop Barrett's esophagus (see Other Causes of Esophageal Inflammation, page 595).

In infants with esophageal reflux, complications are rare. These complications include pneumonia (due to the aspiration of stomach contents into the lungs), delayed growth and weight gain, and iron-deficiency anemia (see page 478).

Treatment.   There are several life-style changes that can help prevent or relieve heartburn.

First, if you are a smoker, stop smoking. Cigarettes relax the lower esophageal sphincter and predispose you to heartburn.

Eat three balanced meals a day but cut down on the size of the portions. Do not eat anything in the 2 to 3 hours before you go to bed. Retiring on an empty stomach decreases the amount of acid your stomach produces and lessens the chance for nocturnal reflux.

If you are overweight, lose weight. A leaner abdomen decreases the pressure on your stomach, which in turn may lessen reflux.

Elevate the head of your bed at least 6 inches by using blocks. This assists gravity in keeping your stomach acid where it belongs.

Avoid tight clothing and tight belts.

Decrease the amount of alcohol, chocolate, fats, and peppermints you consume. These substances relax the lower esophageal sphincter.

Be aware that medications such as birth control pills, antihistamines, antispasmodics, some heart medications, and asthma

---

HIATAL HERNIA

Your chest is separated from your abdomen by a domed sheet of muscle called the diaphragm. To reach your stomach, your esophagus has to pass through an opening (the hiatus) in the diaphragm.

When the tissue around the hiatus weakens, part of the stomach may protrude through the opening into the chest cavity. This is termed hiatal hernia. Hiatal hernia is believed to be caused by a weakening of the anchoring tissues of the gastroesophageal junction to the diaphragm, perhaps due to increased pressure within the abdomen such as sometimes results from obesity or, rarely, trauma.

Hiatal hernias are common. Half of all persons over age 50 have a hiatal hernia. Because the majority of such hernias produce no symptoms, they usually go undetected. For many years, physicians thought hiatal hernias were the cause of heartburn. Although they are frequently found in patients with the symptoms of heartburn who undergo barium x-ray studies, they often are an incidental finding. It is unlikely that a small hiatal hernia will cause you any problems and, by itself, is not a dangerous ailment.

Large hernias (a substantial part of the stomach is above the diaphragm) can cause slow bleeding and iron-deficiency anemia (see page 478). Strangulation of the stomach in large hernias is uncommon, but surgical repair may be advisable to avoid emergency operations in more risky circumstances.

An uncommon type of hernia is known as a paraesophageal hernia. In this situation, part or almost all of the stomach protrudes through the diaphragm into the chest cavity. Paraesophageal hernias also can cause slow bleeding and iron-deficiency anemia. One potential danger of a paraesophageal hernia is strangulation. Sometimes the herniated portion becomes so tightly constricted that the blood supply to those portions of the stomach and esophagus is severely compromised. If this occurs, you will feel persistent chest pain and have difficulty swallowing. This is a medical emergency and may require prompt surgery.

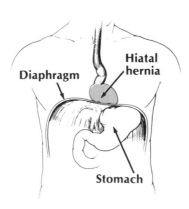

In hiatal hernia, a portion of the stomach protrudes through the diaphragm into the chest cavity.

medicines may aggravate heartburn because they decrease the strength of the lower esophageal sphincter.

For many who experience heartburn occasionally, the use of liquid antacids whenever heartburn occurs, especially after meals and at bedtime, gives significant relief.

If your infant has a mild case of reflux, the condition may improve by keeping the child on his or her stomach with the head and shoulders elevated. It also helps to reduce the volume in each feeding. Try feeding your baby more often and thicken the feedings with cereal. In more severe cases, the baby's head should be kept elevated at all times.

For more significant reflux in adults, drugs such as cimetidine, ranitidine, famotidine, or a new medication called omeprazole, which block acid production in the stomach, may be necessary. Another strategy your physician may try is to increase the strength of the esophageal sphincter with a drug such as bethanechol or metoclopramide. However, no prescription drug should be used until the other methods have been given a chance.

Surgery. Few adult heartburn sufferers require surgery. Only about 5 percent continue to have severe symptoms or have complications despite medication and lifestyle changes. In these cases, surgery is a viable alternative. The procedure, called fundoplication, involves creating a high-pressure zone in the lower esophagus which prevents reflux.

When an infant fails to respond after 6 weeks of intensive medical treatment and has complications of reflux, surgery may be indicated. Consult your infant's physician.

OTHER CAUSES OF ESOPHAGEAL INFLAMMATION

In addition to heartburn from a weakened lower esophageal sphincter, many other disorders can result in inflammation of your esophagus.

Barrett's Esophagus. Persistent reflux of acid from the stomach may damage the normal skin-like lining of the esophagus, which is then replaced by a lining that resembles the lining of the stomach. This new lining usually can resist the gastric reflux, but inflammation at the upper end of the new lin-

ing may narrow (stricture) the interior passageway of the esophagus.

Ulcers may occur in the stomach-like lining and these can bleed and perforate the esophageal wall. In addition, there is a slightly increased risk of cancer occurring in Barrett's esophagus. Your physician may want to evaluate the lining of your esophagus periodically by upper gastrointestinal endoscopy (see page 611) and biopsy to increase the chance of detecting and treating abnormal cells at an early stage.

Herpes Simplex Esophagitis. Infection by herpes simplex virus can cause inflammation and ulcers in the esophagus. People who have such a viral esophagitis are usually debilitated from another disease or, for other reasons, their immune system is exceptionally depressed. Herpes blisters coupled with other symptoms of an esophageal infection strongly suggests a viral esophagitis.

Antibiotics are not effective in treating viral esophagitis, but the antiviral drug acyclovir may be helpful in herpes simplex esophagitis.

Candida Esophagitis. A fungus, *Candida* or *Monilia,* growing in the esophagus can produce an inflammation of the esophagus with associated pain on swallowing. This is called *Candida* esophagitis. This type of infection is often seen in people whose immune systems are depressed as a result of drugs used to fight cancer. There are several antifungal medications that can be used in treatment.

Radiation Esophagitis. This inflammation of the esophagus occurs commonly as a result of radiation treatment for lung (see page 937) or esophageal cancer (see Esophageal Tumors, page 600). The symptoms are heartburn and pain on swallowing. The likelihood of this disorder increases in direct relation to the amount of radiation you receive. With the help of medication, the inflammation usually resolves once the radiation treatment is stopped.

Scleroderma of the Esophagus. Scleroderma is a disease characterized by an overgrowth of scar-like tissue; the result is a stiffening and hardening of tissues. The esophagus is commonly affected. (Besides the gastrointestinal tract, scleroderma can affect organs such as the lungs, heart, and kidneys, as well as the skin; see also Scleroderma, page 1007.)

Scleroderma can weaken the lower esophageal sphincter, allowing acid to reflux into the esophagus and cause the symptoms and complications associated with reflux (see Esophageal Reflux, page 593). At times, a stricture (narrowing) develops in the esophagus, making it more difficult to swallow.

Your physician may prescribe an acid-reducing medication such as cimetidine, ranitidine, famotidine, or omeprazole, which may lessen the amount of reflux. He or she will also instruct you in measures to prevent reflux (see page 594). If the narrowness of the esophagus prevents or retards the passage of food, an esophageal dilation may be performed (see Esophageal Dilation, page 599).

SWALLOWING PROBLEMS

Signs and Symptoms
- Liquids and solid foods stick in the throat or chest;
- Regurgitation of food;
- Gurgling sound in the throat;
- Chest discomfort on swallowing.

Emergency Symptoms
- Complete blockage—unable to swallow liquids or solids (drooling saliva).

Swallowing problems produce different symptoms for different reasons. Food may get stuck in your throat, or it may take longer than normal to swallow your food. You may experience what seems to be heartburn, or you may have a severe chest pain.

The causes of persistent swallowing problems vary. Damage or malfunction of the muscles in the wall of the throat or esophagus will cause swallowing difficulties. Ulcers or scar tissue (stricture) in the esophagus as the result of stomach acid reflux (see Esophageal Reflux, page 593) may make it difficult and sometimes painful for you to swallow. Pouches, called diverticula, may form in the esophageal lining and interfere with the movement of food down the esophagus.

Swallowing problems are also associated with certain diseases such as myasthenia gravis (see page 525) or esophageal cancer (see Esophageal Tumors, page 600).

Swallowing problems may be transient and unimportant; but it is always possible that such problems could be an indication of a serious medical problem. Therefore, see your physician if you continue to have pain or any difficulty swallowing. Early diagnosis *is* important.

Here are some of the kinds of swallowing problems.

Achalasia. This is a rare disorder of the esophagus. It is caused by the lack of coordinated movement (peristalsis) of the muscles of the esophagus and by the failure of the sphincter muscle at the lower end of the esophagus to relax. This makes it very difficult for food to pass into the stomach. The

---

HICCUPS

Holding your breath . . . swallowing water from the "wrong" side of the glass . . . breathing in and out of a paper bag . . . inhaling pepper or ammonia . . . eating a spoonful of sugar . . . having someone startle you.

These all are common—and not consistently successful—methods of getting rid of the hiccups, a generally minor complaint that has afflicted almost everyone at one time or another.

For the most part, hiccups are a harmless, minor annoyance. Sometimes, however, hiccups persist for days or even weeks. When this occurs, they can interfere with eating and sleeping. After major surgery, a prolonged case of the hiccups can impede the healing of an abdominal wound. In rare instances, persistent attacks can be a symptom of a serious disorder.

Although almost everyone has had hiccups, few people know exactly what they are. Very simply, hiccups are repeated, involuntary contractions of your diaphragm. The abrupt closure of your voice box checks the inflow of air: the result is a hiccup.

The phrenic nerves control the smooth, coordinated, normal contraction of the two leaves of the diaphragm, the membrane that separates the chest from the abdomen. The phrenic nerves extend from the neck to the chest. Hiccups may result from irritation anywhere along the path of a phrenic nerve. Reflex contraction of the diaphragm similarly can be the result of irritation to nerves.

Hiccups are more likely to occur when your stomach is distended, typically after eating a big meal or drinking an overabundance of alcohol.

As for a cure, try this: massage the back portion of the roof of your mouth with a cotton-tipped swab, moving the swab gently back and forth for a minute or so. We cannot guarantee this method, but it does work much of the time.

underlying reason for the condition is not fully known.

The primary symptom of achalasia is failure of liquids and solid foods to pass through the esophagus. Food is often regurgitated. Sometimes, particularly in the early stages, drinking a large amount of liquid helps to "push" the food into the stomach. Eventually, however, this fails to provide relief (in fact, in some people certain liquids, especially if very hot or very cold, also may seem to stall in the esophagus from the start). Some chest discomfort or pain may also occur.

If you have the symptoms of achalasia, your physician will order a series of tests including a barium x-ray (see The Barium X-Ray of the Esophagus, Stomach, and Intestine, page 613) or an esophageal motility study (see page 598) to determine whether the esophageal muscles are functioning properly. Often, upper gastrointestinal endoscopy (see page 611) is done to be sure there is no cancer present that may be causing the symptoms of achalasia.

If left untreated, over the course of several decades esophageal cancer may develop in a person with achalasia. Malnutrition, weight loss, and aspiration of food into the lungs, which can lead to pneumonia, are other problems associated with achalasia.

Medication may be somewhat helpful in some cases of achalasia, but it often has little effect.

Another treatment for achalasia is mechanical stretching of the muscles. A slender tube with a balloon attached is passed down the esophagus to the narrowed area. Then it is filled with air or water under pressure to expand the balloon and open (dilate) the passageway. To lessen the discomfort when the tube is inserted, you will be sedated with a medication injected into a vein; also, a spray will be applied to your throat and pharynx to anesthetize them. The balloon dilation weakens the lower esophageal sphincter so that food can pass down the esophagus by gravity. After this treatment, coordinated contractions in the esophagus do not return to normal but most people can swallow adequately.

Also, a surgical procedure called esophagomyotomy can be used. In this procedure, the surgeon opens the chest to reach the esophagus. The muscles at the lower end of the esophagus are then partially cut to allow the food easier passage. The risks of this operation are low and long-term results generally are excellent.

Diffuse Spasm. Multiple, high-pressure, poorly coordinated contractions of the esophagus are referred to as diffuse spasm. They usually occur after a swallow. This is another rare disorder of the esophagus that affects the smooth (involuntary) muscles in the walls of the lower esophagus. The cause for diffuse spasm is not known.

Initially, the diagnosis may be difficult. The symptoms can be mild and even may disappear without treatment. It is possible that you might mistake its symptoms for simple heartburn. But if the cause of the apparent heartburn is diffuse spasm, the symptoms often continue intermittently over a period of years. They may become more severe with time. The symptoms almost invariably are associated with food and liquids being delayed in the esophagus.

Esophageal dilation (see page 596) may produce relief initially. Surgery occasionally may be necessary.

Pharyngeal Diverticula. When muscles in the wall of the pharynx weaken, especially with aging, pouches called diverticula are formed. They can become large enough to trap food.

If pouches form, you may regurgitate food particles shortly after eating. Your throat will become irritated, and you may notice a gurgling sound. As the pouches grow larger, the

If the muscular wall of your pharynx weakens, a small pouch, called a pharyngeal diverticulum, may form and trap food.

Pharyngeal diverticulum

food that is retained for days may give you bad breath.

There is the risk that fluid and undigested food will be regurgitated and passed into the lungs during the night (aspiration), increasing the risk of a lung infection.

Surgery is the treatment for diverticula that are producing uncomfortable symptoms. Pouches or diverticula can also occur in the esophagus but they rarely cause any problems in this location.

Pharyngeal Paralysis. The principal symptoms of pharyngeal paralysis are weakness and incoordination of the muscles of the pharynx which cause difficulty in swallowing. Persons with this problem have difficulty in getting food from their mouth into their throat and esophagus. In addition to swallowing difficulty and throat discomfort, this disorder also may result in inhalation of food (aspiration) into your windpipe or regurgitation of food into your nose.

As with so many swallowing disorders, it is believed that the symptoms are the result of a faulty transmission of nerve impulses to the muscles in the pharynx. This occurs in various neuromuscular disorders such as myasthenia gravis (see page 525) and amyotrophic lateral sclerosis (see page 523) and neurological conditions such as some types of brain tumor or stroke (see Brain Tumor,

page 537, and Stroke, page 508). Food poisoning in the form of botulism may cause the rather abrupt onset of pharyngeal paralysis (see Botulism, page 534).

Tests to establish the diagnosis of pharyngeal paralysis may include a barium x-ray (see The Barium X-Ray of the Esophagus, Stomach, and Intestine, page 613) and an esophageal motility study (see page 598). Upper gastrointestinal endoscopy (see page 611) also may be done to eliminate other possible causes.

If the paralysis is due to a disease such as myasthenia gravis, it usually will respond to treatment for the disease. People recovering from a stroke often experience improvement over time.

Many people with pharyngeal paralysis require temporary feeding and therapy through a nasogastric tube (a tube running through the nose to the stomach). Surgery is rarely effective. Sometimes, a tube is placed directly through the abdominal wall into the stomach for feeding (see Gastrostomy, page 612). This bypasses the affected area in the pharynx or esophagus and allows use of the remaining intestine for proper digestion.

Other Disorders. Swallowing difficulties may result from other conditions such as tumor, scar tissue, or congenital disorders. Some people experience the sensation of a lump in their throat without having any actual problem in swallowing their food. This disorder is called globus. At times, this particular swallowing problem may be the result of stress.

If your physician suspects that the problem is globus, as part of the examination he or she may ask you to identify any possible source of stress that could be responsible. In most cases, relief of your emotional distress will eliminate the problem.

ESOPHAGEAL STRICTURE

Signs and Symptoms
• Difficulty swallowing.

Esophageal stricture is a narrowing of the passageway of the esophagus so that solid food or even liquids cannot pass through without difficulty. In most adults the principal cause of a stricture is excessive exposure of the esophagus to gastric acid as a result of reflux of stomach contents into the espoha-

---

ESOPHAGEAL MOTILITY STUDIES

If your swallowing problem is thought to be caused by abnormal contraction of the muscles of your esophagus, your physician will arrange for an examination called an esophageal motility study. This diagnostic test records movement and pressures in your esophagus. After the recording tube is passed through your mouth or nose into your esophagus, continuous recordings of the pressures are made over a period of 10 to 15 minutes. These recordings demonstrate the strength and coordination of the peristaltic waves along your esophagus when you swallow.

These studies can show whether there is excessive pressure in the esophageal sphincter, if it is functioning properly, and if there are poorly coordinated peristaltic waves that can cause high-pressure readings in several areas of the esophagus at the same time. These studies can confirm the presence of achalasia, esophageal spasm, or pharyngeal paralysis (see Swallowing Problems, page 596).

gus (see Esophageal Reflux, page 593). Reflux causes scar tissue to form, and this tissue narrows the passageway. Scar tissue also can result from previous esophageal surgery or ingestion of caustic chemicals. The swallowing of caustic chemicals is preventable. Proper identification and storage of caustic materials in the household will help prevent such accidents (see Preventing Poisonings, page 301).

An esophageal web also can narrow the upper end of the esophagus. For unknown reasons, these webs are more likely to appear in middle-aged women and may be associated with iron deficiency. The difficulty in swallowing usually is restricted to solids.

Another esophageal constriction is a mucosal ring. This may occur near the lower esophageal sphincter. Again, this disorder causes occasional difficulty in swallowing solids.

The Diagnosis.   Your physician may perform a barium x-ray (see The Barium X-Ray of the Esophagus, Stomach, and Intestine, page 613) and may follow this with an endoscopic examination (see Upper Gastrointestinal Endoscopy, page 611) to be sure that an esophageal or stomach cancer is not the cause of your swallowing difficulty.

Treatment.   If the stricture is a result of chronic esophagitis or previous ingestion of caustic material, of esophageal webs, or of mucosal rings, the restricted passageway may be opened up with an esophageal dilator. The dilator stretches open the stricture, web, or ring (see Esophageal Dilation, page 599). Rarely, a surgical procedure is needed for these disorders.

FOREIGN BODIES

Signs and Symptoms
- Difficulty in swallowing;
- Complete inability to swallow liquids or solids, often accompanied by drooling of saliva.

Emergency Symptoms
- Inability to breathe or to utter a sound;
- Pale and clammy skin.

If you swallow something and it becomes lodged in your throat, your esophagus may be partially or totally obstructed. The likelihood of an obstruction occurring is increased among those who have problems with esophageal strictures (see page 598),

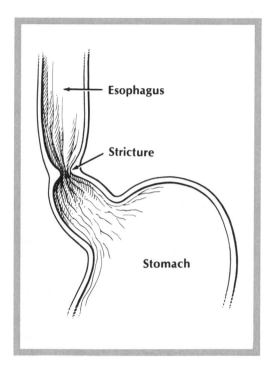

Narrowing of the passageway of the esophagus is called an esophageal stricture. This can cause difficulty in swallowing.

ESOPHAGEAL DILATION

A narrowed or constricted esophagus can be opened or dilated by stretching the tissue that is causing the blockage. This is sometimes called esophageal bougienage.

Prior to this procedure, you will be required to fast for at least 6 to 8 hours. A topical anesthetic will be applied to the lining of your throat. You may also receive a sedative. A thin, flexible instrument called a fiberoptic endoscope is inserted into your esophagus (see Upper Gastrointestinal Endoscopy, page 611). In one commonly used method, a guide wire is inserted through the endoscope and then the endoscope is withdrawn. Progressively larger dilators are threaded along the length of the wire and through the stricture, to force open the passageway. At times, balloons are attached to the guide wire and are moved to the point of the narrowing. There they are inflated, which may help open the passageway.

An esophageal dilator usually is quite safe, but you may feel a little tightness or discomfort in your chest or some pain when you swallow for a few hours after the procedure. The benefit of dilation is that it permits blocked food and fluids to move freely through the esophagus and into the stomach.

tumors (see below), or abnormal muscle contraction (peristalsis) of the esophagus.

When the esophagus is narrowed by any of these conditions, the risk of food, especially a large piece of meat or bone, becoming lodged is increased. Others who have problems with foreign body obstructions are elderly denture wearers and those who have difficulty in chewing their food properly. Children are prone to swallowing pins, coins, pieces of their toys, or other objects that can obstruct their esophagus.

Blockage of the throat by a large piece of meat lodged in it may cut off the airway and is a medical emergency. This situation may result in inability to breathe or to utter a sound. You may turn blue and lose consciousness in a minute or two. The Heimlich maneuver may dislodge the offending piece of food (see The Heimlich Maneuver, page 269). This event sometimes is called a café coronary in that it occurs in a restaurant after a person has eaten a large piece of meat (and, often, has consumed alcoholic beverages).

The more common situation occurs when food is stuck further down your esophagus, at a point where it can block the passage of food into your stomach. If the obstruction is total, you will keep on spitting out saliva. Go to your local emergency room to have the foreign body removed (see Upper Gastrointestinal Endoscopy, page 611).

Whatever its size or shape, a lodged foreign body always is a serious matter. If stuck in the lower pharynx, it can inhibit your ability to breathe. Farther down your esophagus, the object can block the passage of food into your stomach. It also may create swelling at the spot in which it is lodged, which aggravates the obstruction. If an object manages to reach your small intestine before becoming stuck, it can cause an infection, ulceration, or hemorrhage.

Many foreign objects actually may pass into the stomach and through the gastrointestinal tract without delay. However, if the object is sharp-edged, it may scratch or perforate the esophagus, stomach, or intestine on the way through.

Depending on the location and degree of obstruction caused by the lodged object, you may have virtually no symptoms or you may find it almost impossible to swallow. In addition, other symptoms may occur including sweating, nausea, rapid pulse, and cold, pale, or clammy skin.

These symptoms suggest the possibility of perforation or hemorrhage.

The Diagnosis. Your physician may perform a barium swallow examination (see The Barium X-Ray of the Esophagus, Stomach, and Intestine, page 613) followed by an endoscopic examination (see Upper Gastrointestinal Endoscopy, page 611).

Treatment. A foreign object in the esophagus usually is removed with a fiberoptic endoscope. Before the instrument is inserted, you may receive a sedative, and your pharynx will be anesthetized. Through the endoscope your physician can retrieve most objects in the esophagus.

Your physician may elect to push the object into the stomach if he or she thinks that it will pass all the way through the digestive tract. Once the object has been removed from the esophagus and the swelling subsides, your physician will want to inspect your esophagus and to treat any identifiable abnormality that may have contributed to the obstruction.

ESOPHAGEAL TUMORS

Signs and Symptoms
- Progressive difficulty in swallowing;
- Unexplained weight loss;
- Regurgitation;
- Vomiting of blood.

Most esophageal tumors form in the middle or lower part of the esophagus; nearly 90 percent of esophageal tumors are malignant.

The principal symptom of an esophageal tumor, whether benign or malignant, is progressive difficulty in swallowing. The difficulty will begin with solid foods, but eventually it will be difficult to swallow even liquids. As the condition worsens, you will probably lose weight, your breath may become foul-smelling, and you may begin to regurgitate food.

Malignant tumors are twice as likely to occur in men as in women; heavy smokers and drinkers between the ages of 50 and 60 are at the highest risk.

For reasons not fully understood—possibly fear or denial—many people who have these symptoms delay seeing their physicians. Consequently, in many cases by the time help is sought, the cancer has spread beyond the esophagus. Successful treatment depends on early detection.

The Diagnosis.   Any difficulty swallowing requires immediate attention from your physician. The diagnostic tests may include a barium x-ray (see The Barium X-Ray of the Esophagus, Stomach, and Intestine, page 613) followed by an endoscopic examination (see Upper Gastrointestinal Endoscopy, page 611). The latter test will ensure that the barium x-ray did not miss anything and will confirm whatever the barium x-ray may have revealed. In some cases, your physician may take a sample from the esophagus for laboratory analysis (see Biopsies, page 1284). Your physician also may order a CT scan (see page 1286) to determine the extent of the tumor beyond the esophagus.

How Serious Is an Esophageal Tumor?
Most tumors in the esophagus are malignant. Because the disease usually is far along in its development before the diagnosis is made, the survival rate is poor.

Treatment. *Surgery.* If you have a malignant tumor of your esophagus that has not spread beyond that organ, surgery (at times combined with radiation therapy) or radiation therapy alone may be the initial treatment. However, if surgery is ruled out, there are a number of treatments that can relieve the obstruction caused by the tumor. These include frequent dilation (see Esophageal Dilation, page 599), removing part of the obstructing tumor with a laser directed through an endoscope (see Upper Gastrointestinal Endoscopy, page 611), or inserting a prosthesis, a hollow plastic tube, into the esophagus past the cancer. Although these procedures do not cure the tumor, they often temporarily relieve the inability to swallow by increasing the opening through the obstructing cancer.

ESOPHAGEAL VARICES

Emergency Signs and Symptoms
• Vomiting of blood;
• Faintness, sweating, and pallor (shock).

An esophageal varix is a rare condition in which blood vessels (veins) become abnormally dilated or enlarged in the wall and lining of the esophagus. The pressure within the expanded blood vessels may cause them to rupture. If they hemorrhage and the bleeding is heavy, you can go into shock.

Varices frequently occur in those who suffer from liver disease (see Cirrhosis, page 653).

How Serious Are Esophageal Varices?
Bleeding from a varix is a life-threatening situation.

Treatment.   After an endoscopic examination (see Upper Gastrointestinal Endoscopy, page 611), your treatment will depend in large part on the location of the bleeding and how severe it is. Often, drugs are used initially to control variceal bleeding.

Your physician may choose to place a special tube into the stomach. This tube (often called a Sengstaken-Blakemore or Minnesota tube) has balloons attached at the levels of the esophagus and the stomach.

Barium x-ray reveals narrowing of the esophagus (see arrows) caused by a malignant tumor.

When the tube is in place, one or both balloons may be inflated to compress the varices. This may temporarily stop the bleeding, and then the tube with the attached balloons can be removed.

Through the endoscope, your physician may inject a solution into the vein, which initially obliterates and then inflames and scars the varix. This procedure is called variceal sclerotherapy. It often stops the bleeding but needs to be repeated periodically.

Your physician may refer you to a surgeon who may advise an operation to shunt blood away from the ruptured varices (see also Cirrhosis, page 653).

ESOPHAGEAL RUPTURE

Emergency Signs and Symptoms
- Chest pain;
- Rapid and shallow breathing;
- Sweating;
- Blood in vomitus.

The lower esophagus can be torn by an episode of forceful vomiting. This is called esophageal rupture and is a medical emergency.

It is also possible that the lining of the esophagus can be injured during a diagnostic procedure in which an instrument is inserted into the esophagus (see Esophageal Dilation, page 599). You might sustain the same sort of injury swallowing a foreign object (see Foreign Bodies, page 287).

An esophageal rupture may produce some blood in your vomit, and you may think you are having a heart attack because of the pain in your chest. Your physician can diagnose the problem with a chest x-ray, possibly after you swallow contrast material to show the point of the rupture radiographically (see The Barium X-Ray of the Esophagus, Stomach, and Intestine, page 613).

Treatment. Treatment generally is surgical repair of the rupture. Often, the esophageal rupture leaks food into the tissue around the esophagus or into the chest cavity. This area needs to be examined and cleaned out during the operation.

In some situations, the tear is not extensive and the wound will heal without surgery. Antibiotics are given in these situations to prevent bacterial infection. A tube is inserted through your nose into your esophagus or stomach to assist in draining secretions. You will receive nourishment through a vein (intravenous feedings) until the tear has healed.

STOMACH PROBLEMS

Shaped like a gourd, the stomach rests in the left central section of your upper abdomen, just below your rib cage. The stomach receives food from the esophagus, and its churning, mixing action reduces the food to a semi-liquid mixture. In addition, the stomach secretes acid which in turn activates some enzymes that aid in the digestive process.

Most of the stomach's contents trickles into the small intestine for further digestion and absorption.

The stomach does not always function smoothly. We all experience occasional indigestion and painful heartburn. These discomforts usually pass without requiring special medical attention. However, if such commonplace problems persist, they can indicate a more serious underlying problem.

Such problems often involve the lining of the stomach, which generally is remarkably resistant to injury. However, at times its resistance may break down and a small hole (ulcer) may develop in the lining. Ulcers, gastritis, and other stomach problems are discussed in the following pages.

INDIGESTION

Signs and Symptoms
- Discomfort or feeling of fullness in the upper abdomen;
- Heartburn;
- Nausea;
- Bloated sensation, often relieved by belching.

Indigestion (dyspepsia) is a nonspecific term used to describe many symptoms associated with abdominal distress, particularly after eating.

Indigestion itself is not a disease. Rather, it is a common symptom that most people have at one time or another. Some have indigestion only when they eat certain foods or drink excessive amounts of alcohol. Others have episodes daily. Often, despite diagnostic tests, no specific cause of the indigestion is ever found.

However, this does not mean that you should ignore your indigestion, particularly if it occurs often. Indigestion can be a symptom of a serious disease such as peptic ulcer, gastritis, gastric cancer, or gallbladder disease.

The Diagnosis.   Indigestion is a vague description—that is why it is so important for you to be specific about your symptoms. Your physician will ask you to describe the discomfort. Where does it typically occur? Does it occur before, during, shortly after, or several hours after a meal? Because indigestion can be caused by problems anywhere in the digestive system, these questions are your physician's initial attempt to pinpoint the affected area.

For example, if the discomfort is below your umbilicus (navel), it is unlikely to be a problem in your esophagus, stomach, duodenum, or gallbladder. However, if the discomfort is above the umbilicus, these sites may need to be considered further to elimi nate disorders that may be mimicking the symptoms of indigestion.

The timing of the symptoms also may offer a clue. If the discomfort occurs when you are eating, this suggests esophagitis or gastritis (see pages 611 and 608). A discomfort that occurs several hours later may suggest an ulcer in your duodenum (see page 604).

Once your physician has determined the pattern of your symptoms, he or she may want to check for blood in your stool (see Screening for Colon Cancer, page 641). Whether or not other tests are done depends on your age, the duration of your symptoms, and their severity. Because of the risk of cancer, older people with symptoms are more likely to have further diagnostic tests. If you are under 30, your physician may want to try antacids or other medications for a short time to see if your symptoms are relieved. If they are not, your physician may order additional studies.

Abdominal symptoms can be evaluated with barium x-ray studies of the esophagus, stomach, small intestine, and colon (see The Barium X-Ray of the Esophagus, Stomach, and Intestine, page 613). Your physician also may consider an ultrasound or CT scan of your pancreas, liver, and gallbladder (see Ultrasonography, page 1287, and CT Scan, page 1286). Another test that may be helpful is an endoscopic examination (see Upper Gastrointestinal Endoscopy, page 611). The particular tests your physician orders depend on your specific symptoms.

How Serious Is Indigestion?   In itself, indigestion is more a discomfort than a serious problem. However, because it can be a symptom of a major underlying disease, indigestion should be taken seriously, particularly if it is of new onset or is not responsive to medication.

Treatment. *Medication.*   At times, no cause for your indigestion may be found in spite of extensive testing. Your physician may elect to try a few weeks of treatment with antacids or an acid-reducing medication such as cimetidine, ranitidine, or famotidine, or he or she may try to use a medication such as sucralfate that probably works by coating and thereby protecting the lining of the stomach. Another possible medication is metoclopramide which enhances the emptying of the stomach. These medications have various degrees of success.

Lifestyle Adjustments.   Your physician also might advise elimination of certain foods, such as alcohol, that may be causing your indigestion. He or she also might discourage the use of cigarettes, which may be contributing to indigestion. In addition, your physician may inquire as to whether tension or stress in your life may be contributing to your symptoms. If so, efforts should be directed at changing those factors, which, in turn, may relieve your symptoms of indigestion.

If a specific cause such as peptic ulcer, gastritis, or duodenitis is found, your physician will recommend specific therapy.

PEPTIC ULCER

Signs and Symptoms

- Burning, aching, gnawing, or hunger discomfort in the upper abdomen or lower

chest that is relieved by milk, food, or antacids;
• Black, tarry, foul-smelling stools;
• Bloated feeling after meals;
• Nausea and vomiting.

Emergency Symptoms
• Shock: Cold, clammy skin and fainting, suggesting excessive blood loss;
• Vomiting of fresh blood (bright red).

Peptic ulcers are holes or breaks in the inner lining of the esophagus, stomach, or duodenum. Peptic ulcer generally occurs in the lower part of the stomach or in the initial portion of the duodenum.

The cause of ulcers is not fully known. Normally, the linings of the esophagus, stomach, and duodenum are kept intact by a balance between the acid and stomach juices and the resistance of these linings to injury. When the balance breaks down, the result may be a peptic ulcer.

If your stomach produces a great deal of acid, you may not necessarily develop an ulcer; likewise, if you have low acid production, you are not necessarily guaranteed that you will never have an ulcer. What appears to be decisive is the balance between the amount of acid and the quality and quantity of the protective lining.

A peptic ulcer that occurs in the duodenum is called a duodenal ulcer.

Peptic ulcers commonly are found in the three areas where the digestive tract comes in contact with gastric juices: the esophagus,

the stomach, and the duodenum. The most common peptic ulcer, a duodenal ulcer, is one that appears in the duodenum, the initial portion of the small intestine. A gastric ulcer (stomach ulcer) is usually found on the lower portion of the stomach, and an esophageal ulcer is usually located in the lower section of the esophagus.

Peptic ulcers are not uncommon in our society. Statistics suggest that 1 of every 10 people will have a peptic ulcer during his or her lifetime. Typically, the age at diagnosis peaks between 40 and 50 for duodenal ulcers and between 60 and 70 for gastric ulcers. Frequently, ulcers recur within 1 year after healing, sometimes without symptoms.

There is some evidence that some people may have an inherited disposition to ulcers. Peptic ulcers are three times more likely to occur in families of duodenal ulcer patients than in the general population. And relatives of people with gastric ulcers are likely to have the very same kind of ulcer as well.

Contrary to popular belief, there is no clear evidence that people who are under a lot of stress or eat hurried, irregular meals are more likely to have ulcers. Furthermore, ulcers do not affect primarily high-level business executives any more than those in other occupations. Ulcers affect people of all socioeconomic levels.

Duodenal Ulcer.   There is no one symptom that will tell you that you have a duodenal ulcer. A relatively reliable indication, however, is a burning, aching, gnawing, or hungry sensation in the upper middle section of your upper abdomen or a pain under your breastbone that comes and goes. If the ulcer is located on the back wall of your duodenum, it is possible that you will feel pain up in your mid-back. At times, you may feel bloated and nauseated after meals. If the scarring that results from a long-standing ulcer obstructs the pylorus (the opening from the stomach to the small intestine), you may feel distended after meals and even vomit or regurgitate.

In some cases, you may not experience any pain with your ulcer. Bleeding may be the initial sign. The stools may be black, tarry, and foul-smelling. Less common is vomiting of red or coffee-ground material or passing maroon stools.

A condition in which tumors form in the pancreas or duodenum, Zollinger-Ellison syndrome, will cause excessive production

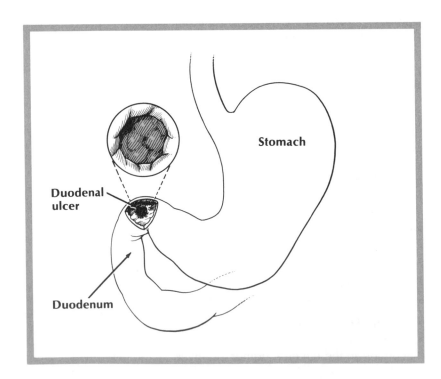

Stomach

Duodenal ulcer

Duodenum

of a hormone (gastrin) that stimulates gastric acid secretion in the stomach. Peptic ulcer may develop in the stomach and duodenum or other areas of the small intestine. These tumors are sometimes malignant (see Zollinger-Ellison Syndrome, page 607).

Cigarette smoking may be associated with duodenal ulcers. Heavy smokers not only are more likely to develop these and other ulcers, but the ulcers are less likely to heal as quickly as in nonsmokers. The relationship between smoking and ulcer formation is not fully understood, but it is thought that the nicotine somehow inhibits the alkaline secretions of the pancreas that are partially responsible for neutralizing stomach acid.

Whether or not psychological factors play any role in duodenal ulcers is a controversial issue. It is no longer believed that there is an ulcer personality type; however, it is thought that chronic anxiety may aggravate an existing ulcer and retard its healing.

Gastric Ulcer. Excessive gastric acid may contribute to the formation of a gastric ulcer. However, in most cases it is believed that a gastric ulcer develops because the mucus and protective lining of the stomach are defective and unable to resist the usual amount of stomach acid. Because excess acid secretion is not the primary cause of a gastric ulcer, smaller doses of either liquid antacids or acid-reducing medications than are required for duodenal ulcers may be effective. Certain medications, including analgesics such as aspirin, can cause gastric ulcer or gastric erosions. The reason why they do this is unclear but may involve a weakening in the protective lining of the stomach.

It is not easy to distinguish between a duodenal and a gastric ulcer on the basis of pain symptoms. The pain from a gastric ulcer may be less likely to be relieved by eating; in some cases, eating actually may make the pain of a gastric ulcer worse.

There are several potentially dangerous complications associated with peptic ulcers. Sometimes an ulcer will hemorrhage, necessitating hospitalization. One danger of severe hemorrhage is shock (see Recognizing and Treating Shock, page 304). Another is that, if the bleeding is only slight but continues over a period of time, an iron-deficiency anemia may develop (see page 478).

Perforation, another serious complication, occurs when the ulcer erodes through the wall of the stomach or duodenum into the abdominal cavity. This produces the sudden onset of an intense and persistent pain. If this occurs, see your physician at once. Most often, emergency surgery is required.

Obstruction at the outlet of the stomach is a complication in individuals with longstanding duodenal or pyloric channel ulcers. This results in dilatation or enlargement of the stomach. Vomiting of easily recognized food ingested hours earlier may occur.

The Diagnosis. If your physician suspects that you have an ulcer, he or she may conduct several diagnostic tests. The two major tests are a barium x-ray (see The Barium X-Ray of the Esophagus, Stomach, and Intestine, page 613) and an endoscopic examination (see Upper Gastrointestinal Endoscopy, page 611). If the barium test is negative yet your symptoms continue, an endoscopic examination may be performed. If the ulcer is in your stomach, your physician may take a sample of tissue for laboratory analysis (biopsy) to rule out a malignancy. Duodenal ulcers are rarely malignant.

How Serious Are Peptic Ulcers? With early detection and proper treatment, most people recover from their ulcers within a few weeks. However, early treatment does not guarantee a cure because more than half of all persons treated for ulcers have a recurrence within 2 years.

Treatment. The goals of treatment are to relieve symptoms, heal the ulcer, prevent relapse, and avoid complications.

Medication. The vast majority of persons with peptic ulcer disease respond well to medication. The key to treatment is either decreasing the amount of acid present or strengthening the protective lining of the stomach or duodenum. The mainstay of treatment for many years has been the use of antacids. For an ulcer in the stomach or duodenum, the most effective treatment is a liquid antacid taken frequently—1 hour before and 2 hours after meals and at bedtime.

In recent years, a new class of drug that decreases the amount of acid produced in the stomach has been made available. These drugs are called H_2 blockers. These medications include cimetidine, ranitidine, and famotidine. Studies have shown these medi-

PEPTIC ULCER SURGERY

In recent years, the number of operations performed for peptic ulcer disease has steadily decreased, primarily because the availability of more effective medications has alleviated the need for surgical treatment in many cases.

However, if you have an ulcer that does not respond to medical treatment or you have serious complications such as hemorrhage, obstruction, or perforation, you may be a candidate for surgery. Understand, however, that surgery is not a panacea. There are many side effects associated with this operation.

The Procedure

Various procedures are used in the surgical treatment of ulcers. If you have an acute perforation, most likely you will need an immediate operation. Depending on his or her evaluation at the time of the operation, your surgeon may only close the hole (perforation) in the stomach or duodenal wall

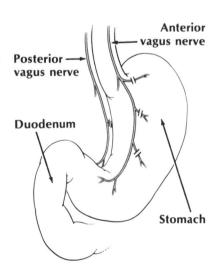

If treatment of your ulcer requires surgery, the surgeon may sever nerves that control acid secretion in your stomach. There are several surgical options; one is called proximal gastric vagotomy (shown above), in which branches of the vagus nerve are severed.

where the ulcer eroded through into the abdominal cavity.

For uncontrollable acute bleeding, the small artery that is the source of the bleeding is identified and tied off. Generally, this is at the base of an ulcer. The entire ulcer also may be cut out.

In addition to these emergency steps, if your surgeon thinks your condition is safe enough to warrant a more extended operation, he or she will perform a surgical procedure to decrease acid production in your stomach. This is similar to what he or she would perform if operating in a non-emergency situation.

Potential Complications

There are several complications associated with peptic ulcer surgery.

Ulcer Recurrence

Ulcers recur in about 5 percent of those who have undergone surgery. The vast majority of these recurrences are seen with duodenal ulcers. The most common symptom of a recurrent ulcer is abdominal pain. Sometimes, a recurring ulcer does not respond well to medication, and a second surgical procedure may be necessary.

Alkaline Reflux Gastritis

A small number of people experience abdominal discomfort, loss of appetite, and vomiting of bile-colored (yellowish or greenish) material that is thought to be due to the reflux of duodenal contents back into the stomach. Often, a severe iron-deficiency anemia is present (see page 478). Medical treatment of this problem generally is not successful. Sometimes, additional surgery is recommended.

Dumping Syndrome

After peptic ulcer surgery, some

persons experience one or more of the following symptoms: light-headedness, sweating, abdominal discomfort vomiting, and diarrhea after meals. This is called the dumping syndrome. The dumping syndrome occurs within 60 minutes after a meal and is thought to be the result of the too-rapid emptying of stomach contents into the small intestine.

Treatment of the dumping syndrome includes the elimination of liquids at mealtime (consume liquids between meals), limiting sweets, and eating frequent small meals rather than three large meals.

Diarrhea

Some people who have undergone peptic ulcer surgery have diarrhea unrelated to dumping, usually within 2 hours after a meal. The cause is not clear.

Hypoglycemia

Palpitations, light-headedness, and sweating may occur more than 1 hour after eating and are thought to be due to a decrease in blood sugar concentration caused by the insulin produced in response to rapid absorption of sugar.

To avoid these symptoms, reduce your intake of sweets at meals. The symptoms of hypoglycemia respond to sugar taken by mouth, best in the form of a fruit juice.

Hematologic Complications

Patients who have all or part of their stomach removed invariably have malabsorption of certain food elements. Iron deficiency is the most common deficiency after peptic ulcer surgery and may be the result of blood loss or iron malabsorption (see also page 621). The anemia that results from iron deficiency usually takes several years to develop, except when it is caused by blood loss. Iron deficiencies can be treated orally or with injections of iron.

In addition, the stomach produces a substance (called intrinsic factor) that is necessary for the absorption of vitamin B_{12}. If this factor is missing or significantly decreased in amount because of the removal of a portion of your stomach, you may have pernicious anemia (see Pernicious Anemia, page 479). Treatment is a monthly injection of vitamin B_{12} underneath your skin. Oral preparations of vitamin B_{12} are not helpful because they will not be absorbed.

General Malabsorption
Mild malabsorption is common after ulcer surgery. Weight loss is more likely to occur in those who have part of their stomach removed.

---

cations to be as effective as the frequent use of liquid antacids in decreasing stomach acid. The usual course of therapy lasts approximately 6 weeks.

Once your ulcer has healed, your physician may advise you to take a smaller dose of one of these medications on a daily basis, particularly if you have had recurrences in the past. Other useful medications include sucralfate which may coat the lining of your stomach and duodenum. Another recently released drug is misoprostil which is believed to have similar properties. Antacids sometimes are used to supplement these medications.

Surgery. Surgery is seldom required unless the ulcer does not heal with medication or there are complications (see Peptic Ulcer Surgery, page 606).

Nutrition. One traditional treatment approach, the bland diet with plenty of milk, is no longer considered important or effective in the treatment of ulcers. Drinking large quantities of milk is discouraged, in fact, because foods rich in protein and calcium tend to stimulate acid production.

Another change from past dietary rules is that your physician may allow you to eat spicy and fatty foods, unless, of course, you find that they increase your discomfort. At the same time, your physician will probably caution you about eating peppers, garlic, cloves, chili powder, caffeine, and alcohol. Avoid even decaffeinated coffee because it promotes acid production.

Prevention. The delicate balance between the acid and the protective lining in your gastrointestinal tract can be disrupted by alcohol, aspirin, and some other medications. Aspirin and certain other anti-in-flammatory drugs have this disruptive effect, but acetaminophen does not (see Drug-Induced Stomach Problems, page 609).

If you smoke, stop. Smoking probably contributes to the development of an ulcer and retards or prevents healing.

If you have a history of ulcer, mention this problem whenever a physician prescribes a medication for you. If aspirin or a potentially ulcer-provoking drug is absolutely necessary, the danger of an ulcer developing can be greatly lessened by the simultaneous use of either an acid-reducing medication such as cimetidine, ranitidine, or famotidine or a protective agent such as sucralfate or misoprostil.

ZOLLINGER-ELLISON SYNDROME

Signs and Symptoms
- Ulcer-like symptoms in the upper abdomen (see Signs and Symptoms of Peptic Ulcer, page 603);
- Symptoms may be severe, persistent, and not relieved by antacids;
- Diarrhea.

Zollinger-Ellison syndrome is a condition in which tumors, called gastrinomas, form in the pancreas or duodenum. The tumors secrete a substance called gastrin that causes excessive acid secretion in the stomach.

As a result, between 90 and 95 percent of those with Zollinger-Ellison syndrome have peptic ulcers at some point during their disease. Ulcers associated with this syndrome are typically more persistent and respond less well to treatment than typical peptic ulcers do (see Peptic Ulcer, page 603). It is estimated that this syndrome is responsible for up to 1 percent of all peptic ulcers.

Zollinger-Ellison syndrome may occur at any age, but the symptoms are more likely to appear between ages 30 and 60.

The Diagnosis.   If you have the symptoms of Zollinger-Ellison syndrome, your physician will perform blood tests to see whether the gastrin level in your blood is increased. Generally, a person with Zollinger-Ellison syndrome has an abnormally high serum gastrin level. Your physician may also order a barium x-ray of your stomach, duodenum, and, sometimes, jejunum (the middle section of the small intestine) or upper gastrointestinal endoscopy to detect the presence of ulcers (see The Barium X-Ray of the Esophagus, Stomach, and Intestine, page 613, and Upper Gastrointestinal Endoscopy, page 611).

How Serious Is Zollinger-Ellison Syndrome? Zollinger-Ellison syndrome may be a serious disease. In half to two-thirds of the patients, the gastrinomas are malignant and slowly spread, most commonly to the lymph nodes and liver. Moreover, the ulcer disease associated with this syndrome usually is severe and not easily treated with conventional ulcer medication or surgery. As with most serious diseases, the earlier the condition is diagnosed, the better the chances of a favorable outcome.

Treatment.   Typically, the ulcer disease in Zollinger-Ellison syndrome is resistant to standard doses of ulcer medication and conventional surgery (see Peptic Ulcer Surgery, page 606). Especially if you are young, your physician may elect to perform an operation to identify the tumor responsible for the excess production of acid. Often, these tumors are small or multiple in nature and therefore cannot be located or removed.

If your surgeon is unable to remove the gastrinoma, he or she may elect to do no further surgery or may consider a conventional peptic ulcer operation (see page 606).

If the production of acid remains a problem despite a conventional peptic ulcer operation, you will need to take an acid-reducing medication. These include cimetidine, ranitidine, and famotidine. Often, you will need to take doses of these medications that are much larger than the usual doses and to take them more often than you would need to for an ordinary peptic ulcer. A new medication, omeprazole, has recently become available. It has the advantage of virtually eliminating acid production for a period of time with small doses. These medications generally need to be taken indefinitely to prevent recurrence of symptoms.

At times, despite the use of high doses of these medications, excess acid production and subsequent ulceration continue and your physician may need to consider removal of your entire stomach. If the gastrinoma is malignant, your physician will need to watch carefully for growth of this tumor in addition to treating its effects on acid production.

GASTRITIS

Signs and Symptoms
- Upper abdominal discomfort;
- Nausea and, occasionally, vomiting;
- Diarrhea.

Emergency Symptoms
- Bleeding.

Gastritis is a general term that means inflammation of the lining of the stomach. It can result from a number of causes, each of which may produce somewhat different symptoms.

Gastritis can occur as a result of acid-induced damage to the lining of the stomach when no ulcer is present. Excessive smoking or alcohol consumption both are known to produce mild gastritis or to aggravate existing gastritis symptoms.

Gastritis also can be a side effect of a number of prescription drugs (see Drug-Induced Stomach Problems, page 609). One form of the ailment, erosive gastritis, is often associated with the ingestion of aspirin or similar medications. Severe stress due to burns, trauma, surgery, or shock may produce gastritis. In some people, gastritis may be caused by a microorganism called *Campylobacter pylori*.

In most cases, the symptoms of gastritis are relatively mild and short-lived, pose no real danger, and have no lasting effect. Oc-

DRUG-INDUCED STOMACH PROBLEMS

Drugs have been, and continue to be, an indispensable part of the medical treatment of many ailments. The federal government and the pharmaceutical industry try to ensure that the drugs marketed in this country are effective and relatively safe. Part of this task involves identifying what, if any, are the potential hazards of the use of prescription and over-the-counter medications.

The obvious goal of drug therapy is to obtain the greatest possible relief with a minimum of side effects. Yet, virtually all drugs produce some unwanted effects. Terms such as "side effects" and "adverse reactions" are used to describe these harmful effects. Therefore, when taking a medication it may be necessary to accept the minor annoyance of some unwanted side effects in order to gain the more important therapeutic effect.

Side effects range from very mild to extremely severe. Some are very common and can be tolerated if the benefits outweigh the discomfort or harm. Others are rare and may be severe enough to be life-threatening. Your physician may want you to either decrease the dosage of the drug or to stop taking it altogether in the event of such unwanted effects.

Stomach and digestive complaints are common side effects of many drugs. Among the most common are heartburn, indigestion, constipation, and diarrhea. In most cases, the problems resolve quickly but, if they persist, consult your physician.

Perhaps the principal offenders are anti-inflammatory drugs, of which many are used to treat the inflammation characteristic of arthritis. These include aspirin and a class of medications known as nonsteroidal anti-inflammatory drugs (NSAIDs) that include indomethacin, ibuprofen, naproxen, tolmetin, sulindac, piroxicam, diflunisal, and fenoprofen.

Aspirin (acetylsalicylic acid is its generic name) is one of the most effective and safest drugs available when it is used prudently. However, persons who take more than two or three tablets a day may experience microscopic gastrointestinal bleeding.

If you are susceptible, aspirin and the other anti-inflammatory drugs may cause an erosion or gastric ulcer in your stomach—despite the fact that you may have no history of stomach ulcer. However, generally these medications do not cause duodenal ulcer.

It is not clear how aspirin and similar drugs produce gastric ulcers. These medications appear to decrease the protective properties in the lining and mucus of the stomach.

Early signs of drug-induced stomach problems might be the symptoms of indigestion (see page 602) or a change in the color of your stool that occurs while you are taking doses of aspirin or an anti-inflammatory drug regularly (see Gastrointestinal Tract Bleeding, page 610). The stools may become black, sticky, and foul-smelling, signs of bleeding in the upper gastrointestinal tract. At other times, the first sign of blood loss may be your physician's discovery of iron-deficiency anemia (see page 478).

In addition to causing gastrointestinal problems, aspirin can inhibit the function of platelets which serve as plugs to stop bleeding every time you cut yourself or sustain any type of laceration. Because of this interference, you should discontinue the use of aspirin prior to any operation. Moreover, pregnant women should not take aspirin because it increases the likelihood of significant bleeding during pregnancy, particularly during delivery.

casionally, gastritis may cause bleeding, but it is rarely severe.

Paradoxically, gastritis is also seen in some persons whose stomachs do not produce acid. In these cases, the lining of the stomach is atrophied (hence the name atrophic gastritis). This condition may be associated with vitamin B_{12} deficiency (see Pernicious Anemia, page 479) and is seen in many older people.

Gastritis affects virtually everyone at some time in their lives. Even very healthy people may experience gastritis with some regularity. The incidence of gastritis increases with age, and more women than men are affected.

The Diagnosis. Your physician may be able to make the diagnosis on the basis of your description of your symptoms. He or she may obtain a barium x-ray of your stomach (see The Barium X-Ray Study of the Esophagus, Stomach, and Intestine, page 613). Often, the results of this study are normal. The diagnosis normally can be con-

GASTROINTESTINAL TRACT BLEEDING

The most common sign of gastrointestinal bleeding is blood in the stool; the most dramatic and grave sign is vomited blood.

The Cause

The most common causes of gastrointestinal bleeding are peptic ulcer, gastritis (often associated with alcohol abuse or the overuse of drugs such as aspirin or other anti-inflammatory drugs, see page 609), variceal bleeding in the esophagus, small tears in the lower esophagus (Mallory-Weiss tears) and upper stomach, tumors, polyps and diverticula in the colon, and hemorrhoids.

Vomited blood clearly suggests that the bleeding is from the esophagus, stomach, or duodenum. Any blood that enters the intestines below the duodenum usually does not reflux back into the stomach but passes in the stool. One of the most common explanations for blood in the stool in patients over age 60 is a painless hemorrhage from a diverticulum in the colon (see page 631).

Vomiting of bright red blood indicates that the bleeding began shortly before you vomited. If the blood is dark red or appears brown and has the texture of old coffee grounds, the blood has been in your stomach for a longer time. Bleeding that occurs in the stomach or duodenum and exits through the rectum often results in black, sticky, and foul-smelling stools that resemble tar. (Licorice or ingestion of iron or Pepto-Bismol may also turn your stool black.)

Often, blood in the stool can be detected only by diagnostic tests because the amount is too little to see (occult blood) (see Screening for Colon Cancer, page 641). Over time, the undetected microscopic bleeding can produce an iron-deficiency anemia that may leave you tired and weak due to the loss of hemoglobin and iron in the stool (see Iron-Deficiency Anemia, page 478).

Red or maroon stool can indicate a number of problems such as colonic polyps (see page 635), cancer of the colon (see page 639), and ulcerative colitis (see page 628). It may also mean blood from the stomach or duodenum, particularly if the bleeding is considerable. If you see blood in your stool or in the toilet, consult your physician. The source of the blood simply may be hemorrhoids (see page 645) but other potential sources should be evaluated.

If your physician suspects that the bleeding is from the upper part of the gastrointestinal tract, he or she may pass a nasogastric tube into your stomach to see if there is blood in it. Endoscopy (see Upper Gastrointestinal Endoscopy, page 611) may be done to find the source of bleeding. If your physician believes that the bleeding is from the colon, he or she may obtain an angiogram of the colon (see page 805) or perform colonoscopy (see page 637), depending on the amount of blood found at the site.

Treatment

Often, the bleeding stops spontaneously; sometimes blood transfusions are necessary. Treatment depends on the cause and severity of the hemorrhage.

If the bleeding is due to an esophageal varix, the continuous intravenous infusion of a drug such as vasopressin is often successful, at least in stopping the loss of blood temporarily. Sometimes delivery of a sclerosing (scarring) agent into the vein via an upper gastrointestinal endoscope may stop the bleeding.

If the bleeding is from a diverticulum in the colon, a drug injected directly into the artery that supplies that portion of the colon may stop the bleeding. At times, the use of an electrical current or laser light delivered through an endoscope may stop bleeding in the stomach, duodenum, or colon. If the bleeding resists these treatment methods, surgery may be required.

firmed by gastroscopy (see page 611) which reveals the typical lesions.

How Serious Is Gastritis?   Gastritis generally is not serious except for the discomfort it produces. Rarely, it results in gastrointestinal bleeding.

If you appear to suffer from gastritis, your physician will inquire about your eating habits. Your physician also will want to know if you are a heavy drinker or smoke regularly. If the gastritis appears to be a side effect of drug use, your physician may recommend that the medication be taken at very specific times of the day or be replaced with other drugs.

Treatment. *Medication.* Antacids in liquid or tablet form are a suitable and common treatment for mild gastritis. If you are troubled by excessive acid and antacids fail to provide relief, your physician may give you a prescription drug such as cimetidine, ranitidine, or famotidine which decreases the amount of acid produced by your stomach.

UPPER GASTROINTESTINAL ENDOSCOPY

Upper gastrointestinal endoscopy (esophagogastroduodenoscopy), sometimes shortened to gastroscopy, gives your physician a direct view of the upper part of your digestive tract. A device called a fiberoptic endoscope is inserted through your mouth into your esophagus, stomach, and duodenum. This thin, flexible tube equipped with a lighting and lens system enables the specially trained physician to examine the interior of your digestive tract. A channel within the gastroscope permits the passage of instruments that allow the physician to take samples of tissue (biopsies) and fluid and to perform certain treatments.

Before the physician inserts the tube, a local anesthetic may be sprayed into your mouth and throat to dull the gag reflex that may be produced by the pressure of the tube on the back of your tongue and throat. You also may be given an intravenous injection of medication to sedate you partially. You may feel some mild discomfort or fullness as the tube is inserted or when air is introduced.

Your physician will pass the instrument through the esophagus, into the stomach, and then into the upper portion of the small bowel (duodenum) in order to examine the upper gastrointestinal tract. Some air will be passed through the instrument to open these regions for an adequate examination.

to sclerose or scar bleeding varices (see page 611). Also, devices can be passed through the channels of the gastroscope that allow electrical current or laser light to be used to stop bleeding lesions or destroy tumor tissue. Narrowed areas (strictures), especially in the esophagus, may be stretched (dilated) to improve swallowing (see also Esophageal Dilation, page 599).

Complications

Gastroscopy is very safe. However, it should be done only by physicians experienced in the use of the endoscope. Very rarely, bleeding or perforation injuries may occur.

Conditions for which endoscopy is often used include the following.

Esophagitis

This is one of the most common benign diseases of the upper gastrointestinal tract (see page 593). It occasionally cannot be diagnosed with an x-ray but can be seen clearly with an endoscope. Obviously, not everyone who complains of heartburn needs to undergo endoscopy. However, when symptoms persist despite treatment, when swallowing is a problem, or when an x-ray reveals a narrowing, mass, or ulcer in the esophagus, endoscopy is advised. The abnormal area can be assessed better through the gastroscope and biopsy specimens can be obtained.

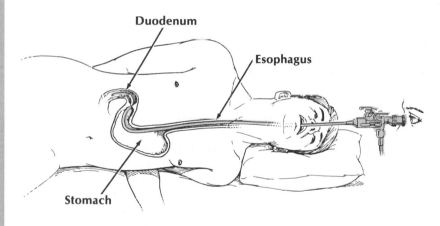

Duodenum

Esophagus

Stomach

A fiberoptic endoscope can give your physician a direct view of your upper gastrointestinal tract (esophagus, stomach, and a portion of your duodenum).

The Procedure

As with the barium x-ray examination (see The Barium X-Ray of the Esophagus, Stomach, and Intestine, page 613), you must fast or restrict yourself to liquids for several hours prior to the examination. This procedure often can be done on an outpatient basis. However, if a sedative is used, do not drive that day.

The Uses

In recent years, endoscopy has proved its usefulness in the diagnosis of many gastrointestinal diseases by permitting both direct observation and biopsy. The channels in the endoscope also allow the passage of devices that can remove small growths, polyps, or swallowed foreign bodies. Special catheters can be inserted

Swallowing Difficulties

Besides scarring of the esophagus, other problems of the esophagus also can affect swallowing. These include motility problems caused by inability of the esophagus to propel food normally into the stomach. Your physician may perform an endoscopic examination in order to obtain a better understanding of the nature of your problem.

Peptic Ulcer

Endoscopy is more accurate than a barium x-ray in detecting most peptic ulcers and may be used as the first test when ulcers are suspected. However, because it is less expensive and not as uncomfortable, many physicians still use a barium x-ray for persons whose symptoms suggest an ulcer. Endoscopy usually is then performed when the barium x-ray is either inconclusive or shows a definite abnormality, especially in the esophagus or stomach. When bleeding from an ulcer or cancer is suspected or ulcer surgery is going to be performed and there is need to see if there are other lesions, endoscopy may be recommended.

Cancer

When cancer is suspected, the endoscope may be used both to examine suspicious-looking masses seen on the barium x-ray and to take a biopsy sample of that tissue. Persons who have gastric ulcers should have follow-up endoscopic examinations to ensure that the ulcer has healed. Gastric ulcers are more likely to be cancerous than other types of ulcers, and an x-ray cannot always correctly identify whether an ulcer is indeed cancerous.

Upper Gastrointestinal Bleeding

Endoscopy is the most accurate method of determining the actual site of upper gastrointestinal bleeding. Many physicians believe that endoscopy should be done on anyone who has continued gastrointestinal bleeding (see page 610) that may require surgery. Although in the majority of cases the upper gastrointestinal bleeding stops spontaneously, there is no way of predicting the cases in which hemorrhage will continue. Thus, endoscopy is usually recommended.

In addition, in persons who continue to bleed or who are suspected to be at risk of bleeding again soon, the use of devices inserted through an endoscope to permit electrocautery, laser treatment, or injection of a sclerosing (scarring) agent may slow or stop the bleeding and eliminate the need for surgery.

Surveillance Examination

Certain chronic conditions of the upper gastrointestinal tract, such as Barrett's esophagus (see page 595), may predispose to the development of cancer. In such individuals, regular endoscopic examinations may be helpful to look for the earlier signs of malignancy.

GASTROSTOMY

Sometimes you are unable to swallow foods properly, such as when the swallowing mechanism of your throat or upper esophagus is disabled. The result is an inability to consume sufficient food for adequate nutrition. If the cause is the result of a neurological problem (such as stroke) or of surgical removal of the swallowing apparatus because of a cancer of the pharynx or larynx, you will need another way to deliver food into your small bowel.

This can be done by the surgical placement of a tube into the stomach. The tube bypasses the swallowing mechanism of the pharynx and esophagus. Nutrients can be infused directly through this tube into the stomach from where they pass into the small bowel for digestion and absorption. With this

A gastrostomy tube allows you to receive food directly into your stomach.

type of feeding mechanism, adequate calories can be instilled to maintain growth and nutrition.

In recent years, gastrostomy feeding tubes have been placed by using upper gastrointestinal endoscopy (see Upper Gastrointestinal Endoscopy, page 611), eliminating the need for surgery and anesthesia. At times, these feeding gastrostomy tubes can be placed while you are an outpatient. Your physician or dietician will instruct you in proper feeding techniques, including the amount of calories to be infused in specially prepared formulas to ensure adequate nutrition.

In some people, the ability to swallow returns and these feeding gastrostomy tubes can be easily removed.

THE BARIUM X-RAY OF THE ESOPHAGUS, STOMACH, AND INTESTINE

The barium x-ray permits your physician to examine your upper gastrointestinal tract and small bowel for the presence of ulcers, tumors, strictures, and other abnormalities. It also allows visualization of motor or motion abnormalities of the esophagus, stomach, and small bowel and assessment of gastroesophageal reflux.

A *barium enema* permits better display of the lining of your rectum, colon, and often the terminal portion of the small bowel (ileum) on the x-ray, aiding in the diagnosis of diseases such as colon cancer (see page 639), Crohn's disease (see page 626), ulcerative colitis (see page 628), and polyps (see page 635).

The Preparation
Prior to the examination, you will fast overnight. For the ingestion of barium, you will be asked to drink a chalky liquid that may be flavored to make it more pleasant tasting.

If you are having a barium enema, you will probably be given

Normal stomach

Normal colon

Stomach cancer (arrow)

Colon cancer (arrow)

a laxative the night before to help empty your colon. You also will be instructed to take a cleansing enema an hour or two before the procedure.

For the barium enema, the material is infused into your rectum. Although you will feel the urge to run to the bathroom, it is important that you hold the barium in so that x-rays can be taken.

The Procedure

X-rays do not pass through the barium mixture. Once the mixture coats and fills in the hollows of your digestive tract, an x-ray picture reveals a clear silhouette of the shape and condition of these organs.

A fluoroscope is used to visualize this image. This device contains a fluorescent screen that converts the x-ray image into visible light. The fluoroscope is also capable of providing a conventional x-ray picture at any point during the procedure.

After the barium is ingested, it moves down the esophagus into your stomach and small bowel. The fluoroscope permits the examining physician to watch this process. A narrowing of the column of barium in the esophagus usually means that the passageway has been narrowed due to stricture, tumor, or varices (see Esophageal Problems, page 593). If the column appears to be abnormal in its contour, it suggests a muscular dysfunction in the esophageal walls. If the barium leaks out, it means that the esophagus has been perforated, which is a very serious matter.

For an even clearer picture of the stomach, occasionally you might be asked to take a powder or pill that releases gas into your stomach. The gas will expand your stomach to provide a more detailed picture of the digestive tract.

The examination may last several hours if your small intestine is to be examined as well (an upper gastrointestinal examination, involving only your esophagus, stomach, and duodenum, takes about 15 minutes). The extra time is required because the additional x-rays of the small intestine will be taken at 15- to 30-minute intervals.

For the barium examination of the colon, the radiologist delivers the barium through the rectum. He or she will place you in various positions and palpate your abdomen as the barium flows through your colon. He or she will attempt to force the barium into the small bowel at the time of this examination. At times, the radiologist may instill some air into your colon to obtain better delineation of fine features of its lining. This is particularly effective in detecting changes of ulcerative colitis or Crohn's disease or in finding very small polyps. The radiologist also may take an x-ray of your colon after you have expelled the barium, to see how the colon empties.

Side Effects

The barium suspension is excreted in the stool and normally should cause no ill effects. Taking a laxative is commonly advised after a barium study of the small bowel to ensure prompt passage of the barium. However, a barium enema has been known to aggravate ulcerative colitis or even precipitate a perforation in the colon, so the test should never be taken lightly.

For several days after the test, your stool will be light pink or white. You should be able to eat a normal diet immediately after the examination, but drink plenty of liquids during the remainder of the examination day.

Medication to protect the lining of the stomach, such as sucralfate or misoprostil, also may be used. If you are deficient in vitamin B_{12}, you will need to take vitamin B_{12} shots (under the skin) on a monthly basis indefinitely.

STOMACH TUMORS

Signs and Symptoms
* Discomfort in the upper or middle region of the abdomen not relieved by milk or antacids;
* Black, tarry stools;
* Vomiting of blood;
* Vomiting after meals;
* Weight loss;
* Anemia;
* Bloated feeling after meals.

Emergency Symptoms
* Shock: Cold, clammy skin and fainting suggest excessive blood loss.

The majority of gastric tumors are malignant. They affect twice as many men as women, usually between the ages of 50 and 70. It is rare to find this type of cancer in people under the age of 40.

As few as 1 of 10 stomach tumors are nonmalignant or benign. Like the malignant tumors, the most common early symptom of a benign tumor is microscopic bleeding that can be detected only by laboratory examination of your stool.

The cause of malignant gastric tumors is unknown. Genetic factors may have some influence. They are 2 to 4 times more common in members of the immediate family of people with the disease. Stomach cancer is much more common in some countries, such as Japan. However, the children of Japanese who migrate to the United States have a much lower incidence of stomach cancer, suggesting that environmental influences such as diet may be potential causes.

The Diagnosis. There is no one symptom that will suggest that you have a malignant gastric tumor. One of every four persons with a malignant tumor has the same symptoms as someone with a peptic ulcer (see page 603). Approximately 5 percent of stomach cancers are lymphomas. The symptoms of lymphoma are very similar to those of stomach cancer (see also Lymphomas, page 489).

If persistent indigestion develops for the first time in your life along with unexplained weight loss and nausea, your physician may want to obtain a barium x-ray (see The Bar-ium X-Ray of the Esophagus, Stomach, and Intestine, page 613) or an endoscopic examination (see Upper Gastrointestinal Endoscopy, page 611).

In most cases, these procedures will determine whether your symptoms are due to a malignant tumor or to some other abnormality such as a peptic ulcer (see page 603). If your physician believes it is warranted, he or she may remove a small piece of tissue from your stomach with the endoscope for laboratory analysis (biopsy). If a malignancy is found, your physician may also want to do a CT scan (see page 1286) to determine if the disease has spread to other organs.

How Serious Are Malignant Tumors?
This form of cancer is difficult to treat. If the cancer is confined to the stomach, the chance of cure is good. However, the disease often has spread, which significantly decreases the chance of cure.

Treatment. *Surgery.* If the tumor is malignant, surgical removal offers the only chance for a cure. The likelihood of success

OTHER GASTRIC DISORDERS

Stomach Dilation
This is an uncommon condition in which the stomach becomes extremely bloated (dilated). The most obvious symptom is a distended abdomen with a constant feeling of fullness.

Dilation occurs most often after a person has had gastric surgery or from an obstruction at the pylorus (see Pyloric Stenosis, page 58). It also can be a complication of some diseases such as pneumonia (see page 917) and diabetes (see page 707), or it may occur for no discernible reason. In any case, the most effective treatment for stomach dilation is nasogastric suction, a procedure in which a tube is inserted through the nose into the stomach. The underlying cause needs to be treated.

Menetrier's Disease
This is a disease of unknown origin in which the lining of the stomach grows to the point that it creates large folds which may contain tiny breaks (erosions). The most likely symptom will be stomach pain, but vomiting, nausea, and weight loss may occur. The erosions can develop into ulcers, and some people experience intestinal bleeding. Protein may be lost from these folds. As a consequence, swelling in your extremities may occur.

If you have Menetrier's disease, x-rays will reveal the enlarged stomach folds. To rule out any possibility of cancer, your physician may perform upper gastrointestinal endoscopy and biopsy (see page 611). Under certain conditions, your physician may opt to perform a laparotomy (a surgical opening of the abdomen) to confirm the diagnosis.

There is no single treatment for this disease, although in all likelihood your physician will urge you to eat only small meals. If you suffer from associated problems such as ulcers or protein deficiency due to the disease, they will be treated separately. The use of acid-suppressing medications may be helpful, particularly if erosions or ulcers are present (see Peptic Ulcer, page 603). These drugs also may decrease the protein loss in the stomach. In some cases, surgery may be necessary to remove all or nearly all of your stomach.

Eosinophilic Gastroenteritis
This is a rare gastric disease in which the lining of the stomach and the intestinal tract becomes infiltrated with eosinophils (a type of white blood cell). The diagnosis can be made by biopsy, and treatment with corticosteroids usually is effective.

depends almost exclusively on whether the cancer has spread (metastasized) to other areas of the body. If the cancer is caught early and it is determined that surgery can remove all of the affected areas, full recovery is possible. Even when surgery may not be able to effect a cure, it still may be recommended to help alleviate pain, bleeding, or obstruction.

Medication.   In addition to surgery, your physician may choose chemotherapy as a treatment, using a number of anti-cancer medications. Radiation is sometimes used, but both radiation and chemotherapy can only relieve the symptoms; they do not cure the cancer. If the cancer is too far advanced for surgery to be effective, drugs may be used to reduce pain and obstruction.

DISORDERS OF THE SMALL AND LARGE INTESTINES

The small intestine consists of three parts: the duodenum, the jejunum, and the ileum. It is in this approximately 20 feet of thin tubing coiled in the abdomen that most of the nutrients are absorbed from the food you eat.

Before food can be absorbed, it must be digested. The food that was broken down into smaller particles in the stomach and thoroughly mixed into a semi-liquid material slowly flows into the small intestine in small portions. There the digestion process goes into full swing and the nutrients are absorbed.

The breakdown products of digestion are absorbed into the bloodstream mainly through the lining of the small intestine. This lining has numerous small projections called villi, and these projections significantly increase the surface area available for food to be absorbed. Bile (from the liver) and pancreatic juices assist in the process of digestion.

In the large intestine, the waste from the digestive process is solidified and prepared for excretion. Also referred to as the colon, the large intestine is about 4 to 6 feet long.

The large intestine is connected to the small intestine at the ileocecal valve. Through this valve, the semi-liquid waste material passes into a chamber of the large intestine called the cecum. Attached to the cecum is the appendix; its function is unknown but it causes problems when it becomes inflamed (see Acute Appendicitis, page 624).

The shape of the large intestine resembles a bridge in that it runs up, across, and down in the abdomen. The ascending colon section of the large intestine starts on the right side of the abdomen in the cecum and moves up toward the liver. The portion of the colon that crosses the abdomen from right to left is referred to as the transverse colon. The descending colon is the section that moves downward into the sigmoid colon. Shaped like the letter "S," the sigmoid colon curves toward the pelvis where it joins the rectum. The rectum is a relatively straight 5-inch tube that leads to the anus.

The nutrients of the food you eat are almost all absorbed in the small intestine, so what passes through the ileum into the large

The wall of your small intestine is lined with many small projections called villi (see inset). Villi serve to increase the surface area available for food to be absorbed by the small intestine.

intestine is a mixture of the unabsorbed nutrients, fiber, water, and electrolytes such as sodium. As this mixture continues through the large intestine, much of the water and salt is reabsorbed through the lining of the large intestine. Once the water is removed, the waste becomes a semi-solid mass which is more easily passed through the anal canal and out the anus. By the time the waste products reach the anus, more than 90 percent of the liquid that originally entered the colon has been reabsorbed.

This reabsorption of water and sodium is critical to good health because both the water and the sodium are required in the functions of the body. If the body's need for water increases or the body's stores become depleted, more water may be reabsorbed, leaving the stool uncomfortably hard. The value of dietary fiber is especially important because it not only increases the bulk of the feces but also keeps the feces relatively moist because the fiber absorbs fluid.

Microorganisms in the colon break down some of the dietary fiber and other waste products in the stool that are not digested by the stomach and small intestine. A part of the waste product of this digestive action is rectal gas.

The large intestine on occasion may become inflamed or infected. For various reasons, this part of the digestive tract is also subject to more tumors and polyps than any other.

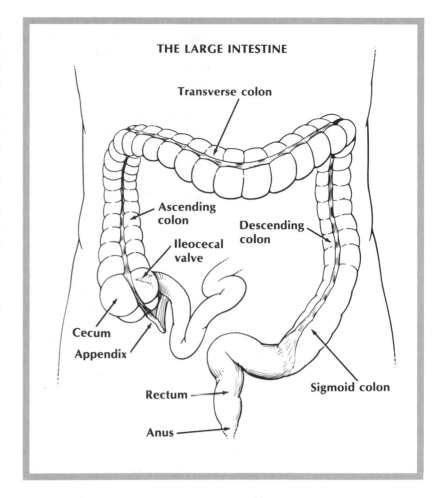

THE LARGE INTESTINE

Transverse colon

Ascending colon

Descending colon

Ileocecal valve

Cecum

Appendix

Rectum

Sigmoid colon

Anus

INFECTIONS OF THE GASTROINTESTINAL TRACT

Signs and Symptoms
- Watery diarrhea, at times bloody;
- Cramping, abdominal pain;
- Low-grade fever;
- Nausea or vomiting or both;
- Occasional muscle aches and headaches.

Emergency Symptoms
- Profuse diarrhea to the point of causing light-headedness.

Infections of the gastrointestinal tract are extremely common throughout the world. In developing countries, diarrhea caused by infection is the leading cause of death in children.

Improvements in sanitation and hygiene have had a significant impact in preventing many of these infections, particularly those transmitted by contaminated food and water. Even so, the Centers for Disease Control estimates that over 25 million infections of the gastrointestinal tract occur each year in the United States and cause over 10,000 deaths.

Viruses account for well over half of the infections of the gastrointestinal tract. In addition, there are infections by bacteria and infestations by parasites. In this section we will describe the common causes of infections of the gastrointestinal tract.

Viral Infections. Acute viral gastroenteritis is the second most common disease in the United States, upper respiratory tract infections being the most common. Normally, the symptoms consist of diarrhea, nausea, vomiting, low-grade fever, abdominal cramps, and muscle pains.

Acute viral gastroenteritis may be severe and may cause death in infants, in elderly or debilitated persons, or in persons whose immune systems are suppressed by disease or certain medications. Viral gastroenteritis also may occur in older children and adults and may be the cause of considerable discomfort and of time lost from school or work.

Generally, in these persons the disease resolves over time. Antibiotics are not effective. The use of antidiarrheal drugs is to be avoided because these medications may prevent elimination of the virus and, thus, may prolong the infection.

Many types of viruses can cause acute viral gastroenteritis. However, the most common are those caused by the rotavirus and the Norwalk virus.

Rotavirus.   Rotavirus is the most common cause of infectious diarrhea in developed countries such as the United States. It is a frequently identified cause of diarrhea in children under age 2. It also is the most common source of diarrhea in children attending day-care centers. Rotavirus occasionally causes epidemics of infection among the elderly in nursing homes. The peak frequency of rotavirus infections in the United States is during the winter. The virus is transmitted from one person to another.

The incubation period is 1 to 3 days. Typical symptoms include watery (non-bloody) diarrhea, vomiting, and low-grade fever lasting 5 to 8 days.

There is no specific treatment for rotavirus gastroenteritis. Current research centers on the development of a vaccine.

Norwalk Virus.   The Norwalk virus is an important cause of outbreaks of gastroenteritis in families and communities, particularly in older children and adults. This disorder also is called winter vomiting disease, a reflection of the most common accompanying symptoms (vomiting) and the time of the year when most cases occur. In addition to diarrhea, nausea, and vomiting, many persons with this disorder experience muscle aches.

This virus usually is found in contaminated food or drinking water. The incubation period from the time of ingestion of the contaminated food or water to the onset of symptoms ranges from 4 to 72 hours.

Other Causes of Viral Gastroenteritis.
Cytomegalovirus is a common cause of diarrhea in immunosuppressed persons. This

virus is not uncommon in those with AIDS (see AIDS, page 848). Gancyclovir, a recently developed medication, is sometimes effective in treating cytomegalovirus-induced diarrhea.

Gastrointestinal infections with herpes simplex virus are frequent in homosexual men, heterosexual women who engage in anal intercourse, and immunosuppressed individuals. Generally, persons infected with the herpes simplex virus experience anal pain, constipation, and bloody diarrhea. These persons also may have neurological symptoms, particularly posterior thigh pain or numbness or tingling of the buttock or anal area. Treatment generally is supportive, consisting of analgesics, warm sitz baths, and stool softeners. The antiviral drug acyclovir can decrease the severity of the initial attack and the chance of later relapses.

Bacterial Infections.   Bacterial causes of infectious diarrhea often are easier to identify than viral causes. Most outbreaks of infectious gastroenteritis caused by bacteria are self-limiting and do not need specific treatment. In some cases, antibiotics are useful.

Many kinds of bacteria can cause diarrheal disease. In this section we will discuss some of the more common varieties.

Campylobacter.   *Campylobacter* infections occur in all age groups, but the largest percentage occurs in children less than 1 year of age and in young adults. *Campylobacter* may be the most common bacterial cause of infectious diarrhea in young adults. Infections with this organism generally occur in the summer and fall.

The most common source of *Campylobacter* appears to be contaminated food, particularly raw milk and poultry.

The incubation period from exposure to onset of symptoms is 2 to 4 days. The illness may have an abrupt onset with the appearance of abdominal pain, nausea, low-grade fever, headaches, and muscle pains. If you become infected, you may experience up to 15 to 18 bowel movements per day. In severe cases, the stools may be bloody.

This illness rarely lasts longer than 1 week. Occasionally, you may experience a relapse or a prolongation of your illness. Because the illness is self-limited, antibiotic treatment often is not necessary. Antidiarrheal agents should not be used because they may delay clearing of this organism from your system and thus prolong the symptoms. If the symptoms are severe, an antibiotic such as erythromycin or tetracycline can be given.

Salmonella. *Salmonella* has been implicated as responsible for about a third of the cases of diarrhea from contaminated food. *Salmonella* generally is within the food itself (as opposed to being on infected food handlers). The population thought to be at greatest risk are those at the extremes of age—the very young and the very old. *Salmonella* infections generally occur in the summer and fall.

Recently, some evidence has been found to suggest that *Salmonella* occurs in animals treated with antibiotics. The use of tetracycline for growth promotion in animals may increase the risk of a *Salmonella* infection in individuals who consume meats from these animals. The potential risk to consumers is now an area of intense investigation.

The *Salmonella* bacteria commonly are found in meats, poultry, eggs, unpasteurized cheese and milk, chocolate made from contaminated cocoa beans, and contaminated marijuana. Pet turtles also are a common source of infection. The disease can be passed by the fecal-oral route. For example, if you change your infected baby's diaper, fail to wash your hands properly, and then sit down to dinner, you could become infected. When *Salmonella*-infected food is not cooked adequately or thawed properly, you may acquire the infection. The symptoms of *Salmonella* include abdominal cramps, diarrhea, nausea, vomiting, and fever.

If you have the symptoms of *Salmonella* infection, your physician may test your stool for the organism. In most cases, the infection clears on its own and only supportive treatment (hydration) is needed. In some people, *Salmonella* can cause a severe and prolonged illness, and antibiotic treatment is necessary. In these cases, the stool is tested to make sure that an effective antibiotic is chosen for the particular type of *Salmonella.*

Shigella. Shigella is an important cause of bacterial gastroenteritis in the developing world and in travelers to these areas. It also occasionally occurs in outbreaks in the United States. This disorder is most common in children ages 1 through 5.

Shigella is transmitted primarily from person to person by the fecal-oral route. Outbreaks can occur in day-care centers. Occasionally, outbreaks can be caused by contamination of food by infected food handlers.

The usual symptoms are watery diarrhea associated with cramping, abdominal pain, and fever. Occasionally, you may pass blood and mucus.

Generally, the disease is self-limited. Antibiotics may be effective in shortening the duration of the diarrhea and in eliminating *Shigella* from the gastrointestinal tract. The usual drug of choice is ampicillin, and it can be given orally after appropriate stool cultures have been obtained. Alternative medications include trimethoprim-sulfamethoxazole and tetracycline.

Escherichia coli. There are various subgroups of the organism called *Escherichia coli (E. coli).* The source for this infection usually is contaminated food and water.

If the diarrhea is mild, generally no treatment is necessary other than rehydration. For more severe or prolonged symptoms, an antibiotic such as trimethoprim-sulfamethoxazole often is prescribed. As an alternative, tetracycline may be used. Antidiarrheal medications should not be used because they delay elimination of the organism.

Parasitic Infestation. Parasitic infestations are the least common of the three major causes of diarrheal diseases.

Giardia lamblia. This parasitic organism causes giardiasis which is probably the most common parasitic cause of diarrhea in the United States. Outbreaks of giardiasis can occur in communities where the water supply is contaminated by raw sewage. Giardiasis also may be contracted by drinking water from lakes or mountain streams far from human habitation, in which case beavers are often thought to be the source of infection.

As many as two-thirds of the persons with giardiasis have no symptoms. However, they may pass the infestation to others. Those who do develop symptoms typically have watery diarrhea, abdominal cramps, and weight loss. Generally, these symptoms occur 1 to 3 weeks after exposure. The stools may be foul-smelling, greasy-looking, and floating. Bloating and distention also may occur. Low-grade fever may be present. These symptoms usually last for 5 to 7 days, although some people have problems for months.

This infestation can be diagnosed by examining the stool under the microscope to look for the characteristic organism. Giardiasis is treated with metronidazole or quinacrine hydrochloride. Follow-up stool examinations are important because the medications frequently do not eliminate the parasite entirely.

Entamoeba histolytica. *Entamoeba histolytica* is a common cause of diarrheal disease throughout the world, although it is relatively uncommon in the United States. Infection generally occurs from person to person through the fecal-oral route. This organism is a common cause for diarrhea in homosexual men.

If this organism is identified as the cause of diarrhea, your physician may recommend

treatment with metronidazole. Other drugs sometimes are used.

Cryptosporidium. *Cryptosporidium* is a common cause of diarrhea in patients with acquired immune deficiency syndrome (AIDS) (see page 848). It can also cause illness in otherwise healthy persons. If you are infected with this parasite you can experience prolonged watery diarrhea with up to 25 bowel movements per day. The diagnosis is based on examination of the stool. In otherwise healthy individuals, the infection resolves without treatment in 1 to 2 weeks. In persons with AIDS, the infection usually is chronic. There is no effective treatment, although several promising drugs currently are undergoing study.

Treatment. As noted in the descriptions above, most of these infestations of the gastrointestinal tract are self-limited. The primary danger is the loss of fluids and electrolytes in the stool. Therefore, the primary goal of treatment is replacement of fluids and these essential electrolytes.

Recently, it has been learned that replacement of fluids orally may be more effective than replacement of fluids through a vein. Thus, your physician may recommend fluid replacement by mouth if this can be tolerated. At other times, particularly if there is severe dehydration or vomiting, he or she may recommend intravenous therapy.

For most infections, the use of antidiarrheal agents is not appropriate. These agents may retard the elimination of the causative organism and thus prolong the disease. However, there are some situations, particularly in mild diseases, in which your physician may recommend their use (see also Prevention of Traveler's Diarrhea, page 340).

ANTIBIOTIC-ASSOCIATED DIARRHEA

Signs and Symptoms
- Diarrhea occurring during antibiotic therapy or within a few weeks after it;
- Abdominal cramps;
- Fever.

Antibiotics, most commonly clindamycin, ampicillin, cephalosporins, and the aminoglycosides, can cause an inflammatory re-

---

FOOD POISONING

Food poisoning is caused by the ingestion of contaminated food. Its symptoms usually include diarrhea and nausea. Vomiting, loss of appetite, and stomachache also may occur.

The most common cause of food poisoning is due to the toxin produced by the bacterium *Staphylococcus aureus.* When this organism contaminates certain foods (often via the hands of a food handler), it multiplies rapidly. This explains why staphylococcal food poisoning often occurs in outbreaks, especially when cream pastries, mayonnaise-containing foods, or potato salad is the vehicle for the bacterium.

Other potential causes of food poison include *Bacillus cereus, Clostridium botulinum* (see Botulism, page 534), *Salmonella, Escherichia*

coli, Campylobacter jejuni, and Norwalk virus (see Infections of the Gastrointestinal Tract, page 617).

What To Do
In most cases, the discomforts of food poisoning pass in a few hours. After the vomiting ends, consume clear liquids for the first 12 hours; then, limit food intake to bland foods for the following 24 hours. For very young children, the elderly, or persons who are ill with other ailments, consult your physician.

Prevention
The best strategy is to avoid food poisoning. Keep all meats and leftovers refrigerated. Beware of any food contaminated by uncooked poultry juices; wash it thoroughly before eating it. Do not eat foods contaminated with molds.

sponse in the intestines, the result of which is diarrhea.

Antibiotic-associated diarrhea is fairly common, affecting up to 25 percent of clindamycin users and up to 10 percent of those who take ampicillin. The most serious form of antibiotic-associated diarrhea is pseudomembranous colitis. Usually, the diarrhea is a result of the antibiotic therapy's altering the environment of the bowel which permits certain bacteria to flourish. This may cause inflammation of the colon.

Typically, the symptoms of diarrhea begin 4 to 10 days after the antibiotic treatment is begun. However, in as many as 25 percent the symptoms do not develop until the antibiotic has been discontinued. The symptoms usually abate after the drug is discontinued.

The Diagnosis.   If your physician suspects that your diarrhea is related to the use of antibiotics, he or she will perform tests on a sample of stool. If you have pseudomembranous colitis, a toxin from a common causative organism, *Clostridium difficile,* may be found.

How Serious Is Antibiotic-Associated Diarrhea?   Many people do well after discontinuing the antibiotic; others become extremely ill and have persistent diarrhea and dehydration. On occasion, pseudomembranous colitis may develop into a life-threatening situation.

Treatment.   Your physician will stop treatment with any antibiotic that may be causing your diarrhea.

If your symptoms are mild, your physician may prescribe cholestyramine which binds to and therefore eliminates the offending toxin of the *Clostridium difficile* organism. For more severe cases, either vancomycin or metronidazole can be used.

Relapses are not unusual and usually require one or more additional courses of treatment.

MALABSORPTION PROBLEMS

Signs and Symptoms
- Weight loss;
- Diarrhea;
- Abdominal cramps, gas, and bloating;

- General weakness;
- Foul-smelling or grayish stools that may float.

If the process of digestion is to go smoothly, the nutrients contained in the food you eat must be broken down (digested) into molecules that can be absorbed into your bloodstream. Sometimes, for various reasons, these nutrients are not completely digested or their absorption is impaired. When this occurs, vital nutrients that should be used by your body instead are eliminated in the stool. The result of this malabsorption can be malnutrition.

Malabsorption can be caused by many different problems. If there is disease of the pancreas, enzymes necessary to digestion may be absent, and malabsorption may be the result. This is often called maldigestion. Because most of the absorption takes place in the small intestine, a disease here may lead to the loss of vital nutrients in the stool.

A principal sign of malabsorption is steatorrheal stools. This results from an excessive loss of fat in the stool. The stool may be gray or pale and somewhat larger than normal. The excessive fat content may cause the stool to float and to be more malodorous than normal. In addition to fat, protein is also lost in the stool, resulting in wasting of the body's tissues.

Malabsorption may cause a deficiency of vitamins A, B_{12}, D, E, and K and folic acid because these valuable nutrients are lost in the stool. Low blood levels of vitamin B_{12} and folic acid strongly suggest malabsorption. With continued loss of fat in the stool, calcium may be lost in excessive amounts and two rather unexpected consequences may occur: urinary stones of calcium oxalate form (see page 898), and a demineralizing state of the bones called osteomalacia develops (see page 985).

Some of the most likely causes of small bowel malabsorption are discussed below. For another common cause of malabsorption, see Chronic Pancreatitis, page 668.

Celiac (Nontropical) Sprue.   Celiac (nontropical) sprue is a common cause of malabsorption. This disease is caused by a sensitivity to gluten, a protein found in wheat, rye, oats, and barley. The intolerance to gluten causes the lining of the intestine to lose its tiny folds (villi) through which nutrients are absorbed. In addition, digestive enzymes are no longer produced in the intestinal lining in adequate amounts. The common symptoms are foul-smelling diarrheal stools, bloated abdomen, and anemia.

Celiac sprue is often seen in children. In these children, the most dramatic symptoms are weight loss and failure to grow. The bony changes of rickets may be seen in children; in adults, osteomalacia may occur with bone pain and tenderness (see Osteomalacia and Rickets, page 985).

In addition to examining your stool to see if it contains excessive amounts of fat and protein, if your physician suspects celiac disease, he or she may order a barium x-ray of your small bowel (see The Barium X-Ray of the Esophagus, Stomach, and Intestine, page 613). Biopsy of the lining of the small intestine is also usually done by using a device inserted through the mouth. The specimen is examined under the microscope for the characteristic changes of nontropical sprue.

Celiac disease usually is treated by eliminating from the diet those foods containing gluten. To correct certain nutrient deficiencies, initially you may be given vitamin and mineral supplements. Your physician or dietician will instruct you in a proper gluten-free diet. They may also give you the names of gluten-free diet cookbooks and of support groups in your area.

If a gluten-free diet is carefully followed, the villi of the small intestine will resume their normal shape and absorption ability over a period of several months. Your stools will return to normal, and you will stop losing weight. The gluten-free diet must be followed indefinitely or the symptoms will return (see page 373).

Tropical Sprue. This is another disease that causes malabsorption. It affects visitors to tropical regions of the world. The symptoms can appear many months or even years after the affected person returns from the tropics. The cause of this disease is uncertain but it may be an infectious microorganism.

People with tropical sprue may suffer from diarrhea, weight loss, anemia, and inability to gain weight.

The diagnostic tests are basically the same as those for celiac sprue.

Treatment for tropical sprue generally consists of a folic acid and vitamin supplement and an antibiotic such as tetracycline. Usually, no special diet is required. Depending on the severity of the disease, you may be on antibiotics for as long as 6 months.

Bacterial Overgrowth. Normally, overgrowth of bacteria in the small intestine is not a problem because the constant movement of the intestine (peristalsis) removes the bacteria. However, under certain conditions, intestinal bacteria may grow to a point such that they cause malabsorption. This condition may be a factor contributing to the diarrhea in diabetics with bowel involvement.

The cause of bacterial overgrowth most often is an impairment of peristalsis (muscular movement of the bowel), which allows bacteria to accumulate. Bacterial overgrowth also is seen after bowel surgery in which segments of the small bowel are bypassed. The diagnosis is made by cultures of samples taken from the small bowel or sometimes by indirect tests that involve collections of blood, breath, or urine. The treatment is antibiotics, often given in a cyclical fashion such as 1 week out of each month.

Scleroderma. When scleroderma affects the intestine, it causes atrophy of its muscular walls, which can impair both absorption of nutrients and movement of the intestine. Scleroderma also may affect the muscular lining of the esophagus and cause heartburn (see Scleroderma of the Esophagus, page 595).

Because the disease is progressive and can spread to other organs, clinically it is known as progressive systemic sclerosis (PSS) (see page 1007). The cause of this chronic disease is unknown. It may be associated with severe diarrhea caused by bacterial overgrowth. Antibiotics given in cyclical fashion (such as 1 week of each month) may be helpful.

AIDS. Another disease that produces problems of malabsorption is AIDS, acquired immune deficiency syndrome (see page 848). The primary symptoms, diarrhea and weight loss, in AIDS patients are thought to be the result of infections in the small intestine and colon.

Whipple's Disease. This malabsorption disorder primarily affects men over age 45. The disease is thought to be caused by an infectious organism that has not yet been conclusively identified. Symptoms such as diarrhea, abdominal pain, progressive weight loss, and a darkening of the skin may occur. The bacterial infection also may produce a low-grade fever. The diagnosis is made by a biopsy of the small bowel.

The long-term use of antibiotics typically is effective in correcting malabsorption due to Whipple's disease.

Amyloidosis. This is a disease produced by the presence of a protein, called amyloid, that has starch-like qualities. Depending on where the unwanted deposits of this protein appear in the body, the consequences can be either insignificant or severe. For example, a buildup of amyloid in the small intestine will make the lining rubbery, firm, and waxy and result in serious malabsorption. The diagnosis of this condition is made by small bowel biopsy.

There is no known method of preventing the formation of amyloid deposits. Treatment is geared toward relieving symptoms or treating an underlying disorder that may be responsible for the amyloidosis (see page 495). Such disorders are tuberculosis, Hodgkin's disease, and rheumatoid arthritis.

Lactose Intolerance. Lactose, the principal sugar in cow's milk and found only in milk and dairy products, requires the enzyme lactase for its digestion. Lactose intolerance occurs when the lining of the walls of the small intestine does not produce normal amounts of this enzyme.

Lactose intolerance causes abdominal cramps, bloating, diarrhea, and excessive gas when more than a certain amount of milk is ingested. Small amounts of milk usually do not produce symptoms. A low level or absence of lactase in the lining of the small intestine actually may be the normal state in that 70 percent or so of the world's population is affected. Northern and Western European whites and their descendants in the United States have a relatively low frequency of low lactase level. Thus, lactose intolerance is uncommon in these persons. Lower levels of lactase occur more commonly in the United States among people of Mediterranean, African, or Asian origin. It is believed that more than 30 million Americans suffer from some degree of lactose intolerance.

Low lactase levels may occur in association with other malabsorptive diseases such

---

DIABETIC INTESTINAL DISORDERS

Long-standing diabetes may result in decreased function of the nerves that control the muscular activity of the stomach and the remainder of the intestinal tract.

A condition called diabetic gastroparesis results, and there is diminished mixing in and propulsive activity by the stomach. Over time, the stomach begins to resemble a limp bag and gradually enlarges. If affected, periodically you may vomit rather large amounts of fluid and partially digested food that has been consumed as much as a day or two before. The unpredictability of the movement of food from the stomach into the intestine makes regulation of the diabetes very difficult. A drug called metoclopramide sometimes is effective in treating this disorder.

When the intestines are the primary site of deterioration of nerves, the propulsive action of the intestine is impaired. The diarrhea tends to occur at night and, because of impaired sensation and function of the anal sphincter, there may be fecal incontinence during sleep. Some degree of malabsorption may be seen, but this may be the result of the simultaneous occurrence of bacterial overgrowth (see page 622), nontropical sprue (see page 621), or pancreatic insufficiency (see Chronic Pancreatitis, page 668).

In some instances, administration of antibiotics in a cyclical fashion (such as 1 week of each month) will control the diarrhea. This suggests that bacterial overgrowth in the poorly moving small intestine is responsible.

At other times, the diarrhea may be the result of impaired function of the nerves to the gut. Occasionally, a medicine called clonidine is effective in this situation.

---

as nontropical or tropical sprue, viral or bacterial infection of the small intestine (see pages 621 and 622), and cystic fibrosis (see page 933).

If you have lactose intolerance, you need not eliminate dairy products totally from your diet. Rather, decrease your consumption of milk products, drink milk only during meals, and try to get your calcium from cheese and yogurt, dairy products that are lower in lactose than milk is. Another alternative is to buy a commercial lactase preparation that can be mixed into your milk. These preparations convert lactose into simple sugars that can be easily digested.

Short-Bowel Syndrome. After surgical removal of a significant portion of the intestine, some persons have malabsorption problems. This condition is referred to as short-bowel syndrome. Because different nutrients are absorbed in different areas of the small intestine, the effect surgery has on nutrient absorption depends upon how much and what part of the intestine was removed. Unless some critical part of the bowel was removed, the remaining portion usually is capable of adapting to accommodate more absorption and thus prevent the malabsorption of nutrients.

ACUTE APPENDICITIS

Signs and Symptoms
* Pain starting in the upper abdomen or around the navel and settling in the lower right side of the abdomen;
* Nausea and vomiting;
* Urge to pass stool or gas;
* Lack of appetite.

The appendix, a worm-shaped structure that projects out from the first section of the large intestine, is about 3½ inches long and has a cavity running down its center. It has no known function or importance in humans. It is not clear as to why on occasion the appendix will become inflamed, swollen, and filled with pus, producing appendicitis.

Those most likely to have an acute appendicitis attack are between the ages of 10 and 30, although it can strike at almost any age. Death due to acute appendicitis is rare. Ap-

The worm-shaped appendix is attached to the cecum; it has no known function in humans. The appendix can become inflamed and lead to a medical emergency.

pendicitis often is more difficult to diagnose in infants and the very old.

The Diagnosis. Your physician will ask you questions about your symptoms, including whether you have lost your appetite, have discomfort on urination, or have an unusual urge to pass gas or move your bowels. Your abdomen will be examined carefully, and a rectal examination will be performed. Abdominal tenderness is an important sign.

If your physician thinks that you may have acute appendicitis, you will be admitted to a hospital immediately. Depending on your symptoms, a blood test and a urine analysis may be done. It is not unusual to have an abdominal x-ray as part of the diagnosis.

How Serious Is Appendicitis?   Peritonitis, a serious infection of the lining of the abdominal cavity (peritoneum), may develop if the appendix bursts.

Treatment. *Surgery.*   The standard procedure is to remove the infected appendix surgically.

MECKEL'S DIVERTICULUM

A diverticulum is a sac or pouch that forms in a weakened section of the wall of the bowel. Meckel's diverticulum is an example of a congenital type of diverticulum. This pouch generally forms in the lower part of the small intestine (ileum). Typically, such diverticula are about 2 inches long.

Although this common disorder frequently presents no symptoms, the diverticulum can become inflamed and bleed. In some cases, especially among young children, bleeding may occur as the result of an ulcer that has formed at the same site. If inflammation of a Meckel diverticulum becomes severe, it can obstruct the intestine or perforate the intestinal wall. The treatment of any of these complications is surgical removal of the diverticulum.

INTUSSUSCEPTION

Signs and Symptoms
* Sudden severe abdominal pain;
* Weakness and lethargy;
* Vomiting, often with bile;

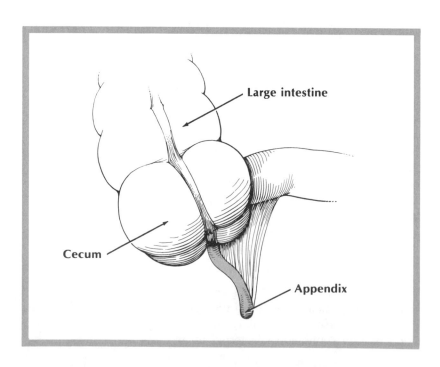

Large intestine

Cecum

Appendix

- Bloody stools which may resemble currant jelly;
- Shallow breathing;
- Shock.

Intussusception is a rare disorder in which a portion of the intestine, usually of the small intestine, telescopes into another segment of the intestine. This is the most common cause of intestinal obstruction in children between the ages of 3 months and 6 years.

The cause is unknown but in some cases there has been a correlation between intussusception and certain viral infections.

Typically, intussusception strikes abruptly in a previously well child. The child suddenly has a severe pain which occurs at frequent intervals. At first, the child may play normally between the pains but soon becomes weaker and lethargic.

The Diagnosis. If your child has these symptoms, do not delay in calling your physician. The symptoms and physical findings may be sufficient to establish the diagnosis. Often, however, further tests such as an abdominal x-ray or a barium x-ray may be done (see The Barium X-Ray of the Esophagus, Stomach, and Intestine, page 613).

How Serious Is Intussusception? If left untreated, intussusception may be very serious. The majority of children recover, however, if treatment is begun within 24 hours after the initial symptoms.

Treatment. The barium enema used for diagnosis may be sufficient to push the telescoped intestine back into its proper place. The recurrence rate after this "treatment," however, may be as high as 10 percent. In many cases, surgery is necessary; generally there is no recurrence after surgery.

OTHER SMALL BOWEL CONDITIONS

Protein-Losing Enteropathy. Some gastrointestinal disorders cause protein in the blood (plasma protein) to be discharged into the gastrointestinal tract and excreted in the stool. Plasma protein may pass into the gastrointestinal tract through an inflamed or ulcerated intestinal lining such as in cases of regional enteritis and ulcerative colitis (see page 628).

Intestinal lymphangiectasia is a type of protein-losing enteropathy in which swelling of the lymph channels of the small intestine leads to loss of protein and fat from the lymph channels into the gut. Children and young adults are most commonly affected by this disorder.

The principal treatment is a low-fat diet.

Primary or Idiopathic Intestinal Pseudo-obstruction. As the name implies, this condition is not truly an obstruction but is an inability of the intestines to function properly, as if they were obstructed. The intestines become distended and you may experience acute attacks of abdominal pain with nausea and vomiting. Malabsorption (see also page 621) may accompany this disorder, with subsequent weight loss. When an underlying disease such as scleroderma (see page 1007) or diabetes (see page 707) is the cause, the term secondary pseudo-obstruction is used.

Treatment of intestinal pseudo-obstruction is difficult. Special diets are ineffective. At times, if the disorder is severe, a fluid containing the nutrients you need can be infused into a vein, thus bypassing your stomach. This can be done on a temporary or even a permanent basis (home parenteral nutrition).

Carcinoid Syndrome. Carcinoid tumors are slowly growing malignancies, usually in the ileum, the lower section of the small intestine. These tumors may spread to the liver and also may metastasize to the lungs, pancreas, spleen, ovaries, and other organs.

Detection of excessive levels of a normal body chemical in the urine is an important biochemical indicator of this type of tumor. This may be associated with a flushing of the skin, diarrhea, and sometimes malabsorption.

The objective of treatment is to decrease the mass of the tumor by either chemotherapy or surgery. Depending on how soon the cancer is detected and where it is located, some people fully recover after surgical treatment. Many live 5 to 10 years after the cancer has been detected because the tumor grows slowly. Death usually results from heart or liver failure when the cancer reaches these organs.

CROHN'S DISEASE

Signs and Symptoms
- Chronic diarrhea;
- Low-grade fever;
- Fatigue;
- Weight loss;
- Abdominal cramps and pain around the navel or on the right side of the abdomen;
- Joint pain;
- Skin lesions.

Inflammatory bowel disease is a term generally used to describe two disorders that involve the gastrointestinal tract and for which no cause has been found. These disorders are Crohn's disease and ulcerative colitis (see page 628).

Crohn's disease, often referred to as ileitis or regional enteritis, is a chronic inflammation of the intestine. It mainly involves the ileum (the lower part of the small intestine). However, it also can affect your colon or other parts of your digestive tract. The inflammation often involves the entire thickness of the bowel wall.

Crohn's disease is relatively rare, occurring in about 1 per 50,000 persons. That number, however, appears to be increasing. The typical patient is white and between the ages of 15 and 35.

Heredity or environmental influences may play a role in the development of Crohn's disease because as many as 1 of every 20 patients has a relative with either Crohn's disease or ulcerative colitis.

The Diagnosis. The symptoms of Crohn's disease may include persistent diarrhea, abdominal pain, fever, and general fatigue. Occasionally, there may be blood in the stool. Often, a significant weight loss occurs.

Barium x-rays of the small intestine and of the colon usually reveal abnormal areas. Segments of intestine appear narrowed and less flexible than normal (see The Barium X-Ray of the Esophagus, Stomach, and Intestine, page 613). Sometimes your physician may use a colonoscope (see page 637) to visualize the lining of your colon and the last several inches of your ileum.

How Serious Is Crohn's Disease? The course of Crohn's disease varies greatly from one person to another. Many people with Crohn's disease remain completely without symptoms (asymptomatic) after the initial one or two episodes of disease. However, many others have recurrent episodes of abdominal pain, diarrhea, and low-grade fever.

The diarrhea itself can be debilitating to the point of significant malnourishment. Episodes of abdominal pain, reflecting gradually increasing bowel obstruction, may reach the point such that you avoid eating because of discomfort.

The complications of Crohn's disease are many and varied. Progressive obstruction, particularly of the small bowel, is the most common reason for surgical treatment in Crohn's disease. Obstructive symptoms generally develop gradually over a long period of time.

Fistulas and fissures in and around the anal and rectal areas also are common. A fistula is an abnormal passage between two segments of the intestine or from the intestine to the skin. An anal fissure is a crack or cleft in the anus or skin around the anus (see also Anal Fissures and Fistulas, page 645). When fistulas develop, food bypasses areas of the bowel necessary for absorption. Bleeding also may occur with Crohn's disease, although it generally is not massive in nature.

Often, the progressive obstruction, the inflamed mass of tissue, or the fistula do not

Barium x-ray shows Crohn's disease. Arrow indicates narrowing of the lower portion of the small intestine (ileum).

respond to medical therapy and may require surgery. Perforation of the bowel or massive bleeding is rare.

If you have Crohn's disease, it is not uncommon to have symptoms and signs unrelated to the bowel. These may involve arthritis, particularly of large joints, or inflammation involving the eye or skin. Occasionally, inflammation of the bile ducts may be associated with Crohn's disease (see Primary Sclerosing Cholangitis, page 665). In addition, the development of kidney stones is common with Crohn's disease. Crohn's disease generally is progressive.

Treatment. *Medication.* If your Crohn's disease is asymptomatic or in remission, treatment may be unnecessary. If your symptoms are mild, perhaps involving several loose stools per day, your physician may prescribe an antidiarrheal pill or a bulk former which contains vegetable fibers.

If your disease is more active, your physician may consider anti-inflammatory medications such as sulfasalazine and corticosteroids. Sulfasalazine is particularly effective if your colon is involved.

If the inflammatory process is confined to the rectum, a corticosteroid enema may be useful in suppressing the inflammation and alleviating symptoms. New enema preparations containing aspirin-like drugs have been used in the last several years to suppress inflammation in the rectum. They appear to work quite well.

Corticosteroids are reserved for more significant flare-ups of the disease. They are effective for both colonic and small bowel involvement. Some physicians may recommend a course of immunosuppressive therapy with drugs such as azathioprine. Often, it takes a number of months before these medications are effective.

Metronidazole may be effective, particularly if there is evidence of fistulas or fissures in the anal region. Generally, this medication needs to be taken indefinitely not only to heal the fistula or fissure but also to prevent recurrence. At times, metronidazole is used for Crohn's disease of the colon. Metronidazole may cause numbness or tingling of the leg if used for a long period of time. If this occurs, discuss it with your physician.

None of these medications cure Crohn's disease. They are used as anti-inflammatory agents to provide relief from symptoms.

Currently, investigators are studying the use of aspirin-like compounds which can be given orally and are not absorbed by the small intestine. Thus, their anti-inflammatory properties can work directly at the site of inflammation. Other drugs are also being investigated.

Nutrition. The ability to absorb adequate nutrients often is limited in people with Crohn's disease, particularly if the disease affects significant portions of the small bowel or if portions of the small bowel have been removed surgically.

Your physician may advise specific replacement of certain vitamins or minerals if there is evidence of deficiency. It is not uncommon that persons with Crohn's disease have a deficiency of vitamin B_{12} which is absorbed in the lower segment (ileum) of the small bowel. If this occurs, vitamin B_{12} can be easily replaced with monthly injections through the skin.

Bile salts also are absorbed in the lower portion of the small bowel. If this absorption is impaired, your physician may recommend a special low-fat diet. If the bile acids are not absorbed in the small bowel, they may cause diarrhea by interfering with the absorption of water in the colon. At times, the use of a bile acid binder, such as cholestyramine, is effective in decreasing the amount of stool.

Some physicians advocate the use of elemental diets consisting of liquid preparations which contain simple sugars, amino acids, and minerals, particularly for active Crohn's disease. Although long-term proof of the effectiveness of this form of feeding is lacking, it occasionally may decrease the inflammation in the gut to allow for more absorption of nutrients. Some affected persons need to receive their nutrition intravenously for weeks, or even months, during severe bouts of Crohn's disease. Avoiding oral intake of food allows the bowel to rest.

Surgery. Approximately 70 percent of those with Crohn's disease require at least one operation at some point. These operations usually are performed for complications such as obstruction, abscesses, or perforation. Although surgical treatment may alleviate the symptoms for several years, it is not a cure and recurrence of the disease is very common.

In people with disease limited to the colon area, the removal of the large intestine may be recommended, particularly if medical treatment fails. In this operation, the entire colon, rectum, and anus are removed, and the end of the ileum (the last section of the small intestine) is brought out through the abdominal wall for the passage of stool. This is called an ileostomy. A pouch into which the stool is evacuated is worn over the opening (stoma) (see Ileostomy and Colostomy, page 638).

When the disease is limited to the small intestine, surgery typically involves removing the diseased segment of bowel and rejoining the two ends of healthy intestine.

ULCERATIVE COLITIS

Signs and Symptoms
- Bloody diarrhea that may contain pus;
- Abdominal pain;
- Painful, urgent bowel movements;
- Fever;
- Weight loss;
- Joint pains;
- Skin lesions.

Ulcerative colitis is one of two disorders that are termed inflammatory bowel disease (see also Crohn's disease, page 626). The causes of inflammatory bowel disease are unknown. Unlike Crohn's disease, which can involve any portion of the intestinal tract, ulcerative colitis is confined to the colon.

Ulcerative colitis is a chronic condition in which an inflammatory reaction characterized by tiny ulcers and small abscesses is limited to the inner lining (mucosa) of the colon. The inflammatory reactions almost always involve the rectum and extend into the rest of the colon. The amount of colon affected by the inflammatory process varies from person to person. If the inflammation is limited to the rectum, the term ulcerative proctitis sometimes is used.

Although this disease can strike at any time of life, its peak incidence is between the ages of 15 and 35. It is more common among whites. Like Crohn's disease, ulcerative colitis tends to run in some families.

The Diagnosis.   If you have the symptoms of ulcerative colitis, your physician will per-

form a flexible proctosigmoidoscopy, a procedure in which an instrument is inserted into the rectum to allow the examiner to see the lining of the lower portion of the colon and rectum (see Screening for Colon Cancer, page 641). The area then can be biopsied. A barium x-ray (see The Barium X-Ray of the Esophagus, Stomach, and Intestine, page 613) or colonoscopy (see page 637) may also be done.

How Serious Is Ulcerative Colitis?   At times, ulcerative colitis may be without symptoms. At other times, inflammation of the colon may occur, causing bloody diarrhea. Such flare-ups may alternate with periods of remission.

For approximately 15 percent of those with ulcerative colitis, the disease process may be quite serious, with inflammatory changes involving the entire colon. The symptoms are severe bloody diarrhea, fever, and abdominal pain. These symptoms even may constitute a medical emergency because there is a risk of dilation of the colon (toxic megacolon) or perforation of the markedly inflamed colon.

Ulcerative colitis also may be associated with various symptoms in other areas of your body. These may include pain or inflammation of large joints, most often the knees, ankles, and wrists. In some cases, ankylosing spondylitis (see Ankylosing Spondylitis, page 1001) may be associated with ulcerative colitis. At other times, acute inflammation of the eye may develop, or flow of the bile from the liver is partially obstructed (see Primary Sclerosing Cholangitis, page 665).

In addition, for people whose colons are completely or almost completely involved by ulcerative colitis, there appears to be a risk of cancer of the colon after the disease has been present for at least 8 to 10 years. In those persons who have lesser degrees of involvement (such as colitis involving only the left side of the colon) the risk is diminished and does not begin until 15 to 20 years after the onset of colitis. The risk of cancer increases with time. However, this risk is not dependent on the degree of inflammation. That is, cancer can develop despite the symptoms of ulcerative colitis being minimal.

Treatment.   The goal of treatment is to control the inflammation process, replace

ILEO-ANAL ANASTOMOSIS

It was not long ago that those who underwent operation for ulcerative colitis had no choice but to have an ileostomy, a procedure in which the entire colon, rectum, and anus are removed and an opening in the abdominal wall is created for the passage of stool. After an ileostomy, these people need to wear a pouch over the opening at all times.

Now, the most common surgical procedure for ulcerative colitis is the ileo-anal anastomosis. During this procedure the entire colon and rectum are removed but the anal sphincter muscles are preserved. A pouch is made in the ileum (the last segment of the small intestine) and is brought down and sutured to the anus.

A temporary ileostomy (see Ileostomy and Colostomy, page 638) usually is created to allow the ileal pouch and its attachment to the anus to heal. After a period of time, this temporary ileostomy is closed and the feces are then expelled through the anus. This eliminates the need for wearing an external bag to collect the feces.

It should be noted that ileostomy is still done for some people with ulcerative colitis, particularly in elderly persons or those with weak anal sphincters.

The Procedure
During an ileo-anal anastomosis, the colon and rectum are removed through an incision in the abdomen. Then your surgeon removes the inner lining from the anus but carefully preserves the sphincter muscles.

A small pouch is then made at the end of the ileum to collect the fecal material to decrease the number of bowel movements you have. This creation of a pouch

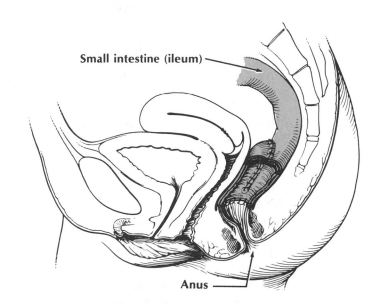

In the surgical procedure known as ileo-anal anastomosis, the diseased colon and rectum are removed but the anal sphincter muscles are left intact. The small intestine (ileum) is then stitched directly to the anus. This procedure allows for near normal passage of stool rather than the permanent use of an ileostomy bag.

may not be necessary in children and young adults because the ileum can often adapt itself.

A temporary ileostomy is necessary to allow time for your intestines to heal. In this procedure, an opening (stoma) is made through the abdominal wall and a loop of the ileum is brought out. Fecal material will then be expelled through this opening and into a pouch that you will wear around it. Unlike a permanent ileostomy, the temporary one is closed in 2 to 3 months. Then, you will be able to go to the bathroom as you always did.

The Recovery
After some initial pain, you should start feeling better soon. Many patients who have been debilitated from their disease are surprised to gain weight and strength so quickly following their operation. By the time they return to the hospital to have the ileostomy closed, they often feel better than they have in years.

Once the ileostomy is closed, expect to have frequent bowel movements for several months. Usually, the first bowel movement occurs about 3 days after the stoma is closed. The pouch made at the end of the ileum slowly increases in size. As this pouch becomes larger, it can store more stool and the number of bowel movements per day will decrease.

Initially, you may get discouraged. During the first few weeks, it may seem like you are spending all your time in the bathroom, and your anus may become sore from frequent bowel movements. You may even have episodes of incontinence. Your physician may prescribe a medication to slow down your bowel and thicken the consistency of the stool if that is a problem.

Usually, determination and patience will pay off. The number of stools will decrease and the incontinence will go away. Then, you will be able to lead a healthy, normal life.

the nutritional losses that occur because of severe diarrhea, and prevent complications.

Medication.   The principal drugs used in the treatment of ulcerative colitis are the anti-inflammatory agents sulfasalazine and corticosteroids.

Sulfasalazine is generally used for minor flare-ups of the disease and also in maintaining remissions. Corticosteroids (see page 1005) are used for more severe episodes of bloody diarrhea. If the inflammatory process is confined to the rectum, a corticosteroid enema may be useful in suppressing the inflammation and alleviating symptoms. New enema preparations containing aspirin-like drugs have been used in the last several years to suppress inflammation in the rectum and appear to work quite well. In addition, investigators are studying the use of aspirin-like compounds that can be given orally and are not absorbed by the intestine. Thus their anti-inflammatory properties can work directly at the site of inflammation.

When the diarrhea is massive, hospitalization may be required to begin medical therapy, to provide hydration through a vein, and to place the bowel at rest by not using oral feedings.

Immunosuppressive therapy with medications such as azathioprine is used occasionally with careful supervision by your physician.

Nutrition.   Some severely ill patients need to have their nutrients infused intravenously when their colon is too diseased to tolerate food. In those who are not as severely ill, a liquid food supplement that can be taken by mouth is often recommended to compensate for the nutrients lost in diarrhea.

Surgery.   Approximately 20 to 25 percent of those with ulcerative colitis require surgery at some time. These are the people who do not respond to medication or who have severe complications. The present trend is to perform surgery earlier in the disease process, when it appears that the inflammation of the colon is unresponsive to medication, instead of waiting until the patient becomes debilitated. The operation most commonly done is the ileo-anal anastomosis (see page 629). Unlike prior techniques, this is not disfiguring, preserves the passage of stool through the anus, and usually is well-tolerated by most of those selected for the operation.

If you have had extensive ulcerative colitis for more than 8 to 10 years, your physician may recommend the elective removal of your entire colon for prevention of cancer (see Ileo-anal Anastomosis, page 629). As an alternative, he or she may suggest periodic examination of your colon by colonoscopy (see page 637) to look for changes suggesting a transformation to malignant cells in your colon and to biopsy suspected areas.

TUMORS OF THE SMALL INTESTINE

Signs and Symptoms
* Abdominal cramps and pain;
* Bloody stools;
* Nausea and vomiting;
* Weight loss.

Tumors of the small intestine are relatively uncommon—they represent only 3 to 6 percent of all abnormal growths in the gastrointestinal tract. Intestinal tumors can be benign or malignant.

Most intestinal tumors are benign and usually are discovered during ages 40 through 60. The most frequent symptoms are pain, nausea and vomiting, and bleeding. There are several types of benign tumors, including lipomas, leiomyomas, angiomas, and adenomas. These tumors do not spread. They often are an incidental finding on an x-ray made because of another problem, although some benign tumors can cause bleeding.

A small percentage of tumors of the small intestine are malignant. The most common malignant types are adenocarcinoma, leiomyosarcoma, carcinoid tumor, and lymphoma.

If you have a malignant tumor in your small intestine, your symptoms may include weight loss, abdominal pain, nausea and vomiting, and bleeding. Your physician may feel an abdominal mass.

Bleeding, perforation, and obstruction are common manifestations of a leiomyosarcoma, whereas a carcinoid tumor may cause no symptoms before it spreads (see page 625).

The Diagnosis.   The diagnosis of a tumor in the small intestine is often made with a barium x-ray (see The Barium X-Ray of the

DIVERTICULOSIS AND DIVERTICULITIS

The development of multiple small pouches that project outward from the wall of the colon is termed diverticulosis. Most often, these pouches produce no pain or other symptoms; however, when inflammation occurs in or around these pouches, the condition is called diverticulitis.

What Is the Cause?

The cause is unknown, but diverticular problems are much more common in industrialized nations such as the United States, leading some physicians to speculate that the relatively low intake of fiber in the Western diet may be a major factor. The risk of diverticular disease increases with age, with the incidence in Western countries ranging from 20 to 50 percent in persons over age 50.

The Symptoms

Most people with diverticulosis have no symptoms. Typically, diverticulosis goes undiscovered or is an incidental finding during a barium enema performed for other reasons (see The Barium X-Ray of the Esophagus, Stomach, and Intestine, page 613).

Diverticulitis is more likely to occur in the lower (sigmoid) portion of your colon. A diverticulum becomes inflamed or infected probably as a result of undigested food and bacteria lodging in it. This compromises the blood supply to the diverticulum, making it susceptible to an invasion by bacteria. The result can range from a small abscess to a massive infec-

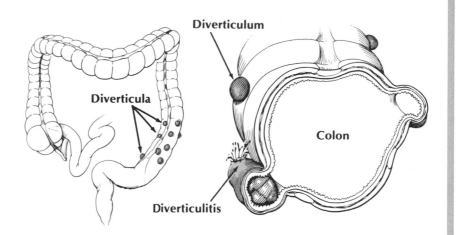

Diverticula are small pouches of the large intestine (left drawing). When these pouches produce no discomfort, the condition is termed diverticulosis. If the diverticula become inflamed, or if they rupture, the problem is called diverticulitis (right).

tion or perforation. The process resembles that of appendicitis (see Acute Appendicitis, page 624) except that it occurs in the lower left side of your colon.

If you have diverticulitis, you may have severe cramping pains, usually more severe on your left side. The pain may be severe or it may be mild for several days before getting worse. Fever and nausea commonly are present.

Sometimes the inflamed diverticulum ruptures, spilling intestinal material into the abdominal cavity. This causes peritonitis, a medical emergency. Hemorrhage is a less frequent complication (see Peritonitis, page 642).

The Treatments

Treatment for diverticulitis may involve simple bed rest, stool softeners, a liquid diet, and antibiotics when the inflammation is mild and the diverticulum has not ruptured. When rupture or widespread infection has occurred, intravenous

antibiotic therapy may be necessary. Hospitalization usually is required.

If you experience a series of attacks, surgical removal of the involved segment of the bowel at a time when no symptoms are present may be advised. Surgery also may be required if you do not respond to intravenous antibiotic treatment during an acute attack. Often, in these more acute situations a temporary colostomy (see Ileostomy and Colostomy, page 638) is performed. At a later date the bowel may be reattached during a second operation.

In regard to diverticulosis, many physicians believe that treatment is unnecessary when there are no symptoms. Others prescribe a high-fiber diet and, if there are some minimal symptoms, an antispasmodic medication. Often, symptoms of an irritable bowel (see Irritable Bowel Syndrome, page 632) are incorrectly blamed on diverticulosis.

Esophagus, Stomach, and Intestine, page 613).

How Serious Are Tumors of the Small Intestine?   Benign tumors are not life-threat-

ening but they can cause dangerous symptoms such as bleeding and obstruction. Like any malignancy, cancer of the small intestine is a dangerous and life-threatening illness and requires prompt treatment.

IRRITABLE BOWEL SYNDROME

Many Americans periodically have an attack of irritable bowel syndrome. Because people with irritable bowel syndrome often suffer in silence without taking their complaint to a physician, the number with this disorder is unknown.

What Is a Spastic Colon?

Irritable bowel syndrome often is called "spastic colon." It probably is the result of abnormal muscular activity of the intestinal wall. The causes of this abnormal activity vary. At times it may be aggravated by a specific food, but in many who suffer from irritable bowel syndrome, chronic stress and depression may be the primary cause or at least contribute to flare-ups of symptoms.

Irritable bowel syndrome often begins in adolescence or in young adulthood. It is seen more frequently in women.

The Diagnosis

How do you know if you have irritable bowel syndrome? Abdominal pain and a change in bowel habits are the main symptoms. The pain can occur anywhere in your abdomen, and it can be severe. Indigestion, heartburn, and nausea also may occur.

Typically, the symptoms occur after a meal and are temporarily relieved by a bowel movement. Persons with irritable bowel syndrome frequently complain of feeling bloated and passing an excessive amount of gas, which also relieves the discomfort.

Constipation also is a frequent complaint. The bowel movement may be pellet-like or in small balls or ribbons. Often, those with irritable bowel syndrome abuse laxatives because of chronic constipation. Diarrhea also may occur but is a less-frequent symptom.

Minimizing Your Symptoms

Irritable bowel syndrome is a chronic condition that may occur on and off throughout your life, but there are things you can do to minimize the symptoms.

1. See your physician. The symptoms of irritable bowel syndrome may mimic the symptoms of a serious disease. It is important that you undergo a complete examination, particularly if the symptoms have appeared only recently, to be sure your problem is not being caused by something more serious. An examination of your rectum (see Screening for Colon Cancer, page 641) and a barium enema (see The Barium X-Ray of the Esophagus, Stomach, and Intestine, page 613) may be done. Knowing that your symptoms are not due to a dangerous disease may ease your mind—and possibly decrease the stress that may make your irritable bowel syndrome worse.

2. Select foods carefully. If a specific food appears to bring on your symptoms, eliminate it from your diet. Sometimes a high-fiber diet including consumption of fresh fruits, vegetables, and fiber supplements is helpful; in some people, however, it can increase bloating and gas.

3. Do not eliminate a food just because it appears to cause symptoms on a single occasion. Be sure that the food produces symptoms consistently before giving it up. Many persons with irritable bowel syndrome restrict their diet to just a few selections and feel the worse for it. They often feel better when they return to a more varied diet. Some foods will seem to cause distress when consumed in larger amounts but do not when taken in small helpings or as part of a meal.

4. Bulk formers, which contain the natural vegetable fiber psyllium, are available without a prescription and may help relieve your constipation and diarrhea. Your physician also may want to try an anti-spasm medication occasionally. This medication may improve your problem temporarily but should not be used for a long period.

   Biofeedback techniques also may be helpful in relieving stress.

   Remember, irritable bowel syndrome does not predispose you to more serious disorders.

Treatment. Surgery is usually recommended for all benign tumors that cause symptoms and for malignancies that have not become too widespread for surgical treatment. At times, the x-ray examination of the intestine cannot distinguish a benign from a malignant tumor, and surgical exploration of the abdomen and removal of the tumor is necessary before the diagnosis can be made. When a tumor has metastasized to such an extent that surgery will not be effective, steroid medications, chemotherapy, and radiation—either individually or in combination—may be used.

CHRONIC CONSTIPATION

Many people believe that constipation is the inability to have a bowel movement daily. In fact, it is not necessary to have a bowel movement every day. For some, regularity means having a bowel movement three times a week; for others, it is part of their daily routine.

True constipation is the passage of hard stools less than three times a week. Accompanying symptoms may include abdominal bloating and discomfort.

What Causes Constipation?

As your colon removes water from the waste products, a stool is formed and moved through the intestine by muscular contractions. Alterations in the speed at which the waste passes through the colon or in the amount of water removed can affect normal bowel function.

If the constipation is a recent development or your stool habits differ from what you consider normal, see your physician. He or she first will rule out such causes of constipation as obstruction (see Intestinal Obstruction, page 643) and hypothyroidism (see page 730). In addition, consideration will be given to your medications. Some medications may cause constipation, including those used to treat Parkinson's disease, depression, hypertension, or some heart disorders.

Your physician may want to obtain a flexible proctosigmoidoscopic examination (see Screening for Colon Cancer, page 641) and a barium study of your colon (see The Barium X-Ray of the Esophagus, Stomach, and Intestine, page 613) to rule out other causes of disease within the colon.

Are Laxatives the Answer?

Many constipation sufferers rely heavily on laxatives to relieve their problem. Paradoxically, laxatives can lead to constipation when not used properly. They also can damage the bowel and disrupt your body's normal balance of minerals.

If constipation is a problem, instead of resorting to a daily dose of laxative, try these steps.

1. Drink at least six to eight glasses of water or other liquids every day.
2. Increase the fiber content of your diet by eating more fresh fruits and vegetables.
3. Consider adding a fiber or bran supplement to your diet.
4. Add to your diet a bulk former which contains the vegetable fiber psyllium.
5. Set aside a specific time every day for trying to have a bowel movement.
6. Do not resist the urge to move your bowels.
7. Incorporate regular physical exercise into your daily regimen.
8. If constipation continues, it may be reasonable to use milk of magnesia or mineral oil occasionally at bedtime, but avoid regular use of it.
9. Avoid irritating enemas such as those containing soapsuds. Such enemas are advised in preparation for certain x-ray or endoscopic examinations of the colon but have no place in daily life.
10. Avoid enemas in general. A thorough "cleansing" of the colon, by either an enema or a laxative, actually contributes to the problem of constipation.
11. If your constipation is not improved, see your physician.

LAXATIVE ABUSE

It is rare for anyone to need a laxative on a daily basis; yet many people find reasons to overuse laxatives.

Some have an irrational fear that they will be ill if their bowels do not move each day and so they take laxatives daily to ensure a daily bowel movement. Others take large amounts of laxatives regularly as a preventive measure, even though they have no evidence of constipation. Still others take laxatives in an attempt to purge their systems in order to lose weight.

Kinds of Laxatives

The best-known laxative is castor oil; it undergoes chemical transformation within the colon to become an acid that prevents the intestinal wall from absorbing water. Prolonged use of castor oil can damage the cells that line your intestinal tract. Phenolphthalein is another laxative that acts by irritating the bowel wall; it is the active ingredient in many of the small chocolate or candy-like tablets that are laxatives. Other laxatives work by increasing the water content within your colon and are less irritating to your bowel; these include milk of magnesia.

Bulk-forming laxatives or so-called natural laxatives expand when they come into contact with water in the colon. These laxatives prevent the formation of hard stools.

What Are the Risks of Overuse?

Excessive use of laxatives is harmful. When taken in excess, laxatives will flush out necessary vitamins and other nutrients before they can be properly absorbed. Laxatives also contribute to an excessive excretion of water, sodium, and potassium. Furthermore, habitual use of laxatives tends to weaken the muscles in the intestine and make them flabby and less able to function properly. As a result, once you stop taking a laxative on a regular basis, your constipation will not only return but also it may be worse.

Excessive use of laxatives can bring about diarrhea or real constipation by inducing lazy bowel syndrome. This is a condition in which the bowels fail to function properly because they have begun to rely on the laxative to do the work of elimination. Laxatives also can interfere with the effectiveness of other medications your physician might prescribe.

INTESTINAL GAS

Everyone produces gas in their colon. In fact, most intestinal gas (flatus) is produced in the colon. Usually the gas is expelled during a bowel movement. However, some people produce an excessive amount of gas that bothers them throughout the day.

What Are the Components of Intestinal Gas?

Intestinal gas is composed primarily of five substances: oxygen, nitrogen, hydrogen, carbon dioxide, and methane. The foul odor usually is the result of small traces of other gases such as hydrogen sulfide and ammonia and other substances.

Nitrogen and oxygen are in the air we breathe and may be in intestinal gas when swallowed air travels through the digestive system. Some carbon dioxide is produced by a chemical reaction in the small intestine. Hydrogen, carbon dioxide, and, in many persons, methane are produced in the large intestine by bacterial fermentation of carbohydrate that has not been digested and absorbed in the small intestine.

What Foods Cause Intestinal Gas?

Foods that may cause excessive gas include peas and beans, wheat, oats, bran, brussels sprouts, cabbage, corn, and rutabagas. People who are deficient in the digestive enzyme lactase also may have problems with milk products (see page 623). Increased intestinal gas can be anticipated as a part of a high-fiber diet and with the use of bulk formers.

What Should I Do About Excessive Intestinal Gas?

Sometimes excessive gas is attributable to a disease of the digestive tract, and treatment for that disease often decreases the amount of gas produced in the intestines. In most cases, however, excessive gas is not the result of disease.

While potentially embarrassing and certainly annoying, excess intestinal gas is not a serious condition. Some people find that the condition improves when they avoid certain "gassy" foods, especially beans and milk. The over-the-counter remedies advertised for the problem rarely are effective.

What Is Swallowed Air?

Swallowed air makes up a small fraction of intestinal gas. On the other hand, the bloating gas you feel in your stomach is almost entirely a consequence of swallowed air. Air may be swallowed with or without the swallowing of food or liquid. Eating too fast, wearing false teeth, and using chewing gum may contribute to the problem. Often, the swallowing of air is part of the act of trying to belch or to relieve the feeling of pressure in the upper abdomen. You may not even be aware that air has been swallowed. This is sometimes called "Yo-Yo" belching because the air goes down and comes right back up. Carbonated drinks may release carbon dioxide in the stomach and so may be a source of gas.

Some swallowed air may travel with the food into the small intestine. Some of the air may be dissolved in the body fluids and ultimately lost from the body via the lungs.

FIBER IN THE DIET

In recent years, Americans have become increasingly aware of the need for more fiber in their diet. Not only does a high-fiber diet decrease the chance of constipation but also many physicians believe that it may decrease the risk of colon cancer.

But before you buy one of the high-fiber supplements on the market, look in your refrigerator and cupboards. The chances are that you have everything you need right in your kitchen to increase the fiber content in your diet.

What Are High-Fiber Foods?

High-fiber foods—often referred to as bulk or roughage—include whole grain products, fruits, vegetables, and legumes. These all are better sources of fiber than anything you can buy at the drugstore.

What is fiber and why does it aid in the digestive process?

Unlike foods that are broken down and absorbed during digestion, fiber is not affected by the digestive enzymes. Thus, it passes virtually unchanged through the stomach and small intestine and into the colon. In the colon, some forms of fiber are fermented by bacteria and others resist fermentation and are expelled in the stool unchanged.

Role of Fiber

Fiber increases the weight and size of the stool, in addition to softening it. The bulky stool is easier to pass, lessening the chance of constipation.

The Benefits

As to why fiber may decrease the risk of colon cancer, some physicians believe that it may help to clear the colon of substances that may be changed by bacteria into cancer-promoting chemicals. They base this belief on the low incidence of colon cancer in countries where a high-fiber diet is the norm. Others argue that fiber itself does not protect against colon cancer but that people who eat high-fiber diets tend not to consume as much fat; and, they believe, animal fat may promote colon cancer.

Many forms of dietary fiber promote bowel regularity. Fiber may decrease the chances of complications in the event of diverticular disease. In addition, fiber may decrease the size of hemorrhoids and prevent hemorrhoidal bleeding. If you have loose, watery stools, fiber may help to solidify the stool, because it absorbs water.

Other benefits of eating fiber include a possible lowering of cholesterol level and, in diabetics, a slowing of the absorption of sugar which may decrease the need for insulin in some people with diabetes.

The Disadvantages

Fiber can produce excess gas. Some sources of fiber—oat bran and wheat fiber, for example—can remove minerals such as calcium, iron, and zinc from your body. If you eat a balanced diet and take a reasonable amount of milk with your oat bran and high-fiber cereals, however, this usually is nothing to worry about.

The Strategies

If you want to make sure you are getting adequate fiber, follow these suggestions.

1. Get your fiber from food. Sometimes people assume that if they take a fiber supplement, they need not pay attention to their diet. In fact, a supplement is no substitute for the fiber from your food.
2. Eat a varied diet, including high-fiber foods such as grains, vegetables, fresh fruits, and legumes. High-fiber snack foods include nuts, seeds, popcorn, fresh and dried fruits, and whole-grain crackers.
3. Try to limit your consumption of processed foods which often have little fiber. The refining process removes the outer coat (bran) from grain; thus, this highly desirable form of fiber is lost. This is why whole-grain products are higher in fiber content than those made of the refined flour. In a similar fashion, removing the skin from fruits and vegetables decreases their fiber content. An orange contains considerably more fiber than the juice squeezed from it. So think twice before peeling fruits and vegetables or even squeezing the juice from them if you want to increase the fiber content of your diet.
4. Increase your fiber intake gradually.

COLON POLYPS

Signs and Symptoms
• Often none are apparent;
• Recent change in bowel movements;
• Blood in the stool;
• Mucus discharged from the anus;
• Microscopic amounts of blood in the stool.

Benign (nonmalignant) tumors of the large intestine are not uncommon. It is believed that two of every three Americans over the age of 60 has some type of growth (or lesion) in their colon.

Most of these tumors are polyps which arise from the lining of the colon. They usually are harmless and are discovered accidentally, often during a screening test for colon cancer (see Screening for Colon Cancer, page 641) or during a test to diagnose another disorder.

There are several different varieties of polyps found in the colon. The most common is a hyperplastic polyp that generally is less than ¼ inch in diameter. These tiny polyps are not a health risk although, if such polyps grow to be larger than ½ inch in diameter, they should be removed for an accurate diagnosis under the microscope.

Juvenile polyps occur during childhood. Your child may experience rectal bleeding or the polyp may even be seen to drop down through the anal canal during defecation. These polyps can be easily removed with a colonoscope (see Colonoscopy, page 637). These polyps also do not degenerate into a malignancy.

Inflammatory polyps are thought to result from injury to or inflammation of the lining of the colon such as after a bout of ulcerative colitis (see page 628). These also are not a significant health risk.

The other major category of polyps are adenomas. These are classified into three varieties based on features seen under the microscope: tubular, tubulovillous, and villous. The most common are tubular adenomas which generally are less than ½ inch in diameter. Villous adenomas are less common. More than half of them are at least 1 inch in diameter. Often, with these tumors you may experience significant mucus discharge in the stool along with blood. Tubulovillous adenomas contain characteristics of the two other types.

The adenomatous polyps have the potential for malignancy, and this potential usually increases as the size of the polyp increases and when more villous characteristics are present. Thus, these polyps should be removed, most often via colonoscopy (see Colonoscopy, page 637), to prevent the development of a cancer. At times, even if the polyp shows microscopic cancer in a few cells, the removal via colonoscopy is curative. At other times, if there is concern about the spread of cancer from the polyp itself, your physician may recommend an operation to remove a section of the colon that includes the polyp and surrounding tissue and lymph nodes.

Most colonic polyps are not considered hereditary, but there seems to be a tendency for them to appear in several members of a family. Also, if a colonic polyp develops in a person, he or she may have others later in life.

One type of disorder in which colonic polyps are present is believed to be strongly hereditary. Called familial colonic polyposis, this rare disorder is characterized by the appearance of numerous (often 1,000 or more) polyps throughout the entire colon. These polyps can be asymptomatic (without symptoms) or may cause rectal bleeding. Typically, this condition appears during childhood or adolescence.

Gardner's syndrome refers to the existence of multiple colonic and other intestinal polyps along with other nonmalignant tumors such as lipomas, fibromas, and osteomas in other regions of the body.

Cancer of the colon inevitably occurs in these hereditary forms of colonic polyposis. Therefore, removal of the colon (total colectomy) is advised as soon as the diagnosis is established. It is also important for blood relatives to be examined at a relatively young age (approximately 10 to 12 years) so that appropriate treatment can be carried out if they also have colonic polyposis.

Polyps are small growths that may appear in the large intestine. In most cases, they are benign (nonmalignant). They may assume a variety of shapes. Pedunculated and lobulated (strawberry) are two common forms.

Colon

Lobulated (strawberry) polyp

Pedunculated polyp

COLONOSCOPY

Colonoscopy is the examination of the entire colon by using a fiberoptic endoscope. This flexible instrument transmits light, allowing the specially trained physician to examine the lining of the colon from the anus to the cecum, the junction of the small and large intestines. Sometimes, the last several inches of the small intestine can be examined as well.

Applications
Colonoscopy represents the most accurate method of examining your colon for polyps or other small lesions. In persons known to be at risk for these abnormalities, periodic colonoscopy may be very useful.

Other common uses include biopsy and removal of polyps (polypectomy) that have been detected during a barium enema or proctoscopy; for searching for a cause of chronic or acute bleeding when a cause cannot be established by other tests; to screen for cancer when there is a history of other diseases or a family history that increases a person's risk of colon cancer; for differentiating colitis caused by Crohn's disease from ulcerative colitis; for assessing the extent of involvement due to colitis prior to surgery; and to identify the cause of diarrhea when other tests or examinations offer no clear diagnosis.

A laser beam can be directed through a channel of the colonoscope and applied to a bleeding lesion or one that has the potential to bleed. Electrocoagulation through the colonoscope can be used for similar purposes.

The Procedure
If you are scheduled to have colonoscopy, you will need to adhere to special dietary instructions, usually beginning the day prior to the test. You will be given a laxative or liquid solution the night before the procedure and often an enema that morning. You also may be given a sedative just prior to the examination.

The Risks
The main complications of the test are hemorrhage and perforation, but the risk is very low. Colonoscopy is not recommended if you are having an episode of acute diverticulitis (see page 631), have vascular disease in the bowel, or are in the midst of an acute phase of colitis.

A   **B**

In performing a colonoscopy examination, a fiberoptic colonoscope is gently inserted into your rectum and large intestine. This instrument provides a direct view of your lower gastrointestinal tract. Inset A: normal colon. Inset B: colon cancer.

ILEOSTOMY AND COLOSTOMY

Ileostomy and colostomy are operations in which a major portion of the intestine is removed, usually because of diseases such as cancer or Crohn's disease. This removes the normal route for the elimination of waste, so an opening (stoma) is created in the abdominal wall, a portion of intestine is brought out through the opening, and the stool is eliminated into a pouch worn securely over the opening.

The main distinction between the two procedures is that during a colostomy a portion of the colon or large intestine is pulled through the abdominal wall whereas an ileostomy involves bringing the end segment of the small intestine (ileum) through the opening.

Colostomy

During a colostomy, the surgeon makes an incision that permits him or her to examine the colon and to remove the diseased areas. Sometimes the anus and rectum are also removed and the anal area is closed with stitches. An opening in the abdomen is then made and a section of colon is pulled through. A pouch is then securely fastened over the opening. The feces then flow into the pouch which is emptied periodically.

There are different types of colostomies, depending on what section of the colon is removed. The consistency of the stool also depends on where the digestive process has been interrupted. For example, if the initial portion of the colon empties into the pouch, the stool will be loose; if the lower end of the colon is brought through the stoma, the stool will be formed because more of the liquid has been absorbed in the colon.

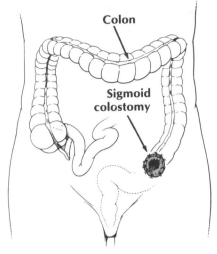

In performing a sigmoid colostomy, the surgeon removes the diseased portion of the colon, which eliminates the normal route for waste excretion. The remaining intestine is brought through an opening (stoma) in the abdominal wall. Stool can be eliminated into a pouch worn securely over the opening.

Although many colostomies are permanent, sometimes a temporary colostomy is done to allow a part of the bowel to heal after injury or disease. After the area is healed, the stoma is closed and the bowel is reconnected so that the normal elimination process can continue.

Ileostomy

This procedure is done when the entire colon and rectum are removed, often because of Crohn's colitis.

During the conventional ileostomy, a portion of the small intestine is brought out through the opening created in the abdominal wall. As in the colostomy, the ileostomy requires that a pouch be worn over the stoma to collect the waste, which in this case has a liquid consistency because the digestive process has been halted before the colon where much of the liquid normally is absorbed.

A relatively new variation of the ileostomy is now being done in some medical centers. Called a continent ileostomy or Kock pouch, this operation involves the creation of an internal pouch and valve for waste, the pouch and valve being constructed of a portion of the small intestine. This pouch can store your waste internally for several hours at a time, eliminating the need for an outside pouch. At your convenience, you insert a catheter (a thin tube) into the opening that has been created in your abdomen and drain the liquid feces from the internal pouch. The valve prevents the pouch from leaking at any other time.

Although most patients are squeamish at first about using the catheter, they soon get used to it, and it is painless. Initially, the pouch is emptied every few hours but after a while two to four times a day usually is adequate. The time required for the emptying usually is no more than if you were having a bowel movement.

The ileal pouch or Kock pouch procedure is done in some situations if you have ulcerative colitis (see page 628) or hereditary polyposis (see Colon Polyps, page 635) and an ileo-anal anastomosis (see page 629) cannot be done. This procedure is not done if you are known to have Crohn's colitis.

Adjusting to the Change

No matter what type of colostomy or ileostomy you require, it can be a traumatic experience, requiring a period of adjustment, both physically and emotionally.

Physical Activity

In the 6 to 8 weeks immediately after the operation, avoid lifting, pushing, or pulling more than 5 to 10 pounds. As you begin to resume normal activities, the best single guide for what to do and not to do is what you were comfortable with prior to your operation.

In general, walking, swimming, and simple exercise are good activities that will help firm your muscles and keep your digestive tract working properly.

Bathing

You may bathe or shower with or without the appliance over the stoma. However, long, hot baths or showers are to be avoided with the appliance attached. You may find that keeping the appliance above the water level in the bath or covering the area with a border of tape in a picture-frame shape will be helpful.

Sexuality

Most physicians advise abstention from sexual activity for a while after this operation. Sexual relations can be resumed thereafter: do not assume that your partner no longer cares for you sexually. Be patient and talk about the feelings each of you has.

You may find that certain positions are more comfortable than others. Sexual dysfunction is not uncommon immediately after the operation. If pain in the vagina or inability to achieve erection occurs, it may be temporary. If the problem continues after several months, discuss it with your physician.

Guidelines for driving a vehicle and other activities will be discussed with you by your physician. Once they get accustomed to the change, most people feel much better than they did before and adjust to the minor inconveniences.

The Diagnosis. Most frequently, colonic polyps are discovered during an examination for another colon problem or during evaluation of microscopic blood in the stool (see Screening for Colon Cancer, page 641). Then, you may have a barium enema (see The Barium X-Ray of the Esophagus, Stomach, and Intestine, page 613) and a proctosigmoidoscopic examination (see Screening for Colon Cancer, page 641). Alternatively, colonoscopy may be performed to examine your colon and to treat any detected lesions.

How Serious Are Polyps? An adenomatous polyp has the potential to become cancerous. Most, if not all, colon cancers seem to develop from polyps. Moreover, sometimes they may cause problems such as bleeding and obstruction. The removal of polyps may play a significant role in the prevention of colon cancer.

Treatment. The removal of most of these benign polyps is a relatively simple procedure. They usually are removed when detected because this eliminates the chance that they will ever become malignant. Commonly, the polyp is removed during colonoscopy. If the tumor cannot be removed by this means, a laparotomy (a surgical opening of the abdomen) and opening of the colon will be required to remove the polyp.

If an adenomatous polyp is found at the time of colonoscopy, your physician will recommend periodic examination of the colon because of the likelihood of further adenomatous polyps developing.

If you have multiple colonic polyposis, the likelihood of colon cancer is virtually 100 percent by age 40. Thus, physicians usually recommend that the entire colon be removed to prevent cancer. The procedure normally done is a colectomy with ileostomy (see Ileostomy and Colostomy, page 638) or an ileo-anal anastomosis (see Ileo-Anal Anastomosis, page 629).

COLON CANCER

Signs and Symptoms
- Rectal bleeding;
- Altered bowel habits;
- Abdominal cramps or pain;
- Microscopic amounts of blood in the stool;
- Unexplained anemia;
- Unexplained weight loss;
- Sometimes, none.

Cancer of the colon and cancer of the rectum are two of the more common forms of cancer among adult men and women. These two cancers are jointly referred to as colorectal cancer or colon cancer.

Factors that increase your risk of colorectal cancer include a family history or prior history of adenomatous colon polyps (see Colon Polyps, page 635), of colon cancer, or of ulcerative colitis (see page 628).

Although the precise cause of colon cancer is unknown, some studies suggest that diet plays an important role. It has been suggested that the higher proportion of animal fat in our diet may account for the large amount of colorectal cancer in the United States compared with countries such as Japan where the dietary emphasis is on vegetables, poultry, and fish.

The Diagnosis.   If you are over the age of 40 and have rectal bleeding, do not assume that you just have hemorrhoids. Your physician will want to perform a rectal examination using a gloved finger. You also may be examined by barium enema (see The Barium X-Ray of the Esophagus, Stomach, and Intestine, page 613), proctosigmoidoscopy (see Screening for Colon Cancer, page 641), or colonoscopy (see Colonoscopy, page 637), depending on the results of the other tests and your symptoms. The diagnosis of colon cancer sometimes is made after investigation of the cause for anemia or for the finding of microscopic blood in the stool (see Screening for Colon Cancer, page 641) or a change in bowel habits.

How Serious Is Colon Cancer? Colon cancer accounts for about 20 percent of the deaths due to malignant disease in this country. When detected and treated at an early stage, these cancers are considered to be curable. Unfortunately, many people do not seek medical attention when such warning signs as rectal bleeding or a change in the shape and size of their stool become evident.

Treatment. *Surgery.* The present approach to the treatment of colon cancer is surgery. In about half of the cases, surgery can cure this form of cancer.

Before the operation, you may have a blood test and a CT scan (see page 1286) to help determine whether the cancer has spread (metastasized) beyond the location of the tumor. If the cancer has spread, surgery may be ruled out unless the cancer causes bowel obstruction or bleeding.

Other Treatments. After surgery, your physician may recommend additional treatment, especially if you are at high risk for a recurrence. For example, your physician may recommend chemotherapy with the drugs 5-fluorouracil (5-FU) and levamisole. These drugs decrease the chance of tumor recurrence and improve survival in persons with colon cancer that has spread only to

nearby lymph nodes. However, to be effective, this treatment must begin within 4 weeks after surgery. (When combined with radiation therapy, these drugs also can be effective as treatment for rectal cancer.) If a bowel obstruction is present or if there is bleeding, laser therapy through a colonoscope may help relieve symptoms. Your physician will advise you as to whether this additional treatment may be useful.

MEGACOLON

Signs and Symptoms
• Severe constipation;
• Malnutrition.

From either congenital or acquired causes, the colon can become so enlarged that it becomes unable to move feces. This condition is referred to as megacolon or giant colon. Nerve damage in the colon or rectum frequently is the cause of megacolon.

Hirschsprung's disease is a congenital disorder in which babies are born without ganglion nerve cells in a segment of their rectum. These infants are unable to have a bowel movement because the segment of the colon nearest the anus is unable to relax to permit the passage of feces. Symptoms are massive abdominal distention, absence of bowel movements, and impaired nutrition. Hirschsprung's disease occurs more often in males and often runs in families. The diagnosis is made by biopsy of the rectum under general anesthesia.

A type of acquired megacolon is psychogenic megacolon which develops usually at the time of toilet training. It creates severe and chronic constipation.

In Central and South America, an infection called Chagas disease causes megacolon. The infection destroys the ganglion cells of the colon to create a condition similar to Hirschsprung's disease (see page 59) except that it occurs in adults rather than in children.

Some other conditions that can cause megacolon are severe neurological disorders such as spinal cord injury and Parkinson's disease (see page 520) and use of some medications including narcotics.

The Diagnosis.   Your physician will examine your rectum with a proctoscope (see

SCREENING FOR COLON CANCER

Cancer of the rectum and colon is the second leading cause of cancer deaths in the United States. Almost 150,000 Americans each year are found to have this disease; roughly 60,000 die.

Often, colorectal cancer is discovered too late for cure. However, this does not always have to be the case. When discovered in its early stages, colorectal cancer usually is curable by surgery. Thus, it is important that you be aware of symptoms of this disease and the diagnostic tests that can detect colorectal cancer in its early, and most curable, stage.

Family History

If a parent or sibling has had colon cancer or an adenomatous polyp (see Colon Polyps, page 635), you also may be at an increased risk for colon polyp or cancer. In this situation, your physician may wish to perform regular examinations of your colon.

Recognize Changes in Bowel Habits

Early detection starts with being aware of the signs of colon cancer. This includes any change in your normal bowel movement, especially the shape of your stool, rectal bleeding, lower abdominal pain, and unexplained, persistent urges to defecate. The latter symptom may be caused by a mass in the rectum.

Undergo Periodic Tests

In addition to seeking medical attention for symptoms, have periodic screening tests.

Although many of the more invasive and expensive tests are not feasible for everyone, there are simple and inexpensive tests that could save your life. These tests screen for excessive blood in the stool. The most accurate such test, called the HemoQuant, measures quantitatively any traces of blood in the stool, such as blood that may be lost from the surface of a cancer or a polyp. A small sample of stool is collected and analyzed in a laboratory to measure the amount of blood. Everyone over the age of 50 should have this test periodically. Unlike earlier tests, this one is quite accurate. Ask your physician about this test. In another version of this test, the stool is smeared onto a piece of paper that has been sensitized to detect hidden (occult) blood. Sometimes these papers can be mailed to a laboratory or to your physician for interpretation of results.

Home test kits are available at the drugstore for those who prefer to do the test themselves. However, these tests are not as accurate as the HemoQuant.

Before taking the test, avoid eating turnips, horseradish, red meat, and vitamin C supplements for 2 days. Substances found in these foods and supplements may affect the test results.

Proctosigmoidoscopy

Another test that often is recommended is a flexible proctosigmoidoscopic examination. This test examines the lower portion of the colon (sigmoid) and rectum by using a flexible, lighted tube called a flexible proctosigmoidoscope. Almost 50 percent of all colorectal cancers or polyps can be seen during such an examination. In addition, diagnosis of other diseases such as Crohn's or ulcerative colitis can be made with this instrument. Samples of tissue can be taken through the instrument for later examination under a microscope (biopsy).

The frequency with which this test should be performed has been a subject of some debate. Our recommendation is that, in the absence of any family history of colon cancer, this examination should be done initially at age 45 and every other year thereafter. For those who have had a previous polyp or have a family history of polyps, more frequent examinations by colonoscopy (see page 637) may be appropriate.

In some situations, an inflexible hollow instrument is used to inspect the rectum and the lower portion of the sigmoid colon. Often, this is done in conjunction with a barium examination of the colon or to diagnose specifically, and at times treat, anal disorders. This procedure commonly is called rigid proctoscopy.

A flexible fiberoptic proctosigmoidoscope allows your physician to examine a portion of your colon (rectum and sigmoid). This is a common screening exam for colon cancer.

page 641) and probably with a barium enema (see The Barium X-Ray of the Esophagus, Stomach, and Intestine, page 613). For the diagnosis of Hirschsprung's disease, the physician will obtain a biopsy specimen of your infant's rectum under general anesthesia. For most cases of acquired megacolon, no biopsy is needed.

Treatment.   The best treatment for Hirschsprung's disease is surgery because it usually will restore normal bowel movements. In the case of acquired megacolon, the key is education on proper bowel habits (see Chronic Constipation, page 633).

Your physician also may suggest the use of enemas or laxatives (such as mineral oil) to help retrain your bowel. Treatment of any underlying problem or decreasing the use of narcotic-containing medication may be appropriate.

PERITONITIS

Signs and Symptoms
- Increasing abdominal pain;
- Distended abdomen;
- Nausea and vomiting;
- Inability to pass feces or gas;
- Fever;
- Low blood pressure;
- Thirst.

Peritonitis is an inflammation, either confined to one area or widespread, of the peritoneum, the membrane that covers the abdominal organs.

Peritonitis most often is due to bacteria in the peritoneal cavity. Typically the bacteria enter from a perforation in the gastrointestinal tract or from trauma of the abdomen, as with a penetrating wound. Peritonitis also can be the result of a severe reaction from the release of enzymes from the pancreas, digestive enzymes, or bile due to injury or perforation.

Persons with systemic lupus erythematosus (see page 1006) also may have bouts of peritonitis due to inflammation without perforation.

The most frequent causes of peritonitis are perforations due to appendicitis (see page 624), diverticulitis (see page 631), or peptic ulcer (see page 603). Obstruction of the small bowel with subsequent gangrene and

bowel perforation (see Intestinal Obstruction, page 643) may cause peritonitis.

The Diagnosis.   If your physician suspects peritonitis, you will be hospitalized; peritonitis is a medical emergency that must be treated immediately. Blood tests and x-rays may be done to help establish the diagnosis.

Treatment.   Surgery usually is necessary, either for the removal of the tissue that has caused the problem (such as diverticulitis) or to repair an injury such as a perforation in the stomach or intestine.

To fight the infection, antibiotics are given through a vein. Because the intestines temporarily do not function during an episode of peritonitis, a tube will be placed through your nose into your stomach to drain secretions or air that accumulates and is not spontaneously passed. This tube is called a nasogastric tube. It can be removed when the bowel resumes its normal function.

FAMILIAL MEDITERRANEAN FEVER

Signs and Symptoms
- Fever;
- Abdominal pain;
- Chest pain;
- Pain in the joints;
- Skin lesions on the lower part of the legs.

Familial Mediterranean fever is an inherited intestinal disorder that is characterized by recurrent fever and inflammation. Because of the inflammation in the abdominal cavity seen with this disorder, familial Mediterranean fever is also called periodic peritonitis.

In most people with familial Mediterranean fever, symptoms begin between the ages of 5 and 15. Fever is present during most attacks. In addition, there may be inflammation of the lining of the abdominal cavity, chest cavity, or joints, producing symptoms that resemble those of peritonitis (see page 642), pleurisy (see page 925), or arthritis (see page 995), respectively. Approximately one-quarter of people with familial Mediterranean fever have a painful red area of swelling in their lower legs. Persons affected by this disorder generally have recurrent attacks that may vary in severity and site from one episode to another.

The cause of familial Mediterranean fever is unknown.

Most affected persons are symptom-free between attacks.

The Diagnosis. Your physician will need to know if any member of your family has ever been found to have this disorder. He or she also will want to know how long your attacks last and how often they occur because familial Mediterranean fever episodes usually last between 24 and 48 hours and occur at intervals of 2 to 4 weeks.

There is no one laboratory test that will be decisive in the diagnosis, although your physician probably will have your blood analyzed. In fact, diagnosis is a process of elimination in that your symptoms may initially suggest a number of other possible diseases, such as appendicitis (see page 624), acute pancreatitis (see page 667), or intestinal obstruction (see page 643).

Treatment. Many different treatment programs, including the use of antibiotics or corticosteroids, have been tried but none has proven effective. The use of colchicine has resulted in a dramatic decrease in the number of attacks in many persons. Your physician will discuss with you the potential side effects of the chronic use of colchicine.

INTESTINAL OBSTRUCTION

Signs and Symptoms
* Abdominal distention;
* Spasmodic pain or cramping in the mid-abdomen;
* Vomiting;
* Inability to pass feces or intestinal gas.

Intestinal obstruction is partial or complete blockage in either the small intestine or the colon. This obstruction prevents the products of digestion from completing the journey through the intestines.

If you have a blockage in your small intestine, you may feel cramp-like pain in the middle of your abdomen and have bouts of vomiting. Failure to pass feces can occur no matter where the obstruction is located. If your lower colon is totally blocked, you will not even be able to pass gas. A partial intesti-

nal obstruction may stimulate your intestine to secrete fluid, which may result in diarrhea.

A dramatic feature of intestinal obstruction is abdominal distention. The abdomen will protrude more and more as the condition worsens. The swelling is produced by intestinal gas and fluid trapped within the obstructed segment of the intestine.

Several things can cause an obstruction. The most common cause of obstruction in the small intestine is adhesion (scar tissue) from a prior operation. Hernias (see page 671) and volvulus (a knotted or twisted intestine) are also common causes of obstruction in the small bowel. In the colon, a cancer and other disorders can cause obstruction.

Sometimes the obstruction is nonmechanical and results from failure of the intestines to move material along. This is called adynamic ileus and sometimes occurs after injury to or operation on the abdomen.

The Diagnosis. No one symptom is a sure sign of intestinal obstruction, nor will any one symptom reveal the precise cause of the obstruction. However, a significant sign of complete blockage would be your inability to pass gas or have a bowel movement.

If your physician believes that your symptoms point to an intestinal obstruction, he or she will arrange for an x-ray that may detect the obstruction. He or she may also conduct a sigmoidoscopic examination (see Screening for Colon Cancer, page 641), colonoscopy (see page 637), or a special x-ray study of the colon (see The Barium X-Ray of the Esophagus, Stomach, and Intestine, page 613) to see where the obstruction is located. Sometimes just these test procedures will relieve the obstruction.

How Serious Is Acute Intestinal Obstruction? If the obstruction blocks the blood supply to the intestine, the tissue may begin to die. This will increase the possibility of gangrene or a perforation of the intestine. These are both life-threatening situations.

Treatment. If your physician suspects an intestinal obstruction, he or she may place a tube through your nose into your stomach or initial portion of your small bowel. Suction will be applied to remove intestinal secretions and air through the tube. Called nasogastric suction, this technique often will relieve the distention of the abdomen. Lost fluids must be replaced with intravenous feedings.

At times, the cause of an obstruction will resolve spontaneously after the distention has been relieved. If the obstruction does not resolve after nasogastric suction, an operation may be necessary. In most cases of adynamic ileus, correction of the underlying disorder will correct the obstruction.

VASCULAR PROBLEMS OF THE BOWEL

The abdomen is fed by a vast network of blood vessels. Unfortunately, sometimes this necessary blood supply is interrupted or decreased. When this happens, the affected area becomes deficient in nutrients and oxygen, and the result can be tissue death.

The vascular disorders of the bowel include the following.

Mesenteric Ischemia. In this disorder, there is partial or complete lack of blood flow to the gut. This commonly occurs over a period of time as a result of the accumulation of cholesterol on the lining of the arteries leading to the intestines (see Atherosclerosis: What Is It?, page 786). This deposition of cholesterol is similar to what happens in the coronary arteries of persons who have angina; thus, it is hardly surprising that coronary artery disease may be found in persons who have impaired arterial blood supply to their intestines.

The main symptom of partial blockage is severe, cramping abdominal pain, most often around the navel, which is aggravated by eating and relieved by fasting. This is analogous to angina pectoris (see page 803) and is sometimes called abdominal angina.

A clot (embolus) that passed from the heart to the arteries supplying the intestine can cause sudden, complete blockage of the supply of blood to a portion of the gut. If you have a complete blockage of the arteries in the intestine, severe pain will begin immediately. You may pass bloody stools.

Examination of the blood vessels, called an angiogram (see page 805), determines the site of obstruction. This generally is followed by an emergency operation to remove the segment of intestine that has lost its blood supply. If there has not been permanent damage to the intestine, the clot can be removed or the affected artery can be reconstructed.

Ischemic Colitis. In ischemic colitis, the blood supply to the colon is decreased, although usually the affected vessels are not major arteries. This condition most often affects the elderly. The symptoms include lower abdominal pain and rectal bleeding.

Surgery may be required in severe cases, but most often the problem resolves spontaneously. Later, a narrowing of the colon (stricture) may occur at the site of the episode of ischemia.

Angiodysplasia of the Colon. This is dilation, distortion, or thinning of blood vessels in the colon. It is more common in the elderly. Rectal bleeding is a common symptom. The diagnosis of angiodysplasia of the colon requires an angiogram of the colon (see page 805) or direct visualization of the lesions at colonoscopy (see page 637). The hemorrhage can be halted by blocking the affected vessel during a diagnostic procedure called arteriography (see page 513) or by cautery or laser treatment of the lesion through the colonoscope (see page 637). When there is massive bleeding or bleeding is from multiple sites, surgical removal of the affected part of the colon may be necessary.

ANORECTAL DISORDERS

The anus is the 1½-inch-long canal that is the outlet for the rectum. A ring of muscles, the anal sphincter, controls the movement of the solid waste products of the digestive process through the anus and thus out of the body.

The anus is a relatively simple structure in contrast to the other parts of the digestive system. Generally, the anorectal disorders are hemorrhoids, inflammations, abscesses, and crack-like sores (fissures).

HEMORRHOIDS

Signs and Symptoms
- Bright red blood on the toilet paper, in the water of the toilet bowl, or on the stool itself;
- Protrusion of soft tissue at the anus;
- Tenderness, especially during a bowel movement.

Hemorrhoids (often referred to as "piles") are clusters of veins located in the anus, just under the membrane that lines the lowest part of the rectum and anus. Sometimes, often as a result of straining during a bowel movement, these veins become swollen. This forms the hemorrhoid. Because these veins are thin and easily ruptured, bleeding may occur during a bowel movement. Hemorrhoids are also common during pregnancy.

Hemorrhoids can occur internally (near the beginning of the anal canal) or externally, outside the orifice itself. Both types are common, and both may bleed.

Hemorrhoids can become especially painful if a blood clot forms. These hemorrhoids are referred to as thrombosed (from thrombosis, for clot). These generally occur

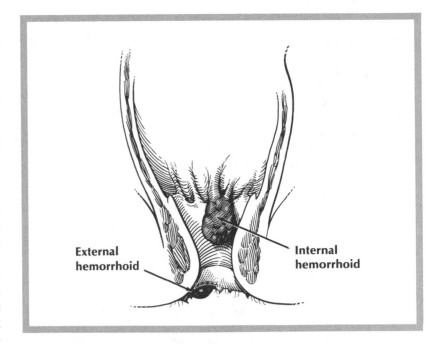

External hemorrhoid

Internal hemorrhoid

in external hemorrhoids and feel as if they have a small pebble in them.

Itching and anal pain generally are not symptoms of hemorrhoids unless associated with a complication such as thrombosis or erosion of the overlying surface.

The Diagnosis. Visual examination of your anus by your physician usually reveals

Hemorrhoids can occur internally (in the anal canal) or externally.

ANAL FISSURES AND FISTULAS

An anal fissure is a relatively minor and uncommon erosion that extends from the anal sphincter up into the anal canal. It may cause some pain during defecation and leave some blood streaks on your stool. This condition is more common in women.

An anal fissure often heals after the addition of fiber to the diet; a medication that softens the stool also may help. If the erosion is an ulcer, the pain may be more intense, both during and after defecation, because the ulcer may

cause the anal sphincter muscle to go into spasm. Again, the addition of fiber, a stool softener, or a bulk former containing psyllium will help relieve the pain (see Chronic Constipation, page 633). A warm bath will relax the muscle and reduce the spasm that causes the pain.

If the pain continues, your physician may decide to operate. This is usually a minor surgical procedure that does not require an overnight stay in the hospital.

An anal fistula is an abnormal tube-like passageway from the anal canal to a hole in the skin around the opening to the anus. An abscess may form in the skin around the anal opening (see Ano-

rectal Abscess, page 647). The skin becomes itchy and irritated because pus and water are discharged through this hole. These fistulas usually result from abscesses beneath the lining of the rectum.

At times, an anal fistula or anorectal abscess indicates the presence of Crohn's disease (see page 626) or is the result of previous operation in this area. A rectal examination (proctoscopy) and a barium enema (see The Barium X-Ray of the Esophagus, Stomach, and Intestine, page 613) may be done.

Treatment consists of the surgical removal of the fistula and drainage of the abscess.

ANAL ITCH

Anal itching, also called pruritus ani, is a distracting, potentially embarrassing, and common problem; almost everyone is afflicted at one time or another.

A persistent anal itch is a more common problem for children and the elderly. In children, it may be due to the presence of a common parasite called pinworms (see page 870). Among the elderly, the cause usually is aging dry skin.

For most of the rest of the population, the problem is not always easily diagnosed. In evaluating your anal itch, your physician will look for signs of a skin ailment such as psoriasis, of skin cancer, or of a yeast infection. He or she will also examine you for hemorrhoids, anal fissure, or anal fistula, each of which may cause itching and irritation. These disorders rarely are a cause of anal itching. In fact, often the precise cause remains a mystery.

Here are some additional factors that may predispose you to anal itching.

Overzealous Hygiene

Some people, in an effort to be squeaky clean, scrub their rectal area with a harsh soap and rough washcloth, which causes itching, burning, and irritation.

Medication Reactions

Some people use over-the-counter medication to relieve the itching. These drugs, in fact, may sensitize the skin and cause irritation, with itching and burning.

Stress

Some physicians believe that stress may be a factor, although this has not been proven.

Loose Anal Muscles

The muscles that normally keep the anal canal closed tightly can become lax, allowing stool-containing mucus to seep out and irritate the surrounding skin.

Poor Hygiene

If the anal area is not cleansed adequately after a bowel movement, bits of stool will cling to the skin and cause irritation and itching.

It used to be that those who suffered from chronic anal itching underwent irradiation of the anal area, injections of alcohol, and even surgery to remove the skin and nerves surrounding the affected area. Given the problem, these measures seem a bit extreme, and most physicians now would not prescribe such treatments.

Instead, try the following.

1. Stop scratching. As hard as this may be, summon your will power and try it. Continued scratching leads to persistent inflammation and damage to the delicate tissue. The more you scratch, the more you itch. Try a cold pack and a 0.5 percent hydrocortisone cream or ointment (available without a prescription) to relieve the discomfort.
2. Keep the area clean. Cleanse the area gently in the morning, in the evening, and after a bowel movement. Use moistened, unscented, white toilet paper or cotton balls.
3. To prevent skin irritation from the leakage of mucus, place a cotton pad between your buttocks, up against the anus. Replace the pad as necessary.
4. Taking an antihistamine tablet at bedtime may lessen the itch. Drugs such as diphenhydramine or chlorpheniramine are available without a prescription.

If these measures do not relieve your problem, see your physician for a thorough evaluation.

whether you have external hemorrhoids. The anus can be examined with a rubber-gloved finger but, because a hemorrhoid is very soft, a definite diagnosis may not be made. Your physician may also examine the area with a proctoscope or anoscope (see Screening for Colon Cancer, page 641). Your examination may also include a barium enema (see The Barium X-Ray of the Esophagus, Stomach, and Intestine, page 613) or colonoscopy (see page 637).

All episodes of rectal bleeding should be investigated. Do not assume that rectal bleeding is from hemorrhoids until other potential sources of bleeding, such as a colon polyp or colon cancer, have been ruled out.

Treatment. Most people with hemorrhoids are so little bothered by the problem that they ignore it. For others, however, the symptoms are too bothersome to be easily dismissed.

If your hemorrhoids are producing only mild discomfort, your physician may advise you to use a cream containing witch hazel or a topical anesthetic. This, in combination with frequent warm baths, may relieve your symptoms. Emphasis on more fiber in

ANAL PAIN

Have you ever had a sharp, stabbing pain in your rectum awaken you from a sound sleep?

This painful condition is called proctalgia fugax. The cause is not well understood, but it is believed to be due to an intense spasm of the muscles in the lower pelvis and rectum. The pain resembles the discomfort you experience from a cramp in your calf.

Typically, the pain occurs at night while you are asleep. You awaken to this intense and unrelenting pain. Within a few minutes to half an hour the pain subsides. It can recur at irregular intervals, with the frequency varying from twice a week to a few times a year. Sometimes the spells disappear entirely.

Although this can be very frightening, rest assured that the pain is not serious. It is not caused by cancer, hemorrhoids, or other diseases of the rectum.

What should you do? First, see your physician. He or she can perform the diagnostic tests that will rule out any serious disease. This will help ease your mind; intense pain is not necessarily equated with serious illness.

Here are some tips to try the next time you have the pain.

1. Sit in a bathtub full of warm water.
2. Try to have a bowel movement; this sometimes eliminates the pain.
3. Drink warm water or eat crackers; this may stimulate normal contractions in the intestine that will relieve the spasm.

---

your diet may make constipation less likely, which may decrease the chances of further hemorrhoids developing.

In some cases, your physician may gently push the protruding hemorrhoid back up inside the rectum, eliminating the swelling and pain. For some sufferers, however, treatment is more involved.

If you have persistent or recurrent protruding internal (inside the anal canal) hemorrhoids, your physician can perform a corrective procedure right in his or her office. This involves tying the hemorrhoid off with rubber bands. In a few days, the hemorrhoid painlessly falls off. This method is effective in about 75 percent of cases.

When a blood clot has formed within the hemorrhoid, your physician can remove the clot, which should render prompt relief.

Other techniques include injecting a shrinking agent into an internal hemorrhoid or destroying the hemorrhoid by photocoagulation, a technique in which the affected tissue is destroyed.

Sometimes hemorrhoids are removed surgically in a procedure called hemorrhoidectomy. The more extensive the removal of hemorrhoidal tissue, the less chance of recurrence but the greater the discomfort in the several days after the operation.

ANORECTAL ABSCESS

Signs and Symptoms
• Discharge of pus;

• Fever;
• Discomfort in or around the anal opening;
• Tenderness or discomfort with the passage of stool.

Anorectal abscesses affect the area immediately around the anus. Some are infections caused by fissures or by sexually transmitted diseases (see page 875), but most anal abscesses are the result of blocked anal glands.

An abscess that is easily accessible near the anus can be lanced and drained, either in

VENEREAL INFECTION OF THE RECTUM

A number of infectious diseases are transmitted sexually through anal intercourse (see Sexually Transmitted Diseases, page 875). Specifically, proctitis caused by gonorrhea (see page 875), herpes simplex virus (see page 877), and anal warts (see page 879) usually is communicated through rectal intercourse (see also Proctitis, page 648).

Sexually transmitted rectal infections can be serious because of the risk of complications, particularly bleeding, the later development of a narrowing or stricture of the rectum, or, rarely, cancer.

Many such bacterial infections are clinically considered to be mild and pose no threat to other systems of the body. However, if you experience the symptoms of any sexually transmitted infection, see your physician for proper treatment. Your physician may want to screen for the AIDS virus if a sexually transmitted infection of the rectum is present.

your physician's office or at a hospital outpatient service. On the other hand, if you have a fever and sharp pains accompanied by a sense of pressure between your anus and coccyx (the coccyx is the tailbone, at the base of your spine), your physician may suspect an abscess higher up into your rectum. These deep abscesses are less accessible, their diagnosis is more difficult, and their potential complications are more serious.

Deep rectal abscesses warrant careful attention because they could be caused by an intestinal disorder such as Crohn's disease (see page 626), ulcerative colitis (see page 628), or diverticulitis (see Diverticulosis and Diverticulitis, page 631).

The Diagnosis.   If there is a possibility of a deep anorectal abscess, your physician will perform a thorough examination of your rectum, which may include proctosigmoidoscopy (see Screening for Colon Cancer, page 641) and a barium enema (see The Barium X-Ray of the Esophagus, Stomach, and Intestine, page 613).

Treatment.   Surgery.   Once the abscess has been identified, you will be hospitalized and the abscess will be lanced and drained. In addition, you will be given an analgesic for your pain and sometimes antibiotics for the infection.

PROCTITIS

Signs and Symptoms
- Blood, mucus, or pus in the stool;
- Constipation;
- Diarrhea;
- Severe rectal pain;
- Fever.

Proctitis is an inflammation of the rectum that may result from an infection (bacterial or viral). It also may be a feature of ulcera-

---

FECAL INCONTINENCE

Fecal incontinence refers to the inability to control bowel movements. When this disorder occurs in any healthy adult, the problem is usually due to some type of underlying condition (see also Encopresis, page 1016), for a discussion of a similar condition in children).

Your physician will question you carefully to determine if there is a precipitating cause of your incontinence, such as sneezing or coughing, if it occurs only at night, and if there are any associated symptoms. He or she also will examine your anal sphincter to determine whether the muscles in this area are intact. Your physician may also order special studies including electromyography (EMG, see page 1294) or the use of special devices to determine various pressures in your rectal and anal regions.

Fecal incontinence may be secondary to an abscess or inflammation in the rectum, anus, or perianal area. It can be the result of a previous operation in this area or of trauma or complications occurring at the time of delivery of an infant. Particularly if the anal sphincter is intact, fecal incontinence can be secondary to an injury or a disorder of the nervous system, particularly one affecting the spinal tract.

Fecal incontinence occurs often in the elderly. As you age, the muscles and ligaments that control urination and defecation become less efficient and thus are more readily disturbed by a physical ailment. However, incontinence is not an inevitable part of getting older.

In addition, particularly in the elderly, fecal impactions are more common. This generally occurs in people who experience constipation. However, the fecal mass generally does not totally obstruct the bowel so that the more liquid portions of the stool seep past the area of impaction, causing incontinence.

In the case of some adults with fecal incontinence, a bowel retraining program can be begun, particularly if the anal sphincter is intact. At times, this may include the use of a bulk former (see Chronic Constipation, page 633). Your physician may advise you to sit for a certain period of time each day for defecation; this often results in continence during the remainder of the day. He or she also will advise you to increase your hydration and emphasize eating fresh fruits and vegetables. This sometimes helps to produce a more normal stool and decreases the number of times you have to defecate.

At times, your physician may recommend a surgical procedure on the anal sphincter, particularly if the sphincter has been damaged by trauma.

tive colitis (see page 628) or Crohn's disease (see page 626). In some instances, proctitis is due to anal intercourse. A person with proctitis due to a sexually transmitted infection can spread the disease to other sexual partners (see Sexually Transmitted Diseases, page 875).

Some of the symptoms associated with proctitis are a clue to the possible cause of the infection. Mucus, blood, or pus in your stool suggests an inflammation caused by gonorrhea. If herpes simplex virus has caused the proctitis, you may find ulcers or blister-like elevations around your anus. In both cases, the skin around your anus may burn and itch.

A repeated urge to defecate or an inability to move your bowels may develop. If the source of the infection is not just in the rectum but deeper in your bowel (proctocolitis), the symptoms are likely to be more severe anorectal pain and fever.

The Diagnosis. Your physician will examine the skin around your anus, analyze the mucus in your stool (if any), and conduct a proctosigmoidoscopic examination (see Screening for Colon Cancer, page 641). The examination also may include a blood test for syphilis (see page 876).

How Serious Is Proctitis? Depending on the cause, the infection may or may not be easily treated. Bacterial infections respond to antibiotics but viral infections do not.

Treatment. *Medication.* The initial treatment for bacterial proctitis is an antibiotic, frequently with tetracycline hydrochloride. There is no medication available that will cure proctitis caused by herpes simplex virus, although your physician will prescribe agents that can control the spread of the infection and ease the symptoms.

LIVER DISEASE

Apart from the digestive tract itself, the organs of the digestive system include the liver, the gallbladder, and the pancreas (see Gallbladder and Bile Duct Disorders, page 661, and Pancreatic Diseases, page 666).

The liver not only is the largest single internal organ in the body but also is the most complex. Weighing as much as 4 pounds, the liver performs many complicated tasks that are essential to the proper functioning of the entire body. These functions may be grouped into three categories: regulation, metabolism, and detoxification.

The liver regulates the composition of your blood, in particular the amounts of glucose (sugar), protein, and fat that enter the bloodstream. The liver also removes from the blood a substance, called bilirubin, which is a residue from the breakdown of red blood cells. Once the bilirubin enters the liver it is chemically changed so that it becomes soluble in water. Then it is added to the bile, enters the intestinal tract, and is eliminated.

If, for any reason, the liver is unable to remove the bilirubin from the blood, the bilirubin level will build up and the bilirubin eventually will be deposited in the skin,

causing a yellow appearance known as jaundice.

The liver processes most of the nutrients that are absorbed from the intestine. Besides converting many of these nutrients into forms that can be used by the body, the liver also serves as a storage center for some nu-

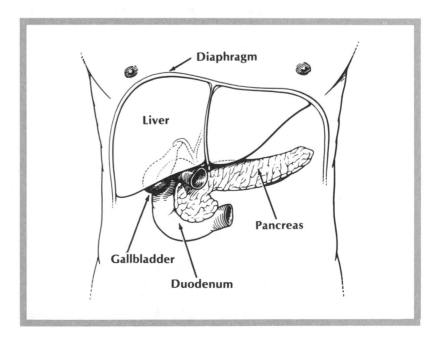

trients such as vitamin A, iron, and other minerals. It manufactures cholesterol, vitamin A, blood clotting substances, and specific proteins.

The liver also detoxifies the blood. This means it removes drugs, alcohol, and potentially harmful chemicals from the bloodstream and treats them chemically so they can be excreted in the feces and urine.

Daily, the liver manufactures about a quart of bile, a yellow fluid. The bile travels through the liver ducts and then through the cystic duct to the gallbladder where it is stored temporarily. After you eat a meal, the gallbladder expels the bile so that it travels through the common bile duct and empties into the duodenum. The bile acids in the bile facilitate the digestion of fats. Spicier fatty meals tend to cause more vigorous contraction of the gallbladder and common bile duct.

Because of the complexity of the liver and its exposure to so many potentially harmful substances, it would be reasonable to believe that it is especially vulnerable to disease. However, nature protects the organ in several ways. First, the liver is capable of regeneration—it can heal itself by repairing or replacing injured tissue. It also is constructed so that many units are responsible for the same task. Thus, if tissue in one section of the organ is injured, by trauma or disease, other cells will perform the functions of the injured section indefinitely or until the damage has been repaired.

Despite this built-in protection, the liver does suffer from many diseases, especially inflammatory conditions that can threaten its health and the health of its host.

ACUTE VIRAL HEPATITIS

Signs and Symptoms
- Jaundice (yellowing of the skin and eyes);
- Fatigue;
- Lack of appetite;
- Nausea and vomiting;
- Alterations in senses of taste and smell;
- Low-grade fever.

Hepatitis is an inflammation of the liver caused by a virus or, less commonly, by certain medications or toxins (see Alcoholic, Toxic, and Drug-Related Hepatitis, page 651).

Three main types of viral hepatitis have thus far been identified: hepatitis A; hepatitis B; and non-A, non-B hepatitis. The symptoms are similar. The delta agent, a recently described cause of hepatitis, requires the presence of the hepatitis B virus.

An acute viral hepatitis can range from being without any symptoms whatsoever to being fatal; the latter is rare. If you have hepatitis, you may feel better within a few days after your initial symptoms disappear, but it may take months for your liver to recover completely.

Acute Hepatitis A.   This is a highly infectious form of hepatitis and is the most common form. The disease is transmitted mainly by contaminated food or water. If you have hepatitis A, the virus will be in your stools, blood, and bile for 2 to 3 weeks before any symptoms develop. The virus disappears once jaundice develops or within 2 to 3 weeks afterward. Thus, anyone who comes into contact with your blood or feces, even before you have symptoms, may become infected with the virus.

The symptoms of hepatitis A often are similar to those of intestinal flu. But because the infected liver is unable to filter bilirubin from your blood, your skin and eyes may become yellow, and the bile excreted in your urine may turn it tea-colored.

The vast majority of persons with hepatitis A recover completely. Within 1 to 2 months, your liver is completely healed. Hepatitis A does not develop into chronic hepatitis (see page 652) or cirrhosis (see page 653), nor does the hepatitis A virus remain in your body even if no symptoms are present (carrier state).

Acute Hepatitis B.   Hepatitis B is potentially a more serious form of viral liver infection. Its symptoms are much the same as those of hepatitis A but can be more severe and last longer. As a result, there is a greater possibility of liver damage. A complication in up to 10 percent of hepatitis B cases is the development of chronic hepatitis.

The hepatitis B virus commonly is acquired through exposure to contaminated blood. Those most likely to contract the virus are intravenous drug users who share contaminated needles. Sexual contact with a person who has hepatitis B also can spread the disease. Other persons who may acquire hepatitis B virus include health-care workers exposed to blood and persons who need repeated transfusions of blood products (for example, hemophiliacs; see Hemophilia, page 496). However, testing of donor blood before transfusion has virtually eliminated the risk of acquiring hepatitis B from a blood transfusion.

A pregnant woman may pass the virus to her developing fetus. There are some infected people (carriers) who never have symptoms but are capable of passing the virus to others. And some persons who have had hepatitis B remain carriers. Ninety percent of those with uncomplicated cases of hepatitis B recover within 3 to 4 months.

Non-A, Non-B Hepatitis.   Non-A, non-B hepatitis produces symptoms that resemble those of hepatitis A and B except that they may be less severe and jaundice may not be present. This disease may be caused by more than one type of virus.

One distinctive feature of non-A, non-B hepatitis is that the virus or viruses responsible for this condition cannot be identified in blood tests. Thus, it is common for this hepatitis to be acquired after a blood transfusion. In fact, this form of hepatitis was discovered in hospitalized patients whose hepatitis developed after blood transfusions. In addition to being transmitted during blood transfu-

---

ALCOHOLIC, TOXIC, AND DRUG-RELATED HEPATITIS

Hepatitis can occur after excessive and chronic use of alcohol; it also can occur immediately after the inhalation or ingestion of a toxin or the use of certain medications.

In general, the symptoms and signs of alcoholic, toxic, and drug-related hepatitis are indistinguishable from those of acute viral hepatitis (see Acute Viral Hepatitis, page 650). The key difference is that the offending agent that caused the hepatitis must be identified and eliminated.

Treatment generally is supportive rather than specific and is designed to give the liver time to heal. This may involve just observation of your health and symptoms; at other times, you may be required to avoid eating protein (which cannot be broken down and eliminated by the liver during the acute phase of injury), and nutrients will be delivered through a vein to maintain calorie support and prevent dehydration.

Alcoholic Hepatitis
This form of hepatitis may produce virtually no symptoms or it can begin with mild flu-like symp-

toms. Sometimes it can lead to liver failure.

Someone with a severe case of alcoholic hepatitis may run a high fever and develop an enlarged liver (see page 659). Recovery often is slow. Even after complete abstinence from alcohol, recovery may take weeks, and abnormalities in the liver tissue can persist for 6 months or more (see Cirrhosis, page 653).

The development of fluid retention, particularly in the abdomen (characterized by an enlarging abdomen), and difficulty in maintaining your mental concentration are worrisome features and may indicate liver failure. It is imperative that, if you are to recover, you must abstain from alcohol permanently. In addition, during the healing phase, the person with alcoholic hepatitis should refrain from using any medication that is broken down and eliminated through the liver.

Toxic and Drug-Induced Hepatitis
The liver can be damaged by chemical agents and industrial toxins such as carbon tetrachloride. But drug-induced hepatitis is a more common problem. Both prescribed medications and those purchased over-the-counter can

produce hepatitis in susceptible persons.

A number of widely used drugs can produce an adverse liver reaction. Isoniazid (used for the treatment of tuberculosis), α-methyldopa (a treatment for high blood pressure), and the pain reliever acetaminophen have been clearly associated with hepatitis. The anesthetic halothane is another.

Certain other drugs have been found to interfere with the flow of bile in some instances. Among them are the antibiotic erythromycin, the tranquilizer chlorpromazine, oral contraceptives, and anabolic steroids. Such liver complications usually subside within a few days or weeks after use of the drug is stopped. Do not use oral contraceptives if you have a history of jaundice during pregnancy. Both oral contraceptives and anabolic steroids have been associated with liver cancer in a small percentage of cases.

Because of these risks, inform your physician if you have any history of liver disease or liver problems before taking any medication. Furthermore, if you have any symptoms or laboratory findings that suggest hepatitis, your physician will want to know if you have been taking any medication in the previous 2 months.

sion, it is believed that non-A, non-B hepatitis is spread through sexual contact. This type of hepatitis may cause chronic liver disease (see Chronic Hepatitis, below).

A recent test shows promise in detecting a virus responsible for non-A, non-B hepatitis. This virus has been called hepatitis C virus. There may be other viruses in the non-A, non-B hepatitis category.

The Diagnosis.   If you notice that your skin is becoming jaundiced or that you have any other symptoms of hepatitis, your physician may conduct a blood test. In addition to a careful medical history, your physician will ask you a number of questions about your sex life, the medications you have taken in the past few months, and whether you have had any blood transfusions (or contact with fresh blood) during the same period.

How Serious Is Hepatitis?   Virtually all patients who were healthy prior to contracting hepatitis A recover completely; 90 percent with hepatitis B also recover. If you are elderly or have medical problems such as diabetes, congestive heart failure, or severe anemia, recovery is apt to take longer and the risk of complications is greater. Although rare in this country, death does occur from non-A, non-B hepatitis. Your physician may advise treatment at a medical center specializing in liver disorders.

Treatment.   There is no specific treatment for hepatitis. Bed rest is not essential, although you may feel better if you restrict physical activity. It is important to maintain an adequate intake of calories. You may find you feel better if most of your day's calories are consumed in the morning.

You will be asked to abstain from any alcohol, at least during your recovery, because both alcohol and drugs make excessive demands on the already damaged liver.

In severe cases, hospitalization may be required, particularly if you are unable to eat solids or drink fluids needed for adequate nutrition and hydration. Generally this is only for several days.

After hepatitis B or non-A, non-B hepatitis, your physician may draw blood periodically for a few months to check for continuing inflammation of the liver or a return to normal.

Although it is not necessary to isolate a person with hepatitis from the rest of the family, the entire household should be aware how the virus spreads. Thus, stringent hand washing after going to the bathroom is important, as is thorough cleansing if there is any contact with the affected person's feces, blood, or any body fluid.

Prevention.   See Hepatitis Vaccine, page 653.

CHRONIC HEPATITIS

Signs and Symptoms
- Often, none;
- Fatigue;
- Lack of appetite;
- Nausea and vomiting;
- Persistent or recurring jaundice;
- Low-grade fever.

Chronic hepatitis comes in two major forms: chronic persistent hepatitis, and chronic active hepatitis.

Chronic persistent hepatitis (which is simply a mild form of chronic active hepatitis) sometimes is the result of hepatitis B or non-A, non-B hepatitis. Often, the cause is not apparent. Generally, this form of chronic hepatitis is nonprogressive. Liver failure does not occur, and cirrhosis of the liver rarely results.

Most people with chronic persistent hepatitis have no symptoms. However, some complain of fatigue, lack of appetite, and, occasionally, vomiting and nausea.

Chronic active hepatitis, on the other hand, is a progressive disease that may lead to liver failure, cirrhosis, or death. Chronic active hepatitis has various causes, the most common of which seems to be hepatitis B and non-A, non-B hepatitis. A reaction to certain medications may cause this condition as well. In some cases, no specific cause is found. With chronic active hepatitis, fatigue is a common symptom, although there may be virtually no symptoms or there may be all of those associated with acute infectious hepatitis (see page 650).

The Diagnosis.   At first, you may appear to have acute viral hepatitis but, if your symptoms do not respond to rest and your blood test results continue to be abnormal, your physician may suspect chronic hepatitis. Besides blood tests, he or she may obtain a liver biopsy (a small sample of liver tissue is removed for microscopic analysis; see page 657). Chronic active hepatitis is a serious disease and can be fatal. Chronic persistent hepatitis generally is well tolerated and may resolve spontaneously, although many months may be required for recovery.

Treatment. No specific treatment is required for chronic persistent hepatitis.

The treatment for some cases of chronic active hepatitis is corticosteroids. Your physician may consider the use of corticosteroids if your chronic active hepatitis was not the result of a virus and you have evidence of severe inflammation in your liver. As many as 60 to 80 percent of those treated with these drugs have a complete remission. You should begin to feel stronger and your appetite should return to normal within a few days to weeks after the treatment is begun. You may have no symptoms after a month or so of treatment, but it may be as long as 6 months to 2 years before your blood is free of all signs of the hepatitis. Even so, relapses are common after the corticosteroid regimen is discontinued.

At times, azathioprine is used in association with corticosteroids. These drugs are most effective when the chronic hepatitis is not caused by hepatitis B virus.

Although suppressing inflammation, the corticosteroids may not prevent progression to cirrhosis (see Cirrhosis, below). Occasionally, if the disease is severe and fails to respond to treatment, your physician may consider liver transplantation (see Liver Transplantation, page 660).

HEPATITIS VACCINE

If a member of your family has hepatitis B or if you work in a profession that exposes you to the hepatitis B virus, your physician may suggest that you be immunized. Americans considered to be at high risk for hepatitis B virus infection include illicit drug users who inject their drugs with needles, sexually active homosexual men, sexual partners of those with hepatitis B, people who undergo hemodialysis for kidney failure, dental and medical health professionals, and male prison inmates.

It has only been in the past few years that a vaccine for hepatitis B has been widely used. One version of the vaccine is made from the blood plasma of recovered hepatitis patients; the other version is made by recombinant genetic technology (not from formerly infected persons). The vaccine produces long-lasting immunity.

The Centers for Disease Control estimates that 200,000 Americans are infected with hepatitis B each year, and an estimated 5,000 die of complications from the disease. Thus, if you are in a high-risk group for hepatitis, your physician may recommend that you receive the vaccine.

Because hepatitis B is widespread in China, Southeast Asia, sub-Saharan Africa, the Amazon basin in South America, and the islands of the Pacific, ask your physician about the vaccine if you plan to travel to any of those parts of the world (see also Immunizations, page 338).

Protection against the most common type of the disease, hepatitis A, is injection of an immune globulin which contains protective antibodies against hepatitis A virus. It is usually given immediately after (within 2 weeks) known exposure to contaminated food or contact with an infected person or before possible exposure to hepatitis A (for example, immediately before a trip to an area where the disease is common). Sometimes it does not actually prevent the infection but does make the disease state mild enough that you have no serious symptoms. The protection given by the immune globulin injection lasts for only a few weeks.

CIRRHOSIS

Signs and Symptoms
*   There may be none;
*   Loss of appetite;
*   Weight loss;
*   Nausea and vomiting;
*   General fatigue and weakness;
*   Jaundice (yellowing of the skin and eyes);
*   Abdominal pain;
*   Intestinal bleeding;
*   Small red spider-like blood vessels under the skin or easy bruising;
*   Loss of interest in sex; men may become impotent, and women cease to menstruate;
*   Itching;
*   Swelling of the abdomen and legs.

Emergency Symptoms
*   Vomiting or passing blood through the rectum;
*   Mental confusion.

Cirrhosis is a condition in which liver tissue has been irreversibly and progressively destroyed as a result of infection, poison, or some other disease. The normal liver tissue is replaced by scarring and areas of regenerating liver cells.

As liver cells die, thick scar tissue may grow in their place. With the death of these cells, more and more of the complicated functions of the organ are handled by fewer and fewer cells. The liver initially may increase in size to compensate for cells no longer able to carry out their normal function. In time, with more scarring, the liver becomes smaller.

A healthy liver performs its various functions on the nutrients that have been absorbed in the gut and sent to it by the bloodstream. If the liver cells die and the liver itself contracts, it becomes increasingly more difficult for blood to flow to the liver. The blood flow may then reverse (portal hypertension) and actually bypass the liver, robbing it of important nutrients. Reversal of blood flow may cause the spleen to enlarge, and varices may develop in your esophagus,

which are prone to bleed (see Esophageal Varices, page 601).

If the scarred or cirrhotic liver is unable to process the blood and remove breakdown products properly, these breakdown products may have an adverse effect on your brain. Often these products are excessive amounts of protein that normally are broken down and removed by the liver. Blood levels of these substances increase and may cause a tremor of the hands, mental confusion, and, finally, coma (encephalopathy).

Another cause of portal hypertension is development of a blood clot in the vein that brings blood into the liver (portal vein thrombosis). In some situations, there may be no discernible cause for the obstruction of this vein.

A blood clot that blocks blood flow out of the liver, a disorder called hepatic vein thrombosis or Budd-Chiari syndrome, is a far less likely cause of portal hypertension. This obstruction also causes the liver to become enlarged and extremely tender to the touch. It usually produces a serious form of water retention in the abdomen (ascites).

There are various causes and forms of cirrhosis.

Alcohol-Induced Cirrhosis. In the United States, alcoholic cirrhosis is the most common type. It usually occurs after many years of heavy drinking and develops in as many as 15 percent of alcoholics. Typically, people who develop cirrhosis from alcohol abuse have consumed a pint or more of whiskey or several quarts of wine daily for at least 10 years. As little as 3 ounces of 100-proof whiskey (45 grams of alcohol) every day for several years may be sufficient to cause liver damage.

Symptoms of cirrhosis are often silent in the alcoholic. For others, the symptoms begin slowly. These include lack of appetite, weight loss, easy bruising, weakness, and fatigue. Jaundice and esophageal bleeding may follow.

Treatment is directed toward the complications of the disease, such as bleeding or the accumulation of excess fluid in the abdomen (ascites). It is imperative that the alcoholic give up alcohol. This will not reverse the damage already done to the liver, but it will lessen further liver damage. The person who has cirrhosis and has stopped drinking will feel better and may live longer.

Shown in cross section, the normal liver (top) shows no sign of scarring, while the cirrhotic liver (bottom) reveals extensive scarring.

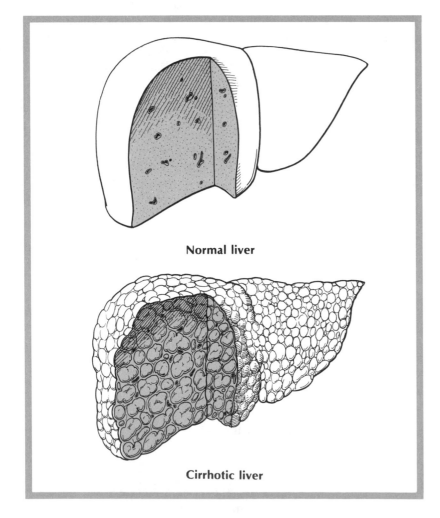

Normal liver

Cirrhotic liver

Cryptogenic Cirrhosis. Also known as post-hepatitic cirrhosis, this is the final stage of chronic liver disease that occurs as a result of hepatitis B virus, non-A, non-B hepatitis virus, or unknown causes. Most of the unknown causes are probably viral.

The symptoms are similar to those of other forms of cirrhosis. At times, people with cryptogenic cirrhosis have no symptoms, and the diagnosis of the disease is made at the time of an operation for another disorder or from a liver biopsy performed for unexplained liver enlargement (see Liver Biopsy, page 657).

Biopsy of the liver is used to confirm the diagnosis. There is no specific treatment for the cirrhosis itself. Rather, attention is directed to controlling fluid accumulation and to avoiding medications or excess protein that may contribute to mental confusion.

Primary Biliary Cirrhosis. The biliary tract consists of the ducts, within and leading from the liver, that deliver bile to the intestine. Primary biliary cirrhosis is characterized by chronic inflammation and scarring of the microscopic bile ducts within the liver. The cause is unknown. The result is that the liver is progressively destroyed and scarring (cirrhosis) develops.

Many people with primary biliary cirrhosis initially have no symptoms. Their condition usually is discovered during a routine physical examination that includes blood tests that relate to various liver functions. For unknown reasons, this form of biliary cirrhosis affects mostly women between the ages of 35 and 60.

The symptoms of primary biliary cirrhosis include severe itching (pruritus) on the hands and feet and eventually the entire body. Jaundice, dark urine, and darkening of skin exposed to the sun occur as the liver disease progresses. This slow progression results eventually in portal hypertension (see page 656), the accumulation of fluids, and eventually liver failure and death. Small collections of fat are often seen in the area around the eyes, a reflection of the high cholesterol values in these persons (see Xanthelasma and Xanthoma, page 1168).

The diagnosis usually is suspected on the basis of your clinical history and appearance and abnormal blood test results. A liver biopsy should be performed to confirm the diagnosis (see page 657). In addition, your physician may want to examine the bile ducts themselves by using x-rays, to exclude any obstruction in this area (see X-Raying the Bile and Pancreatic Ducts, page 664).

There is no specific therapy for primary biliary cirrhosis, but the goal generally is to relieve the symptoms. The drug cholestyramine may be effective in decreasing the itching. In addition, your physician may prescribe vitamin supplements because vitamins are inadequately absorbed in this particular disorder.

Increasingly, liver transplantation is being used for persons with severe liver failure from primary biliary cirrhosis.

Secondary Biliary Cirrhosis. Secondary biliary cirrhosis results from prolonged obstruction of the common bile duct or one of its branches. This may result from a previous operation that produces narrowing (stricture) in the bile duct area. In other cases, a chronic inflammation of the bile ducts (Primary Sclerosing Cholangitis, see page 665) may be the cause of chronic obstruction and the ultimate development of cirrhosis.

The signs and symptoms are similar to those of primary biliary cirrhosis. At times, fever and pain in the right upper portion of your abdomen may be present, reflecting an infection originating from the impaired flow in the bile ducts.

Your physician's diagnosis will be based on identifying the obstruction of the bile ducts. This is done either by using a combined endoscopic and x-ray approach or by inserting a long, thin needle into the liver and then into the bile ducts to introduce a contrast medium that will be visible on the x-ray and so show the obstructed duct (see X-Raying the Bile and Pancreatic Ducts, page 664).

The goal of treatment is to relieve the obstruction. This sometimes can be done with surgical reconstruction, although the recurrence rate is high. If the obstruction is in the portion of the bile duct within the liver, surgery may be quite difficult. A small hollow tube (stent) may be inserted to keep the strictured area open, perhaps at the time of percutaneous transhepatic cholangiography (see X-Raying the Bile and Pancreatic Ducts, page 664). If episodic bouts of infection persist, your physician may consider the use of antibiotics.

Hemochromatosis. This is an inherited disease that causes the body to store excessively high amounts of iron. The liver is most directly affected because it is the primary storage site for iron, and the accumulation of iron in the liver may cause cirrhosis. The excess iron also may affect the pancreas, endocrine glands, and heart.

Hemochromatosis primarily affects men between the ages of 40 and 60. The loss of iron in the menstrual flow tends to protect women from hemochromatosis. The disease may be accompanied by diabetes mellitus (see also page 707) and increased skin pigmentation—thus the nickname "bronze diabetes."

The symptoms are weakness, lassitude, weight loss, and impaired sexual performance. Often, the disease is detected by blood tests in a person who is symptom-free.

If your physician suspects hemochromatosis, he or she will examine your blood for excessive iron content. Biopsy of your liver (see page 657) may be done.

Generally, the best treatment is to remove the excess iron by withdrawing blood (phlebotomy) once or twice a week. Sometimes this treatment may be required for 1 to 2 years until the iron in the blood reaches a normal level.

When the disease is detected early, the outcome usually is good. However, if the disease is left untreated, cirrhosis will develop. If you have hemochromatosis, your blood relatives should be screened for the disorder.

Wilson's Disease. This is an inherited disorder in which copper accumulates in various organs of the body, especially the brain, eyes, kidney, and liver. This rare disease is characterized by tremors, liver disease, pigmentation of the cornea of the eye, and symptoms of chronic hepatitis (see page 652). If untreated, the liver disease leads to cirrhosis.

The treatment involves removing the deposits of copper by use of a medication called penicillamine. This treatment usually is continued for life. With proper treatment, the prognosis is good. If you have Wilson's disease, your blood relatives should be screened.

Alpha-1-Antitrypsin Deficiency. People with a deficiency of the enzyme inhibitor alpha-1-antitrypsin tend to have emphysema and liver disease in adult life. When liver disease develops during infancy, it is often related to this deficiency.

People with this disease often have cirrhosis with no apparent symptoms.

The Diagnosis. The more visible signs of cirrhosis—jaundice, water retention (edema), and spider-like vessels on the skin—are not always present. (See page B-15 for color photograph of spider-like veins.) Even without these more recognizable symptoms, your physician may find an enlarged liver or spleen during a routine medical examination.

Based on these findings, your physician probably will order blood tests. The results may be normal or may reveal minor changes that are not necessarily definitive signs of cirrhosis of the liver. But a long history of heavy drinking would make such a diagnosis more likely. A definitive diagnosis would require a liver biopsy (a sample of liver tissue is examined microscopically; see page 657). This will reveal the extent and nature, and possibly the cause, of the liver damage.

How Serious Is Cirrhosis? Cirrhosis is very serious because the damage is irreversible. There is no cure for cirrhosis. Annually, at least 30,000 people die from alcohol-related liver disorders alone.

There are several serious complications that may occur.

Portal Hypertension. This occurs in more than two-thirds of people with cirrhosis. It causes impairment of flow in the portal vein which supplies the liver. The pressure within the portal system increases, causing enlargement of the spleen and the development of dilated veins in the esophagus and stomach (see Esophageal Varices, page 601).

Esophageal Bleeding. This may result from rupture of esophageal or gastric varices. This is a life-threatening emergency. Initial treatment may involve infusion of a drug (vasopressin) that may reduce the pressure within the varices and stop the bleeding, at least temporarily. In addition, a tube often is inserted through the nose into the stomach. Attached to this tube are both a stomach balloon and an esophageal balloon. These can be inflated to compress the varices in an attempt to stop the bleeding. If bleeding stops or slows, an irritating or sclerosing agent can be injected, by using a catheter placed through an endoscope (see Upper Gastrointestinal Endoscopy, page 611), directly into the vein. This is called esophageal variceal sclerotherapy. In other cases, surgery is necessary to stop the bleeding, although the risk from death during surgery for acute esophageal or gastric variceal bleeding is very high.

Ascites.   Ascites is an accumulation of excess fluid within the abdominal cavity. Treatment often includes a salt-restricted diet and the use of diuretics to eliminate water and salt through the urine.

Spontaneous Bacterial Peritonitis.   This occurs when ascites fluid becomes infected. Abdominal pain along with a low-grade fever may be present. The diagnosis is made by inserting a catheter into the abdomen and removing fluid for laboratory examination to identify the infecting organism. The treatment is with antibiotics.

Hepatic Encephalopathy.   This is a complication in which the brain is poisoned by the toxic elements from the liver which is no longer capable of properly filtering the blood to remove toxins. Blood tests will be conducted to determine ammonia levels which are an index of the degree of accumulation of such toxins. The persons who develop this may experience a change in their personality and may become mentally confused, drowsy, and tremulous (see Liver Disease, page 649).

Treatment.   There is no specific treatment for cirrhosis. Treatment is largely confined to the complications of cirrhosis (see above).

If you have fluid retention, your physician will advise a salt-restricted diet. This needs to be followed carefully because even small increases in the amount of salt in your diet may produce a considerable amount of swelling. In addition, the amount of water in your diet may be somewhat restricted. Diuretics may be prescribed to hasten the removal of fluid from your system.

If there are signs of encephalopathy, your physician also may advise a low-protein diet. Your dietary instructions will provide adequate calorie intake.

Your physician also may prescribe vitamin supplements, particularly vitamins K, A, and D.

If itching becomes particularly troublesome, the drug cholestyramine may be prescribed. This medication may interfere with the absorption of other drugs and therefore should be taken separately.

Abstain from the use of alcohol and any other medication that is broken down by and eliminated through the liver. If some of these medications are absolutely needed, your physician may adjust your dosage.

In some situations, your physician may wish to refer you to a medical center that specializes in liver diseases for consideration for liver transplantation (see page 660).

LIVER TUMORS

Signs and Symptoms
- There may be none;
- Loss of appetite and weight;
- Abdominal pain;
- Nausea and vomiting;
- General fatigue and weakness;
- Enlarged liver;
- Ascites (swelling in the peritoneal cavity);
- Jaundice (yellowing of the skin and eyes).

Most tumors that form in the liver are malignant. Usually they are cancers that have spread (metastasized) to the liver from another part of the body; this is termed sec-

---

LIVER BIOPSY

In the course of diagnosing liver disease, your physician may perform a liver biopsy. This is a simple diagnostic procedure that is used in various liver disorders including cirrhosis, hepatitis, and tumors.

The Procedure
You will be given a local anesthetic to prevent discomfort and will be positioned flat on your back. Your physician will insert a thin needle between or below your ribs into your liver and then will remove a small sample of tissue for laboratory analysis.

The Risks
Liver biopsy is quite safe and unlikely to have any complications. Occasionally, there is some pain or bleeding after the procedure.

The Results
The laboratory tests conducted on the tissues may reveal the presence (or absence) of certain disorders. If you are already known to have a liver disorder, the biopsy can be helpful in evaluating the progress of the disease.

ondary liver cancer. The liver is especially vulnerable to invasion by tumor cells and, with the exception of lymph nodes, it is the most common site of metastasis.

The malignant liver tumor that originates in the liver or bile ducts is called primary liver cancer (hepatocellular or cholangiocarcinoma). In the United States, primary liver cancers account for only 1 to 2 percent of the malignant tumors found during autopsy. Liver cancer occurs 2 to 4 times more frequently in men.

Certain factors tend to predispose a person to primary liver cancer. These include chronic liver disease such as cirrhosis, hepatitis B infection, and exposure to certain toxins.

Benign or nonmalignant liver tumors also occur. The most common is the hemangioma. These are often discovered incidentally during study of the liver for another reason. Normally, treatment is not needed for these benign liver tumors. Hepatic adenomas (another benign tumor) occasionally occur in women who take oral contraceptives over a long period. These tumors may regress or become smaller when use of the birth control pill is discontinued. Hepatic adenomas may cause pain and even may rupture and require surgical removal. Another condition, focal nodular hyperplasia, sometimes occurs with the long-term use of oral contraceptives. This disorder generally has no symptoms.

Cysts commonly occur in the liver. Most often they are harmless.

Liver cysts are very common and usually are found incidentally when the liver is examined by CT or ultrasonography (see page 1287). Liver cysts carry no risk of malig-

nancy, and symptoms are rare. Treatment is unnecessary except in the rare instances when they cause significant abdominal discomfort.

The Diagnosis. Many benign tumors of the liver are asymptomatic and thus are never discovered. If they grow large enough, however, they may cause pain, liver tenderness, or internal hemorrhage.

If the tumor is cancerous, the symptoms are more evident because a person with liver cancer may become debilitated over time. If you have a history of liver dysfunction or liver disease and your health is failing, your physician may consider the possibility of liver cancer.

If a liver cancer is suspected, a thorough physical examination and blood tests may be the first step. In addition, you will probably have a CT scan (see page 1286) or an ultrasound examination (see page 1287); either can reliably detect a mass in the liver. Liver biopsy, in which a sample of liver tissue is removed for laboratory analysis, provides more information (see page 657). An exploratory abdominal operation may be required if the liver biopsy does not provide a definitive diagnosis.

How Serious Is Liver Cancer? Liver cancer usually is fatal. Most patients do not live beyond 6 months to a year after the diagnosis.

Treatment. In some cases, chemotherapy is used to relieve the symptoms, but this treatment only infrequently improves the outcome.

In the case of multiple, spreading (metastatic) tumors, surgery is of little or no value. However, it may be recommended if a benign tumor is very large and causes discomfort or when a primary liver cancer is small and localized.

If a solitary metastatic tumor nodule from a distant site (such as the colon) is found and there is no evidence of spread of the cancer to other locations, surgical removal may be attempted in hope of a cure.

LIVER ABSCESS

Signs and Symptoms
- Persistent fever;
- Chills;

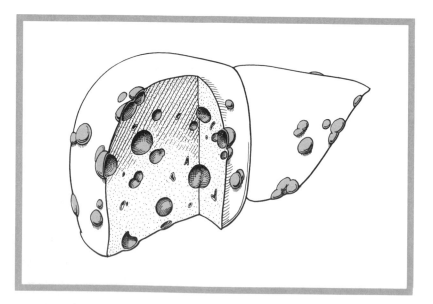

ENLARGED LIVER

Enlargement of the liver is called hepatomegaly.

The Signs

Persons with hepatomegaly may have no symptoms other than a mild tenderness over their liver. Depending on the cause of the enlargement, others may have pain in the upper right section of the abdomen and varying degrees of jaundice.

Enlargement of the liver is usually discovered during an examination of the abdomen by your physician. The normal liver is rather soft and is located beneath the ribs on the right side of your body. Your physician sometimes can feel your liver by placing his or her hand just below your rib margin and asking you to take a deep breath (the deep breath causes your liver to descend so that your physician can feel its edge).

An enlarged liver or one that is firmer than normal often can be felt readily during this maneuver. This is the same technique used to detect enlargement of the spleen (splenomegaly) which is located beneath the left rib margin. Enlargement of the liver or the spleen is more difficult to detect in an obese person.

A CT scan (see page 1286), ultrasound examination (see page 1287), or MRI scan (see page 1287) of the liver will reveal the size, configuration, and texture of the liver and also will determine whether a tumor is present within the organ.

The Causes

Perhaps the most common cause of an enlarged liver is the accumulation of fat. In this country, a fatty liver commonly is part of chronic alcoholism or sometimes of ordinary obesity. This condition also can occur as a complication of prolonged corticosteroid use. Reye's syndrome (see page 531), an acute illness almost exclusively of children, has as one of its features the presence of fatty deposits within liver cells.

The liver may increase in size because of too much glycogen, as a result of a glycogen storage disease. Glycogen is a starch that is stored in and transformed by the liver into glucose, a form of sugar that the body is able to use for energy. Accumulation of glycogen results from many of the disorders that cause fatty infiltration of the liver. In addition, excessive glycogen accumulation may be seen in children and teenagers with poorly controlled diabetes (see page 707).

Amyloidosis is a disorder that deposits an excess of a protein called amyloid in the liver and other parts of the body. The amyloid makes the liver enlarged, pale, and rubbery in consistency; swelling due to water retention (edema) is also a frequent problem with this disorder. The principal means of diagnosis of amyloidosis is a blood test and biopsy of the liver (see page 657).

The liver is vulnerable to infiltration by tumors or lesions caused by other diseases. One example is miliary tuberculosis (miliary refers to the seed-like tumors it generates). Another such disease is sarcoidosis, a disease of unknown origin that causes lesions in many organs of the body including the liver.

The Treatment

Treatment for enlarged liver generally is determined by the underlying cause. The elimination of alcohol intake and the loss of weight, if necessary, are advised.

- Nausea and vomiting;
- Weakness;
- Weight loss;
- Liver tender to the touch;
- Jaundice.

Abscesses sometimes form within the liver as a result of infection by bacteria or ameba. Those of bacterial origin generally have a more rapid course with fever and chills; those from amebiasis progress more slowly.

The Diagnosis. If your physician believes that you may have a liver abscess, he or she may arrange for a CT scan (see page 1286) or an ultrasound examination of your liver (see page 1287). From the image that is produced, he or she may be able to determine the size, location, and number of the abscesses. Blood tests also may be helpful, particularly if your physician suspects that the cause of the abscess is a parasite.

Insertion of a needle into the abscess, using the CT scan or ultrasonogram for guidance, will allow withdrawal of some of the fluid for laboratory analysis. However, if your physician suspects that the cyst is caused by a parasite *(Echinococcus),* he or she may refrain from inserting a needle.

How Serious Are Liver Abscesses? A liver abscess, particularly from a bacterial cause, is a potentially fatal problem. Even

GENETIC LIVER PROBLEMS

Some inherited liver abnormalities cause high concentrations of bilirubin in the blood, a condition called hyperbilirubinemia. This produces jaundice (yellowing of the eyes and skin).

Gilbert's Syndrome

Gilbert's syndrome is an inherited disorder in which bilirubin is not properly processed in the liver for excretion in the feces. Bilirubin has to combine (conjugate) with another substance in the liver in order to make the bilirubin water-soluble and capable of being excreted through the bile. Bilirubin is usually unconjugated or unprocessed in Gilbert's syndrome because of a deficiency of the enzyme necessary to accomplish this conjugation

Gilbert's syndrome may be the most common cause of hyperbilirubinemia. The jaundice it causes is rather mild but may be aggravated by fasting. In some cases, the disorder is only detected during a routine blood test. Gilbert's syndrome does not lead to liver damage; treatment is unnecessary.

Crigler-Najjar Syndrome

This rare, inherited disorder causes two types of hyperbilirubinemia: type I and type II. Type I, the most severe form, is due to an absence of the enzyme needed to conjugate the bilirubin. Type II is less severe because there is only a partial enzyme deficiency.

There is no treatment that will cure type I Crigler-Najjar syndrome. The infant born with it usually dies within the first year. Type II hyperbilirubinemia, however, can be treated successfully with medication, usually phenobarbital.

Dubin-Johnson Hyperbilirubinemia

Some disorders cause both conjugated and unconjugated hyperbilirubinemia. One such inherited disorder is Dubin-Johnson syndrome, otherwise known as chronic idiopathic jaundice. People with this disorder often will have no symptoms or only vague gastrointestinal symptoms. In some cases, their liver is enlarged. This disorder can be successfully treated with medication.

LIVER TRANSPLANTATION

The first liver transplantation in a human was performed in 1963. For the next 20 years, few of those who had their diseased livers replaced by healthy organs survived more than a few months. Since 1981, however, the survival rate for liver transplant patients has improved steadily, and now about three-quarters of the transplant recipients survive a year or more.

Better methods of preserving donated organs, improvements in surgical techniques, and advances in postoperative care are largely responsible for this increase in survival. An important development has been the use of the immunosuppressive drug cyclosporine. Developed in 1980, the drug decreases the body's natural rejection response to a donated organ. Specifically, cyclosporine prevents the lymphocytes (one of your white blood cells) from rejecting the transplanted liver. Better antibiotic drugs have also been perfected that are more effective in the prevention of new infections after the operation.

Who Is a Candidate?

The improving risk-versus-benefit ratio makes the operation appropriate for those people who have potentially fatal liver disease. The most likely candidates for a transplant are children and adults under age 60 whose liver disease is progressive, nonmalignant, and not correctable by any other therapy. People with alcohol-related liver disease, many forms of liver cancer, or viral hepatitis B are poor risks for transplantation. Recurrence rates are high in the latter two conditions. Previous surgery in and about the upper abdomen may make liver transplantation unduly difficult and risky.

Many transplantations are performed to treat congenital liver abnormalities. The most successful operations have been conducted on young children with untreatable liver disease as a result of congenital abnormalities in their bile ducts (see Bile Duct Atresia, page 59). More than half of the children who have had a liver transplant survive beyond the first 2 years.

The Procedure

Liver transplantation is a very difficult operation. It takes between 8 and 10 hours, and it is done only at a few large medical centers. Because of the high risk, a decision for transplantation will require the consent of the patient, the family of the patient, or an authorized representative. Lifelong therapy with immunosuppressive drugs will be needed to prevent rejection of the new organ.

when the liver abscess is correctly diagnosed and properly treated, many affected persons do not survive.

Treatment. If the liver abscess is caused by a bacterium, your physician may advise catheterization for drainage and the use of antibiotics given through a vein for several weeks. At times, surgical exploration and drainage of the abscess or even removal of the portion of the liver containing the abscess is required.

If the cause is ameba or *Echinococcus,* your physician may advise specific medications.

GALLBLADDER AND BILE DUCT DISORDERS

The gallbladder is a pear-shaped sac 3 to 4 inches long and roughly 1 inch in diameter that generally lies underneath the liver on your right side. The gallbladder stores the bile that is produced in your liver and then discharged through the bile duct into the duodenum, usually after a meal. Bile facilitates the digestion of fats.

GALLSTONES

Signs and Symptoms
- Intense and sudden pain on upper right side of the abdomen that moves around to the right shoulder blade;
- Fever;
- Nausea and, sometimes, vomiting;
- Loss of appetite.

Gallstones are a common problem; an estimated 1 million new cases are diagnosed yearly in the United States.

Gallstones are crystalline structures that can be as small as a grain of sand or as large as a golf ball. They can be smooth and round or irregular with many edges. Some people have only one gallstone; others may have several.

The stones that collect in the gallbladder may produce no symptoms. But a gallstone that obstructs the cystic duct (leading from the gallbladder to the bile duct) or the bile duct itself (the conduit into the duodenum for both the liver and gallbladder) may produce a painful spasm and inflammation at the site of the obstruction.

The pain of a gallbladder attack (biliary colic) normally begins quite suddenly and may persist for several hours. It then may subside over the period of the next few hours. The pain is severe and constant, often accompanied by nausea and vomiting. After the pain subsides, there may be a mild aching sensation or soreness in the right upper abdomen, which may last for up to a day.

True pain from a gallbladder attack is infrequent, generally occurring no more than one to three times per year. Belching, bloating, intolerance of fatty foods, or frequent abdominal pain should not be attributed to gallstone disease.

If you become jaundiced, especially if the yellowing of your skin is accompanied by pain, this suggests migration of a stone into the common bile duct (see Bile Duct Obstruction, page 663). The presence of a high fever or shaking chills usually implies an underlying complication such as inflammation of the gallbladder (cholecystitis), acute pancreatitis (see page 667), or infection in the bile duct secondary to obstruction (cholangitis). Sometimes the symptoms of gallblad-

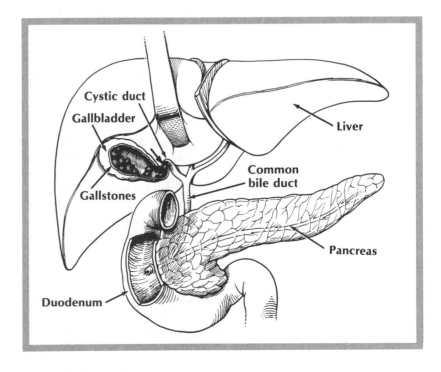

Gallstones may form in your gallbladder. If a stone obstructs your cystic duct (see arrow), you may experience a painful gallbladder attack.

Cystic duct

Gallbladder

Gallstones

Duodenum

Liver

Common bile duct

Pancreas

der disease (biliary colic) may be precipitated by eating a fatty meal.

Not all gallstones are made of the same material. Eighty percent of the stones common in the United States are composed primarily of cholesterol; the remaining 20 percent contain mostly calcium salts of bile pigment. Normally, the bile acids in bile keep cholesterol from becoming too concentrated and thus forming gallstones. However, if the amount of cholesterol in the bile increases beyond the ability of bile acids to maintain this balance, the cholesterol crystallizes and, in some people, a stone eventually will form.

About 1 in 10 Americans has or will have gallstones. Autopsies show that probably 20 percent of all women have gallstones, more than 3 times the number found in men. And the likelihood of gallstones increases with age. It is estimated that, among the elderly, one of five may have gallstones, although many of these people are without symptoms. Obviously, gallstones develop in many people without causing symptoms. The chance of symptoms or complications developing from these stones is probably less than 20 percent over a long period of time.

The need to remove the gallbladder (cholecystectomy) surgically is more likely in persons who have symptoms of gallbladder pain. Those who are young are more likely to have symptoms from gallbladder disease than are persons more than 60 years old at the time of the initial diagnosis. Persons who have diabetes mellitus and gallstones may be slightly more at risk for the development of an infection and thus should consider removal of the gallbladder with its stones soon after the diagnosis is made.

The Diagnosis. If a severe and lasting pain develops in the right side of your abdomen and radiates around to your shoulder blade, your physician may suspect gallbladder difficulties. Your physician will conduct a physical examination to look for jaundice and will palpate your abdomen to see if your gallbladder has become distended due to an obstruction.

If your physician believes the cause is gallstones, you may have a blood test and an ultrasound examination (see page 1287).

Treatment. If you have gallstones and no symptoms that can be attributed to the stones or gallbladder itself, your physician may elect only to observe and not recommend any specific treatment. If you are diabetic or if you are young, your physician may choose to remove the gallbladder even if you have no symptoms.

Surgery. If you are having gallbladder pain (biliary colic or acute cholecystitis) your physician may recommend the surgical removal of the gallbladder (cholecystectomy). This is a very safe operation with a very small risk of complications and is the preferred approach for treating most persons with gallbladder disease. The procedure generally is done after an acute episode has resolved.

Stone Dissolution. An option that has been developed in the last decade is stone dissolution. This applies only to cholesterol stones. A bile acid (chenodeoxycholic or ursodeoxycholic acid) is given in tablet form. The medication works by increasing the bile acid concentration within the gallbladder, which brings the solid cholesterol stone back into solution. This drug works best if the cholesterol stones are small and are the floating type.

If you have a pigment stone, you are not a candidate for this type of medication, nor is this drug recommended for pregnant women with gallstones because of possible damage to the fetus.

The dosage is based on body weight. If you are obese, you may require a larger dose and thus may be more prone to side effects. It generally takes many months or even years for the bile acid treatment to dissolve the stone. Thus, this is not a practical approach if you are having frequent bouts of gallbladder pain. In addition, after the drug therapy ends, there is a 25 to 50 percent chance of another gallstone developing because the underlying problem of excess secretion of cholesterol into the gallbladder is still present.

Alternative Treatments. Alternative treatment methods have been developed in the last several years, especially for those persons who have other serious medical problems and for whom surgery might be dangerous. One involves localization of the gallbladder by ultrasonography and infusion of the drug methyl *tert*-butyl ether (MTBE) via a catheter directly into the gallbladder.

For this to be effective, the stones have to be cholesterol in nature and not contain calcium. Often, this may dissolve the stones after 1 to 2 days of constant perfusion. The gallbladder remains in place, and your physician may prescribe chenodeoxycholic or ursodeoxycholic acid tablets indefinitely to prevent formation of new stones within the gallbladder.

New methods under investigation include stone fragmentation with high-frequency sound waves (biliary lithotripsy) and removal of gallstones via laparoscopy. The latter approach appears to be more promising than the former.

BILE DUCT OBSTRUCTION

Signs and Symptoms
- Jaundice (yellowing of the skin and eyes);
- High fever with chills;
- Clay-colored stools;
- Tea- or coffee-colored urine;
- Abdominal pain in the upper abdomen.

Emergency Signs
- Shock: cold, clammy, pale skin with weak or rapid pulse;
- Mental confusion.

The presence of gallstones in the common bile duct (the conduit into the duodenum for bile from both the liver and the gallbladder) is the most common cause of bile duct obstruction (see Gallstones, page 661). After the surgical removal of the gallbladder (cholecystectomy), in a small percentage of cases a stone remains in the common bile duct. These stones may obstruct the narrow common bile duct and cause episodic pain in the right upper quadrant of your abdomen. Often, spiking fevers with shaking chills (cholangitis) and jaundice also are symptoms of acute bile duct obstruction.

Because the common bile duct and pancreatic duct are joined in most persons, an obstruction in the common bile duct may lead to an obstruction in the pancreatic duct and subsequent pancreatitis (see Acute Pancreatitis, page 667). Obstruction of the common bile duct is an emergency situation requiring immediate relief of the obstruction.

Obstruction of the bile duct also can be caused by a stricture or narrowing of the duct, inflammation of the duct, or cancer.

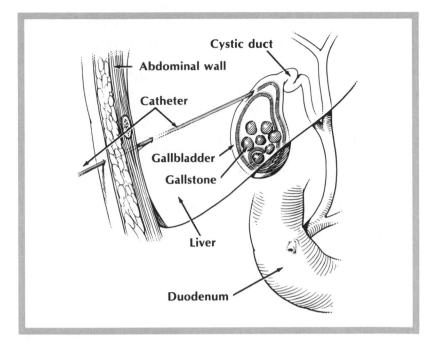

In people for whom gallbladder surgery is inappropriate, a catheter may be inserted into the gallbladder. Then a drug, methyl *tert*-butyl ether (MTBE), is infused to dissolve the stones.

Trauma. Narrowing (stricture) of the common duct is a potential complication of gallbladder surgery. The stricture may develop immediately after gallbladder surgery or may be delayed for several years. In either event, an additional operation often can correct the problem.

Hemobilia. Blood in the bile duct (hemobilia) can lead to a clot that can obstruct the

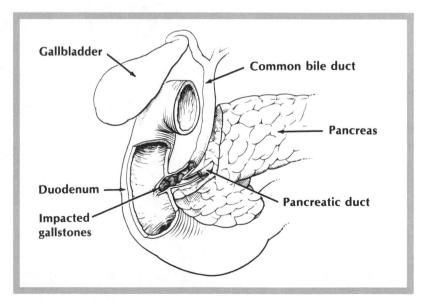

Gallstones can become impacted in the common bile duct at the entrance to the duodenum. This obstruction is a potentially life-threatening condition requiring immediate treatment.

X-RAYING THE BILE AND PANCREATIC DUCTS

There are two principal approaches to x-raying these areas.

Endoscopic Retrograde Cholangiopancreatography (ERCP)

This method involves x-raying the bile and pancreatic ducts through their opening into the intestinal tract by using an endoscope. The purpose of ERCP is to identify bile duct stones (gallstones), long-standing inflammatory disease of the pancreas, or obstruction of either of these two ducts. The obstruction may be from scar or inflammatory tissue or from tumors, usually cancers.

The Procedure

You will be asked not to eat or drink for 8 to 12 hours prior to the test. Just before the procedure begins, an intravenous tube will be placed into a vein in your hand; a sedative and a medication that relaxes your stomach and intestines will be given through this tube. An anesthetic drug will be sprayed into the back of your throat to eliminate gagging when the endoscope is passed into your throat. You will be lying on your left side. At this point, the flexible endoscope is passed into your mouth, down your throat, through the length of your stomach, and into your duodenum. Throughout this entire process the physician views the passage of the endoscope.

Air is used to inflate the intestinal tract in order to identify the tiny opening through which the bile and pancreatic ducts drain their fluids into the duodenum. Once this opening is found, you will be placed on your stomach. A fine hollow tube or catheter is passed through the endoscope and into the bile and pancreatic ducts. A dye or contrast solution is injected through this catheter into the ducts to fill them. X-ray pictures are then taken.

Other types of catheters can be placed through the endoscope to treat specific abnormalities identified in the x-rays. A catheter fitted with an electrical cautery wire can be used to enlarge the opening of the bile duct to permit the extraction of a stone. The extraction can be performed with a specialized balloon or basket catheter. Another type of catheter can be placed into the bile duct to allow delivery of drugs to dissolve stones. Finally, strictures (narrowings) from scarring or tumors can be stretched or opened with a dilating balloon catheter, and a hollow tube (stent) then can be inserted through the endoscope into the narrowing to maintain free passage of bile into the duodenum.

Side Effects

The medications given to you during the procedure may make you feel tired, dizzy, dry-mouthed, and sometimes slightly nauseated. The air placed into your intestines may leave you feeling gassy and bloated for several hours. Do not eat or drink anything until your gag reflex returns. Your throat may feel sore for a day or so; for this you may use lozenges or salt-water gargles.

The entire ERCP procedure takes 30 minutes to 1 hour. It can be done on an outpatient basis so you return home the same day.

ERCP studies, showing (left) a normal common bile duct (white arrow) and pancreatic duct (black arrow). At right is a dilated common bile duct with a stone (white arrow).

Percutaneous Transhepatic Cholangiography (PTHC)

This is another contrast x-ray procedure that provides pictures of the bile duct. It is used to diagnose the cause of upper abdominal pain after gallbladder surgery or unexplained jaundice when a bile duct obstruction (such as from a gallstone) is suspected.

The Procedure

You will be asked not to eat for 8 hours prior to the test. You will lie down on a tilting x-ray table that can be rotated into vertical and horizontal positions. A tube will be inserted into a vein in your arm for administration of medication for sedation and of an antibiotic. Then, the skin over your liver will be cleansed with an antiseptic and a local anesthetic will be injected into the skin. The rest of the procedure begins when you feel numb where the anesthetic was injected.

A long, flexible needle is inserted into your liver. In most instances you will not feel the needle pass into the liver. However, if you should, the feeling of fullness or pain will be only temporary. When the x-ray image indicates that the needle has reached the bile duct, contrast medium is injected through it.

At this point, a series of x-rays are taken as you and the table are rotated to different positions to provide different views of your liver. When the procedure is completed, the needle is removed and a dressing is applied. Your physician probably will ask that you lie in bed on your right side for at least 6 hours after the test. In addition, you may be given pain medication.

The procedure takes between 45 minutes and 1 hour and is usually done in a hospital. Many physicians prefer that you stay in the hospital overnight for monitoring in case bleeding or infection should develop.

---

duct. Hemobilia may occur as a result of trauma to the liver or bile duct during surgery. People with hemobilia often have abdominal pain, jaundice, and occult blood in their stool. Often, the clot dissolves spontaneously. At other times, surgical removal is needed.

Primary Sclerosing Cholangitis. In some people a chronic disorder called primary sclerosing cholangitis (PSC) develops. Sclerosis is hardening and thickening of tissue, in this case of the bile duct wall. PSC can produce a partial blockage of the duct. This obstruction produces much the same symptoms as gallstones in the bile duct, including jaundice, pain in the right side of the abdomen, episodes of fever and chills, itching, and fatigue. In addition, sclerosing cholangitis may cause cirrhosis, liver failure, or hemorrhage from esophageal varices (see Cirrhosis, page 653). Frequently, sclerosing cholangitis is associated with an underlying disease such as chronic inflammatory bowel disease (see Crohn's Disease, page 626, and Ulcerative Colitis, page 628).

Bile Duct Cancer. A malignant tumor in the bile duct can cause obstruction. If you have the symptoms of bile duct cancer (which include jaundice, itching, weight loss, and clay-colored stools), your physician may order an ultrasound examination or CT scan (see page 1286) which then may be followed by cholangiography (see X-Raying the Bile and Pancreatic Ducts, page 664).

Other Disorders. Sometimes the bile duct can become partially or completely obstructed if it is subjected to pressure on its outside wall. This often can be caused by a complication of either acute or chronic pancreatitis (see pages 667 and 668, respectively), cancer of the pancreas (see Malignant Pancreatic Tumors, page 669), lymphoma (see Lymphomas, page 489), or cancer from another part of the body that has metastasized (spread). The principal symptom is jaundice. Treatment is directed at the underlying disorder. At times, it may be necessary to cut the bile duct and place it in another location on the small bowel to bypass an obstructed segment of intestine.

The Diagnosis. Because the initial symptoms of a bile duct obstruction are similar regardless of the cause, your physician will conduct many of the same diagnostic tests that would be used for gallstones. He or she also may inject a contrast material into the bile duct for either endoscopic retrograde cholangiopancreatography (ERCP) or percutaneous transhepatic cholangiography (see X-Raying the Bile and Pancreatic Ducts, page 664).

How Serious Is Bile Duct Obstruction?
Bile duct blockage is a serious and often life-threatening problem and requires prompt treatment. Cultures of your blood during episodes of fever may reveal the presence of bacteria that have leaked into the bloodstream from the obstructed bile duct. Blood infection (sepsis) can lead to shock.

Treatment.   The principle of the treatment is to relieve the blockage of your bile duct.

Surgery and Endoscopic Treatment.   If the cause of the obstruction is stones within the bile duct and, in addition, you have stones in the gallbladder, your physician may recommend surgical removal of both the stones and the gallbladder. At other times, particularly if the risk of operation is great or if you have had your gallbladder removed previously, your physician may recommend a special procedure called an ERCP (see X-Raying the Bile and Pancreatic Ducts, page 664). At the time of the ERCP, a cutting device can be inserted through the entrance of the bile duct at the level of the small intestine. This entrance can then be enlarged to permit the passage of the obstructing stone.

At other times, a catheter can be inserted into the bile duct for delivery of a drug in an attempt to dissolve the stones. This often takes many days of constant infusion.

If the obstruction is the result of a stricture or narrowing of the bile duct, a surgeon skilled in biliary tract repair can reconstruct the bile duct. At other times, particularly if previous unsuccessful attempts at bile duct repair have been made or if there are multiple strictures, an alternative approach may be recommended. A hollow tube (stent) can be inserted into the bile duct across the narrowed area to permit the free passage of bile.

If the cause of the obstruction is bleeding in the bile duct, surgery is often required to tie off the bleeding vessel.

There generally are multiple strictures in primary sclerosing cholangitis. Thus, attempts at operation or placement of a stent often are unsuccessful. There is currently no specific treatment for primary sclerosing cholangitis that will reverse or remove the multiple strictures. If this disorder results in severe liver failure, liver transplantation may be considered (see Liver Transplantation, page 660).

If the cause of the bile duct obstruction is external pressure such as from a malignant tumor, treatment initially will be directed at the primary disorder. At times, the placement of a stent (see above) also is effective in relieving this obstruction.

Medication.   Itching is often a predominant symptom with chronic obstruction of the bile ducts. It can be managed by use of the drug cholestyramine. Your physician also may prescribe vitamins, such as vitamins K, A, and D, that are poorly absorbed in persons with bile duct obstruction.

If fever and chills are present, your physician may wish to treat these symptoms with antibiotics, often given through a vein.

CHOLEDOCHAL CYSTS

Cysts sometime form in the bile duct, leading to an abnormal expansion of the duct (choledochal cyst). As a result, the secretions from the pancreas may return (reflux) into the common bile duct, causing inflammation and, at times, narrowing (stricture) of the duct.

Because the process is gradual, many people have occasional symptoms of abdominal pain and irritation for years before an obstruction develops. The cyst and the associated complications can be diagnosed with such tests as ultrasonography, CT scan, or cholangiography (see X-Raying the Bile and Pancreatic Ducts, page 664).

Treatment.   Once it has been identified, the cyst is removed surgically. People who have had a choledochal cyst have an increased risk of biliary duct cancer developing later.

PANCREATIC DISEASES

The pancreas lies horizontally behind the lower part of the stomach. Its head rests against the wall of the duodenum; its tail reaches toward the spleen.

The pancreas is a gland, meaning it has the ability to manufacture a secretion that is used in another part of the body. In fact, it actually is two glands.

As an exocrine gland (exocrine glands secrete into ducts), it produces and secretes digestive enzymes and alkaline material (sodium bicarbonate) directly into the pancreatic duct. Then these materials flow into the duodenum. The alkaline secretion makes it possible for the enzymes from the pancreas and small intestine to break down nutrients in the gut to smaller units, enabling the nutrients to be absorbed through the small bowel into the bloodstream. The endocrine gland (endocrine glands secrete into the bloodstream) of the pancreas primarily produces the hormones insulin and glucagon. These are important in the metabolism of carbohydrates and fats.

Infections, injury, and tumors can cause enough damage to the pancreas to affect its functions. If the secretion of the hormone insulin is diminished, diabetes mellitus occurs (see page 707). Another disorder that may affect the pancreas, cystic fibrosis, is discussed at length on page 933.

ACUTE PANCREATITIS

Signs and Symptoms
- Abdominal pain that is intense and lasting and may radiate to the back and chest; it often begins 12 to 24 hours after a large meal or bout of heavy drinking;
- Low-grade fever;
- Nausea or vomiting;
- Clammy skin;
- Abdominal distention and tenderness.

Pancreatitis is an inflammation of the pancreas. The inflammation may be acute or chronic (see Chronic Pancreatitis, page 668).

Many factors are associated with or may be a cause of acute pancreatitis, such as alcohol use, gallstones, increased triglyceride or calcium level in the blood (found in blood tests), viral and bacterial infections, and drugs. The mechanisms by which any of these conditions triggers pancreatic inflammation are not well known. Nevertheless, there are a number of theories as to what happens and why.

The principal theory is that the enzymes of the pancreas eat away at the gland itself.

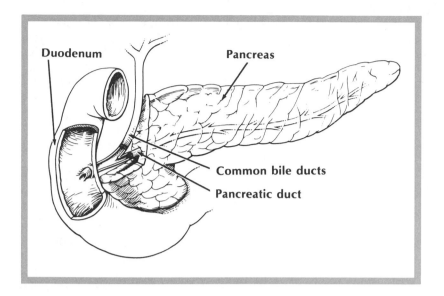

This process is called autodigestion. These powerful digestive enzymes normally are secreted by the pancreas in inactive forms but somehow may be activated inside the gland rather than in the intestine. As a result, the enzymes begin to digest the tissue of the pancreas.

In addition to digesting pancreatic tissue, it is believed that certain enzymes, especially trypsin, set off a chain reaction by activating other enzymes. These reactions then increase the number of enzymes that are digesting the gland.

Autodigestion causes swelling (edema), hemorrhage, and damage to the blood vessels. The process also releases certain substances (histamines) that cause the blood vessels to enlarge. If unchecked, this series of reactions can produce a very serious case of acute pancreatitis.

The Diagnosis. If you have an intense, constant pain in your upper abdomen that may radiate through to your back, chest, or flank, your physician may suspect acute pancreatitis. The pain is often worse when you lie flat and relieved when you sit up or stand. You may notice that you do not pass gas and that your abdomen is tender to the touch and is distended.

During your physical examination, your physician may elicit pain by palpating the abdominal area. He or she also will look for low-grade fever, low blood pressure, and accelerated heartbeat.

A sample of your blood may be taken for analysis for specific abnormalities such as excessive levels of certain enzymes from the pancreas, a high white blood cell count (leukocytosis), high blood sugar (hyperglycemia), and low calcium level (hypocalcemia). You may also have an x-ray taken of your abdomen and chest. An ultrasound or CT scan (see page 1286) of the abdomen may be obtained to examine the pancreas and to look for a bile duct problem or stone.

How Serious Is Acute Pancreatitis?

In most cases, the symptoms of acute pancreatitis subside within a week. However, severe acute pancreatitis can be life-threatening. The major complications of acute pancreatitis include development of an abscess in the pancreas, a cyst in the pancreas (pseudocyst), and leakage of pancreatic fluid into the abdomen.

Treatment. *Medication.*

Treatment of mild acute pancreatitis centers on quieting your pancreas and decreasing the flow of pancreatic enzymes. To ease the pain, an analgesic usually is prescribed. If an abscess develops, you will be given antibiotics through a vein.

Part of the overall strategy is to prevent or reduce the release of pancreatic enzymes and thus protect the pancreas from further damage. Because eating may increase gastric secretion, you may be given nourishment intravenously while the pain is present. In some cases, it may be necessary to drain your stomach through nasogastric suction (by inserting a tube through your nose). Consumption of alcohol is to be stopped.

Surgery.

If the underlying cause of the pancreatitis is gallbladder disease or an obstructed pancreatic duct, surgery may be necessary, but only after the pancreatitis has been brought under control. At times, an operation may be needed if complications of acute pancreatitis develop.

If a stone is present at the common entrance to the small intestine from the common bile duct and pancreatic duct, your physician may consider a procedure in which the duct is enlarged (sphincterotomy). An endoscope is inserted into the opening of the duct (see X-Raying the Bile and Pancreatic Ducts, page. 664) and the duct can then be enlarged so that the obstructing stone can be removed.

CHRONIC PANCREATITIS

Signs and Symptoms

* Abdominal pain that is intense and lasting and may radiate to the back and chest;
* Fever;
* Excessively foul, bulky stools;
* Nausea or vomiting;
* Weight loss;
* Clammy skin;
* Abdominal distention;
* Onset of diabetes mellitus;
* Symptoms appear periodically over a period of years in a pattern of acute attacks.

This type of pancreatic inflammation differs from acute pancreatitis (see page 667) in that it develops over a period of years. A person with chronic pancreatitis has had periodic attacks of acute pain that eventually damage the pancreas. Many people with chronic pancreatitis often have a history of alcohol abuse. In some, the cause is unknown. Chronic pancreatitis may produce acute attacks of pain, which complicate treatment.

If you have chronic pancreatitis, over time your pancreatic gland becomes less able to secrete the enzymes needed for proper digestion and absorption of dietary fats. This inability to perform properly is called exocrine insufficiency and is a principal characteristic of chronic pancreatitis. Among adults, alcoholism is the most common cause of pancreatic exocrine insufficiency; in children, cystic fibrosis is the most common cause (see page 933).

The pain of acute pancreatitis is steady and persistent for many hours or several days. The pain of chronic pancreatitis may be constant and daily, indefinite or occasional, intermittent or absent altogether.

Pancreatic insufficiency (the failure to produce enzymes necessary for digestion and absorption of nutrients) results in weight loss, pale-colored stools (these are fat-containing stools, a condition called steatorrhea), and other signs of malabsorption. In addition, with severe scarring of the pancreas, diabetes mellitus (see page 707) may develop.

Apart from steatorrhea, the key sign of chronic pancreatitis is small, hard deposits that form in the pancreatic duct or tissue. This condition is called pancreatic calcification and can be seen on an x-ray. Alcohol-induced pancreatitis is a common cause of this kind of calcification. Obviously, excessive drinking should be avoided, but even moderate but consistent social drinking over the years may produce significant pancreatic calcification.

The Diagnosis. To confirm the diagnosis of chronic pancreatitis, your physician will take a sample of your blood and your stool. Patients with chronic pancreatitis often have a high fat content in their feces because fat is not being absorbed by the intestine. The analysis of your blood may not show the same high levels of certain enzymes characteristic of acute pancreatitis, but your physician will look for other blood abnormalities associated with chronic pancreatitis.

Your physician may have you undergo endoscopic retrograde cholangiopancreatography (ERCP; see X-Raying the Bile and Pancreatic Ducts, page 664) to look for evidence of an obstruction of the pancreatic or common bile duct. Your physician also may inject a solution to stimulate the pancreas and then measure the gland's ability to discharge secretions into the duodenum. Called a stimulation test, this is important in determining whether your pancreas is the cause of your malabsorption of nutrients and weight loss.

Treatment. The therapy for chronic pancreatitis usually centers on two problems: pain and malabsorption.

Medication. If you have intermittent pain, you may be given a pain reliever (analgesic). It is important to use only as much analgesic as is really necessary, in order to avoid becoming addicted to the medication.

In addition, your problem of malabsorption may be treated with pancreatic replacement therapy. This therapy requires that you take an enzyme preparation with every meal. This preparation replaces the enzymes that are not being secreted into the duodenum by your pancreas. Generally, eight tablets with meals are prescribed (two after eating a few bites, four during the meal, and two at completion of the meal). Three such tablets may be taken with snacks.

Diet. You may be told to avoid fatty foods and alcohol.

Surgery. If the pain cannot be relieved by drugs, surgery may be necessary to remove the damaged pancreatic tissue or to deaden nerves that are transmitting the pain.

MALIGNANT PANCREATIC TUMORS

Signs and Symptoms
- Abdominal pain that may radiate to the back;
- Lack of appetite and weight loss;
- Jaundice (yellowing of the skin and eyes);
- Itching (pruritus);
- Nausea and vomiting;
- Intestinal bleeding.

Cancer of the pancreas ranks just behind lung cancer, colon cancer, and breast cancer as the most common cause of death by cancer. It is more common among men, and men between the ages of 60 and 70 are most at risk. The cause of pancreatic cancer is unknown.

The most common symptoms are weight loss, abdominal pain, and jaundice. Weight loss, the causes of which are not fully understood, usually is significant. The average loss is about 25 pounds. Jaundice occurs if the cancer blocks the common bile duct.

The Diagnosis. If you have an unexplained loss of more than 10 percent of your normal body weight and upper abdominal pain with unexplained back pain, see your physician. Among other things, your physician will be looking for signs of an enlarged liver and abdominal tenderness.

If pancreatic cancer is suspected, he or she may order an ultrasound (see page 1287) or CT scan (see page 1286). Your physician also may arrange for endoscopic retrograde cholangiopancreatography (ERCP; see X-Raying the Bile and Pancreatic Ducts, page 664). A biopsy of the pancreas may be done by using the ultrasound or CT scan for guidance to obtain tissue for examination under a microscope. At times, surgical exploration may be required to make the diagnosis.

How Serious Is Pancreatic Cancer? The survival rate with pancreatic cancer is poor. By the time the malignant tumor is identified, it often has spread (metastasized) to other parts of the body. The median survival

Illustration shows cancer of the pancreas. Computed tomography (CT) scan (inset) is cross-sectional image of body, revealing large, malignant tumor in pancreas (black arrow) that has spread (metastasized) to the liver (white arrow).

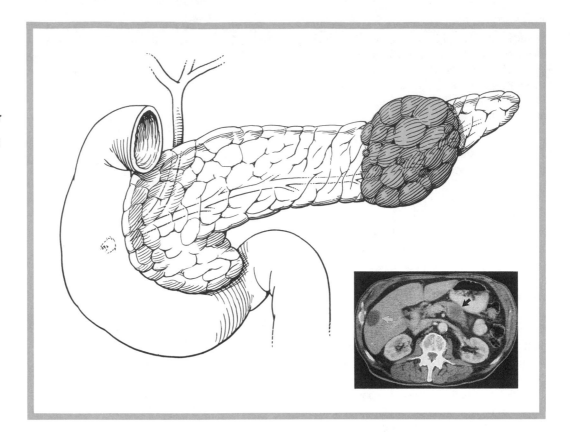

is little more than 6 months from the time of diagnosis.

Treatment. *Surgery.* Surgical removal of the tumor often is required. However, at the time of operation, your surgeon may not be able to remove the tumor, either because it has invaded vital structures that cannot be removed or because it has spread to distant sites.

Your surgeon may elect to bypass a portion of the intestine if he or she is concerned that the tumor may be causing an obstruction in this area. In addition, if you have jaundice, he or she may also bypass the area of obstruction in the common bile duct.

Other Therapies. If it is judged impossible to remove the tumor, your physician may advise an ERCP (see page 664) to insert a thin, hollow tube (stent) to relieve the obstruction and allow the resumption of bile flow into the small bowel.

Chemotherapy may be considered. Pain can be relieved with strong analgesics or by destruction of nerves that lead to the pancreas (celiac ganglionic block). Pancreatic enzymes can reduce malabsorption and weight loss.

CONGENITAL PANCREATIC ABNORMALITIES

Annular Pancreas. An annular pancreas is a ring-shaped formation of pancreatic tissue that grows around the duodenum and may cause intestinal obstruction. Annular pancreas occurs in both children and adults.

This pancreatic abnormality will make you feel exceptionally full after meals, and later you may have pain in the pit of your stomach that might bring on nausea and vomiting. Because the symptoms are mild and tolerable, many people go for years before this condition is properly diagnosed.

Your physician will consider other possible disorders in evaluating your condition because people with an annular pancreas often have complications such as pancreatitis (see page 668) and peptic ulcer (see page 603). The potential for these complications makes it necessary that the problem be corrected surgically once it has been diagnosed.

Pancreas Divisum. This is a congenital defect in which parts of the pancreas fail to grow together. In this event, the pancreas must drain its secretions through a smaller secondary duct which cannot accept the total pancreatic secretion. What may result is a partial obstruction that causes pain and a possible inflammation of the pancreas (see Acute Pancreatitis, page 667); however, at other times this condition may have no apparent symptoms.

Pancreas divisum is suspected in someone who regularly has pancreatitis without any apparent cause or who has pancreatitis after drinking only a small amount of alcohol. It is still somewhat controversial, however, as to whether pancreas divisum is the cause of pancreatitis.

HERNIAS

In the popular mind, a hernia is most often thought to be the result of heavy lifting and the hernia sufferer to be a man who has lifted too much. In fact, hernias often have no apparent cause; anyone—even a newborn baby—can have one.

Our internal abdominal organs are held in place by a thin sheet of muscle. If any part of an organ projects or protrudes through a weak point or tear in that muscular wall, it is considered to be a hernia. Below we discuss the various types of hernias and the method of repair.

TYPES OF HERNIAS

Signs and Symptoms
• Discomfort while bending over or lifting;
• Tender lump in the groin.

There are three types of hernias that commonly affect the general area of the abdomen: inguinal, femoral, and umbilical. Another hernia, called a hiatal hernia, is a protrusion of part of the stomach through the esophageal opening of the diaphragm (see page 594). If the blood supply to the loop of trapped intestine is cut off, it is said to have become strangulated.

Inguinal Hernia. In men, a hernia commonly develops at the point where the spermatic cord that suspends the testis passes out of the abdomen into the scrotum. If the ring of tissue around this opening (the external inguinal ring) becomes weakened, part of the intestine may push through, producing a noticeable bulge in the groin area. This is a direct inguinal hernia (inguinal refers to the groin).

A loop of intestine that passes out of the abdomen and follows the course of the spermatic cord down into the scrotum is an indirect inguinal hernia. This hernia can be very painful and cause the scrotum to swell. Both indirect and direct inguinal hernias probably account for four of every five hernias in men. Less often, an inguinal hernia can develop in a woman at the point where the connective tissue binding the uterus exits from the abdomen to join with the tissue surrounding the vaginal opening.

Femoral Hernia. In women, especially overweight or pregnant women, a hernia develops more often in the upper part of the thigh. This is a femoral hernia and it forms along the canal that carries the principal blood vessels (femoral artery) into the thigh (the femur is the thigh bone). This hernia usually produces a bulge that is slightly

An inguinal hernia occurs commonly in men at the point where the spermatic cord that suspends the testes passes out of the abdomen into the scrotum.

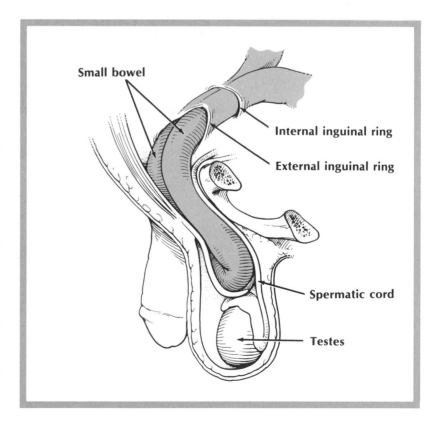

Small bowel

Internal inguinal ring

External inguinal ring

Spermatic cord

Testes

HERNIA SURGERY

Surgery is the preferred treatment for most abdominal hernias, with the exception of an umbilical hernia in an infant (a condition that occurs as a result of incomplete development of the abdominal wall), which usually corrects itself in a year or two.

The Procedure

Hernia surgery is relatively simple. It consists of pushing the protruding intestine back into the abdomen and then surgically repairing the weakened or torn muscle or tissue to prevent the intestine from breaking through again.

Surgery may be postponed if you have a cold and cough because the spasmodic pressure in the abdomen may weaken the incision before it can heal properly.

Before the operation you will be given an anesthetic—local, spinal, or general, depending on the type and severity of the hernia. A small incision is then made in the groin and the herniated tissue is returned to the abdominal cavity. If the herniated intestine is strangulated and gangrenous, that section of the intestine will be removed (resected) and the nongangrenous ends will be sutured together. The operation is concluded by closing the defect in the tissue or muscle of the abdominal wall. The operation usually takes less than an hour.

Your surgeon may elect to strengthen a weakened abdominal wall with a prosthetic or synthetic material (such as Dacron or Gore-Tex). At times this operation can be done as outpatient surgery.

The Recovery

After the operation you will be urged to move about as soon as you are able, usually within the first day. You will be permitted to eat whatever food and liquids agree with you. However, if you notice any redness or discomfort around the site of the incision, report it to your physician. It may be a sign of an infection.

---

lower than where an inguinal hernia usually appears. A femoral hernia is more likely to become strangulated than is any other type of hernia.

Paraumbilical Hernia. A far less common type of hernia is the paraumbilical hernia. In this instance, a bulge appears at the navel because of a weakness in the abdominal wall surrounding the umbilicus. Some newborn children are found to have a similar problem, called umbilical hernia, because part of their bowel has remained within the umbilical cord rather than returning to the abdominal cavity (see page 19). These hernias often are without symptoms (asymptomatic).

Incisional Hernia. A surgical incision in the abdominal wall that did not heal properly can produce a hernia. Such hernias usually pose a relatively small risk of causing any problems although, at times, portions of your intestine may exit (prolapse) through the hernia and cause discomfort.

The Diagnosis. Your physician will look for evidence of a hernia if you report abdominal pain or a bulge in your groin when straining. If the bulge persists and is accompanied by nausea and vomiting, the hernia may have become obstructed or strangulated. Many minor hernias are uncovered during routine physical examinations.

How Serious Is a Hernia? A hernia that cannot be forced back into the abdominal wall by application of pressure is possibly trapped or strangulated. Without treatment, the strangulated or pinched section of the intestine dies because it cannot get any oxygen through the flow of fresh blood. The result can be gangrene, a life-threatening condition requiring immediate surgical attention.

Treatment. *Surgery.* The best treatment for most hernias is an operation in which the intestine is pushed back into the abdomen and the weakened muscles in the abdominal wall are sewn together. After surgery, it will be about a month before you will be able to return to any strenuous activities.

Other Therapies. Wearing a corset or truss is not an acceptable form of treatment for a hernia. Your physician may have you wear one prior to operation as a precaution against the problem growing worse. But this is not a permanent solution.

CHAPTER 25

THE EARS, NOSE, AND THROAT

CHAPTER CONTENTS

Despite the small areas they occupy, the ears, nose, and throat are responsible for a remarkable number of functions. The ear and its associated nerve mechanisms enable us to hear and to keep our balance. The nose makes it possible for us to inhale air and filter it and also, simultaneously, to smell our surroundings. The throat enables us to eat and drink, to speak, and even to sing.

The ear, nose, and throat are interrelated in their functions and in the disorders that affect them. An infection of the throat or nose can spread to the ear. A cold or hay fever may affect nose, throat, and ears. So it is not surprising that the ears, nose, and throat all are treated by the same specialist who is known as an otorhinolaryngologist (from the Latin terms for ear, nose, and throat). This medical discipline, known as ENT, is a subspecialty of surgery. Otologists are otorhinolaryngologists who are specifically interested in the ear.

ANATOMY

THE EAR

The two main responsibilities of the ear are hearing and balance. The ear has three parts: outer ear, middle ear, and inner ear. The outer ear, the part that we see, is composed of the pinna or auricle (the folds of skin and cartilage that we usually refer to as the ear) and the outer ear canal which delivers sound to the middle ear. Within the outer ear canal are wax-producing glands and hairs that protect the middle ear.

STRUCTURES OF THE EAR

Hammer (malleus), Anvil (incus), Stirrup (stapes), Eardrum, Outer ear, Middle ear, Inner ear, Semicircular canals, Cochlea, Eardrum, Middle ear cavity, Outer ear canal, Eustachian tube

The function of the middle ear is to deliver sound to the inner ear where it is processed into a signal that our brain recognizes. The middle ear is a small cavity with the eardrum (tympanic membrane) on one side and the entrance to the inner ear on the other. Within the middle ear are three small bones known as the hammer (malleus), anvil (incus), and stirrup (stapes) because of their shapes. These bones act like a system of angular levers to conduct sound vibrations into the inner ear. The hammer is attached to the lining of the eardrum, the anvil is attached to the hammer, and the stirrup links the anvil to the oval window, the opening to the inner ear.

The middle ear is connected by a narrow channel, the eustachian tube, to the throat. Ordinarily, the eustachian tube is closed but when we swallow or yawn it opens briefly to allow an exchange of air, thus equalizing the air pressure within the middle ear and the air pressure outside.

The inner ear contains the most important parts of the hearing mechanism—two chambers called the vestibular labyrinth and the cochlea. The vestibular labyrinth consists of elaborately formed canals (three semicircular tubes that connect to one another) which are largely responsible for our sense of balance. The cochlea, which begins at the oval window, curves into a shape that resembles a snail shell. The curves of the cochlea are lined with tiny hairs. Both the labyrinth and cochlea are filled with fluid.

When sound waves from the world outside strike the eardrum, it vibrates. These vibrations from the eardrum pass through the bones of the middle ear and into the inner ear through the oval window. They then are disseminated into the cochlea where they are converted into electrical impulses and are transmitted to the brain by the auditory nerve.

THE NOSE

The nose is the gateway to the respiratory system. Air that enters the nasal passage runs along the top of the palate (the structure that separates your nose from your mouth). As you inhale, the air passes through to the intersection of your mouth and throat and continues its journey to the rest of your respiratory system (see page 914).

Your nose is divided into two identical chambers, the nostrils, which are separated by a partition composed of cartilage and bone and covered by a layer of mucous membrane. This wall is known as the septum. Thin pieces of bone, called turbinates, covered by mucous membrane curve in from the outer part of the nose toward the septum and act as baffles in the nasal passage. The nasal passage is also connected to the sinuses, air-filled cavities in the skull. The adenoids are aggregations of tissue in the very back of the nasal passage.

Inside the front of your nose are protective hairs that filter the air you breathe. The main cavity of your nose is lined with a mucous membrane that warms and moistens the air.

In addition to warming and filtering air, the nose is responsible for your sense of smell and, to a large degree, for your sense of taste. In fact, most of your ability to taste depends on your sense of smell. Smell begins with the olfactory nerve which is found in the upper portion of the nose. This nerve contains very fine, sensitive fibers that transmit signals to the olfactory bulb, a structure located at the front of the brain, just behind the nose.

THE THROAT

The throat (pharynx) is part of the system that delivers air to the lungs, food and drink to the stomach, and sounds from the vocal cords to the mouth. Each time you inhale, air passes through the throat on its way to the windpipe (trachea) and lungs. When you swallow food, the muscles at the top of the throat help move the food from the mouth to the esophagus on its way to the stomach.

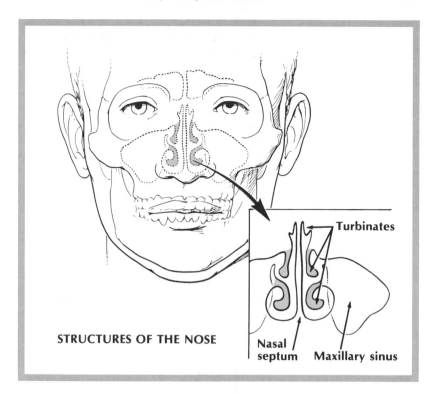

STRUCTURES OF THE NOSE

Turbinates

Nasal septum   Maxillary sinus

Several organs are located in the throat. The voice box (larynx) in the trachea contains the vocal cords which are responsible for most of the sounds of speech (when you speak, the throat also helps you shape the sounds you make). The tonsils are on both sides of the back of the mouth along with the adenoids; these structures help protect children from infections. The epiglottis acts as a sort of lid for the trachea, closing when you swallow in order to keep water and food from entering the windpipe.

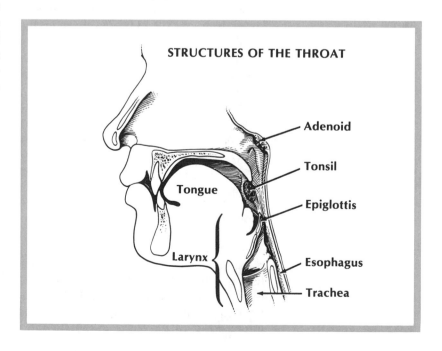

STRUCTURES OF THE THROAT

Adenoid

Tonsil

Tongue

Epiglottis

Larynx

Esophagus

Trachea

DISORDERS OF THE EAR

The ear is a biological marvel. It transfers sound waves from the air through elaborate channels into the inner ear and turns them into signals that the brain can interpret. The complex mechanisms, particularly in the middle and inner ear canals, allow us not only to hear but also to keep our balance.

The ears are connected with the nose and throat through the eustachian tube. The middle ear is linked to the mastoid, a honeycomb- or sponge-like part of the skull. Therefore, an infection in the middle ear can extend into the mastoid. This complexity makes the ear susceptible to infections, congenital disorders, and damage due to accident or occupational exposure.

SWIMMER'S EAR

Signs and Symptoms
- Itching of the outer ear canal;
- Pain in the ear;
- Oozing of yellowish or yellowish green, foul-smelling pus from the ear;
- Pain in the ear produced by movement of the head;
- Hearing loss.

Swimmer's ear (external otitis) is a state of persistent irritation and inflammation of the outer ear canal. An infection also may be present. Eczema, the scaly shedding of skin layers (see page 1155), develops in the canal. The skin breaks, often as a result of scratching the itch of the eczema, and bacteria and fungi invade the tissues of the ear canal.

Swimming in polluted water is only one way to contract external otitis. It also may develop after attempts to clear wax from the canal, by using hairpins or similar "tools," have caused irritation and itching or tears in the skin. This, in turn, may lead to more manipulation with one's favorite "tool"; an added risk is that such instruments can perforate the eardrum. Hair spray and hair dyes also can irritate the ear canal.

External otitis occasionally is caused by a fungus, usually *Aspergillus niger*. The symptoms are the same as for furunculosis, a condition of recurring boils (see page 1174). In furunculosis a hair follicle in the ear canal

becomes infected. People who have furunculosis tend to experience it repeatedly.

External otitis occurs most commonly in young adults.

The Diagnosis.   If you experience ear itching, flaking skin inside the ear, or a pain in the ear canal, you may have external otitis. Yellowish or yellowish green pus often oozes from the ear, and sometimes this oozing seems to relieve the pain. Occasionally, hearing will be affected if the pus or swelling blocks the ear canal.

A physician diagnoses the presence of external otitis by using an otoscope, a hand-held instrument that allows examination of the ear canal. If pus is present, a sample may be taken for laboratory analysis.

While most outer ear infections are bothersome, they are not usually dangerous to general health if treated properly. Left untreated, particularly in diabetic persons, this infection can spread and damage underlying bones and cartilage.

Treatment.   If you suspect that you have swimmer's ear, there are some things you can do to relieve the pain before you see your physician. Placing a warm (not hot) electric heating pad over your ear may help, as will taking aspirin or another analgesic.

After the diagnosis is made, your physician probably will clean the ear canal with a suction device or a cotton-tipped probe. This will help relieve irritation and pain. The physician then will prescribe treatment by one of various methods.

Often, eardrops containing a corticosteroid preparation (to relieve itching and decrease inflammation) and an antibiotic (to control infection) are prescribed (see page 1233). Occasionally, drugs that are taken orally will be prescribed. A painkiller may be prescribed for severe pain. Take care that no water gets into the ear while the condition is healing.

If the external otitis shows no marked improvement after 3 or 4 days, your physician may prescribe an antibiotic to be taken orally. The drug can be selected specifically for the organism causing the infection if the organism is identified by a laboratory test. External otitis caused by a fungus is often treated with a dusting of sulfanilamide powder. Furunculosis is treated with antibiotics, taken either by mouth or as eardrops.

The condition may recur a number of times over a period of months, especially if it is caused by a fungus.

Prevention.   External otitis often can be prevented. Avoid swimming in polluted water. Dry your ears after bathing and swimming, because moisture in your ear canal can make it susceptible to infection. Place balls of lamb's wool, which repels water, in your ears while applying hair spray or hair dye.

BENIGN CYSTS AND TUMORS

Signs and Symptoms
- A lump in the ear canal or in front or behind the ear;
- Accumulation of wax;
- Discomfort in the ear;
- Hearing loss.

Sebaceous cysts are thick sacs filled with cheesy material produced by skin glands. One of the common sites for their development is behind the ear or in the scalp. Sebaceous cysts are benign and usually are not even noticeable.

Benign tumors of the ear canal (exostoses) that are caused by an overgrowth of bone also may occur. Such tumors can grow large enough to block the ear canal and thus trap wax and interfere with hearing. Such exostoses grow very slowly, however, and often present no problem.

The Diagnosis.   Frequently you are not aware that you have a cyst. You may feel a semi-soft lump on the mastoid (the bony protrusion behind the ear) or in front of the ear. Such cysts outside the ear rarely cause any sort of discomfort, although they can become infected. If such a cyst becomes sore, a visit to your physician is in order, and treatment with an antibiotic is likely to be prescribed.

In the case of benign tumor, people are often unaware they have one, and the bony or wart-like growth usually poses no problem. Occasionally, however, such a growth may partially obstruct the ear canal. If your ear hurts or you experience hearing loss, consult your physician. Your physician will examine your ear canal with an otoscope, which allows full viewing of the outer canal.

Treatment.   When a benign tumor grows enough to block the outer ear canal, your physician will recommend that it be removed surgically. The procedure is a minor operation but is tricky in that the skin covering the exostosis must be left intact because it is more resistant to infection than the skin that would grow in its place. Benign cysts and tumors pose no general health problem.

FOREIGN OBJECTS IN THE EAR

Signs and Symptoms
- Pain in the ear;
- Hearing loss;
- Sensation of something present in the ear.

The assortment of objects that physicians remove from ears is astonishing—from marbles, tiny toys, and jewelry to insects, seeds, bits of paper and plastic, and even earplugs. Because of the complicated structure of the ear, any small object that a person puts into the ear can become lodged there.

The Diagnosis.   Usually, you know when something has gotten stuck in your ear. Your ear hurts or feels full, and your hearing may be affected. The problem can be a little harder to diagnose when a small child is affected. Ask the child if the ear hurts and if he or she was playing with any small objects. Look into the ear for a foreign body. If you do see the object, *do not try to remove it.* Your efforts can damage the delicate tissues of the ear or may force the object deeper. See your physician or go to a hospital emergency room for treatment.

How Serious Are Foreign Objects in Ears?
Most foreign objects do not cause a lasting problem. However, if an object is pushed into the eardrum, the eardrum may rupture and the middle ear may be damaged, a potentially serious situation.

Treatment.   After examining the ear, perhaps with an instrument that allows full viewing of the ear canal, the physician will remove the object by using a tiny tool called alligator forceps. Sometimes, gentle suction is used to withdraw the object or the ear is flooded with fluid to flush the object out. If the object is an insect that is still alive, you can try adding a few drops of mineral oil to the ear to immobilize the insect. This may decrease the discomfort until you get to a physician.

RUPTURED OR PERFORATED EARDRUM

Signs and Symptoms
- Earache;
- Partial hearing loss;
- Slight bleeding or discharge from the ear.

One reason for the advice that you should never put anything into your ear is the risk of breaking the eardrum. Sometimes the eardrum is punctured when a person cleans or scratches the ear with cotton-tipped swabs or with a small, sharp object. Other causes of puncture of the eardrum are a slap on the ear and explosions; both of these produce a sudden change in the air pressure in the ear.

An infection of the middle ear (otitis media, see page 680) may cause inflammation and even destruction of part of the eardrum. This is the most common cause of a hole in an eardrum. Small holes may heal, but larger ones stay open and permit infectious agents to enter the middle ear.

Pain in the ear, hearing loss, and a discharge from the ear may indicate a rupture (perforation) of the eardrum (tympanic membrane).

The Diagnosis.   If you experience increasing pain and hearing loss in your ear over a period of a day or so followed by a discharge of blood or fluid (with subsequent relief of the pain), you may have a ruptured

eardrum as a consequence of otitis media. See a physician promptly.

Your physician will examine the ear with an otoscope, an instrument that allows full viewing of the ear canal. If the eardrum is punctured, the physician will see the torn area or the bones of the middle ear behind it.

How Serious Is a Ruptured Eardrum?
Ruptured eardrum can be a painful condition, particularly at first. Sometimes the rupture heals by itself without complications and with little or no permanent hearing loss. Larger perforations may cause recurring otitis media.

Treatment.   If you suspect that you have ruptured an eardrum, see your physician as soon as possible. In the meantime you can relieve the pain with aspirin or other analgesic drugs. Placing a warm (not hot) electric heating pad over the ear will help also.

Your physician may prescribe an antibiotic to make sure that no infection develops in your middle ear. Sometimes a plastic or paper patch is placed over the eardrum to seal the opening while it heals. Also, keep your ear dry until the eardrum heals.

The eardrum will often heal within 2 months. If it has not healed in that time, your physician may recommend a minor surgical procedure to repair the tear.

OCCUPATIONAL HEARING LOSS

Signs and Symptoms
- Progressive hearing loss.

The human ear can be damaged by prolonged exposure to noise at 90 decibels (db) or louder. The intense vibration caused by the loud sound waves damages the hair cells that line the cochlea of the inner ear. This kind of damage causes a condition known as sensorineural hearing loss because it affects the workings of the inner ear. Sensorineural hearing loss usually cannot be corrected.

The noise level of normal conversation typically is about 60 db; the level in a noisy restaurant is nearer 70 db. Other noise levels are about 90 db for the sound of a large diesel truck about 5 yards away, 120 db for a jackhammer at work 3 feet away, and perhaps 130 db for a jet engine 100 feet away.

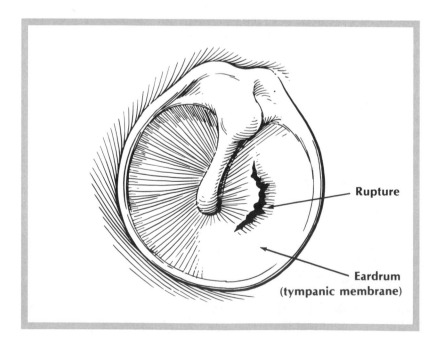

Rupture

Eardrum
(tympanic membrane)

NOISE AND SOUND LEVELS

The ear interprets waves of varying air pressure as sound. These waves, composed of alternating peaks of high pressure and troughs of low pressure, can produce sounds that are loud or soft and of high or low pitch. When these sounds become unpleasant or interfere with other activities, we call them noise.

The loudness of sound is measured in units called decibels (db). Soft sounds are barely audible; very loud ones can cause pain in the ear. Between these levels is the range of sounds that we are exposed to on a regular basis.

We take for granted most of the everyday sounds we hear. Only when they interfere with what we are doing do we notice noise as a problem. Loud noise such as a heavy truck passing by is annoying, but after it is gone we think no more about it. However, very loud noise, such as the continuous operation of a nearby jackhammer, chainsaw, or other tool, can cause pain and ringing in the ears.

As a rule, if you have to shout to make yourself heard, the noise can damage your hearing. Under such conditions, decrease the noise, leave the area, or wear ear protectors. The following charts show the average decibel levels for certain activities and the maximum job noise exposure per day allowed by law.

Maximum Job Noise Exposure Allowed by Law

Duration, Hours per Day	Sound Level, Decibels
8	90
6	92
4	95
3	97
2	100
1½	102
1	105
30 min	110
15 min	115

Sound Levels of Common Noises

Decibels	Noise
	Safe range
20	Watch ticking; leaves rustling
40	Quiet street noise
60	Normal conversation; bird song
80	Heavy traffic
	Risk range
85–90	Motorcycle; snowmobile
80–100	Rock concert
	Injury range
120	Jackhammer 3 feet away
130	Jet engine 100 feet away
140	Shotgun blast

HOW TO PROTECT YOUR EARS

You cannot control the world around you, but you can take steps to protect your ears from unnecessary damage. If you work with or near heavy machinery or are bombarded by other loud or continuous noise, you are at risk of developing sensorineural hearing loss. Because this kind of loss generally is irreversible, it is very important to prevent it. Use the following strategies if you are at risk of hearing loss.

Wear Protective Plugs or Earmuffs in the Workplace
Proven methods include protecting your ears with specially designed earmuffs that resemble earphones. These bring most loud sounds down to acceptable levels. They can close out the outside world, or they can be fitted with miniature speakers and a microphone so that you can communicate with others. Commercially available or custom-molded earplugs made of plastic or rubber effectively protect against excessive noise. Cotton balls are not adequate and can become lodged deep in the ear canal (see Foreign Objects in the Ear, page 677).

Have Your Hearing Tested
Do this regularly if you work in a noisy environment. Early detection of hearing loss will allow you to take precautions to prevent further damage. Your employer may be responsible for providing ear protection. Ask about the kind of protection the company provides.

Beware of Recreational Risks
Sensorineural hearing loss related to recreation is becoming more common. Activities with the greatest risk are trapshooting, driving snowmobiles and some other recreational vehicles, and, in particular, listening to extremely loud music. Music noise can be a factor beyond attending too many rock concerts or cranking up the stereo so that it shakes the walls. Many people now use earphones to listen to music, often from small portable tape cassettes or radios that, despite their small size, can produce extremely high sound levels.

Protect your ears from loud music by turning down the volume on the stereo or tape player. If you attend rock concerts, wear earplugs.

The roar of a subway train also can damage your ears. Again, wearing earplugs or even covering your ears with your hands can help protect you.

Thus it is not surprising that some jobs carry the risk of hearing loss.

Noisy work in heavy construction is a common cause of hearing loss. Airline ground crew members who refuse ear protection are at high risk, as are farm tractor operators. Rock musicians are at great risk, too, and so are the people who listen to rock music played very loud.

The Diagnosis. If you notice that your hearing has become less sensitive, see an ear, nose, and throat specialist and an audiologist. The physician will examine your ears, and the audiologist will perform a series of tests to determine the nature of your hearing loss. From these examinations, a proper course of action can be recommended.

Treatment. If your hearing loss appears to be the result of an occupational hazard, wear proper protective equipment to prevent further deterioration of your hearing (see How To Protect Your Ears, page 679).

If your hearing loss is causing problems in communicating, your physician or audiologist may have suggestions to help you overcome the difficulties. This may include use of a hearing aid (see page 686).

BAROTRAUMA

Signs and Symptoms
- Moderate to severe pain in the ear;
- Stuffy feeling in the ear;
- Slight hearing loss;
- Dizziness;
- Tinnitus (noise in ear).

The air pressure in the middle ear usually is the same as that in the outer ear, because of the eustachian tube. This tube is a narrow channel that connects the middle ear to the back of the nose. When you swallow or yawn, it opens and allows air to flow into or out of the middle ear.

If the eustachian tube is blocked, differences in pressure can occur between the two sides of the eardrum. This condition is known as barotrauma or barotitis media.

The Diagnosis. If you fly or scuba dive while you have a congested nose (allergy, cold, or throat infection), you may experience the symptoms of barotrauma. Pain in one ear, slight hearing loss, or a stuffy feeling in the ears may be caused by the eardrum's pressing inward as a result of a change in air pressure.

A more serious problem can occur if the air pressure change is great or if the eustachian tube is entirely blocked. The small capillaries of the middle ear may rupture and bleed, filling the ear with blood and producing a hearing loss and a feeling similar to that of being underwater.

The symptoms of barotrauma usually disappear within a few hours after they begin. Barotrauma is not a serious condition and does not produce permanent hearing loss. However, if you think you have barotrauma consult your physician, who will examine your ear and monitor your condition to help prevent an infection.

Treatment. If you must fly when you have a congested nose, try taking a decongestant or antihistamine an hour before takeoff and an hour before landing. This may prevent blockage of the eustachian tube. During the flight, suck candy or chew gum to encourage swallowing, which helps keep the eustachian tube open. Another way to open the eustachian tube is to inhale and then gently exhale while you hold your nostrils closed and keep your mouth shut.

If the symptoms do not disappear within a few hours, see your physician. The treatment may involve a surgical incision in the eardrum (myringotomy) and removal of the fluid that is there. Your physician also may prescribe a course of antibiotics to prevent infection within the middle ear.

ACUTE EAR INFECTION

Signs and Symptoms
- Feeling of fullness in the ear;
- Severe earache;
- Fever and chills;
- Nausea and diarrhea;
- Hearing loss.

Acute ear infection (otitis media) occurs in four basic forms: serous otitis media, otitis media with effusion, acute purulent otitis media, and secretory otitis media. In the mildest form, serous otitis media, fluid gathers in the middle ear as a result of blockage of the eustachian tube or excessive production of fluid in the middle ear. There may be discomfort and temporary hearing loss, but usually no infection is present.

The second form, otitis media with effusion, includes both fluid accumulation and an infection. This often develops in conjunction with an upper respiratory infection, enlarged adenoids, or both. This form of otitis can lead to the third, and most serious, form, acute purulent otitis media.

In acute purulent otitis media, pus fills the middle ear. The pressure of the pus may burst the eardrum, causing a discharge of blood and thick pus. Acute purulent otitis most often affects children. The infection can be viral or bacterial.

Occasionally, recurrent or prolonged episodes of otitis media may cause a change in the kind of cells lining the middle ear. These cells then produce a thicker fluid in great quantities. This results in secretory otitis media.

The Diagnosis. When there is a sharp continuous pain in the ear with hearing loss and fever, the chances are good that an infection of the middle ear is present. (In addition to crying often, infants tug at their ear if an ear infection is present.) See your physician without delay. If fluid or pus is visible in the ear canal, your physician may take a sample of it for culture in the laboratory to determine the kind of organism that is causing the infection.

How Serious Is Acute Otitis Media?
Serous and secretory otitis media are inconveniences but usually do not cause permanent hearing loss. If not properly treated, the more serious forms of otitis media can produce infections that can spread to the mastoid process and, on rare occasions, to the inner ear. Permanent hearing loss can result from damage to the eardrum, middle ear bones, or inner ear structures.

Treatment.   Until you see your physician, you can relieve some of the pain of acute otitis media by taking aspirin or some other analgesic and by placing a warm (not hot) heating pad over your ear.

Medication.   In the case of serous otitis media, your physician may only prescribe decongestants to improve nasal breathing and increase the flow of air into and from the middle ear through the eustachian tube. A course of antibiotics may be prescribed to

fight the infection that is present in otitis media with effusion and acute purulent otitis media. This antibiotic treatment may be extended if the infection fails to clear up.

Your physician may prescribe nasal decongestants or antihistamines if nasal congestion or nasal allergies seem to be contributing to the development of the otitis media.

Surgery.   If there is great pressure on the eardrum, a surgical incision in the eardrum (myringotomy) may be needed to relieve the pressure. In children, the myringotomy is likely to be performed in a hospital under general anesthesia. The eardrum heals within a week or two.

CHRONIC EAR INFECTION

Signs and Symptoms
- Earache;
- Periodic seeping of pus from the ear;
- Hearing loss.

Any of the forms of acute otitis media—serous, otitis media with effusion, purulent, or secretory (see page 680)—can become chronic. A chronic ear infection (chronic otitis media) can be more dangerous than an acute one because its slow, long-lasting effect can result in permanent damage. An acute infection develops suddenly and usually is treated quickly. A chronic condition may not cause enough discomfort to warrant immediate action and thus may not be noticed until it is well established.

Chronic serous otitis media occasionally can be due to a persistent swelling or inflammation of the adenoids in the very back of the nasal passage. The swelling blocks the eustachian tube. Problems with adenoids most often occur in children. When adults have the condition, it usually is the result of recurrent blockage of the eustachian tube or scarring of the eustachian tube from previous infections, nasal allergies, or masses in the back of the nose and throat.

Chronic otitis media with effusion and chronic purulent otitis are more serious. It appears that in some cases an initial acute infection never completely clears, and a low-level infection survives even after treatment. Such an infection can spread to the mastoid process, the honeycomb-like bone behind the ear. Infection in the mastoid is more difficult to eradicate.

Sometimes an initial acute infection clears up but leaves the site more vulnerable to future infections. When a chronic infection then takes hold, the pus it produces can cause perforation of the eardrum or damage to the small bones in the middle ear.

The Diagnosis.   If pus is seeping from your ear canal and there is pain in the ear or hearing loss, see your physician. He or she will examine your ear with an otoscope to identify the source of infection and also may arrange for x-rays or a CT scan (see page 1286) of your head to determine if the infection has spread to your mastoid process.

How Serious Is Chronic Otitis Media?
Chronic secretory otitis media is uncommon and, although uncomfortable and inconvenient, it rarely causes permanent harm. Left uncorrected, chronic purulent otitis media can cause permanent damage to hearing.

Treatment.   *Medication.*   Chronic secretory and serous otitis media usually are treated with antihistamines and decongestants if associated with nasal congestion or nasal allergies. Chronic otitis media with effusion and purulent otitis media usually are treated with oral antibiotics. If the eardrum is intact, eardrops are of no benefit because they cannot reach the site of the infection.

Surgery.   If the situation does not improve and adenoids are the cause of the problem, your physician may recommend surgical removal of them.

Another method for treating the problem is to insert a small plastic tube through the eardrum to allow the middle ear to drain (See The Pros and Cons of Ear Tubes in Children, this page). The ear must not become wet for the entire period of treatment, which may be several months to years. This can be difficult for anyone but is particularly so for children.

If you have chronic serous or purulent otitis media and the mastoid process becomes infected, your physician may recommend a mastoidectomy, an operation in which the mastoid process is removed surgically to prevent recurrence and spread of the infection.

THE PROS AND CONS OF EAR TUBES IN CHILDREN

One way of treating otitis media is to surgically insert a small plastic tube through the eardrum, which allows pus to drain out of the middle ear. However, discuss this procedure in detail with your ear, nose, and throat physician. Among the arguments for and against the procedure are the following points.

For the Procedure

1. The procedure usually results in a decrease in the frequency and severity of episodes of otitis media.

2. Hearing is restored.
3. The operation allows ventilation of the middle ear, thereby decreasing the risk of permanent changes in the lining of cells that might occur with prolonged infection.

Against the Procedure

1. The procedure requires brief general anesthesia, although on an outpatient basis.
2. You must avoid getting water in the ears while the tube is in place.
3. In rare cases, severe scarring or a permanent hole in the eardrum may result.

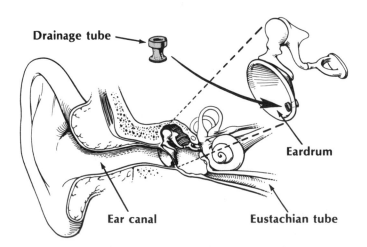

Drainage tube

Ear canal

Eardrum

Eustachian tube

In persistent cases of ear infection, your child's physician may elect to insert a small tube into the eardrum to allow drainage of pus.

CHOLESTEATOMA

Signs and Symptoms
- Hearing loss;
- Pus seeping from the ear;
- Headache or earache;
- Dizziness;
- Weakness of facial muscles.

Cholesteatoma is a disorder of the mastoid process and the middle ear. It occurs when, as a result of a blocked eustachian tube, the air pressure in the middle ear lessens and the eardrum bends inward. It can also occur when ear canal skin grows into the middle ear through a hole in the eardrum. In the middle ear, the skin cells (epithelial tissue) that would normally be shed are caught and form a cyst or tumor known as a cholesteatoma. The cholesteatoma then erodes the bone that lines the cavity and damages the small bones of the middle ear.

In some cases this is a congenital problem in which skin cells have become trapped behind the eardrum during development. When a cholesteatoma develops in the ear of a child, it may grow quickly. In adults the problem usually develops more slowly.

The Diagnosis.   Your physician will examine your ear with an otoscope, a small instrument that allows a full view of the ear canal, and also will inquire about a history of ear infections. If a cholesteatoma is suspected, you may be referred to an ear, nose, and throat specialist who will perform a more complete examination and may give you a hearing test.

How Serious Is Cholesteatoma?   A cholesteatoma is benign and will not spread to other sites. But it can cause permanent hearing loss. It can also affect the facial nerve and, in rare cases, can cause meningitis if left untreated.

Treatment.   The condition is chronic and can only be treated by surgery. If the cholesteatoma is very small, it may be removed in a minor operation. A larger or more advanced cholesteatoma may require a more extensive operation or series of operations to correct damage to the bones of the middle ear. The procedure requires meticulous care to remove every bit of the cyst. Repeat operations may be required because the cyst can grow back.

The operation also may include rebuilding of the bones of the middle ear to restore hearing. Transplanted ear bones from other people or artificial (prosthetic) devices may be used to reconstruct the middle ear.

An alternative procedure in severe cases may be to perform a radical mastoidectomy which leaves a cavity that can be cleaned out periodically. This does not restore damaged bones or lost hearing.

MASTOIDITIS

Signs and Symptoms
- Redness, swelling, and tenderness of the mastoid process behind the ear;
- Earache;
- Fever;
- Discharge of pus from the ear.

If acute otitis media is left untreated (see page 682), the infection may spread to the mastoid process, the bone that is behind the outer ear and is connected to the middle ear. When mastoiditis occurs, the infection moves from the middle ear to the mucous membrane lining the mastoid process and the honeycomb-like bones within. If the infection is severe, it can destroy this bone and may spread.

The Diagnosis.   If any of the symptoms of otitis media or mastoiditis are noted, consult your physician. Your physician will examine

HEREDITARY DEAFNESS

Deafness can be caused by inherited abnormalities. It may accompany hereditary nephritis (Alport's syndrome, see page 888), a kidney disorder that runs in families. There are numerous other forms of deafness that run in families. These include: deafness with goiter (Pendred's syndrome); deafness associated with malformation of the external ears, face, or neck; deafness associated with skin abnormalities; deafness associated with mental retardation; retinitis pigmentosa (see page 776); and peripheral neuropathy.

There also are unusual forms of deafness that are not associated with other abnormalities. These forms of deafness are not common. If one has been or is identified in your family or in your child, seek genetic counseling (see page 45). Appropriate treatment and training should be initiated for any deaf infant or child.

A mother who has rubella (see page 862) during pregnancy runs a high risk that the developing infant will also be affected. If rubella (German measles) occurs during the first 3 months of pregnancy, the child is likely to be born deaf as well as having several other serious defects such as cataracts, heart problems, and brain or nervous system impairment. Rubella occurring later in the pregnancy also can cause hearing loss but is less likely to cause some of the other defects.

Prematurity, lack of oxygen during or shortly after birth, blood incompatibilities, and meningitis can cause hearing loss early in life.

your ear, take a sample of any pus apparent in your ear canal, and may arrange for head x-rays to determine how far the infection has spread. You may be referred to an ear, nose, and throat specialist.

Before the availability of antibiotics, acute mastoiditis was a leading cause of death in children. Now, it can be treated successfully with antibiotics and is a vastly reduced health risk.

Treatment.   Your physician will prescribe antibiotics to cure the infection of the mastoid. Lack of easy drainage of infected material from the mastoid cells makes it difficult to cure this infection. High-dose antibiotic therapy often must be continued for several weeks in order to eradicate the infection. If antibiotic treatment does not solve the problem, your physician may recommend a mastoidectomy, in which part or all of the mastoid bone is removed surgically.

OTOSCLEROSIS

Signs and Symptoms
- Gradual hearing loss in one or both ears;
- Tinnitus (noise in the ear).

In a stapedectomy, the malfunctioning stirrup (stapes) of the middle ear is replaced with a tiny wire or a stainless steel prosthesis to transmit sound vibrations.

In otosclerosis, the bony wall of the inner ear becomes disorganized and an abnormal growth of spongy bone occurs at the entrance to the inner ear. The stirrup, the tiny bone that vibrates to pass sound waves into the inner ear, may become involved and become immobile, causing conductive hearing loss. Conductive hearing loss is failure of the mechanism that passes vibrations through the middle ear via its connective bones. Unlike sensorineural hearing loss (see page 678), conductive hearing loss often can be reversed.

Otosclerosis is the most frequent cause of middle ear hearing loss in young adults, affecting about 10 percent of the American population to some degree. Otosclerosis tends to run in families and is more common in women than in men. It appears more often in whites than in blacks, Native Americans, or Asians.

Symptoms usually become apparent between the ages of 15 and 35. The condition tends to be slowly progressive and can affect one or both ears. The hearing loss may be slight or pronounced. In women with otosclerosis, the rate of hearing loss may increase during pregnancy.

The Diagnosis.   If you notice that your hearing seems to be gradually decreasing, see your physician. He or she will examine your ears, conduct hearing tests, and ask if any close relative experienced early hearing loss.

How Serious Is Otosclerosis?   Otosclerosis does not endanger general health, and it often can be corrected. However, the isolation and emotional distress that deafness can cause may require difficult mental and lifestyle adjustments.

Treatment. *Surgery.*   In most cases, otosclerosis can be treated successfully by an operation called stapedectomy. This is a surgical procedure in which the skin of the ear canal is cut and the eardrum is lifted out of the way so that the stirrup (stapes) can be removed and replaced with a tiny wire or stainless steel prosthesis. The eardrum is then replaced and usually heals in a week or two. In some instances a laser may be used to create a small hole (stapedotomy) in the bottom of the stirrup (stapes) bone to allow for placement of the prosthesis.

You may experience dizziness for some hours after the operation, but that disappears. Hearing usually improves quickly, and you will be back to normal activities within a couple of weeks. Occasionally, a blood clot will form in the middle ear, which

Anvil (incus)   Stirrup (stapes)
Oval window
Hammer (malleus)   Stirrup removed
Eardrum
Ear canal   Eustachian tube   Oval window

blocks sound conduction. Such clots usually disappear within a few weeks.

Stapedectomy can help most people with otosclerosis, but 1 to 2 percent of those who undergo the procedure lose all hearing in the ear. This is a matter for consideration before proceeding with the operation. If you have otosclerosis in both ears, you might consider having one ear operated on and then waiting a year to gauge the results before having the other one done. If your inner ear is damaged, a stapedectomy may not help the problem.

Medication.   Treatment with tablets of sodium fluoride, calcium, and vitamin D is commonly used to prevent the progressive bony changes and further hearing loss by hardening the spongy bone, but there is continuing debate as to their value.

Hearing Aids.   Hearing aids are another effective means of overcoming the hearing loss associated with otosclerosis. If you have otosclerosis in one or both ears, your physician may refer you to an audiologist for fitting of a hearing aid (see page 686).

AGE-RELATED HEARING LOSS

Signs and Symptoms
- Gradual hearing loss;
- Tinnitus (noise in the ear).

Hearing impairment is common among people over age 65. Almost a third of the people in this age group have a noticeable hearing loss; some lose very little hearing, and others become quite hard of hearing.

When hearing loss is severe, it is known as presbycusis (from the Latin *presby* meaning old and *cusis* meaning hearing). Typically, it begins between ages 40 and 50 and often worsens progressively. The hearing in both ears is affected, particularly the perception of high-frequency sounds. Men are affected more commonly and more severely than women.

Presbycusis is a kind of hearing loss caused by changes in the cochlea or in nerves attached to it. Cells within the cochlea, the snail-shaped cavity in the inner ear, carry thousands of tiny hairs that convert sound vibrations into electrical signals. These signals are sent to the brain where they are interpreted as sound. When some of these hairs are damaged or other changes take place in the cochlea, the signals are not transmitted as efficiently, and a loss of hearing results.

This form of hearing loss is known as sensorineural, referring to damage in the inner ear. Hearing loss as a result of aging is permanent and cannot be reversed surgically.

The Diagnosis.   If you or a family member notices that you are hearing less well, see your physician. He or she will conduct a series of tests to determine whether the loss is sensorineural or conductive (see page 684). Often, the person affected will deny that a problem exists. Occasionally, irritating tinnitus (noise in the ear, see page 687) encourages a person to consult a physician.

Many people with presbycusis find that conversations with women and children, whose voices are of higher frequency, are more difficult to understand than those with men, whose voices are lower. You also may find that conversation in a group is more difficult to understand than conversation with someone one-to-one. Severe hearing loss is not a health threat, but it can cause isolation and be socially debilitating.

COMMUNICATING WITH A HEARING-IMPAIRED PERSON

Here are a few tips for communicating effectively with a hearing-impaired person.

- Speak at a normal conversational level if the person is wearing a hearing aid. If the person is not, speak a little louder than normal, but *do not shout*—it is irritating and unnecessary.
- Speak naturally but more slowly than you usually do. Add more pauses than normal in your speech pattern. Rapid speech is more difficult for a hearing-impaired person to follow.
- Before speaking, make sure you have the attention of your listener. If he or she is watching your face, the visual clues can help in understanding your words. Also, watch your listener's face for signs of incomprehension.
- Decrease competing background noise. Turn off the television set or stereo, and close the window to traffic noises.
- Move within 2 to 3 feet of the person you are conversing with so that your speech will be louder than most of the background noise.
- If background noise cannot be decreased, move to a quieter area to talk.

HEARING LOSS AND HEARING AIDS

An estimated 25 million Americans could benefit from using hearing aids—yet only a fifth of that number wear them regularly. Some people do not realize, or refuse to believe, that their hearing is impaired. Others are skeptical that a hearing aid would help them or feel that the cost of a hearing aid is prohibitive. Still others are wary of hearing aids because of the experience of a friend for whom a hearing aid did not work out well or who may have been taken advantage of by an unscrupulous hearing aid dealer.

Set aside your fears. Today, hearing aids are not intimidating. Current models are technologically advanced, simple to operate, and smaller than those of only a few years ago. You must shop carefully to find the hearing aid best suited to your needs but, for most kinds of hearing loss, a hearing aid can be helpful.

Get an Examination

If you suspect that you have a hearing loss, begin by seeing your physician. You may be referred to an otorhinolaryngologist (a physician specially trained in ear, nose, and throat problems) or an audiologist (a professional trained in hearing evaluation) who will conduct a complete examination and a series of hearing tests. Sometimes a hearing problem can be corrected with medical treatment or surgery, particularly if the problem is in the outer or middle ear. However, if the problem is in the inner ear, it usually is not treatable medically. A hearing aid cannot make the problem disappear, but it can improve your hearing.

The Range Is Wide

Hearing aids now are compact and capable of providing a wide range of power. Most people wear in-the-ear aids, although behind-the-ear styles are still common. Models that fit completely in the ear generally are capable of providing as much power as those that fit behind the ear. Even people with severe to profound hearing loss can use behind-the-ear models. Only rarely and in special circumstances are body-mounted hearing aids used. For those units, the earpiece is attached, by a cord, to a microphone and amplifier located in a small box that is carried in a pocket.

Children and adults with a profound hearing loss, including those with nerve deafness, may benefit from a cochlear implant. The surgeon implants an electrode into the inner ear for direct nerve stimulation. Implant recipients gain the ability to hear and recognize speech and many environmental noises. A majority show

Today's hearing aids are more versatile and less obtrusive than ever. A variety of models, including in-the-ear or behind-the-ear aids, are available.

Speech processor

Transmitter coil

Internal receiver/stimulator

Electrodes

Cochlear implant includes external and internal parts. Sounds enter microphone (not shown); speech processor codes the sounds and sends them, by means of a transmitter coil, to an internal receiver/stimulator and then on to electrodes in the inner ear (cochlea).

improved ability to understand speech when hearing through the implant is combined with lip reading. A few can understand speech without lip reading.

The cost of hearing aids varies, but if cost is a problem, check with local civic and community groups. Some have programs to help people meet this cost.

Hearing aids must be custom-fitted to ensure comfort and performance. First, a mold is made of your ear canal so that the earpiece will fit exactly and be both comfortable to wear and capable of passing sound efficiently into the ear.

When you select a hearing aid (or two hearing aids, one for each ear), make sure there is a trial period before the purchase becomes final. Such periods usually are 30 days, which should give you enough time to try the hearing aid. If the hearing aid is uncomfortable or does not seem to improve your ability to hear, ask the dealer to adjust it. If your hearing aid does not help you enough to warrant the purchase, return the unit for a refund. A rental fee may be deducted for the time you used the hearing aid.

When learning to wear the hearing aid, remember that your hearing will not return to normal. A hearing aid can only amplify the sounds around you. For this reason, it may take a bit of adjusting on your part before you feel comfortable with your hearing aid.

Most likely you will need to practice tuning out background noise. Try wearing your hearing aid in quiet surroundings at first. This will allow you to become accustomed to the "new" sounds you are hearing. Wear your hearing aid daily. Make it a part of your routine.

Treat your hearing aid carefully. Avoid exposure to chemicals, such as hair spray, or to extremes of heat or cold. Wipe the ear mold portion daily with a dry tissue. Never immerse your hearing aid in water (it is not waterproof).

If you have any doubts about a hearing aid dealer, check the credentials of the business with the Better Business Bureau. Beware of high-pressure sales techniques and "free" consultations. If for any reason you are unsatisfied with your hearing aid or hearing aid dealer, ask your otorhinolaryngologist or audiologist for additional recommendations.

Treatment.   Presbycusis cannot be treated surgically or medically. A hearing aid is the only method of treatment. Your physician will send you to an audiologist who will conduct a thorough series of tests and fit you for a hearing aid.

You may also learn certain techniques that are useful. These include lipreading, facing the speaker, decreasing background noise (for example, turning off the television set or dishwasher or shutting the window to avoid street noise), and making maximum use of nonauditory clues such as gestures and facial expressions to help understand what people are saying.

TINNITUS

Signs and Symptoms
- Noise in the ear, such as ringing, buzzing, roaring, whistling, or hissing;
- Hearing loss.

Tinnitus, the annoying sensation of noise in the ear when no sound is present, is a common complaint. It can be a symptom of almost any ear disorder as well as other diseases including cardiovascular disease and anemia. The mechanism that causes you to hear the sounds is not understood. Tinnitus is usually associated with hearing loss.

The Diagnosis.   If you hear ringing, buzzing, whistling, or other sounds when there is no apparent source of such noises, you probably have tinnitus. Such noises can be continuous or intermittent, and they can vary in loudness. They may be in synchrony with your heartbeat.

When testing for tinnitus, your physician will be looking for signs of ear disorders such as infectious diseases, ear obstructions, otosclerosis (see page 684), Meniere's disease (see below), acoustic trauma, hereditary deafness, or occupational hearing loss.

Your physician may conduct a series of tests to determine the cause of noise in your ears. Your ears may be examined and your hearing tested. A CT scan may be recommended as well.

Treatment.   Ear noise can be very annoying but is not in itself a threat to health. In some cases the cause of tinnitus can be treated easily, and the noise stops. Such is the case when ear wax, a foreign object, or mild middle ear infection is the cause. Hearing loss then is often reversed.

In many cases, however, treating the underlying cause of the symptom may or may not have an effect on the ear noise. When the tinnitus cannot be controlled by other means, one form of treatment is to cover up the unwanted sound with competing music (for example, with a clock radio at night) or, in some cases, by using a tinnitus masker (a device worn like a hearing aid that produces noise more pleasant than that in the ear). Among those whose hearing is impaired, hearing aids also help decrease ear noise while amplifying outside sounds. If you have tinnitus, you should avoid loud noises, nicotine, caffeine, and alcohol, all of which may aggravate the condition. Often, you just must learn to tolerate this annoying symptom.

ACOUSTIC TRAUMA

Signs and Symptoms
- Hearing loss;
- Tinnitus (ear noise).

Acoustic trauma is a common form of hearing loss. It is most often the result of a blow to the ear or an explosion in which the air pressure changed drastically and sud-denly, causing damage to the delicate bones and other mechanisms of the ear. It also can be caused by long exposure to loud machinery or excessively loud music (see Occupational Hearing Loss, page 678).

The Diagnosis.   Hearing loss after a nearby explosion or a blow to the ear is fairly common. The partial deafness may be accompanied by high-pitched tinnitus (ringing or other sounds in the ear). Your physician will determine what kind of hearing loss you have sustained by using a series of tests.

Treatment.   The only effective treatment for severe sensory hearing loss caused by trauma is a hearing aid (see page 686). However, other strategies can help in making the adjustment to partial deafness easier. These include the use of visual clues (like facial expressions) and lipreading.

Prevention.   If you know you will be exposed to loud noise such as that from a jackhammer at a work site, protect yourself with specially designed earmuffs. These devices block out almost all external sound and can be fitted with microphones and receivers to let the wearer communicate with others.

MENIERE'S DISEASE

Signs and Symptoms
- Severe attacks of vertigo accompanied by nausea and vomiting;
- Tinnitus (ear noise);
- Muffled or distorted hearing;
- Hearing loss.

The symptoms of Meniere's disease were described over a century ago by a Frenchman, Prosper Meniere. The typical symptoms he described included episodic vertigo with fluctuating hearing loss, a ringing in the ears (tinnitus), and a sensation of pressure in the affected ear.

Meniere's disease usually affects one ear first, and in about 25 to 50 percent of the cases it eventually affects the other ear. Its cause is not yet understood. There seems to be an increase of fluid in the part of the inner ear called the labyrinth. This excess fluid causes pressure within the membranes of the labyrinth, distorting and occasionally rupturing them. This produces severe disruption in the sense of balance and often in the sense of hearing.

The Diagnosis. Meniere's disease is marked by periodic attacks. Between attacks—periods that may range from several hours to months or even years—there are no symptoms. The attacks themselves may last from a few hours to most of a day or longer.

The symptoms may range from mild to serious but, in varying degrees, usually involve vertigo (often so severe as to cause nausea and vomiting), tinnitus (ear noise such as buzzing or ringing), and muffled or distorted hearing or hearing loss, particularly in the low frequencies. The attacks can become increasingly severe.

If you experience any of these symptoms, consult your physician without delay. Your physician will conduct a test to measure how well you hear sounds of various frequencies. If this test is inconclusive, further tests may be needed to diagnose the problem.

One such test (called electronystagmography) involves flooding the ear with cold or warm water. Normally, when this is done you feel a whirling sensation that makes your eyes flicker. This flicker is studied. The procedure is repeated with water of different temperatures. The responses to the flooding of each ear are recorded and compared with each other and with normal responses to determine if the balancing function of the inner ear is operating normally.

How Serious Is Meniere's Disease? For most people the disorder is primarily an inconvenience and they have only rare attacks. For a few, however, Meniere's disease can cause complete deafness, and the vertigo and accompanying nausea can be frequent and debilitating.

Treatment. If you experience the symptoms of Meniere's disease, lie as still as possible to ease the symptoms. When the immediate symptoms have subsided, consult your physician.

Medication. Your physician probably will prescribe medication to combat the vertigo and its accompanying nausea and vomiting. Other treatments that seem to help some people include the use of diuretics and a low-salt diet to decrease the fluids in your body. Cutting down on use of caffeine and nicotine may help. Also, avoid alcohol.

Sedatives are sometimes prescribed to relieve the severe anxiety that a serious attack can cause. It is difficult to tell when drug therapy has been useful over long periods because Meniere's disease tends to go into remission and spontaneously disappear.

Surgery. When medical treatment fails to control the frequency and severity of attacks, surgery may be recommended. The operation may involve a procedure to relieve the pressure within the inner ear and its distended inner ear membranes. Sometimes the nerve that controls balance is cut.

When hearing loss is severe or complete in the affected ear and the vertigo is very serious, a procedure in which the entire inner ear is destroyed may be recommended. The balance function is then handled by the other ear and by muscle impulses and sight.

If you have Meniere's disease in both ears, the treatment is more difficult. Surgery may be performed on the poorer of the two ears in an effort to stop the most debilitating attacks. Streptomycin, an antibiotic that is toxic to the ear, may be administered in carefully controlled amounts to disrupt the balance portion of the inner ear while preserving the hearing function.

LABYRINTHITIS

Signs and Symptoms
- Extreme vertigo (loss of balance and a sensation that either you or the room is spinning);
- Nausea and vomiting;
- Involuntary movements of the eyes.

Labyrinthitis is an infection of the labyrinth, the fluid-filled chamber of the inner ear that controls balance and hearing. The infection may be either bacterial (the result of spread from acute otitis media or purulent meningitis) or secondary to a viral meningitis (see pages 680, 527, and 528, respectively). With a bacterial infection, the hearing loss in the affected ear usually is total.

The Diagnosis. If you experience sensations such as nausea and vertigo, your eyes move slowly to one side and then flick back to their original position, and you have lost all hearing in one ear, you may have labyrinthitis. Your physician will examine your ear and ask questions including whether you recently had a middle ear infection.

The symptoms of labyrinthitis can be frightening, but the condition itself is not dangerous when treated properly.

Treatment.   Your physician will prescribe antibiotics if you have bacterial labyrinthitis. For both bacterial and viral labyrinthitis, an anti-nausea drug and a sedative also may be recommended to combat the effects of the vertigo. You will need to rest in bed for several days.

The severe symptoms of vertigo usually pass within a few days to a week. Feelings of imbalance may persist for several weeks or even months, particularly with quick movements. Recurrence of episodes of labyrinthitis is rare.

ACOUSTIC NEUROMA

Signs and Symptoms
- Mild dizziness;
- Tinnitus (ear noise);
- Hearing loss.

An acoustic neuroma is a very slow-growing benign (noncancerous) tumor of the eighth cranial nerve, usually near the point at which the nerve leaves the cranial cavity and enters the bone structures of the inner ear. Because this site is in an angle formed by some of the brain structures (cerebellum and pons) and a part of the skull, it is sometimes called an angle tumor.

The Diagnosis.   If you experience mild dizziness, loss of balance, ringing or other noises in one ear, and gradual hearing loss, you may have an acoustic neuroma. The dizziness does not occur in discrete episodes as it does in Meniere's disease.

Your physician will conduct an audiometry test and a neurological examination and likely will order x-rays or CT scans of the skull to discover if a neuroma is present.

Treatment.   Although benign in character and slow in growth, this tumor can be a serious threat because it is located within the skull adjacent to a number of vital brain structures. As it grows, it creates pressure on these structures that can damage them. The only treatment is removal by surgery.

BENIGN POSITIONAL VERTIGO

Signs and Symptoms
- Abrupt onset of vertigo (sensation that either you are spinning or the room is spinning) lasting less than a minute when you move your head to certain positions;
- Involuntary eye movements accompanying the vertigo.

This disorder is characterized by sudden, extreme vertigo when you lie on one side or another, or when you lean your head back to look at something above. Unlike other forms of vertigo, it is the position of the head, not the movement, that causes the vertigo. The problem lies in the vestibular labyrinth, the fluid-filled chamber of the inner ear that controls balance. The cause is unknown.

The Diagnosis.   If your surroundings seem to be spinning or you seem to be floating while lying on one side or another or with your head tipped back, and your eyes move from side to side involuntarily when this is happening, you may be experiencing positional vertigo. The symptoms usually decrease in less than a minute. See your physician, who may conduct a series of tests to determine what form of vertigo you have and whether your disorientation is a symptom of another disorder.

Treatment.   Positional vertigo is an inconvenience but rarely a serious problem unless you are in an occupation in which even short episodes of vertigo may be disruptive. The most common treatment is avoiding those positions or activities that cause the symptoms.

PROTRUDING EARS

Signs and Symptoms
- Ears which project out an abnormally large distance from the head.

Ears that protrude from the sides of the head are neither more efficient nor less efficient for hearing than are ears that lie flat against the head. Thus, the problem is largely cosmetic. It is fairly uncommon. The protrusion may vary from slight to extremely obvious. In some cases, such ears become the basis of an emotional problem when a sense of shame, ridicule, or unattractiveness results.

Treatment. One of the popularly held misconceptions about protruding ears is that they can be trained to grow closer to the head by taping or strapping them to the side of the head at night. While the practice may bring comfort because something is being done about the problem, it doesn't work. For people with mildly protruding ears, a change of hairstyle that calls less attention to the ears is a more effective approach to the problem.

Surgery. Protruding ears can be corrected by a simple surgical procedure. The surgeon makes an incision near the fold of skin behind the ear. A strip of skin and, in some cases, cartilage, is removed, the ear is then pulled flat against the head, and the incision is closed. The scars are hidden behind the ear. However, the procedure should not be done in children under age 4; their ears are still developing. Usually the procedure is done just prior to beginning school—to avoid teasing.

WAX BLOCKAGE

Signs and Symptoms
- Partial hearing loss;
- Ringing in an ear or ears;
- Earache;
- Sensation that ear or ears are plugged.

The outer ear canal is lined with hair follicles and glands that produce a wax called cerumen. These hairs and wax trap dust and other foreign particles to prevent them from entering the ear, thus protecting the delicate mechanisms of the ear.

Normally, the small amount of wax that is formed makes its way, over time, to the opening of the ear, where it falls out or is removed in the course of washing. New wax is produced in the canal. In some people, however, an excessive amount of wax is produced. This extra wax hardens and blocks the ear canal. Wax blockage is one of the most common causes of hearing loss among people of all ages.

The Diagnosis. If you experience progressive hearing loss over a period of a few weeks or months, if your ears feel full, if you have an earache, or if you hear constant or occasional noises such as ringing in your ears, contact your physician. The first thing he or she will do is look for signs of earwax blockage.

Treatment. There is an old but wise saying: "never put anything smaller than an elbow into your ear." The ear canal and eardrum are very delicate and can be easily damaged by poking around with instruments, including such common items as cotton-tipped swabs, bobby pins, paper clips, and twisted pieces of paper. These usually do not remove problem wax and, more importantly, can easily damage the ear canal. There are better methods for removing wax buildup.

A few drops of baby oil, mineral oil, or glycerin placed in the ear with an eyedropper generally will soften the wax in a normal ear. Use a few drops twice a day for several days. Over-the-counter preparations are available but are more expensive and often less effective.

Once the wax is well softened you can proceed to remove it in the following way. Fill a bowl with water that is about at body temperature (if the water is much cooler or warmer, this procedure may cause severe, but brief, dizziness). With your head upright, grasp the top of the ear and pull upward. With the other hand, squirt the water into the canal by using a rubber bulb syringe. Then, turn your head to allow the water to drain into a sink or bowl. You may need to flush the ear several times before the wax, usually in the form of a plug, will fall out. Dry the outer ear with a towel. A hand-held hair dryer can be used to dry any water that remains in the outer canal.

Your physician uses a similar procedure to cure wax blockage or may scoop the wax out with an instrument called a curette; sometimes, a suction device is used.

DISORDERS OF THE NOSE AND SINUSES

The nose is the main gateway to your respiratory system. Normally, the nose filters, humidifies, and warms the air as it moves from the nasal passage into the throat and lungs, 12 to 15 times a minute.

Occasionally, your nose malfunctions, as when you have a nosebleed, cold, hay fever, or sinus infection. Luckily, most disorders of the nose and sinuses are temporary or are easily cured. Even loss of smell is rarely permanent. In the following pages, we will consider the common disorders of the nose and its adjacent cavities, the sinuses.

NOSEBLEED

Signs and Symptoms
• Sudden bleeding from one nostril.

Most people experience a nosebleed at one time or another. Sometimes the cause is a hard impact on the nose, but often a nosebleed is simply the result of a cold, sinus infection, dry air, or a scab being knocked off. Sometimes there may be no apparent reason.

Among children and young adults, most nosebleeds begin on the septum, the cartilage that separates the two nasal chambers. This form of nosebleed is not serious and usually is easy to stop. The front of the septum, just inside the nostril, contains many fragile blood vessels. These vessels are easily damaged, either directly as from a blow or indirectly from crusting in the nose produced by breathing very dry air. Crusting also can be caused by a head cold or an allergy.

In older people, nosebleeds may begin on the septum or deeper in the nose. These deeper nosebleeds, which are rare, often are harder to stop.

The Diagnosis. In most cases, a nosebleed is easily stopped and there is no need for further examination. However, when the bleeding is hard to stop or occurs frequently, a visit to your physician is in order.

Your physician will examine your nose with a special instrument and light to see precisely where the problem lies. If the problem appears to be deep in the nose, your physician will look for other, more serious, problems such as a tumor in the back part of your nose.

Treatment. The common nosebleed is easy to stop by using the following steps.

First, sit up or stand—don't lie down. An upright position decreases the blood pressure in the veins of your nose, which slows the flow of blood.

Second, pinch your nose near the tip with your thumb and index finger and breathe through your mouth. Do this for 5 to 10 minutes; during this time the pressure on the bleeding septum should stop the flow of blood.

Some people apply an ice bag to the nose in an effort to constrict the blood vessels and stop the bleeding. This method is harmless but it does not help to stop the bleeding—the cold reaches the vessels on the outside of the nose, not those on the septum.

When a nosebleed is difficult to stop or occurs frequently it must be treated by a physician. The treatment may involve several steps. First, excess blood is removed with a suction device; then a medicated cotton ball is placed in the nose. The medication anesthetizes and shrinks the nasal membrane.

Cautery. If the bleeding still continues, your physician may recommend chemical or electric cautery. In this procedure, a topical anesthetic is applied to the inside of the nose and then the affected blood vessels are burned with a chemical or with a tiny electric instrument (cauterized) to promote coagulation of the blood.

If the bleeding persists after cautery, your physician will gently pack the nostril with medicated gauze. The packing, which is left in place for several days, exerts pressure on the bleeding site to stop the blood flow. When the packing is removed the vessels may be cauterized again to discourage recurrence of the bleeding.

Surgery. Nosebleeds caused by an underlying disease, such as hypertension or arteriosclerosis, or that occur far back in the nose are often the most difficult to stop. Your physician will probably recommend the help of a specialist who can place a special pack in your nasal cavity. Its placement requires a special technique and sedation, and this procedure is done in a hospital. A 2- or 3-day stay for observation will be necessary. This procedure may be uncomfortable, but it usually is effective in stopping the bleeding.

In rare instances, the standard techniques do not work and you may lose a large amount of blood. This can be dangerous and may require surgery to block the arteries that supply blood to the nosebleed site. The operation requires a hospital stay of several days.

Prevention. If you have frequent nosebleeds, you can take steps to prevent or decrease the frequency of their occurrence. Apply petroleum jelly to your nasal septum once or twice each day. Increase the humidity of the air you breathe by using a humidifier or vaporizer. Don't pick your nose, and avoid blowing your nose for several hours after a nosebleed. Blowing your nose increases pressure on the damaged vessels and can lead to another bloody nose.

Deviated septum

Your nasal septum separates your nasal chambers. A deviated septum (arrows) may be a cause of nasal obstruction.

NASAL OBSTRUCTION

Signs and Symptoms
• Inability to breathe through the nose.

Nasal obstruction is a physical blockage of the air passageways of the nose. Everyone experiences a certain amount of temporary blockage when suffering from a cold or an allergy. A real obstruction is more than a passing occurrence, however, and usually results from one of two causes: a deviated septum of the nose, or chronic use of over-the-counter nasal sprays. Nasal polyps, nasal tumors, and enlarged adenoids are other potential causes.

The septum is the cartilage and bony partition that separates the two nasal chambers. It generally is thought to divide the nose equally, but few people have a septum that runs perfectly straight. Most variations are small, but in some people the septum veers significantly to one side or the other, creating the blockage. Such deviations are most often the result of an injury such as a blow to the nose. The deviation can also cause a disposition to nosebleeds (see page 692) or sinusitis (see page 696).

The other common cause of nasal obstruction, overuse of nasal decongestant sprays, often begins when a person starts using these as a way to unblock a congested nose. However, the long-term result of frequent use of decongestants is a tendency to more congestion. A cycle results in which you use more spray more frequently to keep your nasal passages clear. This is sometimes called nose-drop addiction or rhinitis medicamentosa.

The Diagnosis. A suspicion of nasal obstruction is warranted when you find that you have trouble breathing through your nose in the absence of a cold or an allergy. When you consult your physician, he or she will examine your nose for the cause of the obstruction and will ask questions regarding possible injury, allergies, and other symptoms as well as your use of nasal sprays.

Treatment. For many people, a deviated septum poses little or no inconvenience. In this case nothing needs to be done. However, for those in whom the condition causes a blockage that makes it difficult to breathe normally, a septoplasty is the answer. Septoplasty is a surgical procedure that realigns the septum. It can be done either under local anesthesia on an outpatient basis or under general anesthesia during a brief hospital stay.

POSTNASAL DRIP

Mucus produced in your nose and sinuses travels in a thin film to the back of your throat. It serves to protect your lungs by trapping dust and other particles that are inhaled. Generally, we are unaware of this process and we swallow the mucus and the impurities it captures. Swallowing this mucus does no harm. It does not need to be spit out.

Normally, your nose and sinuses produce a cupful or more of mucus daily. However, when your nose is irritated by smoke or other irritants, the amount of mucus will increase. This extra mucus, secreted to remove more irritants, is often the cause of the discomfort commonly referred to as postnasal drip.

In a sense, mucus is nature's ointment because it helps soothe an irritated nose. You may become more conscious of it when the air is dry because then the mucus in your nose and throat may become lumpy.

A SIMPLE REMEDY FOR A RUNNY NOSE

While in the throes of a cold, who doesn't yearn for a foolproof method to cure a congested nose? Dozens of ads tout products that promise magical cures, but such products rarely match up to their billings. Even when they do decongest your nose, they may produce unpleasant side effects such as drowsiness or dry mouth.

Sometimes your nose becomes too dry, making it hurt more than the runny nose. When the remedy contains an antihistamine, the mucus in your head may thicken, becoming a better trap for virus particles that can be passed along to the ear or throat. When you have a cold, you need to keep the mucus as liquid as possible. This is one reason it is important to drink lots of fluids.

One of the best temporary remedies for a stuffy nose does not cause complications or cost money. Breathing steam can loosen the mucus and clear your head. To set up a steam source, bring a kettle or pan of water to a boil and inhale the steam for several minutes, taking care not to get so close that it scalds you. Some people like to make a tent of a towel over their heads while inhaling the steam. This method is useful for loosening the mucus in the chest, too. Similarly, people often report feeling their heads clear when they take a steaming shower.

If your blockage is caused by overuse of nose drops or sprays, the treatment is simple: stop using these medications. The condition may become worse for a while, but over a period of weeks your breathing should become more nearly normal as the ill effects of the nose drops wear off (see Beware: Nose-Drop Addiction, page 695).

If chronic nose congestion remains a problem, your physician can examine your nose and sinuses and recommend a program of therapy. You may be referred to an allergist who will conduct a series of tests to determine if you are allergic to specific elements in your environment. If an allergy is found, a course of therapy which may include antihistamines to help combat the problem may be prescribed (see page 462).

JUVENILE ANGIOFIBROMA

Signs and Symptoms
- Frequent nosebleeds.

An angiofibroma is a benign tumor of the nose that occurs at puberty in boys and, in rare instances, in girls. It may shrink on its own accord after puberty, but it can grow rapidly, producing obstruction of nasal passages and sinuses and causing frequent and often severe nosebleeds. Rarely, it may put pressure on the brain.

The Diagnosis. If juvenile angiofibroma is suspected, your physician will examine the inside of your nose for evidence of a tumor. A CT scan (see page 1286) may be conducted to determine the size and location of the tumor. If the tumor does not shrink on its own, treatment can be considered.

Treatment. Tumors that obstruct the airway or cause nosebleeds usually are removed surgically. Occasionally, a procedure called embolization may be used, either alone or just before the surgical removal. During embolization, small pellets of a glue-like substance are injected into blood vessels of the tumor. The pellets help block the blood supply to the tumor.

RHINOPHYMA

Signs and Symptoms
- Large, bulbous, ruddy appearance of the nose.

To judge from his large red nose, W. C. Fields probably had rhinophyma. An exaggeratedly large and distended nose once was thought to result from heavy drinking. Now we know that alcohol consumption has nothing to do with it. People who drink moderately and those who abstain completely can have rhinophyma.

Rhinophyma involves the upper layer of skin—the epithelium—on the nose. This skin thickens greatly, causing the nose to appear large and bulbous. The reason rhinophyma occurs is not clearly understood. Rhinophyma is not a threat to breathing or to general health.

The Diagnosis. If the skin of the nose gradually becomes excessively thick, causing the nose to take on a large, bulbous shape, rhinophyma is probably the cause.

Treatment. The only effective treatment for rhinophyma is surgery. In this procedure, the excess tissue is sliced off the outside of the nose, under general or local anesthesia in a hospital setting. The nose usually resumes its normal shape when healed.

LOSS OF SENSE OF SMELL

Signs and Symptoms
- Decreased ability to detect odors;
- Difficulty breathing through the nose.

While suffering from a head cold, most people temporarily lose their sense of smell. When it is lost without any apparent cause, however, the condition is known technically as anosmia. The latter condition occurs when an obstruction in the nose prevents odors from reaching delicate nerve fibers in the nose that lead to the olfactory area (the area of the brain dealing with smell); when the nerves in the olfactory area are damaged; when the olfactory nerves and fibers are destroyed; or when the area of the brain dealing with smell is damaged.

Obstructions are caused most often by nasal polyps, tumors, or swelling of the mucous membrane. Damage to the nerves of the olfactory area is commonly caused by viral infections (a major cause of anosmia in older adults) and chronic nose infections or allergies (see page 461). Damage to the olfactory nerves and fibers also can be due to a head injury, nasal surgery, or tumor.

Most people with anosmia can distinguish salty, sweet, sour, and bitter tastes (which

---

BEWARE: NOSE-DROP ADDICTION

Your local drugstore sells many products designed to relieve nasal congestion, including nasal sprays and nose drops. These products reach a large area of the mucous membrane directly, so they provide quick decongestion. But use them carefully and only for a limited period, if at all. They can be addicting.

Use nonprescription nasal sprays or nose drops no more than three or four times a day over a period of no more than 3 to 4 days. When used frequently over several weeks, they can have a rebound effect, causing your nose to become even more congested between applications of the medication. The result is the need for greater and more frequent doses of the spray or drops.

Prolonged use of nasal sprays and drops can cause irritation of your mucous membrane, a stinging or burning in your nose, and a chronic inflammation of the mucous membrane known as rhinitis medicamentosa.

The only way to treat the problem of nose-drop addiction is to stop using nose drops. Your nose may become more congested than ever at first, but after a few weeks the congestion should gradually wear off as the inflammation subsides. If the initial problem of congestion remains, consult an allergist or an ear, nose, and throat specialist (see Allergic Rhinitis, page 461).

---

are sensed on the tongue) but cannot distinguish more subtle flavors (sensations provided by taste and smell).

The Diagnosis. If you lose your sense of smell and you do not have a cold, consult your physician. Nasal polyps (see page 463) and chronic nasal allergy are the most common causes of anosmia. You will be checked for tumors of the nasal passages.

Most often, anosmia is an inconvenience. Occasionally it can be a symptom of a more serious condition. Rarely, people experience brief episodes during which they smell odd or foul odors. In such cases, upon finding no relevant nasal condition, your physician may refer you to a neurologist for an examination and diagnostic tests to discover if the problem is in the brain.

You may need to have a CT scan (see page 1286) to check for a brain tumor or signs of a head injury. Trauma can damage the olfactory nerves—the nerves that carry smell sensations from the nose to the brain. If you lose your sense of smell after a concussion or other head injury, the blow may be the cause of your anosmia.

Treatment.   If the cause is a nasal condition such as allergic rhinitis (hay fever) or nasal polyps, it can be treated easily, and the sense of smell is restored. Allergic rhinitis is usually treated with antihistamines; nasal polyps and tumors can be removed surgically.

When the cause is not readily apparent, as is often the case when a virus is involved, the sense of smell may return when the tissues of the olfactory area regenerate on their own.

SINUSITIS

Signs and Symptoms
- Pain about the eyes or cheeks;
- Fever;
- Difficulty breathing through the nose;
- Toothache (uncommon).

The sinuses are cavities in the bone around the nose. There are four pairs of sinuses: the frontal (in the forehead), ethmoid (between the eyes), sphenoid (deeper in the head behind the eyes), and maxillary (in the cheek bones). They are connected to the nasal cavities by small openings. Normally, air passes in and out of the sinuses and mucus drains through these openings into the nose.

Sinusitis is an infection of the lining of one or more of these cavities. Usually, when a sinus is infected, the membranes of the nose itself also swell and cause a nasal obstruction. Swelling of the membranes of the nose

may close off the opening of the sinus and thus prevent drainage of pus or mucus. Pain in the sinus may result from inflammation itself or from the pressure within the sinus that results from closure of the opening.

The infection can be bacterial, viral, or fungal. A common cold is the most frequent precipitating factor in sinusitis. Because the mucous membranes of the nose extend into and line the sinuses, a bacterial infection in the nose easily spreads into the sinuses.

Secondary infections from colds are the most common causes but not the only ones. Chronic allergic rhinitis (hay fever) can cause sinusitis because infections can easily form in the mucus present in the nose and spread to the sinuses (see page 461). A severely deviated septum can lead to sinusitis by obstructing the sinus openings. A dental abscess can extend from the root of an upper tooth to infect the sinuses (see page 567).

There are two forms of sinusitis, acute and chronic. Acute sinusitis is more common by far and usually is a bacterial infection; examples include an infection after a cold, a dental abscess, and a deviated septum.

Chronic sinusitis is most often the result of repeated or untreated acute infections. The opening of the sinus becomes narrowed or closed due to scarring from previous infections, making it difficult for the sinus to drain.

Some people never get sinusitis; others seem to get it every time they have a cold. In some it develops as a result of jumping into water so that their noses and sinuses are

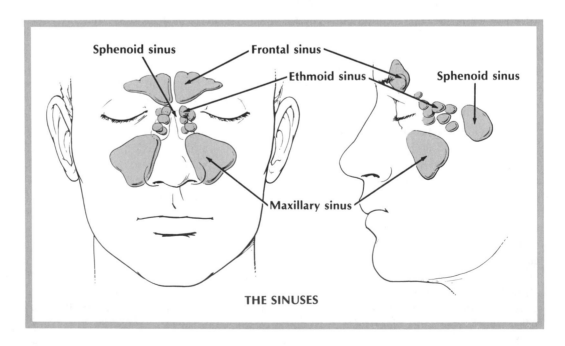

THE SINUSES

suddenly flooded. The irritation and contamination result in sinusitis.

The Diagnosis. If you experience symptoms of sinusitis, see your physician. If you have persistent sinusitis your physician may recommend x-rays or a CT scan (see page 1286) to discover how serious your infection is. A sample of the mucus or pus, if present, may be taken for laboratory analysis.

How Serious Is Sinusitis? Before the advent of antibiotics, sinus infections were known to spread into the bones of the face and occasionally into the brain. Today, sinusitis is unpleasant but it rarely is a threat to general health. If left untreated, however, sinusitis can become chronic, making it more difficult to treat.

Treatment. There are a few things you can do yourself to lessen the symptoms. Stay indoors in an even temperature. Refrain from bending over with your head down; this movement usually increases the pain. Inhale steam from a kettle or basin of boiling water (be careful not to scald yourself). Drink plenty of liquids to help dilute the secretions.

Medication. If the infection is bacterial, your physician will prescribe a course of oral antibiotic therapy lasting 10 to 14 days. Over-the-counter decongestants in the form of drops, sprays, or tablets may be taken to open the passages and encourage drainage of the sinuses. However, take care when using decongestants. They can do more harm than good by drying out your nose too much. Use them only on recommendation of your physician, and follow instructions carefully.

Surgery. Occasionally, sinusitis will persist despite medical treatment. If this happens, your physician may perform a minor surgical procedure under local anesthetic to improve the drainage. A small opening may be made in the bone between the nose and infected sinus. The sinuses are then flushed out with sterile water.

When a severely deviated septum causes recurring or chronic sinusitis, a surgical procedure to correct the deviation may be recommended.

In rare cases of stubborn, chronic sinusitis, a surgical procedure may be performed to reopen the natural openings of the sinuses or to create an artificial opening.

DISORDERS OF THE THROAT

The throat is in constant use, carrying food to the digestive tract and air to the lungs and making it possible for us to speak. With this load, it is subject to occasional problems.

Like other parts of the respiratory system, it is susceptible to infection, both bacterial and viral. Such infections occasionally are limited to the throat, as in the case of laryngitis. More commonly, they affect the entire system, as in pharyngitis or tonsillitis.

The throat also is susceptible to abuse, ranging from heavy alcohol consumption or smoking to improper use of the voice while singing or speaking. These can cause a range of problems from chronic laryngitis to growths on the vocal cords.

PHARYNGITIS

Signs and Symptoms
• Sore throat;

• Difficulty swallowing;
• Fever.

The pharynx is the segment between the tonsils and the voice box—what we commonly think of as the throat. Thus, pharyngitis is another name for a sore throat, an inflammation that can be either acute or chronic.

Acute pharyngitis is caused by a bacterium (most often, beta-streptococcus) or a virus. If caused by the beta-streptococcus bacterium, the infection is commonly called strep throat. The chronic form can be caused by a continuing infection of the sinuses, lungs, or mouth that spreads to the pharynx. Chronic pharyngitis also can be caused by constant irritation such as from smoking, breathing heavily polluted air, or consuming too much alcohol.

The Diagnosis. Your throat will be red and raw, making it difficult to swallow and sometimes even to breathe. Pus may be present. You may feel feverish. If the sore throat lasts more than a few days, consult your physician.

Your physician will examine your throat and will use a swab to take a specimen for laboratory analysis (culture) to determine if the infection is bacterial. You will also be examined for signs of other illness such as nasal or respiratory infection.

Treatment.   Most often, treatment is unnecessary. However, if you have a bacterial infection, your physician will prescribe a course of antibiotic therapy. If it is viral, antibiotics will not help.

Get plenty of rest. You can relieve the pain of pharyngitis with aspirin or an aspirin substitute and by gargling with warm salt water (one-half teaspoon of salt in a glass of warm water) several times a day. Throat lozenges can provide relief as well. You may want to switch to a soft or liquid diet to avoid irritating your throat.

TONSILLITIS

Signs and Symptoms

- Sore throat;
- Headache;
- Fever and chills;
- Sore glands of the jaw and throat.

Tonsils are lymph nodes. They are located at the back of the mouth, one on either side. Among other functions, they filter out harmful microorganisms that could infect the body. Occasionally, however, when they become overwhelmed by a bacterial infection, they swell and become inflamed. This infection is known as tonsillitis. It is common, particularly among children.

The Diagnosis.   Symptoms of tonsillitis are similar to those of the flu. The primary symptom is a sore throat that makes it difficult to swallow; others are headache, fever, and chills. The tonsils become visibly red and swollen. You may also notice specks of white discharge on the infected tonsils. The lymph nodes in the area, such as those under the jaw and in the neck, may be enlarged and tender, too.

If the symptoms last more than 48 hours or you or your child has a history of tonsillitis, see your physician. He or she will examine the throat and take a culture to determine if the infection is caused by the beta-streptococcus bacterium (strep throat).

These days, tonsillitis is primarily an uncomfortable nuisance. Do not leave it untreated, however, because it can lead to formation of an abscess in or around the tonsils.

Treatment.   If you or your child has the symptoms of tonsillitis, rest is in order. Drink plenty of soothing fluids. Gargling with warm, salted water several times a day often

---

TONSILLECTOMY AND ADENOIDECTOMY

The tonsils and adenoids are lymph nodes of the throat. (For a discussion of the lymph system, see page 476.) The tonsils are located at the back of the mouth; the adenoids are in the top of the throat. Each acts to filter infections from the body. The tonsils and adenoids are particularly useful in infants and children up to about 3 years old. As you grow through childhood, the glands shrink so that by puberty the adenoids have almost disappeared and the tonsils have shrunk to the size of almonds.

Often, children over age 3 (and occasionally adults) come down with tonsillitis, a bacterial infection (see this page). Occasionally, the adenoids swell, too, giving the child's voice a nasal quality. When the glands become infected frequently and severely, say three or more times a year, your physician may recommend tonsillectomy and perhaps an adenoidectomy.

In the past, practically every child had his or her tonsils removed (often the adenoids as well) whether or not they became infected frequently. Now, the use of antibiotics makes the treatment of tonsillitis much easier. Most often, surgery is unnecessary. However, in rare cases the tonsils will become so enlarged that they may affect breathing and swallowing. In addition, the back of the nose and the eustachian tube may be blocked by enlarged and inflamed adenoids, thus causing middle ear infection (see page 680) as well as nasal obstruction.

Tonsillectomy and adenoidectomy are simple surgical procedures in which the tonsils and adenoids, respectively, are removed. Tonsils do not grow back, but adenoids can, although they rarely cause a second problem. Your child may be observed for several hours and then sent home (or perhaps hospitalized for a day or two) and will experience a very sore throat that will last for several days after the operation.

Tonsillectomy and adenoidectomy do not guarantee freedom from throat infections. The same organisms that cause tonsillitis, usually streptococci, can infect the throat. However, the frequency of throat infections usually is lessened after removal of these glands.

helps lessen the pain. Aspirin, or an aspirin substitute such as acetaminophen for children, may be helpful.

Medication. If a bacterial infection is the cause of the sore throat, your physician will prescribe a course of oral antibiotic therapy (usually for 10 days). The symptoms should disappear within a few days after the first tablets are taken.

Certain strains of streptococci that can cause tonsillitis and pharyngitis (see page 697) can also cause nephritis (see page 893) or rheumatic fever (see page 823). This is an important reason for completing your course of antibiotic medication as prescribed and not just stopping when the pain is relieved.

EPIGLOTTITIS

Signs and Symptoms
• Sore throat;
• Fever;
• Difficulty swallowing;
• Hoarseness.

Emergency Symptoms
• Difficulty breathing.

Epiglottitis is an inflammation of the lid-like cartilage that covers the windpipe. The condition is most common among children between the ages of 2 and 5, although adults can get it, too. It is more common among males than females and among whites than other races.

Epiglottitis usually is the result of a bacterial infection. Certain conditions, such as Hodgkin's disease, leukemia, and immunosuppressive diseases, can predispose adults to epiglottitis.

The Diagnosis. The symptoms of epiglottitis can be similar to those of pharyngitis (see page 697) and tonsillitis (see page 698) in that you or your child will have a sore throat and swallowing will be painful. Children often are feverish and hoarse. If the sore throat lasts more than a few days, see your physician. Your physician will examine your throat and take a specimen for culture. If the result of culture is positive for bacterial infection, the physician will prescribe an appropriate course of antibiotics. Also, an x-ray of your throat may be taken.

The infection can begin swiftly, reaching an acute stage in hours. When the epiglottis swells, it can obstruct the windpipe, making it difficult to breathe. It is quite common for the person who has epiglottitis to sit leaning forward, neck outstretched, in an effort to make breathing easier. If you or your child has difficulty breathing, call an ambulance or seek emergency treatment.

Treatment. Most cases of epiglottitis are treated with antibiotics to destroy the bacterial organism that causes the inflammation. Severe difficulty in breathing is treated as an emergency, requiring insertion of a tube into the trachea for breathing (tracheostomy).

PERITONSILLAR ABSCESS

Signs and Symptoms
• Sore throat and sore soft palate;
• Severe pain on swallowing;
• Fever;
• Tendency to hold the head on one side, away from the pain.

Peritonsillar abscess, also known as quinsy, is associated with tonsillitis. One of the tonsils becomes infected, and an abscess (a collection of pus) forms between this tonsil and the soft tissues around it.

The infection may spread over the soft palate (the soft area at the back of the roof of the mouth) before the abscess forms, making it possible for the abscess to cover a large area. The infection can spread to the neck and even down into the chest. Peritonsillar abscess is most common in young adults.

The Diagnosis. If your throat becomes sore and the discomfort spreads to the soft tissues at the back of the roof of your mouth (the soft palate), you may have a peritonsillar abscess. Your physician will examine your tonsil and palate, looking for an inflamed tonsil that has been displaced by swelling of the soft area of the palate.

How Serious Is a Peritonsillar Abscess?
If not treated properly, peritonsillar abscess can be serious because the infection can move to the neck and eventually into the chest where it can infect the membrane covering the heart or the tissue between the lungs. Occasionally, the swelling can be so

severe that the roof of the mouth is pushed against the tongue, blocking air flow and making swallowing very difficult.

Treatment.   Your physician will treat the infection with antibiotics. If pus is present and does not drain quickly as a result of the antibiotics, your physician may drain the abscess surgically. Abscesses can recur, thus a tonsillectomy may be recommended. This usually is performed soon after the antibiotic treatment is started or about 6 weeks after the acute infection has healed.

LARYNGITIS

Signs and Symptoms
- Hoarseness;
- Tickling and rawness of the throat;
- Constant need to clear the throat.

Laryngitis is an infection or irritation of the larynx (voice box) which is located at the top of the trachea (windpipe). When the vocal cords of the larynx become inflamed or irritated, they swell, and this distorts sounds produced by the air passing over them. The voice then sounds hoarse; in some cases, the voice can become so soft as to be undetectable.

There are two forms of laryngitis, acute and chronic. The symptoms and treatment are often the same for both forms. Acute laryngitis is caused most often by a virus but can be the result of a bacterial infection. When caused by a virus, it usually disappears without treatment.

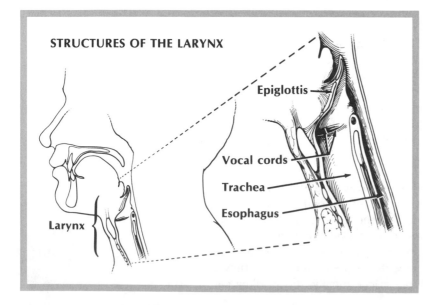

STRUCTURES OF THE LARYNX

Epiglottis

Vocal cords

Trachea

Esophagus

Larynx

Laryngitis can occur in the course of another illness such as an ordinary cold, bronchitis, flu, or pneumonia. Irritations such as excessive talking or singing, allergic states, and breathing of irritating substances such as certain chemicals also can cause hoarseness and loss of voice. Chronic laryngitis is caused most often by constant irritation such as excessive drinking of alcohol or heavy smoking.

The Diagnosis.   The primary symptom of laryngitis is hoarseness. Changes in voice can vary with the degree of infection or irritation, ranging from mild hoarseness to almost total loss of voice so that vocalization becomes little more than the sound of a soft whisper. Your throat may tickle or feel raw, and you may have a frequent urge to clear your throat.

Simple viral laryngitis usually clears up within a few days. If your laryngitis persists for more than 2 to 3 days or you have other symptoms, see your physician.

How Serious Is Laryngitis?   For most people, laryngitis is a temporary problem that either resolves itself or can be treated with antibiotics. When the hoarseness is due to alcoholism, chronic bronchitis, or workplace exposure, the underlying problem should be corrected.

Treatment. *Medication.*   Your physician will determine whether your laryngitis is bacterial or viral by taking a throat specimen for laboratory analysis. If the cause is bacterial, a course of antibiotics may be prescribed. The symptoms should disappear shortly after the first tablets are taken.

Laryngitis caused by a virus or inhaled irritant substance cannot be treated with antibiotics. The best treatment: rest your voice as much as is practical, inhale steam (from a bowl of hot water or a teakettle), and drink warm, soothing liquids. This program of rest, steam, and liquids is useful for treating all forms of laryngitis.

The underlying cause of chronic laryngitis must be treated for the problem to be solved. If you smoke, stop. If chronic bronchitis is the underlying cause (see page 927), antibiotic treatment should resolve the problem. If alcoholism is the cause, that must be treated. In the case of allergy, it can be treated with antihistamines.

VOCAL CORD PROBLEMS

The production of sounds by the larynx is called phonation. Within the larynx are two vocal cords that produce sound (phonate) by vibrating. The muscles of the larynx control the length and tension of the cords which transmit their vibrations to the column of air that passes through the larynx. The vocal cords also help to prevent food and water from entering the lungs during swallowing.

The vocal cords are one vital element in the act of speaking or singing. They are susceptible to problems including those caused by misuse or abuse. Such problems range from polyps to nodules to ulcers.

Polyps

Polyps are small swellings in the mucous membranes covering the vocal cords. As they grow, they take on a rounded shape. They may run the full length of the vocal cords or be localized.

A polyp can develop on your vocal cords as a result of abusing your voice through prolonged or repeated screaming, shouting, or speaking in a very low, unnatural tone. A polyp can also develop as a chronic allergic reaction or as a result of breathing irritants such as cigarette smoke or industrial fumes.

Polyps can make your voice become breathy-sounding and harsh. They sometimes are removed during the course of a special examination called laryngoscopy. Biopsy of the polyp may be performed in order to be certain that there is no cancer. Removal of a polyp should be followed by voice therapy to correct the underlying cause.

Singer's Nodule

People who use their voices a great deal, such as professional singers, teachers, auctioneers, and members of the clergy, are prone to have nodules on their vocal cords. Like polyps, nodules develop as a result of excessive use of the voice.

If you have such nodules, your voice will become breathy and hoarse. A nodule differs from a polyp in that it is a growth of the epithelium that covers the mucous membrane, not of the mucous membrane itself. Thus, it has a structural resemblance to a corn on a toe or a callus on the hand.

Resting the vocal cords by allowing little or no speaking for several weeks may permit the nodules to shrink. Sometimes biopsy and surgical removal are necessary. Voice therapy is essential in eliminating the vocal abuse and habits responsible for nodule formation. Children occasionally have screamer's voice nodules; these usually can be treated with voice therapy alone.

Contact Ulcers

The vocal cords also are subject to development of sores called contact ulcers. This ailment often results from improper use of the voice. Damage to the vocal cords (for example, due to the frequent regurgitation of gastric juices or following intubation for general anesthesia) is another common cause.

Contact ulcers appear where the two pieces of cartilage that

A small, angled mirror is used in performing indirect laryngoscopy, which provides a direct view of the vocal cords. (A) depicts a vocal cord polyp. (B) shows a contact ulcer. (C) reveals vocal cord cancer (see page 702).

hold the vocal cords in place touch each other. Symptoms include mild pain when swallowing or speaking and hoarseness.

Your physician will ask a series of questions to determine how you use your throat and what your eating patterns are. He or she also probably will take a sample of the ulcerated tissue for laboratory testing to be certain there is no cancer present.

The primary treatment for contact ulcers is rest of the voice—often for 6 weeks or more—to allow the sores to heal. Retraining of the voice may be needed to prevent the ulcers from recurring. If gastric juices are the cause of the ulcers, there are several techniques for avoiding recurrence. Your physician may recommend

an antacid medication, eating at least 2 to 4 hours before retiring, and having the head of your bed raised on 4- to 6-inch blocks (see Esophageal Reflux, page 593).

Leukoplakia

Leukoplakia, literally white *(leuko)* patches *(plakia)* in Latin, can appear on one or both vocal cords. They can be associated with cancer. When discovered, they are removed for laboratory study. Leukoplakia is often caused by smoking. (For further discussion of leukoplakia, see page 578.)

Juvenile Papillomas

Many children have warts, benign growths believed to be caused by

viruses. A few children, primarily boys, develop them on their vocal cords (juvenile papillomas).

They are not malignant, and they usually disappear at puberty. In the meantime, however, these warts can be troublesome. They can grow in clusters, making them difficult to remove without damaging the larynx. On rare occasions they can grow very fast and in a large quantity, thus obstructing breathing. When this happens, they must be treated quickly to keep the air supply from being cut off entirely.

Laser treatment has become the preferred procedure. It is more effective and less harmful than excision with a blade. Juvenile papillomas frequently recur, making repeat treatments necessary.

PROPER USE OF YOUR VOICE

Here are a few practical recommendations that may help you avoid vocal cord problems.

Excessively loud or raucous talking, yelling, screaming, or singing at a pitch that is too high for you can cause contact ulcers and vocal cord nodules. Lowering the pitch and speaking in a more normal range will lessen the strain on your voice.

Also, a prolonged, hacking cough or persistent throat tickle that requires frequent vigorous throat clearing can cause damage to your vocal cords. Have these conditions treated promptly.

Some men and boys try to lower the pitch of their voices in an effort to sound more

masculine. When you speak for any length of time in this manner, your throat quickly becomes tired, causing pain and even contact ulcers.

A less obvious recommendation regarding the use of your voice has to do with overall health and well-being. Everyone experiences the effects of physical fatigue and emotional stress at one time or another. When emotional stress or fatigue occurs, the muscles of your larynx and neck may become tense. Occasionally, vocal cord problems such as hoarseness, breathiness, or even loss of voice result from such stress. Thus, your voice can be a clue to your emotional health. Examine your life. If necessary, make changes to reduce unnecessary stress. It can contribute to the way you live—and sound.

CANCERS OF THE THROAT

Signs and Symptoms
- Hoarseness;
- Pain or difficulty swallowing;
- Swelling in your neck.

Almost everyone experiences occasional hoarseness. It may be only one symptom of a cold or tonsillitis. If you have laryngitis, hoarseness may be your only symptom. Whether you have a cold or laryngitis, your voice usually returns to normal within a few days.

Hoarseness is also the key symptom of most other vocal problems and the only early symptom of vocal cord cancer. Most throat cancers occur as tumors on the vocal cords or in or around the larynx. Difficulty and pain on swallowing are signs of other forms of throat cancer, as is a large swelling in the neck.

People who smoke cigarettes, cigars, or pipes are at greater risk of developing throat cancers than those who do not. People who drink large quantities of alcohol are at greater risk as well. The combination of drinking and smoking is particularly conducive to the development of cancer of the larynx. Throat cancers usually develop at around age 60, and men are 10 times more likely to develop them than women.

When hoarseness is your only symptom, if it has no obvious cause, and if it lasts more than 2 weeks, consult your physician without further delay. If swallowing is difficult or painful for several weeks or if you notice a swelling in your neck, see your physician.

The Diagnosis.   Your physician will examine your throat and conduct an examination called a laryngoscopy. There are two kinds of laryngoscopies, direct and indirect.

VOICE AIDS AFTER LARYNGECTOMY

Anyone who has had a laryngectomy has to learn to speak again without the aid of a larynx. Not having a voice box does not mean you must remain speechless, but your new speech will not sound the same as your voice did before.

Esophageal Speech
Many laryngectomees learn to speak again by a technique called esophageal speech. You swallow air to force it into your esophagus, lock your tongue to the roof of your mouth, and then expel it. The walls of the pharynx and esophagus vibrate, making a low-pitched sound similar to a burp. This sound is formed into words by using the tongue, palate, lips, and teeth. With training by a speech pathologist and practice, most laryngectomees learn esophageal speech.

Artificial Voice Aids
Esophageal speech is not the only method of vocal communication for laryngectomees. People who have trouble learning the techniques or who are unable to produce sounds that are loud enough to be easily understood can use artificial voice aids. These devices produce sounds that can be transmitted to the vocal tract. They often can be used in conjunction with esophageal speech.

The two main kinds of artificial larynx are neck type and intra-oral. Neck-type devices are hand-held, battery-driven electronic vibrating machines. The head of the device is held against the neck. The vibrations penetrate the neck tissues and resonate in the throat, mouth, and nose where they are converted into speech by using the tongue, teeth, lips, and palate. Intra-oral devices deliver sound directly into the mouth. Many of these devices use only air from the lungs.

A tone generator delivers sound into the mouth through a flexible tube. The sound is then manipulated by the tongue, lips, teeth, and palate to produce speech. Neck-type electronic aids can often be adapted for intra-oral use as well.

A third method of vocal communication is a voice prosthesis. This essentially provides a bridge between the trachea and the esophagus. The surgeon makes small openings in the rear wall of the trachea and the front wall of the esophagus. A small tube is placed into these openings to allow air to pass into the esophagus and to keep the opening clear and the trachea free of food and liquid. A valve sometimes can be placed on the stoma and when this valve is closed the air that passes through the device and into the esophagus permits esophageal speech to be produced in the mouth.

The two main types of artificial voice aids are the neck type (A) and the intra-oral device (B).

Indirect laryngoscopy is a method of looking at the throat by using a mirror. This simple procedure usually can be done in the physician's office. You will be asked to open your mouth and breathe through it. Your tongue will be pulled forward gently to help open your airway. A local anesthetic may be sprayed on the back of your throat and soft palate, particularly if you have a strong gag reflex. Your physician will then place the mirror toward the back of your throat. As you say "ah" and "eee," your larynx will rise and its interior can be viewed in the mirror. The presence of tumors or other abnormalities can be viewed easily in the mirror. Small, flexible fiberoptic instruments may also be used to view the voice box area.

Direct laryngoscopy is a more elaborate procedure that allows a more complete inspection of the larynx. It is performed by a throat specialist and requires local or general anesthesia, so it usually is done in a hospital. During a direct laryngoscopy, an instrument is inserted into your throat and a tissue sample is often removed from a vocal cord for laboratory analysis.

How Serious Are Throat Cancers?   Most cancers of the throat can be cured if detected early. They must not be ignored because they can spread to other parts of the throat and, ultimately, to other parts of the body.

Treatment.   Tumors of the throat are treated in one of several ways. Cancers detected early often can be cured by radiation therapy or surgery limited to only part of a vocal cord or the larynx. Usually, the tumor can be removed without removal of the larynx, but more advanced forms may require complete removal of the larynx, a procedure known as a laryngectomy.

If laryngectomy is required, your voice can be restored by the surgical placement of a prosthesis (see Voice Aids After Laryngectomy, page 703) or by working with a speech therapist to learn a new method of speaking.

CHAPTER 26

THE ENDOCRINE SYSTEM

CHAPTER CONTENTS

THE ENDOCRINE SYSTEM AT WORK

The endocrine glands function as a control system for the human body. Unlike other organs and body parts that enable us to move, breathe, eat, or sense the world around us, the endocrine system influences the body's processes. Along with the nervous system, it coordinates the body's activities and responses to usual and unusual events.

The key mechanism of the system is the hormone. Different types of endocrine hormones are secreted by different glands.

Most of these hormones are released into the bloodstream so that they can deliver instructions to various organs and tissues. The pancreas, for example, secretes the hormone insulin, which enables the body to regulate the amount of sugar in the bloodstream. In response to stress or other stimuli, the adrenal glands secrete adrenaline (also called epinephrine), which produces a sudden and remarkable burst of energy. Similarly, the pituitary, thyroid, parathyroid, and gonadal glands each influence certain body functions.

A hormone is a chemical messenger (the name itself comes from the Greek verb that means urge). Although hormones circulate throughout the body via the bloodstream, each influences only certain organs (target organs) or tissues.

As a rule, the greater the amount of a particular hormone in the bloodstream, the greater the activity of the target organ or organs of that hormone. Some hormones (such as several of those produced by the pituitary gland) control other glandular activity, but virtually every system in the body is subject to the influence of the hormones, either directly or indirectly. Reproduction and growth patterns are established by hormonal activity, as are the body's fluid and salt balances.

The endocrine system consists of several separate but interrelated glands or tissues that produce hormones. In most people, the pancreas, the adrenal, pituitary, thyroid, and parathyroid glands, and the ovaries or testes work in tandem, controlling the ebb and flow of hormones so efficiently that the body's glandular activity remains virtually unnoticed. Occasionally, however, the endocrine system malfunctions.

Because of the complexity of the endocrine system, many problems, great and small, can result from a malfunction. For example, in diabetes, the most common endocrine disorder, there is an excess of a sugar, called glucose, in the blood. This may produce various symptoms, including constant thirst and excessive urination. When a child's pituitary gland malfunctions, he or she may be at risk of gigantism or dwarfism if the disorder is not properly diagnosed and treated.

Glands that constitute the endocrine system include the pituitary, the thyroid and parathyroid glands, the pancreas, the adrenal glands, the ovaries, and the testes (not shown).

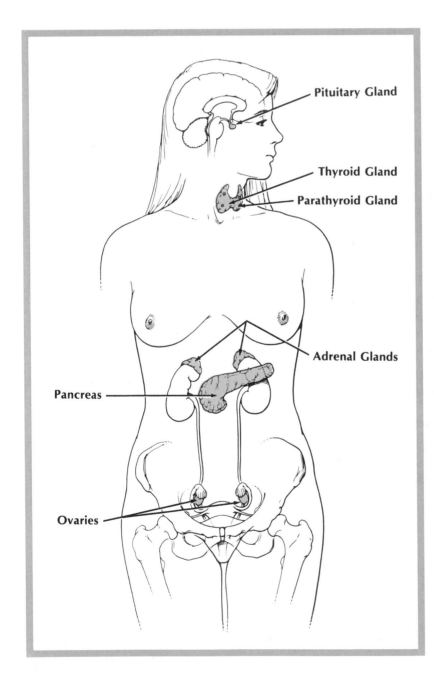

Pituitary Gland

Thyroid Gland

Parathyroid Gland

Adrenal Glands

Pancreas

Ovaries

The physician whose principal concern is the function of the endocrine system is the endocrinologist. In the following pages, we will consider the hormonal problems that endocrinologists commonly encounter. These ailments involve the pancreas and the adrenal, pituitary, thyroid, and parathyroid glands. (The testes and ovaries are discussed in the chapters Health Problems of Men and Health Problems of Women, pages 1111 and 1053. Also, breast disorders, although sometimes hormonally caused, are discussed in the chapter Health Problems of Women.)

PANCREATIC DISORDERS

Located behind your stomach, the pancreas is a long, thin organ roughly the length of your hand. It plays a key part in the digestive process, producing enzymes essential to the digestion of food (see The Digestive System at Work, page 590). The other role of the pancreas, which might best be described as "fuel control," is the one that affects persons with diabetes.

The hormones produced by the pancreas enable your body to break down (metabolize) the food you eat. They regulate your body's use of glucose, a simple form of sugar that is an energy source for much of the daily activities of all of your cells. When your pancreas is functioning normally, the glucose concentration in your blood changes in response to a wide variety of events including meals, exercise, stressful situations, and infections, but it remains within set limits.

Three hormones are produced by the pancreas. The first is insulin which is produced when the concentration of glucose in the blood increases. This normally occurs shortly after you eat a meal. Muscle and fat cells, among others, are stimulated by insulin to absorb the glucose they need as fuel for their activities. Surplus glucose is stored by the liver in the form of a starch called glycogen.

The second pancreatic hormone is glucagon. When needed, it breaks down the glycogen stored in the liver, causing it to be released as fuel into the bloodstream. In effect, this raises the concentration of sugar in the blood.

The third hormone produced by the pancreas, somatostatin, is thought to be a factor in regulating the production and release of both insulin and glucagon.

Sometimes this balanced system of control fails. The amount of glucose in the bloodstream becomes increased at the same time that the cells are unable to draw on it.

The result is hyperglycemia (from the Greek *hyper* for "above," *glyk* for "sugar," and *emia* for "blood"). This condition is easily diagnosed by measuring the concentration of glucose in the blood. If it is high enough, some glucose will spill into the urine, where it can be detected easily.

When your body's cells are unable to use the glucose in the bloodstream because of a lack of insulin activity (absence of enough hormone or resistance to the hormone), diabetes results.

DIABETES MELLITUS

Signs and Symptoms
- Increased thirst;
- Increased urination, both in volume and frequency;
- Weight loss despite increased appetite;
- Fatigue, nausea, vomiting;
- Vaginitis, skin infections, blurred vision, frequent bladder infections;
- Occasionally, impotence in men and cessation of menses in women.

Emergency Symptoms
- Diabetic ketoacidosis: Increased thirst and urination, nausea, deepened and more rapid breathing, abdominal pain, and a slightly sweet-smelling breath are the symptoms that precede a gradual loss of consciousness from diabetic ketoacidosis. This condition is most likely to occur in insulin-dependent diabetics, often after a dose of insulin is missed or when they have an infection.
- Hypoglycemic coma (insulin reaction): Trembling, weakness, or drowsiness followed by headache, confusion, dizziness, double vision, or lack of coordination are hallmarks of an insulin reaction.

An intoxication-like state, and eventually convulsions or unconsciousness, may follow. Emergency care is essential.

- Hyperosmolar coma: This is a gradual loss of consciousness, most often in an older person whose diabetes usually does not require insulin injections. Hyperosmolar coma often occurs in conjunction with some other illness, such as stroke.

More than 10 million Americans have been diagnosed as having diabetes mellitus. It is estimated that at least another 5 million are unaware that they have the ailment. Often, mild diabetes causes no outward symptoms for years. The origins of the name are Greek, referring to sweetness or honey *(mellitus)* that passed through *(diabetes)*.

About 1 in 10 diabetics have insulin-dependent diabetes mellitus (IDDM), and the rest have non-insulin-dependent diabetes mellitus (NIDDM). Insulin-dependent diabetes mellitus is also known as type I, juvenile, ketosis-prone, or juvenile-onset diabetes. We will refer to it as IDDM, a name that most accurately describes the disorder.

IDDM can develop in anyone at any age. Persons typically affected are children and young adults (young males are at somewhat greater risk than young females). Most diabetics who are diagnosed before age 19 years have the insulin-dependent variety of diabetes. Apparently, heredity is a factor in the development of diabetes—about two of every three diabetics are from families with some history of the disease. Although genetics is an important factor, inherited characteristics alone are not sufficient to produce the disease without the influence of other factors that are not yet completely understood.

As the names suggest, IDDM is distinguished from NIDDM by the fact that insulin is needed for treatment. In the person with IDDM, the pancreas usually produces little or no insulin. The symptoms of IDDM usually develop rapidly, in a matter of months or even weeks. During the first year after diagnosis, there may be a time of improvement, called the "honeymoon period," during which insulin is not needed or its dosage may be greatly decreased. In the fully developed state of IDDM, insulin injections are needed to prevent ketoacidosis and ultimately death.

The various terms also used for NIDDM include adult-onset, stable, and type II diabetes. Typically, persons with NIDDM are more than 40 years old.

The problem faced by persons with NIDDM is not an absence of insulin. Although they may have a modest shortfall of the hormone, they are equally likely to have normal or even elevated concentrations of insulin in their blood. Rather, much of their problem is their body's resistance to insulin. Greater amounts of insulin are needed to maintain normal amounts of glucose in the blood.

Most persons with NIDDM are overweight or obese. Excess weight worsens the state of the diabetes, and weight reduction has a favorable effect. In some instances, insulin injections will be required to keep blood glucose concentrations within satisfactory limits but, unlike the situation in IDDM, omission of these injections will not result in ketoacidosis. Medicines taken by mouth, called oral hypoglycemic agents, often are helpful in NIDDM but are of no value for treating IDDM. As a result of a weight-loss program, insulin or an oral hypoglycemic medication often may be decreased or eliminated.

Because most pregnant women are young adults, diabetes occurring during pregnancy usually will be of the IDDM variety. Therefore, if you are pregnant and you develop diabetes, see a specialist.

A third, but much less common, type of diabetes is called secondary diabetes. This may behave like either IDDM or NIDDM, but it is distinguishable from them because its cause is another disease altogether. Secondary diabetes can occur as a consequence of disorders such as acromegaly (see page 723), Cushing's syndrome (see page 719), hyperthyroidism (see page 727), or surgical removal of the pancreas.

The Diagnosis.   If you experience frequent urination and thirst, consult your physician, who will determine the concentrations of sugar in your blood and urine. Glucose in the urine is a condition called "glycosuria"; a high glucose concentration in the blood is termed "hyperglycemia." These findings are evidence of both forms of diabetes, IDDM and NIDDM.

Testing the urine for substances called ketones may help distinguish between IDDM and NIDDM. Unless insulin is given in appropriate amounts, the person with IDDM may frequently have substantial amounts of ketones in the urine, whereas in NIDDM only small amounts of ketones will be found from time to time.

If the person with IDDM fails to receive insulin for a few days, ketoacidosis will almost certainly develop. This condition involves an accumulation of ketones in the blood and urine, deeper and more rapid breathing, and gradual loss of consciousness. If prompt and vigorous treatment is not undertaken, death is likely.

NIDDM may develop gradually over a period of years. Often, it is discovered unexpectedly during a routine urine or blood test conducted at the time of a physical examination. A substantial amount of glucose in the urine is required to produce the classic triad of symptoms of increased thirst, increased volume of urine, and weight loss.

How Serious Is Diabetes?   Until the discovery of insulin in 1921, the almost inevitable result of IDDM was death. However, modern medications administered in a carefully monitored program have made possible the effective management of both IDDM and its less severe variant, NIDDM.

Some insulin-dependent people experience extremes of high and low concentrations of sugar in the blood, a condition variously termed "brittle," "unstable," or "labile" diabetes. These individuals ultimately may require hospitalization in order to have their condition stabilized. "Intensive insulin therapy" consists of three to four insulin injections per day, and it is often used for unstable diabetes. However, a carefully controlled lifestyle, including proper dietary controls and a less-demanding schedule of insulin or oral medications, will, in most cases, enable the diabetic to live a normal, productive life despite the diabetes.

Both IDDM and NIDDM have potential short- and long-term risks. Short-term dangers are posed by insulin reactions (very low concentrations of glucose) and by very high concentrations of glucose in the blood, but these complications usually are resolved when a satisfactory program of diet, exercise, and, if necessary, adjustment in medication dosage is developed. Ketoacidosis is another short-term danger that the diabetic must avoid.

Diabetes has two types of long-term effects. These develop slowly and have few early symptoms. One type is associated with blood vessel involvement. Damage to the large vessels puts the diabetic at greater risk of stroke, heart attack, and gangrene of the feet; when small blood vessels sustain long-term damage, problems with the eyes, kidneys, and nerves may occur. Nerve damage (diabetic neuropathy), the second type, may also result directly from prolonged elevation of the blood glucose concentration (see pages 508, 558, 777, 835, and 909).

Ketoacidosis.   This acute complication of IDDM most often occurs when the diabetic fails to receive scheduled insulin injections or is under stress from illness or injury. (Mayo Clinic physicians believe that psychological factors or emotional stress has little or no effect on the blood glucose concentration in the diabetic.) Glucose accumulates in the blood and the amount of ketones in the blood increases, causing it to become more acidic.

Increased urination and an unquenchable thirst will develop over the course of several hours (it may happen more quickly in a child). Weakness and drowsiness may follow, along with a flushed complexion and even vomiting, diarrhea, or abdominal pain. Sometimes the breath assumes a sweet, fruity smell that may be confused with the odor of alcohol (it's actually another waste product, acetone, being expelled via the lungs). At an advanced stage, breathing becomes deeper and more rapid. If consciousness is lost, the condition is described as diabetic coma.

These symptoms demand immediate treatment because death can result (government statistics suggest that ketoacidosis is the cause of about 1 in 10 deaths in diabetics). Ketoacidosis is most likely in the undiagnosed diabetic or in a person whose diabetes is not well controlled. However, any diabetic is subject to ketoacidosis under such circumstances as accidental injury, infection, or loss of large quantities of fluid through vomiting or diarrhea. In these situations, it is important for the diabetic to monitor closely the glucose concentrations in the blood and urine and the ketone concentration in the urine.

Emergency medical treatment is required for ketoacidosis. It involves the administration of insulin and intravenous injection of salt solutions to replace lost body fluids. Close monitoring of the blood glucose concentration and fluid status is needed until stability is established. If treatment is prompt, recovery from ketoacidosis usually is rapid and complete.

Hyperosmolar Coma. Older persons with NIDDM who also have another illness (such as stroke) and who fail to consume enough water may develop very high concentrations of glucose in the blood. Ketones are found only in small amounts, if at all.

The result may be a loss of consciousness requiring hospital care. It is extremely important for persons who have even mild diabetes to consume a generous amount of water during illnesses. Nursing home patients who may become confused and fail to ask for water are particularly vulnerable to hyperosmolar coma.

Hypertension, Atherosclerosis, and Coronary Artery Disease. In the person with high blood pressure (hypertension), the blood is pumped through the body under

HYPOGLYCEMIA AND THE INSULIN REACTION

Hypoglycemia is not a widespread phenomenon, contrary to much of the press devoted to it in recent years. It develops most frequently in people who are taking insulin or oral hypoglycemic drugs.

Hypoglycemia is the name given to the situation in which the concentration of glucose in the blood is below normal. When too little glucose is circulating to the nervous system and other cells, they become energy-starved. Hypoglycemia can occur if the dose of insulin or oral hypoglycemic agent is too large, if a meal is missed, or in the event of extended or vigorous physical activity. In nondiabetics, the circumstances that may produce hypoglycemia include certain kinds of tumors and ingestion of alcohol with minimal intake of food.

Symptoms
Insulin reactions occur most often in diabetics who take insulin by injection, although such reactions also may occur in diabetics who take antidiabetic tablets by mouth—"oral hypoglycemic agents." The symptoms vary from one person to another, but common early symptoms include weakness, trembling, and dizziness. Often, heavy, cold perspiration may occur. The skin appears pale or ashen. Nervousness, hunger, blurred vision, and a tingling sensation in the hands and feet may accompany the other symptoms.

If hypoglycemia is not corrected in the diabetic patient, other sensations may follow, including headache, confusion, dizziness, and difficulty in walking. Nausea and rapid heartbeat are other common symptoms. To the observer, the diabetic experiencing hypoglycemia—also called an "insulin reaction"—may exhibit unusual behavior patterns, most often appearing to be confused and sometimes stubborn or uncooperative. As the condition worsens, the lack of coordination may become more exaggerated, and the diabetic may seem to be intoxicated. Unconsciousness may occur in extreme cases. Convulsions also may result, particularly in children. In elderly people, strokes may occur but are extremely uncommon.

Solution
In most cases, ingestion of a source of sugar (simple carbohydrate) will alleviate the symptoms in 10 or 15 minutes. A glass of orange juice or a soft drink containing sugar will suffice, as will two or three sugar cubes or a piece of candy. If the symptoms do not disappear, consume a second helping of the sweet food. When the symptoms have subsided, consume additional food to prevent recurrence. Because panic attacks may closely resemble insulin reactions, testing the blood for sugar before consuming any food will help you determine whether anxiety or an insulin reaction is causing the symptoms.

Recognizing the Signs
Part of the education process for diabetics who take insulin or oral agents is to alert them to the possibility of the hypoglycemic reaction and to train them to deal with it. Your physician may even induce an episode of hypoglycemia under supervised conditions to help you recognize the feeling.

When symptoms begin to appear, stop all activity—bring the car to a halt, turn off the lawnmower, cease jogging. It is also important to carry a concentrated source of sugar with you at all times in case a candy or soda machine isn't within easy reach when symptoms appear. Alert family and friends to the symptoms and the usual course of your hypoglycemia attacks. They should never attempt to feed you sweet substances if you have lost consciousness, but they may help you in the earlier stages or summon help if you lose consciousness. Sometimes syrup can be given to a semiconscious person a teaspoonful at a time without danger when drinks that are more liquid may "go down the wrong way."

Emergency Assistance

Insulin reactions must be taken seriously, but if recognized early and treated promptly, they are usually dealt with easily and are more annoying than dangerous. However, if unconsciousness oc-

curs, it will be necessary to administer an injection of either glucagon under the skin (as if it were an insulin injection) or glucose into the vein. Because of the risk of an insulin reaction, wearing a medical-alert necklace or bracelet or carrying a card that identifies you as a diabetic is a sensible precaution.

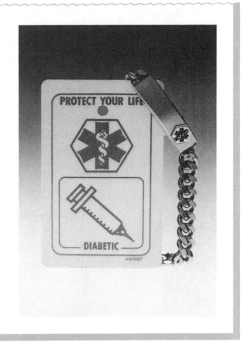

An alert-bracelet or identification card can be a life-saver in an emergency. This identification will make medical personnel aware of your condition, helping them to reach a correct diagnosis and to provide you with appropriate treatment.

abnormally high pressure. This can damage blood vessels, tissues, and organs through which the blood passes. Atherosclerosis produces fatty deposits that thicken the lining of the arteries, eventually resulting in smaller, less flexible pathways for the blood. Coronary artery disease involves atherosclerosis of the blood vessels that supply the oxygen and nutrients required by the heart.

All three of these complex, long-term disorders are substantially more likely to occur in diabetics than in other persons. Refer to the detailed discussions of hypertension (see page 796), atherosclerosis (see page 786), and coronary artery disease (see page 801) for their usual courses and approaches to treatment and prevention.

Occasionally, diabetics experience a cramping of the calves when walking or climbing stairs. The cramps cease when the activity is stopped. This symptom (called "claudication") or any unusual discoloration of the foot, skin ulcers, or wounds that do not heal should prompt a consultation with the physician immediately (see page 834).

Vision Problems. When blood glucose concentrations are high, a refractive error in the eye may result and produce blurred vision. This blurring may become much worse when treatment causes rapid lowering of the blood sugar concentration. Glasses should

not be fitted until the blood sugar value has been stabilized for 6 to 8 weeks. The diabetic also faces potential long-term vision problems as the result of disturbances of circulation within the retina (see page 773).

At the root of these diabetes-induced vision problems are changes in the small arteries that provide blood for the retina (the retina is the light-sensitive lining at the rear of your eye). Approximately half of all diabetics may experience eye problems after having the disorder for 10 years, and such problems are almost universal in those who have had diabetes 30 or more years. Diabetic retinopathy (see page 777) is the most common such problem, although cataracts (see page 768) and glaucoma (see page 765) are somewhat more likely in the diabetic than in the nondiabetic. Because diabetic retinopathy often is symptomless until well advanced, it is important that you schedule regular eye examinations if you have diabetes. If diabetic retinopathy occurs, a laser treatment may retard its progression (see page 773).

Other Long-Term Complications. Many diabetics experience kidney disease due to long-term deterioration of the small blood vessels (see Chronic Renal Failure, page 909). Diabetic neuropathy (a deterioration of nerve fiber function) also may occur, especially in the feet and sometimes the hands. In such cases, a painful burning sensation may be felt. Over time, the affected areas become less sensitive and more subject to injury and infection. Ulcer formation and secondary gangrene on the soles of the feet also may result from neuropathy. When gangrene is a result of atherosclerosis, it usually begins in the toes or at the site of an injury. In addition, impotence is a frequent complication in diabetics (see page 1141).

Treatment.   Although medications are essential for people with IDDM and for many with NIDDM, the treatment of either disorder involves all-important life-style components. Unlike certain other diseases that have no demonstrable link to patterns of physical activity and diet, the management and progress of diabetes are inextricably linked to behavior. Patients with diabetes must be prepared to confront the disorder in three ways: an appropriate diet and weight control plan, a sensible approach to physical activity, and medication (if necessary).

Various health-care professionals may be involved in the care of the diabetic. The family physician, general pediatrician, general internist, or an endocrinologist or diabetologist will probably supervise the medical care, but consultations with podiatrists, oph-

thalmologists, and other professionals may also be needed if complications result. Yet, your role is as vital as that of any of the care-givers.

If you have diabetes, you must assume responsibility for the day-to-day management of your illness. This includes not only administering the insulin or ingesting oral hypoglycemic agents but also helping to control the blood sugar concentration through close adherence to the dietary and exercise regimens recommended by your physician.

Nutrition.   A proper diet is essential. In fact, for many with NIDDM, a program of weight control alone is sufficient to treat the disorder. A specific diet is tailored for each person, but the basic approach of dietary therapy involves weight reduction for the overweight individual and the establishment of regular eating patterns for the lean patient. (For guidance regarding the ideal weight for your height and frame size, consult the chart on page 350. If your weight is 20 percent or more in excess of the number given and you are not unusually muscular, you are overweight.)

Alcoholic beverages tend to aggravate diabetes; therefore, you may need to limit your alcohol consumption. Furthermore, alcohol is a concentrated source of calories.

Over a period of years, diabetes can result in a deterioration of nerves and blood vessels in your extremities. In such cases, minor wounds sometimes can lead to development of neurotropic ulcers (A). In some instances, the deterioration of blood vessels can severely limit flow of blood, leading to gangrene (B).

A   B

Its consumption may complicate your weight-control program.

The goal of any such diet is twofold. First, it will help control the glucose concentration. Second, and equally important, it will help you control or reduce your weight. Obesity increases the body's need for insulin because the extra food contributes greater amounts of glucose to the system. The result is that controlling the blood sugar concentration becomes even more difficult, and the likelihood of serious complications also increases.

Diabetics must carefully regulate their consumption of carbohydrates (sugars and starches), fats, and proteins. Your dietician will devise a program that is satisfactory. Avoid simple sugars, such as those in candy and cookies and sugary drinks. Include in your diet fiber-rich foods such as whole-grain breads, fruits, and vegetables. (See page 372 for a discussion of a diet for diabetics.)

Exercise.   Exercise is another part of the treatment program for diabetes. Regular exercise helps maintain overall health but, more important to the diabetic, it benefits the heart and blood vessels and may improve circulation. It also can be valuable in a weight-reduction program.

The muscles use more glucose during vigorous exercise. Therefore, exercise helps to decrease the blood glucose concentration. In addition, exercise makes the cells throughout the body more sensitive to insulin, enabling them to use the available supplies of it more efficiently.

Your physician will help you establish guidelines for how frequently and how vigorously you should exercise. In Chapter 14, exercise programs in general are discussed (see page 377), but diabetics have several special concerns. Because exercise functions much like insulin in decreasing the blood glucose level, you have to be alert to the possibility of an excessively low concentration (see discussion of hypoglycemia, page 710). Consuming a light carbohydrate snack and drinking milk about 30 minutes before exercising is a good practice. Carrying a fast-acting carbohydrate or glucose tablets is also recommended in the event you feel the nervousness, weakness, hunger, or other characteristic symptoms of hypo-

glycemia. If you have IDDM, try to time your physical activity so that it doesn't coincide with the times at which your injected insulin has its maximal effect—this practice will lessen the risk of hypoglycemia.

Medication.   In principle, insulin is the drug used for diabetics younger than age 40 years. Oral hypoglycemic medications may be used by people who develop the disorder after age 40 years. However, there are exceptions to the general rule.

As the name suggests, those with IDDM require insulin; alternatively, those with NIDDM may or may not require medication. However, in all diabetics, a key factor in the use and dosage of a drug or insulin is the individual's willingness to follow the dietary and exercise guidelines discussed above.

The decision to use insulin or an oral hypoglycemic medication is based on the type and severity of the diabetes. For an obese person with NIDDM, careful regulation of food intake, accompanied by an exercise regimen, may be the solution. If such measures cannot control the disease, your physician may prescribe either oral medication or insulin injections. If you have IDDM, insulin shots are necessary. Dosage will depend, in part, on how carefully you follow your guidelines for diet and exercise.

Insulin.   Insulin is available in various types and strengths (see Table IV-26-1, page 714). Some is obtained from the pancreas of cattle or hogs. In recent years, recombinant DNA technology has made possible the production of synthetic insulin.

Some varieties of insulin act quickly, and others act for longer periods. The type of insulin, its amount, and the timing of administration are tailored to each diabetic's needs and readiness to undertake a disciplined program. A single injection of intermediate insulin in the morning is the most common initial approach, although a mixture of regular insulin with intermediate insulin and additional injections at other times of the day may be needed. Your physician will help determine which approach is best suited to your needs.

For those with very unstable diabetes who are ready to undertake a more elaborate program, an injection of rapidly acting insu-

TABLE IV-26-1. Insulins

Name	Description	Origin
Intermediate-acting insulins: Greatest effect is during first 12 to 18 hours; total duration is 20 to 24 hours. All types are cloudy.		
NPH	Isophane suspension	Beef-pork mixture, pork, beef, human
Lente	70% Ultralente and 30% Semilente	Pork-beef mixture
Mixtard	70% Isophane suspension and 30% regular insulin	Beef-pork mixture
Short-acting insulins: Greatest effect is during first 4 to 5 hours; total duration of action is about 8 hours. Semilente forms act for 12 to 18 hours.		
Regular	Solution, clear	Beef-pork mixture, pork, human
Semilente	Suspension, cloudy	Beef-pork mixture, pork, beef, human
Long-acting insulins: When given daily, they provide nearly equal action throughout the 24 hours. All types are cloudy.		
Ultralente	Suspension	Beef, beef-pork mixture
Protamine zinc	Suspension	Beef-pork mixture

Pork insulin resembles human insulin more nearly than beef; therefore, sometimes it is preferred to beef-pork mixtures or beef. Human insulins are made both by a recombinant DNA technique (synthetic) and by replacing one amino acid of pork insulin (semisynthetic). Trade names of human insulins are Humulin and Novolin. All cloudy insulins require careful mixing before being drawn into the syringe.

TABLE IV-26-2. Oral Hypoglycemic Agents*

Trade Name	Generic Name	Tablet Size	Maximum Dose per Day	Usual Dose per Day
DiaBeta or Micronase	Glyburide	1.25, 2.5, and 5.0 mg	20 mg	1.25–20 mg
Diabinese	Chlorpropamide	100 and 250 mg	500 mg	100–500 mg
Dymelor	Acetohexamide	250 and 500 mg	1,500 mg	250–1,500 mg
Glucotrol	Glipizide	5 and 10 mg	40 mg	5–20 mg
Orinase	Tolbutamide	250 and 500 mg	3,000 mg	1,500–2,000 mg
Tolinase	Tolazamide	100, 250, and 500 mg	1,000 mg	250–500 mg

*Medications taken by mouth in tablet form that lower the concentration of sugar in the blood.

The dose should be adjusted to your needs. Side effects are rare except that Diabinese (chlorpropamide) and Orinase (tolbutamide) sometimes can cause nausea and flushing shortly after the ingestion of alcohol. Diabinese also can decrease the serum sodium concentration in association with persistent weakness. Usually, an oral hypoglycemic agent is given once daily, but with larger doses your physician may prefer to have you take it twice a day. The effects of Diabinese may persist as long as 4 or 5 days after the last dose, but the other agents usually will have little effect by 24 hours after the last dose. In rare instances, any of these agents may cause unusually severe and prolonged lowering of the blood sugar value.

lin before each meal can be very helpful. The dose depends on measuring the blood glucose concentration at the time. This regimen is called intensive insulin therapy. The use of an insulin pump may be helpful for the person with very unstable diabetes (and not just as a convenience to avoid the injection of insulin). An insulin pump is a battery-operated device that holds a supply of insulin for delivery continuously and automatically through a needle under the skin of the abdomen. Mayo Clinic physicians recommend the multiple-injection approach (intensive insulin therapy) rather than use of a pump.

Oral Hypoglycemic Agents.   These drugs stimulate the pancreas to increase the output of insulin and are appropriate for use in about a third of patients with NIDDM. They are most suitable for diabetics who are unable to control the glucose concentration with diet alone (see Table IV-26-2, above).

Prevention.   There is no known prevention for IDDM, but obesity is closely associated with the development of NIDDM in persons older than 40 years. As a result, weight reduction may help forestall its development in some cases; thus, if your weight is 10 percent or more over that recommended for your height and frame size, a weight-reduction program is in order, especially if you are older than 40 years and have a family history of diabetes (see page 790 for a discussion of obesity).

Once you have been diagnosed as having diabetes, there are measures you should take to limit the development and progression of possible complications. A good exercise program is crucial. If you are a smoker, the onset of diabetes may provide the impetus you require to quit; smoking is an especial hazard to the diabetic and significantly adds to the long-term risk of heart disease and other side effects (see Smoking, page 788).

Care of the feet is very important for diabetics because of the frequent problems caused by impaired nerve function and narrowing of arteries in the lower half of the body (atherosclerosis), which limit the flow of blood to the feet. Wear shoes that fit properly. This minimizes your chance of developing calluses, corns, and blisters. If circulation is impaired, minor injuries such as blisters or ingrown toenails may lead to serious infection and gangrene. If the nerve supply is damaged, sensation is poor and burns or other injuries may not be felt until serious

THE INSULIN INJECTION

All insulin is administered by injection (when taken orally, the digestive system destroys the hormone before the body can put it to use). It is important that this simple procedure be conducted properly.

1. Remove the protective covering from the needle. Draw the plunger back to the mark on the syringe corresponding to the exact dosage of insulin you require.
2. Hold the bottle of insulin upright in one hand, and push the needle through the rubber stopper. Push the plunger down to empty the air from it.

3. Turn over the bottle and syringe together. Check that the tip of the needle is covered by the solution, then slowly pull the plunger back, drawing in fractionally more than your prescribed dose.
4. Remove any air bubbles by tapping the syringe until the bubbles rise to the needle end, then push the plunger until they return to the bottle. Adjust the solution in the syringe to your exact dose, and remove the needle from the bottle.
5. Using an alcohol swab or a cotton ball soaked with alcohol or soap and water, clean the area of the injection.
6. Hold the syringe as you would a writing utensil. With your other hand, pinch a 1- to 2-inch fold of skin.
7. Push the point of the needle straight into the fold. Release

your grasp of the flesh and, using that hand, hold the syringe in place. With your other hand, pull up on the plunger 3 or 4 units.
8. If no blood enters the syringe, push the plunger all the way down and then withdraw the needle. However, if blood does enter the solution, withdraw the needle immediately and discard the syringe. Prepare a new dose, find a second injection site, and repeat the first three steps.
9. After injecting the insulin, cover the area of the injection with a cotton ball dampened with alcohol. Apply pressure to the area for a few seconds, but do not rub it as that could cause the insulin to be absorbed into the bloodstream too quickly.

Although direct reading strips are available, blood glucose meters can automatically analyze the sample and provide a single numerical reading rather than an estimated range.

Determining the proper insulin dosage is essential to properly controlling diabetes. The most accurate measurements involve blood rather than urine analyses. Many people find it simpler to use spring-loaded devices like this one. The needle is activated by a button or other mechanism. These devices are quick and easy to use, and reduce discomfort of the pinprick to a minimum.

In the glucose monitoring test, a drop of blood is applied to the chemically treated portion of a test strip.

Limit injection sites to your abdomen and change the sites systematically. Formerly, the thighs, arms, and buttocks often were used. Because insulin injected into the abdomen is absorbed more consistently than that injected into other areas, current opinion advocates use of the abdomen exclusively. This is particularly true during periods of physical activity. If too many injections are given in a small area, however, scarring of the fatty tissue under the skin may occur and absorption of the injected insulin into the bloodstream can become erratic.

injury has occurred. Also, if the nerves are damaged, difficult-to-heal ulcers may occur as a result of calluses. Your physician may advise you to see a podiatrist for instructions about frequent inspections of the foot, proper nail care, and other reasonable precautions (see page 1187).

ISLET CELL TUMORS OF THE PANCREAS

Signs and Symptoms

Insulinoma
- Episodes of weakness, sweating, rapid heart rate, and confusion relieved by consumption of food.

Gastrinoma (Zollinger-Ellison Syndrome)
- Stomach pain that is relieved temporarily by food and antacids but grows more severe over periods of weeks and months;
- Watery diarrhea.

Glucagonoma
- Skin rash that occurs on various areas of the body;
- Sore tongue;
- Weight loss.

Most pancreatic tumors do not manufacture hormones, and many of them are malignant (see page 669). Some uncommon or rare tumors arise out of the islets of Langerhans, the clusters of cells in the pancreas that normally secrete the hormones insulin and glucagon. These tumors often secrete a hormone in excessive amounts which, in turn, may produce serious effects.

The tumor may be named after the hormone it produces. The islet cell tumor that produces insulin is called an insulinoma and

---

GLUCOSE SELF-MONITORING

The key to treating diabetes is controlling the blood glucose concentration, and in order to manage it, you must monitor it. Glucose self-monitoring offers a way to determine whether adjustments in diet, medication, or exercise are necessary for dealing with your diabetes.

Glucose monitoring is especially important to the diabetic who requires medication, whether it is insulin or an oral agent. Pregnant diabetics and diabetics whose glucose value is unstable would also do well to check their concentration several times daily. In general, both urine and blood tests should be routinely conducted before meals and at bedtime. At these times, glucose levels should be relatively normal. In addition, your physician may order a special blood test (called a "glycosylated hemoglobin test") to determine how your sugar has been controlled during the previous 6 to 8 weeks.

Keep careful records of the results of each test. These results, taken individually and together, will help you and your physician determine the effectiveness of your treatment program and determine when changes in medication, diet, and exercise are necessary.

Your physician will advise you as to which type of test is best for you (urine or blood) and also will help you determine the timing, frequency, and methods to be used.

Urine Tests
These tests are convenient, easy to use, and inexpensive. However, their use is usually best confined to persons who have NIDDM and whose glucose values are not subject to extreme highs or lows.

Various urine tests are on the market; some use chemically treated strips, whereas others use tablets. Each of the forms will change color when in contact with urine. The degree of change indicates the amount of glucose in the urine, which in turn is an indirect reflection of the amount of glucose in the blood. Other urine tests are available to measure acetone and other ketones in the urine.

Blood Tests
Blood tests provide direct readings, but they are more expensive and less convenient than urine tests. However, for diabetic babies or adolescents, persons with IDDM or kidney disease, or anyone who is pregnant, blood testing is more suitable.

Several types of blood tests are available. Each involves drawing a large drop of blood (usually from a fingertip) and dropping it onto a chemically treated strip. You should follow the manufacturer's and your physician's instructions as to the procedure and schedule for such testing.

Glucose monitoring can be important before and after exercise. You will learn more about the effects of exercise on the state of your diabetes by recording your glucose concentration before and after your workout, along with the medication and food taken before, during, and after exercise.

causes periods of hypoglycemia (low concentration of sugar in the blood). The symptoms are the same as those of insulin reactions that occur after insulin injections (see page 710). These symptoms tend to develop gradually over a period of several months to a year and often occur with exercise, on an empty stomach, or before breakfast. Dietary therapy is of no permanent value, although frequent consumption of food may alleviate symptoms temporarily. Treatment is surgical removal of the tumor.

A second type of hormone-producing islet cell tumor is gastrinoma. Gastrin is a hormone that stimulates secretion of acid and digestive juices in the stomach. A tumor that overproduces gastrin will cause severe ulcer symptoms that respond poorly to standard ulcer treatments. The condition associated with such a tumor is called Zollinger-Ellison syndrome. The diagnosis is confirmed by finding excessive amounts of gastrin in the blood and acid in the stomach. Treatment options are discussed in the chapter on the digestive system (see page 607).

A third type of tumor that arises in the pancreas secretes glucagon and is called glucagonoma. The skin symptoms are the key for identifying glucagonoma, but your physician also will conduct blood tests to determine whether your glucose concentration is abnormally high.

There are still other hormone-producing tumors, but these are rare and have a wide range of manifestations including watery diarrhea (even during fasting), weight loss, and a low potassium concentration in the blood. If you are experiencing severe watery diarrhea accompanied by fatigue and weight loss over a period of several weeks, your physician probably will want to do special stool, blood, and radiological tests to rule out those rare conditions.

How Serious Are Pancreatic Tumors?

Like all tumors, pancreatic tumors demand immediate treatment. When diagnosed promptly, however, they often can be removed.

Treatment.   Surgical removal of the affected tissues is usually the key component of treatment.

ADRENAL GLAND DISORDERS

There are two adrenal glands, each located on top of a kidney and each about the size of the end section of your thumb. An adrenal gland consists of two portions: the inner core, called the medulla, and the outer layer, called the cortex.

The medulla produces two hormones—adrenaline (also called epinephrine) and noradrenaline (norepinephrine). The brain controls the production of these hormones. When secreted into the bloodstream, they increase your heart rate and blood pressure and affect other body functions. Physical and emotional stresses usually trigger the release of these hormones.

The cortex produces a group of hormones called corticosteroids, of which there are three kinds. One kind, the sex hormones, includes male hormones (androgens) and female hormones (estrogens) which affect sexual development and reproduction. (Note that sex hormones also are produced elsewhere in the body, by the testes and ovaries, and that both male and female hormones are found in men and in women.) Another kind includes the hydrocortisone family of hormones (glucocorticoids). These influence the conversion of starchy foods into glycogen, a storage form of sugar, in the liver. The third kind, the mineralocorticosteroids, controls the body's use of the minerals sodium and potassium; aldosterone is the principal member of this group. All of the corticosteroids are under the control of a hormone from the pituitary gland, except that aldosterone mainly is controlled by a different hormone, renin, produced by the kidney.

The hormones of the adrenal glands affect virtually every system in the body to some degree. Their effects are complex, and there are overlaps in the actions of some of the adrenal hormones. In this intricate system, disturbances and failures can occur, and these lead to the following disorders.

CUSHING'S SYNDROME

Signs and Symptoms

- The face becomes rounder and more red over a period of several months to years;
- Hump-like collection of fat between and above the shoulder blades;
- Striations on skin of lower trunk;
- Fatigue and muscle weakness;
- Water retention (edema);
- Hypertension;
- Excess growth of hair;
- Mood swings;
- Impotence or cessation of menstruation;
- Osteoporosis, especially in the spinal and pelvic bones;
- Beginning of diabetes;
- Easy bruising.

This disorder occurs when excess glucocorticoid hormones circulate in the bloodstream. The excess may be the result of an overproduction by the adrenal gland or of extended use of steroid drugs for treating another ailment. The disease is named for Harvey Cushing, an early 20th-century American surgeon.

The Diagnosis.   During the physical examination, the physician looks for characteristic changes in the head and shoulders. Roundness and redness of the face and an excess of fatty tissue above the collar bones and between the shoulder blades are clues to diagnosis. Frequent, or even spontaneous, bruising on the arms and legs is another symptom.

If you are taking a corticosteroid drug to treat another ailment (such as rheumatoid arthritis, asthma, or a skin disorder), the cause should be obvious to your physician. However, if the cause is overproduction of the hormones by the adrenal glands, hospitalization may be required for further testing. This overproduction may be due to a tumor of one adrenal gland, to enlargement of both glands, or to overactivity of the pituitary gland because it contains a tumor. Occasionally, a malignant tumor of the lung or some other organ will cause Cushing's syndrome. Tests include examination of blood and urine for the presence of greater than normal amounts of steroid hormones. Computed tomography (CT) of the pituitary and

Cushing's disease occurs when an excess of adrenal hormones is secreted. If untreated, the face can assume an exaggerated roundness, the back has a characteristic hump, and skin on lower trunk shows striations.

adrenal glands also may be done (see page 1286).

How Serious Is Cushing's Syndrome?

The successful removal of a benign pituitary or adrenal tumor is likely to result in a full recovery, although long-term hormone therapy may be required. Accelerated atherosclerosis with heart attacks and fractures of the spine is common. If left untreated, this disorder ultimately may result in death.

If the cause is an excessive dose of steroid medication, the symptoms will gradually disappear as the dosages of steroid hormones are reduced.

Treatment. *Medication.* When the symptoms result from taking steroid hormones as a medication, treatment consists of stopping their use or decreasing the dosage. However, do not discontinue this medication without consulting your physician because sudden termination of steroid treatment can aggravate the underlying disease (asthma or other ailments for which the steroid was prescribed). Your physician will prescribe a gradual reduction in the dosage of steroids. In some cases, another drug may be used in place of the steroid originally prescribed. For as long as a year after steroid medication is stopped, a physical stress such as injury, infection, or surgery may produce a dangerous insufficiency in production of adrenal hormone so that emergency treatment may be needed (see Addison's disease, below).

Surgery.   When Cushing's syndrome is the result of a tumor in the adrenal gland, pituitary gland, or lung, removal of the tumor, or even of the entire gland if it is in the adrenal, may be the best treatment. Radiation therapy may be an option for tumor in the pituitary gland. If the treatment renders the adrenal glands incapable of providing the hormones your body needs, your physician will prescribe drugs to be taken orally to replace the missing hormones.

ADDISON'S DISEASE

Signs and Symptoms
- Weakness, lethargy, and anemia;
- Weight loss and decreased appetite;
- Darkening of the skin;
- Low blood pressure;
- Hypoglycemia;
- Abdominal pains accompanied by diarrhea, indigestion, vomiting, or constipation;
- Decreased sexual interest.

Emergency Symptoms
- Acute adrenal failure (addisonian crisis): dehydration (precipitated by severe diarrhea and vomiting), shock, and loss of consciousness.

In contrast to Cushing's syndrome (see previous entry), Addison's disease occurs when the cortex of the adrenal gland fails to produce enough steroid hormones. The disorder is named for the 19th-century English physician who identified it, Thomas Addison. Sometimes it is called adrenocortical hypofunction.

This failure of the adrenal glands may be the result of the body attacking itself (as in an autoimmune disease) or a consequence of some other disease such as tuberculosis. The disorder may occur at any age, including infancy, and is equally likely in males and females.

The Diagnosis.   Usually, the symptoms of Addison's disease develop slowly, perhaps over a period of months, but they may appear suddenly. If your physician thinks you have this disorder, samples of your blood and urine will be analyzed to measure the amounts of corticosteroid hormones present.

How Serious Is Addison's Disease?   Immediate hospitalization is essential for acute adrenal failure, which may be provoked by physical stress, infection, injury, vomiting, diarrhea, or use of diuretic drugs. Adrenal failure is a life-threatening condition that requires immediate medical care including injections of salt solutions and steroid hormones. However, when Addison's disease is diagnosed early, treatment requires only daily doses of steroid tablets and salt supplements, taken orally, for a normal, healthy life. The symptoms will disappear. Often, the skin will lose its dark color.

Treatment. *Medication.* If you have Addison's disease, your physician will prescribe one or more steroid drugs for use on a regular basis. Take this medication faithfully according to your physician's instructions. It is your body's only source of these essential steroid hormones. Without these hormones, acute adrenal failure can result.

A typical routine for taking the replacement hormones, usually one of the prednisone or hydrocortisone drugs, involves a dose in the morning and one in the late afternoon (to mimic your body's normal rhythm of steroid production). A second drug, called fludrocortisone (Florinef), controls your body's sodium and potassium needs and is necessary to maintain a normal blood pressure. Too large a dose of this drug may result in excessive salt retention which causes high blood pressure and swelling in the feet. The amounts of these drugs used to replace lacking adrenal hormones should not cause stomach ulcer problems, and so these drugs do not need to be taken with antacid medication.

The body's reliance on artificial steroids means that it is not able to respond to stressful circumstances that require additional amounts of hormone. These stresses include events such as an operation, an infection, or even a minor illness. In the event of an unusually stressful situation, consult your physician about a possible change in dosage of the steroids. It is imperative that any person taking this type of steroid medication regularly should wear a necklace or bracelet that states the need for the hormones in case of emergency with loss of consciousness.

Nutrition. Moderate amounts of salt should be consumed in the diet daily. A low-salt diet could provoke symptoms of acute adrenal failure.

TUMORS OF THE ADRENAL GLAND

Signs and Symptoms
- High blood pressure;
- Excessive sweating;
- Increased heart rate;
- Weight loss;
- Constipation;
- Personality changes.

There are four types of tumors of the adrenal gland that secrete hormones. One, pheochromocytoma, develops in the medulla (core) of the adrenal gland and overproduces the hormones adrenaline and noradrenaline (or epinephrine and norepinephrine, respectively). The second type of adrenal tumor occurs in the adrenal cortex and causes overproduction of the hormone aldosterone—Conn's syndrome. The third type causes Cushing's syndrome (see page 719). The fourth type manufactures male or female hormones and can cause feminization in men or masculinization in women.

These tumors of the adrenal gland are uncommon.

The Diagnosis. *Pheochromocytoma.*
Pheochromocytoma often occurs in several members of a family (familial occurrence) and may be associated with cancer of the thyroid. The disorder is often diagnosed when the family of an affected patient is studied to find relatives who also might have it but do not yet have obvious symptoms.

High blood pressure (hypertension) is the key symptom. When a person has high blood pressure in episodes or constantly and, after a minor emotional upset, exposure to cold, or a limited period of physical exercise, has such symptoms as fainting, exaggerated heartbeat, or severe headache, the physician may suspect an adrenal tumor. If a urine analysis reveals high concentrations of adrenaline or noradrenaline or their by-products, the diagnosis of pheochromocytoma is strongly suggested and further tests are needed.

Conn's Syndrome. The presence of high blood pressure, increased urination, extreme thirst, and muscle weakness or cramps may suggest Conn's syndrome. In this case, a blood test is needed. If the test shows too much sodium and too little potassium in the blood, Conn's syndrome indeed may be present.

Feminizing and Masculinizing Syndromes. The symptoms of these extremely rare syndromes involve the development of sexual characteristics of the opposite sex.

To confirm the presence of either type of adrenal tumor, CT scanning (see page 1286) and further blood and urine tests will be done.

How Serious Is an Adrenal Tumor? Tumors of the adrenal gland ordinarily can be removed surgically. In most cases, symptoms disappear after removal of this unwanted tissue. However, if not diagnosed or not treated properly, pheochromocytoma can be life-threatening, as can the rare malignant adrenal tumors.

Treatment. *Surgery.* If a tumor is found in either the medulla or cortex of an adrenal gland, it can be removed surgically.

Medication. If increased hormone levels are found, the physician may prescribe medications to block the effects of the hormones until the appropriate surgical or other treatment is selected. Usually, removal of the tumor will eliminate the symptoms and the medication can be discontinued. In a few patients, a daily medication to control hypertension may be necessary even after the operation.

IDIOPATHIC HIRSUTISM

In some women, hair may begin to grow on the face, chest, ears, and other locations where typically only men have hair. Such hairiness, called hirsutism, can be caused by the use of certain drugs such as phenytoin (better known by its brand name Dilantin), which is used to treat epilepsy, and some agents used to control hypertension. Certain tumors and other disorders of the adrenal glands and ovaries also can cause hirsutism.

However, in many cases, after tests and examinations, the physician finds no apparent explanation. These patients have what is known as idiopathic hirsutism—that is, hairiness of unknown cause.

Physicians believe that in most cases the cause of idiopathic hirsutism is a slight increase in production of androgen (male hormone), a change that occurs for no known reason. Women with idiopathic hirsutism experience normal menstrual cycles, have normal ovaries, and have no evidence of tumors or abnormal adrenal gland function. With such causes ruled out, the condition poses no health risk but is a matter of cosmetic concern.

Potential drug treatments are available. No one drug has been approved specifically for the purpose of treating excess hairiness, but several—including cortisone-like hormones, a diuretic called aldactone, and oral contraceptives that contain the hormones estrogen and progestin—may prove effective for suppressing androgen levels and controlling hirsutism.

However, keep in mind that these are powerful drugs. They have possible side effects. Also, they are not uniformly effective in treating hirsutism and, even when successful, they may take several months to produce an effect. Therefore, cosmetic methods of control may be preferable (see page 1184).

When women develop excess hair on the face and other locations, the condition is termed hirsutism. It can occur as a side effect of certain prescription drugs, but often occurs for no known reason.

When actual changes in the adrenal cortex, rather than a tumor, have caused an increase in aldosterone level, a drug may be prescribed to decrease the excessive amount of salt in the body.

Nutrition. When removal of the tumor does not restore adrenal hormone levels to normal, it may be necessary to restrict the dietary intake of salt to help control hypertension (see page 800).

CONGENITAL ADRENAL HYPERPLASIA

Signs and Symptoms

- Enlargement of the penis in male infants and of the clitoris in female infants;
- Sometimes, acute adrenal failure (see page 720);
- High blood pressure (rarely);
- Growth accelerated in early childhood but ceases early, resulting in short adult stature.

This condition is the most common adrenal gland disorder in infants and children (it is rare in adults). It is the result of a genetic abnormality that causes the adrenal glands to produce a distorted pattern of steroid hormones.

The Diagnosis. When the presence of congenital adrenal hyperplasia is suspected, the physician will examine the genitalia carefully and conduct blood and urine tests to measure the hormones produced by the adrenal gland.

How Serious Is Congenital Adrenal Hyperplasia? The first step is to rule out other causes for the symptoms. Once this disorder has been diagnosed in a child, it usually can be treated with medication. The principal long-term risk is the side effects of the medication, so the physician will closely monitor skeletal and other growth patterns in young patients.

Treatment. In most cases the therapy consists of corticosteroid drugs taken orally on a daily basis.

PITUITARY GLAND DISORDERS

Located at the base of the brain behind the nasal passages, the pituitary gland is roughly the size and shape of the last two segments of your little finger. Despite its diminutive size, it is the most important of the endocrine glands. It functions as a control center for the body's long-term growth, day-to-day functioning, and reproductive capabilities.

The pituitary consists of two parts, the front (anterior) lobe and the rear (posterior) lobe. The anterior lobe is responsible for producing six distinct hormones, including prolactin to stimulate the production of breast milk and growth hormone to regulate the body's physical growth. The other hormones in the anterior lobe influence other parts of the endocrine system, stimulating activities in the thyroid gland, ovaries, testes, and adrenal glands.

The posterior lobe produces two hormones: oxytocin and antidiuretic hormone. Oxytocin acts in women to stimulate the breasts to release milk during breast-feeding. Also, it prompts contractions during childbirth. Antidiuretic hormone acts on the kidneys to control urine output.

PITUITARY TUMORS

Acromegaly.   This chronic disease occurs in adults and is the result of increased secretion of growth hormone after normal growth has been completed. It is characterized by gradual overgrowth of the bones of the hands, feet, jaw, and skull. Because the bones cease to increase in length after adolescence, acromegaly produces a thickening of the skeleton. The most noticeable change in a person with acromegaly is the exaggerated growth of the forehead and jaw bones, which results in enlarged and coarsened facial features and widely separated teeth.

Gigantism.   Like acromegaly, this rare ailment results from excess production of growth hormone (by the pituitary gland). Unlike acromegaly, gigantism results in accelerated growth so that adult height is excessive. The differences between the two disorders is the age at which the person is affected: gigantism occurs in people who

have not yet reached adulthood. Relatively few tall children, however, suffer from gigantism (also referred to as giantism).

Prolactinoma.   This pituitary tumor causes an overproduction of the hormone prolactin. In women, it may cause irregularity or cessation of menstruation. In men, infertility or impotence may result.

Craniopharyngioma.   Visual field impairment, headaches, and sexual retardation are the symptoms of this pituitary tumor.

Cushing's Syndrome.   An adrenal gland tumor can also cause this disorder (see page 719).

Acromegaly and gigantism result from an overactive pituitary gland—the gland pro-

Acromegaly is caused by an excess of growth hormone in adulthood. The condition may result in an overgrowth of the hands, jaw, skull, and other bones, producing exaggerated body size and coarsened features.

duces too much of a hormone known as growth hormone (also called somatotropic hormone). This overproduction usually occurs when a tumor develops in the gland. The disorder is called hyperpituitarism (the Greek prefix *hyper* means above or over).

Two types of tumors can develop in the pituitary gland. One is called a craniopharyngioma. As it grows, it exerts pressure on the pituitary gland. This can result in decreased hormone production, and ailments such as hypopituitarism (see page 725) or diabetes insipidus (see page 726) result. The second type of pituitary tumor is an adenoma. Such a tumor is not likely to spread, but it can produce an excess of various hormones, resulting in disorders such as acromegaly, gigantism, or Cushing's disease (see page 719). Some tumors may not produce an excess of a hormone but can cause harm through mechanical pressure on the adjoining optic nerves and on the normal adjacent pituitary tissue.

The Diagnosis.   The physician will conduct a physical examination and will look for and ask about physical changes: overall aches and pains, tingling sensations in the hands, headaches, and increased perspiration. In the adult patient, the physician will be concerned with whether an increase in shoe or glove size was necessary recently. The person will be asked whether vision is failing—an enlarging tumor may press on the optic nerve and interfere with vision to either side. A more elaborate test of vision called a visual field measurement may be performed if the physician suspects that vision to the sides is diminished. Other questions are whether you are tired much of the time, whether your skin is oily, and whether your tongue seems unusually large.

Special blood and urine tests will be used to determine the amounts of hormones circulating in the bloodstream and being excreted. If abnormal values are found, a CT or MRI scan of the head (see page 539) may be obtained to pinpoint a tumor in the pituitary gland. If acromegaly is suspected, x-rays may also be useful for indicating if changes have occurred in the bones of the skull.

How Serious Is a Pituitary Tumor?   The key to treatment depends on how far the tumor has developed. The earlier it is diagnosed—and the smaller it is—the better the chances for a complete cure. In some cases,

the pituitary gland itself is damaged in the course of destroying or removing a tumor. When that occurs, lifelong hormone replacement therapy usually will become necessary.

Acromegaly.   Acromegaly results from excess growth hormone and causes growth not only of the skeleton but also of the internal organs. An enlarged heart can result in heart failure or high blood pressure. If left untreated, acromegaly can also cause diabetes, eye problems, and disfiguring changes in one's appearance.

Surgical treatment should prevent any worsening of eye complications and stop the progress of the disease. However, the changes in appearance generally are not reversible. The patient with acromegaly is also at increased risk for diabetes and long-term heart, artery, and lung disease; thus, sensible preventive measures (such as not smoking) should be taken to minimize the risks of these disorders.

Gigantism.   Gigantism can also be treated effectively. In most cases the progress of the ailment can be halted once the tumor has been removed or its overproduction of growth hormone has been blocked.

Prolactinoma.   The most common symptom of prolactinoma in women is irregularity or absence of menses and infertility. In men, impotence or infertility may result. Galactorrhea (the production of milk by the breasts of a woman who is not about to give birth) is another sign of prolactinoma; infrequently, this can occur in a man. (See discussion of galactorrhea, page 1078.)

Excess prolactin can result from several causes, including the use of certain oral contraceptives and tranquilizers and overproduction by a pituitary tumor (prolactinoma).

Cushing's Disease.   A pituitary tumor can also cause Cushing's disease by stimulating overproduction of the hormone that stimulates the adrenal glands (see page 719).

Treatment.   Most often, pituitary tumors are removed surgically. Because the gland itself is small, the procedure requires great skill. If the tumor is not removed surgically, the drug bromocriptine often is used to treat prolactinoma or as an adjunct to other treatments of acromegaly. Bromocriptine lessens the overproduction of certain hormones. In most cases of pituitary tumors, however, medication is not the principal treatment.

In some patients, radiation treatments may be appropriate when an operation is not feasible. Combination therapies to reduce the chance of the tumor recurring also are common.

HYPOPITUITARISM

Signs and Symptoms

In Children
- Slowed growth and sexual development;
- Hypoglycemia (see page 710).

In Adults
- In women, cessation of the menses, infertility, or inability to lactate after childbirth;
- In men, decreased sexual interest and loss of beard or body hair;
- Fine wrinkling of the skin adjacent to the eyes and mouth;
- Fatigue;
- Decreased appetite and sometimes weight loss.

Emergency Symptoms
- Fever and a decrease in blood pressure to low levels in response to stressful situations or infection.

Hypopituitarism is a disorder in which the pituitary gland produces insufficient quantities of one or more of the pituitary hormones. The name is derived in part from the Greek prefix *hypo,* which means under. Some people inherit a tendency toward hypopituitarism. Others acquire the ailment for unknown reasons. In many instances, however, the cause is identifiable.

The condition may be caused by a tumor in the gland, or it may develop after a serious head injury. Some women experience hypopituitarism after childbirth because the gland, which normally increases in size during pregnancy, grows so large that the body is unable to provide it with the oxygen and other blood-delivered products it needs; some or all of the pituitary tissue then dies.

Because the pituitary gland also produces hormones that activate other glands, underproduction of those hormones can also result in the symptoms of other disorders, including hypothyroidism (see page 730) and Addison's disease (see page 720).

The Diagnosis.   Dwarfism will result in a child with hypopituitarism. The key indication is abnormally slow growth. Pediatricians monitor the growth of infants, and this exaggeratedly slow growth pattern will be observed at the baby's regular checkups. This ailment is rare, and very few children who are shorter than average have the hormone insufficiency.

If hypopituitarism is suspected in a child or adult, the physician will conduct tests to measure hormone concentrations in the blood and urine. Subsequent testing may involve injection of insulin into the body to induce low blood sugar concentrations (hypoglycemia; see page 710). This condition stimulates the pituitary gland to produce its hormones, and they can then be measured.

If test results indicate a shortage of pituitary hormones, further tests are done to determine the underlying cause. A tumor is one possibility (see Pituitary Tumors, page 723).

How Serious Is Hypopituitarism?   The shortage or absence of pituitary hormones can be life-threatening because the adrenal gland may then be unable to respond to powerful stresses or infections. In such an instance, the physician prescribes corticosteroid replacement therapy.

A child with dwarfism is given injections of growth hormone to produce more nearly normal growth patterns. Without the therapy, the child will not reach full maturity in physical size. Sexual maturity may depend on the administration of other hormones as well.

In adults, similar hormone therapies are necessary.

Treatment. *Medication.*   Treatment of hypopituitarism may require various hormone replacement therapies depending on the degree of dysfunction in the pituitary gland.

Growth Hormone.   This medication may include hormones to replace those secreted by the pituitary gland. In addition to growth hormone replacement, adrenal and thyroid hormones and even ovarian hormones (for women) or testosterone (for men) may be needed.

Corticosteroids.   When the function of the adrenal glands is reduced, the natural hormone cortisol must be replaced by a drug taken orally, usually prednisone or hydrocortisone. In circumstances of high stress or surgery, these or other steroid drugs may also be administered in large amounts.

Other Hormones.   If estrogen, testosterone, or thyroid hormones are insufficient, they may also be prescribed.

DIABETES INSIPIDUS

Signs and Symptoms

- Excessive thirst;
- Increased urination.

Emergency Symptoms

- Dehydration, physical collapse, and low blood pressure may precipitate a comatose state.

Despite the similarities in symptoms and in name, this disorder should not be confused with diabetes mellitus. In contrast to diabetes mellitus, the result of a deficiency of insulin (the hormone that enables the body to use and maintain glucose to provide its cells with energy), diabetes insipidus results from a deficiency of antidiuretic hormone (ADH). This hormone is secreted by the posterior lobe of the pituitary.

If there is a shortage of antidiuretic hormone, the body loses control of its water balance. Rather than reabsorbing the water required to maintain proper fluid levels, the kidneys simply pass the water out.

In almost half of the cases of diabetes insipidus, the cause of the disorder is unknown, although a pituitary tumor may become evident several years after the onset of symptoms. Identifiable causes include damage to the pituitary from a head injury or from surgery for pituitary tumors.

The Diagnosis.   The key symptom is the large volume of urine that is excreted. A urine output of between 5 and 20 quarts within 24 hours is not uncommon. Urination throughout the day and night will be the rule, as frequently as every 30 minutes. The dehydration that results from such increased urination may also result in dry skin and almost certainly will result in an insatiable thirst.

If diabetes insipidus is suspected, your physician probably will conduct a water-deprivation test. In this test, the person consumes no fluid for several hours. Urine produced during that time is analyzed. The volume of urine will decrease in a person with normal amounts of antidiuretic hormone, whereas substantial volumes of water will be eliminated by a person with diabetes insipidus. Your physician may also conduct blood tests to determine water and salt balance.

How Serious Is Diabetes Insipidus?   Diabetes insipidus is treated effectively with hormone replacement. Except for cases in which the underlying cause—a tumor or disease—presents difficulties, a person with diabetes insipidus can expect to lead a normal life.

Treatment.   Your physician will have three goals: to determine the cause, to eliminate it (if possible), and to control the symptoms.

Medication.   Antidiuretic hormone will be administered either in a nasal spray or by injection of a synthetic form of the hormone.

This hormone therapy usually is lifelong. However, for cases in which the known cause is an injury to the head or the result of surgery, the gland may regain its normal function over a few months to a year; if so, the medication can be discontinued.

A diuretic drug in the thiazide family may also be prescribed. Despite the fact that diuretics ordinarily are used to increase urination, thiazides are effective for treating diabetes insipidus in some people.

Surgery.   If a tumor in the pituitary gland is the cause, surgery or radiation therapy may be appropriate (see Pituitary Tumors, page 723).

Nutrition.   Because sodium restriction helps in some cases, your physician may advise limiting dietary salt intake.

THYROID DISORDERS

Shaped like a bow tie, your thyroid gland is located at the base of your neck. The gland wraps around your windpipe (trachea), and its pair of lobes are connected by a crossbar (isthmus).

This gland helps in setting the rate at which your body functions. It responds to instructions from your pituitary gland by secreting the hormone thyroxine, whose actions control the pace of chemical activity in your body. Such activities vary directly with the quantity of thyroxine present: the more of the hormone that is circulating in the bloodstream, the greater the speed at which chemical reactions occur. Calcitonin, a hormone that affects the amount of calcium in your blood, also is produced by the thyroid gland.

HYPERTHYROIDISM

Signs and Symptoms

- Weight loss despite increased appetite;
- Increased heart rate and blood pressure;
- Nervousness and sweating;
- Swelling at the base of the neck (goiter);
- Increases in the frequency of bowel movements, sometimes diarrhea;
- Muscle weakness.

Emergency Symptoms

- Thyrotoxic crisis: This medical emergency is characterized by fever, very rapid pulse, agitation, and even delirium. Immediate care is required.

Hyperthyroidism (also known as overactive thyroid disease) occurs when the thyroid gland produces excessive amounts of thyroid hormone. Its name is derived from the Greek *hyper,* which means over, and *thyreos,* for shield-shaped, describing the appearance of the thyroid gland. (Hypothyroidism, or underactive thyroid disorder, is discussed on page 730.)

The two forms of hyperthyroidism are Graves' disease (also known as toxic diffuse goiter) and hyperfunctioning nodular goiter (sometimes called Plummer's disease, named for an early physician at the Mayo Clinic). Both forms involve the excessive

manufacture and release of the thyroid hormone thyroxine.

Graves' Disease. The functions of the thyroid gland ordinarily are controlled by a hormone secreted by the pituitary gland. In Graves' disease, the thyroid gland is stimulated excessively by an abnormal antibody, and the normal thyroid-stimulating hormone (TSH) from the pituitary cannot be detected in the blood. The production of thyroid hormones is abnormally high. The amount of thyroxine in the blood also is high.

Hyperthyroidism involves an increase in the body's normal energy expenditure (that is, its basal metabolic rate). One manifestation of this change is an increased appetite because the body will demand more fuel for its added activity. The body generates excessive heat, so that patients with hyperthyroidism feel warm when others may be cool or comfortable. They may have a tremor of the hands with warm, sweaty palms. The heart pounds forcibly at a rapid rate. Occasionally the heart develops a rapid irregularity (atrial fibrillation) (see page 817). They also may have difficulty sleeping.

If you have hyperthyroidism, your thyroid gland will be enlarged, but often so slightly that it isn't noticeable. The abnormal antibody that stimulates the thyroid also has effects on the eyes and may cause protrusion, widening of the lids, excessive tearing and redness, and sometimes double vision.

The result of an excess of thyroid hormone, Graves' disease can produce a variety of symptoms, including a tremor of the hands, rapid heartbeat, and difficulty in sleeping. The most evident visual symptom is pictured here: the characteristic protruding eyes.

Hyperfunctioning Thyroid Nodules.

This form of hyperthyroidism results from excessive production of thyroxine by one or more adenomas of the thyroid. An adenoma of the thyroid is a portion of the gland that has walled itself off from the rest of the gland. It can be felt, and sometimes seen, as a lump, often half an inch or more in size.

Most adenomas of the thyroid produce little or no thyroid hormone, but occasionally an adenoma will begin to manufacture an excessive amount of the hormone. This overproduction results in all of the symptoms of hyperthyroidism found in Graves' disease except that the eyes are not affected.

The Diagnosis.

Your physician will try to detect a slight tremor when you stick out your tongue and extend your fingers and may inquire whether you have experienced diarrhea or other changes in your toilet habits. You may be asked whether you find yourself sensitive to increases in temperature and whether your symptoms are lessened in cooler temperatures.

Because anxiety can cause symptoms like those of hyperthyroidism, psychological causes for the symptoms must be ruled out. Blood tests will be used to detect an increase in the thyroxine concentration and low to absent amounts of TSH. A radioactive iodine tracer test usually is done to help establish the diagnosis and to aid in planning treatment. In Graves' disease the thyroid gland usually has an abnormal "hunger" for iodine. A greater-than-normal amount of the radioactive iodine given with this test will collect in the thyroid within 24 hours. The amount of radioactive iodine used in the tracer test is much smaller than the amount used in treatment.

In the case of hyperfunctioning thyroid nodules, blood test results are similar to those in Graves' disease. Radioactive iodine tracer tests show that the iodine goes almost entirely to the overactive adenoma.

How Serious Is Hyperthyroidism?

Hyperthyroidism varies in severity. In some people, a brief cycle of treatment produces a complete and permanent cure. In others, relapses occur and a second or even third round of treatment is necessary.

If left untreated, the disorder is potentially fatal. In most cases of hyperthyroidism, however, normal health can be restored.

Treatment.

Three types of treatment are available: a liquid form of radioactive iodine, an antithyroid medication in tablet form, and surgery. The proper course of treatment for you will be determined by your physical condition and age and by the nature and severity of your hyperthyroidism.

Medication.

The most common treatment for hyperthyroidism involves drinking a liquid form of radioactive iodine. Your body will deliver the iodine (which is a key component of thyroid hormone) to the thyroid gland, and the concentrated radioactive iodine will cause the tissue in the gland to slow its production of hormones. The dose of radioactive iodine depends on the size of the thyroid gland and the findings on the tracer test.

The status of the thyroid will need to be reassessed in 2 to 3 months. At that time, a second dose of radioactive iodine may be required or thyroid replacement therapy is initiated (see Hypothyroidism, page 730). If thyroid function is normal, reassessments at

---

GOITER

The term goiter, which is derived from the Latin *guttur* for throat, is used to describe a wide variety of conditions. In fact, goiter means simply an enlargement of the thyroid gland. This enlargement can be a small, localized lump or it can be a more general swelling of both lobes.

The enlarged thyroid gland can produce normal, subnormal, or excessive amounts of its hormone. In rare instances the enlargement

Goiter is an enlargement of the thyroid gland, most often due to a shortage of iodine in the diet. After iodized table salt was introduced, goiter became an uncommon ailment in the United States.

will grow around the trachea (windpipe), causing it to narrow. This enlargement can interfere with swallowing. Surprisingly, goiters generally produce little discomfort. In most instances in which a person has a feeling of pressure or the sensation of a lump in the throat, the discomfort results from emotional tension.

In the past, the most common cause of goiter was a shortage of iodine in the diet in areas where the soil was deficient in iodine. Goiter became much rarer after iodized salt was introduced; also, our food supply now is such that even if one does not use iodized salt there is little or no likelihood of iodine deficiency. Taking iodine supplements is unnecessary and therefore undesirable, although in other parts of the world iodine deficiencies are not uncommon.

Simple Goiter

Simple goiter is characterized by a soft, widespread enlargement of the gland. It is most common during pregnancy or adolescence, although it is relatively uncommon today. If the simple goiter enlarges to the degree that it becomes a cosmetic problem, thyroid hormone can be given to decrease its size.

Graves' Disease

Graves' disease usually produces a slight but generalized swelling of the thyroid, although the gland may become large. It is the result of excessive stimulation of the gland (see Hyperthyroidism, page 727).

Adenomatous Goiter

Adenomas are aggregations of more or less normal thyroid tissue that wall themselves off from the rest of the gland. Infrequently, one or more adenomas will produce excessive amounts of thyroid hormone, and hyperthyroidism results. Also, rarely, an adenoma partially blocks the windpipe (trachea) and produces breathing difficulty that superficially may resemble asthma (see Hyperfunctioning Thyroid Nodules, page 728).

Thyroid Cancer

Most thyroid cancers grow slowly. They tend to occur somewhat more frequently in persons who have had radiation therapy to the neck. The common types are papillary and follicular. The papillary type tends to spread to the lymph glands in the neck. The follicular type may go to the lungs and other more distant parts of the body.

As a thyroid cancer develops, it is initially a small lump in the thyroid and cannot be distinguished readily from an adenoma. Tissue from a lump suspected of being cancerous can be obtained through a needle for microscope examination. Although this test does not always produce a clear answer as to whether the lump is cancerous, the information often is a good guide to the need for surgical removal of the lump.

If the lump proves to be malignant at operation (the pathologist can tell the surgeon within a matter of minutes whether the removed lump is malignant), the surgeon will remove most of the thyroid gland. Under certain circumstances, radioactive iodine can be given after the operation to supplement surgical treatment. Thyroid hormone medication also is thought to retard growth of the remaining cancer cells.

Medullary Cancer of the Thyroid

This is an unusual form of thyroid malignancy. The cells of this cancer secrete a hormone called calcitonin, and the progress of the cancer can be followed by measuring calcitonin concentrations in the blood. Medullary carcinoma frequently occurs in members of the same family, and a person who has it also may have pheochromocytoma (see page 721).

Lymphocytic Thyroiditis

This type of goiter is sometimes called Hashimoto's disease, named for the Japanese pathologist who described it. In this condition, an abnormal antibody causes the thyroid gland to lose function—an effect that leads to hypothyroidism (see page 730). The gland is usually moderately enlarged and rather rubbery in texture.

Usually, thyroid hormone treatment will cause the gland to shrink so that surgical removal is not needed. This is one of the most common of all thyroid disorders. Blood tests for the antibody are helpful for diagnosis, and a thyroid needle biopsy usually will confirm it.

Subacute Thyroiditis

This is an uncommon condition causing thyroid pain that is aggravated by swallowing. The gland is slightly enlarged and very tender. A special test called the sedimentation rate test may be conducted (see page 1283). In cases of subacute thyroiditis, the sedimentation rate may be very high, and thyroid hormone values may be either high or low.

The thyroid generally returns to normal in a few months. Often, aspirin will control the symptoms, although your physician may prescribe corticosteroid medications if the symptoms are more pronounced.

6- to 12-week intervals will be needed to monitor the gland's function.

Another treatment involves taking antithyroid drugs in tablet form. Within 6 to 8 weeks after this therapy is started, the symptoms of hyperthyroidism ordinarily will disappear. However, the usual course of treatment requires that the tablets continue to be taken for at least 9 to 12 months. When the year-long course of treatment is completed and the drug is discontinued, there is a substantial chance that the hyperthyroidism will return and another course of treatment will be needed.

Surgery. Treatment of hyperfunctioning thyroid nodules consists of surgical removal in most instances, but radioactive iodine and antithyroid drugs are also used in the same manner as for Graves' disease. During surgery, most or a portion of the thyroid gland may be removed, especially if symptoms recur after two or three courses of radioactive iodine therapy or of an antithyroid drug. In rare cases, the abnormality of the eyes is so severe that vision is threatened and an operation may be needed to relieve the pressure behind the eyes.

Nutrition. For cases in which severe weight loss and muscle wasting have occurred, a diet providing supplemental calories and protein may be necessary.

HYPOTHYROIDISM

Signs and Symptoms
- Lethargy characterized by slowed physical and mental functions;
- Slowed heart rate;
- Intolerance to cold temperatures;
- Constipation;
- Dry skin and hair;
- Goiter (in some patients);
- Heavy and prolonged menstrual periods;
- Decreased sexual interest.

Emergency Symptoms
- Myxedema coma: This is characterized by a sensation of intense cold intolerance and drowsiness followed by profound lethargy and unconsciousness. A myxedema coma may be precipitated by sedatives and requires emergency medical treatment.

An underactive thyroid gland causes hypothyroidism (the opposite of hyperthyroidism, page 727). Its name comes from the Greek *hypo* for under and *thyreos* for shield-shaped. The group of symptoms and findings that develop after several years of untreated hypothyroidism is termed myxedema.

The thyroid hormone has such significant effects on growth and development that deficiencies can lead to various health problems. In extreme cases, deficiency states can lead to mental retardation in infants and young children and to a slowing of mental processes, an inability to maintain normal body temperatures, and even heart failure in adults.

In hypothyroidism, the body's normal functioning rate, its basal metabolic rate, is slowed. The shortage of thyroid hormone causes the body to slow down, leaving the patient feeling mentally and physically sluggish.

In some cases, failure of the pituitary gland to produce a hormone called thyroid-stimulating hormone (TSH) causes hypothyroidism. More often, the thyroid gland gradually is destroyed by an abnormal antibody. In other cases, the cause of the hypothyroidism is unknown. In still others, the treatment for hyperthyroidism may produce hypothyroidism by working too well. In these cases the thyroid hormone status is reversed (from an excess of the hormone to a deficiency); this condition may be temporary or permanent. In some rare instances, infants are born without thyroid glands.

Hashimoto's disease (lymphocytic thyroiditis) may also be a cause of hypothyroidism.

Although it is not a common ailment, hypothyroidism is not unusual. It can occur in anyone of either sex or any age. However, middle-aged women are most commonly affected, and it is most likely to remain undiagnosed in elderly persons.

The Diagnosis. Hypothyroidism usually develops slowly over months or even years. Although the person who has it may not notice some of the changes, a friend or relative who has not seen the patient for some months may find the apparent deterioration remarkable.

At first, a constant tiredness with muscle aches and an inability to stay warm in cool or cold temperatures may be the only symptoms. Constipation may also occur. The face will become puffy, and the skin will be lusterless and assume a dry and thickened quality. The voice may grow hoarse, and there may be hearing loss. Although weight gain often is considered to be a common symptom of hypothyroidism, the increase in weight is only slight, if present at all.

The most effective way to diagnose hypothyroidism is with laboratory tests. Blood samples are analyzed for different forms of the thyroid hormone and for thyroid-stimulating hormone (TSH) and antibodies (low thyroid hormone and high TSH values suggest hypothyroidism, and a high antibody value suggests that Hashimoto's disease is the cause of the hypothyroidism).

How Serious Is Hypothyroidism? In most people, hypothyroidism is neither chronic nor progressive, and its treatment results in a normal life. However, treatment is especially important in infants and in people with severe hormone deficiencies.

Myxedema Coma. Hypothyroidism is unlikely to be life-threatening, except when myxedema coma occurs. This rare condition is usually the result of long-term, undiagnosed hypothyroidism, and it may be provoked by illness, exposure to cold, accident or injury, or surgery. Myxedema coma requires immediate treatment, usually with hormone injections.

Cretinism. In infants, untreated hypothyroidism can result in dwarfism and mental retardation (cretinism). If the condition is diagnosed within the first several months of life (as it often is because of routine blood tests conducted immediately after birth), the chances of normal development are excellent. In a child with the arrested development characteristic of cretinism, typical signs include a tendency to drool constantly, a swayback and potbelly, short stature, and irregularly placed, poorly formed teeth.

Treatment. *Medication.* The key treatment is the daily consumption of thyroid hormone. Mayo Clinic physicians prefer to prescribe a synthetic thyroid hormone, although medication derived from animal thyroid glands can also be used. In most cases, the condition improves noticeably within a week after the hormone therapy is begun. All symptoms disappear within a few months. However, the individual must continue this treatment for the rest of his or her life.

Nutrition. In some people, the lack of thyroid hormone results from a long-term shortage of iodine in the diet. The thyroid gland then increases in size in an attempt to compensate, and goiter, a swelling at the front and base of the neck, results. This condition is extremely rare in the United States because our table salt is supplemented with iodine and our food supply is generally rich in iodine. However, in parts of the world where the soil lacks iodine, iodine deficiency is a common cause of goiter. In such areas, the use of iodized salt is an effective public health measure (see page 728).

PARATHYROID GLAND DISORDERS

The thyroid gland is at the front and base of the neck, and the parathyroid glands are located on its four corners. The parathyroid glands are small—each is about the size of a grain of rice. They produce parathyroid hormone. When too much of this hormone is produced, the resulting disorder is called hyperparathyroidism (the Greek prefix *hyper* means above), and an underproduction is hypoparathyroidism (the Greek prefix *hypo* means below).

Increased hormone secretion by one or more of the parathyroid glands increases the amount of calcium in the blood, mainly by releasing it from the bones and by increasing absorption of it from the small intestine. The parathyroid glands maintain the level of calcium in the blood within very narrow limits by turning their secretion off or on (just as a thermostat controls a heating system to maintain a constant air temperature). Vitamin D is also necessary for regulating the amount of calcium in the blood. Another hormone, called calcitonin, which is manufactured in the thyroid gland plays an uncertain role.

Located on your thyroid gland, the rice-sized parathyroid glands produce a hormone that controls the level of calcium in your blood.

HYPERPARATHYROIDISM

Signs and Symptoms

Hyperparathyroidism may be symptomless at first, unless pain from kidney stones develops. However, over several years, symptoms may appear:

- Kidney stones;
- Indefinite fatigue;
- Increased urination and thirst;
- Indigestion or ulcer symptoms.

When one or more of the parathyroid glands produce an excess of their hormone, the resulting disorder is termed hyperparathyroidism (the reverse disorder is hypoparathyroidism, in which too little of the hormone is produced; see next entry). When there is too much parathyroid hormone circulating in the body, the calcium concentration becomes exaggeratedly high and the phosphorus concentration is low.

In more than 80 percent of cases, the cause is a small growth in one of the parathyroid glands. In other instances, all four of the glands become enlarged and overproduce the hormone. The growths are usually localized and are unlikely to spread to other organs.

Once thought to be rather rare, this ailment is not uncommon among middle-aged

people. Women are about twice as likely to have hyperparathyroidism as men.

The Diagnosis. In about half of patients with hyperparathyroidism, there are no symptoms and the diagnosis is often the result of a routine blood test showing a high concentration of calcium in the blood rather than a search for the cause of any of its symptoms.

Blood tests that reveal excessive amounts of calcium and parathyroid hormone in the blood suggest the presence of hyperparathyroidism. Frequently, the diagnosis is made almost accidentally: the abnormally high calcium and hormone values are discovered during routine tests for some other disorder. Low amounts of phosphorus in the blood are suggestive of the disorder.

Direct measurement of the amount of parathyroid hormone in the blood helps confirm the diagnosis. Over the next several years, considerable improvement in the tests for this hormone is expected, and so more reliance can then be placed on them.

Once the preliminary diagnosis of hyperparathyroidism is made, the patient is asked whether he or she consumes excessive amounts of vitamin D. The use of certain diuretic drugs, called thiazides, is another possible cause of an increased blood calcium value. The physician may also conduct an ultrasound examination of the thyroid region in an attempt to locate tumors in the parathyroid glands. A condition called sarcoidosis (see page 934) can also increase the amount of calcium in the circulation and must be excluded. Some cancers of the lung, breast, and other organs sometimes secrete a substance that closely resembles parathyroid hormone and will thereby increase the blood calcium concentrations.

How Serious Is Hyperparathyroidism?

In some cases, treatment is unnecessary and your physician will simply monitor your condition. The condition of your kidneys will be followed closely to determine whether kidney stones are appearing and whether the kidney is disposing of waste substances normally. There is a long-term danger to your bones: too much calcium in the blood means that much of the mineral is being liberated from the bones, which are the storage area for calcium in the body. The bone changes become a problem only infrequently, however, because the presence of active kidney stones or deterioration of kidney function will require surgical attempts at removal of the tumor before the skeleton deteriorates significantly. Occasionally, patients have peptic ulcers with hyperparathyroidism.

Treatment. A surgeon experienced in parathyroid surgery will be able to find and remove the tumor in most cases. If the tumor is not found in the usual location of the parathyroid glands, more elaborate techniques to locate the tumor and even surgical exploration of the region behind the breastbone (sternum) may be needed.

HYPOPARATHYROIDISM

Signs and Symptoms
- Muscle spasms or numbness, especially in the hands, feet, and throat;
- Breathing difficulty;
- Dry skin;
- Yeast infections;
- In children: vomiting, convulsions, and headaches.

When the parathyroid glands produce too little of their hormone, the disorder that results is termed hypoparathyroidism. (The opposite disorder is called hyperparathyroidism, in which too much hormone is produced; see previous entry.)

Parathyroid hormone is crucial to your body's use of calcium. Without sufficient quantities of it, the amount of calcium in the blood falls below normal and the amount of phosphorus rises. A low blood calcium concentration can produce various problems, particularly muscular spasms and cramps; over several years, cataracts and, rarely, convulsions may develop.

Hypoparathyroidism is rare and is far less likely to occur than hyperparathyroidism. There are two types of hypoparathyroidism. Spontaneous hypoparathyroidism of unknown cause may be associated with a susceptibility to yeast infections and a failure of the ovaries or adrenal glands. Children are affected more often than adults.

The second type results from inadvertent removal of the normal parathyroid glands during surgery for goiter or as a surgical complication after removal of multiple overactive parathyroid glands.

The Diagnosis. The key finding in the diagnosis of hypoparathyroidism is abnormally low concentrations of calcium in the blood (a condition known as hypocalcemia) and abnormally high concentrations of phosphorus.

How Serious Is Hypoparathyroidism?
The muscle spasms associated with hypoparathyroidism can be uncomfortable, and breathing difficulty can result from spasms of the muscles controlling the vocal cords. If the amount of calcium in the blood is low for many years, cataracts and convulsions can occur.

Treatment. Your physician will prescribe vitamin D and calcium supplements. If certain symptoms are especially severe (in particular, the muscle spasms), you may be given an intravenous injection of calcium to provide immediate but temporary relief.

Calcium and vitamin D supplements must be taken for life. They must be taken in amounts considerably larger than those required for ordinary nutrition. Also, because the blood calcium concentration must be monitored, your physician will establish a schedule of blood tests for you. The supplements should restore satisfactory health, but the regularly scheduled tests are important for maintaining normal levels of the essential calcium in your blood.

If your physician suspects a parathyroid tumor, he or she may conduct an ultrasound examination. Directed through a wand, sound waves are used to generate an image of your parathyroid glands, thus revealing any abnormal growths.

CHAPTER 27
THE EYES

CHAPTER CONTENTS

THE EYE IN SYSTEMIC DISEASES
The Eye and Diabetes
Third Nerve Palsy
Graves' Disease and Eye Problems

Hypertension and Vision
The Eye and Warning Signs of
Stroke
Cranial Arteritis and Vision

HOW YOU SEE

Your eye is a singular instrument, able to receive in an instant millions of disparate pieces of information about the world outside your body. The eye is often compared with a camera, but the comparison is hardly fair to the eye. True, as with the camera, an image enters your eye by passing through a lens. And the image is in some sense recorded at the back of both devices: on film in the camera and by a complex communication system in your eye that transmits the image to your brain. The eye is like a camera, but it is more sophisticated than any machine imaginable.

Thousands of times a day, your eyes move and focus on images near and far, picking out objects for interpretation within a vast available field. Instantaneously, your eye records what a dozen cameras could not, providing you with an ever-changing, incredibly detailed chain of three-dimensional pictures of the world around you.

PARTS OF THE EYE

The complex structure of the eye is compact: each of your eyes, lying within protective sockets formed by the skull and surrounding tissues, measures about 1 inch in diameter. The delicate workings of your eye are protected by the bridge of your nose, your eyebrow, and your cheekbone. The bones and tissues surrounding your eye are known collectively as the orbit.

Your eye is also protected by your eyelid. The eyelid opens and shuts involuntarily, shielding the eye from intense light, impact, and foreign particles.

Tears serve to lubricate, clean, and nourish your eye. Tears are secreted by glands in your upper eyelids and in the orbit above and to the side of the upper lid. Tears are drained into your nose from two tiny openings located in your upper and lower eyelids, very close to where the lids join adjacent to your nose (inner canthus). The ducts that convey tears from your eyes to your nose are called the nasolacrimal ducts.

When you blink, which happens every few seconds, your eyelid acts like a windshield wiper complete with fluid, washing away dirt and particles and putting on lubricant. During sleep your eyes are protected from drying out by being closed.

The movement of your eye is controlled by six muscles attached to the outside cov-

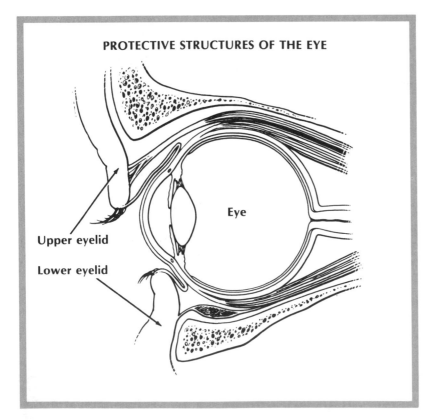

PROTECTIVE STRUCTURES OF THE EYE

Eye

Upper eyelid

Lower eyelid

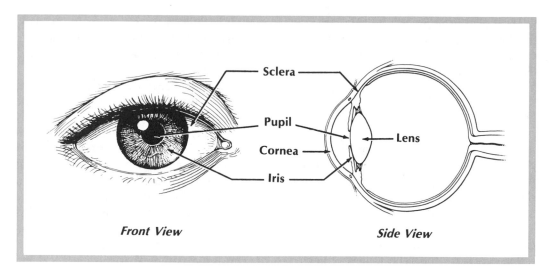

Front View

Side View

ering (sclera) of the eye. They act in concert to move both eyes up, down, around, and from side to side so that your two eyes will center on exactly the same point. (When the centering mechanisms are impaired, the eyes are said to deviate from one another.)

The eyeball itself is composed of several layers of tissue. The conjunctiva runs along the inside of the eyelid and the outermost portion of the eye. It meets the sclera, the tough white membrane that covers most of the eyeball. Both contain tiny blood vessels that nourish the eye.

Inside the conjunctiva at the center of the eye lies the cornea. This layer of clear tissue with its overlying film of tears provides about two-thirds of the focusing power of the eye. The cornea is shaped to refract light as it enters the eye, directing it through the lens and to the retina at the back of the eye.

The pupil and iris lie behind the cornea. The pupil is the opening through which light passes to the back of the eye. Muscles controlling the iris (the colored part of the eye) allow it to change the size of the pupil to adjust to the amount of light. The pupil becomes larger in dim light to allow more light in and smaller in bright light to protect the delicate retina from excessive light. The pupil also opens (dilates) in response to excitement and as a reaction to certain drugs.

Between the cornea and the iris lies the anterior chamber. This space is filled with aqueous humor, a transparent fluid. This fluid is manufactured in the posterior chamber of the eye close to the attachment of the iris. The fluid passes into the anterior chamber through the pupil and then is absorbed into the bloodstream through Schlemm's canal in the angle where the iris meets the

cornea. Your body regulates the pressure of the aqueous humor.

Behind the iris and posterior chamber is the lens. This transparent, colorless tissue is enclosed in a capsule and suspended in the middle of the eye by a net of fibers. The lens can change shape in order to focus light rays on the retina. When an object is nearby, the lens thickens to best perceive the image; when an object is farther away, the lens thins in order to focus the image clearly on the retina. Throughout one's life the lens accumulates more fibers. These added fibers gradually make the lens less elastic, so that generally by middle age you become less able to focus on near objects.

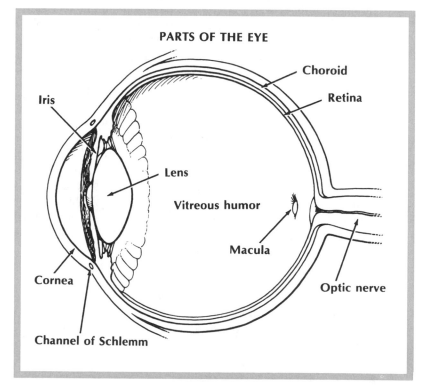

PARTS OF THE EYE

The bulk of the eyeball, which is behind the lens, is formed by the round vitreous chamber. It is filled with a colorless, gelatin-like substance known as the vitreous humor. You may notice that occasionally you see spots or what look like tiny bits of string or lint in your vision. Suspended in the vitreous humor, these are known as "floaters" and are usually leftover bits of material from the growth of the eye before birth. Occasionally they can be a sign of a more serious eye disorder.

Behind the vitreous chamber is the retina. The retina of the eye is equivalent to the film of the camera. Composed of 10 layers, the retina processes the light images projected from the cornea and lens.

Rod cells within the retina perceive light, and cone cells perceive light and color. Rod cells outnumber cone cells 20 to 1, and they can respond to faint light. Cone cells need more light to function, which is one reason why it is difficult to see colors in the dark. The responsibility of the rods and cones is to transform the light that they perceive into electrical impulses.

A small depression in the center of the retina, known as the fovea, provides the most acute vision. This section contains only cones and is the most visually sensitive part of the eye. The small area surrounding the fovea is known as the macula lutea, and as a whole it is responsible for central vision.

The retina is nourished primarily by the choroid. This multilayered tissue, which lies between the retina and the sclera, is composed of veins and arteries.

The optic nerve takes the electrical impulses recorded by the retina and transmits them to the brain. The point at which the optic nerve leaves the retina on its way to the brain is known as the optic disc. The optic nerve carries impulses to the visual cortex at the back of the brain. The brain

HEREDITARY DISORDERS OF THE EYES

Conditions and diseases affecting the eyes can be passed from generation to generation. Such conditions range from simple far-sightedness (which can be corrected with glasses or contact lenses; see page 742) to more serious eye diseases such as retino-blastoma (see page 762). Certain systemic diseases, including diabetes and hypertension, also can produce eye complications.

Refraction errors such as near-sightedness, farsightedness, and astigmatism are due to the shapes and characteristics of the cornea, lens, and eyeball, and often they are present from birth. The cause of such abnormalities is unknown but, because the deformity often recurs generation after generation, genetics is thought to play a key role. Often, however, only certain members of a family inherit a disorder and others are entirely free of the problem.

Heredity seems to play a part in the incidence of strabismus (habitual squint; see page 750) and amblyopia (poor vision, usually secondary to misalignment of the eyes; see page 750). If your eyes were misaligned as a child, you have a greater chance of having a child with the same problem.

Defects of color vision, commonly and often wrongly termed color blindness, usually are present from birth, having been passed along through the mother, usually to her sons. Most people who have defects of color vision cannot distinguish between reds and greens in dim light; some people cannot separate the colors even in bright light. Only a minority of so-called color-blind people see everything in tones of gray, and only they are truly color-blind. Color vision defects are common. They are caused by a lack of one or more of the light-sensitive substances found in the cones of the retina.

Certain eye diseases also seem to have a genetic factor. People with glaucoma (see page 765) often have a family history of the disease, as do people with cataracts (see page 768). Retinitis pigmentosa is a serious threat to sight, and often there is a pattern of recurrence of the disease within families (see page 776). Retino-blastoma, a cancerous tumor of the eye that occurs in young children, seems to have a genetic component in 30 percent to 40 percent of cases (see page 762).

Other general disorders that affect the eyes and have a hereditary component include diabetes and hypertension. Diabetes affects eyesight after many years (see Diabetes Mellitus, page 707, and Diabetic Retinopathy, page 777). Hypertension (high blood pressure) affects eyesight when the disease is particularly severe, and it can even be diagnosed on the basis of changes seen within the eye (see High Blood Pressure, page 796, and Hypertension and Vision, page 779).

interprets these messages into what we perceive as sight.

THE MECHANISM OF SIGHT

The listing of all of the eye's parts may make the device seem complicated indeed. Yet the basic mechanism of sight is relatively simple.

Rays of light project through the cornea, the pupil, and then the lens. The internal eye muscles help adjust the shape of the lens to focus the light rays on the back of the retina. There, the rods and cones turn the light into electrical impulses that are carried by the optic nerve to the brain.

Once the brain receives the electrical impulses, it must interpret them. The image received by the retina is upside-down, a characteristic of a simple convex lens. The brain reinterprets the image, however, so that what you perceive is right-side up. The brain also must coordinate the images from each eye, which are slightly different. The merging of the two images produces three-dimensional (stereoscopic) vision.

THE EYE EXPERTS

Because the eye is such a complicated and delicate instrument, anything more than the most routine care must be handled by physician specialists. A physician specially trained to treat eyes is known as an *ophthalmologist.*

Formerly known as an *oculist,* an ophthalmologist specializes in the treatment of eye diseases and conditions. He or she is a medical doctor (M.D.) who has, in addition to medical school training, at least 4 years of specialized training in the care of the eyes and the diagnosis and treatment of eye ailments. An ophthalmologist can prescribe eyeglasses and contact lenses; complete eye examinations and eye care can be provided by ophthalmologists. An ophthalmologist also treats injuries to the eye and performs various surgical procedures when they are required.

An *optometrist* is a person trained to diagnose refraction errors and to prescribe corrective lenses. Optometrists graduate from a school of optometry and earn a doctor of optometry (O.D.) degree. They can conduct certain simple tests, and often they detect signs of eye disease or other kinds of disease apparent from examination of the retina. In some states, optometrists can diagnose and treat eye diseases.

An *optician* is a technician who fills the prescriptions of ophthalmologists and optometrists. Opticians grind and fit lenses, but they do not examine eyes for disease or refraction problems.

REFRACTION PROBLEMS

The most common eye problems—myopia (nearsightedness), hyperopia (farsightedness), astigmatism (asymmetrical cornea), and presbyopia (the inability to focus on an object at close range as one ages)—are all due to errors of refraction of the lens and cornea of one or both eyes.

If you are to see an object clearly, its well-focused image must reach your retina, the light-sensitive membrane at the back of your eye. As light rays enter your eye, your cornea and lens refract (bend) them to converge on your retina.

For the image to be clear, the focusing power of the lens and cornea must be coordinated with the length of your eyeball. In normal eyesight, the image then appears focused.

When the focusing elements and the eyeball are not properly coordinated, however, the image will not reach the retina in focus, and the light will then be focused in front of or behind the retina. When the shape of the eyeball is such that light is focused in front of the retina, the condition is known as *nearsightedness* because only objects at near range are focused on the correct part of the retina. *Farsightedness* is the result of light being focused correctly on the retina only at long range. When the cornea is irregularly shaped, thereby misdirecting some of the light rays, the condition is known as *astigmatism.*

Nearsightedness, farsightedness, and astigmatism may be the result of heredity or other causes. However, another refraction

THE EYE EXAMINATION

How Often Do I Need to Visit the Ophthalmologist?

Everyone should have their eyes examined from time to time. If you do not have eye problems, have your eyes examined every 3 to 5 years up until about age 50 years. After 50, have them checked more frequently for signs of glaucoma and other eye disease. If you have refraction or other eye problems, have your eyes checked every 2 years, or as recommended by your eye specialist.

Children should have their first examination at around age 3 or 4 years, unless you have reason to believe there may be a problem earlier. If you do, tests are available that can be performed on toddlers.

The Examination

Your eye specialist may begin by asking a series of questions about your family's medical history and your personal medical history. Then a series of tests will be conducted. One simple test involves passing a light in front of your eyes in a set pattern in order to check the movements of the eyes, both separately and together. Your eye doctor will check peripheral vision by moving an object at the edge of your field of vision.

The Snellen Chart

You will be asked to read letters on a chart known as a Snellen chart. In this test you usually are asked to read the letters on each line of the chart from 20 feet away. If you can read the letters that people with perfect eyesight can read at 20 feet from the chart, you are said to have 20/20 vision. If you read at 20 feet what most people can read 40 feet from the chart, you have 20/40 vision. For children who are too young to recognize letters, another similar test using shapes can be conducted.

Color Testing

Color vision usually is tested by asking whether you can discern figures in a series of illustrations made up of numerous colored dots or circles.

The Ophthalmoscope

The back of the eye is examined with an instrument known as the ophthalmoscope. The device has a magnifier and a light that shines through to the back of the eye, allowing the examiner to see clearly the rear (posterior) portions of the eye, particularly the retina.

The back of each eye (known as the fundus) provides many clues to your general health. The region is unique from other portions of your body in that tiny blood vessels and nerve tissue of the retina can be seen directly.

The condition of the retinal vessels often has a tale to tell. For example, if you have hypertension (high blood pressure), the changes in these vessels often indicate the severity of your problem and the urgency with which treatment should be started. Clues to circulatory disturbances in the brain sometimes are provided by the small particles appearing in the blood vessels of the fundus, which indicate the formation of cholesterol-containing plaques or clots of other material. Changes in the blood vessels characteristic of diabetes also can be visible, as can holes or tears in the retina and a host of other problems.

The optic nerve head (optic disc) is also visible with the ophthalmoscope. The optic disc is actually an extension of your brain. If the nerve is swollen it may indicate that you have a disorder, even a problem as serious as a brain tumor, causing increased pressure within your skull.

For the ophthalmoscope examination, a few drops are placed in your eyes to dilate the pupils so that more of the fundus can be seen. The lights of the room are dimmed also so the pupils will widen. Then the bright light of the ophthalmoscope is shone in and each eye is examined.

The use of dilating eye drops is a routine part of most eye examinations. They can make it temporarily difficult for you to focus on near objects or to tolerate bright light. If you are being checked for signs of cataracts or retinal problems, however, eye drops are necessary.

People older than 50 years should be tested regularly for signs of glaucoma. A simple test to measure the pressure inside the eyeball is done with a device called a tonometer (see Glaucoma, page 765).

error is a basic part of aging. This is known as presbyopia, and it is the result of changes in the lens of the eye. The lens hardens with age, reducing its ability to change shape and focus light at close range. This hardening results in a difficulty with focusing on near objects.

Most errors of refraction are treated easily with corrective glasses or contact lenses. For most people, a pair of glasses or lenses prescribed and fitted by an ophthalmologist or optometrist provides the necessary correction for them to function easily in daily activities. Also, a new operation may prove useful for people with mild or moderate myopia (see page 742).

NEARSIGHTEDNESS

Signs and Symptoms
• Blurred vision of distant objects.

Nearsightedness (myopia) is a common vision problem, affecting about 20 percent of the population. If you are nearsighted, your eye is slightly out of round. It probably is too long from front to back, so that the light rays that are refracted by the cornea and lens meet in front of (rather than at) the retina. The result is that distant images are blurry.

You may be able to focus on nearby images, although the degree of your myopia determines the focusing ability. If you are severely nearsighted you may be able to see clearly only objects that are a few inches from your eyes; if you are mildly nearsighted, you may see clearly the objects that are several yards away.

Occasionally, nearsightedness results not from an elongated shape of the eye but from too much focusing power in the lens and cornea. The result is the same in that, again, the light rays focus in front of the retina.

Nearsightedness often is observed during childhood, from the early school years through the late teens; it affects boys and girls equally. It can develop rapidly during this time, requiring new lenses every few months. It tends to stabilize during young adulthood, so that during your 20s and 30s you may not require a change of eyeglasses or contact lenses. At about age 40 years, however, the normal effects of aging may begin to change your vision. Nearsightedness tends to run in families.

The Diagnosis. If you notice that your child persistently squints, sits close to the television, movie screen, or class blackboard, holds books very close while reading, and seems to be unaware of distant objects, have your child's vision tested by an ophthalmologist or optometrist.

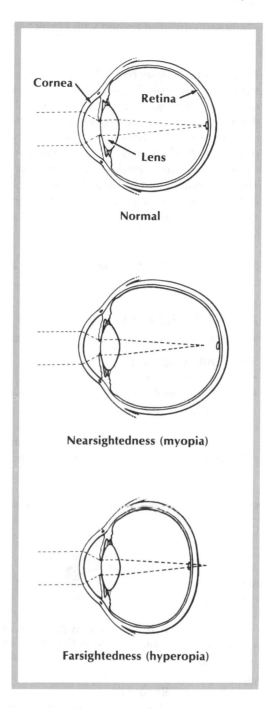

Normal

Nearsightedness (myopia)

Farsightedness (hyperopia)

For clear eyesight, the lens and cornea must be coordinated with the length of your eyeball.

The examination will begin with your child reading a chart of letters to determine the vision in each eye (visual acuity). Special charts are available for young children who are unable to read letters (see The Eye Examination, page 740). Your physician also will perform a series of tests to determine the extent of correction needed.

How Serious Is Nearsightedness? Nearsightedness in children can be socially, emotionally, and educationally debilitating if not diagnosed early and treated with corrective lenses.

Treatment. *Corrective Lenses.* Nearsightedness is treated easily with eyeglasses or contact lenses. Your eye specialist will determine a specific prescription to suit your child's needs. This prescription, a specially made concave lens for one or both eyes, can correct vision to normal or nearly normal. The prescription can be made for glasses or contact lenses in various forms, although contact lenses are usually unsuitable for preteen children.

Surgery. Another possible treatment is a procedure called radial keratotomy.

FARSIGHTEDNESS

Signs and Symptoms
• Blurred vision at close distance;
• Eyestrain, including aching eyes and headache.

Farsightedness (hyperopia) is a common refraction problem. In most cases it is the result of the eyeball being too short from front to back. Thus, the rays of light converge on the retina short of the focal length at which they would be in focus. The angle between the iris and the interior surface of the cornea is narrowed in the farsighted individual, making him or her more vulnerable to closed-angle glaucoma later in life (see Chronic Glaucoma, page 766).

Farsightedness also can be caused by a weakness in the ability of the lens and cornea to focus. Whatever the cause, however, close images appear blurry, although distant ones may appear clearly.

Farsightedness usually is present at birth and tends to run in families. Young people can often overcome mild farsightedness naturally as the eyes accommodate to the condition; the ciliary muscles contract and change the shape of the lens to bring the focal point forward to meet the retina. Thus, they do not need corrective glasses for their hyperopia. However, with age, the ability of the eyes to ''correct'' the condition is lost, and glasses or contact lenses are required.

The Diagnosis. You may not have symptoms for several years, if ever, depending on

---

RADIAL KERATOTOMY

A new surgical technique to correct mild to moderate myopia, called radial keratotomy, is currently under evaluation. The process, developed in the Soviet Union, seems simple, but it requires careful microsurgical technique.

The Procedure
A series of delicate incisions is made in the cornea of each eye in a radial or spoke-like pattern. Each eye is done separately, on different days. The center of the cornea flattens and the outer downward-sloping portion becomes steeper. This changes the way light rays are bent, focusing them more on the retina.

Radial keratotomy is a series of surgical incisions in the cornea to correct nearsightedness (myopia).

Recovery
The procedure is done on an outpatient basis—it takes only 15 to 30 minutes—and with the person under local anesthesia. The individual wears a patch or dark glasses for several days, although recovery can take several months.

The Results
Radial keratotomy in principle seems like a good solution to nearsightedness. A long-range follow-up study of individuals who have

had the procedure suggests that slightly more than half reported that their vision was fully corrected. Approximately a fourth reported partially corrected vision but still needed glasses or contact lenses, and about 15 percent had their vision overcorrected so that they became farsighted. One percent experienced serious complications.

Other drawbacks to radial keratotomy include the potential for fluctuating vision, late infections of the cornea, and slightly increased risk of traumatic corneal rupture.

Most eye surgeons remain uncertain of the usefulness of radial keratotomy. At this point it is impossible to know who might have long-term benefits from the procedure. We advise caution when considering it.

the severity. You may, however, find it difficult to focus on objects close at hand. You may have headaches or general eye discomfort after doing close tasks such as reading, writing, or drawing.

If you have such problems, consult an eye specialist, who will conduct a series of tests to determine the nature and extent of the problem and who will then prescribe eyeglasses or contact lenses precisely suited to your needs (see The Eye Examination, page 740).

Treatment. Farsightedness is treated easily with eyeglasses or contact lenses made to suit your needs. Your eye specialist will determine the precise prescription needed to correct one or both eyes with convex lenses. The shape of the lens serves to refract the light at an angle that brings the convergence forward to meet the retina. The prescription can be made for glasses, which are appropriate for all ages, or contact lenses, which are best suited to adults and teenagers.

Surgical techniques to treat farsightedness are available but are not in widespread use.

PRESBYOPIA

Signs and Symptoms
- Decreased ability to focus on objects at close range;
- Eyestrain which may include a feeling of tired eyes and a headache.

When functioning correctly, the lens in your eye changes shape in order to focus on objects: when looking at something at close range, the ciliary muscles contract and thicken the lens to bring the object into focus. However, as you age, the lens becomes harder and less elastic, making it more difficult to see nearby objects clearly.

The resulting condition is known as presbyopia. This hardening process is a normal part of life, and it happens to everyone to some degree.

The Diagnosis. Many people begin to notice a change in their vision around age 40 years. Close-up objects that were once easy to see become blurred. The print in newspapers and books begins to seem smaller, and you instinctively hold them farther away from your eyes to read them.

REFRACTION ERRORS DUE TO CHANGING BLOOD SUGAR CONCENTRATION

A prolonged increase in the blood sugar concentration (a problem characteristic of poorly controlled diabetes) tends to cause a metabolic change in the lens of the eye, altering its shape.

When diabetes develops, often the blood sugar concentration gradually increases over a period of weeks or months. The subsequent change in the shape of the lens causes a slow change in focus, which often is not noticeable immediately. However, when the diabetes finally is discovered and treatment produces a rapid decrease in the blood sugar concentration, a rapid change in focus toward farsightedness (hyperopia) often occurs, a change that may be alarming.

It is worthwhile to postpone fitting of glasses until your blood sugar concentration has been well controlled for at least a month. Subsequent minor fluctuations in the blood sugar concentration from day to day or week to week are unlikely to cause perceptible changes in vision or the strength of glasses required (see Diabetes Mellitus, page 707).

If you are already farsighted you may notice the changes somewhat earlier and will need to have stronger corrective lenses made. Even if you are nearsighted you will experience the effects of presbyopia, and you may find yourself taking off your glasses to read small print. You may find that your eyes seem increasingly tired after reading, or you may experience frequent headaches as a result of eyestrain.

When close work such as sewing and reading becomes difficult to do at a normal distance or if you experience frequent eyestrain and headaches, see your ophthalmologist or optometrist, who will test your eyes and prescribe appropriate lenses (see The Eye Examination, page 740).

Treatment. Presbyopia usually is treated with glasses and only occasionally with contact lenses. Your eye specialist will fit you with a prescription for convex lenses to help adjust the focal point more narrowly. As your own lenses lose the ability to adjust, you may need new prescriptions every few years until about age 65 years. At that point the lenses of your eyes will have lost most of their ability to accommodate, and so changes in your prescription are less frequent.

If you are already nearsighted or astigmatic, you will probably find yourself needing a second pair of glasses to counteract the effects of presbyopia. Some people require a third set for middle distances (2 to 4 feet). You need not constantly shuffle glasses, however, for they can be made with two or even three lenses. The double lens, known as a bifocal, was first introduced by Benjamin Franklin. The top portion of each lens (upper segment) is corrected for distance; the bottom portion (lower segment) is corrected for near objects. Trifocals include a third (middle) lens for focusing at arm's length.

Some practice is needed to become accustomed to bifocals and trifocals. Be certain that the frames are adjusted to your head: it is important that, as you tilt your head up and down, your line of vision will move from one segment to another in both eyes at precisely the same time.

ASTIGMATISM

Signs and Symptoms
- Portions of your visual field are blurred, typically vertical, horizontal, or diagonal lines.

Astigmatism is a refraction error due to an uneven curvature of the cornea, blurring some of what you see. In a normal eye, the cornea is symmetrically curved, but an astigmatic eye typically has areas of the cornea that are steeper or flatter than normal, a shape that produces the distorted vision. In some instances, astigmatism may result from abnormalities of the lens inside the eye although the cornea is normal.

Astigmatism is usually present from birth and may occur in combination with nearsightedness or farsightedness. It is a condition that tends to remain constant, neither improving nor deteriorating considerably with age.

The Diagnosis.   You may notice that horizontal lines appear less clear and that vertical lines are clear, or vice versa. Diagonal lines may or may not be blurred. If you notice that your child seems able to see some things clearly but not others, in a seemingly random pattern, consult your eye doctor for complete testing (see The Eye Examination, page 740).

Treatment.   Astigmatism can be treated readily with corrective glasses or contact lenses. After careful examination, your eye specialist will determine your needs. Lenses then can be made to counteract the unevenness of the cornea of one or both eyes or to correct for a combination of astigmatism and nearsightedness or of astigmatism and farsightedness.

WHAT YOU SHOULD KNOW ABOUT CONTACT LENSES

Recent advances in contact lens technology have almost doubled the number of people wearing such lenses during the past 10 years. The newer lenses, such as gas-permeable hard lenses, soft lenses, and extended-wear soft lenses, are far more comfortable for long-term wear than any previously available. However, with the increase in the types available and their rapidly expanding use, more problems are reported, some of them serious.

WHO SHOULD WEAR CONTACT LENSES?

Contact lenses are most useful for people with refraction errors such as nearsightedness, farsightedness, and astigmatism. In addition, certain unusual conditions such as keratoconus (conical cornea) are better treated with contact lenses than with glasses. Some people who have had artificial lenses implanted during cataract operations find contact lenses preferable to glasses.

In all cases, however, only people who are highly motivated to wear contact lenses should consider them. Learning to wear them requires varying periods of adjustment, during which your eyes may be uncomfortable. You also need a certain amount of manual dexterity to put these tiny lenses in and remove them. Also, most contact lenses require daily care, varying from minimal for some kinds to fairly elaborate for others.

For these reasons, contact lenses are not for everyone. They generally are not suitable for small children or for people with certain diseases that limit mobility of the hands, such as arthritis or Parkinson's disease. In addition, contact lenses are not suitable for people with certain eye diseases and disorders. Your eye specialist can advise you.

HOW DO THEY WORK?

As its name implies, a contact lens is worn in contact with the eye. The specially shaped plastic disc sits on the cornea of your eye. (The cornea is the transparent window that lies in front of the pupil, like the crystal of a watch.) The lens floats on the tears that bathe the eye when you blink. This liquid also allows necessary oxygen to reach the cornea.

Each contact lens is made according to a prescription to focus light on the retina of your eye, just as each lens for a pair of eyeglasses does. However, in contrast to the situation with eyeglasses, with contact lenses your entire field of vision is corrected because all images reaching the eyes pass through the lenses. The outer and inner surfaces of each lens are ground to correct your particular refraction error and to fit the curvature of your eye.

TYPES OF CONTACT LENSES

The two basic types of contact lens are hard (rigid) and soft. Hard lenses are small plastic discs that fit just over the cornea. Soft lenses are made of a thin plastic polymer and fit over a slightly larger portion of the eye.

Hard Contact Lenses. These are the sturdiest contact lenses, but they are the least comfortable. Because they are rigid, they do not scratch or tear easily. They also need less maintenance than the delicate, soft variety. However, the rigid plastic is more water resistant and so it is harder to keep wet and more difficult to keep fixed in position on the eye.

Soft Contact Lenses. Soft contacts are indeed delicate because the polymer can tear easily. But they are usually much more comfortable to wear than rigid lenses because the soft plastic causes less friction on the eyelid than do hard lenses. Soft lenses require more care than hard ones because they must be cleaned and often soaked in special solutions. They tend to stay on the eye better than hard lenses.

Other Types. Two other types of lenses are gas-permeable hard lenses and extended-wear soft lenses. One of the problems with all contact lenses is getting enough oxygen to the cornea. Soft lenses have a varying amount of water in them that allows oxygen to pass through the medium. Hard lenses move a little each time you blink, allowing oxygen to reach the cornea. Gas-permeable hard lenses also have pores in the rigid plastic to allow more oxygen to reach the cornea when you blink.

As their name suggests, extended-wear soft lenses can be worn for greater lengths of time because they have sufficient water in them to allow oxygen to pass into the cornea, even while you sleep. They are even thinner than daily-wear soft lenses, a feature that makes them more comfortable but also more fragile.

Tinted soft lenses are a popular choice among fashion-conscious people. These lenses are tinted in the portion of the lens that covers the iris. They come in shades of blue, brown, and green and provide an intense color to the eyes. They are also useful for disguising defects of the iris, corneal scars, and irregularly shaped pupils.

Bifocal Contact Lenses. Bifocal contact lenses are available for people needing corrections for near and far distances. However, because they move with the eye, in some individuals it is difficult for the eye to adjust for near and far vision. Often, a more satisfactory solution is reached by correcting one eye for distant vision and the other for close vision with regular soft lenses.

Combination Contact Lenses. Piggyback contact lenses are designed for people with certain eye disorders. These lenses are a combination of hard and soft lenses. A soft lens with a central excavation is fitted for comfort, and then a hard lens is placed to correct for vision. People with corneal malformations are particularly helped by these lenses.

GET THEM FITTED PROPERLY

Good vision, comfort, and the overall health of your eyes depend on properly fitted contact lenses. Whichever form of lens you choose, make sure that you have them custom-fit by a professional who can determine your exact needs.

BE ALERT FOR PROBLEMS

If you receive a careful fitting of your lenses and are free of other eye problems, expect good results from your contact lenses. Be aware, however, that on rare occasions potentially sight-threatening problems can develop.

Several of these problems are related to the amount of oxygen your cornea receives. One of the more common of these rare problems is overuse. If you wear contact lenses for too long at a time, your corneas may become starved for oxygen. The symptoms are blurry vision, pain, tearing, redness, and sensitivity to light.

Remove your lenses immediately. If the pain persists, see your eye doctor.

Corneal vascularization is another response of the cornea to inadequate amounts of oxygen. In this condition, tiny blood vessels grow into the clear tissue of the cornea. In extreme cases your vision can become clouded. Should this occur you may need to switch to another type of lens or stop wearing contact lenses altogether.

Corneal warpage is yet another problem of too little oxygen reaching the cornea, and it involves a gradual change in the cornea's shape. The result is uneven or fluctuating vision for hours or days after removing your lenses. The problem is infrequent for wearers of gas-permeable hard lenses or soft contact lenses, but it is more common among those who use standard hard lenses.

Giant papillary conjunctivitis is a relatively common allergic disorder among wearers of soft lenses. It evolves gradually. You may find it increasingly difficult to wear your lenses for long. Your sight may be blurry when you blink (one or both contacts ride up under your eyelids), or one or both eyes may itch and ooze soon after you remove your lenses. The condition is more common among people whose soft contact lenses are fairly old or whose lenses have developed a layer of protein on the surface. See your ophthalmologist; it may be necessary to stop using your lenses until the problems subside. Switching to a newer type of soft lens or a gas-permeable hard lens may be helpful.

Sensitivity to the cleaning solution is another fairly common problem. Some people develop a reaction to chemicals found in contact lens solution, particularly the preservative thimerosal. If you experience discomfort, see your eye specialist. He or she may advise you to switch to another solution that uses different chemicals.

A bacterial or fungal infection of the cornea resulting in a corneal ulcer is rare but

---

CARING FOR YOUR CONTACTS

Proper care of your contact lenses is vital to your comfort and the overall health of your eyes. Each kind of lens has its own requirements, but no matter what variety you wear, the first rule is keep them clean.

Wash your hands before handling your lenses. Keep your lens case clean and readily available so you can remove and safely store your lenses if your eyes begin to hurt or become red or if your vision blurs.

Hard Lenses
These are the easiest to care for because they are less fragile than other kinds. Use only a commercial contact lens wetting solution to moisten them for insertion (never use saliva). Clean the lenses each day with a commercial cleaning solution.

Gas-Permeable Hard Lenses
These hard lenses have pores in them to allow oxygen to reach the cornea. Wash them each day in a commercial cleaning solution and store them overnight in a conditioner. Clean them each week with an enzyme solution. When rinsing, use distilled water because tap water leaves a residue.

Soft Lenses
These lenses require careful maintenance. They must be cleaned each day with a surface cleaner designed specifically for soft lenses. Disinfect them either daily with a disinfecting solution or every other day with heat (be sure to follow the manufacturer's instructions for temperature and duration).

Do not use a mixture of salt tablets and distilled water for cleaning because it can allow infections to develop. Use a bottled or aerosol saline solution without preservatives. *Never* use tap water. Apply an enzyme treatment weekly, rinse with saline, and disinfect to neutralize the enzyme.

Extended-Wear Soft Lenses
Remove your lenses most nights and clean them in the same manner as for regular soft lenses.

serious (see Corneal Ulcers and Infections, page 764). You may notice a loss of vision, and your eye becomes red, very painful, and sensitive to light. Such infections are sometimes the result of improper cleaning of contact lenses. Extended-wear soft lenses are associated with the problem most frequently. If you suspect you have a corneal ulcer, see your ophthalmologist immediately.

Acanthamoeba keratitis is a rare but dangerous infection. The cause is an amoeba organism that lives in stagnant water, certain tap water, and occasionally saliva. It causes a painful, red eye that is difficult to treat. It usually develops as a result of improperly cleaned soft contact lenses and can be avoided by using commercial saline solutions or by heat-sterilizing the lenses.

Finally, if you are a contact-lens wearer, have a pair of glasses available as a backup in case an eye problem develops that requires you to stop wearing your contacts temporarily.

TRAUMA TO THE EYE

From time to time, eye injuries of one kind or another happen—whether they result from an errant foul ball at a Little League game, a grain of sand at the beach, a splash of household chemical, or some other cause.

Many such injuries can be avoided by properly protecting the eyes with goggles or glasses when participating in hazardous activities: for example, make it a habit to wear safety glasses when using tools. If an accident occurs and your eye is injured, immediate, careful examination and proper medical care are required (see Eye Emergencies, page 314).

Trauma to the eye can result from objects striking or entering the eyes (see page 747) or from chemical burns (see page 749). Injury can lead to infections such as orbital cellulitis (see page 761) or acute iritis (see page 760). The following pages also discuss proper eye protection. (For a full discussion of first aid for eye injuries, see Foreign Bodies in the Eye, page 287.)

FOREIGN BODIES

Signs and Symptoms
- Sudden pain in the eye;
- Sudden worsening of vision;
- Redness of the eye.

Everyone occasionally gets a speck of dust in the eye; usually, all that is required is that you blink until your tears wash the particle away. However, you may find that this does not work or that something more serious has entered your eye.

The injury may be limited to the conjunctiva and cornea (these are the most frequent sites), or it may affect the eyeball. Whenever pain and redness persist, the injury should be treated professionally to ensure that vision is not lost (for emergency treatment, see Foreign Bodies in the Eye, page 287).

The Diagnosis. If severe pain develops suddenly in an eye and your vision is suddenly worse, you may have a foreign object in your eye. If the pain is severe, go to a hospital emergency room or arrange to see your ophthalmologist as soon as possible.

Do not try to remove the object yourself. Your physician will examine your eye under good strong light to see whether the cornea has been scratched (abraded) by the foreign object. An injury to the cornea can be very painful. A local anesthetic may be administered to lessen the pain.

If the object has entered the eye itself, an x-ray or a CT scan may be obtained. You will be asked a series of questions to determine the nature of your activities at the time of the accident and thus what substance might have entered the eye.

How Serious Are Foreign Bodies in the Eye? A foreign body in the eye can be a serious threat to sight, particularly if the object enters the eye itself or damages the cornea or lens. Professional emergency treatment is required.

Treatment. If the object can be seen on the eye surface under strong light, your ophthalmologist may be able to remove it with surgical tweezers. If the object is no longer

PROTECTING YOUR EYES

Myths about care of the eyes abound. For example, the warnings that reading in dim light or watching television while sitting close to the screen will damage your eyes are not true. Reading by flashlight is a harmless activity, too, as are sitting in the front row of a movie theater, doing close work with your eyes, and driving or doing other things in bright sunshine without sunglasses. These activities may make your eyes feel tired or strained, but they do not harm them.

Grease and Chemical Hazards

However, many situations *can* seriously harm your eyes. Some of the most common injuries are the result of accidents while doing everyday tasks such as cooking, cleaning house, or working in the garden or yard. Spattered grease, splashed household chemicals, or sprayed garden chemicals are common causes of serious eye injuries.

Use Safety Goggles

Protect yourself by wearing safety glasses or goggles. Make sure your children also get in the habit of wearing protective eyeglasses when helping with hazardous housework, cooking, or gardening tasks. Teach children early to wear goggles when using tools.

The Hazards of Makeup

A scratched or abraded cornea can be the result of hastily applying mascara or accidentally squirting hair spray in the eyes. Be careful when using anything near your eyes, from brushes to fingernails. Shield your eyes when applying hair spray.

Sports Risks

Sports carry their share of eye risks. If a hockey puck or racquetball contacts your eye, it easily can cause internal damage. Protective eyeglasses or shields can help prevent such injuries. Basketball players frequently suffer corneal abrasions from finger pokes, and football players sometimes sustain broken bones near the eye. More and more professional athletes now wear protective shields or goggles. You should, too.

Workplace Practices

Anyone whose job carries a risk of eye injury is required by law to have protective glasses provided by the employer and to wear them.

Should I Wear Sunglasses?

There is increasing concern about the effects of ultraviolet radiation from the sun on the eyes. Generally speaking, you do not need to wear sunglasses every time you step outside. However, if you spend a great deal of time in the sun, wear sunglasses designed to screen ultraviolet radiation.

Such sunglasses are available in inexpensive and expensive models. Be sure to wear them if you use an ultraviolet sunlamp. Never look at the sun directly, even through sunglasses or x-ray film, because it can cause permanent damage.

Safety goggles are available in a wide variety of styles.

present but has scratched the cornea, your eye will be treated topically with an antibiotic. Then a patch will be placed over the eye to protect it overnight. Generally, this treatment will allow the cornea to heal itself.

If the object has entered the eye, it must be removed by an ophthalmic surgeon. In the meantime, emergency treatment usually is begun. The pupil may be dilated and antibiotics may be prescribed. A metal shield is placed over the eye to protect it until surgery is performed.

CHEMICAL BURNS

Signs and Symptoms
- Pain in the eye;
- Decreased vision;
- Increased sensitivity to light.

Chemical burns of the eye can endanger your vision. If your job entails the use of hazardous chemicals, be aware of the dangers and protect your eyes with goggles. Household cleaning products, particularly those that contain ammonia or bleach, and garden chemicals also can cause serious harm.

Direct contact (chemicals splashed in your face, for example) is most hazardous, but concentrated fumes and aerosols also can be dangerous. Wear goggles or protective glasses and try to work in well-ventilated surroundings. Be careful not to splash when mixing and pouring chemicals.

The Diagnosis. You probably will know when a chemical is burning your eyes. They hurt and may be more sensitive to light, and your vision may be blurred. If pain is present, seek prompt medical care: chemical burns to the eyes are to be regarded as a medical emergency and should be treated promptly by an ophthalmologist.

Treatment. Before you do anything, flush the eye immediately with water, and continue doing so for 15 to 30 minutes. Hold your head under a water faucet or pour water into your eye from a clean container. Keep your eye open as widely as possible during flushing.

Go to the emergency room of your local hospital or contact your ophthalmologist. The physician examining and treating the eye may use a local anesthetic to lessen the pain. Depending on the extent of injury, the eye may be bandaged, treated with an antibiotic, and left to heal.

Serious damage to the conjunctiva, cornea, or eyelid may require surgical repair at a later date.

BLACK EYE

Signs and Symptoms
- Bruising around the eye;

- Broken blood vessels in the white of the eye;
- Swelling of the lid and tissue around the eye.

Perhaps you were in an accident and a blunt object hit your eye, or maybe your child encountered the schoolyard bully. Whatever the cause, there is a bruise about the eye—the so-called black eye.

If you sustain such an injury, it may be limited to a small amount of bleeding beneath the skin that gives you the characteristic black-and-blue bruising about the eye. You might also incur more serious damage to the eye itself. Sometimes a black eye will indicate a more extensive injury, even a skull fracture, particularly if the area around both eyes is bruised. In any case, such an injury should be examined by an ophthalmologist to be sure the eye itself has not been hurt.

The Diagnosis. If the area around your eye bleeds under the skin, the lid and nearby tissues also may swell. The eye itself can become red and swollen. The injury may not be serious, but recurrent bleeding within the eye can reduce vision and damage the cornea. In some cases, glaucoma also can result (see page 765).

Treatment. Apply ice to the injured eye, taking care not to press on the eye itself. Your ophthalmologist can determine whether more serious damage has occurred. If so, the eye may be bandaged, bed rest will be prescribed, and you may be sedated to lessen the pain and anxiety. In addition, your physician may prescribe medication to reduce pressure within the eye.

HYPHEMA

Signs and Symptoms
- Bleeding within the front portion (anterior chamber) of the eye.

Bleeding into the front portion (anterior chamber) of the eye may follow trauma to the eye. This may occur from either a blunt blow to the eye or a perforating injury. At times, hyphema may occur from severe inflammation of the iris, a blood vessel abnormality, or a cancer within the eye itself.

Generally, the blood is absorbed completely within a few days.

Treatment.   In some cases of hyphema, an ophthalmologist may recommend hospitalization. Repeat bleeding may occur, and it is a serious complication. Medication may be prescribed to decrease the risk. If the bleeding is severe, your ophthalmologist may elect to evacuate the blood through a small opening in the eye. This drain can be re-opened on subsequent days if further bleeding occurs.

STRABISMUS AND AMBLYOPIA

Strabismus and amblyopia are usually first observed during early childhood. Strabismus, from the Greek word for squinting, is the general term for crossed eyes or those that in some other way are misaligned. Amblyopia, often called lazy eye, can be a consequence of strabismus.

Normal vision depends on the eyes focusing together, producing what is known as binocular vision. However, when the eyes do not function in tandem, double vision results. In a young child with strabismus, however, one of the images will be ignored and the development of nerve connections between that eye and the brain will fail to take place normally.

The resulting single vision will lack the depth perception of binocular vision. The affected eye probably will not develop good vision unless it is made to "work"; this is accomplished by surgery (to bring the eyes into alignment) or perhaps by wearing a patch over the unaffected eye.

Amblyopia (literally, dull eye) is a condition in which the vision in the nondominant eye is poor, usually as a result of strabismus. It also can be caused by a greater degree of farsightedness, nearsightedness, or astigmatism in one eye; it can even be caused by the rare occurrence of a childhood cataract. The more-affected eye is then "turned off" by the brain, and the stronger eye becomes dominant and retains good vision.

Six muscles are attached to the outside of each eye. If an object is to be perceived properly, these muscles must work in unison to focus the image on the center of the retina (macula) in the back of each eye. From the retina, the images then are relayed by the optic nerve to the vision reception area of the brain. Your brain "translates" these electrical messages from your two eyes into a single three-dimensional image which provides the depth perception of binocular vision.

No one knows why some children's eyes are misaligned, although it has been observed to run in families. Strabismus seems to affect boys and girls equally.

The eyes of some children are misaligned, a condition called strabismus. Two common forms of strabismus are esotropia (cross-eye) and exotropia (walleye).

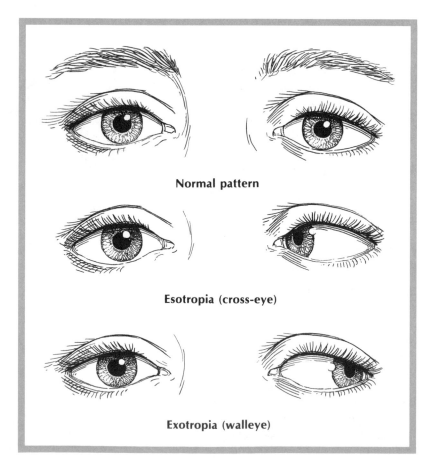

Normal pattern

Esotropia (cross-eye)

Exotropia (walleye)

EARLY RECOGNITION

About 4 percent of children are affected by strabismus; if not treated before age 5 or 6, they risk permanent loss of visual acuity in the nondominant eye. Thus, the key to curing strabismus and amblyopia is early detection of the problem.

Strabismus is usually easy to recognize, but amblyopia may not be evident because the child usually does not realize that vision is poor in the eye. Tests of visual acuity may be needed to discover the amblyopia (see The Eye Examination, page 740).

The most common forms of strabismus in children are esotropia and exotropia. Esotropia (cross-eye) is characterized by the eye turning inward. Exotropia (walleye) occurs when the eye turns outward. Occasionally the eye will turn down or up. The deviation may be constant or occasional, such as when the child is tired and the muscles weakened.

Babies are born with the ability to see, but at first they are unable to focus. The nerve connections between the eyes and the brain have not yet become organized. During the first few weeks of life, your baby's eyes may appear to wander. At times they may appear to work independently, sometimes crossing and at other times roving outward. This is normal. By the end of the third or fourth month, however, your baby's eyes should appear to be working in parallel, and they should be able to focus on small objects.

Infants and toddlers often have a wide, flat nose and an extra fold of skin where the eyelids join the nose. These features may make your child appear cross-eyed. As the shape of your baby's features changes, however, the fold may disappear. Before you become alarmed that your child may have misaligned eyes—and before you dismiss the possibility—check carefully.

Begin by looking intently at your child's eyes. Is the point of light that you see in each eye symmetrically positioned with the other? If so, your child's eyes probably are aligned correctly.

The following is a list of other things to look for.

Do your child's eyes seem to work together? Test this ability by passing your hand across your child's field of vision. Look to see whether the eyes seem to move as one.

Does each eye seem to follow objects, such as your face or a toy, if the opposite eye is covered?

Does one eye squint when your child is in the sun?

Does your child seem cross-eyed when playing with toys or other close objects but normal when looking into the distance?

Does your child tend to tilt his or her head to one side?

Is your toddler unable to gauge depth when handling or playing with objects?

If you think that your child might have misaligned eyes, see your family physician or an ophthalmologist. It is never too early to have a child's vision tested for alignment—even newborns can be diagnosed.

The key to diagnosing amblyopia in a young child is to identify a difference in vision between the eyes. Your child's physician or ophthalmologist can test your baby by covering one eye and observing the baby's responses to the movement of various objects. If one eye is amblyopic, your child may try to remove the patch or otherwise object to its presence when it covers the favored eye.

By age 3 years, vision usually can be measured accurately. Poor vision in one eye does not necessarily mean that it is amblyopic. Reduced vision in one eye may be due to nearsightedness, farsightedness, or astigmatism, which your physician will test for. At the same time, your physician will examine

DOUBLE VISION

Because of a nerve or muscle problem in the eyes, one eye may deviate from the other. The eyes will not focus in unison, and the images the brain receives from your eyes will be different from one another. This condition is called diplopia (double vision).

If the eye and brain connections have become well established (which usually happens by age 1 or 2), when a misalignment of the eyes occurs, the brain interprets the signals just as it receives them and produces two sets of images. Strabismus is the medical term used to describe eyes that deviate. The effect can be confusing and debilitating because objects appear twice in the field of vision.

Sometimes double vision is a sign of a more serious underlying problem such as diabetes mellitus (see The Eye and Diabetes, page 777), myasthenia gravis (see page 525), multiple sclerosis (see page 522), Graves' disease (see page 778), or brain injury.

In these cases, the underlying disease affects the nerves between the brain and eye muscles or the nerves of the eye muscles themselves. Double vision is usually only one of several symptoms of any of these disorders. If you develop double vision, contact your physician for a thorough examination.

In the meantime, you can alleviate the sensation temporarily by placing a patch over one eye. Treatment of an underlying disorder may resolve the double vision. If it does not, the condition sometimes may be corrected with prescribed eyeglasses. Occasionally, the condition is treated surgically to correct muscle misalignment.

VISION THERAPY

Are your children doing as well as possible in school? Perhaps they find time spent at a chalkboard or with books stressful. If your child shows trouble concentrating on schoolwork, you naturally want to help.

In such situations, many people consider the possibility of a vision problem. If you suspect that your child may not be seeing as well as possible, have his or her vision checked by a qualified professional. Beware, however, of promoters offering "vision therapy" or "vision training." Ophthalmologists recently issued a statement that these programs are of little value.

The Promises
Vision therapists claim to strengthen a child's eyesight through a series of exercises and the use of eyeglasses. They emphasize methods of hand-eye coordination, watching a series of blinking lights, focusing on a string of objects, and even sleeping in a certain position.

Promoters say this regimen will improve scholastic and athletic performance, will increase a student's IQ, and may help keep youngsters from juvenile delinquency. They also claim that it can help with the problem of dyslexia (inability to interpret written language, see also page 134).

Vision training sessions are time-consuming—often once or twice a week over the course of a year—and expensive. There is no evidence that such training has any benefit.

Know Your Professionals
Eye professionals are classified into two main groups, optometrists and ophthalmologists. Optometrists have at least 6 years of training after high school and graduate from a school of optometry. They are not physicians, but they are qualified to prescribe eyeglasses and contact lenses. Behavioral optometrists are a subgroup within the profession. They are the chief supporters of vision therapy.

Ophthalmologists are physicians who have had special training, at least 4 years after both college and medical school, in the treatment of eye disorders and eye diseases. Ophthalmologists are qualified to diagnose and treat eye diseases medically or surgically. Ophthalmologists and some optometrists dismiss the value of vision therapy.

What Should I Do?
If you suspect that your child has trouble seeing properly, arrange for an eye examination. Consult an ophthalmologist, or contact your child's school because many schools offer visual acuity tests free of charge. Testing is important because children often do not realize that blurred vision is unusual. If your child does have a vision problem, appropriate action (from corrective glasses to medical therapy) can then be taken.

If your child is having difficulty learning, discuss the problem with his or her teacher or your family physician or pediatrician. One of these professionals can arrange for specific educational and psychological testing to determine whether a specific learning disability is present (see also Learning Disorders, page 132). But "vision therapy" almost certainly is not the answer.

---

the interior of the eye for signs of a cataract, tumor, inflammation, or other disorders.

CORRECTIVE MEASURES

Contrary to what many people believe, children do not outgrow strabismus and amblyopia, so prompt treatment is essential to prevent permanent vision impairment in the affected eye. Optical, medical, and surgical methods, alone or in combination, may be recommended.

Optical Approaches. If your child has strabismus associated with farsightedness (the eyes become crossed only when looking at close objects), eyeglasses may be enough to solve the problem. Sometimes the lenses are bifocal or have special prisms designed to compensate for the particular defect in the eye.

Medical Treatment. The nonsurgical form of treatment for amblyopia involves placing a patch over the normal eye in an effort to improve vision by forcing use of the weak eye. This stimulus seems to aid in the organization of the nerve connections between the eye and parts of the brain that process visual perception. Normally, this organization and coordination takes place for both eyes in the first year of life. If the stimulus of focusing an image is absent (such as in the nondominant eye of the child with strabismus), this organization fails to take place.

The same result sometimes can be achieved by treating the normal eye with medicated drops, called cycloplegics, which blur its vision temporarily and dilate the pupil. Some children with strabismus also may be treated with eye drops called miotics which cause the pupil to constrict. These methods are most effective with young children.

Once vision in the weaker eye has improved, the treatment program will concentrate on bringing the eyes into parallel position.

Some practitioners advocate eye exercises for strabismus and amblyopia, but most ophthalmologists believe them to be of little value and thus do not recommend them (see Vision Therapy, page 752).

In some cases, eyeglasses or surgery may be appropriate.

Surgical Treatment.   Many children, particularly those with strabismus, require an operation to realign their eye muscles. The operation usually takes place on an outpatient basis in a hospital setting with the child under general anesthesia.

The surgeon will make a small incision in the tissue that covers the eye. One or more of the muscles of the eye are then repositioned to allow proper alignment. Depending on the complexity of the problem, more than one operation may be needed to bring the eye to normal position.

When treatment is completed before age 5 or 6, vision often is improved to near normal. The child not only will see better than before but also will appear normal. Looking like all the other kids can be of considerable importance during the impressionable years of personality development.

EYELID DISORDERS

Our eyelids, although thin and delicate, are extremely important protectors of the eyes. Quick and powerful reflexes make the eyelids close when an object nears or when irritating particles are in the air. The eyelids also lubricate the eyes and wash foreign particles from them.

Lacrimal glands located above each eyeball produce tears, which are fed beneath the eyelids as a thin film. The tears drain away from the eyes through lacrimal ducts whose openings are located at the inner edge of each lid. The lacrimal ducts carry the tears to the nose, which is why whenever your eyes water or you cry, your nose waters too. The lids are lined with a transparent mucous membrane called the conjunctiva which also covers the white surface (sclera) of the eye.

Occasionally the eyelids can be the site of problems. Most often such problems are infections, but they can be the result of muscle or nerve damage (see Eyelid Laceration, page 315).

STYES AND LUMPS

Signs and Symptoms
- Painful swelling on the eyelid margin;
- Slightly blurred vision.

A stye is an infection near the root (follicle) of an eyelash. A sore similar to a boil or pimple develops as a result of bacterial infection. You may get more than one stye at a time or several in succession because the bacteria that initially infect one hair follicle spread and infect others.

Another form of swelling on the lid is a chalazion, which, unlike a stye, is relatively painless. A chalazion is the result of a blockage of one of the small glands (meibomian glands) that produce part of the tear layer. Bacterial growth may take place within the blocked gland. The chalazion is essentially an internal stye.

The Diagnosis.   A stye usually develops gradually, forming a painful red lump. Eventually the lump fills with pus and bursts. The release of pus relieves the pain, and after a few more days the stye usually disappears.

A chalazion develops a little farther up on and within the structure of the eyelid. In most instances it is only mildly uncomfortable, but it may be unsightly.

Styes and lumps are almost always harmless to the eye and general sight. However, if a stye interferes with your sight or does not disappear of its own accord or if you have successive infections, see your ophthal-

A stye is an infection near the root of an eyelash. A blockage in one of the small glands in the eyelid can produce a similar swelling, called a chalazion.

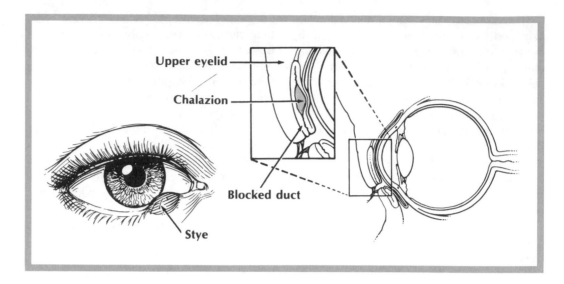

Upper eyelid

Chalazion

Blocked duct

Stye

mologist. A chalazion probably will need to be treated by an ophthalmologist, although it might disappear without treatment. A presumed chalazion that persists despite treatment rarely is a tumor. A biopsy (in which a sample of the tissue is removed for laboratory analysis) may be required to make the diagnosis. (See color photograph, page B–11.)

Treatment.   You can treat a stye by applying a warm compress to the sore for about 10 minutes four times a day. To make a compress, soak a very clean cloth in warm water and wring it out before applying it to your eye. Using warm compresses will help relieve the pain.

Do not squeeze the stye in an effort to remove the pus. Let the sac burst on its own, then wash it thoroughly.

If the stye is stubborn, or you have successive infections, your physician may prescribe a topical antibiotic cream to apply to the eyelid. A particularly stubborn stye may be lanced and drained by your ophthalmologist.

A chalazion often will disappear without any treatment over time, perhaps a month or two. Applying warm compresses may help to speed the healing, as may application of an antibiotic corticosteroid ointment as prescribed by your physician.

If these methods prove unsuccessful or if the chalazion continues to enlarge, it can be removed in a simple surgical procedure. The operation can be performed in your physician's office with local anesthesia. After the procedure, the eye usually is covered with a patch for several hours.

PROBLEMS OF TEARING

Tears often are thought of as a result of intense emotion. However, every time you blink—which you probably do every few seconds—tears lubricate your eyes. The fluid is essential for the proper functioning of your eyes.

When your eyes become irritated, extra tears form to help wash away foreign bodies. Occasionally, however, problems develop with the tear glands, and the results can be continuously watering eyes or dry eyes. Infection of the tear ducts also can cause tearing problems.

Dry Eyes.   Dry eyes, caused by a lack of tears, can be a most uncomfortable sensation. The eyes may feel hot and gritty and may appear swollen and red. The condition is usually present in both eyes.

Dry eyes can be due to the presence of Sjögren's syndrome, a connective tissue disorder often found among people with rheumatoid arthritis (see Sjögren's Syndrome, page 1008). Dry eyes may be a result of an allergy to eye drops or ointment used for another condition; they also can occur for no apparent reason. They are most common among women after menopause. Although the condition is generally not a threat to sight, the sensation is so uncomfortable that medical treatment is usually necessary.

Treatment.   If your eyes feel dry, if they swell, and if they feel hot and gritty, especially when you blink, consult your ophthalmologist. He or she will examine your eyes to determine the cause.

Your ophthalmologist probably will prescribe artificial tears that you can use to bathe your eyes whenever you want. If an allergic reaction to eye drops is the cause, discontinue using them. However, the problem may not resolve and you may need to use artificial tears indefinitely.

Watering Eyes. Too much tearing can result from excessive tear production or improper drainage of the tear ducts. Other causes include irritations of the eye due to abrasion from foreign bodies, infection of the eyelid, inward-growing eyelashes, allergies, or nasal problems.

Improper drainage often is caused by blockage of a tear duct or drain, which occurs mostly among adults. However, about 5 percent of babies are born with a tear duct that has failed to open. Usually only one eye is affected by continuous tearing.

If your eye or your child's eye tears constantly over a period of several days, see your ophthalmologist. The physician will examine the eye carefully for signs of blockage of a tear duct or of excessive tear production and ask you a series of questions to isolate other possible causes. Such causes include scarring of the tear duct caused by chronic sinusitis, chronic allergy, or injury to the nose.

Treatment. Your ophthalmologist may begin treatment by probing and irrigating the tear ducts. This method is most useful in infants and children. In some cases, an operation may be needed.

Infection of the Tear Duct. Occasionally the tear duct that leads to the nose can become blocked and infected. This condi-

---

EYE DROPS

Many brands of eye drops can be purchased at your drugstore without a prescription. These fall into two general categories: those that act as artificial tears, and those whose active agent is a vasoconstrictor such as tetrahydrozoline.

Artificial Tears
These preparations contain substances, such as methylcellulose, that hold water and, indeed, resemble your own tears. One or two drops of these in each eye usually will provide lubrication and comfort for several hours. You may use artificial tears as often as you like.

Vasoconstrictors
In contrast, the products in this category contain a drug that causes the tiny blood vessels within the conjunctiva to constrict. If you have bloodshot eyes—redness and visible blood vessels—one or two drops in each eye will relieve the redness for several hours and often give comfort also. They may be useful for relieving the itchy eyes of hay fever sufferers, but they must not be used habitually.

Some of the eye drops in this category also contain an antihistamine to provide added relief if you have hay fever. Use this type of eye drop no more than two or three times a day, unless otherwise directed by your physician.

Reducing the Risks of Complications
Each person has a different tolerance for drugs, and drugs affect different persons in different ways. Therefore, the risks of an unexpected response vary. Also, it is not possible to eliminate completely all of the effects from helpful and necessary eye medications. You can take a few steps to minimize the effects, however.

To begin, use only the recommended dosage. It is easy to overdose by adding an extra drop or two. Over time, this increase can lead to problems. After placing the medication in your eye, follow these simple steps.

Keep your eye closed for 30 to 60 seconds. This encourages absorption of the drug by your eye and minimizes drainage of the medication through your tear outflow canal into your nose.

Do not blink. Blinking tends to move the medication from your eye into your tear outflow canal.

Use your index finger to apply firm pressure for a minute or two over the junction of your lower eyelid and nose. This blocks the opening of your tear outflow canal and minimizes drainage.

Follow the Directions
Read the directions carefully for whatever sort of eye drops you use. Your pharmacist can help you understand the uses of these medications and also help you select the type that you need.

tion is called dacryocystitis. When this occurs, the tissues between the inner angle of the eye (canthus) and the bridge of the nose become swollen, red, and tender. Tears then can no longer find their way into the nose and there will be excessive tearing. If you have these symptoms, see your ophthalmologist.

Treatment. Try applying a warm compress several times a day to the eye to relieve the discomfort. Soak a clean, lint-free cloth in warm water, wring it out, and place it over the affected eye for about 10 minutes.

Your physician may prescribe antibiotics. Once the acute infection has been treated, a new tear duct may need to be created surgically.

BLEPHARITIS

Signs and Symptoms
- Sticky, crusty, and reddened eyelids;
- Itchy, burning, swollen eyelids;
- Conjunctivitis (see page 759);
- A granular feeling with blinking;
- Loss of lashes.

Blepharitis is an inflammation of the eyelid edges that involves both seborrheic dermatitis (see page 1157) and a bacterial infection. When excess oil is produced in glands near the eyelashes, an environment favorable for the growth of bacteria develops. The result is a crusty inflammation that is uncomfortable and unsightly, but it is rarely threatening to sight.

A drooping of the upper eyelid is known as ptosis.

People with blepharitis often have a history of recurrent styes and chalazions (see page 753). In severe cases a corneal ulcer may develop as a result of the irritation (see page 764).

The Diagnosis. If your eyelids become red and irritated and secrete an ooze that becomes crusty, you may have blepharitis. Do not be alarmed if you have to pry your eyes open in the morning, because the sticky secretions of the eyelids during the night often act to seal the eyes shut. In severe cases, small ulcers may develop on the edges of the lids, and the cornea can be scarred. Consult your ophthalmologist, who will examine your eyes and prescribe an appropriate course of action.

Treatment. *Self-Help.* Cleaning your eyelids carefully is important for treating blepharitis. In the morning, soak a clean lint-free cloth in warm water, wring it out, and place it over the eyes as a compress. This will loosen the scales. Then gently scrub your eyelids with a cotton-tipped swab that has been soaked in dilute baby shampoo. This will help remove the crusts and restore the normal lid environment.

Medication. Your physician may prescribe an ointment or eye drops containing both antibiotic and corticosteroid medications to clear the infection and reduce the swelling. If local treatment is unsuccessful, a course of antibiotics taken orally may be recommended.

DROOPING EYELID

Signs and Symptoms
- Drooping of one or both upper eyelids.

Drooping eyelid (ptosis) is a condition caused by a weakness of the muscle responsible for raising the lid. Some children are born with the condition, and for them surgical correction may be necessary to prevent amblyopia (see page 750). When present from birth, the condition usually affects only one eye. Drooping eyelid often runs in families.

In adults the condition usually is a normal effect of aging as the eyelid muscles lose tone; less often, it also can be the result of an injury or disease such as diabetes (see

The Eye and Diabetes, page 777), myasthenia gravis, stroke, brain tumor, or cancer at the base of the neck or the apex of the lung, all of which can affect nerve and muscle responses.

The Diagnosis. If you notice that your child's eyelids are noticeably uneven, especially to the degree that vision out of one or both eyes is obscured, see your ophthalmologist. Your physician will examine the eye and ask a series of questions regarding your child's general health. A complete physical examination may be recommended if a general health problem seems to be present.

If you suddenly notice that one or both of your own eyes droop, see your physician. Again, a complete physical examination may be in order to determine whether a more general health problem could be the cause. If you notice the problem developing over a number of years, it may be due to the effects of aging.

Treatment. If your eyelid interferes with vision, see your physician. If the drooping is the result of a congenital abnormality, aging, or injury, an operation to strengthen the muscle may be performed. If a more general health problem such as myasthenia gravis, stroke, or diabetes is the cause, treatment of the underlying problem may help relieve the drooping eyelid.

ENTROPION AND ECTROPION

Signs and Symptoms
- Scratching of the eye by lashes;
- Excessive tearing;
- Eye irritation and matter in the eye on arising.

Entropion and ectropion are problems often related to aging. In entropion, the upper or lower lid turns in, allowing the lashes to scratch the eye. In severe cases, an ulceration or scarring can occur on the cornea.

Ectropion is the reverse problem, and it is often the result of muscle weakness. The lower lid turns out, sometimes causing the tears to flow out instead of lubricating the eye.

Although entropion and ectropion are usually the result of the aging process, ectro-

ABOUT THAT TWITCHY EYELID

From time to time you may experience the discomfort of a twitch in an eyelid. The involuntary quivering of the eyelid usually lasts only a few seconds but it can be irritating, and it can make you wonder whether something is wrong with your eyes.

Generally there is no need for concern because a twitch is almost always a minor ailment. The occasional twitch of a muscle in a hand, forearm, leg, or foot is a common experience, and eye twitches are closely related. These flutters, called fasciculations, last only a few seconds, although their occurrence can be frequent.

No one knows exactly what causes most twitches, although many people report that they seem to be related to fatigue and stress. Many people find them worrisome because they can be distracting, and some people fear that the condition may signal a more serious problem. Some people have eyelids that close involuntarily because of an unusual disorder called essential blepharospasm. Only very rarely are eye twitches a symptom of a serious disease. Serious facial tics, facial muscle spasms, and multiple sclerosis (see page 522) do involve the eyelids, but symptoms of those ailments are different enough that your physician will not confuse them with the ordinary twitchy eyelid.

Eye twitches are almost always harmless, but they can be irritating. Try gently massaging the affected eyelid. Many people find that this relieves the twitch significantly.

pion can be due to an underlying condition such as atopic dermatitis (see page 1157) or lupus erythematosus (see page 1006).

The Diagnosis. One of the first signs of entropion is excess matter and irritation of the eyes in the morning. It usually clears later

ITCHY EYELIDS

Itching about the eyes often accompanies hay fever—but itchy eyelids may be a manifestation of contact dermatitis (see page 1155). If your fingers come in contact with some irritating or allergy-causing substance, it may be carried to your eyelids by your fingers. Cosmetics also may cause allergic reactions on the sensitive skin of the eyelids.

Do not rub or scratch your eyelids excessively because rubbing ultimately can result in lichen simplex chronicus (see page 1156), with thickening patches of skin and persistent itching. If the skin of your eyelids is sensitive to certain cosmetics or other materials, avoid using them.

COSMETIC SURGERY OF THE EYELID

If your eyelids droop and the bags beneath your eyes sag, the problem may have developed as a result of heredity or as a natural part of aging. But whatever the cause, you may imagine that you always look tired. Perhaps the sagging skin even interferes with your peripheral sight. You decide to take action: you want the excess skin removed.

Blepharoplasty is a surgical procedure to remove excess skin and fat from the upper and lower eyelids. It is done routinely on an outpatient basis with a local anesthetic.

The Procedure

Your surgeon makes an incision in the fold of the lid and just below the lower lash line. Excess skin and fat are removed, and the incision is stitched.

The Recovery

One of the most important elements in recovery is your follow-up care. This means you must follow directions from your surgeon in every detail.

The Results

Blepharoplasty should not interfere with your vision, and you may wear your eyeglasses the day after the procedure. Wearing glasses can also help protect your eyelid from injury.

The recovery time is usually 2 to 4 weeks, by which time most swelling, tenderness, and pain should have subsided.

Complications

Blepharoplasty has fewer complications associated with it than most other forms of cosmetic surgery. However, you may experience some temporary problems. Because many tiny blood vessels become disturbed during the operation, hematomas (blood under the skin) are always possible. These usually subside after a few days and leave no permanent sign.

During the operation the muscles of the eye may be disturbed slightly and cause temporary double vision, as can swelling of the conjunctiva. This usually subsides within the first few hours after operation. Many people report excessive tearing for a few days, but this usually disappears quickly.

Although rare, more serious complications can occur. One problem is ectropion, caused by removing too much skin from the lower eyelid. The eyelid turns out, causing tears to fall from the lid rather than passing over the conjunctiva and lubricating the eyeball. If severe, ectropion can be corrected surgically.

Signs of Infection

If you experience any of the following symptoms after your eyelid operation, report them to your physician.

1. Excessive swelling that does not disappear gradually.
2. Redness that becomes worse over several days.
3. Tenderness or pain in the eyelid that does not disappear gradually.
4. Problems with vision.

Blepharoplasty is a surgical procedure to correct drooping eyelids. Top: condition prior to surgery. Bottom: results of corrective surgery.

in the day. As the disorder advances, the irritation may become more frequent, if not constant. You may notice the lashes turning in toward the eyes.

With ectropion, you may notice the lower eyelid seeming to sag away from the eye, causing tears to run out of your eye rather than lubricating it and being absorbed by the eye.

In either case, see your ophthalmologist, who will examine the eye. In the early stages, entropion may not be obvious when you are sitting or standing, so one of the tests your doctor may recommend may involve lying back and blinking forcibly.

Treatment.   When ectropion causes tears to flow from the eyes, there are fewer tears to serve as lubrication, and the cornea may need to be kept moistened with artificial tears and lubricating ointments. A protective plastic shield often is worn at night to keep moisture in the eye.

Both entropion and ectropion can be treated surgically to tighten the muscles holding the lids in place. The procedures are fairly simple and are usually performed on an outpatient basis with a local anesthetic.

When an underlying condition is the cause of ectropion, treatment of the ailment is the first consideration.

DISORDERS OF THE EYE

Considering what a delicate and precise instrument the eye is, it is surprisingly tough. We tend to take our eyes for granted because most of the time they function flawlessly. However, the eye is susceptible to various disorders that, although not seriously affecting your ability to see, can be annoying or, over time, may present more serious risks.

These disorders include infections or inflammations of the conjunctiva (the mucous membrane that covers the inside of the eyelid and most of the outside of the eyeball itself), the iris, or the uveal tract within the eye. Other potential problems include eye hemorrhage and tumors (see also Corneal Problems, page 763).

CONJUNCTIVITIS

Signs and Symptoms
* Redness in the eyes;
* Gritty feeling in the eye;
* Itching of the eye;
* Discharge in the eye that forms a crust during the night;
* Blurred vision and sensitivity to light.

Conjunctivitis is an inflammation of the transparent membrane (the conjunctiva) that lines the eyelids and the eyeball up to the margin of the cornea. Conjunctivitis can be caused by a bacterial or viral infection (commonly known as pinkeye), by an allergic reaction, or, in newborns, by an incompletely opened tear duct. Newborns are also susceptible to certain bacteria that can infect the birth canal. This form of conjunctivitis is known as ophthalmia neonatorum and must be treated without delay if sight is not to be threatened.

Both viral and bacterial conjunctivitis are common among children and are extremely infectious. Conjunctivitis can spread through a whole classroom of children in a matter of a few days.

The Diagnosis.   All forms of conjunctivitis share certain symptoms. The white of the eye becomes red or pink, and the eye feels gritty when you blink. The eye also produces a yellowish discharge that forms a crust during the night. This sticky crust can seal the eyes shut and you may have to pry the lids gently apart or to soak off the crusts.

Viral conjunctivitis usually produces a small amount of watery discharge, whereas bacterial conjunctivitis often produces a good deal of thicker matter. Some conjunctivitis also can be associated with a respiratory infection or with a sore throat.

Allergic conjunctivitis is a response to an allergen rather than an infection. When you come into contact with a substance to which you are sensitive, such as pollen, your body produces an immune response to ward off what it perceives as an invader. The result is usually intense itching, tearing, and inflammation of the conjunctiva. You will likely also experience some degree of itching and watery discharge from the nose.

If you have any of the symptoms of conjunctivitis, see your physician immediately. Your physician may take a sample from the conjunctiva for laboratory analysis to determine which form of infection you have.

(See page B-11 for color photograph of conjunctivitis.)

How Serious Is Conjunctivitis?   The inflammation of conjunctivitis makes it an irritating condition, but it is usually harmless to sight. However, because it can be highly contagious, it must be diagnosed and treated early. Occasionally conjunctivitis can cause corneal complications in adults (see Corneal Problems, page 763).

Treatment.   You can soothe the discomfort of conjunctivitis by applying warm compresses to the affected eye or eyes. Soak a clean, lint-free cloth in warm water, squeeze it dry, and apply it to the eyes. Allergic conjunctivitis in particular is often effectively soothed with cool compresses. It also may be helped by specially formulated eye drops that contain both an antihistamine and an agent that constricts blood vessels (see Eye Drops, page 755).

Medication.   Your physician may prescribe antibiotic eye drops if the infection is bacterial. Viral conjunctivitis disappears on its own.

Prevention.   Because bacterial and viral conjunctivitis spread easily and quickly, good hygiene is the most useful method for controlling them. Once the infection has been diagnosed, the following steps may be useful.

1. Keep your hands away from the eye.
2. Wash your hands frequently.
3. Change your towel and washcloth each day.
4. Wear clothes only once before washing them.
5. Change the pillowcase each night.
6. Throw away eye cosmetics, particularly mascara, after a few months.
7. Do not use other people's eye cosmetics.
8. Do not share towels or handkerchiefs with others.

SCLERITIS AND EPISCLERITIS

Signs and Symptoms
- Pain in one or both eyes;
- Patchy redness on the eye;
- Blurred vision.

The outer part of the eyeball is composed of several parts. The sclera is a tough layer of tissue that covers most of the eyeball—the part commonly referred to as the white of the eye. The sclera, in turn, is covered by the episclera, a transparent tissue that stands between the sclera and the outer membrane

(the conjunctiva). Occasionally, either the episclera or the sclera can become inflamed. (The conjunctiva is also subject to inflammation or infection; see Conjunctivitis, page 759.)

Inflammation of the episclera (episcleritis) is a mild and localized inflammation that most often occurs among young adults. Inflammation of the sclera (scleritis) is a more uncommon and serious disorder, one often associated with certain systemic autoimmune diseases such as rheumatoid arthritis (see page 997) or inflammatory bowel disease (see page 628). Scleritis occurs primarily among people between the ages of 30 and 60 years.

The Diagnosis.   Both scleritis and episcleritis are characterized by a red or violet patch on the eye. In both disorders, tiny blood vessels of the tissue become inflamed. Scleritis may be accompanied by a dull pain. When scleritis occurs at the back of the eye, vision may be blurred. If you suspect you have either scleritis or episcleritis, consult your ophthalmologist for an eye examination. If you have scleritis, a more general examination also may be conducted because the ailment often is associated with another systemic disease.

Treatment.   Episcleritis tends to disappear on its own after a week or two; it also tends to recur episodically. Your physician may prescribe steroids in drop or ointment form to help reduce the inflammation.

If you have scleritis, your physician likely will prescribe a course of corticosteroids in oral form or as eye drops to help reduce the inflammation. A cycloplegic drug can be used to dilate the pupil by relaxing some of the muscles inside the eye, which lessens the chance for injury to the iris and reduces discomfort.

UVEITIS AND IRITIS

Signs and Symptoms
- Redness of the eye;
- Blurred vision;
- Sensitivity to light.

Uveitis is an inflammation of the uvea, the layer of the eye immediately beneath the sclera. The uvea consists of the iris (the colored portion of the eye), the ciliary body (which produces the fluid inside the eye and also helps control the movement of the lens), and the choroid (which lies just within the sclera and lines the eyeball from the iris all the way around the eye; see also Choroiditis, page 775). Thus, inflammation of the uvea may include the area at the back of the eye in addition to the sides and the iris.

When the inflammation involves mainly the iris and the ciliary body, it may be called anterior uveitis. When it involves mainly the choroid, it may be called either choroiditis or posterior uveitis.

Uveitis may be a disordered immune reaction provoked by a systemic disease such as rheumatoid arthritis (see page 997), Crohn's disease (see page 626), ulcerative colitis (see page 628), sarcoidosis (see page 934), or another disorder. Uveitis also can occur in the presence of herpes simplex or herpes zoster (see Shingles, page 1176) infection.

Iritis is inflammation that primarily involves just the anterior portion of the eye.

An unusual but very serious form of uveitis is called sympathetic ophthalmia. If a seriously injured eye shows persisting inflammation for several weeks, there is a chance that an immune reaction may occur in the uninjured eye with inflammation of the uvea and, ultimately, a substantial loss of vision in both eyes. This is the reason that an ophthalmologist may advise removal of an injured eye (enucleation) if the inflammation caused by the injury is not subsiding as expected.

The Diagnosis. In uveitis, the eye is somewhat red, vision is blurred, and the eye is sensitive to light. Should you have any of these symptoms, see your ophthalmologist for an eye examination. A general examination also may be recommended to rule out the possibility of an underlying disorder.

Treatment. Uveitis and iritis can be treated medically with several drugs. Your physician likely will prescribe a cycloplegic drug to keep the pupil dilated. This relieves pain by preventing motion of the inflamed iris and lessens the chance of scars or adhesions between the lens and the posterior surface of the iris. Topical steroid ointment or drops may be prescribed to reduce swelling. Aspirin or an oral course of corticosteroids also may be prescribed to reduce swelling in more severe cases.

Proper treatment will lessen the chances of some of the potential complications such as glaucoma (see page 765), cataracts (see page 768), and fluid within the retina.

ORBITAL CELLULITIS

Signs and Symptoms
- Pain in the eyes;
- Decreased vision;
- Displacement of the eyes;
- Swelling of the eyelids;
- General malaise.

Orbital cellulitis is a rare, acute infection of the eye socket. It affects primarily children, and its onset is rapid and severe. Bacteria enter the orbit of the eye, often from an infection in the sinuses, a boil on the eye or eyelid, or a foreign object. The soft tissue lining becomes infected. In most cases, only one eye is affected.

The first signs of orbital cellulitis are usually swelling and redness of the eyelids, followed rapidly by pain and decreased vision. There may be noticeable displacement of the eye due to the swelling, resulting in an apparent protrusion of the eye from its socket. If your child exhibits these symptoms, call your physician and go to the nearest hospital emergency room.

The Diagnosis. Your physician will conduct a series of tests to determine the nature of the infection. He or she will begin with an eye examination. Blood tests will be performed and specimens will be taken for

Orbital cellulitis is an infection that produces swelling and redness of the eyelid and eye socket. This requires immediate medical attention.

EYE HEMORRHAGE

The conjunctiva is filled with tiny blood vessels. Occasionally one of them may break, appearing as a red spot or speck of blood on the white of the eye. This is called a subconjunctival hemorrhage, and it can be alarming when you first see it. It is nothing to worry about, unless your eye also hurts. If it does, see your ophthalmologist without delay.

Most simple eye hemorrhages disappear after 2 or 3 weeks. If hemorrhages recur, see your physician, who may recommend a more thorough physical examination to detect a possible underlying blood disorder or an excess of blood anticoagulant medication.

laboratory analysis. A CT scan may be recommended to determine if the sinuses are involved or if a foreign object is present.

Treatment. Because orbital cellulitis is an acute and dangerous infection, your child most likely will be treated in a hospital. Your physician will determine a course of antibiotic treatment based on the particular infectious organism. Surgical drainage of any abscess may be necessary.

RETINOBLASTOMA

Signs and Symptoms
- A white reflection visible in the pupil;
- Crossed eyes;
- Red, painful eye;
- Poor vision;
- Bleeding inside the eye;
- Iris a different color in each eye;
- White spots on the iris.

A tumor is an abnormal growth of tissue. Tumors can develop anywhere in the body and may be benign (self-limiting) or malignant (those that can spread and threaten life).

Retinoblastoma is a dangerous malignant cancer found in children, usually those younger than 5 years. One or both eyes can be affected. It is estimated that 30 percent to 40 percent of all retinoblastoma cases are hereditary. The prognosis for retinoblastoma is good, particularly when it is treated early. If someone in your family has had retinoblastoma, be sure to have your children tested early in life and then reexamined periodically.

The Diagnosis. If you suspect that your child might have retinoblastoma, see your ophthalmologist immediately. The key to diagnosis is a thorough examination by a specialist experienced in diagnosing and treating retinoblastoma.

Examination is usually done with the patient under general anesthesia in a hospital setting. The eyes are widely dilated to see whether growths are evident. Your ophthalmologist also may conduct an ultrasound examination and probably will recommend a CT scan of the head and eye orbits and globes.

Treatment. The treatment of retinoblastoma depends on the number and size of tumors, their location, and whether both eyes are involved. If the tumor is small, irradiation, laser therapy, or cryotherapy (freezing) may destroy it without damaging the eye. If the tumor has extended outside the eye or has spread to other areas (metastasized), chemotherapy may be used. If the tumor is large and has impaired the vision or if it continues to grow despite other treatment, the eye may be removed.

Prevention. If you have a family history of retinoblastoma, seek genetic counseling before having children.

MELANOMA OF THE EYE

Signs and Symptoms
- Brown or black spot on the iris or conjunctiva (membrane covering the white of the eye);
- Iris a different color in each eye;
- Poor vision in one eye;
- Red, painful eye.

Melanoma usually is thought of as a cancer of the skin (see page 1171), but it can occur in the eye also, especially among elderly persons (see color photograph, page B-11).

Melanoma is often lethal. It is an especially fast-growing and fast-spreading form of cancer, so early detection is essential. However, the signs are not always recognizable, and so early diagnosis is sometimes difficult. The eye can be the primary site of the melanoma, or it may have spread (metastasized) from another location in the body.

The Diagnosis. If you suspect you have melanoma, see your ophthalmologist without delay. The key to diagnosis is a thorough examination by a specialist familiar with the clinical features and variations of eye tumors. In addition to a thorough eye examination, your physician may recommend diagnostic tests to determine the extent of the tumor. These may include ultrasound examination, CT scanning (see page 1286), or MRI scanning (see page 1287).

Treatment. A small tumor often may be treated with radiation. Chemotherapy may be recommended if the tumor has spread. The eye may need to be removed surgically if the tumor continues to grow after other treatments.

CORNEAL PROBLEMS

The cornea is the curved, transparent covering at the front of the eye. It works in concert with the lens to focus images on the retina, which in turn transmits "pictures" to the brain where they are interpreted.

In some sense, the cornea is the window behind which the eye operates. Thus, being the most exposed part of the eye, the cornea is susceptible to a host of problems including various injuries, ulcers, and infections.

CORNEAL INJURY

Signs and Symptoms
- Severe pain in the eye;
- Red eye;
- Swollen eyelids.

Injuries to the cornea are fairly common. It takes little abuse to damage such a delicate tissue. A wind-borne speck of sand or sawdust can scratch the cornea; wearing hard contact lenses for too long also can abrade the cornea. The cornea can be burned from exposure to ultraviolet radiation after sitting in the sun or under a sunlamp for too long without proper eye protection.

The Diagnosis. The moment injury to the cornea occurs, you may realize that something has happened to your eye. The tissue around the eye swells, and the eye itself reddens and begins to hurt intensely. Alternatively, you may not feel the symptoms for several hours after injury, and then suddenly you find yourself in extreme discomfort for no apparent reason (see page 314).

If you experience the symptoms of corneal injury, see your ophthalmologist as soon as possible or go to the emergency room of the nearest hospital.

Your physician will examine the eye for signs of abrasion or burning and will determine the extent of damage. Using eye drops containing a dye will help your physician identify damage to the cornea.

Treatment. Simple corneal injuries are treated by removing the foreign material (if any), covering the eye with a patch, and letting the eye heal itself. The cornea usually heals quickly, and within as little as a day or two your eye should be back to normal. Your physician may also apply an antibiotic ointment to prevent infection and prescribe a painkiller for the first day or two to relieve the discomfort.

A more serious corneal injury may require operation to repair or replace it (see Corneal Transplantation, page 764).

VITAMIN A DEFICIENCY

Severe vitamin A deficiency in infancy and childhood may cause softening and deterioration of the cornea and permanent blindness. Lesser degrees of vitamin A deficiency will impair night vision (see Problems in Night Vision, page 240).

Vitamin A deficiency sufficient to cause eye problems is almost unheard of in the United States, but it is a major problem in some underdeveloped countries.

Prevention. You can prevent future problems by wearing safety goggles when working with power tools and by wearing ultraviolet goggles when working with welding equipment, when sitting under a sunlamp, or when exposed to the sun's rays for long periods (see Protecting Your Eyes, page 748).

To ensure the health of your skin as well as your eyes, it is wise to take proper precautions and to limit the amount of time spent sunbathing either outdoors or under a lamp (see How To Avoid Sunburn, page 1165).

CORNEAL TRANSPLANTATION

Surgical advances now offer a solution to severe corneal injury or scarring. If eyesight is greatly impaired by scarring or opacity of your cornea, transplantation may be possible. However, corneal grafting cannot be done if there is any infection in your eye.

The Preparation

A normal transparent cornea is obtained, usually within a few hours of death, from a person who has made arrangements to be a donor. Often, tissue-typing is done to help ensure a good match between the recipient and the donor cornea. Rejection is much less of a problem than with organ transplants such as kidney or pancreas because the cornea has few blood vessels. However, if evidence of rejection develops in the weeks after the procedure, corticosteroid drops usually will control the problem.

The Procedure

The donor cornea can be preserved in a special nutrient solution for several days, if necessary, before operation. The operation is performed by removing the central part of the injured cornea with a trephine (a circular cutting instrument). Then, a graft of corresponding size is fashioned from the donor cornea. The graft is placed in the hole of the recipient eye and fastened into place with very fine sutures.

Your surgeon will give you detailed instructions in the care of your eye after the operation and will watch closely for signs of rejection in the transplanted cornea.

Warning Signs

If you note any of the following symptoms or signs, contact your physician:

1. Increased discharge or redness in the eye.
2. Pain in the eye other than itching (which is normal).
3. Worsening or any marked change in your vision.
4. Light flashes, multiple new floaters (dark or light spots, specks, or lines in the field of vision; see Spots and Floaters, page 775), or a gray film over your vision.

CORNEAL ULCERS AND INFECTIONS

Signs and Symptoms
- Impaired vision;
- Pain in the eye;
- Reddened eye;
- Visible white patch on the cornea.

A corneal ulcer is an open sore on the cornea. The ulcer can form as the result of an infection or, more commonly, from an abrasion or foreign body (see Corneal Injury, page 763) that may become infected. Eyelid problems, such as entropion (see page 757) and blepharitis (see page 756), also can cause a sore to form. Retraction of the lids, as in Graves' disease (see page 778), may permit exposure of the cornea so that it fails to be bathed in tears. This may result in ulceration of the cornea.

The infection itself can be viral, bacterial, fungal, or protozoan (another type of microscopic infectious organism). Viral infections are most frequently caused by the herpes simplex virus.

The Diagnosis. The discomfort of a corneal ulcer probably will send you to an ophthalmologist. This physician will examine your eye and take a sample of the ulcer tissue for analysis to determine whether the cause is infectious.

The symptoms of a bacterial ulcer are generally more severe than those of a viral one. A bacterial ulcer also may be visible as a whitish patch over the cornea. A herpes simplex viral ulcer is usually invisible unless a test is performed in which a stain is placed on the cornea. The ulcer that appears will resemble the branches of a tree.

Treatment. Corneal ulcers are serious and should be treated as soon as possible by your ophthalmologist. Once your physician has determined the kind of ulcer you have, appropriate treatment will be prescribed.

Bacterial ulcers usually are treated with antibiotic eye drops. If the ulcer is severe, an antibiotic may be injected near the eye for faster absorption. Topical application of corticosteroids sometimes is used to lessen the inflammation.

If your infection is viral, your physician

may prescribe antiviral drops or ointment. These will help control the ulcer but, as with most other herpes infections, the ulcer may reappear.

If your corneal ulcer is caused by a fungus or protozoan organism, your ophthalmologist will prescribe specific drops for the eyes.

If left untreated, an ulcer may permanently damage the cornea. A deep ulcer can even erode through the cornea, thereby infecting the entire eyeball. If this happens, you will need surgery. A severely scarred cornea may require surgical replacement (see Corneal Transplantation, page 764).

DISORDERS OF VISION

Disorders of vision can affect various parts of the eye. Some are refraction problems involving the shape of the cornea or muscular disorders (such as in strabismus and amblyopia; see Refraction Problems, page 739). Still others are the result of injury (due to burns, foreign objects, or abrasions; see Trauma to the Eye, page 747) or are caused by infection or inflammation (iritis, orbital cellulitis, uveitis, and others; see Disorders of the Eye, page 759).

Among the most serious disorders of vision are those related to the functioning of the eye itself. Some are the result of aging, a genetic tendency, or both. Such disorders include glaucoma (increased fluid pressure within the eye), cataract (clouding of the lens), and various retinal problems (detachment, macular degeneration, retinal vessel occlusion, retinitis pigmentosa, and choroiditis).

New techniques and medications for detecting and treating glaucoma and cataract have made these two leading causes of blindness very treatable. In the case of glaucoma, early detection is the key to successful treatment. Today's modern surgical procedures make the treatment of cataracts among the most successful of all operations.

These diseases and disorders can be sight-threatening, particularly if not treated promptly.

GLAUCOMA

In the United States, glaucoma is a leading cause of blindness. About 3 percent of Americans older than 65 years—about 2 million people—are affected. Of those, about 60,000 are legally blind.

If detected and treated early, however, glaucoma need not cause blindness or even severe vision loss. Glaucoma is not a single disease but rather is a group of diseases of the eye. However, the group has a single feature in common: progressive damage to the optic nerve due to increased pressure within the eyeball. As the optic nerve deteriorates, blind spots and patterns develop. If left untreated, the result may be total blindness.

The term glaucoma is derived from the Greek word *glauco* which means bright or sparkling. It may have been used to distinguish blind people with clear pupils from those whose eyes were clouded from cataracts. The term has evolved to mean vision loss associated with increased pressure within the eye.

The space between the lens and the cornea in the eye is filled with a fluid called the aqueous humor. This fluid circulates from behind the colored portion of the eye (the iris) through the opening at the center of the eye (pupil) and into the space between the iris and the cornea. The aqueous humor is produced constantly, so it must be drained constantly. The drain is at the point that the iris and the cornea meet, known as the drainage angle, which directs fluid into a channel (Schlemm's canal) that then leads it to a system of small veins outside the eye.

When the drainage angle does not function properly, the fluid cannot drain and pressure builds up within the eye. Pressure also is exerted on another fluid in the eye, the vitreous humor behind the lens, which in turn presses on the retina. This pressure affects the fibers of the optic nerve, slowly damaging them. Over time, the result is a loss of vision.

The group of diseases known as glaucoma can be divided into two forms, acute and chronic. Of the two, the chronic form is far more common, affecting about 95 percent of people with glaucoma. Both types are discussed in detail below.

There also are several rare forms of glaucoma that do not fit into the two main categories.

ACUTE GLAUCOMA

This sequence of photographs suggests the progressive narrowing of the field of vision characteristic of chronic glaucoma.

Signs and Symptoms
- Blurred vision, usually in one eye;
- Halos appearing around lights;
- Pain in the eye;
- Eye becomes red.

Acute (closed-angle) glaucoma is less common than chronic glaucoma; it occurs primarily among elderly persons who are farsighted (see Farsightedness, page 742). Acute glaucoma often runs in families, as does farsightedness.

As we age, the lens in each of our eyes becomes gradually larger and tends to push the ciliary body and iris forward. This change gradually narrows the angle between the iris and the cornea; eventually, the narrowing is sufficient to close off the passage of aqueous humor to the extent that there is a sudden increase in pressure. Sometimes this closure is provoked by eye drops that are used to dilate the pupil for examination of the interior of the eye. This is the reason ophthalmologists are cautious about dilating the pupil in older, farsighted persons.

The Diagnosis.   Attacks of acute glaucoma can develop suddenly or with warnings (preliminary attacks) weeks or months ahead. The attacks usually occur in the evening when the light is dim (and the pupil is dilated), and they last as long as the angle is closed. Your vision becomes blurred, you may see halos around lights, your eye becomes red, and you may have pain.

In a full-blown attack the symptoms are similar but are more severe and persistent. The pain may be extreme, causing vomiting. The cornea appears hazy, even gray and granular. The eyeball may be painful and hard.

How Serious Is Acute Glaucoma?   An attack of acute glaucoma is an emergency that should be treated immediately. If you suspect that you are having such an attack, contact your ophthalmologist without delay or go to your local hospital emergency room.

Treatment.   Acute glaucoma often is treated with an emergency operation, known as an iridotomy, to create a drainage hole in the iris. New lasers allow eye specialists to form this opening in the iris without making an incision in the eye. The laser iridotomy technique is an office procedure that avoids many of the risks associated with conventional surgical treatment. With laser treatment, you often can resume normal activities the same day.

CHRONIC GLAUCOMA

Signs and Symptoms
• Gradual loss of peripheral vision.

Chronic glaucoma, unlike the acute form, often goes undetected for years. In chronic glaucoma the drainage angle is not blocked by the iris (as in acute glaucoma) and hence it also is called open-angle glaucoma. Still, fluid does not drain properly from the front chamber. As a result, the pressure within the eye increases gradually over months or years and slowly damages the optic nerve and retina.

The cause of the impaired outward flow seems to be some fault in the mechanism of absorption of the aqueous humor. Persons who are vulnerable to chronic glaucoma may have an increase in pressure within the eye after the use of corticosteroid eye drops. (For a more detailed discussion of glaucoma's effect on the eye, see Glaucoma, page 765.)

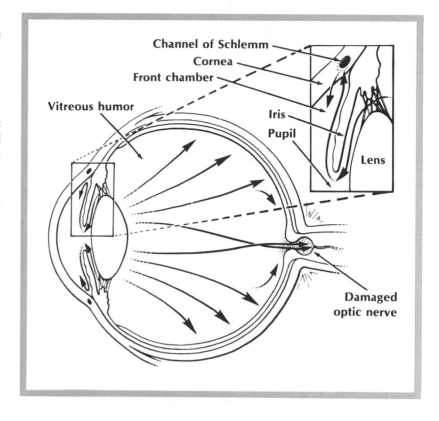

The Diagnosis. Chronic glaucoma has no early warning signs. Your central vision will remain normal until the last stages of the disease. You gradually lose your peripheral vision, so that eventually only a narrow section of your visual field remains clear.

The only way to diagnose glaucoma early is to have regular eye checkups once you reach age 40 years. Certain tests can be performed by a general physician, although others must be performed by an eye specialist.

The earliest detectable abnormality of chronic glaucoma is increased pressure in the eye. A tonometry test is an inexpensive and painless test that allows your physician to determine the pressure within the eye (see Tonometry and Your Eyes, page 769). Your physician may include an ophthalmoscopic examination as part of a routine checkup. The ophthalmoscope, a small hand-held device, allows a clear view of the eye's interior and can show damage to the optic nerve, a sign of glaucoma (see The Eye Examination, page 740).

Your peripheral vision also can be tested. Larger defects in peripheral vision can be detected by asking you to look into the eyes of the physician while he or she moves a hand off to one side and then up and down and asks whether you can see it. More de-tailed testing is done with computer-assisted devices. The tests can reveal optic nerve damage long before you become aware of any vision loss.

This test is not part of a routine eye examination. Rather, it is more likely to be used when your physician suspects glaucoma or another disease of the eye or brain.

How Serious Is Chronic Glaucoma?
Chronic glaucoma is a leading cause of blindness. Because the only symptom is a gradual narrowing of vision, it often goes undetected for years. Early detection through regular checkups can prevent blindness.

Treatment. It is not always necessary to treat slightly increased eye pressure. If no evidence of optic nerve damage is found, a modest increase in intraocular pressure does not necessarily require therapy. Instead, your physician may suggest careful monitoring of the condition by examination several times a year.

Most chronic glaucoma is treated with eye drops to help decrease the pressure in the eye. For years, the most popular eye drops to treat glaucoma were those containing epinephrine or pilocarpine to increase the outflow of fluid. However, these drugs sometimes have troublesome local side ef-

The vision loss of glaucoma results from the pressure of built-up fluid within the eye. Fluid normally passes through a narrow space between your iris and lens (see inset), then drains out of your eye through the channel of Schlemm. If this outward flow is blocked, pressure can damage your optic nerve and reduce vision.

fects. As a result, the most common topical medications prescribed today contain a beta-adrenergic blocker.

Beta-adrenergic blockers are remarkably effective and generally safe drugs. Three such drugs commonly used are timolol, betaxolol, and bunolol. However, if enough of the drug enters the general bloodstream, side effects may result. Rarely, they may aggravate the symptoms of heart failure. They can disturb heart rhythm and worsen bronchial asthma symptoms. In some circumstances, they can leave you feeling fatigued, drowsy, depressed, or confused. They can cause temporary impotence. If you have diabetes and use insulin, a beta-adrenergic blocker may cause your blood sugar concentration to decrease unexpectedly (see also Eye Drops, page 755).

Another form of treatment involves oral medications. Certain drugs, such as acetazolamide, can lower the pressure within your eye by decreasing the formation of normal eye fluid. This type of medicine also can cause general side effects. Long-term use of these drugs typically is avoided.

Your ophthalmologist understands the possible side effects and probably will tell you what you should look for. If you experience such problems, contact your ophthalmologist or your general physician. Your dosage may be adjusted or you may be given alternative treatment. When you see your physician, take the medication with you.

Surgery.   If medical treatment is unsuccessful, your physician may recommend operation. Several options are available. In one, a laser beam is used to open blocked drainage channels in the front chamber of the eye. This fairly simple procedure can be done in your physician's office.

In more severe cases, an operation known as a filtration procedure may be recommended. In this operation, a drainage passage is surgically created between the interior of the eye and the conjunctiva to relieve the pressure within the eye.

CATARACTS

Signs and Symptoms
- Blurred vision;
- Impaired vision at night or in very bright light;
- Halos around lights;
- Second sight (the ability to read without glasses; often occurs with increasing age).

Cataracts are a major cause of vision loss worldwide: almost 20 million people are blind because of the condition. In the United States, over half a million cataract operations are performed each year.

Many people find the idea of cataracts alarming, assuming that if they develop them they will become blind. In truth, however, cataracts are one of the least serious eye disorders because surgery can restore lost sight in most instances.

A cataract is a clouding of the normally clear lens of the eye. The lens, one of the two main focusing mechanisms of the eye, lies just behind the pupil. The clouding of the lens blocks the passage of light needed for sight. Although a cataract often starts in only one eye, usually both become involved. Cataracts are accompanied by changes in the chemical composition of the lens, but the cause of these alterations is unknown.

Everyone develops some clouding in the eye lenses with aging. In this sense, most people older than 60 years have some degree of cataract formation.

RISK FACTORS FOR CHRONIC GLAUCOMA

Many people do not notice any symptoms of chronic glaucoma until significant, permanent damage has occurred. For this reason, it is particularly important to be aware of the risk factors for chronic glaucoma.

Age
After age 40 years your chances of developing chronic glaucoma increase. The disorder is uncommon among children and young adults.

Family History
Glaucoma runs in families. About 20 percent of people with glaucoma have close relatives who have the problem.

Diabetes
If you have diabetes, your risk of developing glaucoma is 3 times greater than that for people who do not have diabetes.

Race
If you are black, your chance of developing glaucoma is significantly higher than that for other races.

The presence of several of these risk factors suggests that you and your physician should be especially alert for indications of glaucoma.

TONOMETRY AND YOUR EYES

Glaucoma is one of the leading causes of blindness in the United States. Early detection of glaucoma cannot restore lost vision, but prompt treatment can arrest deterioration and slow subsequent loss. A simple testing procedure, called tonometry, can alert you and your physician to the possibility that you have glaucoma.

Tonometry is a method of measuring the pressure within the eyeball. Normal intraocular pressure is approximately 8 to 22 millimeters of mercury. If tonometry reveals higher pressure, further tests can be performed to determine whether you have glaucoma.

The Schiotz Tonometer

Several types of tonometry tests are practiced today. Your family physician may perform one, using a Schiotz tonometer, during a general checkup. While you are in a reclining position, anesthetic drops are placed on your cornea. An instrument then is placed directly on the anesthetized cornea. The weight of the tonometer indents the eye: the dimension of the indentation is read from a scale on the instrument and the intraocular pressure is then determined from a conversion table. The amount of indentation is indirectly proportional to the pressure within the eye and can indicate if something is amiss.

The Applanation Tonometer

Your ophthalmologist may perform a more sensitive test with an applanation tonometer. The applanation tonometer is a sophisticated device that usually is fitted to a slit lamp, a common instrument for eye examination. For this test you sit up rather than lie down. Your eyes are anesthetized with drops and the tonometer is placed directly on your eye. The readings from the device denoting eye pressure are very accurate. After the anesthesia wears off, your eyes may feel scratchy for a short time.

The Air-Puff Tonometer

Optometrists, who are not physicians, often use the air-puff tonometer to test for glaucoma. This device, which uses air to measure eye pressure, is not as accurate as the applanation tonometer, but it is useful for glaucoma screening.

Tonometry should become a routine part of your general medical examination after age 40 years. If you have a family history of glaucoma, are nearsighted, or have diabetes, you should also be tested periodically before you reach 40.

Schiotz tonometer (left) measures eye pressure while you lie down. This instrument is satisfactory for glaucoma screening. For a more precise measurement, or to confirm an abnormal eye pressure, your physician may use an applanation tonometer (right). This test, for which you sit upright, is performed by an eye specialist.

Age is not the only factor in the development of cataracts. Certain diseases, such as diabetes mellitus, contribute to the formation of cataracts. People who take corticosteroid drugs for diseases such as rheumatoid arthritis over a period of years may develop cataracts. People who receive high amounts of ultraviolet radiation from the sun over a period of time seem to have an increased risk of developing cataracts.

Occasionally a child is born with cataracts or develops them shortly after birth. Certain eye disorders such as iritis (see page 760) or an injury to the eyeball also can contribute to the development of cataracts. Cataracts tend to run in families.

The Diagnosis. Because everyone experiences changes in eyesight later in life, you may not even notice the gradual clouding of a lens. You may first discover a problem when you have trouble passing a vision test to obtain a driver's license.

You may notice a gradual change in your vision. This change often is described as a film-like covering over one or both eyes; the

Cataracts (clouding of the eye's normally clear lens) are of several forms. Above: a nuclear cataract. Below: wheel-spoke-patterned peripheral cortical cataract. Almost all cataracts can be effectively treated by surgery.

sensation may be rather like looking through fog. Your vision may be worse in dim or bright light (which results in narrowing of the pupil opening).

You may begin to have problems with night vision, particularly when driving. Glare and halos around oncoming lights make driving uncomfortable and dangerous. Some people notice a change in sight when reading. They find that they can read without their eyeglasses, a condition known as second sight. As the degree of clouding increases, the temporarily improved reading ability decreases.

Second sight is caused by a form of cataract known as nuclear sclerosis. Nuclear sclerosis is the most common form of cataract among older people. As the name im-

CATARACT SURGERY

Recent advances in technology have made cataract surgery one of the more successful of all operations. Approximately 95 percent or more of all cataract operations result in improved vision. Today's surgical techniques make the procedure safe, fast, and nearly painless. Recovery time with modern techniques also is quick.

The Procedure

Cataract operation routinely is performed under local anesthesia in a hospital setting on an outpatient basis. The operation usually takes about an hour to perform.

A small incision is made at the outer edge of the cornea (the transparent front portion of the eye). The lens is removed, and an intraocular lens is usually implanted. This is an artificial plastic lens. It is nearly invisible when in place and helps provide excellent vision after surgery. Lens implantation is now the favored method, being used in nearly all routine cataract operations. The incision is closed with fine sutures. There is minimal or no pain during the procedure. You most likely will experience nothing more than a dull discomfort for a few days afterward.

Alternatives to Intraocular Lens Implant

Alternatives to the implantation of an intraocular lens include eyeglasses and contact lenses.

Eyeglasses
Until recently, thick-lensed eyeglasses were necessary. Although they are helpful, they do have significant drawbacks, including excess magnification, reduced side vision, and limited depth perception.

Contact Lenses
Contact lenses provide better vision than thick glasses. They are especially helpful if the lens of only one eye must be removed. Recent advances in the design and manufacture of contact lenses have made them more convenient and comfortable. Extended-wear contact lenses often are prescribed after cataract operation. However, contact lenses often are not recommended for older people, particularly those who have arthritis in the hands, because these lenses can be difficult to insert and to remove. (See also What You Should Know About Contact Lenses, page 744, and Caring for Your Contacts, page 746.)

Cornea

Lens

Eyeball

During cataract surgery, the clouded lens is removed. It is replaced with an artificial lens such as those shown at right.

plies, the cataract is located in the center (nucleus) of the lens. In early stages of development, the cataract serves to increase the focusing power of the lens.

People with nuclear sclerosis may find that they need a change in prescription glasses more frequently than in the past.

If you notice changes in your vision, see your ophthalmologist for a complete examination. Cataracts are often not visible to the observer until they are quite advanced. Your physician will conduct a complete eye examination, including a slit-lamp examination, and may use ultrasonography (see page 1287) to evaluate the posterior part of the eye to discover whether there are other abnormalities that cannot be seen through the ophthalmoscope because of the opacity of the cataract.

Treatment. The most effective treatment for a cataract is surgical removal. However, before such a major step is taken, a few simpler approaches can help temporarily.

Eye drops to widen your pupil may help if you have small cataracts near the back of your lens. Repositioning a workroom light to avoid glare on the clouded lens also may help. Keeping your prescription for glasses up to date may make a difference too.

Surgery. At some point you probably will have to face the question of surgery. An operation usually is appropriate when your failing vision seriously interferes with your normal activities. The decision to have the procedure varies with each person, depending on age, occupation, and lifestyle.

In some instances, surgery may be recommended early if there is risk that the cataract may lead to other eye complications. With earlier surgical techniques you were advised to wait until the cataract had "ripened" (totally clouded the eye). Allowing the cataract to become too advanced also can (rarely) cause complications. With recent advances in the procedure, physicians no longer recommend waiting that long.

Cataract removal is now one of the more successful operations performed. It is usually done under local anesthesia and takes about an hour. The lens is removed from the eye and in most cases is replaced with an artificial one (see Cataract Surgery, page 770). Alternatives to an artificial lens include contact lenses or thick-lensed eyeglasses.

At times, cataracts can be removed suc-cessfully but vision does not improve. This may be the result of macular degeneration (this page), which cannot always be diagnosed initially because of the presence of the cataracts—they preclude your physician from "looking in" in the same way that they affect your ability to "see out."

MACULAR DEGENERATION

Signs and Symptoms
*   Increasingly blurred central vision.

Involutional macular degeneration is the most frequent cause of legal blindness in the United States and Great Britain. (The criteria for legal blindness may vary from state to state. A common standard is a vision of 20/200 or less in the better eye while using well-fitted glasses.) This disorder most often affects the elderly.

The macula, from the Latin meaning spot, is located in the central portion of your retina. The macula is responsible for your central vision. In early stages of macular degeneration, small deposits form and blood vessels grow in the macular region between the retina and its supporting layer of choroid tissue. If these vessels leak plasma or blood, the retinal cells responsible for central vision are damaged. Eventually a scar may develop, producing considerable impairment of central vision.

The Diagnosis. Early diagnosis of macular degeneration is vital to successful treatment. The disease usually develops gradually and painlessly. It typically affects both eyes, either simultaneously or one after the other.

A damaged or diseased macula causes difficulty in reading small print and seeing distant objects such as street signs. Fortunately, side vision is retained, so that if you have the ailment, you can walk about and even cross streets unaided. If you notice any decrease in your central vision, see your ophthalmologist as soon as possible. Better yet, have your eyes examined once a year once you reach age 50 years.

Your physician can test for macular degeneration during a routine examination. He or she may perform a test known as fluorescein angiography to evaluate the blood vessel pattern in the eye and detect the presence of abnormal blood vessels. In this test a special dye is injected into a vein of the arm, and it then flows to the vessels of the eye. A series of photographs of the retina is then taken and the dye identifies any problems with the blood vessels.

Treatment.   The only treatment for macular degeneration is laser therapy to coagulate abnormal (leaking) blood vessels to prevent or slow further loss of vision. Such therapy is useful during only the early stages of the disease.

Your ophthalmologist may ask you to use an Amsler grid to help prevent loss of vision from macular degeneration. By checking the pattern of the grid daily with each eye, subtle changes in your vision may be apparent. These changes may be due to fluid leaking from blood vessels. If changes occur, see your ophthalmologist without delay.

RETINAL DETACHMENT

Signs and Symptoms
- Sensation of flashing lights;
- Many floaters in the eye;
- Blurred vision;
- Shadow over a portion of the field of vision.

The retina is a thin, transparent membrane in the back portion of your eye. The retina contains the rods and cones that are sensitive to light. In addition, the retina contains the nerves that carry impulses from the rods and cones to the optic nerve which, in turn, leads to the brain. The retina is essentially the film that processes the images projected by the cornea and lens.

Behind the retina is a layer of tiny blood vessels. This layer supplies oxygen and nutri-

ents which are essential for your eye to function properly. Retinal detachment results if the retina separates from this layer of blood vessels.

Most cases of retinal detachment are associated with a tear or hole in the retina. This defect, which may be caused by trauma to the eye or by changes in the vitreous fluid of the eye due to aging, allows fluid from the vitreous to leak under the retina and lift it from the underlying layer. Occasionally a tumor or an inflammatory disorder affecting the back portion of the eye is responsible for a detached retina.

Each year approximately 20,000 people in the United States suffer a retinal detachment. There are several risk factors. Nearsighted people are more prone to retinal detachment than others. The condition is more common among men than women, and it is more common among whites than among people of other races. The problem occasionally affects more than one member of the same family, so there may be a genetic factor.

The Diagnosis.   Retinal detachment is a medical emergency requiring immediate attention (see page 315). The condition is painless. However, symptoms almost always appear before the retina detaches. As the vitreous shrinks and sags, it may tug on the retina, producing the sensation of flashing lights. If the tugging is strong enough and causes a retinal tear, small blood vessels may be damaged, allowing blood to seep into the vitreous and causing hazy vision and the sudden appearance of new floaters (dark or light spots or specks or lines in the field of vision; see Spots and Floaters, page 775).

Not all tears or holes in the retina progress to a retinal detachment. If a detachment does occur, however, the portion of your visual field corresponding to the detached part of the retina becomes lost. You will perceive this vision loss as a shadow or curtain moving over your eye.

If you have any of these symptoms, see your ophthalmologist immediately or go to the emergency room of your local hospital. The physician will examine your eye and may use ultrasonography to get a precise picture of the condition of your eye.

Treatment.   Surgery is the only effective therapy for retinal detachment. If a tear or hole is treated before detachment develops

Vitreous humor

Detached retina

Your retina is a thin membrane attached to the back of your eye. If it develops a hole or tear, the jelly-like vitreous may flow behind your retina and detach it (detached retina).

THE USE OF LASERS IN EYE DISEASES

During the past 10 years, advances in laser technology have made possible effective treatment of various eye ailments. Sometimes lasers are used to seal a tear or to cauterize a blood vessel.

Diabetic Retinopathy

One of the more frequent applications of laser therapy is for diabetic retinopathy. This condition seems to be caused mainly by a reduction of the oxygen supplied to the tissues of the retina due to blood vessel deterioration consequent to diabetes.

By making numerous small burns in the periphery of the retina with the laser, the amount of retina that uses up oxygen is reduced and the remaining retina then has an adequate supply of oxygen. At each of the small burns there is, of course, no vision, but because they are mainly around the periphery, they cause only minimal impairment of vision.

For the most part, the results of laser therapy in persons with diabetes have been very good. The treatment should begin as soon as retinopathy threatens vision.

If you have diabetes, be sure to get regular examinations by an ophthalmologist.

Glaucoma

Physicians use a technique called laser iridotomy in treating acute glaucoma (a sudden increase of pressure within the eye). In this procedure, which can be done in a physician's office, a small opening is made in the iris to relieve built-up pressure between the iris and lens. Chronic glaucoma also can be treated with laser therapy to reduce intraocular pressure (see Glaucoma, page 765).

Retinal Reattachment

Lasers are used to treat retinal detachment. Retinal detachment is a very serious disorder in which the retina located at the back of the eye becomes partially detached from the choroid tissue that nourishes it. If the retina is not reattached quickly, severe loss of vision may result. Lasers are now used to help seal the retinal tears that precede detachment (see Retinal Detachment, page 772).

Macular Degeneration

In its early stages, macular degeneration can be treated with laser therapy, although results are often disappointing (see page 771). In this disorder, blood vessels grow between the central portion of the retina (macula) and the choroid tissue. These vessels often leak blood, causing scarring and loss of vision. If the condition is diagnosed early, lasers can seal the blood vessels.

Secondary Cataract

After a cataract operation (see Cataract Surgery, page 770), vision may decrease gradually because a thin membrane within the eye (the posterior lens capsule) sometimes clouds up. The posterior lens capsule is left in the eye during most cataract operations because it is safer for the eye and it supports the intraocular lens implant. If the capsule causes blurred vision, the problem often can be solved with a laser beam. The procedure is usually performed in the ophthalmologist's office or on an outpatient basis at a hospital.

Orbital and Eyelid Tumors

New types of lasers are sometimes helpful for treating tumors around the eye. Your ophthalmologist will advise you as to whether this is indicated.

or if a retinal detachment is treated before the macula (the portion of the retina responsible for central vision) has detached, your vision probably can be saved.

When a retinal tear or hole has not yet progressed to a detachment, your physician may use one of two techniques. A laser procedure is often used to prevent further detachment. In this process, known as photocoagulation, a laser beam is directed to the damaged area of the retina. The treated area then forms a scar which usually holds the retina to the underlying tissue. The other method, known as cryopexy, uses intense cold. An ice probe is applied to the outer portion of the eye that covers the defect. This produces an inflammation that leads to formation of a scar (as in laser therapy) which holds the retina to the underlying tissue.

A major advantage of photocoagulation and cryopexy is that they can be performed on an outpatient basis. If your retina does become detached, however, you will have to be admitted to the hospital for further operation.

Surgical reattachment of the retina is usually performed by pushing the scleral layer of the eye back against the retina with a technique called scleral buckling. In this procedure the wall of the eye (sclera) is indented (buckled) over the defect. Silicone either in the form of a soft sponge or a solid piece is stitched to the outer surface of the sclera. When there are several tears or holes or an extensive detachment, scleral buckles sometimes are placed around the entire circumference of the eye.

Occasionally scar tissue forms in the vitreous, either before or after operation, and prevents reattachment of the retina. When this happens, the scar must be removed surgically and scleral buckling must be performed. In some complicated cases, injection of air or other gases or silicone oil into the vitreous cavity helps push the retina back against the wall of the eye.

You will be able to leave the hospital a few days after the procedure. You may need to avoid strenuous activities for 3 to 4 weeks after the operation.

RETINAL VESSEL OCCLUSION

Signs and Symptoms
- Sudden blurring or loss of vision in a portion or all of the visual field of one eye.

The retina of the eye functions rather like the film in a camera, processing images from without and transmitting the information to the brain. Cells of the retina are nourished by tiny blood vessels. On rare occasions these retinal arteries and veins can become blocked by a blood clot or fatty deposit. If a retinal artery is blocked, the retina stops functioning, and blindness results in part or all of the eye.

Blocking of a retinal artery is an emergency because without a blood supply the rod and cone cells of the retina die. Blockage of a retinal vein is less threatening to sight than blockage of an artery. However, the blocked vein may rupture and spill blood and fluid into the vitreous humor, blurring and clouding vision.

These conditions, known collectively as retinal vessel occlusion, are more commonly found among elderly people. Often they are symptoms of another disorder such as hypertension or diabetes.

The Diagnosis.   An acute blurring of vision is the only symptom of retinal vessel occlusion. If the blockage is in an artery, the upper or lower field of vision may be affected. If a retinal vein becomes blocked, blood and fluid in the vitreous humor may cause blur-

ring and clouding of vision over a period of several hours.

If you experience the symptoms of retinal vessel occlusion, contact your ophthalmologist immediately. This physician will examine the eye to determine an appropriate course of action. He or she probably will recommend a thorough general medical examination to identify any underlying systemic disorder such as hypertension or diabetes.

Regular eye and general examinations are most helpful for early detection of a possible problem.

Treatment.   In many cases, little can be done to treat retinal vessel occlusion. If you are fairly young and experience a retinal vein blockage, the spilled blood may be reabsorbed by the eye and sight will be restored. If the blood is not reabsorbed, the blurred vision will be permanent. Laser therapy may be used to treat glaucoma that may occur after retinal vein occlusion.

If an artery is involved, emergency treatment is the only chance of improving impaired vision. Administration of anticoagulant drugs to prevent further growth of a clot or even an emergency operation to dislodge a blockage in the carotid artery (the major artery in your neck, supplying blood to your eyes and brain) may be helpful. Often, however, vision is only partially restored, if at all.

OPTIC NEURITIS

Signs and Symptoms
- Acute loss of vision in one eye;
- Pain on movement of the eye.

Optic neuritis, an inflammation of the optic nerve, may be the result of a viral illness or of multiple sclerosis. In elderly people the cause may be a condition known as temporal or cranial arteritis (see Cranial Arteritis and Vision, page 780). The condition also can occur for unknown reasons.

When the condition affects the portion of the optic nerve visible through the ophthalmoscope, it is known as papillitis. (An ophthalmoscope is a hand-held instrument that illuminates the back of the eye.) When the inflammation occurs in the orbital portion of the optic nerve, it is known as retrobulbar neuritis.

The Diagnosis.   In optic neuritis, the optic nerve swells, blocking signals to the brain. The result is a gradual or sudden loss of vision. In the case of papillitis, the loss of vision is usually the only symptom. When retrobulbar neuritis is present, the loss of vision may be accompanied by pain on moving the eye. Nearly complete loss of vision in the eye can result within a day or two. When temporal arteritis is present, the condition may involve both eyes.

If you experience any of these symptoms, see your ophthalmologist, who will conduct a series of tests to determine the nature and extent of the problem. Your eyes will be examined with an ophthalmoscope, and you may have your visual field and color vision tested. Because optic neuritis often is associated with multiple sclerosis in young adults, your physician may recommend a complete medical examination. If you are older than 60 years, your physician may recommend testing for temporal arteritis.

Treatment.   In many cases optic neuritis disappears on its own within 2 to 8 weeks, and sight is fully restored. Your physician may recommend corticosteroid medications in the form of tablets. This may hasten the resolution of the inflammation, but such treatment is controversial.

Optic neuritis can recur, especially when associated with multiple sclerosis, and each time more damage may be done to the eye.

COLOBOMA

A coloboma is a congenital defect in the development of the eye. This ailment occurs before birth. Often the iris, ciliary body, and other structures of the eye are absent. If the optic disc is involved, the optic nerve fibers are absent.

Depending on the extent of the defect, there may be partial or even complete loss of vision in the affected eye. Sometimes both eyes are affected. If either partial or complete vision is lost in an eye, it is imperative that protective glasses be obtained for your child as soon as possible to protect the unaffected eye.

CHOROIDITIS

Signs and Symptoms
- Blurred vision in one eye;
- Pain or discomfort in the eye.

The choroid is the layer made up mainly of blood vessels that lie between the retina and the sclera of the eye. Blood vessels in the choroid nourish the retina.

When this layer becomes inflamed (choroiditis), the retina may also become inflamed. This condition is then called chorioretinitis. When the inflammation sub-

SPOTS AND FLOATERS

Just about everyone occasionally sees what appear to be specks, hairs, and transparent strings floating freely in the fluid of the eye. These vitreous floaters dart in and out of your field of vision. They are often leftovers from the prenatal growth of the eye.

Changes in the Vitreous
As you age, you may notice more and different floaters because the vitreous of your eye may partially liquefy. The vitreous is a jelly-like substance located behind the lens of your eye. It is composed almost entirely of water and accounts for three-fourths of the weight of your eye. At the back of the eye, the vitreous is attached to the retina, the light-sensitive part of the eye.

When some of the vitreous liquefies, it creates the appearance of spots, specks, hairs, or strings floating freely in the fluid. Common age-related floaters appear gradually over time and are rarely of medical importance. There is no effective treatment for the condition. The floaters may be annoying, but they tend to become less conspicuous with time.

Vitreous Collapse
If you are nearsighted or elderly, partial liquefaction of your vitreous may cause additional problems. The back portion of your vitreous may sag inward, causing a small portion of it to detach from the retina. This vitreous collapse is a common condition and also may cause the appearance of a floater or flashes of light when your eyes are closed or you are in a darkened room. These "lightning flashes" occur when your eyes move and the shrunken vitreous gently pulls on your retina, initiating a nerve impulse that you perceive as light.

Danger Signs
The sudden appearance of floaters or flashes of light may indicate a serious eye disorder. Possible causes include retinal tear, which can lead to a detachment, hemorrhage, and infection. If floaters or flashes of light appear suddenly, consult your ophthalmologist immediately.

sides, the choroid and retina may be scarred and vision may be impaired.

Because the inflammation tends to occur in a spotty fashion, the loss of vision that corresponds to the scars therefore also is spotty. Each area of scarring will have a corresponding area of blindness, which can be discovered through testing of your visual fields. In many persons, the scarring left from choroiditis poses no handicap to vision because the spots of blindness (scotomas) are small.

The condition occurs among both children and adults. The cause is often unknown, although occasionally it may be associated with infections such as histoplasmosis or toxoplasmosis (see Histoplasmosis, page 925, and Toxoplasmosis, page 193).

The Diagnosis. If you experience blurred vision with or without pain or discomfort in your eye, see your ophthalmologist. Your physician will examine the eye with an ophthalmoscope (an instrument that illuminates the back of the eye) and may recommend testing by fluorescein angiography to identify areas of inflammation. In this test, dye is injected into a vein of the arm, and it then flows to the blood vessels of the eye. A series of photographs of the retina are taken at close intervals.

Your physician also may recommend a general medical examination to rule out the possibility of a serious underlying disorder.

Treatment. Your physician may inject a corticosteroid drug near the eye to reduce the swelling. Treatment of any underlying disorder may help to reduce the inflammation of the choroid.

RETINITIS PIGMENTOSA

Signs and Symptoms
- Difficulty seeing at night or in reduced light;
- Poor central vision;
- Loss of peripheral vision.

Retinitis pigmentosa, most commonly known as night blindness, is sometimes an inherited disorder, but often it occurs for no apparent reason. The retina slowly degenerates in both eyes. The rods in the retina are affected most, causing defective night vision. As the disease progresses, peripheral vision also is lost, producing so-called tunnel vision.

The disease is uncommon. It leads to legal blindness in many cases. (The criteria for legal blindness may vary from state to state, but generally a visual acuity of 20/200 or less in the better eye while wearing glasses is a standard.)

The Diagnosis. Retinitis pigmentosa often can be detected in childhood. Reduced night vision may become evident by age 10 years. If there is a history of the disorder in your family, have your child tested early.

Your ophthalmologist will conduct a series of tests and will ask for a thorough family history. On examination, your physician may see dark pigmentation of the retina, hence the name pigmentosa. Tests to determine the presence and extent of the disease include electroretinography (which records the actions of the retina in response to light stimuli) and dark adaptation (to determine how the eyes adjust to reduced illumination).

As the disease progresses, night vision becomes increasingly poor and both peripheral vision and central vision are gradually lost, particularly during and after middle age.

Treatment. There is no effective treatment for the disease, although use of magnifying lens devices may be helpful.

Some researchers suggest using sunglasses to protect the retina from the effects of visible and ultraviolet light in an effort to preserve vision. Experimental glasses that widen the field of vision may prove helpful in the future.

Genetic counseling is the best hope for preventing retinitis pigmentosa.

THE EYE IN SYSTEMIC DISEASES

The eyes provide a direct view of a portion of the circulatory system when the back of the retina is examined. Changes that take place in the blood vessels of the retina can help in diagnosis of certain systemic diseases such as diabetes and hypertension and even the possibility of stroke. However, these diseases and others also affect sight either in the long-term, as with diabetes and hypertension, or in the short-term, as with stroke, Graves' disease (a thyroid disorder), and cranial arteritis (a circulatory problem).

THE EYE AND DIABETES

Signs and Symptoms
- Blurred vision;
- Fluctuating vision;
- Sudden loss of vision;
- Eye pain, in advanced cases.

Both your vision and the movement of your eye may be affected in diabetes (for a detailed discussion of Diabetes Mellitus, see page 707).

Diabetic retinopathy, the medical term for a deterioration of the blood vessels of the retina, is a leading cause of blindness in the United States. It usually occurs in both eyes.

As the name implies, the disorder is a complication of diabetes, and it is commonly found among people who have had the disease (particularly the insulin-dependent variety) for at least 10 years. Almost all persons with diabetes show signs of retinal damage after about 30 years of living with the disease. The changes of diabetic retinopathy can be seen by your physician with an ophthalmoscope.

In diabetic retinopathy, there are poorly understood metabolic changes that lead to a relative lack of oxygen in the retina. The small blood vessels (capillaries) in the retina leak some of the protein and fats from the blood plasma to form deposits. The capillaries tend to close off, thus contributing to the lack of oxygen. The process of diabetes also weakens the walls of the vessels, which tend to become enlarged (microaneurysms). These microaneurysms appear as tiny red dots at the back of the eye. Sometimes these small blood vessels break, causing hemorrhages within the retina or extending into the vitreous, and these hemorrhages cloud vision. Often the blood is absorbed by the retina, but scars that decrease vision may remain.

New blood vessels also can grow over the retina and into the vitreous humor (the jelly-like material within the back portion of the eye). When this occurs, the disorder is known as proliferative retinopathy. These blood vessels also can swell and burst, causing loss of vision. The blood sometimes is reabsorbed but the retina can detach (see Retinal Detachment, page 772).

The Diagnosis. Diabetic retinopathy is not a symptom of the onset of diabetes but is rather a long-term complication of the disease. It is separate and distinct from the changes in refraction that result from fluctuating blood sugar values (see Refraction Errors Due To Changing Blood Sugar Concentration, page 743). If you have diabetes, your eyes should be monitored and examined by an ophthalmologist annually.

Your physician will examine the retina with an ophthalmoscope (an instrument that shines a bright light into the back of the eye), looking for signs of dilated blood vessels and microaneurysms. He or she also may use fluorescein angiography, in which a dye is injected into a vein of your arm and a series of retinal photographs are taken to detect signs of leaky blood vessels. This test allows your physician to pinpoint areas that threaten hemorrhage.

Treatment. Treatment begins with controlling the diabetes. This may involve insulin or other antidiabetic medications, nutrition, and exercise programs.

Specific treatment for diabetic retinopathy may include laser therapy (see The Use of Lasers in Eye Diseases, page 773). If a vein has leaked into the vitreous humor and scarring has occurred, a vitrectomy may be recommended. In this procedure, a part of the

THIRD NERVE PALSY

Third nerve palsy is a common condition in diabetics. In this disorder there may be a rather sudden onset of pain around the eye and double vision. The affected eye turns downward and outward. The pupil usually continues to react normally, enlarging in darkness and contracting in light. The upper eyelid often tends to droop.

It is easy to think that such symptoms might imply a stroke, and in fact the disorder is the result of a temporary interruption of blood flow to the third cranial nerve which governs the action of some of the muscles that control the position of the eyeball. Ordinarily, there are none of the other symptoms of stroke (see page 508). The pain lasts a few days and the eye recovers its normal function in 2 to 3 months.

vitreous is removed along with the scar tissue. If the retina becomes detached from scarring, an operation may be required to reattach it.

GRAVES' DISEASE AND EYE PROBLEMS

Signs and Symptoms
- Bulging or feeling of pressure about the eyes;
- Blurred or double vision;
- Tearing;
- Sensitivity to light;
- Retraction of the eyelids;
- Increased nervousness and heat intolerance;
- Increased appetite, accompanied by weight loss.

Graves' disease is a disorder of the thyroid gland in which too much of its hormone thyroxine is produced. An excess of thyroxine causes a wide range of symptoms including jitters or nervousness, heat intolerance, weight loss despite a healthy appetite, rapid and irregular pulse, and a fine tremor of the hands (for a more detailed discussion of Graves' disease, see Hyperthyroidism, page 727).

The same abnormal immune mechanisms that stimulate the thyroid to excess activity also may cause eye problems. Changes in the muscles that control your eyes and eyelids can cause double vision and a wide-eyed (or pop-eyed) appearance. The eyes may actually protrude because of an in-

The result of an excess of thyroid hormone, Graves' disease can produce a variety of symptoms, including a tremor of the hands, rapid heartbeat, and difficulty in sleeping. The most evident visual symptom is pictured here: the characteristic protruding eyes.

crease in volume of the muscles, fat, and other tissues in the orbit behind the eye. This condition is called Graves' ophthalmopathy. In some cases, the optic nerve may be compressed by the enlarged tissues and may be seriously threatened. If retraction of the lids is extreme, the cornea may be exposed enough to cause severe drying or even a corneal ulcer (see Corneal Ulcers and Infections, page 764).

Once the disease is diagnosed, drugs or radioactive iodine can slow the gland's production of hormones, or surgeons can remove part of the gland to diminish its function. Sometimes, however, even after the excess production of thyroid hormone is corrected, eye problems persist or become more severe. Until recently there was little to do for people with Graves' ophthalmopathy. Today, however, it can be treated effectively.

The Diagnosis. If you have protruding eyes and the distance between the upper and lower lids seems to be widening, your appearance is likely to be so distinctive that the diagnosis can be made quickly.

Sometimes, however, the eye changes can begin subtly and slowly so that the cause is not readily apparent. At times, only one eye will seem to be affected, giving the appearance of a tumor or infection from a sinus behind the eye. Sometimes irritation of the conjunctiva may be the most apparent symptom, and the problem may at first be regarded as a stubborn conjunctivitis or an allergic reaction.

Occasionally, the eye changes develop a year or more before or after the beginning of the abnormal thyroid action. Ordinarily, if the thyroid has just shown evidence of being abnormal, your physician will automatically look for the eye changes. However, if the thyroid is producing no symptoms, the physician may be less likely to think of Graves' disease as a cause of any eye symptoms. Double vision may be the first symptom, and a neurological disorder, such as myasthenia gravis, may be considered initially.

The degree of protrusion of the eye can be measured by the ophthalmologist with an exophthalmometer. This is of more use for determining whether the protrusion is worsening (or, if it is being treated, whether it is improving) than of establishing the diagnosis.

A CT scan of the orbit (see CT Scanning, page 1286) will show enlarged muscles within the orbit and help eliminate the diagnosis of a tumor or infection as a cause for the protruding eyes.

Treatment. In many cases, Graves' ophthalmopathy is a mild disorder that requires no treatment. Sleeping with the head elevated may lessen eyelid swelling.

If the symptoms are mild, topical ointments and artificial tears may be all that are needed to soothe the eyes. For some people, temporary oral treatment with cortisone drugs can help. Glasses with side guards also can be used to help protect the eyes from dust and drying wind.

In more severe cases, operation may be needed to correct the condition. To accommodate the swollen tissue behind the eyes, a surgeon may create extra space in the nearby sinus cavity. This allows the eye to settle back into a more natural position within the eye socket. This procedure often corrects the optic nerve changes which can seriously threaten vision. The surgeon later may also reposition the enlarged muscles that control eye movement, thus correcting the double vision. Eyelid procedures can usually help the retraction of the eyelids.

Overactivity of the thyroid gland should be treated as soon as it is identified. Although there does not seem to be a clear connection between how the thyroid hyperactivity is treated and the condition of the eyes, it is desirable to eliminate the overactivity of the thyroid promptly and completely. If the treatment results in underactivity of the thyroid, replacement therapy with thyroxine tablets is initiated.

HYPERTENSION AND VISION

The ophthalmologist can make a remarkably accurate assessment of the seriousness of hypertension (high blood pressure) by examining the retina with an ophthalmoscope (for a full discussion of High Blood Pressure, see page 796).

The small blood vessels in the retina constitute a sample of all of the blood vessels in the body and have the advantage of being readily visible for your physician's inspection. Narrowing of the arteries, small hemorrhages, and exudates (accumulation of protein that has leaked from affected blood vessels) are evidence of hypertension. It is very unusual for hypertension to impair

vision, but this can occur as a result of severe constriction of the retinal arteries and swelling (edema) of the retina, which occur in a hypertensive crisis. Treatment of the hypertension is the only way to reverse the loss of vision that may occur in a hypertensive crisis (for a more detailed discussion of treatments for hypertension, see page 799).

THE EYE AND WARNING SIGNS OF STROKE

Signs and Symptoms
- Sudden loss of vision in one or both eyes;
- Double vision.

The term stroke is used to describe several disorders related to a disturbance in the blood supply to the brain. The cause may be an insufficient supply of blood due to a blocked brain artery (known as an ischemic stroke) or a rupture of an artery and subsequent bleeding into the brain (known as a cerebral hemorrhage) (see Stroke and Vascular Disorders, page 507).

In most cases there are no warning signs for stroke. Only when you are experiencing one do you notice the symptoms of headache, paralysis, sudden weakness, and double vision or loss of vision.

However, certain ischemic strokes often are foreshadowed by a series of small incidents known as transient ischemic attacks (TIAs). These attacks, which last for a few seconds or as long as a few minutes, are most often related to the disease atherosclerosis which develops when fatty deposits form inside arteries (see Atherosclerosis, page 786).

Risk factors for stroke or TIAs include hypertension, some types of heart disease, diabetes, smoking, and advanced age. Most strokes occur in people 60 to 80 years old and are a major cause of death (see Transient Ischemic Attack, page 510).

The Diagnosis. If you experience any sudden loss of vision or double vision or any other symptoms such as sudden weakness on one side of the body, speech difficulty, or incoordination in an attack that lasts up to a few minutes, see your physician immediately. You may experience several of these incidents over several days.

Your physician will examine you with an ophthalmoscope, an instrument used to examine the arteries of the retina. Tiny cholesterol-containing plaques in the retinal blood vessels can warn of an impending stroke. Two other tests, known as ophthalmodynamometry and oculoplethysmography, also may be performed to measure the amount of blood flowing through the arteries of the eyes. A general medical and a neurological examination also may be recommended.

Treatment. *Medicine.* If atherosclerosis is found to be causing the attacks, you may be given anticoagulant medication to keep the blood from thickening and forming clots. This may include warfarin (Coumadin) or perhaps a combination of aspirin and dipyridamole. Treatment for hypertension may alleviate the symptoms and prevent a stroke as well (see High Blood Pressure, page 796).

Surgery. In some cases, surgery may be required if a carotid artery appears to be narrowed or blocked. Some of the debris from atherosclerotic plaques in the lining of the affected artery is removed to restore blood flow.

CRANIAL ARTERITIS AND VISION

Signs and Symptoms
* Acute loss of vision in one eye;
* Jaw pain when chewing;
* Pain in the temples;
* Headache;
* Sore scalp;
* Poor appetite;
* Muscle ache, particularly about the neck and shoulders;
* Weight loss.

Cranial arteritis, often known as giant cell arteritis or temporal arteritis, is an inflammation of an artery in the head, often near the temple (see also Vasculitis, page 1009).

The inflammation is probably a form of a disordered immune reaction. This reaction can thicken the lining of the affected artery, blocking blood flow to various parts of the body, most commonly the eyes. If left untreated, the disorder can cause partial or total blindness in one or both eyes.

Until recently, up to 30 percent of those suffering from cranial arteritis became blind in one eye. Today, modern drugs offer effective relief, and blindness and other disabilities can be prevented.

Cranial arteritis is a condition of older people—usually between 60 and 75 years—and most frequently affects women. Blacks and Asians rarely develop the disease.

The Diagnosis. Diagnosis is sometimes difficult because the symptoms of cranial arteritis can mimic the symptoms of other ailments. The symptoms may be vague—some people often feel just "run down." You may have fever and poor appetite or muscle and joint aches (particularly in the morning). You also may have the more usual symptoms of throbbing headache, loss of vision, pain over the temples, a painful jaw when chewing, and sore scalp. If you have any of these symptoms, see your physician for a thorough examination.

There is only one sure way to determine the diagnosis of cranial arteritis. A segment of artery, usually the temporal artery, must be removed for study. The procedure is often done as an outpatient procedure with a local anesthetic. Sometimes more than one biopsy is needed and so the procedure must be repeated.

Treatment. Cranial arteritis can be treated orally with corticosteroid drugs. At first your physician probably will prescribe a large dose of the medication to be taken daily. After several weeks the dosage may be reduced. The symptoms should decrease soon after treatment begins, and the risk of loss of vision is greatly reduced. Treatment often continues for a year or more.

The corticosteroid drug is used in the smallest dose that will control almost, but not quite all, of the symptoms. Occasionally, if symptoms are mild, aspirin can be substituted for the corticosteroid medication.

The disorder will run its course gradually in a year or more and then use of the drug can be discontinued.

CHAPTER 28

THE HEART AND BLOOD VESSELS

CHAPTER CONTENTS

THE HEALTHY HEART AND BLOOD VESSELS

For generations, poets have endowed the human heart with a wide range of emotional abilities. Yet the plain truth is a good deal simpler: The heart is a pump—no more, no less.

But it is an extraordinary pump. Every minute of your life, your heart beats approximately once a second, and considerably more often when you are exercising. It weighs only about a pound but manages to pump 5 or more quarts per minute. In a single day, your heart will pump about 2,000 gallons of blood through your circulatory system.

When functioning normally, your heart pumps blood to the tissues to provide the cells with the oxygen and nutrients they need. This circulatory system consists of arteries and veins. The arteries take the blood to the tissues; the veins bring it back to the heart to be cycled through the lungs before it is returned to the tissues.

When the pumping of your heart, and the resultant circulation of the blood, is interrupted for more than a few minutes, life ends. In fact, all too often the first sign of heart disease is sudden death. It is for this

reason that in recent years so much emphasis has been given to prevention (see Disease of the Heart and Blood Vessels: Living With the Risks, page 785).

THE PARTS OF THE HEART

The heart has two pumps. Each pump consists of a pair of chambers formed of muscles. It is the contraction of these muscles that causes the blood to be pumped. In each pump, the lower chamber is called a ventricle and the upper chamber is called an atrium. The four chambers of the heart are connected by valves.

The tissue of the heart consists of three layers. The exterior layer is the thin epicardium. In the middle is the myocardium, the heart muscle itself (from the Greek *myo* for muscle and *kardia* for heart). The inner lining of the heart is the endocardium, a thin, smooth structure. Protecting the whole package is the pericardium, a fibrous sac with a very smooth lining. In the space between the pericardium and the epicardium there is a small amount of fluid.

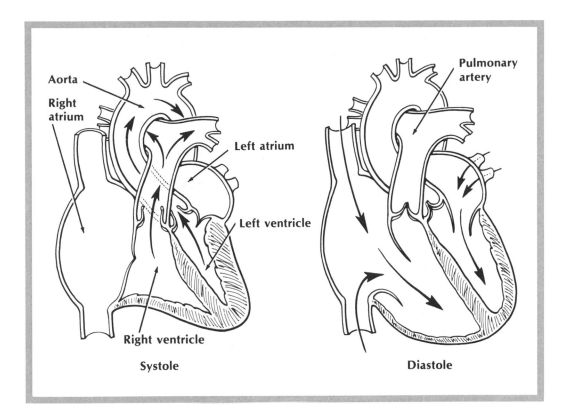

Aorta

Right atrium

Left atrium

Left ventricle

Right ventricle

Systole

Pulmonary artery

Diastole

At its simplest, the pumping of the heart is a two-stage process. During systole, the ventricles are contracting and pumping blood out of the heart; during the relaxation stage, called diastole, the ventricles allow blood to reenter the heart.

THE CARDIAC CYCLE

The blood entering the right side of the heart is returning from the tissues and has been delivered by the veins. The receiving chamber is the right atrium. This atrium also is a low-pressure pump, and it moves the blood into the right ventricle through the tricuspid valve.

The right ventricle has thicker, stronger walls than the right atrium. The right ventricle pumps the oxygen-poor blood through the pulmonic valve into the lungs where the blood gives up the carbon dioxide it has carried from the tissues. At the same time the blood absorbs oxygen. From the lungs, the pumping action moves the blood to the receiving chamber on the other side of the heart, the left atrium, which gently pumps the blood into the left ventricle through the mitral valve. The left ventricle exerts a powerful pumping action to send the oxygen-enriched blood into the aorta, the principal artery that subdivides and delivers the blood to the body's tissues, including the brain, organs, and extremities.

The contraction of the ventricles of the heart that forces blood out is called systole; the relaxation of the ventricles to allow blood to enter is diastole. The right and left sides contract and relax simultaneously.

The rate at which the heart pumps varies, depending on the body's activities at the moment. When you are at rest, your heart pumps more slowly; when you run or climb stairs, the pace of your heart increases to provide your muscles and other tissues with the additional oxygen they need.

The typical heart rate is 72 beats per minute, and at each beat 2 to 3 ounces of blood is pumped into the arterial system. At this rate, the heart beats 104,000 times per day.

THE VASCULAR SYSTEM

The vascular system consists of the blood vessels in your body; its name comes from the Latin *vasculum,* for small blood vessel.

The vessels become smaller as they extend farther from the heart. The aorta delivers its flow to the large arteries; they, in turn, branch into smaller vessels, arterioles. The arterioles supply the tiny capillaries that nourish tissues. The oxygen is given up from capillaries to the tissues, and the carbon dioxide from the tissues is taken up into the capillaries. The arteries have to be strong as well as flexible because of the pressure of the blood being pumped through them.

From the capillaries, the blood begins its trip back to the heart by way of the venous system. The veins increase in size closer to the heart. As part of the venous system, the blood circulates through the liver and kidneys which remove waste products. The veins, under less pressure, are less muscular and less elastic than the arteries.

DISORDERS OF THE HEART AND BLOOD VESSELS

Because of the constant activity of the heart and blood vessels, there is a wide range of potential problems and disorders. The two problems most often discussed in the popular press are coronary artery disease (see Coronary Artery Disease, page 801), the principal cause of heart attack, and hypertension (see High Blood Pressure, page 796). Yet there are other kinds of problems that can affect the health of the valves (see Dis-

orders of the Heart Valves, page 822), the heart muscle (see Diseases of the Heart Muscle and Pericardium, page 830), the rhythm of the heart (see Disorders of Heart Rate and Rhythm, page 816), or the ability of your blood vessels to circulate the blood to your tissues (see Circulatory Problems, page 834). Some problems, called congenital, are present at birth; others occur as the result of infection, hereditary factors, problems with the action of thyroid hormone on your heart, lung diseases that affect your heart, or trauma.

In the following pages, we will consider individually several dozen heart and blood vessel disorders, as well as some of the remarkable advances made in recent years in diagnosis and treatment for heart and circulatory problems. (Certain congenital heart ailments are discussed elsewhere in this book; see Congenital Heart Disorders, page 54.) But before considering the problems, it is important to understand something about

---

LISTEN TO YOUR HEARTBEAT

For most of us, the feel of the cold stethoscope on our chest is familiar. Less familiar is the bass-drum thumping your physician hears through the other end of that hearing device. The interpretation of that drumbeat can provide your physician with considerable knowledge about your heart and your health.

When listening to your heart, your physician will ask you to breathe in and out naturally or perhaps in a deliberately rhythmic fashion. He or she will move the stethoscope in small steps from one location to another over your heart.

During this examination, your physician can interpret the sounds he or she hears. The normal heartbeat has a consistent pattern represented by the syllables "lubb" and "dubb." These sounds correspond to closure of the heart

valves. "Lubb" is followed by a short pause; "dubb" is followed by a longer pause. Differences in the intensity of these heart sounds may provide clues to disease involving your heart or lungs. Obesity, emphysema, or fluid around the heart may seem to muffle the heart's pumping sounds.

Other sounds also may be detected. Murmurs are the result of turbulence in the blood during the heartbeat. Depending on the location, the character, and the relationship of the murmur to the lubb-dubb sounds, your physician often can identify the structural change in the heart valve that is responsible for the turbulence.

The presence of abnormal sounds (known as gallop sounds) during the relaxation phase (diastole) while the ventricles are filling suggests an alteration in the function of the heart muscle. Sounds heard during contraction (systole) of the ventricles, called clicks, combined with a murmur identify specific types of valve alterations.

A murmur may be a symptom of anemia, a leaky valve, or a heart infection such as endocarditis (see Infective Endocarditis, page 824). In children, murmurs often are heard that are not the result of a structural abnormality. Called innocent murmurs, these typically are very faint, often are heard only intermittently, and usually are detected in only a small area of the chest. Innocent murmurs are harmless and often disappear by adulthood.

The echocardiogram (see The Echocardiogram: Images Made With Sound, page 827) has improved the physician's ability to interpret what he or she hears through the stethoscope by allowing frequent comparison of what is heard to the actual flow of blood through the various compartments of the heart.

When your physician listens to your heartbeat, he or she is gathering clues to the health of your heart or to understanding what ails it.

the basic interaction between our health and the lives we lead.

What we eat, our exercise patterns, whether we smoke, and a number of other lifestyle considerations have an impact on the health of our hearts as well as on other organ systems. So we will begin with the risk factors for coronary artery disease and what we can do to use that knowledge for longer, healthier lives.

Your primary-care physician may treat minor heart and circulatory disorders. However, your physician may refer you to a cardiologist, a specialist who has had additional training in the diagnosis and management of heart and blood vessel disorders.

CONGENITAL HEART DISEASE

There is a range of minor to serious heart ailments that are evident at or shortly after birth. Some involve malformations of the heart itself, and some involve malformations of the connections among the lungs, the major blood vessels, and the heart itself.

For a detailed discussion of Congenital Heart Disorders, see page 54.

DISEASE OF THE HEART AND BLOOD VESSELS: LIVING WITH THE RISKS

Whether you are 80 years old and have survived a heart attack or are 18 years old and have no signs of heart disease, a sensible strategy of avoiding, minimizing, and living with the various risk factors for coronary artery disease may be important to your future.

Our century has seen a rapid increase in the prevalence of coronary artery disease. Today coronary artery disease is the leading cause of death in the United States, accounting for about 590,000 deaths a year—about one of every two deaths in the United States is the result of heart disease. Another 6 million or more of us have symptoms of coronary artery disease.

The positive side of the recognition that coronary artery disease is our principal killer is that a tremendous amount of research has been and is being done on understanding, treating, and, perhaps most important, preventing heart disease in its various forms.

Since World War II, many scientists have been investigating the cause-and-effect relationships between our behavior, genes, and aging processes and the ways our hearts function (or malfunction). The Multiple Risk Factor Intervention Trial, the Framingham Heart Study, and many others have brought us to a new level of understanding.

The findings are persuasive. A remarkably high percentage of heart attack victims have a history of exposure to certain *risk factors.* A risk factor is a behavior or condition that places you at greater risk of having a disease than if you were not exposed. The fact is that people with high blood pressure, smokers, diabetics, and those who consume quantities of foods high in fats are more likely to have a heart attack than are those who avoid those risk factors.

Your sex, age, and heredity are other factors that also are in the equation. Rarely, acute, overwhelming stress can also result in a heart-related death (see Sudden Cardiac Death, page 821). In general, however, chronic stress probably does not cause coronary artery disease, although it can make you feel that life is not worth living. Contrary to earlier ideas about "type A" behavior, there does not appear to be any specific type of personality or behavior that predisposes you to coronary artery disease.

As you read the discussions of risk factors that follow, remember that they are to be considered together rather than separately. In fact, the different risks have a multiplier effect on one another. One finding of the Multiple Risk Factor Intervention Trial conducted by the National Heart, Lung, and Blood Institute makes the point effectively. According to this study, of about 13,000 white men between 30 and 60 years old, only 2 percent had a heart attack if they kept their cholesterol and blood pressure levels within reasonable limits and did not smoke. If one of these behavior controls was abandoned, the risk of heart attack increased to 5 percent; two risk factors produced an increase to 10 percent; and among those who smoked *and* failed to maintain healthy cholesterol *and* blood pressure levels, 20 percent had a heart attack.

There are few absolute answers, however. There are conflicting findings. Some studies suggest that there are causal relationships between certain dietary habits or laboratory findings and heart attacks; others conclude that the evidence is not so clear-cut. Yet, one message is paramount: the data suggest that how you live your life may have an important impact on your cardiovascular health.

In the following pages we will discuss the key risk factors. They are divided into two categories: those that you can do something about, and those that you cannot change, such as having a parent who experienced a heart attack at an early age. However, recognizing the uncontrollable risk factors can be valuable. If you know your risks are high, you can take special measures in regard to the other risk factors that you can control.

ATHEROSCLEROSIS: WHAT IS IT?

Healthy arteries are like healthy muscles. They are flexible, strong, and elastic. Their inside lining is smooth so that the flow of blood through them is unrestricted.

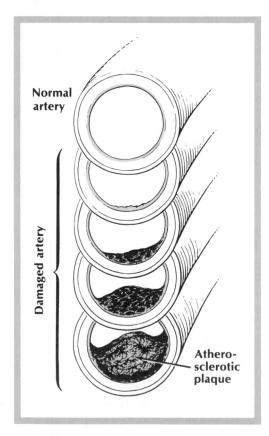

Normal artery

Damaged artery

Athero-sclerotic plaque

Atherosclerosis is an accumulation of plaque deposits in the lining of the arteries. This sequence of drawings illustrates a gradual build-up of atherosclerotic plaque, which, in the long term, reduces circulation of blood. This increases the risk of heart attack, stroke, and other serious arterial diseases.

Atherosclerosis describes the condition in which fatty deposits accumulate in and on the lining of the artery walls. The name comes from the Greek word *ather* meaning porridge, because the fatty deposits are soft and resemble porridge.

Blood cells called platelets often clump at microscopic sites of injury to the inner wall of the artery. At these sites, fat deposits also collect. Initially, the deposits are only streaks of fat-containing cells but, as they enlarge, they invade some of the deeper layers of the arterial walls, causing scarring and calcium deposits. Larger accumulations are called atheromas or plaques and are the principal characteristic of atherosclerosis.

The greatest danger from these deposits is the narrowing of the channel through which the blood flows. If this occurs, the tissues (heart muscle, brain, muscles of the legs, or others) that the artery supplies will not receive their full quota of blood. Pieces of the fatty deposits also may be dislodged, travel with the blood flow, and finally obstruct an artery at some distant point (see Arterial Embolism, page 836).

The term arteriosclerosis means hardening of the arteries (from the Greek *sklerosis* for hardening). This often accompanies atherosclerosis and is not clearly separated from it. The walls of the artery become more rigid and often contain calcium deposits. Sometimes, the arteries in the forearms can be felt and may resemble small, hard pipes. In combination with atherosclerosis, arteriosclerosis also may lead to weakening and enlargement of an artery, a condition called an aneurysm (see page 837).

Atherosclerosis may be discovered in the course of a routine physical examination. During your physician's stethoscope examination of your neck, abdomen, or groin area, he or she may hear a blowing sound (a bruit) if a narrowing and roughening of the lining of the arteries at one or more of these points causes turbulence of the blood flow. He or she also will estimate the amount of blood flow by feeling for pulsations in the arteries at the wrists, legs, and feet. A decrease in pulsations is a reason to suspect partially obstructed blood flow.

More elaborate tests of circulation using sound waves often help in establishing the presence and degree of decreased blood flow (see Ultrasonography, page 1287). A CT scan of the abdomen (see CT Scanning, page 1286) often is used to identify a suspected aneurysm of the aorta in the abdomen. Another test for locating the sites of plaques that narrow blood vessels is arteriography. In this test, a dye that shows on x-rays is injected into an artery in the groin and a number of x-rays of the organ or limb are taken.

In many cases, the diagnosis is not suspected until the artery is completely obstructed and you have experienced a stroke, heart attack, or arterial embolism.

To some extent, the body can protect itself from narrowing of a particular artery by developing, with time, additional arterial connections that detour blood around the narrowed point. This is called collateral circulation.

If you have a significant amount of atherosclerosis in one part of your body, you are likely to have some degree of impairment of arterial circulation in another part. For instance, the person who has poor arterial circulation in the legs may be vulnerable to angina or a heart attack because of some narrowing of the coronary arteries.

The details as to how atherosclerosis can cause difficulty will be described in the sections on stroke (see page 508), coronary artery disease (see page 801), and arteriosclerosis (see page 834).

CONTROLLABLE RISK FACTORS

There are a number of factors that may contribute to the development of atherosclerosis. These risk factors exert their effects over a period of years. High blood pressure has a multiplying effect on the harm of an increased cholesterol level. Keeping the blood pressure under control by limiting salt consumption and taking prescribed medications regularly lessens the chance of significant atherosclerosis developing. Smoking is a very strong promoter of atherosclerosis and is to be avoided. Diabetes accelerates the development of atherosclerosis and should be controlled as closely as possible. Obesity has an aggravating effect on atherosclerosis, particularly if the excess body fat is located mainly around the middle of the body. You can have at least some control over all of these factors. The precautions you take now should be continued over a long time or,

better yet, indefinitely. Avoid all of these risk factors as far as possible, even if doing so might be inconvenient.

High Blood Pressure.   Hypertension is the term physicians use for high blood pressure. This term does *not* describe a state of emotional tension, and the term should not be applied to brief increases in blood pressure such as those seen with exercise or stress.

There are many causes of high blood pressure and, fortunately, many effective treatments; both are discussed at length later in this chapter (see High Blood Pressure, page 796).

High blood pressure is an important risk factor for heart disease (see pages 797 and 801). Over a period of years, high blood pressure can damage the arteries throughout the body so that the artery walls become thickened and stiff, a condition called arteriosclerosis. In persons with high concentrations of fats in their blood, fatty deposits will further narrow the arteries (see Atherosclerosis: What Is It? page 786).

The result of this arterial damage is a decrease in blood flow to vital organs such as the brain, heart, and kidneys. The body responds to this threat by increasing blood pressure to maintain an adequate flow of blood. This increase in blood pressure will lead to further blood vessel damage, and thus a vicious cycle is set in motion. This cycle exacts a toll on your heart, too, because it is forced to work harder. In some cases, the size of the heart muscle actually increases to accommodate its added load, a condition called cardiac hypertrophy. High blood pressure may eventually lead to congestive heart failure and even heart attack (see Congestive Heart Failure, page 807, and Heart Attack, page 809).

A typical blood pressure reading is 120/80 millimeters mercury (mm Hg). This means that the heart is creating a maximum pressure of 120 mm Hg during its pumping effort; when it is at rest between beats, the blood pressure is 80 mm Hg (see How To Take Your Own Blood Pressure, page 798).

There is considerable disagreement on what value represents the beginning of high blood pressure, but there is some agreement that if you consistently have a reading of 140/90 mm Hg or higher you have high blood pressure.

It is estimated that as many as 50 million Americans have high blood pressure, undiagnosed in many of them. The disorder has no evident symptoms. Having high blood pressure will not make you feel more nervous or tense; nor will it cause headache or nosebleeds (except in some very exceptional circumstances). In many cases, the problem is discovered during a physical examination when your physician routinely measures your blood pressure. Often there is no identifiable cause, although in some cases an association can be made with a family history of hypertension, kidney disease, or, in those sensitive to it, a high consumption of salt.

However, even if you have normal blood pressure, if you have close relatives who do have high blood pressure you would do well to limit your use of salt and to avoid weight gain. Have your blood pressure measured at least once a year.

Rarely, hypertension may be the result of a tumor of the adrenal gland (see page 721) or of an abnormality of the arteries that supply blood to a kidney (see Blood Vessel Damage, page 797). However, 95 percent of those with high blood pressure have no identifiable cause. This form is termed essential hypertension.

There are many effective treatments for high blood pressure. In fact, the long-term complications that affect the kidneys, eyes, brain, and heart can be avoided with proper care which may include drugs, cessation of smoking, reduction of salt, alcohol, and fat intake, and other strategies (see pages 800 and 801).

Smoking.   More than 25 years ago, the Surgeon General of the United States announced that smoking cigarettes is a health hazard. Subsequently, a printed warning of the hazards of smoking was required on every package of cigarettes sold in the United States. In the years since, that warning has been made more emphatic—and an immense amount of clinical, statistical, and other research has reinforced the original point.

Smoking is bad for you—not only because of the association between smoking and lung cancer but also because smoking is near the top of the list of risk factors for heart disease. Smoking doubles the risk of sudden cardiac death (see page 821). It increases the risk of heart attack (see page 809). If a smoker stops smoking, the risk of heart attack returns to that of a nonsmoker within about 2 years.

Smoking a cigarette causes your adrenal glands to secrete a hormone that temporarily increases your blood pressure and makes your heart work harder. Smoking decreases the amount of oxygen available to your heart. As a result, every cigarette places a small but unnecessary load on your heart and blood vessels.

Smokers also have more atherosclerosis than nonsmokers do. This is probably because smoke increases the clumping of platelets and, through a series of steps, this clumping is a stimulus for the deposit of cholesterol in the arteries. Over time, smoking—especially in combination with other factors—can exact a significant toll.

Tobacco smoke contains carbon monoxide gas. When inhaled, the carbon monoxide binds to the hemoglobin in the blood, taking the place of valuable oxygen. The result is that the blood traveling to all parts of your body has less oxygen to deliver to your cells. Often, as much as 8 percent of a smoker's hemoglobin may be occupied by carbon monoxide and thus is unable to carry out its normal function of transporting oxygen.

Other research suggests that carbon monoxide also may have a direct, degenerative effect on the heart muscle itself, on the blood vessels, and perhaps even on the clotting of your blood. Low-tar low-nicotine cigarettes also form carbon monoxide and thus cannot be considered to be safe (see also The Low-Yield Cigarette, page 409).

Because high blood pressure accelerates the process of atherosclerosis and so does smoking, probably as a result of the harmful effects of nicotine and carbon monoxide on blood vessels, a smoker who has high blood pressure is at much greater risk of atherosclerosis.

Recent research suggests that there is a risk to nonsmokers from "passive" or "second-hand" smoking, the inhalation of tobacco smoke from nearby smokers. Even if you are not actually smoking, the presence of the smoke in the air around you can affect your health.

The bottom line is simple: you will be doing your health a favor if you quit smoking. The cumulative effect of smoking on your lungs, heart, and vascular system argues convincingly for quitting. (For specific advice on how to go about breaking the tobacco habit, see How To Stop Smoking, page 412.)

CHOLESTEROL AND DIETARY FATS

We should all be aware of our blood cholesterol concentration because it has a strong influence on whether we will, at some time, experience one of the complications of atherosclerosis. These include coronary artery disease with angina or a heart attack (myocardial infarction) (see also page 801), stroke (see page 508), and arteriosclerosis obliterans (see page 835).

If any of your blood relatives has or had a high cholesterol level, a heart attack, or stroke at an early age, you have a greater chance of having difficulties from atherosclerosis. Men are more at risk than women. There is nothing you can do to change your heredity, but you can take the precautions of having your blood cholesterol measured from time to time, of following a prudent, preventive diet, of controlling your weight, and of avoiding tobacco.

The problem of abnormal blood fat values is often discussed solely under the designation "cholesterol." Actually, there are three blood fats ordinarily measured—namely, total cholesterol, high density lipoprotein (HDL) cholesterol, and triglycerides. Knowing the levels of these three blood fats will help your physician to identify abnormal states, to plan treatment, and to monitor the results of treatment. Still another test, called a lipoprotein profile, may be used to identify some of the uncommon blood fat abnormalities.

Serum total cholesterol and HDL cholesterol values may vary somewhat from day to day, or even from laboratory to laboratory. Tests done on blood obtained from the finger are more likely to give an erroneous result than are those done on blood obtained from a vein in the arm. Do not conclude that you have abnormal blood fats on the basis of a single measurement. Nor should you be completely reassured. Before coming to any conclusion, either that you do or do not have a problem, get at least two sets of measurements that are in essential agreement with each other.

Triglyceride (TG) values vary more widely than do total or HDL cholesterol values. Alcohol use and poorly controlled diabetes tend to increase the triglyceride levels.

A fourth blood fat value, low density lipoprotein (LDL) cholesterol, can be calculated from the three primary measurements by the formula

$$\text{LDL chol.} = \text{total chol.} - (\text{HDL chol.} + \frac{TG}{5})$$

but is more accurately determined by direct measurement.

The LDL cholesterol value roughly parallels the total cholesterol value. High values

WHAT DO MEASUREMENTS OF BLOOD FATS MEAN?

First, one test is not enough. All three measurements of blood fat (total cholesterol, HDL cholesterol, and triglycerides) should be made on two or more occasions. Wide differences in results suggest that a laboratory made a mistake.

Once you have two sets of values that are in agreement, how do you evaluate these numbers?

The National Cholesterol Program published the following guidelines in 1988 for the use of total cholesterol measurements. *Normal* total cholesterol is designated as less than 200 mg/100 mL. If your value is in this range, you need to have measurements made only at 4- to 5-year intervals. *Borderline* cholesterol is in the range 200 to 239 mg/100 mL; dietary measures are advised for those whose value is in this range. If, in addition, you have some of the other risk factors for coronary artery disease or are known to have coronary artery disease, you will need further studies and perhaps your physician will advise more stringent dietary restrictions and possibly drug therapy.

Abnormal total cholesterol is 240 mg/100 mL or above. Drug therapy may be advised if this value remains above 240 mg/100 mL in spite of dietary efforts.

In persons over 60 years of age, an increase in total cholesterol may not be as good a predictor of risk for coronary artery disease as it is in younger persons. A family history of coronary artery disease or the presence of it along with the presence of other risk factors are issues that physicians consider in evaluating older persons. Regardless of age, smoking, diabetes, and high blood pressure should be controlled before any medication for treatment of high blood fat levels, such as total cholesterol, is started.

for these two categories are an indication that you may be vulnerable to atherosclerosis. In simple terms, the LDL cholesterol can be thought of as contributing to atherosclerosis in the same manner that hard water can cause a buildup of lime inside pipes—it is a simple matter of the cholesterol depositing into and onto the lining of the blood vessel.

HDL cholesterol, the so-called good cholesterol, can be thought of as a scavenger or "clean-up" form that decreases the amount of the undesirable form, LDL cholesterol. Higher values of HDL cholesterol mean a good outlook with respect to development of atherosclerosis. The HDL cholesterol level tends to increase with exercise, but considerable amounts of exercise may be needed before definite results are seen.

Higher levels of triglycerides are thought to favor development of atherosclerosis but this relationship is not nearly as clear as that for LDL cholesterol and total cholesterol values (some physicians think that the triglyceride level is of little significance in the development of atherosclerosis). Very high levels of triglycerides can lead to pancreatitis (see page 667).

Hereditary factors can produce abnormal blood fat values. One rare hereditary disorder causes such high levels of cholesterol that the affected person may die of a heart attack in childhood. Those who inherit a lesser form of this disorder have very high cholesterol levels and often have heart attacks in mid-adult life or sooner. The trend to high triglyceride levels may also be in one's genetic makeup.

Associated diseases such as hypothyroidism (see page 730), poorly controlled diabetes (see this page), and kidney failure (see page 906) may influence blood fat levels. Some medications such as beta-adrenergic blockers or thiazide diuretics used for hypertension may have an adverse effect. As a first step in treating high blood fat concentrations, it is necessary to identify and correct, as far as possible, any associated disease.

An exercise program emphasizing aerobic exercise is reasonable if the HDL cholesterol level is low (see Cardiovascular Fitness, page 793). Alcohol intake should be forbidden if the triglyceride level is high. Although some studies suggest a somewhat lower frequency of coronary artery disease among people who take one or two drinks a day than among teetotalers, one should not regard this as a reason to take those one or two drinks per day.

OBESITY

If your weight exceeds your ideal weight (see chart of ideal weights, page 350) by 20 percent or more, you are obese by most definitions. If you are very muscular, you may be an exception because the norms of the height and weight table are not for heavily muscled people with relatively little body fat.

Obesity is not a specific risk factor unless it is associated with or contributes to a high cholesterol level in the blood. In addition, obesity may be associated with other risk factors such as high blood pressure and diabetes. Overweight people tend to have lower levels of the "good" HDL cholesterol, and weight loss tends to increase the HDL cholesterol level.

In short, if you are overweight, you may be increasing your risk of coronary artery disease and heart attack. A sensible program of dietary adjustment and exercise to reduce your weight can help you reduce your risks (see Setting the Pace for Weight Control, page 364).

DIABETES

Diabetes is characterized by a lack of insulin, resulting in the body's inability to process the sugars in the diet. The use of insulin or other anti-diabetic drugs has made the disorder manageable, but diabetes remains an important risk factor for heart disease.

Increased blood sugar level often is accompanied by increased fat level, which leads to atherosclerosis (see page 786) and other blood vessel problems. Male diabetics have about twice the normal risk of coronary artery disease and female diabetics have a *five* times greater risk.

If you are diabetic, careful management of your blood sugar level must be a key component of your strategy to minimize heart and blood vessel problems. A combination of dietary measures, weight control, exercise, and insulin or other anti-diabetic drugs

DIET AND BLOOD FAT LEVELS: WHAT YOU EAT CAN MAKE A DIFFERENCE

To decrease a high blood fat level, start with dietary changes. If your triglyceride level is significantly high, avoid alcohol. If you are overweight, trim down. Try to achieve a distinctly lean weight. Avoid simple sugars such as syrups, table sugar, and sugar-sweetened soft drinks.

If your primary problem is an increase in total or LDL cholesterol, avoid foods that are high in cholesterol and saturated fats (they are often the same), decrease the total amount of fat in your diet, and increase the amount of complex carbohydrates (cereals, vegetables). How stringent your attempts are to do this and the details of how you can change your diet should be determined by your physician working together with a registered dietician.

Know Your Fats

Some oils, such as palm and coconut oil, contain no cholesterol because they are of vegetable origin, but they tend to promote atherosclerosis because they are largely saturated. Hence, the statement "No Cholesterol" on a food label does not necessarily mean that that food is a good choice if your cholesterol value is high.

The process of hydrogenating an oil (such as making margarine from corn oil or safflower oil, or treating peanut butter so that the oil will not separate) will convert some of the polyunsaturated fats to mono-unsaturated fats and, to a lesser extent, saturated forms. The change to saturated forms increases somewhat their tendency to cause atherosclerosis. On the other hand, usually only a small proportion of the polyunsaturated fat is converted to a saturated form, and the margarine of safflower or corn oil origin, for instance, can be used by persons with a high blood cholesterol value in spite of the label "hydrogenated."

There is no advantage to deliberately increasing the amount of polyunsaturated fats in your diet but, if you want to use an oil or fat as a part of a recipe or of a dish on a menu, polyunsaturated or mono-unsaturated forms are preferable to saturated forms. While convenient, such generalizations are not always accurate. For example, stearic acid is a saturated fat found in meats but probably does not cause atherosclerosis. Thus, the relationship between diet and atherosclerosis is not an entirely simple matter.

Myths and Maybes

Folklore has it that garlic and onions are useful in controlling blood pressure and preventing heart attacks, but there is no evidence to support this.

Much has been said and written about the potential benefits of increasing the amount of fiber in the diet. Fiber takes many forms, however, and it is mainly the fiber derived from oat bran and the soluble fibers in guar gum (a filler in ice cream and some other foods) and pectin (found in fruits and vegetables) that may have benefit in lowering blood cholesterol. However, as a practical matter, it takes substantial amounts to cause a decrease in your cholesterol level (see page 367). Also, large amounts of fiber in the diet may bind and lessen the availability of calcium and some essential trace minerals. Calcium, in particular, is bound by the phytate in oat bran and is made unavailable.

No Magic Answers

Consuming fish oils containing a high proportion of omega-3 unsaturated fatty acids recently has been proposed as an easy way to lower the risk of heart attacks. Fish that have a higher proportion of such fat are found in colder waters—the most common examples are tuna and salmon. These oils tend to lower the blood triglyceride level. However, they may increase the total cholesterol level. When consumed in large amounts, such fish oils interfere with the function of blood platelets in starting the process of blood clotting. Eskimos in Greenland who consume large amounts of these oils appear to have fewer heart attacks but have more strokes than do Europeans. They also bruise easily and have a tendency to bleed excessively.

Because fish oils can be considered a food supplement, they escape the ordinary supervision given to drugs by the Food and Drug Administration. Various forms have been widely promoted. Some of these have contained large amounts of vitamins D and A, toxins, or chemical residues. We suggest that you incorporate fish into your diet when convenient and feasible but avoid the use of capsules or other medicinal forms of fish oil.

can help (see Diabetes Mellitus, page 707). The diabetic who smokes is at particular risk. If you are a diabetic smoker, it is doubly important that you quit (see page 788).

LIFESTYLE

If your lifestyle is sedentary—that is, if you get no regular exercise—you may be allow-

DRUGS FOR TREATMENT OF ABNORMAL BLOOD FAT LEVELS

The decisions about the degree of dietary modification and whether or not to use a drug for correction of abnormal blood fat levels must be made by your physician who knows all the aspects of your health. After treatment begins, your physician will monitor your blood fat levels with periodic blood tests to judge effectiveness of the treatment and to determine whether additional measures are needed (such as increasing the dose of or changing the medication).

The following are the principal medications used in lowering abnormally high levels of blood fats.

Cholestyramine and Colestipol

These two drugs are resins that bind bile acids in the intestinal tract, thereby causing the liver to increase its manufacture of bile acids. Because some of the same mechanisms are used to make cholesterol, less cholesterol is made. Like all medicines intended for control of blood fats, these must be used daily, for months and years, to have a favorable effect on atherosclerosis. These resins are somewhat unpleasant to take, are expensive, and tend to cause constipation and bloating.

Nicotinic Acid

Nicotinic acid is one of the vitamin B complex. When taken in amounts many times larger than needed for its vitamin function, it becomes a drug. It has a favorable effect on triglyceride, HDL cholesterol, and total cholesterol. It is inexpensive but has the drawbacks of causing flushing, changes in liver function test results, and a tendency toward diabetes. Taking an aspirin tablet 20 to 30 minutes before taking the nicotinic acid may lessen the flushing.

Gemfibrozil

This medication is more convenient to take and, like nicotinic acid, has a favorable effect on all three types of blood fats. It may have some adverse intestinal effects.

Probucol

Probucol also is convenient to take and lowers total cholesterol. However, it also lowers your HDL cholesterol level and this is an undesirable effect.

Lovastatin

Lovastatin was introduced only recently. Several more years will be required for full evaluation of this medicine. It is a promising drug because it acts directly to interfere with the manufacture of cholesterol. It has only slight effects on the other blood fats. Lovastatin may promote the resorption of cholesterol deposits, which would make possible the reversal of atherosclerosis.

Blood Fat Level and Blood Pressure Drugs

Blood fat level may have a bearing on the selection of a medicine to control high blood pressure. Thiazide diuretics tend to increase total cholesterol and triglycerides. They may decrease HDL cholesterol.

Some beta-adrenergic blockers may increase LDL cholesterol and triglycerides and decrease HDL cholesterol, all adverse effects. If LDL cholesterol increases and HDL cholesterol decreases, there may be no change in total cholesterol. Calcium antagonists and alpha-adrenergic blocking agents may have favorable effects on both LDL and HDL cholesterol.

Aspirin

Through its effects on blood platelet function, aspirin lessens the likelihood of clots to form. Your physician may advise its use if you are at risk for stroke or heart attack (see sidebar on Aspirin, page 812).

Is Age a Factor?

There is some suggestion that abnormal blood fat levels are somewhat less harmful in older persons. However, high values should not be neglected. Discuss a high cholesterol or other blood fat finding with your physician.

---

ing your heart to become deconditioned. Like any muscle, the heart requires exercise to maintain its tone, endurance, and ability to circulate blood efficiently through your body.

As yet, there is no proof that exercise can prevent coronary artery disease. However, exercise does affect other risk factors. Regular exercise can help decrease your normal heart rate, lower your blood pressure, decrease the level of fats in your blood, and help you keep your weight down.

Keep in mind, however, that not all physical activities are equally beneficial. Aerobic exercise—that is, exercise that involves continuous, rhythmic movements like running or swimming and which increases the rate and depth of your breathing—enhances heart health. Isometric exercises (like weight-lifting) that do not increase breathing are not as helpful to the health of your heart, despite the benefits of increasing muscle strength and bulk (see Cardiovascular Fitness, below).

Remember, too, that if you are over age 40, have had a heart attack, are obese or diabetic, or have another serious disease, discuss any exercise program with your physician before embarking on it.

HDL CHOLESTEROL LEVELS: WHAT IS NORMAL?

This table can help you understand the significance of your HDL cholesterol level. The levels shown below are found among apparently normal people.

HDL Cholesterol at Age	Normal Range, mg/100 mL	
	Males	Females
20 and under	30–65	30–70
20–29	30–70	30–75
30–39	30–70	35–80
40–49	30–70	35–85
50–59	30–70	35–85
60 and over	30–70	35–85

UNCONTROLLABLE RISKS

Your gender, age, and genetics cannot be changed: they are part of what you are. Nevertheless, be aware of what these factors mean to you and your risk of heart disease.

Age. The aging process itself does not cause coronary artery disease, yet as you age your risk of heart attack and related disorders increases.

Gender. Men are more likely to have coronary artery disease than women are. But the role of gender in heart and blood vessel problems is complicated.

After menopause women become in-creasingly likely to have heart attacks and other related problems. Some scientists believe that the hormone estrogen has a protective effect, so that after its disappearance at menopause the risks increase. It has also been observed that, until puberty, boys and girls have roughly the same levels of HDL cholesterol. However, during puberty, the levels in men decrease, which may explain the difference in rate of coronary artery disease.

Middle-aged men are the most likely candidates for heart attack; after age 60, the difference in risk between men and women narrows. But, as our society has changed in recent years and as women's roles and behavior have changed (specifically, there has been an increase in smoking in women), women have shown an increased frequency of heart attack, especially at earlier ages.

Heredity. The subject of genetic inheritance is complex. In simple terms, if your father or another close relative had a heart attack at a young age, then your risk of coronary artery disease is significantly greater than that in someone whose family has no history of cardiac problems. In short, the tendency to coronary artery disease runs in families, so you and your physician should be interested in the health of your parents and other immediate relatives. The risk includes not only the risk from genetic inheritance but also the risk from other influences such as smoking and a high-fat diet.

On the other hand, if your father died prematurely of a sudden heart attack, you are not necessarily destined to suffer the same fate. This is simply another piece of information to help you decide how you want to live your life. It argues strongly, however, for taking every preventive advantage offered, especially dietary and exercise regimens intended to minimize risks you can control.

If you do not have a family history of heart disease, you can still have heart disease. Therefore, pay attention to controllable risk factors.

CARDIOVASCULAR FITNESS

Your overall health can be enhanced by regular physical exercise. Whether you have the resilience of youth or are feeling the toll the years take, whether you are male or female, tall or short, rail-thin or heavyset, whether you love competition or fade at any hint of attention, your heart—and virtually all your body systems, including your muscles and bones—will serve you better if you get regular exercise. A program of exercise can help you lose excess weight, decrease tension, become physically stronger, and even feel better about yourself. In addition, it may decrease your risk of cardiovascular disease (see Exercise and Fitness, page 377).

By definition, cardiovascular exercise involves the heart (from the Greek *kardia*) and blood vessels (from the Latin *vasculum* for small vessels). It is exercise that strengthens your heart by making it pump harder. Your muscles increase their ability to use oxygen as well. More oxygen is supplied to the heart muscle itself. More oxygen also is delivered to your muscles and other tissues, and this increases your overall capacity for work. Over time, cardiovascular exercise will make your heart more efficient. Paradoxically, working the heart harder during exercise means it will beat more slowly while you are at rest or exercising.

Another good effect of exercise is that it increases the amount of "good" cholesterol, high density lipoprotein (HDL) cholesterol, in your blood, which seems to protect against heart attack.

AEROBIC AND ANAEROBIC EXERCISE

Not all types of exercise are equal. Aerobic exercise enhances cardiovascular health. It is essentially "exercise with oxygen." See your physician before you begin such an active exercise program.

An aerobic workout is one that causes your body to use extra oxygen and calories continuously. Jogging, bicycling, swimming, and walking are good examples. They increase your rate and depth of breathing (you begin to puff). Your body becomes warm. If the exercise is sufficiently long and vigorous, you will perspire.

Anaerobic exercise can be healthy, too, but it does little for the health of your heart. Anaerobic exercise is intense exercise of short duration. Weight-lifting is a classic example: strong muscles may be the end result of a weight-lifting program, but lifting heavy barbells a few times offers little challenge to your heart and lungs to deliver oxygen in a sustained fashion to your body's tissues. Workouts with light weights of sufficient duration may be aerobic, as evidenced by increased breathing and perspiration.

HOW CHALLENGING SHOULD MY WORKOUTS BE?

There is a direct relationship between your heart rate and the intensity and duration of your exercise. The harder you exercise, the higher your heart rate (pulse) goes, until you reach your maximal heart rate.

Your physician can calculate a target heart rate for you. Your target heart rate is the rate at which you must exercise regularly and continuously if you wish to achieve an increase in cardiorespiratory fitness. It will be lower than your maximal heart rate. Several techniques are used to calculate target heart rate and are based on fitness level, age, and personal interest in an exercise program. For example, exercising at approximately 70 percent of your age-adjusted maximum heart rate for 20 to 30 minutes three to five times a week will improve your fitness remarkably. Your age-adjusted maximum heart rate is calculated by subtracting your age from 220. For example, if you are age 50: 220 − 50 = 170; 70 percent of 170 = 119 beats a minute. (NOTE: Some persons with very irregular heart rates should not use the target heart rate method to regulate intensity of exercise.) (See also How To Measure Your Pulse, page 796.)

The target heart rate calculation gives a heart rate that will fall somewhere within 50 percent to 80 percent of your exercise capacity. Some individuals with very irregular heart rates cannot use the heart rate method to regulate exercise intensity.

Another way of judging how challenging your workout should be is through a rating of perceived exertion. This refers to the total amount of physical effort experienced and takes into account sensations of exertion, physical stress, and fatigue. When using the rating scale, do not become preoccupied with any one factor, such as leg discomfort or labored breathing, but try to concentrate on your total inner feeling of exertion. A rating of 6 indicates a minimal level of exertion, such as sitting comfortably in a chair. A rating of 20 corresponds to a maximal effort—for example, jogging up a very steep hill.

Perceived Exertion Scale

Score	Perceived Exertion
6	
7	Very, very light
8	
9	Very light
10	
11	Fairly light
12	
13	Somewhat hard
14	
15	Hard
16	
17	Very hard
18	
19	Very, very hard
20	

Your physician will prescribe a specific perceived exertion range for you. A rating of 13 generally corresponds to 70 percent of maximal exercise capacity and would be considered near ideal for most people.

Another way of judging your workouts is the simple "talk test." During exercise you should be able to carry on a conversation with a companion. If you cannot do this, you are probably pushing too hard and should slow your exercise pace.

In general, if your exercise heart rate or perceived exertion rating is below the level recommended for you, you may increase your intensity. If your heart rate or perceived exertion level is above the recommended level, you should decrease your intensity. Additional fitness benefits gained from high-intensity exercise are small, and you increase the risk of muscle or joint soreness or injury.

A moderate exercise program should not cause discomfort. Stop exercising and consult your physician if you begin to have chest discomfort or pressure, severe shortness of breath, bursts of very rapid or slow heart rate, irregular heart rate, excessive fatigue, marked joint or muscle pain, or dizziness or fainting.

If you are just beginning, increase the duration and rate of your workout slowly over a period of 4 to 6 weeks. By monitoring your pulse rate, you can achieve this slow increase.

HOW OFTEN DO I NEED TO WORK OUT?

The consensus among cardiologists is that at least three to five vigorous aerobic workouts per week are required to accomplish physical conditioning. Your heart rate should be in your target zone (70 to 80 percent of your age-adjusted maximum heart rate) for the duration of each workout. Each workout should last from 20 to 45 minutes. Include warm-up and cool-down activities (see The Elements of Exercise, page 379).

It does not necessarily follow that this amount of exercise is enough to cause a readily measurable decrease in your total blood cholesterol level or an increase in HDL cholesterol. Nevertheless, an exercise program is likely to have some positive effects on your blood fat levels.

WHAT IS THE BEST KIND OF EXERCISE?

Ideally, you want an exercise program that involves continual activity but as little stress on your muscles and joints as possible. Walking, swimming, cycling, jogging, skating, and cross-country skiing are excellent. Tennis, basketball, and dancing can be aerobic, too, but each involves periods of inactivity, which decreases their aerobic value (see also page 794).

Try to find a form of exercise that you enjoy; if you are bored at the end of the first week, you may not be able to keep at the exercise indefinitely. Establishing a consistent pattern of workouts is essential.

The intensity of exercise in any particular activity or sport can be judged by the increase in pulse rate and the general feeling of needing to breathe more heavily. The faster the pulse and breathing, the greater the intensity of the exercise. You can use walking at the rate of 3 to 4 miles per hour (a moderate degree of exercise) as your basis for comparison.

WALKING AND AEROBIC EXERCISE

Walking appeals to many because it requires no special athletic skills. Best of all, it can be

HOW TO MEASURE YOUR PULSE

Knowing your pulse rate can help you evaluate an exercise program. If you are taking heart medications, recording your pulse and reporting the results to your physician can help him or her determine whether the drugs prescribed are effective. If you have had a pacemaker implanted in your chest, pulse rate is a key indicator of how it is functioning.

These are the steps for determining your pulse in the radial artery in your wrist.

1. Stop your exercise.
2. Using the tips of your index and third fingers, locate the area between your wrist bone and tendon on the thumb side of either wrist. You will feel the pulsing of the artery when you have positioned your fingers properly.
3. Make sure not to press so hard on the blood vessel that the flow of blood is obstructed.
4. Count your radial pulse for 10 seconds and then multiply by 6 for your pulse rate per minute.

fun, convenient, and inexpensive and is a form of exercise that you can enjoy alone or with friends.

Walking briskly on a regular schedule improves your body's ability to consume oxygen during exertion. Thus, it can be an excellent form of aerobic exercise. It can help lower your resting heart rate and reduce your blood pressure. It helps burn calories.

To reap these benefits, you must walk briskly (raising your heart and breathing rates) for at least 20 to 30 minutes without interruption and regularly (at least three days each week) (see Walking for Exercise, page 384).

JUST STARTING OUT?

If you are over 40 years old, sedentary, obese, diabetic, or a smoker, if you suffer from hypertension, a kidney disorder, or other serious health problem, or if a close relative died of a heart attack before age 50, consult your physician before starting an exercise regimen. Your physician may have you undergo an exercise tolerance test (see page 804).

If at any time during a workout you experience chest pain, faintness, shortness of breath, or irregular heartbeat, stop your workout and consult your physician.

WARM UP AND COOL DOWN

Each exercise session should open and close with some stretching exercises, perhaps easy jogging or walking. Your muscles, as well as your heart, need to be allowed to adjust to the change in pace (see The Elements of Exercise, page 379).

HIGH BLOOD PRESSURE

Throughout this book, we identify medical disorders by giving their symptoms: this or that pain or pallor suggests that you may have this or that ailment. With high blood pressure, however, that approach does not work.

Most affected persons have no symptoms. Even a physician cannot readily tell that you have high blood pressure until he or she actually measures the pressure by using an instrument called a sphygmomanometer (cuff and pressure gauge). Some think that headaches, dizziness, or nosebleeds are symptoms of high blood pressure, but this is not necessarily true.

"High blood pressure" and "hypertension" are interchangeable terms that refer to the fact that your blood is traveling through your arteries at a pressure that is too high for good health.

Although high blood pressure generally is symptomless, this does not mean that it is not dangerous. High blood pressure has been termed "the silent killer" because about 60 million Americans have it but half of them do not know they have it. The risk lies in the long-term damage the ailment can cause to your heart, blood vessels, and kidneys, causing problems that can lead to early death.

NORMAL BLOOD PRESSURE

A typical normal blood pressure reading is 120/80 mm Hg. This means that the heart is exerting a maximum pressure (systolic pressure) of 120 mm Hg during its pumping phase; when the heart is at rest between beats, the blood pressure (diastolic pressure) is 80 mm Hg (for a discussion of blood pressure and how to take it, see How To Take Your Own Blood Pressure, page 798).

Blood pressure is determined by two factors, the amount of blood your heart pumps and the diameter of the arteries into which the blood is being pumped. In general, the more blood the heart pumps and the smaller the arteries, the higher the blood pressure. A number of other things can influence these key factors and affect your blood pressure. In practice, a wide range of considerations enter into the equation.

Your kidneys regulate the volume of water circulating in your body and the amount of salt your body contains. These two features have direct effects on your blood pressure. More salt in your body means that more water is being retained in your circulation and may cause an increase in blood pressure. More salt in your body also may increase the tendency for blood vessels to become narrow. Less salt means a trend to lower pressure. In someone who does not have high blood pressure, there is little effect on blood pressure over a wide range of salt intake. Other considerations are your nervous system, the blood vessels themselves (in particular, the smaller arteries called arterioles), and a number of hormones.

CAUSES OF HIGH BLOOD PRESSURE

The principal characteristic in most cases of high blood pressure is an increase in resistance to blood flow. This can occur if your vessels become smaller. Your heart has to work harder to pump the same amount of blood, and the pressure at which the blood is pumped increases.

In general, the diagnosis of high blood pressure is made if your blood pressure is consistently 140/90 mm Hg or higher. Why it reaches or exceeds this level may not be identifiable. In fact, in fewer than 1 case in 10 of high blood pressure can a specific dis-ease or health problem be identified as the cause. When a cause cannot be determined, high blood pressure is categorized as essential hypertension.

When the cause can be clearly established, the term used is secondary hypertension because the increased pressure is the result of some other ailment. Among these specific causes are adrenal gland problems such as Cushing's syndrome (see page 719) or a tumor of the adrenal gland (see page 721) and kidney problems such as renal artery stenosis (see page 905), glomerulonephritis (see page 893), and renal failure (see page 906). In some women, oral contraceptive use or pregnancy results in abnormally high blood pressure.

COMPLICATIONS OF HIGH BLOOD PRESSURE

Over a period of years, the excessive pressure of high blood pressure, left untreated, can lead to damage in various parts of your body. Heart attack, kidney damage, stroke, loss of vision, and other complications can result.

Blood Vessel Damage. When your blood vessels are subjected to high pressure for extended periods of time, they respond by thickening. This condition, called arteriosclerosis, will make the blood vessels less flexible. If excessive amounts of fats are present in the blood, the stiffening arteries will also accumulate the fatty deposits of atherosclerosis (see page 786).

If the blood vessel changes result in a decreased blood flow to the kidneys, the kidneys will respond by releasing renin, a hormone that causes an increase in blood pressure. This further exaggerates the high blood pressure and thus contributes to further blood vessel damage.

Hypertensive Heart Disease. The major cause of death in people with high blood pressure is one or more complications of coronary artery disease. High blood pressure accelerates the process of atherosclerosis (see page 787). This may affect the arteries that supply blood to the heart muscle. If these vessels become obstructed and the heart muscle is deprived of oxygen, a heart attack may occur.

HOW TO TAKE YOUR OWN BLOOD PRESSURE

If you have high blood pressure, monitoring your blood pressure can be a necessary part of your treatment. You can take your own blood pressure at home. Various devices, called sphygmomanometers, are available for measuring blood pressure. There are mechanical models with gauges and electronic ones with digital readouts. Discuss the purchase with your physician; he or she may recommend one model over another.

The most common model measures pressure without using mercury; this design measures the pressure in the cuff by its effect on a metal diaphragm. Another kind, a mercury gauge device, resembles a thermometer and consists of a vertical glass tube with a reservoir of mercury at the base. This is the kind used in many physicians' offices and hospitals. With either type, a rubber inflatable bladder encased in a cuff and a rubber squeeze bulb are the other constituent parts. A stethoscope may be attached or may be a separate element of the package.

An electronic sphygmomanometer enables you to take your own blood pressure without the use of a stethoscope. Your blood pressure appears on a digital readout.

The standard cuff fits most people. However, if you have a large or a small arm, a special cuff may be necessary. If you purchase a blood pressure monitoring device, bring it to your physician and have it calibrated to make sure that it records blood pressure accurately.

Do not take your blood pressure if you have a full bladder, have just consumed coffee, or have smoked a cigarette. These situations increase your blood pressure.

Sit quietly for 5 minutes before obtaining a blood pressure reading. Then follow these steps.

1. Position your arm at heart level, perhaps resting it on a tabletop or the arm of your chair. Right-handed people should measure the pressure in their left arm; left-handers do the reverse.
2. Apply the cuff of the sphygmomanometer to your bare upper arm. It should fit snugly, with its lower edge approximately 1 inch above the bend of your elbow.
3. Place the disc of the stethoscope face down under the cuff and immediately above the bend of your elbow (see illustration).
4. Squeeze the hand bulb rapidly. When the pressure gauge reading is 30 mm Hg above your anticipated systolic blood pressure, stop pumping. You should not hear any pulse sound.
5. Deflate the cuff slowly (the pressure should decrease approximately 2 to 3 mm Hg per second). As the pressure falls, listen for the pulse sound. Note the reading on the gauge when the beating first becomes audible: *this is your systolic pressure* (the highest pressure produced by the contraction of your heart).
6. Continue deflating the cuff. Note the reading when the heartbeat ceases to be audible: *this is your diastolic pressure* (the lowest pressure reached during the relaxation of your heart).
7. Your blood pressure is written as systolic pressure/diastolic pressure.
8. Repeat the procedure at least one more time to confirm the accuracy of your reading.

Proper position for obtaining a blood pressure reading using a mercury-gauge sphygmomanometer.

Electronic sphygmomanometers are becoming increasingly popular these days. They are more expensive but are easier to use because there is no stethoscope. An electronic chip performs the task of detecting your pulse, and a digital readout provides your blood pressure reading.

When the blood vessels narrow, the heart is forced to work harder to maintain blood flow to the tissues. In some cases this results in the heart muscle actually increasing in size in order to keep up with its added load. This increase can result in a stiffening of the heart muscle and a net decrease in efficiency, which in turn adds to the overload on the heart.

In the long term, congestive heart failure may result. This does not mean that the heart stops. Rather, it means that, although pumping as best it can, the heart falls behind in circulating the blood. The result is a congestion of fluids in the body, as the blood "backs up." Excess fluid may accumulate in the lungs, legs, and other tissues (see Congestive Heart Failure, page 807).

Stroke. When a blood vessel in the brain ruptures (cerebral hemorrhage) or, more commonly, a clot or a fragment of atherosclerotic plaque blocks blood flow to part of the brain (cerebral thrombosis), a stroke is the result. High blood pressure is often a factor in the occurrence of such strokes (see Stroke, page 508).

Strokes are much more likely in people with high blood pressure. When the blood pressure is decreased by appropriate treatment, the risk for stroke is decreased as well.

Kidney Disease. About a fifth of the blood pumped by the heart goes to the kidneys. The kidneys filter out waste products and help to maintain proper blood chemistry values. They also control the balance of salts, acids, and water.

The kidneys are especially vulnerable to the variations in blood flow that result from high blood pressure and its complications. They cannot function properly if the flow of blood to them decreases significantly, so decreased blood flow will cause the kidneys to release more of the enzyme renin. This causes blood vessels throughout the body to constrict, further increasing the blood pressure in an effort to restore flow to the kidneys.

This can produce a destructive cycle which, ultimately, results in increasing blood pressure and a gradual failure of the kidneys to remove impurities from the blood. Toxic waste products may then accumulate in the blood (see Kidney Failure, page 906).

DRUG TREATMENTS FOR HIGH BLOOD PRESSURE

Lifestyle changes regarding weight loss, exercise, and dietary adjustments (see What *You* Can Do for Your Hypertension, page 800) are preferred over long-term use of hypertensive drugs. However, in many cases, a combination of therapies is required, including medications. High blood pressure can have a wide range of causes; therefore, there similarly is a wide range of medications used in its treatment.

Your physician will determine which drug or combination of drugs may be best suited for you. There may be several steps in the selection process because the first drug may not lower your blood pressure, so a second, third, or even fourth drug program may be tried.

Among the groups of drugs your physician may choose from in treating high blood pressure are the following.

Diuretics. Usually, the first choice of drug, especially when the abnormal blood pressure is not very high, is a diuretic. This type of drug increases the rate at which your body eliminates urine and salt, which serves to decrease blood pressure. Diuretics decrease the amount of fluid in your blood vessel walls, which decreases resistance to blood flow. However, the thiazide diuretics may increase the cholesterol level in your blood.

Diuretics also have few side effects, although you will urinate more frequently and more immediately after you consume fluids. Most diuretics cause a loss of potassium, so that blood potassium levels must be monitored and supplements of potassium may be needed. Increased consumption of foods such as orange juice or bananas ordinarily is insufficient to correct a potassium deficiency caused by a diuretic. Careful restriction of dietary sodium both increases the effectiveness of the diuretic drug and decreases the tendency to eliminate potassium.

Beta-Adrenergic Blockers. These drugs work by blocking many of the effects of adrenaline (epinephrine) in your body, in particular the stimulating effect that it has on

WHAT *YOU* CAN DO FOR YOUR HYPERTENSION

In the majority of cases, the precise cause of high blood pressure remains unknown. Still, the condition can be effectively treated. In fact, through proper treatment, the pressure can be brought down to manageable or normal levels, and most or all of the potentially dire consequences of hypertension can be avoided. If you have high blood pressure, follow the therapy your physician prescribes. This can decrease your blood pressure to normal—and keep it there. You will have a normal or nearly normal life expectancy.

Many physicians believe that the best strategy is to begin your treatment with changes in lifestyle: shed any extra weight (even to the point of leanness), adjust your diet (decrease salt intake), restrict use of alcohol and caffeine, and increase physical exercise. If, after 3 to 6 months, your blood pressure has not dropped to healthier levels, a program of medication may be required (see Drug Treatments for High Blood Pressure, page 799). Even with drug treatment, however, lifestyle changes continue to be important.

Diet

The food you eat has an impact on your overall health but especially on your heart and blood vessels. In particular, the elimination of one ingredient—salt—can decrease blood pressure almost immediately in sensitive people.

Salt Restriction
Excessive salt in the diet has been the focus of much study in recent years. The evidence is convincing: salt causes the body to retain fluids and thus, in many people, is a factor in causing high blood pressure. If you decrease your total salt intake (the salt contained in foods such as bread and butter as well as salt from a salt shaker) to an amount less than 1 teaspoon each day, you will probably decrease your blood pressure.

Salt (sodium chloride) is found in virtually all plants and animals. Some salt is necessary for the normal functions of your body. We need perhaps half a grain daily (roughly a quarter teaspoon of salt), but the average American consumes between 3 and 4 full teaspoons of salt every day.

Do not add salt to your food at the table; use only limited amounts (less than half a teaspoon a day) in preparing your food. Avoid highly salted foods such as chips and foods that are pickled. Remember that highly processed foods are often high in salt, including: cheeses and cheese products; luncheon meats, bacon, and ham; condiments such as ketchup, mustard, and soy sauce; ''fast foods''; and canned soups.

Get in the habit of reading food labels: monosodium glutamate (MSG), sodium chloride, or baking soda all represent salt. The closer the salt substance is to the top of the ingredients list, the greater the quantity found in that food product.

If your blood pressure is normal, there is no evidence to suggest that limiting salt intake will necessarily protect you from subsequent development of hypertension. If you have relatives with hypertension, you would do well to avoid excess salt consumption; in any case, this dietary recommendation is simple and easy to comply with.

Weight Reduction
If you are overweight and have high blood pressure, shed those extra pounds. The excess weight adds to the strain on your heart. In fact, in some people, weight loss alone is sufficient to avoid the need to take hypertensive drugs (for specific guidance on weight control, see page 346).

Exercise

An appropriate regimen of exercise is good for your heart (see Cardiovascular Fitness, page 793). It also may help you to lose excess weight. Although the exact role aerobic exercise can play in treating high blood pressure has yet to be defined, hypertensive people who exercise regularly *have* had a decrease in their blood pressure. However, before embarking on an exercise program, consult your physician.

Other Factors

Both smoking and drinking liquids containing caffeine can have a short-term effect in increasing blood pressure. There is conflicting evidence that smoking and the use of caffeine contribute to sustained high blood pressure. However, the use of tobacco can accelerate the process of atherosclerosis in people with high blood pressure (see Atherosclerosis: What Is It? page 786). Quitting smoking is the healthiest strategy. If you need help in doing so, see Tobacco (page 407).

Heavy drinking also can lead to high blood pressure. So, limit your consumption of alcoholic beverages to no more than 1 ounce of alcohol daily (see page 422).

your heart. The result is that your heart will beat more slowly and less forcefully while the blocker is active in your body.

A common side effect is lethargy and a sense of fatigue, which limits the usefulness of these drugs. Certain of these classes of

ESTABLISHING YOUR DRUG THERAPY

If your hypertension treatment involves medications, the chances are that you will be taking such medications continuously for the rest of your life.

Because each case of high blood pressure is different, your physician may have to adjust dosages or even change medications several times before finding the right drug combination.

Taking Your Blood Pressure

Because high blood pressure has no symptoms, the only way to be sure your medication is working is to measure your blood pressure.

At first, do it three or four times a day. Blood pressure tends to vary throughout the 24 hours. Sometimes it will increase gradually through the day, decrease while you sleep, and begin to increase shortly before you awaken. When you measure your blood pressure, be sure to record the time of day as well as the date and blood pressure reading. The goal is to keep your blood pressure in a good range around the clock.

Once your blood pressure returns to a satisfactory range, check it once or twice a week but try to do this at different hours (see How To Take Your Own Blood Pressure, page 798).

Do not stop taking your medication when your blood pressure reaches an acceptable level. The drug is needed to help keep your blood pressure at that level. However, if your blood pressure goes up again despite your drug therapy, consult your physician.

Side Effects

If you have side effects, consult your physician before you stop taking the drug. There may be alternatives available, and your physician probably can change the dose or choose another medication to meet your needs with fewer or no side effects.

Make It a Habit

As obvious as it sounds, you must take the drugs regularly and on schedule for them to work properly. At first, it may seem foreign to you, but establish a regimen so that swallowing your pills becomes a part of your daily routine.

It is sometimes helpful to use a plastic pillbox with one to three compartments for each day of the week. You can "load up" once a week for the 7 days to come, and if you are not sure whether you have taken your pill for a given scheduled time, you see what pills are remaining in the box.

---

drugs also may decrease the blood level of HDL cholesterol, the "good" cholesterol (see page 790).

If use of a diuretic drug does not bring your blood pressure down, your physician may prescribe a beta-adrenergic blocker, perhaps in combination with a diuretic.

Calcium Channel Blockers. These drugs function by blocking the entry of calcium into your cells. This decreases the tendency of your small arteries to become narrow.

Angiotensin-Converting Enzyme Inhibitors. Like the calcium channel blockers, these inhibitors help prevent narrowing of arteries. The mechanism is different, however, in that these drugs block the formation of a natural body chemical, angiotensin II. This allows your blood vessels to dilate, and thus your blood pressure is decreased. These may be used alone or in combination with diuretics.

Other Drugs. Hydralazine and diazoxide are used for severe high blood pressure; nitroprusside may be used in emergency situations when an extremely high blood pressure threatens life.

Reserpine, rauwolfia, alkaloids, and guanethidine are other options for therapy. Each drug has circumstances in which it is appropriate as well as situations in which it is not suitable or its usefulness is limited.

CORONARY ARTERY DISEASE

Coronary artery disease is our nation's leading disease killer, accounting for about 600,000 deaths each year. Although the condition may develop slowly over many years, its impact is instantaneous in nearly a third of the cases—death, without warning, is its first manifestation.

The blood vessels (coronary arteries) that

provide oxygen and nutrients to the muscles of the heart are small. These arteries encircle the heart like a crown (hence the name "coronary") and send branches downward to the tip of the heart. In coronary artery disease, there is a buildup of material—cholesterol, scar tissue, calcium, and other substances—in the lining of these arteries. This accumulation, called atheromatous plaque, is the principal characteristic of atherosclerosis (see Atherosclerosis: What Is It?, page 786); its effects vary, from recurring chest pain called angina (see page 803) to the dreaded heart attack (see page 809) and congestive heart failure (see page 807).

Atherosclerosis usually occurs in a somewhat irregular fashion so that there will be considerably more narrowing at some points than at others. The roughening of the lining of the arteries over the atheromatous plaques favors the development of a blood clot. Usually, in a heart attack, the final closure of the narrowed segment occurs as the result of a clot forming in this location.

The same factors (for example, smoking, high blood cholesterol levels, high blood pressure) that contribute to the development of atherosclerosis in other parts of the body also favor occurrence of atherosclerosis in the coronary arteries.

The walls of the coronary arteries include muscle fibers. At times, these may go into spasm—that is, contract and cause further narrowing of the channel. Such spasm may occur without apparent cause, but it also may result from strong emotional stress or exposure to cold.

Coronary artery disease is treated with a wide range of techniques, medications, and lifestyle adjustments. The diagnosis and treatment of coronary artery disease have seen a great deal of innovation in recent years. There are tests to determine if your symptoms suggest coronary artery disease (see The Exercise Tolerance Test, page 804). Other tests are available for those who have already experienced coronary artery problems (see Scans and Coronary Angiogram, page 805). In the operating room, bypass operations can direct blood around narrowed or blocked arteries (see also page 814). In some situations, specialized procedures can open narrowed arteries (see Coronary Angioplasty, page 812).

The frequency of coronary artery disease appears to be decreasing slowly, perhaps because of a growing attention to the controllable risk factors (see page 787). The introduction of medications and new procedures and operations to improve the flow of blood to the heart muscle have proved helpful in minimizing symptoms and, to a lesser extent, have lengthened life in those who have had symptoms of coronary artery disease.

COMMON DIAGNOSTIC TESTS

Narrowing or blockage of arteries in your heart can cause chest pain (angina pectoris), heart attack, or even death. One of the challenges to your physician is to detect coronary artery disease *before* such consequences occur and to help you avoid or minimize consequences.

Your physician cannot detect blocked coronary arteries simply by listening through the stethoscope, but there are clues to be heard (see Listen To Your Heartbeat, page 784). Your physician will also take your pulse and measure your blood pressure. But there are more specialized tests to be used as well.

Electrocardiogram The electrocardiogram—also known as the ECG or EKG (the "K" is for the Greek word *kardia* for heart)—is an important tool in detecting heart disease and in pinpointing where the difficulty lies when a heart problem is present.

An ECG is a graphic representation of the electrical forces at work in your heart. During the cardiac cycle, a pattern of changing electrical pulses precisely reflects the action of your heart. These pulses can be recorded through electrodes attached to the surface of your body. The activity of the heart—represented by characteristic waves—can then be evaluated instantaneously on a television monitor or studied later on graph-paper printouts.

The ECG procedure is painless. While you are relaxing motionless on a bed or examining table, 12 to 15 electrodes are attached to the skin of your legs, arms, head, and trunk. Then, the recording process begins and is over in a few minutes.

The analysis involves looking for indications of heart rhythm abnormalities, of an old or a recent heart attack, or other trouble. Your physician may wish to record an ECG of your heart when you are between 30 and

40 years old and in good health. This will provide a basis for comparison later if any heart problems develop.

Since its invention at the turn of the century, the ECG has proved to be an invaluable tool for the cardiologist. Most often, it is used on stationary, relaxed subjects. It also is a key part of the exercise tolerance test (see page 804). With a portable version, the Holter monitor, an ECG can be recorded from your heart during a 24-hour period while you go about your regular activities. This provides your physician with a day-long "diary" of your heart's functions, an especially useful tool in attempts to diagnose heart rhythm disturbances (see Disorders of Heart Rate and Rhythm, page 816).

Blood Tests   A sample of your blood may be taken for analysis. Among the measurements made will be your cholesterol level. Too much LDL cholesterol or too little HDL cholesterol puts you at greater risk of atherosclerosis, an accumulation of fats in your blood vessels (see also Cholesterol and Dietary Fats, page 789). Other tests will include measurement of blood sugar level (for indications of diabetes) and of thyroid hormone (an overactive thyroid gland can produce heart abnormalities).

Chest X-Ray   A chest x-ray produces a picture of your heart and blood vessels and can be useful in identifying certain results of heart disease including an enlarged heart. A wide range of new scanning methods allow further inspection of your heart (see Scans and Coronary Angiogram, page 805).

ANGINA PECTORIS

Signs and Symptoms
- Heart pain (tight, band-like, crushing sensation, often sharp and suffocating, that usually is centered beneath the breastbone (sternum) and often spreads to the throat or to one arm or the other);
- Sensation of heaviness or tightness that is less than pain;
- Attacks generally brought on by exercise or emotional stress;
- Feelings of anxiety or of impending death.

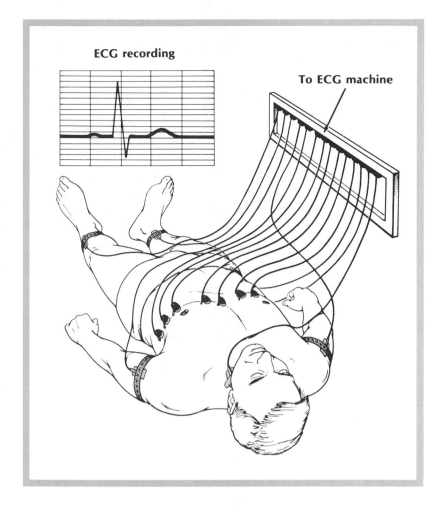

ECG recording

To ECG machine

An electrocardiogram (ECG) records electrical activities of your heart. Electrodes convey impulses of your heart to a device that produces a graphic representation of your heart's activity. This can be studied for patterns and abnormalities.

Angina pectoris gets its name from the nature of the pain: the Latin *angere* for choke describes the characteristic suffocating sensation and *pectoralis* for chest, where it is located.

The discomfort usually lasts for a minute or two; sometimes as long as 10 to 15 minutes. The pain may be severe and may be accompanied by a constricting feeling behind the breastbone (sternum) that may extend into the throat or down one arm or the other. It may also be a mild heaviness, tightness, or burning discomfort.

Angina usually is brought on by exertion such as heavy lifting, sexual activity, or strenuous exercise. It is relieved by rest. Extreme cold can cause it as can ingestion of a heavy meal or emotion such as extreme fear, anger, grief, or frustration.

Angina is the direct result of insufficient blood reaching your heart muscle (ischemia). When you exert yourself, your heart requires more oxygen to do the extra work. When the coronary arteries that serve your heart are narrow and unable to accommodate the increase in flow of blood demanded

THE EXERCISE TOLERANCE TEST

The exercise may be on a treadmill or a stationary bike; the test may be called an exercise tolerance test or a stress test or a treadmill test. Whatever the exercise or the name, the principles are the same.

It is important to take an exercise tolerance test before you embark on a program of vigorous exercise, particularly if there is a history of heart disease in your family or if you are over age 40 and have other heart risks (see Disease of the Heart and Blood Vessels: Living With the Risks, page 785). The test is not done routinely, but your physician may advise it if you have symptoms that suggest coronary artery disease. He or she also may order the test if you already have had a heart attack, to determine the extent of your coronary artery disease.

The test accurately identifies the presence of coronary artery disease in nearly three-fourths of those with the disorder; it also identifies 90 percent of those without significant coronary artery disease.

Electrodes are placed on various parts of your chest and a blood pressure cuff is placed on your arm. Then you mount a treadmill or bicycle. The workout that follows will become progressively more demanding, and your heart rate will increase. The physician overseeing the test will be monitoring your heart rate, blood pressure, and electrocardiographic tracings and also will be watching for symptoms.

The test takes about half an hour, time well invested if you have one or more of the classic cardiac risk factors which include smoking, diabetes, high blood pressure, high cholesterol level, or family history of stroke or heart disease. If you have already had a heart attack, your response on the test can help your physician to devise an exercise program for you that will enhance your recovery. Even if your heart reveals no signs of artery disease, the test can be useful in designing an effective workout program.

If the exercise tolerance test indicates that your heart's activity was constant and strong during the stress, the chances are excellent that your heart will function properly when you work out on your own. If there are signs of problems, the test results will be useful in establishing exercise limits and developing a special fitness program for you. If the exercise produces any abnormal patterns on the electrocardiographic tracings, your physician may advise additional evaluations which may include angiography or a radionuclide scan with exercise (see Scans and Coronary Angiogram, page 805).

A treadmill test measures the activity of your heart while you exercise.

by the exercise, nerves in your heart transmit pain messages to your brain.

Angina is a symptom, not a disorder. It can be the result of arteries narrowed by a passing spasm. More likely, a limitation of blood flow is the result of atherosclerosis (see page 786) in which the arteries are narrowed by an accumulation of deposits of fatty plaque.

Thus, angina often is one of the warning signs of coronary artery disease. When the attacks come frequently and are not linked to physical activity, they may be warning signs of an impending heart attack and re-

SCANS AND CORONARY ANGIOGRAM

In diagnosing coronary artery disease, it often is invaluable to be able to "see" the coronary arteries and the shape and function of the heart chambers. Today, this can be done best by one of two basic approaches, either entirely from outside the body (noninvasive) or by inserting catheters or other instruments into the body (invasive). In general, images made by scanning devices are noninvasive; angiography, however, is an invasive procedure.

If your exercise ECG is abnormal, your physician may suggest conducting a noninvasive radionuclide scan to help confirm the diagnosis of coronary artery disease. These tests are highly accurate, are easy to perform, and do not require a stay in the hospital. The radiation exposure is slight, and such a scan may eliminate the need for an angiogram (see below).

A different approach uses sound waves to recreate the shape of the heart and large blood vessels. Heart ultrasound scans (echocardiograms) allow your physician to see the movement of your heart (see The Echocardiogram: Images Made With Sound, page 827).

Radionuclide Scans

Radionuclide scans can cost up to 4 times the amount of a treadmill exercise test, but they also provide more information. There are two types.

Thallium Exercise Scan
One type of radionuclide examination of the heart is the thallium exercise scan. This procedure involves the injection of a small dose of radioactive isotope into a vein in your arm during a treadmill test. A special scanning device then records a series of pictures of the locations of this isotope in the region of your heart. Dark areas on the scans indicate portions of your heart to which blood flow is impaired. However, this does not provide a picture of the actual blocked artery.

Radionuclide Angiogram
For this procedure, you receive an injection of a radioactive isotope that labels your blood cells. You are then placed on an exercise table (either supine or semi-upright) with your feet on the pedals of a bicycle. As you work the pedals, scans are made to locate the isotope in the region of your heart. A key finding would be impaired expansion or contraction of the heart wall, a signal that narrowed arteries are not carrying sufficient amounts of oxygen-rich blood.

Angiogram

The procedure for making an angiogram involves insertion of a catheter (a hollow, flexible tube) into an artery at your groin or elbow. This catheter is guided through your main artery, the aorta, into your heart. Then it is guided into a coronary artery. A dye that is opaque to x-rays is injected through the catheter to make the inside of the heart and artery visible on an x-ray picture.

Angiography can be done on many blood vessels in the body, but when it is done on heart arteries (coronary arteries) the test is called coronary angiography or cardiac catheterization.

In addition, the catheter can be placed in the left side of the heart where the function of the mitral and aortic valves can be studied; the shape and function of the left atrium and the left ventricle of the heart also can be observed. To study the right atrium and ventricle and its valves (tricuspid and pulmonic), a catheter can be inserted into a large vein and advanced into the right side of the heart.

A variation of this procedure is used to treat narrowed coronary arteries (see Coronary Angioplasty, page 812).

Coronary angiogram outlines major arteries of your heart. Arrow reveals narrowing due to buildup of atherosclerotic plaque.

quire special treatment (see Heart Attack, page 809).

Angina is quite common. In men, it usually occurs after age 30; in women it tends to appear later. The cause in most cases is atherosclerosis.

The Diagnosis.   Most often, the discomfort occurs after strenuous physical activity or an emotional upset. However, it also can occur after mild exercise or even while you are asleep. The nature of the distress has been described as tight, band-like, crushing, burning, and, occasionally, sharp. Sometimes it is mistaken for indigestion.

The duration of the pain is variable, up to a few minutes. If the chest pain is prolonged beyond 5 to 10 minutes, the risk of damage to the heart muscle increases. The pain may also be "referred," a term used to describe pain impulses confused by your brain. It may feel as if your jaw, neck, or arms are in great pain when in fact it may be the pain of angina that is being perceived as stemming from one or more of these locations.

There is no specific laboratory test for the diagnosis of angina. Your physician may want to obtain an electrocardiogram to see if damage has occurred. He or she also may order blood tests to rule out heart damage. In addition, your physician may want to obtain blood tests to make sure hyperthyroidism (see page 727) and anemia (see page 477) are not present. Both of these disorders may force your heart to beat faster, use more oxygen, and, therefore, precipitate angina.

How Serious Is Angina?   The decrease in blood flow to your heart is partial and temporary, so damage does not occur. This is in contrast to the blockage of a heart artery that results in permanent damage to a part of the heart muscle (see Heart Attack, page 809).

Treatment.   If you experience angina, try to stop the activity that precipitated the attack. This should lessen the load on your heart and reduce its need for oxygen. The distress should stop within a minute or two. Then, see your physician. If the discomfort does not cease within a few minutes or if the frequency or severity of the attacks increases, seek immediate medical attention.

If you smoke, stop. Lose the extra pounds if you are overweight. Eliminating obesity or smoking may decrease or even eliminate your symptoms.

Exercise.   Having angina does not need to make you a sedentary person. In fact, exercise is a key part of dealing with your angina. The exercise must be compatible with the limitations imposed by your pain. Your own body and your physician will help you determine how much exercise is appropriate.

Medication.   The classic treatment for acute attacks of angina is the drug nitroglycerin. Nitroglycerin opens (dilates) the coronary arteries, allowing more blood to flow to the heart muscle. It is taken orally as a tablet, usually by letting it dissolve under your tongue. Recently, a form of nitroglycerin that is sprayed under the tongue has become available. In a remarkably short time—perhaps a minute or less—the discomfort will ease.

One side effect of nitroglycerin is that it causes headaches in some people. Usually the headaches are temporary and mild. If your physician prescribes nitroglycerin, keep your drug supply fresh because the tablet form of the drug loses potency in a matter of weeks. Also, keep the tablets out of direct sunlight which causes loss of potency.

Long-acting nitrites also may be helpful in decreasing the frequency of angina attacks.

Calcium channel blockers are drugs that interrupt the normal flow of calcium through channels in your heart muscle. This produces dilatation of the coronary and other arteries in your vascular system, which results in increased blood flow to the heart muscle. The work required of the heart is also decreased and its demands for oxygen are lessened. The calcium channel blockers also decrease blood pressure.

The beta-adrenergic blockers decrease heart rate and blood pressure. Both are useful in reducing the symptoms of angina.

Your physician will select an appropriate medication for your particular symptoms.

Surgery.   If the angina continues in spite of the use of medications or occurs more often or with greater intensity, your physician may consider coronary angioplasty or coronary artery bypass surgery (see pages 812 and 814).

CONGESTIVE HEART FAILURE

Signs and Symptoms
- Swelling (edema) in the ankles; if bedridden, swelling in lower portions of back;
- Breathlessness;
- Weakness and fatigue.

The term heart failure is almost enough to make one's heart stop. But actually, the congested heart rarely ceases to pump. It is really a matter of losing efficiency.

Congestive heart failure is a serious condition and at times is life-threatening. In the most common forms, the heart fails to pump blood effectively. This decreases blood flow to muscles, tissues, and organs throughout the body. The ineffective pumping also causes blood to back up into the veins that return blood to the heart.

With failure of the left side of the heart, blood backs up into the lungs, which causes them to become congested with fluid (see Pulmonary Edema, page 808). This congestion is responsible for the sensation of breathlessness which is common in congestive heart failure.

If the right side of the heart fails, blood backs up into the legs and into the liver, which becomes congested. This produces a swelling (edema) that usually is most obvious in the lower legs and ankles. Often both left and right sides of the heart are failing.

Lack of adequate blood flow to the kidneys leads to accumulation of excess fluid and water in your body, an additional factor that increases the edema. Inadequate blood flow to the muscles reduces endurance. Therefore, people with congestive heart failure often experience early fatigue when they exert themselves physically.

The loss of pumping efficiency of the heart in congestive heart failure may be the result of weakened muscle tissue in the heart due to heart attack; of diseases directly affecting the heart muscle (see Cardiomyopathy, page 831); of a mechanical problem in the valves of the heart (see page 822); or of prolonged high blood pressure.

The Diagnosis. At first, congestive heart failure produces a feeling of weakness and fatigue, and routine physical activities may become more and more difficult to perform.

Breathlessness also occurs. At first, it appears only after exercise, but later the shortness of breath may occur after a long day of work or after going to bed. Breathing may be more difficult when you are lying down. You might need to elevate your head on several pillows in order to be able to sleep.

The breathlessness is a sign of a failure of the left side of your heart. At its worst, the difficulty may seem to attack your breathing and may awaken you at night. Such episodes usually are relieved by sitting up.

If your physician suspects heart failure, he or she will listen to your heart and lungs with a stethoscope to detect the sounds associated with heart failure. Your physician also will look for swollen neck veins, an enlarged liver, and swelling (edema) of the feet, all of which may be signs of heart failure. Blood and urine tests will reveal whether your kidneys are properly removing waste products. An electrocardiogram (ECG; see Common Diagnostic Tests, page 802) will be recorded to investigate the rate and rhythm of your heartbeat and to look for evidence of a previous heart attack and a disturbance in the pathways that conduct electrical messages within your heart. A chest x-ray may reveal enlargement of the heart and congestion in the lungs. Echocardiography will allow your physician to see weakened heart muscle or valve problems (see The Echocardiogram: Images Made With Sound, page 827).

How Serious Is Congestive Heart Failure?
If untreated, congestive heart failure can be fatal. However, lifestyle adjustments and proper drug treatment can improve heart function and relieve symptoms. There is no cure, but medications can be used long-term and often will permit a nearly normal lifestyle.

Treatment. Once your physician has confirmed that you have heart failure, the first new rule of your life is to get plenty of rest to help you conserve energy. However, this does not mean you should retire to your bed. On the contrary, maintaining your mobility or, in some cases, even an exercise regimen, is a key component of the treatment program. Motion helps to keep your circulation moving. Given the effect of gravity, you may also find that a comfortable chair is better than your bed for resting.

Diet. Your physician may give you specific nutritional guidelines to follow but, in general, you should restrict the amount of salt you consume. Sometimes the need to restrict salt consumption is such that a dietician may need to give you special dietary instructions that will include the use of salt-free bread and salt-free margarine or butter. Avoid alcoholic beverages. Reach and maintain a weight appropriate for your height and build (to determine your ideal body weight, consult the chart on page 350).

Medication. Most cases of congestive heart failure are treated with drugs in addition to appropriate dietary measures. The two most commonly used medications are diuretics and digitalis.

Diuretics, which also are often used in treating mild cases of high blood pressure (see page 799), are sometimes called water pills. These drugs increase the rate at which your body eliminates urine and salt. This decreases the load on your lungs (thus relieving the breathlessness) and the swelling in your legs. Diuretics have few side effects, although you may urinate more frequently and more immediately after consuming fluids. In addition to salt loss, potassium is also eliminated. Your physician will monitor your blood potassium level and, if it is found to be depleted, will prescribe a potassium supplement.

Digitalis preparations affect the heart directly. They increase the strength of the heart's pumping action and are especially useful if your heart failure is the result of a heart rhythm disturbance (see page 816).

The newest form of drug therapy for heart failure involves use of drugs that dilate arteries (vasodilators). These drugs also are used for high blood pressure. With heart failure, dilating the arteries reduces the work the heart has to do, which allows it to pump blood more effectively.

Whatever drug you are taking, it is extremely important to take the prescribed doses regularly. The dose is often determined by blood tests, including measurement of the amount of the drug in your blood.

Surgery. Occasionally, surgery is required. For example, if your cardiologist determines that you have a leak between the chambers of your heart or a small area of damaged cardiac tissue, surgical repair may be appropriate. If you have a diseased heart valve, replacement may be necessary (see Heart Valve Surgery, page 830). For persons with myocarditis or cardiomyopathy, heart transplantation may be an option (see Heart Transplantation, page 833).

PULMONARY EDEMA

Emergency Signs and Symptoms
- Severe shortness of breath;
- Restlessness and anxiety, feeling of suffocating;
- Pink, frothy sputum;
- Sweating;
- Pallor.

Pulmonary edema occurs when the back pressure within the veins of your lungs becomes so high that large amounts of fluid are rapidly forced out of the veins and into the air sacs (alveoli) of your lungs. This produces fluid (edema) in the lungs.

Pulmonary edema is usually caused by an extensive heart attack, mitral or aortic valve disease, or, although rare, exposure to high altitude.

The Diagnosis. Severe shortness of breath is the primary symptom of pulmonary edema; you feel as if you are starving for air or are drowning. This feeling of suffocation is accompanied by anxiety and restlessness. Other symptoms including sweating, pallor, and a cough that commonly brings up pink, frothy sputum. Breathing becomes difficult and is often accompanied by a grunting sound; exhaling is prolonged. In some people the fluid causes wheezing. Thus, these people are said to have "cardiac asthma."

How Serious Is Pulmonary Edema? Pulmonary edema is a life-threatening condition. Immediate hospitalization and treatment are required.

Treatment. Treatment consists of receiving oxygen through a mask. If you are having extreme difficulty breathing, it may be necessary to insert a breathing tube into your trachea and provide mechanical ventilation.

Medication. A diuretic usually is given intravenously to remove fluid from your lungs. Morphine sulfate also is effective in relieving pulmonary congestion. If the pulmonary edema is due to a decrease in pumping function of your heart, medications that will strengthen the heart muscle (such as digoxin) may be given intravenously.

HEART ATTACK

Emergency Signs and Symptoms
- Intense, prolonged chest pain, often described as a feeling of heavy pressure;
- Pain may extend beyond the chest to the left shoulder and arm, back, and even teeth and jaw;
- Prolonged pain in upper abdomen;
- Shortness of breath;
- Fainting episode;
- Nausea, vomiting, fainting, and intense sweating may occur;
- Frequent angina attacks that are not the result of physical exertion (unstable angina).

The technical term for heart attack is myocardial infarction. *Myo* means muscle; *kardia* means heart; an *infarct* is an area of tissue that has died because of oxygen starvation.

Heart attack is the unscientific term that is applied to the event that occurs when a blood clot (thrombus) blocks the flow in one or more of your coronary arteries. When the clot blocks the blood supply to a heart muscle region, the oxygen supply to the cells in that area is cut off. Just as in angina pectoris (see page 803), this produces pain. The difference is that the interruption to the blood flow is temporary in angina but in a heart attack the blood supply to a portion of the heart muscle is completely or nearly completely shut off. The result is that the heart muscle in the affected region dies.

Most often the clot that causes a heart attack forms in a coronary artery narrowed by the thickening of its walls by the fatty deposits of atherosclerosis (see page 801).

By definition, a heart attack is a medical emergency: if you think you are having a heart attack or are with someone who is, seek immediate medical attention. If your companion's heart attack has caused him or her to stop breathing, immediate cardiopulmonary resuscitation is necessary (see page 270).

Do not delay in seeking medical help. Delay is a mistake that takes thousands of lives every year. You may think the pain will disappear of its own accord; at times, so-called heartburn (see page 593) can be confused with the chest pain of heart attack. Get immediate help. It may save your life.

The Symptoms.   The powerful squeezing sensation in your chest is the chief symptom. Some describe it as the feeling of an enormous fist enclosing and squeezing their heart; others recall an accompanying sense of doom. The pain is similar to that of angina, but it is sustained and responds little or not at all to nitroglycerin.

A heart attack may be preceded by a series of angina attacks or it may occur suddenly with no advance warning. Unlike angina, however, the pain does not cease when the exercise or stress that caused it is discontinued. However, the pain may be constant or it may come and go.

The pain may be a discomfort or an inexplicable tightening, or it may feel as though an elephant has stepped on your chest.

Occasionally, the pain does not fit any particular pattern. This is especially true in the elderly and in persons with diabetes mellitus. Any prolonged pain in your chest or upper abdomen is cause for concern. Seek prompt medical attention. Do not attribute this pain to indigestion.

In some persons, a primary symptom of a heart attack is sudden onset of shortness of

The pain of a heart attack varies from person to person, but typically there is a profound squeezing sensation in the chest, accompanied by profuse perspiration. Pain may radiate to the left shoulder and arm, to the back, and even to the jaw.

breath, which may or may not be associated with chest pain. In approximately 10 percent of cases, the only symptom of a heart attack is a sudden fainting spell (see Fainting Spells, page 819).

In elderly people and in diabetics, it is not unusual for a heart attack to occur with no accompanying pain or other symptoms. These "silent" heart attacks may be detected only when a routine electrocardiogram reveals a change in the pattern of transmission of electrical impulses through the heart.

The Diagnosis. In the emergency vehicle or when you reach the hospital and profes-sional medical care, your blood pressure will be taken and an electrocardiogram will be recorded (ECG; see Common Diagnostic Tests, page 802). In fact, you may be attached to this machine for much of your hospital stay so that your physicians and nurses can constantly monitor your heart's condition, perhaps within the confines of a special section of the hospital specifically for heart patients called a coronary care unit (see page 811).

At the hospital, other tests may be ordered including blood tests for enzymes that are released by damaged heart tissue. Other tests that may be done include scans and angiograms (see page 805). You will be observed carefully for a period of several days. If there are no setbacks, you will be permitted to increase your activity gradually. The time in the hospital varies but ordinarily is in the range of 7 to 14 days.

How Serious Is a Heart Attack? If the area of the damaged tissue (infarct) is small and the electrical system that controls your heart is not damaged, your chances of surviving a heart attack are good. However, roughly a third of those who suffer heart attacks die before they receive medical care. Only a few years ago, the statistics were much worse—only about one in two survived. This improvement is due in part to the implementation of a wide variety of techniques including cardiopulmonary resuscitation (CPR, see page 270), special tests (angiograms and scans, among others), and improved emergency care in ambulances or emergency vehicles or in cardiac care units designed to meet the immediate and continuing needs of persons having heart attacks.

The frequency of sudden death is a key reason why it is imperative that medical attention and, if necessary, CPR be provided as quickly as possible to the person who is having the heart attack. Most of those still alive 2 hours after a heart attack will survive; however, there is a range of possible complications.

The Complications of a Heart Attack. *Cardiac Arrhythmia.* The system that controls your heartbeat is electrical. In some people, damage to the heart tissue from a heart attack can result in arrhythmia problems such as ventricular fibrillation. In this condition there are very rapid and uncoordinated contractions of the ventricles, result-

---

SEXUAL ACTIVITY AFTER A HEART ATTACK

In short, no, it is not necessary to forgo the pleasures of sexual activity forever. On the other hand, a sensible lapse is in order, perhaps for 30 days after your heart attack.

The demands placed on your heart when you have sexual relations are roughly the same as taking a brisk walk or climbing a flight or two of stairs. Your heart rate, breathing rate, and blood pressure increase, so sexual activities should be approached as any other physical activities: sensibly, with caution but without fear.

At First, Take It Easy
Before the resumption of sexual intercourse, it makes sense to content yourself with lesser contacts, at first confining your intimacies to kissing or caresses. As your confidence grows in the health of your heart, gradually resume your usual sexual patterns.

In order to minimize the stress on your heart, it is sensible strategy to resume sexual relations with your usual partner under your usual circumstances: you will probably feel more relaxed and natural making love in a familiar setting. If you find certain positions less strenuous than others, take the less taxing route, at least at first.

The Importance of Communication
Talk to your partner, too, both before and after, to reassure yourself and that person. Shared fears and concerns may be alleviated if lines of communication are open.

Talk to your physician if you have fears or concerns. It is quite normal for your needs to have changed temporarily: you may experience an increased or reduced desire for sexual activity.

Recognize Warning Signs
If you experience chest pain, extreme shortness of breath, or irregular heartbeat during sexual activity, stop. Do not try to go too far too fast.

Again, it is time to go on with your life, but it is wise to do it sensibly and with the help and guidance of your physician and the loved ones around you.

ing in insufficient blood flow to vital organs (see Heart Arrhythmias, page 816).

In some persons, the arrhythmia may be a heartbeat that is too slow. This may require temporary or, occasionally, permanent placement of a pacemaker (see Artificial Cardiac Pacemakers, page 820).

Congestive Heart Failure. In some cases the amount of damaged heart tissue (infarct) may be so extensive that the remaining heart muscle cannot do an adequate job of pumping the blood out of the heart. This can result in congestive heart failure (see page 807).

Death. In about one of every four people who die suddenly of a heart attack, there were no previous symptoms of heart disease. The immediate cause of death is thought to be underlying arrhythmia such as ventricular fibrillation (see Sudden Cardiac Death, page 821). The vast majority of persons who die had severe disease of more than one coronary artery and the pumping action of their left ventricle was impaired, which, in turn, caused the arrhythmia. If no evidence of coronary artery disease is found, the cause of ventricular fibrillation often remains unknown.

Treatment. If you have symptoms that suggest a heart attack, seek professional medical help immediately. Telephone your physician or call an ambulance. If you think you are having a heart attack, do not try to drive to the hospital yourself.

Once you reach the hospital, the diagnostic tests discussed above will be initiated. You also may be supplied with oxygen.

Medication. In some cases, a drug will be administered to dissolve the clot that is blocking the flow of blood. Clot-dissolving drugs (thrombolytic agents) such as streptokinase or tissue plasminogen activator may be delivered through a vein in the arm or directly to the clot by the use of a catheter. Your physician may also give you an anticoagulant drug orally to prevent further clotting.

There is a wide range of drugs your physician may prescribe depending on your condition and your rate of recovery.

1. *Pain Killers.* If your condition is stable but your pain is great, you may be given

THE CORONARY CARE UNIT

If you have just had, or are about to have, a heart attack, the best place for you is in a hospital coronary or cardiac care unit (CCU).

The combination of constant cardiac monitoring and nursing observation in a CCU allows early detection of signs and symptoms and virtually instant attention when you need it. Such specialized care is required for people who have had a recent heart attack or who have severe angina (see page 803), disturbed heart rhythms (see page 816), or congestive heart failure (see page 807).

The Team
A cardiologist heads the CCU team; in some hospitals, a resident physician is available at all times as well. Highly trained nurses manage the monitoring and other care tasks and, often, the emergency procedures that must be done at a moment's notice.

The Equipment
Electrodes applied to your skin will connect you to a cardiac monitor (ECG, see Common Diagnostic Tests, page 802) which continuously monitors the rhythm and rate of your heartbeat. Your blood pressure will be monitored. Through a needle inserted into a vein in your arm, you may receive fluids and medications intravenously. Oxygen may also be provided.

More dramatic steps may be necessary if you actually experience a "coronary event" while in the CCU. Such events may be a problem with the rhythm of your heartbeat (see Disorders of Heart Rate and Rhythm, page 816), your heart actually stopping (cardiac arrest), or your heart beating rapidly but ineffectively (fibrillation). Electroshock equipment, cardiopulmonary resuscitation (CPR), and specialized drugs may be used in such emergency circumstances.

an analgesic drug such as morphine to relieve the pain.
2. *Nitrates.* These drugs work by decreasing the oxygen requirement of your heart muscle. The best known of them, nitroglycerin, is placed under your tongue at the onset of angina pain (see Angina Pectoris, page 803); other forms are applied to the skin as an ointment or as a medicated patch or taken as long-acting tablets. Nitroglycerin often is given through a vein during or after a heart attack to produce a continuous decrease in oxygen requirements.
3. *Beta-Adrenergic Blockers.* These block the stimulating effect of the hormone epinephrine on your heart. The result is that your heart will beat more slowly and less

ASPIRIN: DOES IT PREVENT HEART ATTACKS?

In a recent study, male physicians took either one aspirin every other day or a placebo. Those who took the aspirin had fewer heart attacks.

Does this mean that taking an aspirin should be an every-other-day event for you, too? *Not necessarily.*

Aspirin and Platelets

Aspirin affects the way your blood clots. When you bleed because of an injury to a blood vessel, blood cells called platelets accumulate at the injury site. The platelets form a sticky plug that seals the opening in the blood vessel. Aspirin decreases the accumulation of platelets and impairs the formation of the clot when bleeding occurs.

Aspirin and Heart Attack

Because a heart attack is the result of blockage of a coronary artery by a blood clot, the effect of aspirin on clotting is beneficial during the first hours of a heart attack. Daily aspirin intake is beneficial for most persons with coronary artery disease, including those recovering from bypass surgery (see page 814).

Aspirin and Stroke

When you have had a bleeding event such as rupture of a small artery in your brain (hemorrhagic stroke, see Stroke, page 799), the aspirin-a-day regimen may be dangerous. The clotting ability of the blood is diminished by the aspirin, so the bleeding will be less likely to be stopped by the clotting of your blood.

Aspirin and Your Health

If you have coronary artery disease or if you have undergone coronary artery bypass surgery, aspirin may help decrease your risk of a subsequent heart attack. However, if you have high blood pressure, a history of stroke in your family, a bleeding disorder, ulcers, or impaired liver or kidney function or if you are taking the drug warfarin (Coumadin), avoid aspirin.

In any case, before taking aspirin regularly, discuss the matter with your physician.

(Note that aspirin—its chemical name is acetylsalicylic acid—is different from aspirin substitutes such as acetaminophen. Aspirin has an effect on clotting; acetaminophen does not.)

forcefully and thus will require less oxygen to continue its work.

4. *Digitalis.* Digitalis preparations work by causing your heart to pump more forcefully. The most commonly used digitalis preparation is digoxin. These drugs are used mainly when there are symptoms of congestive heart failure (see page 807).

5. *Calcium Channel Blockers.* These drugs interrupt the normal flow of calcium through channels in your heart muscle. Although they are not used routinely in treating heart attacks, occasionally physicians will prescribe one of these medications to decrease the demands of the heart muscle for oxygen.

Recovery. When you are hospitalized, your activities will be limited and carefully monitored by the hospital staff. When you are released, follow your physician's instructions exactly.

Every day that passes means that you and your heart are recovering. The longer the time elapsed since your heart attack, the greater your chances of avoiding a second one and living a normal life.

Remember that you are not necessarily disabled. In fact, regular exercise—within the guidelines your physician suggests—can contribute to the return of your good health. Subject to your physician's guidance, you can return to work.

Do not be anxious about the possibility of another heart attack. Instead, try to channel anxiety into positive energy. Quit smoking (an absolute for anyone with heart disease). Establish a sensible exercise program and use it to keep your weight down. Decrease the fat content in your diet. Consider the other controllable risk factors in your life (see Disease of the Heart and Blood Vessels: Living With the Risks, page 785).

CORONARY ANGIOPLASTY

Narrowed or blocked arteries may produce a heart attack, angina, or other problems. In some cases a special diet or medication or both may be the best treatment for such arterial problems; in other cases, bypass surgery (see page 814) or coronary angioplasty may be the best answer.

The full name for coronary angioplasty is percutaneous transluminal coronary angioplasty (PTCA). This means that, through the skin (percutaneous), a procedure is performed inside an artery (transluminal) of the heart (coronary) that reshapes (angioplasty) that artery.

The procedure is simpler than

its name. PTCA is performed with local anesthesia while you are awake. This procedure is quite like the diagnostic procedure called coronary angiography (see Scans and Coronary Angiogram, page 805).

The Procedure

After a local anesthetic is injected into your groin or shoulder area, the physician inserts a hollow, flexible tube, called a guide catheter, into a leg or arm artery. While watching on a TV monitor that displays an x-ray image of the blood vessel and catheter, the physician guides the catheter into the narrowed coronary artery. A small amount of radiopaque dye may be delivered to the area through the catheter, in order to enhance the clarity of the angiogram and help the physician be sure of the exact location of the blockage.

A smaller catheter is then inserted inside the guide catheter. This one has a balloon at its tip. When the catheter tip reaches the area of obstruction in the coronary artery, the balloon is inflated for about half a minute to widen the obstructed part of the artery. While it is inflated, you may feel chest pain; when it deflates the pain will fade. Several inflations and deflations usually are necessary. Then the balloon catheter is removed, and more x-rays (angiograms) are taken to see how blood flow has improved. The entire process usually takes between 30 and 90 minutes.

The procedure also may be used to treat blocked arteries elsewhere in the body, including the legs.

The Results

Improved blood flow, increased blood pressure in the affected artery, compression or splitting

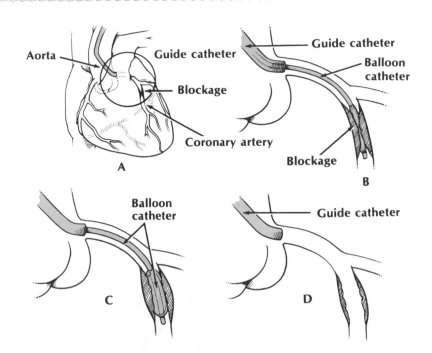

A procedure used to open narrowed or blocked coronary arteries is called **percutaneous transluminal coronary angioplasty (PTCA)**. The technique involves insertion of a guide catheter from an artery in the groin or shoulder. The catheter is threaded to the affected artery (A). A second catheter is then inserted inside the first one (B). When it reaches the narrowed or blocked area, a balloon on its tip is inflated to reopen the artery (C). The catheters are withdrawn following the procedure (D).

apart of the blockage itself, and stretching or enlargement of a portion of the artery wall are the hoped-for results. In a small percentage of cases, the procedure is unsuccessful and bypass surgery is necessary; usually, a surgical team is available to proceed immediately. When the angioplasty alone is successful, the need for major surgery and the use of a heart-lung machine are avoided. The costs are considerably less and the hospital stay is days rather than weeks.

Recovery and Rehabilitation

For 24 hours after the procedure, your heart rate and rhythm and other vital signs will be closely monitored. Because the procedure involves insertion of a small catheter through the skin, the incision is small and many people go

back to work a week after the procedure.

Who Is a Candidate for PTCA?

People whose angina has not been relieved by medications are candidates for this procedure. The ideal candidate has only one narrowed artery, although many persons with several areas of narrowing can undergo PTCA. The decision to recommend PTCA rather than bypass surgery is based on the location, number, and severity of blockages as well as on the overall function of the heart.

However, the procedure does not cure the underlying disease. In fact, the procedure may have to be repeated to reopen the same or another coronary artery that becomes blocked.

In future years, physicians may be able to remove plaque by using laser light or mechanical devices.

CORONARY ARTERY BYPASS SURGERY

Heart attacks, angina, and other problems occur as the result of narrowed or blocked arteries. In most instances, preventive medical treatments should be used initially. These may include dietary changes, weight reduction, treatment of diabetes and high blood pressure, exercise, and avoidance of smoking. However, in certain situations, coronary artery bypass surgery or a coronary angioplasty is appropriate (see also Coronary Angioplasty, page 812). These situations include cases in which the symptoms do not respond to optimal medical treatment or when blockage of the coronary arteries is severe.

The Procedure

Bypass means an alternate route. A coronary bypass operation involves taking a short length of vein, usually from the thigh (the saphenous vein), and using it to allow blood to bypass the blockage in an artery. One or as many as eight or nine segments of these arteries may receive bypasses, although four or five is average.

With time, these saphenous vein segments tend to develop blockages similar to those present initially in the coronary arteries. This may require medical treatment or another operation. More recently, the internal mammary artery has been used as the bypass. This artery lies inside the front of the chest. There is one on each side of the breastbone. The lower end of this artery is freed and sewn to the coronary artery beyond the blockage. The other end is left attached. Blood is thus rerouted into the coronary arteries.

The major advantage of this type of graft is its tendency to resist later buildup of atherosclerosis. Sometimes these arteries are unable to be used and sometimes both can be used.

For the operation, you will be given a general anesthetic. For a portion of the operation, the functions of your heart and lungs will be assumed by a heart-lung machine. The duration of the operation is 2 hours or more, depending on how much work is required.

The Results

Adequate blood flow to the heart muscle is reestablished. This often relieves the angina or other coronary artery problem, but it does not cure the underlying disease. Also, the segments of bypass seem to be more likely to have coronary artery disease than are the natural arteries. Therefore, adherence to a low-fat diet and other preventive changes in lifestyle are especially important after you have bypass surgery.

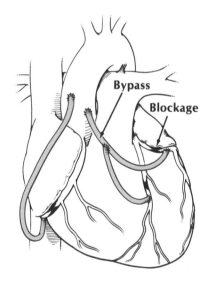

A coronary bypass surgical procedure involves rerouting (bypassing) the flow of blood around narrowed or blocked coronary arteries by surgically implanting lengths of vein taken from another part of the body.

Recovery and Rehabilitation

A 7- to 10-day stay in the hospital is usual. After the operation, you may spend a few days in a special cardiac care unit (CCU; see page 811). There the rate and rhythm of your heart and other vital signs will be closely monitored. Food and water will be provided intravenously; a tube will allow drainage from the site of the surgery. Oxygen or a respirator may be required.

Your physician and surgeon will advise you about your activities for the next several weeks of recovery and the gradual resumption of normal activity.

Bypass operations are done frequently and safely. However, as with any operation, there are risks. In general, if you have a normal left ventricle (the major muscle pump of the heart) and relatively good health, you have less than a 1 percent risk of dying during the operation and hospitalization for coronary bypass surgery.

Who Is a Candidate for Coronary Artery Bypass Surgery?

If you have mild angina or have recovered from a heart attack with no continuing symptoms, you are probably best treated by medication or other means rather than by a bypass or other operation.

Although there have been controversial aspects of coronary artery bypass surgery, especially in the early days of its use, the consensus now favors this treatment in appropriate situations: for those with a blocked left main coronary artery; for those with disease in multiple vessels and poor function of the left ventricle (the main pump of the heart); and for those with debilitating angina. For these persons, a bypass procedure is of clear value in most cases and life is clearly prolonged.

CARDIAC REHABILITATION

Recovery from a heart attack or "coronary event" may require a wide variety of rehabilitation strategies; to help you implement them, an equally varied group of professionals may be needed, including physicians trained in cardiology (cardiologist) and rehabilitation medicine (physiatrist), nurses, dieticians, occupational and physical therapists, an exercise physiologist, a psychologist, a smoking cessation counselor if appropriate, a pharmacist, and a rehabilitation coordinator.

The process of cardiac rehabilitation has three key stages. First are the immediate activities involved in saving your life and over which you have little control. Second is the ongoing medical attention, including medication and perhaps surgery; again, most of the decisions concerning this part of the process are made by your physician.

However, as a cardiac patient, you must take charge of the third stage which includes the life-style adjustments you need to make as you recover. These begin with mental adjustments and carry through to changes in personal exercise, diet, smoking, and other habits. Below are some of the key matters you must address, often in conjunction with the appropriate professional help.

Stress

The psychological component of heart disease is still somewhat of a mystery, but there is a clear consensus that many people exert unnecessary pressures on themselves as they go about living their lives. After a heart attack, avoid such pressures.

Recovering from a heart attack does not necessarily mean you should change your job, avoid all of life's challenges, or make other radical changes. Decreasing the stress in your day-to-day activities, however, may involve rethinking workaholic habits, avoiding frustrating commuting or high-pressure deadlines, and working to minimize stressful events in your life.

Exercise

The prevailing wisdom used to be to advise the heart attack survivor to retire from an active life. This is not the approach today for most people.

As you recover, you may be given an exercise tolerance test (see page 804) to assess your heart's responses to physical activity. Your physician will advise you on what to do and not do, but in general your heart will grow stronger as you recover; exercise will enhance that strengthening process.

You will not go back to full-speed activities on day 1, but enrolling in a cardiac conditioning course may help you get started. If you were sedentary before your heart attack, a carefully planned exercise program is especially important.

While you are still in the hospital, a physical therapist may begin to help you get your body moving again and to regain your confidence in your heart and health. The therapist will instruct you in the initial phases of an exercise program and advance the program during your convalescence. An occupational therapist may provide you with instructions for a home program once you are dismissed from the hospital.

Ask your therapists for help in planning and establishing new exercise patterns appropriate to your lifestyle and condition. Also, outpatient supervised exercise rehabilitation programs are appropriate for many persons who have had a heart problem. Sometimes YMCAs or YWCAs offer them. Ask if one is available in your community.

Diet and Weight Control

If it was true before your heart attack, it is even truer now: keeping your weight down and avoiding saturated fats and cholesterol-rich foods are very important. Losing those extra pounds will decrease the stress on your heart. A change in eating habits to avoid fats will help limit the further accumulation of fatty plaque in your arteries.

Discuss your dietary habits with a registered dietician at the hospital. This professional can help you draw up a plan to decrease intake of fats and to learn to think before you eat in restaurants and as you go about your day (see Nutrition and Health, page 345).

Stop Smoking

The nicotine in every cigarette you smoke affects more than your blood pressure and heart rate. It accelerates the process of atherosclerosis (see also page 788). Use the experience you have just had as an impetus to quit (see How To Stop Smoking, page 412).

Where To Get Help

Ask your physician or other professional helpers about where to turn for further cardiac conditioning programs or counseling after you leave the hospital. Check with the local YMCA or chapter of the American Heart Association in your area.

The message of cardiac rehabilitation is risk factor modification and instruction in exercise to resume a normal lifestyle (see Controllable Risk Factors, page 787). Listen! It may prolong your life.

DISORDERS OF HEART RATE AND RHYTHM

The pumping of your heart must be constant and continuous; if the process becomes disordered or interrupted, your heart may fail to deliver the blood your tissues require for life.

Your heart itself is essentially two pumps, each of which consists of a pair of hollow chambers formed of involuntary muscle. The contraction of the muscle causes blood to be pumped.

The control mechanism for the heart rate involves electrical impulses. One of the four chambers of the heart, the right atrium, contains a group of cells called the sinus node. The sinus node acts as a pacemaker, producing electrical impulses that signal the muscle of the heart to expand and to contract in the pumping cycle.

Your heart rate varies depending on your activity at any given moment. When you are at rest, your heart pumps more slowly and at a regular rate, in the range of 60 to 80 beats per minute. When you run, climb stairs, or otherwise exert yourself, the sinus node issues electrical "instructions" to increase the pace of the heart in order to provide your muscles and other tissues with the necessary additional blood and its supply of oxygen. Your heart rate may increase up to 200 beats per minute if you exert yourself strenuously.

The sinus node, located in the right atrium, acts as your heart's pacemaker, controlling its contractions by issuing nerve impulses along electrical pathways throughout the heart.

If something goes wrong with the functioning of the sinus node and the normal pacing of your heart is disturbed, one of a number of rhythmic disorders of the heart may occur. Too rapid a heartbeat is termed tachycardia; too slow a heart rate is bradycardia.

Your heart rate may be affected by various factors including tobacco use, caffeine-containing foods, alcohol, and a number of drugs, both prescription and nonprescription. In addition, the cardiac disorders discussed in the following pages may produce heart rate problems.

HEART ARRHYTHMIAS

Signs and Symptoms
- None;
- Palpitations or skipped heartbeats;
- Spells of light-headedness;
- Chest discomfort;
- Shortness of breath.

If the rhythm of the beat of the heart is disturbed, the problem is termed arrhythmia. Depending on the nature of the arrhythmia, the symptoms vary. You may be entirely unaware of the problem or you may experience one or more of the symptoms listed above.

Almost everyone experiences an occasional skipped heartbeat or minor palpitation. In general, such an event is not an indication of a problem. However, if the discomfort is great or if the problem recurs, consult your physician. The problem may be quite minor or it may be serious; no treatment may be necessary, or a regimen of medication or other intervention may be required. Your physician's approach will depend on your age, physical condition, presence of underlying heart disease, and the precise nature of the disorder.

Ectopic Atrial Heartbeat. The least serious of the cardiac arrhythmias is an ectopic atrial heartbeat (from the Greek *ektopos* for misplaced). This problem involves a small variation in an otherwise normal pulse. In fact, the old cliché "my heart skipped a beat" may well have been coined to describe an ectopic heartbeat.

Sinus node

An ectopic atrial heartbeat is often termed extrasystole. The extrasystole may show up on a routine electrocardiogram. If there is concern that the ectopic beats are causing some of the symptoms listed above, a 24-hour Holter monitor study may be needed (see Twenty-Four-Hour Cardiac Monitoring, page 818).

In most cases, an ectopic heartbeat is harmless and requires no treatment. Often the problem is precipitated by excessive use of tobacco, alcohol, or caffeine-containing foods and beverages. Try decreasing or eliminating the use of these substances if you have an ectopic heartbeat.

In some cases your physician may prescribe a medication that will control the rhythm of your heart.

Atrial Fibrillation and Flutter. The upper chambers of the heart are the atria (see The Healthy Heart and Blood Vessels, page 782). When functioning normally, the atria contract at a rate coordinated with the rates of the other chambers of the heart, the ventricles. In some people, however, the atria may begin to contract much too often, a condition called atrial flutter. The ventricles tend to beat at every second or fourth atrial beat.

When the muscles making up the atrial walls are contracting in an ineffective and uncoordinated manner, the condition is called atrial fibrillation. In atrial fibrillation, the electrical impulses are transmitted to the ventricles in an irregular fashion, often more rapidly than normal. Both atrial flutter and atrial fibrillation tend to occur in episodes, with occasional attacks separated by long periods of normal heart rhythms. However, atrial fibrillation may become persistent and chronic.

In atrial flutter or atrial fibrillation, the ventricles may fail to pump enough blood. The result is faintness and weakness. With atrial fibrillation, you may be aware of the irregularity of your pulse and heartbeat. The failure of the atria to contract normally (meaning that the chambers fail to empty completely) can allow a clot to form in an atrium. If the clot breaks loose and is carried in the bloodstream to the brain, it may cause a stroke (see page 508).

Occasionally, a dysfunction of the sinus node may occur. Your symptoms may include a combination of dizziness, confusion, fatigue, shortness of breath, and fainting spells. Your physician may obtain a 24-hour Holter monitor recording (see page 218) which reveals episodic atrial arrhythmias. This sometimes is referred to as sick sinus syndrome.

Atrial flutter is most often associated with a heart attack or a lung or heart operation. Atrial fibrillation may occur without heart disease or be produced by one of a number of disorders including coronary artery disease, rheumatic heart disease (see page 823), malfunction of the mitral valve of the heart (see Mitral Valve Problems, page 825), heart infection (see Pericarditis, page 832), and various other lung and heart disorders. An excess of thyroid hormone also can result in the disorder (see Hyperthyroidism, page 727), but there may be no apparent cause, in particular among younger people.

Treatment. In order to establish the diagnosis, your physician or cardiologist will obtain an electrocardiogram (ECG). If the rhythm disturbance is intermittent, you may be provided with a portable electrocardiograph machine, called a Holter monitor, that records your heart rate while you go about your normal activities (see Twenty-Four-Hour Cardiac Monitoring, page 818). Other tests also may be required, ranging from simply taking your blood pressure to performing an echocardiographic examination (see The Echocardiogram: Images Made With Sound, page 827) and, rarely, angiography (see Scans and Coronary Angiogram, page 805).

Once the diagnosis has been confirmed, the treatment depends on the cause. Most often, a medication will be prescribed that will control the rhythm of your heart (see Medications To Pace Your Heart, page 821).

In some cases an electrical stimulus called electrical cardioversion may be given to help restore normal rhythm. First you will receive a drug treatment to limit the risk of an embolism. Then, after you have been anesthetized by a short-acting painkiller, an electric shock will be delivered from two "paddles." This mild shock will interrupt the pattern of arrhythmia and allow your heart to reestablish a normal rate and rhythm.

Paroxysmal Atrial Tachycardia. If you feel your heart suddenly race, you may be experiencing an attack (paroxysm) of tachycardia (the word comes from the Greek words *tachys* for rapid or swift and *kardia* for heart). During such an attack, which may last for minutes or as long as a day or two, your heart rate may range between 140 and 240 beats per minute. Some people report an accompanying sensation of doom or anxiety.

Paroxysmal atrial tachycardia is not a life-threatening disorder, although repeated attacks may increase the risk of heart failure developing (see Congestive Heart Failure, page 807). Consult your physician when an attack occurs because he or she will be able to understand your condition better when able to examine you during an attack. An electrocardiogram examination may also be conducted (see also Twenty-Four-Hour Cardiac Monitoring, below).

Treatment. Several self-help treatments are effective in returning the heartbeat to its normal rate. Holding your breath and straining (exerting pressure as if you were blowing up a balloon) while sitting with your upper body bent forward may help. Your physician can instruct you in other helpful techniques after he or she has examined you to make sure the techniques would be safe.

You also may be able to prevent future attacks by making some small changes in your lifestyle. Excessive use of tobacco and consumption of alcohol and caffeine-containing beverages (coffee, tea, and cola drinks) may increase your risk of such attacks. Try to limit their consumption.

Your physician may use other means to slow down your heart rate during an attack. Certain medications may be used, but other methods may be appropriate. Among them may be the gentle application of pressure to the arteries in your neck. In some cases, an electrical stimulus, called electrical cardioversion, may be given to restore normal rhythms (see Atrial Fibrillation and Flutter, page 817).

Some types of paroxysmal atrial tachycardia, especially those associated with a rare condition called Wolff-Parkinson-White syndrome, may be permanently cured by surgery. This approach would eliminate the need to take medications on a daily basis.

Ventricular Tachycardia and Fibrillation. Ventricular tachycardia is the term used to describe too-rapid contractions of the ventricles. It usually is associated with heart disease (see Coronary Artery Disease, page 801) or occurs in the several days immediately after a heart attack (see page 809).

Ventricular fibrillation describes a condition in which the muscle fibers of the ventricles contract in an uncoordinated and inefficient manner so that the pumping action virtually ceases. If a normal, organized pumping action is not restored in a matter of minutes, death results (see Sudden Cardiac Death, page 821).

Treatment. The first approach is to control the ventricular arrhythmia. Various medications will be administered and in some cases an electric shock may be delivered in a procedure called electrical cardioversion to restore normal heart rhythms. Occasionally, such arrhythmias can be treated surgically or by the use of special

---

TWENTY-FOUR-HOUR CARDIAC MONITORING

The electrocardiogram (also known as ECG) is an important tool in detecting and diagnosing different types of heart rate and rhythm disorders.

An ECG is a graphic representation of the electrical forces of your heart. As the cardiac cycle repeats itself every second or so, there is a pattern of electrical pulses that precisely reflect the action of the heart. These pulses can be recorded by electrodes attached to the surface of your body. The activity of the heart—represented by characteristic waves—can then be read instantaneously on a television monitor or studied later on graph-paper printouts.

The ECG has proven to be an invaluable tool for the cardiologist. A portable version, designed by J.J. Holter and called a Holter monitor, has been in use since 1961. Electrodes attached to your chest are linked to a small box containing a recording device. As you go about your normal ac-

tivities, the device records the activity of your heart.

When you return to your physician a day or two later, he or she will have a day-long record of your heart's activities. The Holter monitor is an especially useful tool for diagnosing heart rhythm disturbances that may occur at odd and unpredictable times. Together with a written diary you may be asked to keep regarding your activities and symptoms, the ECG from the Holter monitor may allow your physician to relate your symptoms to actual variations in your heart's rhythms.

Unfortunately, the suspicious symptoms may not occur while the Holter monitor is attached. Under such circumstances, your physician may choose to provide you with a transtelephonic monitor or event recorder. These devices allow you to send an ECG over the telephone when the symptom, such as a palpitation, is occurring. This increases the chances of making a correct diagnosis about your heart rhythm's relationship to the symptoms.

autonomic defibrillators that can be implanted in the body somewhat like a pacemaker.

Other Arrhythmias. Among other (and usually minor) arrhythmias are ventricular premature complexes (VPCs). These resemble ectopic atrial beats. Ectopic ventricular beats are observed in the electrocardiograms of nearly two of every three adults monitored over a period of hours (see Twenty-Four-Hour Cardiac Monitoring, page 818). VPCs usually require no treatment unless they are associated with other symptoms or are occurring frequently.

However, there is an association between certain patterns of VPCs and sudden cardiac death (see page 821). Thus, if your physician notes VPCs in your electrocardiogram, he or she may recommend use of an anti-arrhythmia drug (see Medications To Pace Your Heart, page 821).

HEART BLOCK

Signs and Symptoms
- None;
- Breathlessness and feeling of exhaustion.

Emergency Symptoms
- Extreme breathlessness and weakness;
- Loss of consciousness, convulsions.

Your heart rate is controlled by electrical impulses issued by the sinus node in the right atrium. These pacemaker cells produce electrical impulses that travel throughout both atria, causing the muscular walls of the atria to contract.

The electrical impulses travel from the atria through a small bed of specialized tissue called the atrioventricular node to specialized fibers (bundle of His) that conduct them to the muscle fibers of the ventricles. These muscles then contract.

In heart block, the electrical impulse passes through the atrioventricular node and bundle of His slowly, intermittently, or not at all. This condition can result from various causes including scarring in the path of the specialized conduction fibers, coronary artery disease (including a heart attack), congenital heart disease, the effects of certain drugs (including heart medications such as digitalis and the beta-adrenergic and cal-

cium channel blockers), infections such as Lyme disease (see page 854) and mononucleosis (see Infectious Mononucleosis, page 852), and other disorders.

The Diagnosis. In many people with heart block, there are no obvious symptoms. On the other hand, in severe cases, there may be a sudden loss of consciousness.

Heart block is classified by degrees. First-

FAINTING SPELLS

A fainting spell can be frightening, both for you and for those around you. Most often, however, there is no reason to panic.

A fainting spell—the medical term is syncope—is a symptom, not a disorder. When you pass out or faint, it means that your brain is not getting sufficient oxygen to function properly. The signs of impending syncope may include nausea, perspiration, or a "graying-out" of your vision. The key sign, however, is a loss of consciousness.

What Are the Causes?
Syncope usually is the result of a malfunction in either the cardiovascular or the nervous system.

Various heart problems can produce fainting spells. Among them are arrhythmias of the heart, especially an excessively rapid heart rate. In this case the heart pumps insufficient blood to the brain, resulting in syncope (see Heart Arrhythmias, page 816). A narrowing of the valve that feeds blood from your heart to your main artery (see Aortic Valve Problems, page 828), sudden decreases in blood pressure, and slowing of the heart also can produce syncope.

The involuntary *(autonomic)* nervous system controls the pumping of your heart and the pressure in your blood vessels. When it fails to function properly or if too little blood is being pumped, the autonomic nervous system may malfunction and fainting spells may occur.

What Are the Risks?
Once you are lying flat, blood flow is quickly restored, and you usually regain consciousness. Recovering consciousness quickly after a fainting spell means that little or no damage is sustained by your brain due to the shortage of oxygen. In fact, the most serious risk of syncope is usually from the fall itself: fractures or head injuries may result.

What Is To Be Done?
If you experience a fainting spell, consult your physician. He or she will first identify the cause of the syncope. Your physician then will treat the cause with appropriate means, which may mean heart medications or, rarely, a pacemaker. If the problem involves the autonomic nervous system, garments that constrict the circulation in your leg veins may help maintain an adequate supply of blood to your heart.

degree heart block is asymptomatic (without symptoms) and is evident only on the electrocardiogram as a delay in the transmission of the impulse from the atria to the ventricles.

In second-degree heart block, some of the impulses fail to reach the ventricles. The result is an irregular pulse. In many cases, second-degree heart block is a result of an excess of certain heart drugs, and the heartbeat returns to normal with the withdrawal of the medication. In others, the use of an artificial cardiac pacemaker is necessary (see Artificial Cardiac Pacemakers, below).

ARTIFICIAL CARDIAC PACEMAKERS

If your heart is unable to maintain a fast enough heartbeat or if it occasionally pauses, the solution may be the surgical implantation of an artificial cardiac pacemaker. This may be short-term treatment or a permanent solution.

Symptoms that may suggest a problem that will require a pacemaker include blackout spells, near faints, shortness of breath (especially during physical activity), and undue fatigue. Slow heartbeat or pauses can occur with various types of heart disease and even in an otherwise apparently normal heart.

An artificial pacemaker is an electrical device that causes the heart to beat by releasing a series of electrical discharges. It replaces the function of your heart's own control system, the sinus node and conduction system (see Disorders of Heart Rate and Rhythm, page 816). The implanted pacemaker mimics the electrical impulses of a healthy heart and restores a sufficiently fast heartbeat. At times, your heartbeat may be fast enough on its own; the pacemaker then automatically goes on standby.

The Equipment
The pacemaker itself is small (weighing about 1½ ounces) and is powered by a lithium battery that lasts up to 10 years. Other models that are generally used only for short periods of time are not implanted but are carried outside the body.

The Procedure
The pacemaker usually is implanted beneath the skin on the front side of your chest just below your collarbone. The pacemaker is connected to one or, occasionally, two insulated, flexible wire leads. These usually are passed, via a large vein beneath the collarbone, into the right side of the heart. There, an electrical contact (electrode) discharges impulses to the inner surface of the right side of the heart to stimulate its contractions when the heart rate slows.

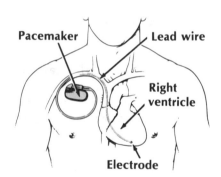

If the sinus node fails to control your heartbeat, an artificial pacemaker may be surgically implanted. The battery-powered pacemaker is located beneath the skin of your chest. Flexible wire leads are threaded into the right side of the heart to deliver controlling electrical impulses.

Applications
The artificial cardiac pacemaker is not a solution to all heart problems, but it can be used to treat a number of heart disorders. Its primary application is to control or prevent slow arrhythmias of the ventricles. Many pacemakers prevent the heartbeat from ever going below a certain rate; this lower limit can be set by the physician even after the pacemaker is implanted. Other pacemakers are designed to increase the heart rate automatically during activity or stress, just as in the normal heart.

Two-wire pacemakers (with one wire in the top chamber, or atrium, of the heart and one wire in the bottom chamber, or ventricle) are called dual-chamber devices. They ensure that the heart beats in a normal sequence—atrium first followed quickly by the ventricle.

Some very specialized pacemaker devices can be used to treat specific types of fast arrhythmias when medicines are not effective.

Living With a Pacemaker
There have been major technologic advances in recent years, but modern pacemakers may still be affected by outside electrical interference. People with pacemakers should avoid powerful electromagnetic fields such as those found near a high-voltage transmission line or substation, arc welder, or magnetic resonance imager. Avoid hard contact to the pacemaker, such as might occur while playing football or firing a rifle from the shoulder near the pacemaker. Modern pacemakers are not affected by microwave ovens, although you may occasionally see such warnings in cafeterias.

In third-degree heart block, no impulses reach the ventricles and the ventricles are forced to beat with their own intrinsic rhythm. The beating of the heart at this intrinsic rate is often so slow that the flow of blood to the brain and other parts of the body is insufficient. Loss of consciousness may result.

Treatment. First-degree heart block and many forms of second-degree heart block are not serious conditions. Only observation or withdrawing or reducing the medication that produced the heart block is necessary.

When the heart is no longer able to pace itself, a procedure to implant an artificial cardiac pacemaker is required (see page 820).

SUDDEN CARDIAC DEATH

Signs and Symptoms
- Immediate loss of consciousness for no apparent cause;
- No pulse.

To many, having a heart attack is their most terrible fear. Yet a different ailment—called sudden cardiac death or cardiac arrest—is actually the leading cause of death in young and middle-aged men (it is more than 3 times as common in men as in women).

Modern medicine is only beginning to understand how the heart of an apparently healthy person suddenly stops beating or beats in an uncontrolled fashion. At times this has been associated with alcohol, the use of illicit drugs such as cocaine, and exercise.

The blood flow to the brain instantly ceases, and loss of consciousness results. Ventricular fibrillation is most often the cause of sudden cardiac death. In turn, the fibrillation is usually caused by coronary artery disease (see Heart Arrhythmias, page 816). However, in a significant number of cases, the cause of sudden cardiac death is unknown.

The ventricles are the lower two chambers of the heart and are largely responsible

---

MEDICATIONS TO PACE YOUR HEART

In treating your heart rhythm disturbance (arrhythmia), your physician may prescribe one or more of a group of drugs. Some work to slow down the pace of the heart; others increase it.

Digitalis
Digitalis preparations (for example, digoxin) may be prescribed to treat atrial arrhythmias. Digitalis slows the transmission of the heart's electrical impulses, thereby helping restore normal heart rate and rhythm. Digoxin also is used to increase the efficiency of the pumping action of the heart.

Quinidine, Tocainide, and Procainamide
These drugs work to control abnormal heart rhythms, including atrial fibrillation, atrial flutter, and paroxysmal tachycardia. Each of these drugs functions by slowing the activity in the heart's control system (the sinus node in the right atrium) and by delaying the rate at which electrical impulses are transmitted to other chambers of the heart.

Calcium Channel Blockers
These drugs decrease the frequency and force of the heart's contractions, resulting in a decrease in its oxygen needs. They function by blocking the entry of calcium into your cells. Two of the calcium channel agents, verapamil and diltiazem, are used to treat arrhythmias.

Atropine
This drug is used to increase the heart rate. It may be used in treating the decreased heart rate (bradycardia) that results from heart attack or other disorders.

Beta-Adrenergic Blocking Drugs
These drugs block the stimulating effect the hormone epinephrine has on your heart. In treating disorders of arrhythmia, the beta-adrenergic blockers slow the speed at which the nerve impulses travel from the sinus node to the rest of the heart muscle.

Other Drugs
When conventional medications for treating ventricular arrhythmia have failed, amiodarone frequently has been effective. There is a likelihood, however, of side effects that may be serious. These will be discussed with you by your physician.

Many new, experimental drugs are now undergoing evaluation and may be available soon. These include mexiletine, aprindine, encainide, flecainide, and propafenone.

for pumping the blood to all parts of the body. When the control system of the heart malfunctions and causes the ventricles to quiver very rapidly and ineffectively (fibrillate), the blood flow stops and sudden cardiac death can result.

When ventricular fibrillation occurs in someone in a hospital and prompt treatment is available, this rhythm disturbance sometimes can be corrected. However, in most cases of sudden cardiac death, the event occurs beyond the immediate reach of appropriate care and the victim dies before treatment can be given.

Treatment.   If the heart ceases to function, cardiopulmonary resuscitation (see page 270) should be used to maintain some oxygenation of the blood and some flow of blood to the brain.

CPR may restore heartbeat but, in the event of ventricular fibrillation, an electrical shock delivered to the heart may be re-quired. A device called a defibrillator is used. It imitates the heart's own method of stimulus, delivering an electrical impulse from the right atrium to the other parts of the heart.

Medication.   After resuscitation, drugs may be used to prevent episodes of ventricular fibrillation from recurring (see Medications To Pace Your Heart, page 821).

Prevention.   As we learn more of the causes of sudden cardiac death, it is becoming apparent that in some cases we can identify persons who are most at risk. Certain arrhythmias and other factors have been shown to produce ventricular fibrillation in some people. This is one reason why many cardiologists recommend having a so-called baseline electrocardiogram at about age 30.

People who have already had one heart stoppage are at increased risk for sudden cardiac death.

Each heart valve consists of two or three folds of tissue. When closed, a valve prevents blood from flowing to the next chamber or from returning to the previous one. When open, blood flows freely.

DISORDERS OF THE HEART VALVES

The human heart consists of four chambers and four valves. Two of the valves (the mitral and tricuspid valves) control the flow of blood from the upper chambers (the atria) to the ventricles (the pumping chambers); the other two valves (aortic and pulmonary valves) control the flow of blood out of the ventricles for circulation to other parts of the body.

The mitral valve links the atrium to the ventricle on the heart's left side; also on the left the aortic valve opens to allow blood into the main artery for the body, the aorta. On the right side, it is the tricuspid valve that controls flow from the atrium to the ventricle and the pulmonary valve that allows blood to exit from the heart to the lungs via the pulmonary artery.

Each valve consists of two or three thin folds of tissue. When closed, the valve prevents blood from flowing to the next chamber or from returning to the previous one.

When the valve opening becomes narrowed and flow through it is limited, the condition is termed stenosis. Each of the heart's valves may be subject to stenosis or obstruction. In some cases, a valve will lose its shape and begin to sag (prolapse) or will fail to close completely, causing a backflow of blood (regurgitation).

Valve problems may occur as a result of infection, congenital abnormality, or other causes. In the following pages, we will discuss a range of such disorders.

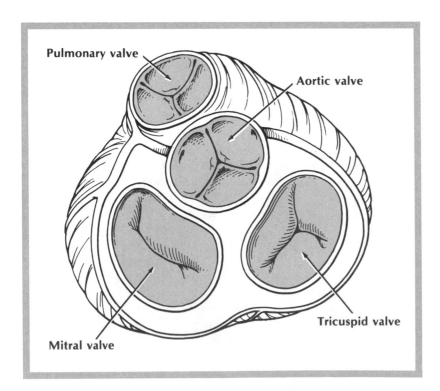

Pulmonary valve

Aortic valve

Mitral valve

Tricuspid valve

RHEUMATIC FEVER

Signs and Symptoms

Major (two of the following must be present for the diagnosis to be made):

- Inflammation of the heart (carditis), sometimes manifested by weakness and shortness of breath;
- Arthritis that tends to migrate from one joint to another;
- Uncontrolled movement of limbs and face (chorea);
- Raised, red patches on the skin;
- Lumps under the skin (subcutaneous nodules).

Minor (presence of one major and two minor criteria and evidence of a throat infection suggest the diagnosis of rheumatic fever):

- Joint aches without inflammation;
- Fever;
- Previous rheumatic fever or evidence of rheumatic heart disease;
- Abnormal heartbeat on electrocardiogram (ECG);
- Blood test indicating presence of inflammation.

A decade ago, many experts were making claims that rheumatic fever had virtually disappeared. Apparently it had; but subsequent outbreaks of rheumatic fever among children in several cities in the United States indicate that the disease has made a comeback.

Rheumatic fever appears to be the result of an immune reaction of the body to specific strains of streptococcal bacteria. A week or two after a streptococcal throat infection, the initial symptoms of rheumatic fever may appear. Vigorous and complete antibiotic treatment of streptococcal sore throats will largely prevent the occurrence of rheumatic fever.

One of the problems in preventing rheumatic fever is that sore throats that result from harmless viral infections are often difficult to distinguish from those caused by streptococci. To be sure that streptococcal throat infections are treated properly, throat cultures are obtained to identify the organisms. If the throat culture result is positive, your physician will institute appropriate antibiotic treatment.

If the antibiotic is administered orally, all of the prescribed drug must be taken, even though the sore throat disappears within the first day or two.

Rheumatic fever still occurs relatively rarely. The vast majority of streptococcal throat infections do not lead to rheumatic fever. When rheumatic fever does occur, it usually occurs in children.

The Diagnosis.   The signs and symptoms detailed above provide quite distinctive criteria for your physician's diagnosis of rheumatic fever.

How Serious Is Rheumatic Fever?   Rheumatic fever can result in inflammation in one or several organs. Most often, several joints are affected with an arthritic swelling, redness, and the sensation of heat.

The heart valves may become inflamed (carditis) so that they fail to close properly. This causes regurgitation and inefficiency of the heart pump. In rare instances, the heart muscle itself is overwhelmed by the inflammation and death from heart failure occurs (see page 807).

The heart inflammation may resolve with no permanent effects. However, there may be permanent scarring of one or more valves, which may result in obstruction to blood flow (stenosis) or reversed (backward) flow of blood (regurgitation or insufficiency). Sometimes, over a period of months or years, serious complications develop and surgery ultimately may be required to repair or replace the damaged heart valve or valves.

If rheumatic fever affects the brain, uncoordinated or uncontrolled movements of the limbs or facial muscles may occur. Such movements are described as chorea, a word derived from the Greek word meaning to dance. In the past, it was common for people to refer to this complication of rheumatic fever as Saint Vitus dance.

Rheumatic fever also can produce disclike raised and red areas on the skin called erythema marginatum. Lumps or nodules may form beneath normal-appearing skin.

Treatment.   *Prevention.* Rheumatic fever is avoidable. Pay close attention whenever your child develops a sore throat, especially if it persists for more than 24 hours and is accompanied by a fever. Consult your physician (see page 89).

The Throat Culture. If your physician suspects the presence of a streptococcal throat infection, he or she will collect a specimen by wiping the back of the affected person's throat with a cotton swab. This specimen then will be used in laboratory tests.

INFECTIVE ENDOCARDITIS: PROTECTION AND PREVENTION

You are susceptible to infective endocarditis if: you were born with a malformed heart or heart valve; your heart valves were scarred by rheumatic fever; or you have an artificial heart valve. Even if the cardiac problem is minor and has never caused any difficulty or if the cardiac defect has been repaired and you feel entirely healthy, you still are at risk for this potentially life-threatening infection.

Antibiotics offer protection from infective endocarditis by destroying or controlling bacteria. Use of such drugs may be advisable before and after certain procedures during which bacteria could enter your bloodstream, travel to your heart, and cause an infection there.

If you are at risk, follow these recommendations which are adapted from the American Heart Association preventive regimens:

Dental Procedures and Oral or Respiratory Tract Surgery
If you are to undergo any procedure on your mouth or throat that may cause bleeding, your physician or dentist probably will prescribe penicillin for oral administration. Take the penicillin 1 hour before the procedure and again 6 hours afterward.

If you are allergic to penicillin, an alternative antibiotic such as erythromycin may be substituted. If you have already had heart valve surgery, an injectable antibiotic may be necessary.

Urological or Gastrointestinal Surgery or Examination With Instruments
The intestinal bacteria (enterococci) often are resistant to penicillin. Appropriate preventive measures may include a combination of injectable antibiotics just prior to and again 8 hours after the procedure.

Lung and Skin Infections
Antibiotic treatment may be appropriate as a prophylactic measure if a lung or skin infection develops.

Think Prevention
Daily oral hygiene is vital. So is regular, professional dental care. Get regular checkups, and routinely brush and floss your teeth and gums (see Tooth Care, page 393).

Be sure your dentist and each of your physicians know that you are at risk for endocarditis.

If certain types of streptococci are detected, your physician can prescribe an appropriate antibiotic drug. In many cases, this will be penicillin.

Treating Rheumatic Fever. Antibiotics are given to eliminate any remaining streptococcal organisms. Usually, some kind of a suppressive schedule of antibiotics is continued for several years to prevent second attacks of rheumatic fever. Large doses of aspirin, and sometimes cortisone-like drugs, may be given to suppress the inflammatory process of rheumatic fever.

Remember, a sore throat is a common, and usually minor, problem. However, if a streptococcal infection is present and left untreated, serious life-long heart complications potentially can result from a bout of rheumatic fever.

INFECTIVE ENDOCARDITIS

Signs and Symptoms
- Fever;
- Unusual fatigue or loss of appetite;
- Heart murmur;
- Night sweats, chills.

The endocardium is the membrane that covers the interior of your heart's four chambers and valves. For infective endocarditis to occur, your heart must have a place where the infecting organism can lodge and reproduce; thus, if you have a normal, healthy heart, you are unlikely to contract infective endocarditis. However, you are at risk for this disease if you were born with a malformed heart or heart valves or if your heart valves have become scarred from rheumatic fever (see page 823). Such problems may mean that you have a roughened and abnormal surface within your heart where the infecting organisms can congregate, multiply, and potentially spread to other parts of your body.

Certain bacteria that commonly inhabit the mouth and upper respiratory tract may cause endocarditis. They may enter the bloodstream during a dental or surgical procedure such as a tooth extraction, tonsillectomy, or other operation that involves bleeding in the mouth or throat. Intestinal bacteria, called enterococci, may enter your bloodstream during an instrumental examination or surgery in areas such as the prostate, bladder, rectum, or female pelvic organs. Drug addicts who inject drugs into a vein with unsterilized needles also are vulnerable.

The Diagnosis. Endocarditis may develop rapidly, usually with fever and chills, but this is not always the case, especially in elderly people. You may experience any one of various other symptoms including night sweats, malaise, fatigue, loss of appetite and weight, and joint inflammation.

When the infection develops more slowly, your physician will look for such symptoms as an abnormally rapid heart rate (tachycardia), enlargement of the spleen, pallor or a yellow-brown color to the skin, tiny red spots on the skin and mucous membranes, and heart murmurs. Your physician will order a series of blood cultures to determine which microorganism is causing the infection.

How Serious Is Infective Endocarditis? Infective endocarditis is fatal without treatment and elimination of the infection. Because the illness usually occurs in people who already have heart disease, the outcome depends largely on whether complications occur. Even if you are cured of the bacterial infection, you may have continued heart symptoms for years after treatment. Complications such as cardiac or renal failure may develop as well.

Treatment. *Prevention.* Even with the availability of powerful modern antibiotics, treatment can be difficult and the results uncertain. Thus, prevention is the best approach (see Infective Endocarditis: Protection and Prevention, page 824).

Medication. Antibiotic therapy depends on the type of microorganism causing the disease. Cultures of the blood are used to determine which antibiotic is appropriate; often, a combination of antibiotics is used, with penicillin commonly being one of them. The medication is often injected directly into a vein and may be given continuously over a period of several weeks to eradicate the infection.

Surgery. If the infection causes major damage to the heart valves, valve replacement may be necessary (see Heart Valve Surgery, page 829).

MITRAL VALVE PROBLEMS

Signs and Symptoms
- None;
- Breathlessness, especially after exercise;
- Easy fatigability;
- Frequent bouts of bronchitis;
- Chest discomfort or palpitations.

On the left side of your heart, the mitral valve links the upper chamber, the atrium, to the ventricle below. When the opening of the mitral valve becomes narrowed and the passage of blood through it is restricted, the condition is termed mitral valve stenosis (from the Greek *stenosis* for narrowing). When the mitral valve fails to close properly and blood flows back into the atrium from the ventricle, the disorder is called mitral valve regurgitation or incompetence.

Each of these problems is most likely to occur in people who have had rheumatic fever that damaged the tissues of their heart.

Mitral Valve Stenosis. Obstruction of the mitral valve results in too much blood accumulating in the left atrium because of the narrowing of the exit valve. The atrium becomes enlarged as the pressure in it increases; blood also backs up into the lungs, leading to lung congestion (pulmonary edema). Mitral valve stenosis commonly leads to atrial fibrillation.

Mitral Valve Regurgitation. A different problem occurs when the mitral valve does not shut tightly during the contraction of the left ventricle. Because blood flows back into the atrium, the flow to the rest of the body is decreased. The heart then pumps harder in an attempt to compensate for this decreased flow of blood. Thus, the heart may become enlarged.

There are several possible causes of mitral valve regurgitation. It can be the result of damage sustained during a bout of rheumatic fever, but mitral valve regurgitation also may be present from birth. Mitral valve regurgitation can result from a ballooning out (prolapse) of the mitral valve (see Mitral Valve Prolapse, page 826).

The Diagnosis. If you experience breathlessness, especially on mild exertion or at night, your physician may suspect mitral valve stenosis. In advanced cases, the backing up of blood may lead to accumulation of fluid (edema) in the ankles, causing them to swell. In cases of mitral valve regurgitation, many of the symptoms are similar to symptoms of mitral valve stenosis.

To confirm the diagnosis, your physician or a cardiologist will listen to your heartbeat to try to detect the sound of a characteristic heart murmur. A chest x-ray and electrocardiogram will be obtained (see Common Diagnostic Tests, page 802). An echocardiogram (see The Echocardiogram: Images Made With Sound, page 827) can define the configuration of the valve along with abnormalities of blood flow through it.

How Serious Are Mitral Valve Problems?
When the valve disease is mild, you may remain well, or have only minimal symptoms, for decades. However, the fatigue and breathlessness that eventually may occur can be disabling over time if the deformity of the valve is severe. There also is the risk of atrial fibrillation in which the atrium beats in a rapid and uncoordinated fashion (see Heart Arrhythmias, page 816). This can lead to the dangerous formation of emboli (see Arterial Embolism, page 836).

Treatment. *Prevention of Complications.* There is no way to prevent mitral valve disorders, but avoiding complications may be possible. Mitral valve problems put you at risk of infective endocarditis, so take proper precautions before undergoing oral or lower gastrointestinal examinations (see Infective Endocarditis: Protection and Prevention, page 824).

Medication. The excess accumulation of fluid (edema) in your lungs or lower extremities may be treated by use of a diuretic drug. Often called water pills, these drugs will increase the rate and volume of your urine formation, helping to decrease excess fluid in your body.

If you experience atrial fibrillation, a drug (digoxin) may be prescribed to slow the rapid heart rate. In addition, an anticoagulant may be prescribed to prevent the formation of blood clots (emboli).

Surgery. In cases of mitral stenosis, when other treatments are unsuccessful, your physician may recommend a procedure called valvotomy. In this operation, the constricted valve opening is enlarged surgically. It is a serious operation, but it has become routine and may alleviate the symptoms for many years. Some cases of mitral regurgitation can be corrected by repairing the valve surgically; other cases require replacement of the mitral valve.

Surgical replacement of the mitral valve can be accomplished with tissue prepared from certain animals or with a man-made mechanical version (see Heart Valve Surgery, page 830). In selected situations, a heart valve valvuloplasty can be done for mitral stenosis (see Heart Valve Valvuloplasty, page 829).

MITRAL VALVE PROLAPSE

Signs and Symptoms
- None;
- Brief episodes of rapid heartbeat (palpitations);
- Chest pain.

Located on the left side of your heart, the mitral valve links the upper chamber, the atrium, to the ventricle below. When functioning normally, the mitral valve, which consists of two leaflets, controls the movement of blood between the chambers. In some people, however, one or both of the valve leaflets balloon out (prolapse).

The prolapse of the valve results in extra clicking sounds that your physician can detect when listening to your heart with a stethoscope. The condition may also result in failure of the valves to close properly, and blood may leak back into the atrium during pumping by the ventricle. This flow of blood back into the atrium produces a sound called a murmur. The combination of these sounds has led to one of the names for mitral valve prolapse, the click-murmur syndrome.

This generally harmless condition may be found in as many as 1 in 10 Americans, more often in women than in men. It also is more common in women who have scoliosis or certain other skeletal abnormalities (see page 994).

The Diagnosis. Your physician probably will diagnose mitral valve prolapse with the aid of a stethoscope. Your physician or a cardiologist may do a confirming test called an echocardiogram (see below).

How Serious Is Mitral Valve Prolapse?
Often, mitral valve prolapse is discovered during a routine stethoscope examination of your heart. Unsettling as such a discovery may be at first, the condition is rarely a cause for concern.

In a small percentage of cases, however, this condition may cause episodes of rapid heartbeat (palpitations), chest pain, and significant valve leakage which may require regular medical attention or even surgery.

Treatment. The vast majority of people with this condition live normal lives, have

---

THE ECHOCARDIOGRAM: IMAGES MADE WITH SOUND

Until the development of echocardiography (sometimes referred to as diagnostic cardiac ultrasound examination), your physician or cardiologist had to rely on physical examination, a graphic display of the heart's electrical activity (ECG), or an x-ray to evaluate the condition and function of your heart. Now it is possible to "look" directly at your heart without ever penetrating your skin.

This device uses reflected sound (echo) of the heart (cardio) to record (graph) an image. Special vibrating crystals generate harmless, high-frequency sound waves (they are inaudible to the human ear) that are aimed at and reflected from the tissues of your heart. The machine records the pattern of the reflection to compose an image of the heart on a monitor screen.

The heart can be seen in action. On the screen of the echocardiograph your physician can observe the heart's external covering (pericardium), the shape and thickness of the walls of the chambers, the valves, and the large veins and arteries that lead into and out of the heart. The direction and velocity of the flow of blood through the valves and in the heart chambers can be determined.

The Procedure
Echocardiography is noninvasive and usually is painless. You will be asked to lie on your back and perhaps turn slightly to your left. Special jelly will be applied to your chest to increase the conductivity of the ultrasound waves.

The transducer (which contains the crystals that produce the waves and receive the echo) will be maneuvered to the best position on your chest. This transducer is linked by a cord to the monitor screen and other electronic components.

The Advantages
No x-ray exposure is necessary; the procedure is safe and noninvasive. The equipment is also portable, so the study can be done at your hospital bedside or in your physician's office.

The Diagnosis
Echocardiography can be used to diagnose various heart ailments. Among them are congenital heart defects in infants as well as in children and adults, tumors or blood clots within the heart, fluid around the heart (pericardial effusion), valve disorders, weakened heart muscles, coronary artery disease, and aneurysm. In addition, it has been particularly useful in evaluating function of the left ventricle, the main pumping chamber of the heart.

In echocardiography, a wand (transducer) is positioned over the heart. Sound waves are generated. The waves are reflected back from the heart tissues, recorded, and processed to produce continuous images on a monitor screen. Above: The image produced by the echocardiogram shows a normal mitral valve (MV).

normal life expectancies, and are not required to make adjustments in their lifestyles. For most, the condition is probably best regarded as nothing more than a harmless variation from normal.

Mitral valve prolapse may put you at greater risk of infective endocarditis. As a precaution, prophylactic use of antibiotics before dental and certain surgical procedures is appropriate (see Infective Endocarditis: Protection and Prevention, page 824).

Medication. If you are among the few people who have mitral valve prolapse that produces frequent and troubling palpitations, your physician may prescribe a beta-adrenergic blocker drug. These drugs block the stimulating effect the hormone epinephrine has on your heart.

AORTIC VALVE PROBLEMS

Signs and Symptoms
- None;
- Weakness on exertion;
- Breathlessness;
- Chest discomfort (angina);
- Fainting spells.

The aortic valve permits the flow of blood from the main pumping chamber (the left ventricle) into the main artery of the body, the aorta, which, in turn, conducts the oxygen-carrying blood to progressively smaller arteries and to the tissues of the body. The valve itself consists of three cusps (cup-shaped folds of tissue) that come together to prevent blood from flowing back from the aorta to the ventricle between contractions.

Aortic Stenosis. When the opening of a valve becomes narrowed and passage through it is limited, the condition is termed stenosis. Such a narrowing in the aortic valve means the left ventricle (the main pumping chamber of the heart) has to pump harder to maintain a normal output of blood. This often results in the muscle of the left ventricle becoming thickened, a condition called left ventricular hypertrophy.

Aortic Regurgitation. A different sort of problem occurs when the aortic valve fails to shut tightly between contractions. Called aortic regurgitation or aortic incompetence, this condition means that blood tends to leak back into the ventricle. Consequently, flow of blood to the rest of the body decreases and the heart must pump harder in an attempt to compensate for the decreased blood flow. As a result, the heart often becomes enlarged.

Both aortic stenosis and aortic regurgitation are the result of damage sustained by the heart muscle from rheumatic fever or the result of a congenital abnormality. Aortic stenosis is much more common among men than among women.

The Diagnosis. Your physician may discover either of these disorders while listening to your heart with a stethoscope. He or she then may order one of several other tests, including a chest x-ray (to determine if your heart has become enlarged), an electrocardiogram (ECG) to look for evidence of left ventricular hypertrophy, and an echocardiogram (see The Echocardiogram: Images Made With Sound, page 827).

How Serious Are Aortic Valve Problems? The most serious risk with aortic valve problems is posed by the overwork of the left ventricle. This may result in angina (see page 803), congestive heart failure (see page 807), or fainting spells (see page 819).

Aortic valve problems are insidious in that they develop without symptoms until they reach a hazardous phase. Prompt treatment (such as aortic valve surgery) may be necessary.

Treatment. In most cases, aortic stenosis or regurgitation does not mean you need to adopt a passive lifestyle. While strenuous activity is to be avoided, reasonable physical activity is usually encouraged.

Prevention. Aortic valve problems may put you at greater risk of infective endocarditis. As a precaution, preventive use of antibiotics prior to dental and certain surgical procedures is appropriate (see Infective Endocarditis: Protection and Prevention, page 824).

Surgery. If your aortic valve is badly deteriorated, the only long-term solution may be surgical replacement or reconstruction of the valve (see Heart Valve Surgery, page 830).

TRICUSPID AND PULMONARY VALVE PROBLEMS

The blood flows out of the four chambers of the human heart through valves. The preceding pages discussed the most common valve problems, those that concern the aortic and mitral valves in the left side of the heart. Rarely, the pulmonary and tricuspid valves also develop malfunctions.

Blood flows from the upper chamber, the right atrium, through the tricuspid valve to the right ventricle below. Then, through the pulmonary valve, it exits from the right ventricle to the pulmonary artery which carries the blood to the lungs for oxygenation.

Both the tricuspid and pulmonary valves (like the aortic and mitral valves) can have problems in which the valve opening narrows, restricting the flow of blood (conditions called tricuspid stenosis and pulmonary stenosis). In some cases, the valve fails to close properly, allowing blood to flow back through the valve when it is supposed to be closed (such disorders are termed incompetence or regurgitation).

Often, these ailments are discovered by physicians during routine examinations; treatment may not be required. However, if the function of the valve is badly deteriorated, valve replacement may be necessary (see Heart Valve Surgery, page 830). In certain situations, the valve may be opened by

---

HEART VALVE VALVULOPLASTY

If you have a narrowed heart valve (stenosis), it may be limiting blood flow, and this could lead to such complications as an enlarged heart. The problem may be treated by open-heart surgery (see Heart Valve Surgery, page 830),

Balloon-tipped catheters

Calcified aortic heart valve

To open a calcified (narrowed) aortic heart valve, one or two balloon-tipped catheters can be guided into the heart and placed through the valve, and then inflated. This procedure, called balloon valvuloplasty, results in improved blood flow.

but another treatment option your physician may recommend is balloon valvuloplasty.

The heart valve valvuloplasty is used when the opening of a heart valve has narrowed. This may occur due to age or to medical conditions that cause calcium deposits to form on the flaps of tissue, the cusps, that form the working parts of the valve.

If you have symptoms of mitral valve stenosis (see Mitral Valve Problems, page 825), mitral balloon valvuloplasty is sometimes used as an alternative to surgery. If you have symptoms of aortic valve stenosis (see Aortic Valve Problems, page 828), aortic balloon valvuloplasty is sometimes used but generally only if aortic valve surgery is thought to be risky for you or if you have some other serious medical problem that requires treatment prior to when the surgical replacement of an aortic valve could be performed.

The Procedure
Balloon valvuloplasty of the aortic valve is a nonsurgical procedure in which a guide wire is inserted through a large artery, most often in the groin area. This wire is advanced through your blood vessels to your heart. A catheter (tube) with an elongated balloon at its tip is threaded over the guide wire. When the tip arrives in the opening of the diseased valve, the balloon is inflated. The narrowed valve is thus enlarged, improving blood flow. Sometimes inflation of two balloons is required to enlarge the opening.

The procedure for mitral valve valvuloplasty is similar except that the balloon-tipped catheter generally is inserted into a vein in the groin area (instead of an artery) and then advanced to the right side of the heart. The catheter is passed from the right atrium, through the common wall shared by the atria, to the left atrium, and then through the mitral valve where the balloon is inflated to widen the valve opening.

The Recovery
As with any heart procedure, there are risks. However, the result may be an immediate relief of such symptoms as breathlessness. The hospital stay and recovery are also substantially less—typically only a few days—than with open-heart procedures.

HEART VALVE SURGERY

In some cases, heart valve problems require no treatment. If treatment is necessary, it may include medications or a procedure called heart valvuloplasty (see Heart Valve Valvuloplasty, page 829). Occasionally, however, open-heart surgery is the best option.

The term open-heart surgery implies opening the chest and using a heart-lung machine to replace the heart while the abnormality of the heart is being repaired. Open-heart procedures include coronary artery bypass surgery (see page 814), correction of congenital abnormalities of the heart (see Congenital Heart Disorders, page 54), heart valve surgery, and removal of some heart tumors.

Valvotomy

Your physician may recommend a surgical procedure called valvotomy. This operation is appropriate when flow through a valve has become restricted (stenosis). Valvotomy is the surgical enlargement of the opening of the valve. It is a serious operation, but it has become routine and may alleviate the symptoms for many years.

Three commonly used replacement heart valves are (A) valve made from animal tissue, (B) tilting disc valve, and (C) caged-ball valve.

Valve Replacement

Another option is surgical replacement of the valve. In the case of aortic valve stenosis, heart valve replacement has proved to be one of the true success stories of modern surgery, with high success rates often regardless of the age of the patient.

The Procedure

You will be given a general anesthetic. Through an incision the length of your breastbone (sternum), your heart is exposed and connected to a heart-lung machine that will assume your breathing and blood circulation during the procedure.

The damaged heart valve will be removed and replaced. The new valve will be one of two basic types: mechanical, made of metal or plastic; or a tissue valve, usually from a pig.

The Recovery

After the operation (which lasts several hours), you will spend one or more days in a coronary or intensive-care unit where your heart function and general recovery will be closely monitored.

During recuperation, which may range from a few weeks to a few months depending upon your overall health and age at the time of the operation, you will be assisted by an assortment of physical and other therapists. Usually the salt content of your diet is restricted for some time after such an operation.

stretching it with a balloon catheter inserted through a vein in the leg and advanced to the heart.

These valve problems also may put you at greater risk of infective endocarditis. As a precaution, preventive use of antibiotics prior to dental and certain surgical procedures is appropriate (see Infective Endocarditis: Protection and Prevention, page 824).

DISEASES OF THE HEART MUSCLE AND PERICARDIUM

There are three layers of heart tissue: the epicardium, a thin, very smooth covering on the outside; the myocardium, the heart muscle itself (the name comes from the Greek *myo* for muscle and *kardia* for heart) in the middle; and the endocardium, the inner lining, a very smooth layer in contact with the blood. Protecting the whole organ on the outside is the pericardium, a fibrous sac.

The heart muscle and its associated lining are subject to disease. Although relatively rare, diseases that damage the heart muscle (cardiomyopathy) do occur, both as an isolated problem and as a consequence of disorders that affect other organs as well. Inflammations of the myocardium (myocarditis) and the pericardium (pericarditis) also may occur.

CARDIOMYOPATHY

Signs and Symptoms
- Brief episodes of rapid heartbeat (palpitations);
- Breathlessness;
- Weakness;
- Chest pain;
- Fainting;
- Fluid retention (edema).

When the muscle of the heart is damaged or defective, the disorder is termed cardiomyopathy, or heart muscle disease (the name cardiomyopathy comes from Greek roots for heart [*kardia*], muscle [*myo*], and disease [*pathos*]). Cardiomyopathy may appear in one of several forms.

Forms of Cardiomyopathy. *Dilated Cardiomyopathy.* In dilated cardiomyopathy (also referred to as congestive cardiomyopathy), the heart muscle is weakened and is unable to pump efficiently. This may produce symptoms of congestive heart failure (see page 807) including breathlessness and retention of water which results in a swelling (edema) that is most evident in the feet and ankles. Dilated cardiomyopathy also causes enlarged heart compartments and may lead to the formation of clots (emboli) within the enlarged compartments. The clots may travel to other parts of the body. It is most common in middle-aged men.

Hypertrophic Cardiomyopathy. If you have this form, the muscular walls of your left ventricle (the main pumping chamber of your heart) become thickened and stiff. This may impair the flow of blood into your heart as well as the ejection of blood out of it. This disorder often runs in families.

Alcoholic Heart Disease. Alcoholics may have a heart muscle malfunction after they have consumed large quantities of alcohol over many years. If the problem has not advanced to the point of heart failure, cessation of the drinking may halt the progression of the disease.

Restrictive Cardiomyopathy. This condition is characterized by stiffening of the heart muscle and a decreased ability to expand and fill with blood between contractions (the portion of the cardiac cycle termed diastole). Development of blood clots within the heart chambers, water retention (edema), and a tender liver are other common signs.

The Diagnosis. In diagnosing cardiomyopathy (heart muscle disease), your physician will consider your symptoms, especially breathlessness and chest discomfort, and may perform x-ray and electrocardiographic examinations. Your physician also may obtain an echocardiogram to observe the motions of your heart at work (see The Echocardiogram: Images Made With Sound, page 827). The echocardiogram often can determine what form of cardiomyopathy is present. In some cases, your physician will obtain a biopsy specimen (tissue sample) from your heart for microscopic examination. This specimen is obtained by passing a flexible instrument through a large vein into your heart.

How Serious Are Cardiomyopathies?
In most cases, there are no symptoms of cardiomyopathy until the disease is quite advanced. Sometimes, sudden death is the first indication of the presence of the problem (see Sudden Cardiac Death, page 821).

Often, drug and other treatments can be used to ease the symptoms, and there may be improvement over time. In some instances when the heart is badly damaged, heart transplantation is an option (see Heart Transplantation, page 833).

Treatment. In learning to live with cardiomyopathy, in general it is wise to avoid all strenuous exertion. Treatment must be individualized to the type of cardiomyopathy.

Medication. The choice of drugs for treatment depends on which type of cardiomyopathy is present. The possible drugs include diuretics (water pills to decrease water retention), calcium channel blockers (see Calcium Channel Blockers, page 821), blood vessel dilators, drugs to control irregular heart rhythm (see Heart Arrhythmias, page 816), and digitalis and beta-adrenergic blockers.

In some cases, heart muscle disease is a secondary result of another ailment, and the symptoms may resolve after effective treatment of the primary problem. Examples of this include specific heart muscle diseases, sarcoidosis, and hemochromatosis (see pages 934 and 656).

Prevention.   Certain of the cardiomyopathies may put you at greater risk of infective endocarditis. As a precaution, prophylactic use of antibiotics prior to dental and certain surgical procedures is appropriate (see Infective Endocarditis: Protection and Prevention, page 824).

Alcohol Consumption.   In cases of alcoholic heart muscle disease, complete and permanent abstinence from alcohol is essential.

MYOCARDITIS

Signs and Symptoms
* Fever;
* Vague chest pain;
* Joint pain;
* Abnormally rapid heartbeat.

The middle of the three layers of heart tissue is the myocardium. As its name suggests, the myocardium is the heart muscle itself (the word comes from the Greek *myo* for muscle and *kardia* for heart).

Acute myocarditis is an inflammation of that muscle and usually occurs as a complication during or after one of various infectious diseases (viral illnesses including polio, influenza, and rubella), rheumatic fever, or exposure to radiation, certain chemicals, or drugs. Accompanying pericarditis also may develop (see this page).

The Diagnosis.   In diagnosing the disease, your physician probably will use an electrocardiogram and an x-ray. Often, a heart muscle tissue examination (biopsy) is performed because this is the only way to confirm a diagnosis. Myocarditis can be very serious, but the outcome depends on the type of infection. Severe cases can lead ultimately to cardiac failure and death, but in most cases the inflammation will clear and good health will be fully regained.

Treatment.   Therapy consists of avoiding vigorous exercise until the pattern of your heart's activity has returned to normal. A proper diet emphasizing salt restriction and treatment of the underlying cause if it can be identified are important. If your physician observes abnormalities in your heart rhythm, he or she may recommend hospitalization, electrocardiographic monitoring of your heart with an ECG, and appropriate anti-arrhythmia medications (see Medications To Pace Your Heart, page 821) until your heartbeat returns to normal. In severe situations, your physician may consider heart transplantation (see page 833).

PERICARDITIS

Signs and Symptoms
* Chest pain radiating to the left side of the neck, shoulder, back, or upper and middle abdomen;
* Breathlessness;
* Swelling of the abdomen.

The pericardium can be described as the bag that encloses the heart. Essentially a sac, it has a very smooth inside surface; outside is the tough (fibrous) parietal pericardium.

Acute Pericarditis.   Pericarditis is an inflammation of the pericardium; it may be caused by bacterial or viral infection. It occurs primarily in men between the ages of 20 and 50, often after a respiratory infection. As a result of the inflammation, pain is felt when the pericardium and the outer layer of the heart rub against each other. There may be an accumulation of excess fluid between the pericardium and the heart.

Cardiac Tamponade.   When a great deal of fluid accumulates in the pericardium and presses on the heart, so that the heart cannot fill properly, the condition is termed cardiac tamponade. Injury to the pericardium at surgery or in an accident can cause an accumulation of blood and cardiac tamponade. Tuberculosis, tumors, or acute viral infections may result in fluid accumulation and also produce cardiac tamponade. The result can be a restriction of blood flow to the lungs and the rest of the body.

Constrictive Pericarditis.   In some cases, a permanent thickening, scarring, and con-

HEART TRANSPLANTATION

Heart transplantation has been performed for more than 20 years with increasing success. It is now performed in many hospitals all over the world.

Who Qualifies for a Heart Transplant?

Heart transplantation is not a solution to all heart problems. In fact, it is suitable for only a few persons with only certain kinds of heart disease. The usual profile for a candidate for heart transplantation is age under 55 to 60 years, psychologically stable, and surrounded by a supportive family. All of the other vital organs must be in excellent health, particularly the kidneys, liver, and lungs. Transplantation may be appropriate for people with heart failure and certain diseases of the heart that are serious enough that life expectancy is decreased to less than 2 to 3 years.

The Procedure

Before the operation, a donor heart must be found. Most often, this heart comes from the body of a healthy person who died in an accident but did not sustain heart injuries.

The donated heart generally is brought to the recipient, transported in a special solution. The recipient's chest cavity is opened and the diseased heart is removed; then, the new organ is put in its place. During this portion of the procedure, the pumping of oxygenated blood to the body is taken over by a heart-lung machine, as is done routinely in many kinds of heart surgery.

What Is Rejection?

All transplanted organs are susceptible to rejection. The body's immune system recognizes the transplanted tissue as foreign and produces antibodies to attack the "intruder."

In order to minimize the risk of rejection of a transplanted heart, you will be given drugs that suppress your body's normal immune response. Some of these "immunosuppressive drugs" will be used for a short term and will be discontinued shortly after the operation. You must take others for the rest of your life. These drugs have side effects; they decrease your body's ability to recognize and resist infectious disease. Therefore, dosages must be adjusted carefully.

The Recovery

Most successful recipients of heart transplants seem to recover to carry on relatively normal lives. Approximately 80 percent of those who have received heart transplants are alive and active 1 year after the operation; some have lived for more than a decade.

Heart transplantation remains a complicated procedure. For success, this procedure requires a well-organized team of experienced transplantation specialists and a motivated recipient. If you have a transplant, you will continue to see members of the transplantation team for the rest of your life. They will carefully adjust medications and perform periodic heart biopsies to monitor rejection, and they will treat any complications.

Transplantation is most appropriate in those cases in which it is the only hope for survival and the possibility of success is high.

---

tracture of the pericardium occurs, often without apparent cause. Occasionally, a previous inflammation such as would be caused by tuberculosis may be responsible. The result again is a decrease in the ability of the heart muscle to expand between contractions and fill with blood (the portion of the cardiac cycle termed diastole).

The Diagnosis. If you have acute pericarditis or tamponade, your physician may take an x-ray and record an electrocardiogram and an echocardiogram in order to differentiate pericarditis from a heart attack. Blood tests also may be obtained. Although recurrences are common, most patients recover completely from acute pericarditis in 2 weeks to 3 months. The diagnosis of constrictive pericarditis may require, in addition, CT scans of the chest (see CT Scanning, page 1286) or heart catheterization (see page 1290).

In cardiac tamponade, a procedure called pericardiocentesis may be required. This involves draining the excess fluid from the pericardium by using a small tube (catheter).

Treatment. *Medication.* Treatment may include analgesics to relieve the pain. If water retention (edema) and swelling are present, diuretic drugs also may be given.

If an underlying cause, such as tuberculosis or other bacterial infection, is identified, anti-tuberculosis or antibiotic drugs may be prescribed to treat that cause.

Surgery. In cases of chronic constrictive pericarditis, surgery may be required to cut out (resect) the portions of the pericardium that have grown stiff and are limiting the working of your heart. The procedure is called pericardiectomy. Although the pericardium is thought to serve various purposes, your heart will continue to function normally even if the entire pericardial sac is removed.

CIRCULATORY PROBLEMS

The vascular system, the circuit through which your blood travels, consists of the blood vessels in your body. Its name is derived from the Latin *vasculum* for small blood vessel.

The circulatory system consists of two loops. The shorter loop (pulmonary circulation) begins at the right side of your heart, delivers blood to your lungs, and then returns the oxygenated blood to your heart. The longer loop (systemic circulation) begins at the left side of the heart, where it receives the blood that was oxygenated in the lungs.

From the left side, the blood is pumped to the tissues of your body through a sequence of smaller and smaller blood vessels: arteries branch off into smaller arterioles, and the arterioles branch into tiny capillaries that deliver blood to the tissues. After the blood in the capillaries collects carbon dioxide and other waste products from the tissues, it begins its trip back to your heart via small venules and, eventually, veins. Blood circulates through your liver and kidneys, where waste products are removed or processed; then it returns to your heart.

The total amount of blood within your body is essentially constant (about 7 percent of your body weight); the distribution of blood within blood vessels varies considerably with exercise and exposure to heat and cold. During exercise, for example, the blood flow to active muscles is increased; after you eat, your stomach and intestines draw more blood to assist in the digestive process. Changes in the surrounding temperature also affect the flow of blood: warmer temperatures produce increased flow to the outer layers of your skin (which helps you to dissipate heat); on the other hand, your body responds to cold by redistributing blood flow into the inner vessels (in order to conserve heat).

This flexible system is subject to a wide range of malfunctions. Some are the result of heart disorders; others occur because of disorders that directly affect the blood vessels, such as diabetes. The problems range from weakened blood vessel walls that balloon out (aneurysm) to blockages or narrowings that limit or stop the flow of blood (atherosclerotic blood vessel disease). These blood vessel problems can lead to life-threatening events such as stroke and heart attack.

ARTERIOSCLEROSIS OF THE EXTREMITIES

Signs and Symptoms
- Leg pain, especially in the calves and feet, which develops during activity and resolves shortly after the activity is stopped (intermittent claudication);
- Numbness or pain in the foot or toes when at rest;
- Ulcers or gangrene on the foot or toes.

The effects of arteriosclerosis are most likely to appear first in your legs or feet (see also Atherosclerosis: What Is It?, page 786, and Disease of the Heart and Blood Vessels: Living With the Risks, page 785). In one of its

The circulatory system consists of two loops. The shorter loop, called pulmonary circulation, begins at the right side of the heart and delivers blood to the lungs before returning the oxygenated blood to the left side of the heart. The longer loop (systemic circulation) begins at the left side of the heart and pumps blood through arteries to tissues of the body, and then returns blood through veins to the right side of the heart.

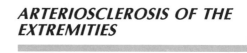

To entire body

To

Lungs

From

From entire body

Left heart

Right heart

forms, arteriosclerosis obliterans, the major arteries that deliver blood to your legs and feet become narrowed and blood flow decreases. Smaller blood vessels assume some of the load, but the physical activity of walking a block or two can produce cramps in your legs or feet; the cramps disappear within a few minutes after you discontinue the exercise. This sequence of walk-pain-rest is also termed intermittent claudication.

When some of the blood vessels actually become blocked (occluded), your foot may become pale, cold, and painful. Sometimes the final blockage develops gradually and your foot becomes vulnerable to even minor injury and infection. Gangrene consists of the actual death of tissue and usually appears as a spot or area of black, shrunken skin near the tips of your toes or about your heel (see Gangrene of the Extremities, page 835).

If the occlusion happens suddenly, as when a fragment of plaque or a clot lodges at a fork of your leg artery (commonly, at your knee), there is sudden and severe pain as well as paleness and coldness below the level of the blockage (see Arterial Embolism, page 836).

The limitation in blood supply often will

GANGRENE OF THE EXTREMITIES

When the supply of blood to any tissue is severely impaired, the supply of oxygen and nutrients is also restricted. If the flow of blood is not restored in time, the tissue may die. Gangrene is the term used for dead (necrotic) tissue.

The blood flow to the legs may cease abruptly (see Arterial Embolism, page 836) or slowly. In either situation, the foot becomes pale and cold. The pain is variable. Calf pain with walking (claudication) is almost always present, and minor injuries tend to cause an infection that may burrow deeply in the foot and involve the bones (see Osteomyelitis, page 987). As the circulation to the extremities ceases, the blood-starved tissues die and gangrene results.

Forms of Gangrene

There are two types of gangrene: wet and dry. Tissue with dry gangrene has died but has not become infected; areas affected with wet gangrene have died and become infected with bacteria.

Dry Gangrene

Tissue affected with dry gangrene is cold to the touch and gradually becomes black. At first, the tissue is painful but, as the affected tissue dies, the pain fades. Over time, the tissues will dry and drop off, but the gangrene will not spread. However, there is some risk of wet gangrene developing (see below).

Dry gangrene may occur in persons who have had diabetes (see page 707) for a long time or who have hardening of the arteries (see Arteriosclerosis of the Extremities, page 834) or frostbite (see page 842).

Wet Gangrene

Also termed moist gangrene, this type involves bacterial infection. At first, the involved tissues may be red and hot to the touch due to inflammation. With time, the tissues become cold and blue; pus may ooze from the area. Eventually, the tissue with wet gangrene begins to fall off.

Because of the bacterial infection, wet gangrene tends to spread rapidly. The bacteria contribute to tissue breakdown. Perhaps the most serious form, called gas gangrene, produces a gas that has a strong, disagreeable odor as it destroys the tissue. If not promptly treated, the person with gas gangrene may die in a matter of days (see Gas Gangrene, page 1180).

Prevention

If you are diabetic or have advanced arteriosclerosis, you must take special care of your feet (see Proper Care of the Feet in Diabetes, page 983). Even minor injuries must be treated with special attention. Careful control of blood sugar level is important in diabetics. If you smoke, stop; every cigarette causes additional damage to blood vessels.

Whether you are diabetic or not, if you sustain a wound or injury, be sure it is properly treated. If virulent bacteria are present, wet gangrene may result from even a minor injury of a limb in which the blood supply is decreased. Proper care early can prevent wet gangrene later.

Treatment

If you think you may have gangrene, consult your physician. Treatment should be initiated immediately. Surgery to open or bypass blocked arteries may be necessary. Tissues affected by dry gangrene may shrivel up and not be a problem, but surgical removal of the dead tissue often is needed.

Antibiotic drugs usually will be prescribed to prevent or to treat wet gangrene. Tissue affected by wet gangrene may have to be removed surgically.

cause inflammation and damage to the nerves (neuritis) which is manifested by burning, pain, and numbness.

These circulation problems are common in persons with diabetes; they also may have diabetic neuropathy. The decreased sensation that often accompanies diabetic neuropathy makes the person more likely to incur injury to the affected foot (see Diabetes Mellitus, page 707).

The Diagnosis.   The key aspect to diagnosis is the nature and timing of your discomfort. Does the pain occur only with exercise? Is it relieved by rest? Does it recur when activity is resumed? If so, your physician may suspect arteriosclerosis of your extremity.

Your physician may take your blood pressure in the vicinity of the pain. The pressure there may become too low to measure during exercise. Other tests, including an ultrasound scan of the area, also may be ordered. An angiogram (the injection of a dye into the affected area during an x-ray examination) will tell your physician exactly where the blockage is and whether surgical repair can be attempted.

How Serious Is This?   For many people, arteriosclerosis of the leg is not a serious problem. For most, conservative care will prevent severe disability or loss of a limb; among diabetics, the problem occurs somewhat more often. If gangrene develops, surgical amputation may be necessary (see Gangrene of the Extremities, page 835).

Treatment. *Self-Help.*   In most cases, physical activity is a useful element in treatment of limited arterial blood supply to the legs. Your physician will help you devise an appropriate regimen of daily walking or other exercise. The basic principle is to intersperse periods of exercise long and hard enough to produce pain with periods of rest. Over time, the amount of activity required to cause pain will increase. The circulation can improve with time because collateral vessels that bypass the blocked segment will develop.

Smoking.   Smokers are at particular risk for arteriosclerosis. Smoking also decreases the blood's ability to carry oxygen to your tissues and constricts the size of your smaller arteries. Smoking also encourages the deposition of platelets on microscopic areas of damage on the inner layer of arteries. Cholesterol then accumulates. If you have limited arterial circulation, stop smoking.

Proper Foot Care.   If you have diabetes as well, foot care is essential. Wear shoes that fit properly. Even minor cuts or scrapes require immediate attention because the decreased circulation means that the tissues heal slowly. If left untreated, even a minor injury to the skin of your lower leg or foot can lead to infection, gangrene, and amputation (see Proper Care of the Feet in Diabetes, page 983).

Medication.   Your physician may prescribe aspirin or another analgesic if the pain continues even at rest. Your physician also may prescribe a drug called pentoxifylline (Trentyl) to improve the blood flow to your limbs, but its effectiveness is controversial.

Surgery.   A surgical approach may be appropriate if one of the larger arteries in your leg becomes blocked. In some cases, a balloon device to expand the narrowed artery (balloon angioplasty) may be used (the procedure is similar to that used in heart surgery; see Coronary Angioplasty, page 812). Occasionally, lasers and other devices are used to open blocked arteries. Surgery to remove the damaged artery or to bypass it with an artificial vessel made of Dacron may be required.

Surgery is usually reserved for persons with severely impaired walking ability, pain, or breakdown of skin or who have the potential for loss of a limb.

ARTERIAL EMBOLISM

Signs and Symptoms
- Pain in the affected area;
- Pale, cool skin;
- Numbness.

An embolus is a clot or perhaps some debris from a buildup of atherosclerotic plaque (see Atherosclerosis: What Is It?, page 786) that has moved from its point of origin, has lodged in a new location, and is blocking the flow of blood. (The embolus is distinguished from a thrombus in that the latter is a clot that forms in the vessel and remains stationary and the former is a clot that travels to another location in the body; see Heart Attack, page 809.)

Emboli may be small and multiple, or they may be single and massive. Emboli can be life-threatening, such as when they lodge in the brain (see Stroke, page 508), or can lead to tissue death in an arm or leg if not treated within a few hours. Arterial emboli may originate in the left atrium if you are experiencing atrial fibrillation (see also page 817) or in the left ventricle after a heart attack.

The Diagnosis. When embolization occurs, the flow of blood to the legs and feet may stop abruptly or can slow gradually over weeks and months. If a clot or some debris from an atheromatous plaque in the aorta is carried with the flow of blood through the arteries in the thigh, it may plug the arteries at the level of the knee where the larger artery splits into several small ones. This obstruction causes sudden pain and pallor in the lower leg and foot.

If the clot or debris is not removed by surgery within a matter of hours, the tissue below that level may die and amputation might be necessary. When embolism happens, it is important to protect the leg from any injury by wrapping it loosely with a soft blanket and gauze. Because the foot is very cold, it is tempting to apply heat but this may damage the already compromised tissue. However, protecting the leg from loss of heat by using a blanket, gauze, or other wrap is important.

Your physician will measure the blood pressure in the affected limb and also may try to localize the embolus by an ultrasound examination or by injecting a dye into the affected blood vessels and taking an x-ray (arteriogram).

How Serious Is an Arterial Embolism? If the flow of blood is not restored within a few hours, the affected limb could be permanently damaged and amputation may be necessary.

Treatment. *Medication.* When your physician concludes that the diagnosis is arterial embolism, he or she may immediately give you a drug to break up the embolus, perhaps delivering it directly to the affected artery through the use of a catheter. This is called thrombolysis. Long-term use of aspirin or a so-called blood thinner (anticoagu-

lant drug) may be appropriate in order to prevent the development of more clots.

Surgery. If the health of a limb is in danger, immediate surgical removal of the clot may be required. This usually can be performed by using a balloon-tipped catheter inserted into the artery. As it is being withdrawn, the inflated balloon pulls the clot out. Occasionally, replacement or bypass of the blocked vessel is necessary.

AORTIC ANEURYSM

Signs and Symptoms
- Often, none;
- Pulsating sensation in the abdomen.

An aneurysm is an abnormal widening of an artery. A weakened wall of an artery is stretched as the blood is pumped through it, often creating an egg-shaped ballooning.

An aneurysm can occur in any blood vessel, including major ones in the brain (see Stroke, page 508) and minor ones anywhere in the body, but it is most likely to occur in the aorta, the main blood vessel that carries blood from the heart. One common site for an aortic aneurysm is immediately below the kidney but above the junction of the

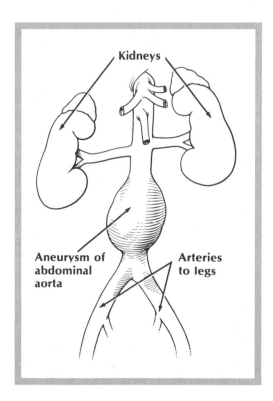

Kidneys

Aneurysm of abdominal aorta

Arteries to legs

An aneurysm is an abnormal widening of an artery. The weakened wall balloons out as blood is pumped through it. A common location: the abdominal aorta, just below the kidneys.

abdominal aorta and the arteries that supply the legs.

Abdominal aneurysms are thought to be largely the result of atherosclerosis. Complicating factors such as high blood pressure (hypertension) may contribute to the development of an aneurysm.

In addition to the expansion of the arterial wall, an aneurysm also characteristically has an accumulation of cholesterol, calcium, and even small blood clots. The weakened muscle fibers of the artery wall become fragmented and are replaced by scar tissue. Despite all these changes, however, the size of the artery's central channel may remain roughly normal.

Abdominal aortic aneurysms most often strike people over age 60, and men are more commonly affected than women.

The Diagnosis.   Often there are no symptoms. However, in advanced cases, pain may be present in the abdomen and lower back. Aneurysms tend to grow at a rate of about ⅛ to ¼ inch per year and often do not cause symptoms until blood begins to leak from the ballooning wall of the artery. If the aneurysm ruptures, shock, loss of consciousness, and death may be the catastrophic result.

Your physician may feel the pulsating vessel on routine examination of your abdomen. In some cases, an x-ray taken for another reason will reveal an aneurysm. Its presence is usually confirmed with an ultrasound examination or a CT scan (see page 1286).

How Serious Is an Aneurysm?   An abdominal aortic aneurysm can be life-threatening; all too often, the ailment is discovered during autopsy. Like heart disease, abdominal aortic aneurysm can be considered a silent killer. However, if discovered in time, there is a highly effective surgical procedure available to treat this disorder.

In some people, the layers of tissue that compose the wall of the aorta separate (dissect). Immediate treatment is required for this disorder; often surgical removal of the affected artery is necessary.

Treatment.   Drugs are not of value in treating an abdominal aortic aneurysm. If the aneurysm is small and no symptoms are apparent at the time it is discovered, your physician may recommend a watch-and-wait approach. No changes will be required

in your physical activities, but periodic ultrasound examinations or CT scans will be done to determine if the aneurysm is expanding.

Surgery.   In an emergency or as a preventive measure, your physician may recommend an operation to replace the diseased portion of aorta with an artificial artery made of synthetic material.

The risk of the aneurysm rupturing—a potentially life-threatening event—increases as the aneurysm grows in size. The operation is relatively safe when performed prior to rupture, but less than half of those operated on after rupture survive.

THROMBOPHLEBITIS

Signs and Symptoms
* Tenderness and pain in the affected area;
* Redness and swelling.

When a clot and associated inflammation occur in a vein, the disorder is termed thrombophlebitis. The name comes from Greek words for clot *(thrombos),* vein *(phleps),* and inflammation *(itis).* Often the name is conveniently shortened to phlebitis; if the inflammatory component is minor, it may be termed thrombosis.

Phlebitis usually occurs in an extremity and is most common in leg veins. It may affect either the deep or the superficial veins. The cause often is traceable to prolonged bed rest after an operation, paralysis, a malignancy, or the use of the female hormone estrogen. Sometimes prolonged sitting during a long car or airplane ride will cause thrombosis of a vein.

The Diagnosis. *Superficial Thrombophlebitis.*   When the clot and inflammation occur in a readily visible vein near the surface of the skin, the diagnosis is superficial thrombophlebitis. Your physician can make the preliminary diagnosis on the basis of the discomfort you have in the area and the hard, usually tender, clot that can readily be felt and seen.

Deep-Vein Thrombosis.   When the phlebitis occurs in a vein deep within the leg (or, more rarely, in the arm), the condition is termed deep-vein thrombosis. To reach this diagnosis your physician may choose to perform one or more special tests including an ultrasound examination and making an x-ray after injection of dye into the veins of the leg (venogram).

How Serious Is Thrombophlebitis? Superficial thrombophlebitis rarely leads to serious complications. However, with deep-vein thrombophlebitis, the principal danger is pulmonary embolism (see page 836). If you have several episodes of deep-vein thrombosis, a permanent obstruction could develop in the vein with persistent leg swelling.

Treatment. Treatment of superficial thrombophlebitis usually is limited to the application of heat to the affected area, elevation of the limb, and use of an anti-inflammatory drug. Deep-vein thrombophlebitis is treated by elevating the leg and using anticoagulant medications (see below). Often, hospitalization is required.

Medication. An anticoagulant drug (most likely heparin) may be prescribed for treating the more serious deep-vein thrombophlebitis. It is likely to be administered intravenously. Later, warfarin (Coumadin) may be given orally, perhaps for several months. The purpose of the anticoagulant therapy is to prevent further growth of the clot. Rarely, drugs to dissolve the blood clots may be used.

Surgery. Your physician may recommend surgical treatment. The affected vein or the main vein in the abdomen (vena cava) may be tied off surgically to prevent the clot from coming free and lodging in the lung, causing a pulmonary embolism (see page 836). Sometimes, filters can be inserted into the veins to prevent movement of a blood clot to the lungs.

VARICOSE VEINS

Signs and Symptoms

- Enlarged veins readily seen under the skin of the legs;
- Brownish gray skin discoloration on the ankle;
- Skin ulcers near the ankles.

Incompetent valve

Varicose veins are enlarged veins that are easily seen beneath the surface of the skin of the legs and feet. These twisted veins may be caused by incompetent valves.

Varicose veins are twisted and enlarged veins close to the surface of the skin. Any vein may become varicose (the name comes from the Latin root *varix* for twisted), but the areas most likely to be affected are the legs and feet.

About 1 in 10 Americans has varicose veins. Women are about twice as likely as men to have this disorder.

A possible explanation for the disparity in the occurrence of varicose veins between men and women is the effect of pregnancy. Varicose veins occur as a result of a malfunction of the valves in the veins. Normally, the valves help propel blood to the heart but, as a result of pregnancy, previous thrombophlebitis (see page 838), congenital weakness, obesity, or other cause, the valves can become stretched. When the valves are weakened and are no longer able to close normally, blood pools in the veins. As a result, the veins enlarge and become varicose.

A condition that frequently occurs with varicose veins is the spider-burst leg vein. While not medically significant, the vein patterns seen through the skin may be of cosmetic concern (see Spider-Burst Leg Veins, page 1166).

The Diagnosis. Superficial varicose veins are dilated, twisted, and usually dark blue.

Spider-burst veins are common and are only of cosmetic importance.

You may or may not have mild aching of your legs. Occasionally, the veins deep within the legs are involved. In such cases, you may see significant swelling of your limbs; occasionally skin ulcers will develop.

Your physician will examine your legs while you are upright and also will look for swelling, another indication of a malfunction of the vein valves.

Sometimes, ulcers form. Ulcers caused by varicose veins or malfunction of the valves within the vein ordinarily are located near the ankles and are the result of long-term "waterlogging" of these tissues as the result of increased pressure of blood within the affected veins. Brownish pigmentation usually precedes the development of an ulcer.

How Serious Are Varicose Veins?   Varicose veins tend to become increasingly prominent over time. However, the self-help measures described below may limit their progression and discomfort. In some cases, surgery may be required to correct varicose vein ulcers.

Treatment. *Self-Help.* Avoid standing or sitting for long periods. If your lifestyle is essentially sedentary, be sure to flex your legs and ankles frequently—get up and walk around. At the end of the day, you will find that elevating your legs at least 12 inches above the level of your heart will help relieve any swelling.

A pattern of regular exercise also is valuable. Walking, biking, or swimming will help decrease the pressure in the veins and ease your discomfort. Another important strategy is wearing appropriate hose or socks (see The Value of Supportive Stockings, below). If a skin ulcer caused by an incompetent vein is present, your physician may place a specially treated piece of gauze over the site to aid in healing.

Surgery.   In severe cases, the skin near the varicose veins may become itchy or ulcerated or the pigmentation may change. If inflammation or bleeding occurs, consult your physician.

Some surgeons recommend a stripping or removal of the veins, which may include removal of the varicose tributaries in addition to the main vein. The long-term benefit of varicose vein surgery in appropriate persons is high; in one study, 85 percent of patients were getting along very well at 10 or more years after the operation. Occasionally, if a skin ulcer fails to heal, your surgeon may elect to remove the ulcer and use a skin graft to assist healing.

RAYNAUD'S DISEASE

Signs and Symptoms

- Fingers or toes turn white upon exposure to cold, with an accompanying stinging pain; the skin may turn blue or red before it recovers.

Named after the French physician who described it more than a century ago, Raynaud's disease results from changes in the

---

THE VALUE OF SUPPORTIVE STOCKINGS

If you have varicose veins or deep-vein malfunction, an important component of your self-help program involves wearing the right clothing. You may find that appropriate support hose provide immediate and lasting relief. Use of supportive stockings also may be appropriate during pregnancy.

Elastic bandages or stockings (support hose) compress the varicosities and provide needed support. Your physician may prescribe specially fitted elastic stockings; they will provide the most pressure in the lower portions of your legs. Put them on first thing in the morning, even before you get out of bed. Make sure, however, that the stockings you wear are not tight around the groin or calf of your leg.

circulation in the hands or feet. It is a normal physiological reflex mechanism for the blood vessels in your extremities to narrow when exposed to cold. However, for unknown reasons, in the person with Raynaud's disease this response is exaggerated.

Not only the fingers and toes but also the cheeks, nose, and ears may be affected. About 1 in 20 Americans has Raynaud's disease. Women are 4 to 5 times as likely to develop the problem as men. Typically, the first episode occurs before age 40.

Raynaud's Phenomenon. Raynaud's disease is an independent ailment and is not associated with any other problem or disease. In contrast, Raynaud's phenomenon may be a consequence of scleroderma (see page 1007), exposure to certain chemicals (especially vinyl chloride, used in the rubber industry), or long-term use of vibrating tools such as pneumatic drills, jackhammers, or chain saws.

(See page B-16 for color photograph of Raynaud's disease.)

Acrocyanosis. Another related disorder, acrocyanosis, involves persistent coldness of the fingers, toes, or other affected tissues. Like Raynaud's disease, it is not a consequence of another disorder but, unlike Raynaud's disease, the affected areas are almost always cold. Excessive perspiration often accompanies the feeling of cold.

Treatment. For most people, Raynaud's disease is more of a nuisance than a disability. Only rarely are there any long-term, serious consequences such as gangrene or ulcers of the fingertips.

Prevention. To avoid attacks of Raynaud's disease, adequate protection from the cold is essential. Dress warmly when exposed to cold, protecting the entire body, head, hands, and feet.

Other preventive measures include the following. Do not smoke. The nicotine in tobacco decreases blood flow in your skin. Use insulated glasses for cold drinks. Keep a pair of mittens or gloves adjacent to the freezer to use when handling cold containers. Run your car heater for a few minutes before driving in cold weather. In cases of acrocyanosis, further treatment is rarely necessary.

Medication. Avoid over-the-counter cold remedies and diet pills containing the drug phenylpropanolamine. If you use birth control pills, switch to another method of contraception because these drugs affect your circulation and may make you more prone to attacks.

If these measures are not sufficient, your physician may prescribe a drug to prevent the blood vessel spasms that lead to Raynaud's disease. In extreme cases, a surgical procedure to cut the nerves that control the blood vessels may be done, but the operation (known as sympathectomy) is not always successful and usually is a last resort. A similar procedure called sympathetic blockade can be performed by using an injection of various chemicals into the sympathetic nerve.

BUERGER'S DISEASE

Buerger's disease, named after the American physician Leo Buerger who identified its symptoms in 1908, is a rare disorder in which the blood vessels of the hands and

---

HYPOTENSION

Hypotension is low blood pressure. If your blood pressure falls to dangerously low levels, which can occur during episodes of shock, loss of blood due to hemorrhage, or as a result of certain infections, fevers, cancers, or other disorders, low blood pressure can be life-threatening. In such cases, one of the goals of emergency treatment will be to bring your blood pressure up to more normal levels.

Chronic low blood pressure (your blood pressure is below average but not hazardously so) is not uncommon. It can result from medications given for high blood pressure or from pregnancy, diabetes, or arteriosclerosis.

Postural Hypotension

One potentially dangerous manifestation of low blood pressure is called postural hypotension. A dizziness or faintness that occurs upon standing up quickly from a seated position is the key symptom.

Typically, this is not a serious problem. Sensible precautions will often avoid future incidents. Stand up slowly from a seated position. If episodes seem to occur when you have been in the sun for prolonged periods or after a time of fasting, avoid such circumstances.

However, if you experience persistent fainting spells, consult your physician. Your physician will determine whether there is some underlying cause of the problem.

CHELATION THERAPY

You may have heard the sales pitch: chelation therapy is a kind of chemical Roto-Rooter that can clear obstructing plaques from your arteries.

The truth is that, while chelation therapy has its uses—for example, for ridding your body of toxic amounts of minerals or heavy metals—it has not been proven to be of value in treating arteriosclerosis, atherosclerosis, or other cardiovascular disorders.

Nevertheless, there are clinics across the country that make such claims. Chelating agents (the name comes from the Greek word meaning claw) are able to attach themselves to some toxic substances. One agent, called edetate disodium (EDTA), proponents say, can bind to the calcium in the plaque in your arteries and then remove it. The treatment cycles typically involve 30 to 40 sessions over a number of weeks during which EDTA is administered intravenously. The cost usually runs to several thousand dollars.

We strongly advise against this "therapy." Neither your insurance company nor Medicare will pay for it. It is of no proven worth in preventing or treating cardiovascular disorders. In addition, it can be hazardous. Serious kidney complications and even death have resulted in some cases.

---

feet become diseased. The skin of the hands and feet becomes tender and, over time, pain and ulcers develop and eventually amputation is needed. This occurs because of blockages that form in the blood vessels supplying the extremities.

The disease characteristically strikes men between ages 20 and 40; for unexplained reasons, there appears to be a direct link between smoking or chewing of tobacco and Buerger's disease.

The avoidance of tobacco use usually results in a cure. However, many men with Buerger's disease seem to find it difficult to quit, and amputation of affected areas is the inevitable long-term result.

FROSTBITE

Signs and Symptoms
- Hard, pale, cold skin after prolonged exposure to cold;
- White patches of skin;
- Lack of sensitivity in the area;
- Flesh is red and painful after thawing.

When your skin and the underlying tissues freeze, the condition is called frostbite. The affected areas of the body most often are the hands, feet, nose, and ears.

Frostbite can occur to anyone exposed to very cold temperatures for a sustained period of time (several hours or more), but people with circulatory problems such as atherosclerosis are at greater risk (see page 834).

How Serious Is Frostbite? In severe cases, the flow of blood to the affected area has stopped and the blood vessels have been damaged. In many cases, immediate treatment can reverse the damage, but in some instances amputation of the frostbitten areas is required.

Treatment. *Prevention.* The wearing of proper clothing in cold conditions can prevent most episodes of frostbite. Be sure to protect your hands, feet, nose, and ears. Avoid consuming large amounts of alcohol when you are exposed to prolonged cold.

If you are arriving in a cold climate and your body is used to a warmer one, your body requires some time to adjust to the change. Try gradual ventures into the colder temperatures, allowing your body, and your circulatory system in particular, time to decrease the blood flow to the surface of your skin and to maintain the heat within.

The Warming Process. If your fingers or other areas are frostbitten, prompt treatment is essential. Seek professional care. Never immerse the affected part in hot water (see Frostbite, page 279, for treatment of less-serious frostbite).

Further Treatment. In severe cases in which infection is present, after the affected area has been warmed, antibiotics may be necessary. Bed rest and physical therapy may be appropriate. Do not smoke cigarettes during recovery.

CHAPTER 29

INFECTIOUS DISEASES

CHAPTER CONTENTS

THE WORKINGS OF THE IMMUNE SYSTEM

Your body has many mechanisms that defend you against infectious organisms (see also Understanding Allergy, page 448). Your skin is the first line of defense. If these organisms get past that barrier, the immune system takes up the challenge of eliminating any unwanted invaders.

There are two general categories of immune mechanisms: humoral and cell-mediated.

Humoral Mechanisms.   These are based on certain body proteins, called antibodies, that are found dissolved in the blood and other body fluids. The antibodies are made by plasma cells which are derived from certain white blood cells called B lymphocytes (or B cells), and this happens in response to exposure to a foreign substance. In birds these plasma cells are derived from a partic-

ular structure called the bursa of Fabricius, and hence the term B cell.

Any foreign substance that enters the body—perhaps by injection or through a wound—and causes the manufacture of antibodies is called an antigen. The antibody produced will "fit" the antigen much like a key fits a lock and will neutralize that foreign substance or render it harmless. Antibodies are specific: each is effective against any antigen that caused its creation.

A good example of how antigens create antibodies to protect our bodies is the immunization for prevention of tetanus. Tetanus toxoid in a carefully determined amount is injected into the muscle. (A toxoid is a toxin that has been rendered harmless to your body but is still capable of producing immunity.) The body recognizes the tetanus toxoid and responds by creating antibodies that will neutralize the toxic substances pro-

Your immune system reacts to foreign invaders (antigens) such as infectious organisms. The immune response aims to neutralize or destroy the antigen, thus rendering it harmless. The antigen may activate a kind of white blood cell, a B cell (lymphocyte), which circulates in the bloodstream. In humoral immunity, B cells produce plasma cells which, in turn, produce antibodies that neutralize the antigen. In other situations, so-called memory B cells "remember" the antigen and rapidly produce antibodies to inactivate the antigen.

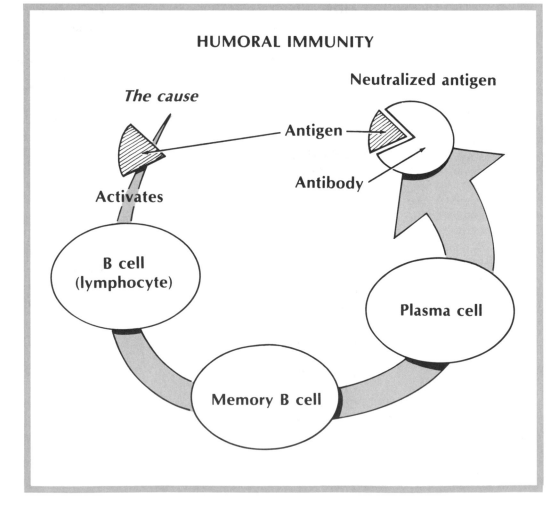

HUMORAL IMMUNITY

The cause

Neutralized antigen

Antigen

Antibody

Activates

B cell (lymphocyte)

Memory B cell

Plasma cell

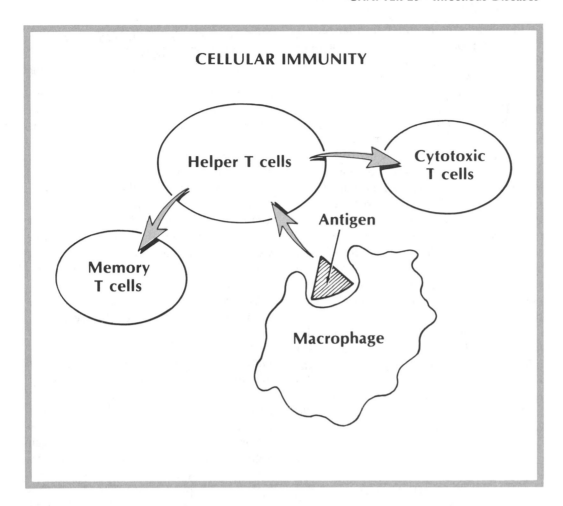

CELLULAR IMMUNITY

Helper T cells

Cytotoxic T cells

Memory T cells

Antigen

Macrophage

A second type of immune response is called cell-mediated immunity. In this type, antigens (foreign invaders) are ingested (engulfed) by macrophages. This activates the helper T cells, which aid in development of cytotoxic T cells (which kill antigens directly) and memory T cells (which stimulate an immune response upon re-exposure to the same antigen).

duced by the tetanus organisms. Within a few weeks, these antibodies begin to circulate in the body's fluids and will persist in measurable amounts for many years.

Once the body has learned to produce a particular antibody, it can resume production of that antibody quite rapidly. Thus, if a person has had the initial series of immunization injections for tetanus, a single injection 5 to 10 years later (booster shot) can stimulate the appearance of protective amounts of antibodies in the blood within a few days.

Cell-Mediated Mechanisms. These are based on the actions of phagocytes and other white blood cells. These cells can dissolve or engulf and destroy viruses, bacteria, fungi, and cells foreign to the body.

The white blood cells that are involved in this defense are a type of lymphocyte called T cells because they are derived from the thymus gland. About 70 percent of the T cells are designated helper-inducer cells and the remaining 20 to 30 percent are cytotoxic cells.

The helper cells function to increase the number of cells (macrophages) that can engulf or dissolve foreign particles in response to an infection. Neutrophils, another type of white blood cell, also function in this fashion. They are greatly increased in number during infections such as pneumonia or appendicitis. The helper-inducer cells also facilitate the production of antibodies by stimulating growth and activity of B cells.

Lymphocytes are found in the bone marrow, in the spleen, circulating in the blood, and in the lymph nodes. The lymph nodes are collections of lymphocytes held together by connective or fibrous tissue. Some nodes are located in the neck, groin, and armpits where they can be felt if they become firm and enlarged in the course of a disease. They often are mistakenly called lymph glands. Other lymph nodes are found in the abdomen and at the roots of the lungs.

Lymph is a nearly colorless fluid that runs in channels in all parts of the body to and through the lymph nodes and, ultimately, into the bloodstream. The lymph nodes constitute a partial barrier to organisms that may be traveling in the lymph. For instance, if a virulent streptococcus bacterium penetrates the skin by way of a crack between the toes of a person with athlete's foot, it can multiply and travel up the leg in the lymph channels. These channels carrying the infection may be seen beneath the skin as red streaks, sometimes incorrectly termed blood poisoning (also called lymphangitis, see page 1175). The lymph nodes in the groin of that leg become swollen and tender while keeping the infection in check at that level. On the other hand, in some diseases that cause multiplication and mobilization of lymphocytes and that involve the entire body, such as infectious mononucleosis, all of the lymph nodes and the spleen may become enlarged and can be felt by the physician during a physical examination.

Your immune system is a complex defense system for suppressing and eliminating infections. At the same time, infectious organisms have complex offense systems. The result is a constant battle between your body and infection—a battle your body usually wins, but not always.

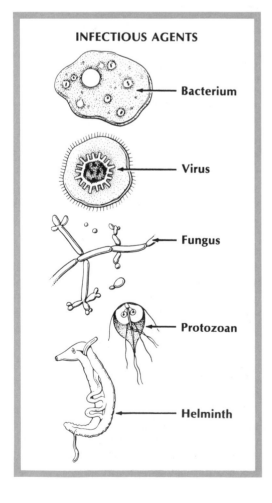

INFECTIOUS AGENTS

Bacterium

Virus

Fungus

Protozoan

Helminth

TYPES OF INFECTIOUS AND PARASITIC AGENTS

Agents that can invade your body live everywhere—in the air; on dust particles, food, and plants; on and in animals and humans; in soil and water; and on virtually every other surface. They range from microscopic organisms to larger parasites.

The vast majority of these organisms do not produce disease, but some do. This majority is usually kept under control by your immune system but, if that system becomes weakened or you encounter an organism to which you have not built up a resistance, illness results.

The following are the basic types of organisms that cause infectious diseases.

Bacteria.   Bacteria are one-cell organisms that are visible only under a microscope. They appear as slender rods or groups of round cells, live without need for other organisms, and are able to live and multiply by subdivision. When infectious bacteria gain entry to your body, they multiply and may produce powerful chemicals, called toxins, that damage specific cells in the tissue they have invaded and that cause you to become ill. A few of the more common groups of bacteria that cause disease are staphylococci, streptococci, chlamydia, haemophilus, gonococci, and rickettsia.

Viruses.   A virus is not able to reproduce on its own. In its simplest form, it is a capsule containing genetic material. When it invades your body, it enters some of your cells and takes them over, instructing these host cells to manufacture the parts the virus needs in order to multiply. In the process, the host cell eventually is destroyed. Polio, AIDS, and the common cold are among the many ailments caused by viruses.

Fungi.   Molds, yeasts, and mushrooms all are types of fungi. Obviously, mushrooms are not infectious, but certain yeasts and molds can be. These single-cell organisms are slightly larger than bacteria. Of the thousands that are harmless or even helpful (yeast causes bread to rise), only about 100 cause disease. *Candida* is one example. It can produce thrush, an infection of the mouth and throat, in infants and in persons who have received antibiotics or have impaired immunity (see page 18).

Protozoa. Protozoa are single-cell organisms that may live within you as a parasite. Often these organisms spend part of their life cycle outside of humans, living in food, soil, water, or insects. The protozoa that cause malaria are an example. Many protozoa reside in the intestinal tract and are harmless, although some may cause disease.

Helminths. The word "helminth" comes from the Greek word meaning worm. These are the larger parasites. If they enter your body, they take up residence in your intestinal tract, lungs, liver, skin, or even brain, where they live off the nutrients in your body. The most common helminths are the tapeworms and roundworms.

ANTIBACTERIAL AGENTS

Before penicillin was discovered, very few medications were available to combat bacterial infections. Now, however, a wide range of antibacterial agents are available to treat infectious diseases, and more are continually being developed.

Most antibacterial agents are antibiotics (substances produced by microorganisms), but not all. Some are synthetic chemicals. All of the antibacterial agents may cause undesirable and sometimes serious effects.

Bacterial Specificity
Each antibiotic works against specific types of bacteria. Some affect only one or two kinds; others affect many. When your physician first suspects you have an infectious disease, he or she may take samples of your blood, pus, urine, stool, or sputum to try to identify the organism and to determine how resistant or susceptible that particular strain will be to different antibiotics.

It usually takes at least 24 hours to get the results of these tests. Therefore, depending on the diagnosis, your physician may prescribe one of the antibiotics that attack a broad array of bacteria. Then, the culture results may suggest a change to a more appropriate antibiotic.

Topically vs. Orally Administered Antibiotics
For certain localized infections of the eye, ear, or skin, antibiotics are applied topically as a solution or ointment. However, in most cases, antibiotics are given orally, intramuscularly, or intravenously. After an antibiotic (or any drug) is administered it enters your bloodstream from your intestine (if taken orally), from muscles (if given intramuscularly), or directly (if given intravenously). Antibiotics are given intravenously or intramuscularly only if the infection is serious or the drug is not properly absorbed when taken orally.

The Antibiotic at Work
Once absorbed into your bloodstream, the antibiotic circulates rapidly through your whole body (it takes only about a minute for your heart to circulate all of the blood in your body). However, the antibiotic will only act where it encounters particular bacteria. It does this by either killing the bacteria or by preventing them from multiplying, depending on the type of antibiotic and the dosage.

Kinds of Antibiotics
Some antibiotics—such as the penicillins and cephalosporins—kill bacteria by interfering with their ability to form cell walls, which ultimately causes their death. Most other antibacterial agents—including the aminoglycosides (such as gentamicin and streptomycin), the tetracyclines, the sulfonamides, and the macrolides (such as erythromycin)—interfere with chemicals the bacteria need to multiply and survive. This allows your body's natural immune system to control and eliminate them.

When bacteria are exposed to an antibiotic they may, over time, develop a resistance or tolerance to that antibiotic. This can happen quickly or slowly. The development of resistance does not change the appearance under the microscope or any other characteristic of that strain of bacteria. Whether or not a given strain of bacteria is resistant to an antibiotic can be determined only by sensitivity tests.

Because antibiotic resistance develops in the bacteria in our environment, some antibiotics have become less useful than they were in the past. Newer antibiotics are constantly being developed but we can expect that they, too, will become less effective in a number of years. Infections that are acquired while a person is in a hospital are particularly likely to be caused by an antibiotic-resistant organism.

ANTIVIRAL DRUGS

In the last 2 decades, drugs that have an effect on viruses have been introduced into medical practice. No drug completely eradicates a viral infection, but it can decrease the severity and duration of the infection. Viruses multiply extremely rapidly, so antiviral drugs must be given very early in an infection or as a preventive measure (prophylactically).

Acyclovir
The most commonly prescribed antiviral drug is acyclovir, which is used in the treatment of diseases caused by the herpes virus, such as genital and oral herpes, encephalitis, chickenpox, and shingles. Usually, the drug is given orally. If the patient has a weakened immune system or a severe infection, it may be given intravenously.

Amantadine
This antiviral drug helps to prevent or to ease the symptoms of influenza (see page 853).

How Antiviral Drugs Work
A virus cannot multiply on its own; it needs to invade the body's cells and cause the host cells to manufacture the components of the virus. Some antiviral drugs work by changing the genetic material of the host cell so that the virus cannot use the host's genetic material for its own reproduction. Other drugs block the enzyme activity of the host cell. Amantadine blocks the influenza virus from entering the host cell. However, antiviral drugs may have adverse side effects, so use caution.

ANTIFUNGAL DRUGS

Infections caused by fungi, such as athlete's foot, jock itch, ringworm, and candidiasis, rarely heal without some drug therapy. There are several drugs that are effective in the treatment of fungal infections. Some only should be applied topically; others may be taken orally or given as an injection.

Antifungal drugs act upon the cell wall of the fungus, damaging it and allowing the contents of the cell to leak out, which kills the cell. When given topically, antifungal drugs rarely have adverse effects.

GENERALIZED INFECTIONS

Among the challenges to your immune system are a wide range of diseases. Some are bacterial; some are viral; and still others have other causes.

In the following pages we will discuss a number of the most common infectious diseases, ranging from such familiar childhood ailments as measles and chickenpox to today's headliner, the deadly AIDS.

Note that in most cases in which an infectious disorder predominately affects only one organ or body system (such as the heart, brain, or skin), the disease is discussed in the chapter devoted to that subject.

AIDS

Signs and Symptoms
- Prolonged unexplained fatigue;
- Unexplained swollen lymph nodes;
- Fever lasting more than 10 days;
- Night sweats;
- Unexplained weight loss;
- Purplish or discolored lesions on the skin or mucous membrane that do not go away;
- A persistent, unexplained cough or sore throat;
- Shortness of breath;
- Persistent colds;
- Persistent, severe diarrhea;
- Oral yeast infection (candidiasis);
- Easy bruising or unexplained bleeding;
- Confusion, dementia, and, finally, coma.

AIDS, which stands for acquired immune deficiency syndrome, is a combination of symptoms that result from destruction of the body's immune system. It was first recognized in the United States in 1981.

Normally, your immune system produces white blood cells and antibodies that attack infectious agents that enter the body. These "attackers" are called T-cell lymphocytes.

In the person who has AIDS, however, a virus called HIV-1 (which stands for human immunodeficiency virus type I) has entered the blood's helper T-cell lymphocytes and has multiplied, destroying these health-promoting cells. (For further discussion of types of lymphocytes, see The Workings of the Immune System, page 844.) In the person who has AIDS, this destruction has proceeded to a point such that the immune system has little ability to defend itself, and various infections and tumors are thus allowed to develop. Other names for this virus are HTLV-III (human T-cell lymphotropic virus type III), LAV (lymphadenopathy-associated virus), and ARV (AIDS-related virus).

The terminology used in this disease is confusing but may be more understandable in light of the sequence of events. The virus enters the body in one of several recognized ways including via shared needles among intravenous drug users, through sexual intercourse, and from mother to unborn child. The virus enters the helper T cells where it multiplies. Within the next several months, the body develops antibodies to the virus. Blood tests (ELISA and Western blot; see page 850) thus become positive. There may be symptoms for 1 to 2 weeks; these begin a few months after the virus enters the body. The symptoms resemble those of infectious mononucleosis and may include swollen lymph nodes, sore throat, fever, malaise, and skin rash. Then, the symptoms subside and, over the next several years, there may be few or no symptoms.

During this period, the amount of virus in the body increases, slowly at first and more rapidly later. Simultaneously, the number of helper T cells decreases. The person is then considered to be infected with the virus that causes AIDS but not to have AIDS. However, this person can infect others at any point in the course of the disease.

As the helper T cells are lost, the body's immune defenses slowly fail and the body gradually becomes vulnerable to various infections and tumors. When symptoms such as swollen lymph nodes and low-grade fever, which herald impairment of the immune system, occur, the stage of the dis-

order is termed AIDS-related complex (ARC). Still later, when the immune defenses are greatly impaired, the full-fledged syndrome, designated AIDS, which includes an "opportunistic infection," is present. (An opportunistic infection is one caused by bacteria or viruses that are able to invade the body only when its immune defenses are severely lacking.)

The full effects of AIDS may appear only 5 to 10 years after the original infection with the virus; death usually follows within 2 to 3 years after the appearance of these effects. This is a newly recognized disease, however, and as further observations are made in the next several years our understanding of the natural course of this disease may change.

AIDS is now epidemic. A decade ago, AIDS was unknown in this country. Today, it is a major public health concern. From June 1981 through June 1990, more than 140,000 Americans were diagnosed as having AIDS. Of this group, more than half have died, most within 4 years of showing symptoms of the disease. Many others now carry the virus in their bodies and will ultimately develop AIDS. According to estimates by the World Health Organization, there are more than 500,000 cases of AIDS worldwide. Currently, 1.0 to 1.5 million people in the United States and 5 to 10 million worldwide are estimated to be carriers of the virus.

It is likely that the number of affected persons will continue to increase considerably. The greatest number of AIDS cases are found in two groups: homosexual or bisexual men; and male and female intravenous drug users who share needles. Others at risk are the sexual partners of those at risk of contracting AIDS, an infant born to a mother who carries the AIDS virus, and persons who received blood transfusions or clotting factor preparations (blood product made from multiple blood donations) between 1977 and April 1985, prior to the establishment of standard screening for the virus in donated blood.

We want to emphasize that the disease can be passed from men to women or from women to men through sexual intercourse. The use of a condom in either homosexual or heterosexual intercourse will help reduce transmission of the virus, but the protection is not perfect.

How Do You Get AIDS? AIDS is not a highly contagious disease. For the virus to be transmitted, it must find its way from the blood or semen of the infected person into the bloodstream of the uninfected one. In sexual intercourse, this transmission occurs when semen comes in contact with mucous membranes (the membranes lining the mouth, vagina, or rectum) of another individual. Then, the virus must be able to enter small abrasions or cuts in the mucous membranes before it is able to reach the bloodstream and infect the lymphocytes. Small quantities of blood may be passed from an infected to an uninfected person when a syringe for administration of an illegal drug is shared. Although the virus has been found in saliva, sweat, and tears, it is present in these fluids at very low concentrations and scientists believe that the virus is not transmitted by exposure to the tears or saliva of an infected person. Physicians, nurses, dentists, and laboratory workers who give injections, who handle blood, or who may experience needle sticks are at some risk, but the number of infections acquired in the care of AIDS patients has been exceedingly small. In fact, the occupational risk to health-care workers for acquiring hepatitis B (see page 650) in this fashion is considerably greater.

The HIV is relatively easy to kill and cannot live very long outside of the body. It is not possible to acquire this virus from contact with inanimate objects such as toilet seats or doorknobs. Mosquitoes do not spread AIDS, just as they do not spread measles.

The Diagnosis. The diagnosis of an infection by HIV is suggested first by the person being in one of the recognized groups of persons known to have a greater frequency of the disease. The diagnosis of ARC (AIDS-related complex) is suggested by a series of debilitating symptoms as listed at the beginning of this section. If, in addition, a defect of the immune system is found and certain opportunistic infections have occurred, the person is then said to have AIDS. The particular manifestation of the diminished capacity of the immune mechanisms will depend on the infectious agents present in the individual and multiple other factors—hence, the variable manifestations of AIDS.

The combination of symptoms that allows a physician to make the diagnosis of AIDS usually appears 5 to 10 years or more after the person acquires the infection.

A common opportunistic infection in AIDS is *Pneumocystis carinii* pneumonia. A wide variety of other infectious diseases also infect AIDS patients.

Kaposi's sarcoma is a rare form of cancer that occurs in elderly people or in persons whose immune system is impaired (see page 1172).

At present, there is no readily available test that directly detects the presence of HIV-1. The tests currently being used detect antibodies produced by the body in response to HIV-1; these do not become positive until the virus has been multiplying in the body for a month or more. Thus, a negative test is no guarantee that the person does not carry the virus. The most common test is the enzyme-linked immunosorbent assay (ELISA) which is performed on a blood sample. This test is very sensitive and detects almost all persons infected with the virus except during the first few months after the virus has entered their body. On the other hand, in a very small percentage of cases this test may indicate the presence of infection but in fact the test result may be the consequence of rheumatoid arthritis or some other unidentified factor (called a false-positive test). Having a false-positive test can be extremely distressing.

Generally, the diagnosis of AIDS is not made until a positive test by the ELISA method is confirmed by the Western blot test. This test is less sensitive than the ELISA method (and thus it may fail to identify the virus in some infected individuals) but it almost never gives a false-positive result.

Before being tested, it is important to discuss with your physician or health authority the arrangements for the reporting of the results in the event that the test confirms the presence of the infection. Most states require a positive result to be reported to the state health department.

Treatment. In treating AIDS or ARC, supportive care, including moral support, good nutrition, and a generally hygienic mode of living, is important.

Medication. The medications available for inhibiting the growth of the virus are largely experimental at this stage. The first drug with some proven effectiveness is azidothymidine (AZT) which seems to in-

WHEN A LOVED ONE HAS AIDS

AIDS is a devastating and debilitating disease. Dealing with the effects and consequences of AIDS is difficult not only for the patient but also for his or her family and friends. Despite the advances being made with new medications such as azidothymidine (AZT), there is no cure for AIDS. So the emotional and physical support of family and friends is vital in helping those with the disease to lead the most nearly normal life possible.

There are many things you can do and should know if you have a friend or relative who is stricken with AIDS. First and most important: know the facts (see page 848); many misconceptions exist about this disease.

Conflicting Feelings Are Natural

Hearing that a friend or relative has AIDS is bound to cause conflicting emotions. It is common to blame a patient or an individual with AIDS for the high-risk behavior of many who have contracted the disease. You may disapprove of his or her lifestyle, or you may be forced to confront that person's lifestyle for the first time. Realizing that someone you care about may die can bring out unresolved pain and problems between you. Especially because most AIDS patients are in the prime of their lives when the disease develops, the effects of the illness and the prospect of death are hard to face.

Try To Be Positive

Try to focus on the positive aspects of your relationship—who the individual is, why you care about him or her, and what you can do to help. Do not feel that you need to keep your feelings to yourself. Discuss them with the patient and others, including perhaps clergy, counselors, or members of support groups.

Do Not Go It Alone

You cannot care for an AIDS patient alone. It is important to establish a network of professionals, friends, and relatives who can provide help and support. Depending on his or her health, the patient should make as many of the personal decisions as possible.

It may be helpful to designate one or two people to serve as contacts for health-care and other professionals, friends, and relatives who are concerned but not as involved in the day-to-day care of the individual. This person, or persons, also can look after the patient's business matters such as bills, insurance, and correspondence. You may want to consult an attorney about having one person assume power of attorney with the right to make decisions on behalf of the patient if he or she is incapacitated.

A diagnosis of AIDS can have an effect on insurance, employment, education, and housing. So respect the person's right to privacy and let him or her decide who should know about the condition. Remember that the disease should not exclude someone from receiving care or services. The American Medical Association, other professional groups, federal law and many state regulations state that you must not discriminate against AIDS patients.

Home Care

In providing home care, create an environment that is pleasant and comfortable.

Maintain the person's personal hygiene. This is vital. Also, the individual should bathe regularly, especially if he or she suffers from fevers or night sweats. Hospital or home health-care workers can teach you the rollover method for bathing a person and changing sheets without getting the person out of bed. Oral hygiene is also important. If a toothbrush causes bleeding, use a washcloth or sponge-tipped swab to clean the teeth and gums, or use a mouth rinse of warm salt water or dilute hydrogen peroxide.

Am I at Risk?

You cannot contract AIDS by coming into casual contact with a patient, but do avoid direct unprotected contact with the individual's blood, semen, vaginal secretions, or other secretions that contain blood because these are infectious. Do not share razors, toothbrushes, or other items that may carry blood. Clothing, sheets, and towels that carry bodily secretions, vomit, or diarrhea should be removed and washed separately in hot, soapy water. If secretions spill onto a hard surface, wash them off with a 1:10 solution of household bleach to kill the virus.

Wash your hands before and after any contact with the patient. When giving injections, cleaning the teeth, or washing the anal or genital areas, use disposable vinyl or latex gloves. If you handle feces, vomit, or urine, wear gloves and a shoulder-to-knee apron. If the possibility exists that secretions may splash into your mouth or eyes, wear a mask or protective glasses. If you use needles and syringes as part of the person's care, use special (puncture-proof) containers to dispose of them and never bend, break, or recap a needle.

Remember that an individual with AIDS is not just a patient. He or she also is a person who needs affection and needs to carry on as normal a life as possible for as long as possible.

hibit the virus at least partially. It slows the production of the virus and thereby relieves symptoms but it does have major side effects. AZT is not a cure but it has prolonged many lives. Other drugs are currently under investigation.

Many unproven treatments are being advocated. This is a most unfortunate situation because most of these treatments will likely prove to be of no value. Meanwhile, considerable money will have been spent, some going to unscrupulous persons who exploit the AIDS victim's situation by selling material with little or no real promise of effectiveness. Furthermore, because the course of AIDS and its manifestations are so variable, a drug that confers no real benefit may falsely acquire a reputation for being helpful. A seeming improvement in condition may actually be a usual variation in the course of the disease but may be mistaken for a curative effect of the drug. This is the reason that it is important to have statistically valid controlled studies—that is, patients on one plan of treatment being carefully compared with comparable patients on another plan (or, if circumstances permit, on no treatment other than supportive measures).

Some of the medications prescribed for the person with AIDS are intended to control the opportunistic infections associated with the disease. For instance, the occurrence of *Pneumocystis carinii* pneumonia can be decreased by use of inhaled pentamidine.

A vaccine is being sought, but the AIDS virus is able to change its characteristics rapidly and this, among other obstacles, makes the development of an effective vaccine difficult. It is doubtful that an effective vaccine will be available for a number of years.

INFECTIOUS MONONUCLEOSIS

Signs and Symptoms
- Fever;
- Sort throat;
- Loss of appetite, fatigue and weakness, sore muscles;
- Swollen lymph nodes;
- Pain on the upper left side of the abdomen.

Infectious mononucleosis (mono) is also called Epstein-Barr virus infection after the herpes virus that causes the disease. This virus may affect anyone, but the infection most often occurs in people between the ages of 10 and 35, especially teenagers. It can occur as an epidemic or in single cases, and it is believed to be spread by infectious saliva. The incubation period for the disease is usually 7 to 14 days in children and adolescents. The incubation period is longer for adults; at times it may be 30 to 50 days.

The Diagnosis. Infectious mononucleosis has a wide variety of symptoms. You may experience fever, sore throat, swollen lymph nodes, or, in some cases, enlargement of the spleen. Nausea, hepatitis, jaundice, headache, stiffness, sensitivity to light, chest pain, cough, difficulty breathing, tachycardia (rapid heartbeat), and arrhythmias also may be caused by the virus. Loss of appetite, muscle pain, fatigue, and weakness often are present, and some individuals have a red rash. This range of symptoms can make diagnosis difficult.

If mononucleosis is suspected, your physician may do a monospot test to verify the presence of the virus in your bloodstream.

How Serious Is Infectious Mononucleosis? Mononucleosis is not a serious disease, except in rare cases in which the spleen becomes severely enlarged and ruptures or when other vital organs such as the brain or heart are infected. Persons with infectious mononucleosis do need support and understanding because, even though most of the symptoms are not severely debilitating in themselves, the disease may cause prolonged fatigue and weakness. In most cases, the fever, swollen lymph nodes, and enlargement of the spleen disappear after 10 days; however, it may take 2 to 3 months before you feel completely back to normal.

Treatment. There is no specific antiviral treatment for infectious mononucleosis. Bed rest is the primary recommendation. Generally, do not expect to return to your normal routine for at least 2 to 3 weeks. Drinking plenty of water and fruit juices helps to relieve the fever and sore throat and keeps you from becoming dehydrated. Aspirin and, for a sore throat, gargling (one-half teaspoon of salt in a glass of warm water) several times a day are suggested.

The sore throat of infectious mononucleosis occasionally is aggravated by a strepto-

CHRONIC FATIGUE SYNDROME

Recently, there has been a renewed interest in people who suffer chronically from fatigue, weakness, decreased ability to concentrate, and poor memory. In some of these cases, tests for the Epstein-Barr virus have been positive, leading some physicians to diagnose chronic infectious mononucleosis.

A number of things can produce fatigue, weakness, and loss of memory, including stress, an unidentified disease, or a psychological condition such as depression. Experts have developed the term chronic fatigue syndrome to designate this vague group of symptoms. (A syndrome is simply a collection of symptoms.) No definite cause for the chronic fatigue syndrome has been found, although emotional and psychological factors may play a role. Usually, there is no underlying viral infection.

Certain criteria have been proposed that should be met before the diagnosis of chronic fatigue syndrome can be made. First, you must suffer from recent and extreme fatigue and weakness that has impaired your ability to work for 6 months. All other known diseases, infections, or psychiatric illnesses that might cause these symptoms must be ruled out. In addition, you must have six of the following criteria: 1) low-grade fever (99.5°F to 100.5°F) or chills; 2) sore throat; 3) painful lymph nodes in the neck or armpits; 4) general weakness; 5) prolonged fatigue following previously tolerated exercise; 6) generalized headaches; 7) unexplained muscle soreness; 8) pain that moves from one joint to another, without evidence of redness or swelling; 9) forgetfulness, irritability, and confusion; 10) sleep disturbance.

Finally, your physician must be able to identify the presence of two of the following physical signs: 1) low-grade fever (99.5 to 100.5°F); 2) small, tender lymph nodes in the neck or armpits; 3) redness of the throat, without evidence of a bacterial infection.

For chronic fatigue syndrome, the symptoms are treated and allowed to run their course.

The key question is whether these symptoms represent a new disease or are a collection of complaints without clear cause. We think that this is not a new disease. Many people who claimed to have symptoms of fatigue underwent tests that showed they had been exposed to the Epstein-Barr virus. However, further analysis has shown that many people exposed to the Epstein-Barr virus are free of symptoms. And not all those who do say they have symptoms have been exposed to the virus.

The chronic fatigue syndrome is just that—a syndrome or collection of symptoms. In most cases, there is no serious underlying disease causing it.

---

coccal infection which requires treatment with an antibiotic.

See your physician immediately if you experience sudden sharp pains in the left upper side of your abdomen. This could mean a ruptured spleen. This is rare, but if it should occur, emergency surgery may be required.

INFLUENZA

Signs and Symptoms
- Fever and chills;
- Sore throat;
- Cough;
- Muscular aches and pains;
- Fatigue and weakness;
- Nasal congestion.

Like the common cold, influenza—or flu, as it is commonly called—is primarily spread between people indoors, especially at schools, nursing homes, and other places where large numbers of people gather. Outbreaks usually occur in the winter and early spring. Unfortunately, many viral diseases that are not influenza also are called flu, which causes considerable confusion.

There are three types of influenza viruses. All of them are spread from person to person by inhalation of infected droplets from the air. Type A, originally found in swine, usually is responsible for the large influenza epidemics. Types B and C are not as widespread: type B causes smaller, more localized outbreaks, and type C is less common and usually causes only a mild illness.

Types B and C are fairly stable viruses. Type A is constantly changing, with new strains appearing regularly. This results in a new epidemic every few years, and the disease arises in a number of areas concurrently. Every 10 to 40 years, influenza breaks out as a pandemic, affecting people all over the world.

The Diagnosis. Influenza usually comes on suddenly, causing fever (usually of 101°F to 102°F, but sometimes reaching 106°F), chills, muscular aches and pains, weakness, malaise, nasal congestion, flushed face, dry cough, and sore throat. All of the symptoms are similar to those of the common cold but usually are more severe. Influenza typically develops after an incubation period of 1 to 4 days, and the fever may last for 3 to 5 days, although it can last as little as 1 day or as long as a week.

Diagnosing influenza with complete certainty is difficult because it is similar to many mild illnesses that are accompanied by a fever. If your physician suspects influenza, he or she may be able to isolate the virus from throat washings or may do a blood test to look for antibodies to the virus. These tests are mainly of value to public health officials who can better advise the public if they know the character and extent of the disease in a community.

How Serious Is Influenza? Influenza itself generally is not dangerous and usually lasts only for 1 day to a week. However, complications can follow influenza, such as acute sinusitis, bronchitis, and pneumonia. Pneumococcal pneumonia is the most common complication; staphylococcal pneumonia is also serious and can lead to death. Elderly people and people with weakened immune systems or severe medical disorders are at a greater risk and should be vaccinated (see Influenza [Flu] Shots, this page).

Treatment. There is no specific treatment for influenza. Bed rest is important, as are proper nutrition and drinking lots of liquids. Inhaling steam or taking a sedative cough medicine may temporarily relieve the cough, and analgesics help to decrease the fever and muscle soreness. The antiviral drug amantadine, which is taken orally, may be helpful in relieving the signs and symptoms of influenza. Antibiotics do not provide relief and should be used only to treat the complications caused by bacterial infection.

Prevention. The primary way to prevent influenza is by use of influenza vaccine each fall. Amantadine hydrochloride often is also effective at greatly decreasing the risk of infection. However, if used for prevention, it must be started before or immediately after exposure to the influenza A virus. It usually is prescribed only for those persons at risk for a severe case of the disease or complications. Note that amantadine only protects against influenza A, but the vaccine protects against both the A and B influenza strains. Neither prevents other types of viral diseases.

LYME DISEASE

Signs and Symptoms
- Characteristic red rash at the site of a tick bite;
- Headache;
- Chills and fever;
- Body aches;
- Joint inflammation and arthritis.

INFLUENZA (FLU) SHOTS

Each year, a vaccine is recommended by the Centers for Disease Control based on a prediction as to which strain of influenza virus will be prevalent. We highly recommend immunization for people with impaired immune systems or with serious illnesses such as chronic heart or kidney disease, lung disease or impaired ability to breathe (including heavy smokers), cystic fibrosis, chronic anemia (such as sickle cell anemia), or severe diabetes. Elderly people, especially those over age 65, also should be vaccinated. Health-care workers, police officers and fire fighters, and others on whom public safety depends should receive immunization.

The vaccine is given as one injection into the shoulder in the early fall, just before the flu season begins. Children may sometimes receive the vaccine in two separate injections, 1 to 2 weeks apart. In subsequent years, only a booster shot each fall is needed. If you are subsequently exposed to the flu, the shot does not guarantee that you will not get the disease, but most likely you will have only a mild illness. Because the virus changes so rapidly, however, protection is not permanent, and you must get a new vaccination each season.

The vaccine may cause some soreness at the site where the shot is given. A very small percentage of people run a slight fever and have minor muscular aches beginning 6 to 24 hours after immunization. These discomforts may last for a day or two, but severe reactions are rare. However, people who are sensitive to eggs and egg products may experience a severe allergic reaction, and they probably should not be immunized. If you are pregnant, wait until after your third month before being vaccinated.

Named after a large outbreak among children in Lyme, Connecticut, this disease is caused by an organism (spirochete) that lives in a certain type of tick. From May to October the tick is found throughout the United States, especially on the east and west coasts and in Wisconsin and Minnesota.

The Diagnosis. Lyme disease is difficult to diagnose because it mimics various other diseases. A characteristic red rash usually occurs at the site of the tick bite, followed by flu-like symptoms such as headache, chills, fever, and body aches and stiffness (see color photograph, page B-14). However, the bite may go entirely unnoticed. A few weeks to months later, muscle paralysis, joint inflammation, various neurological symptoms, and sometimes heart palpitations and heart block (see also page 819) may occur.

Your physician will run a blood test to look for antibodies to the bacteria. However, the test is not always conclusive.

How Serious Is Lyme Disease? If caught in its early stages, the disease can be eliminated with use of antibiotics. If not treated early, complications involving the joints, heart, and brain can occur.

Treatment. *Medication.* Therapy consists of antibiotics. Aspirin helps to relieve joint inflammation.

Prevention. When walking in wooded or grassy areas, wear shoes, long pants tucked into socks, and long-sleeved shirts. Check yourself and your pets often for ticks. If you find any, remove them immediately by using a tweezers. Do not yank or crush the tick, but pull carefully and steadily.

ROCKY MOUNTAIN SPOTTED FEVER

Signs and Symptoms
- Chills and fever;
- Severe headache;
- Widespread aches and pains;
- Restlessness;
- Red rash occurring between days 2 and 6 of fever.

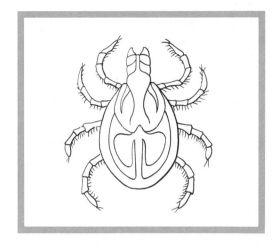

Ixodes dammini **tick carries the Lyme disease bacterium.**

Rocky Mountain spotted fever is caused by the organism *Rickettsia rickettsii* and is transmitted to humans by wood ticks in the western United States, by the dog tick in the eastern United States, and by other ticks in the southern United States and Central and South America. In the United States, it occurs primarily during the late spring and early summer and is most common in the eastern part of the country.

The Diagnosis. Three to 10 days after being bitten by an infected tick, you experience nausea, headache, loss of appetite, and a sore throat. As the disease develops, fever, chills, tenderness and soreness in the bones and muscles, restlessness, insomnia, abdominal pain, nausea, and vomiting occur. You may have a cough and, possibly, delirium, lethargy, and stupor. Between the second and sixth days of the fever, a red rash appears on your wrists and ankles and spreads up your arms and legs to your chest. Your physician may do a blood test to confirm the diagnosis or may stain a specimen of the rash to detect the presence of the causative organism.

How Serious Is Rocky Mountain Spotted Fever? In mild cases and when treated promptly, Rocky Mountain spotted fever is fairly benign. Even without treatment, mild cases will disappear after 2 weeks. However, in severe cases the disease can be serious or even fatal, especially in elderly people.

Treatment. *Medication.* If use is begun early, antibiotics usually eliminate the fever quickly. Prompt treatment is important because the disease may progress rapidly.

TYPHUS

Caused by *Rickettsia prowazekii,* typhus is transmitted to humans by lice or, in a milder form, by rat fleas. It is found primarily in persons in crowded living conditions that favor heavy infestations of vermin. It is very rare in the United States. About 2 weeks after exposure, cough, headache, and chest pain occur, followed by a sudden high fever and chills. The person may become delirious or fall into a stupor.

A positive blood test confirms the diagnosis. In children and young adults the disease is usually benign, but it may lead to death in elderly people. It is treated by antibiotics. If a case is identified, attempts should be made to eradicate body lice in the community.

TYPHOID FEVER

Signs and Symptoms
- Fever;
- Headache;
- Weakness and fatigue;
- Sore throat;
- Cough;
- Diarrhea.

Emergency Symptoms
- Sudden drop in temperature;
- Shock characterized by decrease in urination, light-headed feeling particularly on standing up, lethargy, and change in level of consciousness.

Typhoid fever is caused by the bacterium *Salmonella typhi.* It is contracted by consuming contaminated food or fluids. It is rare in developed countries. The bacteria penetrate the wall of the small intestine and cause inflammation of the lymph nodes and the spleen. Chronic carriers are possible sources of the disease. These are people who carry typhoid bacteria in their intestinal tract for years but have no symptoms. In developing countries with poor sanitary conditions and unsafe water supplies, epidemics of typhoid fever may occur.

The Diagnosis. Although it may come on suddenly with chills and fever, especially in children, the disease usually develops slowly. It begins with headache, cough, weakness and fatigue, general achiness, and sore throat. Vomiting, constipation or diarrhea, and abdominal pain are often present as well. There is fever that usually is higher in the evening than in the morning.

If typhoid fever is untreated, the second stage sets in after 7 to 10 days. The individual becomes extremely ill. The fever becomes continuous and diarrhea the consistency and color of pea soup or severe constipation sets in. In severe cases, the person may fall into "the typhoid state," lying motionless with eyes half-closed and appearing wasted and exhausted. After about the second week, a rash may appear on the chest and back; it disappears in 3 to 4 days.

If there are no complications, the individual begins to improve slowly. The abdominal symptoms disappear gradually and the fever falls in steps, returning to normal after another week to 10 days. However, the disease can recur at any time up to 2 weeks after the fever has subsided. About a third of the patients have complications. Intestinal bleeding, usually during the third week, is manifested by a sudden decrease in blood pressure, increase in pulse, and signs of shock followed by blood in the stool. Perforation of the intestine also may occur in the third week and may cause an increase in body temperature, an increase in pulse, rigidity, and abdominal pain and tenderness. Other, rarer, complications include pneumonia, psychosis, meningitis, and infection of the bladder, kidney, or spine (called typhoid spine).

To diagnose typhoid fever, your physician will take samples of your blood, urine, and stool and the laboratory will attempt to grow the organism from these samples.

How Serious Is Typhoid Fever? Untreated, typhoid fever is very serious; even when treated, a small number of people who have it may not survive. Elderly people and people who are already debilitated are especially vulnerable; in children, the disease usually is milder. When complications develop, the outlook is poor. A few patients become chronic carriers.

Treatment. Because the person can easily become malnourished, ingestion of fluids plus a high-calorie, nonbulky diet is important. At times, administration of fluids through a vein (intravenous feeding) is necessary. Because the bacteria are present in the stool and urine, care must be taken to isolate contaminated clothing and bedding.

Medication. Your physician will prescribe an antibiotic to which the organism is sensitive. The choice depends on the strain of the bacteria.

Prevention. The currently available vaccine is given as two injections not less than a month apart. This vaccine is only partially effective. People who plan to live or to travel in an area where the disease is prevalent, who may have been exposed during an epidemic outbreak, or who come into contact with a carrier of typhoid should be immunized. Proper environmental hygiene is important, and carriers must never be allowed to work as food handlers. A new and more effective vaccine will soon be available.

BRUCELLOSIS

Signs and Symptoms
- Fever, chills, and night sweats;
- Fatigue and irritability;
- Headache;
- Loss of appetite;
- Pain in the joints;
- Swollen lymph nodes.

Brucellosis is uncommon in the United States. It is caused by three bacteria, of the genus *Brucella,* found in cattle, hogs, and goats. The disease is transmitted to humans by contact with infected animals (primarily in slaughterhouse workers) or with the placenta of an infected animal (among farmers and veterinarians) or by drinking or eating contaminated unpasteurized milk or cheese. The bacteria enter the body through cuts or abrasions in the skin or through the digestive tract.

The Diagnosis. Although the disease usually begins suddenly with a fever, it may begin insidiously and weeks may pass before the infected person consults a physician because of the weakness he or she experiences after minimal activity. Other symptoms are headache, abdominal pain, loss of appetite, and constipation. The fever can be low-grade and sustained, but most people experience cycles of evening chills, fever, and early morning sweats. Your physician will do blood tests. If you are tested early, it may be

possible to detect the organisms in your blood.

How Serious Is Brucellosis? The disease is not serious, and most affected persons recover completely within 3 to 6 months. In a few, chronic localized brucellosis develops, causing intermittent illness for longer periods of time. Several decades ago, this disease was often incorrectly blamed for chronic fatigue.

Treatment. Bed rest during the fever and adequate nutrition are important.

Medication. Antibiotics are the preferred medication.

TETANUS

Signs and Symptoms
- Stiffness of the jaw, neck, and other muscles;
- Irritability;
- Spasms of the jaw and neck muscles;
- Painful convulsions.

Tetanus, also known as lockjaw, is caused by bacteria whose spores are found in soil.

FEVER OF UNKNOWN ORIGIN

Fever is the most common body reaction to an infection—but a fever does not necessarily signify that you have an infection. A fever can develop as one of the symptoms of some noninfectious diseases, and sometimes it is not possible to identify the cause. If your body temperature is greater than 100.5°F for more than 3 weeks and there is no obvious cause, even after extensive evaluation, the diagnosis may be "fever of unknown origin."

Some of the tests your physician may use to try to identify the cause of your fever are blood tests, frequent physical examinations, and x-ray examinations. In some cases, a biopsy of your arteries, lymph nodes, bone marrow, liver, or muscles may be necessary.

Sometimes, a medication can cause an adverse reaction, resulting in a fever. If you stop taking the medication, the fever usually disappears within a week.

It is not always possible to determine why you have a fever but, through persistence, the cause usually can be identified and your physician can prescribe an appropriate treatment.

If the spores enter a deep wound beyond the reach of oxygen from the air, they germinate and produce a toxin, tetanospasmin, that interferes with the nerves controlling your muscles. The incubation period from the time of the injury until symptoms appear is 5 days to 3 weeks (average, 8 to 12 days).

The Diagnosis. Although some affected persons may experience only pain and tingling at the wound site and some spasms in nearby muscles, most have stiffness of the jaw and of the neck, difficulty swallowing, and irritability. Spasms of the jaw or facial muscles follow, progressing to spasms and rigidity of the neck, abdominal, and back muscles. Finally, painful convulsions caused by minor stimuli affect the respiratory muscles so that the individual is unable to breathe. The person is usually awake and alert throughout the disease.

How Serious Is Tetanus? If muscle spasms develop early, chances of recovery are poor. Tetanus is quite serious, often leading to death, especially in small children and elderly people. For this reason, prevention is the best treatment.

Treatment. Consult your physician immediately if you incur a wound that is contaminated with soil, particularly if it is deep. If you have had a series of tetanus shots previously, your physician probably will give you a booster shot of the vaccine tetanus toxoid if more than 5 years have passed since your last booster shot. Your body will quickly manufacture the needed antibodies to protect you against tetanus.

Treatment with antibiotics and opening and cleaning of the wound also may be necessary. Often, muscle relaxants are used to relieve the muscle spasms.

Prevention. Active immunization is vital for everyone. It is usually given to children as part of the DTP shot (see page 867), with booster shots every 10 years or at the time of a major injury. Also, be sure to clean and disinfect wounds adequately.

RABIES

Signs and Symptoms
- Pain and then tingling at the site of an animal bite;
- Skin sensitivity;
- Excessive drooling of saliva;
- Inability to swallow liquids;
- Rage alternating with calm;
- Convulsions and paralysis leading to death.

Rabies is caused by a virus that affects the brain. It is transmitted to humans by saliva from the bite of an infected animal. Dogs and cats may be infected, and many bats, skunks, and foxes are infected; rodents are unlikely to be. The incubation period from the time of the bite until symptoms appear is usually 3 to 7 weeks but can range from 10 days to 2 years.

The Diagnosis. Rabies begins with pain followed by tingling at the site of an animal bite. The person is extremely sensitive to temperature changes and air currents and tends to choke whenever he or she tries to swallow liquids. Restlessness, muscle spasms, rage and extreme excitability, and excessive drooling are also present. Finally, convulsions and paralysis ensue.

How Serious Is Rabies? Rabies is almost always fatal. Death due to heart or respiratory failure and paralysis usually occurs within 7 to 25 days after symptoms appear.

Treatment. If you are bitten by a dog, cat, or farm animal, the animal should be caught, confined, and observed by a veterinarian for a week to 10 days. If bitten by a wild animal, the animal should be killed, if possible, and the brain tested for rabies. Wild raccoons, skunks, bats, coyotes, and foxes generally are presumed to have rabies.

Your physician must decide whether or not to treat for rabies. Treatment consists of administration of a passive antibody (half directly to the wound and half injected into a muscle) and a vaccine, given as five injections on separate days.

HOW TO TAKE A TEMPERATURE AND HOW TO READ A THERMOMETER

Normally, your temperature shows a definite pattern: low in the morning, gradually increasing during the day, and reaching its maximum during late afternoon or evening. Ordinarily, body temperature varies by 1°F to 2°F over the course of the day, usually not exceeding 99.9°F.

Thus, the mark at 98.6°F (37°C) on your thermometer is only a general guide. Readings somewhat above this are not necessarily abnormal. Increased body temperature does not become dangerous until it goes above 105°F.

Ordinarily, your body controls its temperature to be within the range 97°F in the morning to 99°F in the evening. When fever is present, the mechanisms that control body temperature are simply set a few degrees higher—for example, 102°F instead of the normal 97°F to 99°F. When a fever begins, you feel chilly and may shiver. You may be more comfortable wrapped in a blanket or huddled with a heating pad because this will help your body gain heat and reach the new set point. Then, when your temperature reaches the new set point (for example, 102°F), you will no longer feel cold and will stop shivering.

If whatever caused the fever disappears or if you take acetaminophen, the set point will return toward the normal range and you will feel warm. Therefore, you will seek cooler surroundings and will perspire profusely, both of which tend to dissipate body heat.

There are three ways to take your temperature. All require the use of a thermometer. Oral and rectal thermometers are essentially glass tubes containing a column of mercury. As the mercury expands, in response to the heat from your body, it moves up the column.

An oral thermometer has a long, slender bulb at one end containing mercury and is used in the mouth or under the armpit. A rectal thermometer has a shorter, stubby bulb of mercury at one end and is used in the rectum, usually in children. Electronic and temperature strip thermometers are also available, but the latter are generally less accurate. When you are purchasing a thermometer, look for one with a column that is easy to see and with degree markings that are easy to read.

Before taking a temperature, make sure that the top of the mercury column is down near the bulb. Hold the thermometer firmly at the end away from the mercury bulb and shake it with several abrupt downward flicks of your wrist. Then, wash the thermometer in cold water. To read the thermometer, hold it near the light and rotate it slowly until you see the silver column of mercury.

In adults and children age 7 or over, the temperature is taken orally by inserting the bulb end of the thermometer under the tongue and having the patient close his or her mouth. After 1 minute, you can remove the thermometer and read it.

In children under age 7, the temperature can be taken by placing an oral thermometer in the armpit and having the child cross his or her arms across the chest. After 3 minutes remove the thermometer, read the temperature, and *add* 1°F to convert to oral temperature. You also can use a rectal thermometer in young children. Insert the bulb end of the thermometer a short way into the child's rectum, while holding the child down with your arm, if necessary. After 1 or 2 minutes, remove the thermometer, read the temperature, and subtract 1°F.

After taking a temperature, rinse the thermometer in cold water or alcohol.

When taking an infant's temperature with a rectal thermometer, the thermometer should be inserted about 1 inch. After 1 minute, remove the thermometer, read the temperature, and subtract 1 degree. Don't let go of the thermometer while it is in your child.

COMMON CONTAGIOUS DISEASES

Many of the most familiar diseases of childhood—chickenpox, measles, mumps—are highly infectious ailments that can be passed easily from person to person. Although many of these ailments are taken for granted as a part of childhood, others, like dreaded polio, are very serious indeed. Still others are likely to be harmless in children but can be serious in adults—for example, mumps in mature men and German measles in pregnant women.

Ordinarily, the diagnosis of these common diseases is made on the basis of their characteristic symptoms and signs and to some extent on the presence of other cases in the community. Blood tests to confirm the diagnosis are usually unnecessary. Occasionally, such tests are obtained to assist public health authorities determine the nature and extent of a disease in a community.

Today, immunizations make it possible to avoid altogether certain of these problems. In the following pages, we will discuss the common contagious disorders and review appropriate procedures and schedules for immunizations.

COMMON VIRAL COLDS

Signs and Symptoms
- Congested nose;
- Sneezing;
- Watering eyes;
- Sore throat;
- Cough;
- Slight fever which may be accompanied by shivering, body aches, and chills;
- Headache;
- Overall malaise.

Everyone experiences a cold now and then. In fact, perhaps as many as half of all short-term illnesses are colds or other acute viral respiratory illnesses which include croup (see page 863), pharyngitis (see page 697), laryngitis (see page 700), bronchitis (see page 916), and some types of pneumonia (see page 917).

Colds are most common in children. They usually have their first cold during their first year of life and are especially susceptible to them until about age 6 when their immunities seem to be established (see Common and Recurrent Colds, page 90).

As we get older, we tend to be less susceptible to colds, but statistics suggest that three to four colds per year per person is typical.

Most colds are caused by a virus. The common cold is not the result of one specific virus. More than 200 different viral strains cause acute respiratory illnesses. These include the rhinoviruses, the group most often associated with the so-called common cold. Most colds primarily affect the nose and throat, although the same viruses can cause bronchitis in the lungs and laryngitis in the larynx. More serious bacterial infections of the throat, ears, and lungs can follow a viral cold.

The method by which colds are spread is still unclear. It seems that direct contact with infected secretions is the most effective method. Shaking hands with a person who has been blowing his or her nose or coughing into his or her hand seems a common way of becoming infected with that person's virus. Open sneezing and coughing also spread the virus into the air to be inhaled by others, but this is a much less efficient method of transfer.

Myths and popular wisdom about catching colds abound—for example, if you get wet in a rainstorm or go out with wet hair you surely will catch a cold, or if you are exposed to cold air you will come down with one. Fatigue and lack of sleep are often cited as sure causes of colds. However, none of these has been proved, in clinical studies, to affect the risk of becoming infected with a cold virus.

Colds do have a seasonal bias. More people have colds during fall, winter, and spring than during summer.

The Diagnosis.   The general symptoms of a cold are fairly standard and include congestion of the head and nose, cough, sneezing, hoarseness, and watering eyes. Because so many different viruses cause colds, the symptoms can vary considerably. For instance, you may have a mild fever and chills during one cold but not during another. In one, the cough may be more troublesome than the running nose.

Onset of a cold usually comes within 1 to 2 days after exposure and may be signalled at first by an itching or sore throat, increasing congestion of the nose, or mild body aches or headache. A watering, running nose is often the first major symptom. After a while, the discharge becomes thick and yellowish green.

A normally healthy person has no need to see a physician for a cold. However, if it lasts for more than 10 days to 2 weeks, see your physician to make sure that no secondary bacterial infection of the lungs, larynx, trachea, sinuses, or ear has set in. If you have a history of any such infections, consult your physician without delay.

How Serious Is a Cold?   Colds are general nuisances that for the most part must just be waited out. Occasionally, however, a more serious secondary respiratory infection can follow a cold and must be treated aggressively by a physician.

Treatment.   Because a cold is a viral infection, antibiotics are useless. The cold usually lasts 3 to 4 days, or a week at most. Therefore, treating a cold is largely a matter of patience.

Self-Help.   There are measures you can take to help you feel better.

Rest at home if you feel tired, are drowsy from medications, or have a bad cough. Staying at home also helps avoid infecting others. Remain in a warm (not hot) room in which the air is moistened by a humidifier or vaporizer. Drink lots of fluids (to loosen the mucus). Adults can take aspirin for aches and pains. Children should use acetaminophen instead.

Nonprescription cold remedies, decongestants, and cough syrups may help to relieve some of the symptoms, but they will not cure the cold or make it any shorter in duration. Many people find cough drops useful to keep their throat lubricated. However, they can upset the stomach after a while, so consider sucking hard candy instead.

Sore throat can be relieved by gargling with warm salty water several times a day or by using a nonprescription topical anesthetic to relieve throat discomfort. Be careful not to use nasal sprays or drops for more than a few days because they can become addicting. Some people ask their physicians for

antibiotics to fight a cold. Unless there is a bacterial infection present, antibiotics are of no use and, indeed, may cause stomach upset, diarrhea, or a rash.

MEASLES

Signs and Symptoms
- Fever;
- Cough, sneezing, swollen eyelids;
- Sore throat;
- Tiny white spots on the lining of the cheek;
- Rash.

Measles, also known as rubeola, is a common childhood illness, although adults also are susceptible. The virus that causes the disorder is transmitted by inhalation of infecting droplets such as from a sneeze. Measles is most contagious before the rash appears, making it difficult to avoid the disease; until the rash disappears you still can pass it on to others. Once you have had measles, you are permanently immune and will not contract the disease again.

The Diagnosis.   Measles begins as a fever, often as high as 104°F to 105°F, with a persistent cough, sneezing, and sore throat. After about 4 days, a red, blotchy rash appears on the face and behind the ears. The rash spreads to the chest and back and, finally, to the arms and legs. By the time it reaches the arms and legs, it has begun to fade from the face (see color photograph on page B-1).

The symptoms usually appear 10 to 14 days after exposure to the virus. The diagnosis ordinarily is made on the basis of the characteristic rash and the small white spots on the inside lining of the cheek.

Occasionally, your physician may obtain a blood sample to test for the presence of antibodies to the virus, but this is usually done only as a part of a public health survey to define the nature and extent of an epidemic.

How Serious Is Measles?   Normally, the infection lasts for 10 days to 2 weeks, and the person recovers completely. In a small number of cases, pneumonia may develop early in the course of the illness, or complications may arise immediately after appearance of the rash. Encephalitis, which causes vomit-

THE DANGERS OF ASPIRIN

Aspirin is an effective drug for treating a wide range of symptoms and disorders. We think of it as mild and harmless, but in certain cases it can be very dangerous. The notable risks are these:

In Children

Do not give aspirin to children who have a fever. Aspirin seems to be related, in some unknown way, to the very serious condition Reye's syndrome (see page 531).

In Adults

Aspirin may cause minor bleeding from the stomach, so it should be used only when necessary. If your stools appear to be black and tarry, you may be having gastrointestinal bleeding. Discuss your aspirin use with your physician; he or she may recommend a coated aspirin or an aspirin substitute such as acetaminophen.

---

ing, convulsions, coma, and brain disorders, or a bacterial infection (such as pneumonia) may develop.

Treatment. *Medication.* Acetaminophen and a sedative cough medicine may be taken. Remain isolated until a week after the rash disappears and stay in bed until the fever disappears. If a bacterial infection develops, your physician may prescribe an antimicrobial medication.

Vaccine. The measles vaccine is effective and is usually given as a combined measles-mumps-rubella inoculation. It should be given to children at age 15 months or older.

GERMAN MEASLES

Signs and Symptoms
- Rash;
- Mild fever.

German measles (rubella) is only moderately infectious. It is transmitted by inhalation of droplets of moisture that are carrying the virus. The incubation period is 2 to 3 weeks, and the affected person is contagious for 1 week before the rash appears.

The Diagnosis. The symptoms of the disease usually are mild and sometimes are hardly noticed. They may include mild fever, enlarged lymph nodes, and a fine, pink rash that appears on the face, the trunk,

and then the arms and legs. The rash usually disappears in 2 to 3 days, lasting no more than 1 day on each part of the body. In many cases, the rash does not even occur. Your physician may take a blood sample to check for antibodies to the virus. (See page B-1 for color photograph of German measles rash.)

How Serious Is Rubella? In itself, rubella is a mild infection. Once you have had the disease, you usually are permanently immune. However, if a woman is pregnant when she contracts rubella, the consequences for her unborn child may be severe. The child may have any one of various problems including growth retardation, cataracts, rashes, deafness, congenital heart defects, and organ defects. The highest risk to the infant is during the first trimester, but exposure during the second trimester is also dangerous.

Treatment. The infection is allowed to run its course, although taking acetaminophen may help to relieve symptoms. Treatment of the child who was exposed to the disease while in the mother's uterus depends on his or her problems and often requires years of medical and surgical care. If a woman contracts rubella while she is pregnant, therapeutic abortion may be considered.

Prevention. Usually, a combined measles/mumps/rubella vaccination is given. Live weakened (attenuated) vaccine should be given to all girls before they begin menstruating. If an adult woman is given the vaccine, she must practice birth control for at least 3 months after vaccination.

ROSEOLA

Signs and Symptoms
- High fever;
- Swollen lymph nodes in the neck.

Roseola is believed to be caused by human herpes virus 6. The route of transmission is unclear. It only affects children, but the infection is not serious and no complications have been reported.

The Diagnosis. The primary symptom is a sudden, high fever (to 104°F) in a child 6 months to 3 years old. The child may be irritable, and his or her lymph nodes become swollen. Convulsions can be caused by the high fever (see page 73). As the fever goes down, a rash appears on the trunk and neck and may last a few hours to a few days (see color photograph on page B-1).

There is no specific test for roseola.

Treatment. Treatment consists of acetaminophen and application of tepid sponges to bring the fever down. The convulsions usually are brief if they occur, but your physician may prescribe anticonvulsant medication.

WHOOPING COUGH

Signs and Symptoms
- Sneezing, nasal congestion, and tearing;
- Loss of appetite;
- Malaise;
- A hacking cough, often followed by explosive coughs that end in a high-pitched whoop.

Emergency Symptoms
- Difficulty breathing, blue lips.

Whooping cough gets its name from the high-pitched "whooping" sound characteristic of the disease. It is also known as pertussis, after the bacterium that causes it, *Bordetella pertussis.*

Whooping cough primarily occurs in infants less than 2 years old and is contracted by inhaling infected airborne droplets, often from an adult with a mild case of the disease. The disease is most contagious early, but it can be transmitted until the infection is completely cleared.

The Diagnosis. Diagnosing whooping cough in its initial stages is difficult because the symptoms are similar to those of a common cold. After 10 days to 2 weeks, the characteristic whooping cough may develop: the person has spasms of rapid, consecutive coughs followed by a strained, hurried, deep inhalation with a high-pitched whooping sound.

Coughing attacks can be set off by a number of stimuli such as fright, anger, crying, and sneezing. The person coughs up large amounts of thick saliva, and vomiting is common. About 4 weeks after the coughing attacks begin, the symptoms gradually disappear.

How Serious Is Whooping Cough? With antibiotic therapy, most children recover from whooping cough without incident. However, whooping cough can lead to pneumonia with subsequent damage to the lungs. Asphyxia (lack of oxygen) or the pressure from coughing episodes may lead to brain damage. If a child's lips turn blue, this means that the child is having difficulty breathing and should be rushed to the hospital immediately.

Treatment. The child should be given small meals frequently and plenty of fluids.

Medication. Antibiotics are given. In severe cases, corticosteroids are given for several days. Cough medicines provide little benefit.

Prevention. Whooping cough is uncommon in the United States because of the widespread immunization (vaccination) of children. In other countries in which immunization against whooping cough has lagged, the consequences have been disastrous, with deaths occurring from the re-emergence of whooping cough.

There are some risks from the vaccine, and your physician can discuss these with you. Immunizations are generally given as a combination of vaccines against diphtheria, tetanus, and whooping cough (pertussis), known as the DTP vaccine. No connection has been found between the DTP vaccine and sudden infant death syndrome.

CROUP

Signs and Symptoms
- A loud, brassy cough;
- Difficulty breathing.

Croup is an infection of the voice box (larynx), windpipe (trachea), and bronchial tubes that usually is caused by a virus. It occurs most often in children between the ages of 3 months and 5 years. Boys are more likely than girls to get croup. An upper respiratory illness of several days' duration usually precedes the symptoms of croup.

Due to a narrowing of the airway, a child with croup has a tight, brassy cough that may resemble the barking of a seal. The child's voice usually is hoarse. It is difficult for the child to inhale. Agitation and crying make the breathing difficulties worse. The child usually is more comfortable sitting up than lying down.

Croup typically lasts 5 to 6 days. During that time it may go from mild to severe several times; usually the condition worsens at night.

Treatment.   If croup is caused by a bacterial infection, antibiotics can be used to treat it. However, antibiotics are not effective against a viral infection.

The majority of children with croup can be cared for at home. Warm, moist air seems to relieve some of the airway swelling and ease the cough. Run the hot water in your shower for 10 minutes with the bathroom door closed. Once the room looks like a steambath, take your child into the bathroom for at least 10 minutes.

A child with croup is often frightened and crying, which exacerbates the problem, so try to both reassure and distract him or her with a cuddle, a book, or a favorite game. Other methods of creating humidity include using a humidifier in the child's room (not a hot vaporizer). Fill the humidifier with warm water and have the child put his or her face in the mist and breathe deeply through the mouth. A wet washcloth placed loosely over the nose and mouth or taking the child out in the fresh air for a few minutes also may relieve symptoms.

If your child has croup, encourage him or her to drink clear, warm fluids, which may help loosen thickened secretions. During the illness, it is a good idea to sleep in the same room with your child, so you will be alert to any worsening of his or her condition. And do not let anyone smoke in the house, because cigarette smoke can make croup worse.

Occasionally, croup may cause complete obstruction of the airway. This is an emergency situation that usually occurs over the course of several hours and can be fatal if the child does not receive immediate medical care. To guard against this dangerous complication, be alert for the following symptoms.

- Your child drools or has great difficulty swallowing;

- Your child cannot bend his or her neck forward;
- Your child is unconscious;
- Your child's lips are blue or dusky;
- Your child is making high-pitched noises when inhaling;
- Your child's coughing worsens and his or her breathing becomes more difficult;
- Your child's heart rate exceeds 160 beats per minute.

If you notice any of these symptoms or if it just seems your child is getting worse, call your child's physician or get emergency help.

CHICKENPOX

Signs and Symptoms
- Fever and weakness;
- Red, itchy rash.

Chickenpox, also known as varicella, occurs primarily in children, although adults who are not immune can contract it. It is quite contagious and is spread by breathing in infected respiratory droplets or coming into contact with the rash where it has ruptured. In persons who have had chickenpox, the virus can cause shingles later in life (see page 1176).

The Diagnosis.   The best known symptom of chickenpox is the itchy, red rash that breaks out on the face, scalp, chest, back, and, to a lesser extent, arms and legs (see color photograph on page B-1). The rash usually appears about 2 weeks after exposure to the virus and begins as superficial spots.

The spots quickly fill with a clear fluid, rupture, and turn crusty. These then slough off in a week or two. The rash continues to break out for the first 1 to 5 days, so spots at various stages of development may be present at the same time. Fever and malaise, mild in children and more severe in adults, also develop.

How Serious Is Chickenpox?   In children, chickenpox is a mild disease, but in adults it is more serious. In adults, pneumonia may develop, which can lead to death, although this is rare. In persons with suppressed immune systems, such as children with leukemia or kidney transplants, the disease is very serious. Although uncommon, encephalitis may occur, but recovery usually is complete.

If a pregnant woman contracts chickenpox during the first or second trimester, there is a small risk that her child will be born with a congenital malformation. When a pregnant woman contracts the disease within 5 days of delivery, there is a high risk of the newborn having serious disease; the child should be immunized immediately with varicella-zoster immune globulin (VZIG).

Chickenpox seldom lasts for more than 2 weeks, from the appearance of the first rash to the disappearance of the last one. Infection of the ruptured rash by bacteria may cause scarring.

Treatment. To prevent spreading of the disease, isolate the person with chickenpox until the rash crusts. Keep the skin clean by frequent baths or, once the fever has subsided, showers. Cool, wet compresses or tepid water baths may help to relieve itching. Complications are treated according to their symptoms; bacterial pneumonia is usually treated with antibiotics.

Medication. Occasionally antihistamines are used to help relieve the itching. Acyclovir is sometimes used for severe varicella infections involving the lungs or the brain and in persons with a depressed immune system.

Prevention. Varicella-zoster immune globulin (VZIG) or a vaccine given to children with suppressed immune systems is effective in preventing the disease.

MUMPS

Signs and Symptoms
- Swollen, painful salivary glands;
- Fever;
- Weakness and fatigue;
- Possibly, inflammation of the pancreas, testes, ovaries, or brain.

Mumps is a childhood disease, but it can occur in adults. Its clinical name is epidemic parotitis. Mumps is caused by a virus and is spread by inhalation of infected droplets. The affected person becomes contagious 1 day before the symptoms appear, is most contagious for another 3 days, and then

---

SMALLPOX

The eradication of smallpox is a success story of modern medicine. Smallpox was once a highly infectious viral disease that would spread in epidemics, causing death in up to 40 percent of its victims. The disease caused severe headache, fever, and a red, blistering rash that often left scars.

At the end of the 18th century, Edward Jenner, an English physician, discovered that inoculation with cowpox virus, which is usually harmless, prevented smallpox. Campaigns were launched in the United States and Europe to inoculate people against smallpox. However, as late as 1967, when the World Health Organization (WHO) launched a global campaign to eliminate this disease, outbreaks still occurred regularly in many countries.

After 10 years of effort, this international campaign was successful and the disease was eradicated. Smallpox vaccination is no longer necessary.

---

becomes less contagious as the swelling goes down.

The Diagnosis. The symptoms of mumps usually appear 2 to 3 weeks after the virus infection begins. The primary, and best known, symptom is swollen, painful salivary glands, causing the cheeks to puff out (see color photograph on page B-1). In small children, fever is usually slight. If the affected person experiences headaches and becomes lethargic, inflammation of the brain and its lining (meningoencephalitis) may be present. Pain in the upper abdomen, nausea, and vomiting may indicate inflammation of the pancreas; lower abdominal pain in women may mean inflammation of the ovaries. This is often difficult to diagnose.

In about a quarter of the men who contract mumps, inflammation of the testicles (orchitis) (see page 1117) develops. Your physician can confirm this diagnosis by identifying the mumps virus in your saliva or by finding a large increase in antibodies in your blood. However, this sort of testing is rarely necessary.

How Serious Is Mumps? Mumps makes you quite uncomfortable but it usually is not a serious disease and rarely lasts more than 2 weeks. In some cases, however, encephalitis may develop, which is a serious complication of mumps and can lead to neurological symptoms and, rarely, death. Orchitis is uncomfortable and occasionally causes sterility.

Treatment. There is no specific treatment for mumps. Your physician may advise bed rest until the fever disappears. Isolation to prevent the spread of the disease also may be appropriate. For most of the complications that may arise, treatment depends on the symptoms. Occasionally, an analgesic such as acetaminophen may be advised.

Prevention. The live virus vaccine against mumps is safe and effective and should be given to all children more than 1 year old. It may be given by itself or combined with other vaccines. Use of this vaccine has greatly decreased the incidence of mumps in the United States.

DIPHTHERIA

Signs and Symptoms
- Sore throat and hoarseness;
- Nasal discharge;
- Malaise and fever;
- Thick gray membrane covering the throat and tonsils;
- Rapid pulse.

Diphtheria is an acute infection caused by the bacterium *Corynebacterium diphtheriae*. It usually attacks the respiratory tract. Infection occurs by inhalation of airborne droplets exhaled by a person with the disease or by a carrier who has no symptoms. The organism also can infect skin wounds or any mucous membrane. The disease is now rare in the United States.

The Diagnosis. After an incubation period of 2 days to a week, a mild sore throat, fever, and malaise develop. Your physician will look for a gray membrane covering your throat and tonsils.

How Serious Is Diphtheria? With proper treatment, the prognosis is good if no complications develop. However, the gray diphtheria membrane can be dangerous because it may obstruct breathing. In addition, the disease may cause a serious heart infection called myocarditis (see page 832).

In some cases, the bacteria may affect the cranial nerves, causing nasal speech, regurgitation of food, and inability to swallow. This is seldom fatal, unless paralysis of the respiratory muscles develops. If the person survives these complications, recovery is slow but complete.

Treatment. A person with diphtheria should be isolated, kept at bed rest for 10 to 14 days, and fed a liquid to soft diet.

Medication. Administration of diphtheria antitoxin is essential. Antibiotics are given to eradicate the infection and the carrier state.

Prevention. Immunization (vaccination), ordinarily carried out in infancy, is by injection of a combination of vaccines that includes whooping cough (pertussis) and tetanus (see pages 863 and 857). The vaccine is very effective. A booster shot every 10 years is appropriate, especially if you are to travel to an area where diphtheria is common.

SCARLET FEVER

Signs and Symptoms
- Sore throat;
- Fever;
- Vomiting;
- Rash on neck and chest.

Scarlet fever was once a common, serious childhood illness but now is quite rare. Caused by a specific type of streptococcal bacteria, scarlet fever usually begins suddenly with sore throat, fever, and vomiting. The bacteria produce a specific type of toxin (erythrogenic toxin) which causes a rash. Within 12 to 36 hours, the rash appears on the neck and chest, but not on the face; then

---

IMMUNIZATION SCHEDULE FOR NORMAL, HEALTHY INFANTS AND CHILDREN

Age	Vaccine
2 months	DTP (diphtheria/tetanus/pertussis) and OPV (oral polio virus)
4 months	DTP and OPV
6 months	DTP
15 months	MMR (measles/mumps/rubella)
18 months	DTP and OPV
2 years	Hib (*Haemophilus* B conjugate vaccine)
4–6 years	DTP and OPV (before entering school)
14–16 years or more	Td (adult tetanus toxoid and diphtheria) given as a booster shot every 10 years to children over 12 years old and to adults

IMMUNIZATIONS

In the United States, nearly all children are vaccinated by age 4 or 5 years because they must be immunized before they are allowed to enter school. Some parents put off vaccination until their child reaches school age. This puts the child at needless risk of contracting potentially severe diseases.

For most vaccines, immunization should begin when a child reaches age 2 to 3 months. The injections of live vaccines—for polio, measles, mumps, and rubella—should be completed by the time the child reaches 18 months of age.

These are available vaccines and when they should be given.

Diphtheria

This vaccine usually is given in combination with tetanus and pertussis (whooping cough) vaccines (DTP shot). The immunization should be started when the child reaches 2 months of age and is given as a series of five shots. Children over 12 and adults should receive tetanus-diphtheria toxoid, adult type. A booster shot should be given every 10 years.

Pertussis (Whooping Cough)

Immunization is begun between 1 and 3 months of age, usually in combination with tetanus and diphtheria. In a few children, a reaction to the shot may occur, in which case no further injections should be given. The vaccine generally should not be given to children more than 6 years old.

Tetanus

Tetanus vaccine usually is given to children in a series of five shots, in combination with diphtheria and pertussis. It is given at ages 2,
4, and 6 months, again at 18 months, and before the child enters school. A tetanus/diphtheria booster is given every 10 years.

Polio

Poliomyelitis vaccine generally is given orally as a live vaccine at ages 2 and 4 months (and at 6 months if polio is prevalent in the area) and again at 18 months at the same time as the DTP vaccine. Although further vaccination is not essential, a final dose has been recommended just before the child enters school (between 4 and 6 years of age).

Measles

A live weakened measles vaccine routinely is given to healthy children at about 15 months of age, usually in combination with mumps and rubella vaccines. If it is likely that a child will be exposed to measles before that age, he or she should be vaccinated earlier, but a second shot may be necessary at age 15 months because the child may not have developed antibodies to the virus after the first vaccination. If the immunization schedule is missed, older children and adults can be safely inoculated with the live vaccine. Children who have leukemia or some other severe debilitating illness or are receiving radiation, corticosteroid, or antimetabolite therapy should not be vaccinated.

Mumps

Mumps vaccine is given in one dose, usually in combination with the measles and rubella vaccines. It should not be given to children less than 1 year old.

Rubella

Usually this vaccine is given at age 15 months, in combination with measles and mumps vaccines. Al-
though rubella is not a particularly serious disease, if a woman is exposed to rubella while she is pregnant, there may be dire consequences for her unborn child in the form of severe birth defects. Therefore, live weakened (attenuated) vaccine should be given to all girls before they begin menstruating. If a woman is given the vaccine, she must practice birth control for at least 3 months thereafter.

Haemophilus Type B

Immunization with the *Haemophilus influenzae* type B conjugate vaccine is recommended for all children at 2 years of age. Children who are at risk of being infected by this bacterium, such as those who attend day-care centers, should be immunized at age 18 months.

Hepatitis B

There are two vaccines available for people who do not test positive for the hepatitis B virus but are at risk of contracting the disease (see page 653).

Rabies

If you are bitten by a rabid animal, you must receive a vaccine, given as five injections on separate days, along with a passive antibody. Failure to get the shots can be fatal (see page 858). If you are traveling to an area where rabies is common (India, parts of South America), consider pre-exposure prophylactic treatment.

Pneumonia

There is a vaccine that gives protection against pneumococcal pneumonia (see page 917). The primary vaccination is very safe. However, because they may cause serious reactions, repeat or booster shots should not be given except in very special situations. Also, very young children may not be protected by the vaccine.

it spreads over the body. The rash has a sandpaper consistency and is flushed (see color photograph, page B-1). Often, the area of greatest involvement is above the armpits and at the groin. The tongue becomes swollen and bright red.

The rash usually disappears after 3 days, and the fever disappears. The tongue may be swollen for somewhat longer, but recovery usually is uneventful.

Treatment.   Your physician probably will prescribe penicillin or another antibiotic for a minimum of 10 days. Drink plenty of liquids, get bed rest, and use acetaminophen to help relieve the symptoms.

PARASITIC INFESTATIONS

Parasites range from the microscopic, single-celled organisms called protozoa to larger parasites called helminths (from the Greek word meaning worm). Protozoa often spend part of their life cycle outside of humans, living in food, soil, water, or insects. The protozoan that causes malaria is a well-known example. Other protozoa are always present in your body but are kept under control by your immune system.

Tapeworms and roundworms are the most common types of helminths, the larger parasites. If they enter your body, they take up residence in your intestinal tract, lungs, liver, skin, or even brain where they live off the nutrients available at those sites.

MALARIA

Signs and Symptoms
- Sequential chills, fever, and sweating;
- Headache;
- Muscle pains;
- Anemia.

Malaria is spread primarily by the female *Anopheles* mosquito, although it also may be transmitted by contaminated blood transfusions, by passage from an infected mother to her unborn child, and by sharing of needles among intravenous drug users. The disease is found primarily in the rural areas of tropical and subtropical countries. Worldwide, more than 200 million people have malaria; in the United States, about 1,000 cases are reported each year, primarily among people returning from areas where this genus of mosquito thrives.

The female mosquito becomes infected with the malarial parasite when it ingests blood containing the sexual forms of the protozoa. After developing in the mosquito, the parasite is transmitted to humans by the bite of the mosquito. In the human, it migrates to the liver. After developing further, the parasite enters the bloodstream and infects the red blood cells. In these cells they multiply and, 48 to 72 hours later depending on the species, cause the red blood cells to rupture, releasing a new generation of parasites.

The Diagnosis.   The symptoms of malaria relate closely to the parasite's life cycle. After an incubation period of anywhere from 8 days to 8 months, chills begin, lasting 15 minutes to an hour, that correspond to the rupture of the red blood cells and to the increase in body temperature. Headache, vomiting, and nausea also may occur.

Body temperature remains high for several hours, and during this time the parasite begins to invade new blood cells. Then, a sweating stage begins as body temperature falls. The cycle may recur every 48 or 72 hours, depending on the species of protozoan.

If you experience any of these symptoms within a year of traveling to an area where malaria is present, see your physician immediately. The usual diagnostic test is examination of a blood smear.

How Serious Is Malaria?   Left untreated, malaria can be fatal. The disease may end after 6 to 8 months, but it can persist for up to 3 years or even longer with certain species.

Treatment.   *Prevention and Medication.* Various drugs are available for the prevention and treatment of malaria. If you are planning to visit a country where malaria is present, start taking medication 1 to 2 weeks before you begin your trip. The medication, usually the drug chloroquine taken once a week, must be continued throughout your stay and for 6 weeks after your departure from the country. The antibiotic doxycycline is an alternative medication for short-term travel.

In certain areas, falciparum malaria, a severe form of the disease that is resistant to chloroquine, is prevalent. If you are going to such an area, your physician may give you a treatment dose of the antimalarial drug Fansidar to be carried during travel and to be taken promptly in the event a feverish illness occurs when professional medical care is not available. Your physician will discuss with you the potential side effects of these antimalarial medications. Note that Fansidar is a sulfa drug, and some people are allergic to this type of medication.

Both malaria and the drugs that prevent it may cause miscarriage or stillbirth in pregnant women.

Taking precautions to avoid being bitten by mosquitoes, such as sleeping under mosquito netting, staying in buildings with screens on doors and windows, staying indoors between dusk and dawn (times when the mosquito feeds), and wearing mosquito repellent may help to avoid the disease.

TAPEWORM

Signs and Symptoms
- Presence of eggs in stool or worm segments in clothing, bedding, or stool;
- Hunger, dizziness, fatigue;
- Loss of appetite, weight loss, vomiting, and irritability.

The tapeworms usually found in humans represent only six species. The beef tapeworm (the largest, up to 75 feet in length), fish tapeworm, and pork tapeworm usually are acquired by eating infected raw or undercooked beef, fish, or pork, respectively. The dwarf tapeworm is transmitted directly from one person to another. The rodent tapeworm (common in rats) is transmitted by accidentally swallowing infected rat fleas, beetles, or cockroaches, usually after they have gotten into cereals or other stored foods. The dog tapeworm is typically found in children who come into close contact with infested dogs or cats and have swallowed infected fleas or lice.

The Diagnosis. Tapeworms usually cause few symptoms. The beef, pork, and fish

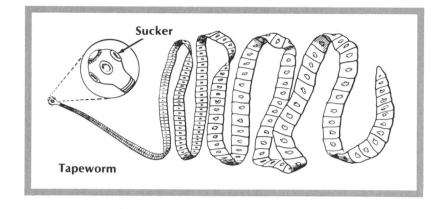

tapeworms may cause hunger, dizziness, and fatigue. The three smaller tapeworms may cause loss of appetite, weight loss, vomiting, and irritability (especially in children). In severe cases, nausea, diarrhea, and abdominal pain may be present. Tapeworms are usually discovered when eggs are found in the stool or worm segments are found in the stool, bedding, or clothing. Your physician will make the diagnosis by obtaining segments and examining them under the microscope.

How Serious Is a Tapeworm Infestation?
The presence of tapeworms in the intestine usually is not a serious situation. However, certain types of tapeworms can penetrate the intestinal wall and spread to various internal organs. The resulting condition then may become very serious.

Treatment. *Medication.* Many drugs are available to treat tapeworm. The worm in the intestine usually begins to disintegrate and is passed out of the body within 24 to 48 hours after start of treatment. It is generally assumed that the worm has been eliminated if no segments reappear after 3 to 5 months.

TRICHINOSIS

Signs and Symptoms
- Diarrhea and cramps;
- Malaise;
- Fever;
- Muscle pain and tenderness;
- Swelling of the face.

Trichinella spiralis lives in the intestines of most carnivores, including marine animals. The female worm releases larvae that enter muscles and form cysts. When the infected muscle is eaten, the cysts develop into a new generation of worms. Humans usually get trichinosis from eating infected raw or undercooked pork or pork products or from eating beef that has been ground in a contaminated meat grinder or mixed with infected pork. The incidence of infection has been greatly decreased by public health measures, but meat from wild animals, especially bear, is one continuing source of infection.

The Diagnosis. Two to 12 days after eating infected meat, you may experience diarrhea, abdominal cramps, and malaise lasting 1 to 7 days, although some people may have no symptoms at all. When the muscles are invaded by the larvae, muscle pain and tenderness, fever, swelling of the face, weakness, sensitivity to light, and conjunctivitis may be present and usually last about 6 weeks.

To diagnose trichinosis, your physician probably will do a blood test and possibly a muscle biopsy to detect the larvae.

How Serious Is Trichinosis? Except in severe cases, trichinosis is not serious and usually disappears on its own.

Treatment. In most cases, treatment is not necessary. During the initial stage, a medication may be prescribed.

Prevention. Trichinosis is easily prevented by thoroughly cooking meat or freezing it at −15°C for 3 weeks.

PINWORMS

Signs and Symptoms
- Severe itching of the anal area at night;
- Insomnia, irritability, restlessness;
- Vague gastrointestinal symptoms.

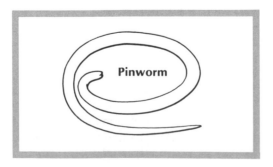

Humans are the only host of the pinworm which lives in the lower intestine. At night, the female worm migrates out through the anus, lays large numbers of eggs, and dies. After a few hours, the eggs can spread to other individuals or can reinfect the host if they are transferred to the mouth by contaminated food, drinks, or hands. After the eggs are swallowed, they hatch in the small intestine and migrate down to the lower intestine. The entire cycle takes 3 to 4 weeks, and eggs are viable for up to 2 to 3 weeks. Pinworm occurs more frequently in children than in adults.

The Diagnosis. The primary symptom is severe itching around the anus, particularly at night, although some patients may experience no noticeable symptoms. Pinworm is diagnosed by identifying eggs taken from the anal area. The most reliable method is to apply a short piece of cellophane tape to the itching area and then spread it on a slide for microscopic examination. The examination must be done in the morning before the affected person has defecated or bathed.

How Serious Is Pinworm Infestation? The infection is annoying, but it is not serious and is easily cured. However, reinfection is common.

Treatment. Persons with symptoms, and often other members of the household as well, should be treated. In addition, affected persons should avoid scratching and should take special care to keep their fingernails clean, to wash their hands after defecating, and to wash the bedding to help prevent the spread or recurrence of the infection.

Medication. Appropriate medications are available and are very effective. One example is mebendazole (Vermox).

STRONGYLOIDOSIS

Signs and Symptoms
- Small, sometimes itchy lesions;
- Diarrhea sometimes alternating with constipation;
- Abdominal pain;
- Flatulence.

Strongyloidosis comes from the scientific name of the small worm, *Strongyloides ster-*

coralis, that causes the disease. Also known as threadworm, it is found in many tropical and subtropical areas, although strongyloidosis sometimes occurs in temperate areas including the United States. It is common in overcrowded, unsanitary conditions such as mental institutions and jails. Most victims also suffer from simultaneous infestation by hookworm (see below).

The Diagnosis. The first sign of infestation is small, red, and sometimes itchy lesions caused by the larvae entering the skin. The larvae travel through the bloodstream to the lungs from which they rise to the throat and are swallowed. They then inhabit the intestine and cause diarrhea (sometimes alternating with constipation), abdominal pain, and flatulence.

The abdominal pain is similar to the dull, burning cramp caused by an ulcer. Nausea, vomiting, and loss of appetite also may occur. In severe cases with diarrhea, the stool contains blood and mucus. While they are in the lungs, the worms may cause a dry cough, irritation of the throat, or a low-grade fever, wheezing, difficulty breathing, and bronchitis. Determining the cause of the disease is difficult because of the wide variety of symptoms, but finding the larvae in the feces or duodenal fluid confirms the diagnosis.

Unless the infection is an overwhelming one, most patients recover completely once the worms are eliminated.

Treatment. *Medication.* Medications are available to treat strongyloidosis.

ASCARIASIS

Signs and Symptoms
- Vomiting, accompanied by stomach pain and bloating;
- Wheezing, coughing, or difficulty in breathing.

Ascaris lumbricoides is the largest of the roundworms and also is the most common intestinal worm. It is found wherever human feces are used as fertilizer or standards of hygiene are poor. The worm only affects humans, and infestation is most severe in children. The eggs are found in the soil and enter humans who consume contaminated food or drink. After migrating to the lungs, the larvae eventually take up residence in

Ascaris lumbricoides

the small intestine where they develop into an adult form that lives for a year or more. In the lungs, they cause wheezing, cough, and difficulty breathing and can cause permanent damage. In the intestine, the worms cause vomiting, upper abdominal discomfort, and distention.

Treatment. Treatment consists of taking antiparasitic drugs.

HOOKWORM

Signs and Symptoms
- Dry cough and difficulty breathing;
- Low-grade fever;
- Weakness and fatigue;
- Loss of appetite;
- Diarrhea and ulcer-like abdominal pain;
- Pallor.

Hookworm is widespread in moist tropical and subtropical areas. The larva lives in damp soil until it penetrates the skin, whereupon it travels in the bloodstream to the lungs. Then, it rises to the mouth, is swallowed, and attaches to the lining of the small intestine where it develops into a half-inch-long adult worm. The disease may affect anyone, but children are particularly susceptible to severe infestations.

The Diagnosis. At the spot where they enter the skin, the larvae cause an itchy rash called ground itch. When in the lungs, they provoke a dry cough, wheezing, difficulty breathing, a low-grade fever, and sputum tinged with blood. Two weeks after entering the skin, they reach the intestine.

Head

Hookworm

You may experience no symptoms, but in people with serious infestations or without adequate iron intake, the worms can cause a loss of appetite, diarrhea (usually with stool containing blood), abdominal pain, weakness and fatigue, pallor, and possibly anemia. Finding eggs in the feces confirms the diagnosis.

How Serious Is Hookworm Infestation? Because the worms do not reproduce in humans, they simply die and disappear in 1 year or in 3 to 5 years, depending on the species. People with mild or severe cases usually recover completely if treated adequately.

Treatment. If you have no intestinal symptoms, treatment is unnecessary; the worms eventually will be passed out of your system. If you have a serious infestation, antiparasitic medication is necessary. A diet high in protein, vitamins, and iron supplements prevents malnutrition and anemia until the infestation is eradicated.

Medication.   Several types of medications may be prescribed. However, certain of them should not be used by pregnant women, so if you are pregnant, be sure your physician is aware of your condition.

Prevention.   Toilet facilities that prevent contamination of the soil will break the cycle of infection. Also, wear shoes when going into contaminated areas. They afford good protection.

INSECT INFESTATIONS

Some infestations are caused by small insects that attach themselves to your skin and feed off your blood. In the United States, these organisms are annoying but most do not cause dangerous illness. However, some insects do transmit viruses or bacteria that can cause serious illness in humans.

SCABIES

Signs and Symptoms
- Itching at night;
- Thin, pencil-like lines on your skin.

In scabies, tiny mites, almost impossible to see without a magnifying glass, cause severe itching. Usually the itching is worse at night. Found worldwide among all groups of people and at all ages, they often infest an entire family. Scabies are spread by close physical contact and, less often, by sharing clothing or bed sheets with an infested person. Canine scabies can be transmitted from dogs to humans. (See color photograph, page B-14.)

The Diagnosis.   Scabies prefer to burrow into certain areas of the skin, such as between your fingers, in your armpits, around your waist, along the insides of your wrists, on the back of your elbows, on your ankles and soles of the feet, around the breasts and genitals, and on your buttocks. They form a characteristic burrow that looks like a thin, irregular pencil mark.

Your physician will look for such a burrow and will remove the mite located at the end of one to confirm the diagnosis. Although not serious, scabies are very annoying.

Treatment. *Medication.*   Treatment involves eliminating the infestation. Several creams and lotions are available and are usually applied all over the body, from the neck down, and left on overnight. Your physician will prescribe the appropriate medication. Because of the high rate of infestation, it may be appropriate that all family members and sexual partners be treated, even if no infestation is apparent.

LICE

Signs and Symptoms
- Intense itching;
- Lice on the scalp and clothing;
- Nits on hair shafts.

Lice are tiny parasitic insects that occur among people who live in overcrowded buildings under conditions of poor hygiene. These insects are transmitted by close contact, including sexual contact. Lice often are spread among schoolchildren; they also can be spread from infested toilet seats. There are three species: head lice, pubic lice (also called crabs), and body lice.

The Diagnosis. The first sign is intense itching. With body lice, some people have hives and others have abrasions from scratching. The surest way to diagnose lice is to detect the tiny yellow-gray insects. Head lice are found on the scalp and are easiest to see at the nape of the neck and over the ears. Small nits (eggs) that resemble tiny pussywillow buds can be found on the hair shafts. Body lice are difficult to find on the body because they burrow into the skin, but they usually can be detected in the seams of underwear. Pubic lice are found on the skin of the pubic area. (See color photograph, page B-14.)

Lice do not cause a serious medical problem; however, they are very annoying and are easily spread.

Treatment. *Medication.* Several lotions and shampoos, both prescription and over-the-counter, are available. One example is lindane (Kwell). Apply the product to all infected and hairy parts of the body. Any remaining nits can be removed with tweezers or a fine comb. Your sexual partner should be examined and treated if infected. Children should be kept at home until at least one treatment has been applied. Sheets, combs, brushes, and hats should be washed in hot, soapy water.

FLEAS

Signs and Symptoms
- Localized rash;
- Severe itching.

Fleas are small insects that suck blood from dogs, cats, humans, and other animals. By using their tremendous jumping ability, they often spread from family pets to their owners. Eggs laid in bedding hatch and remain there to feed off animals or humans.

The Diagnosis. Fleas cause intense itching, and clusters of bites can be seen around the waist, along the ankles, in the armpits, and in the crooks of elbows and knees. Hives may develop in persons who are especially sensitive to flea saliva. The surest way to diagnose fleas is by identifying the tiny insects themselves. In the United States,

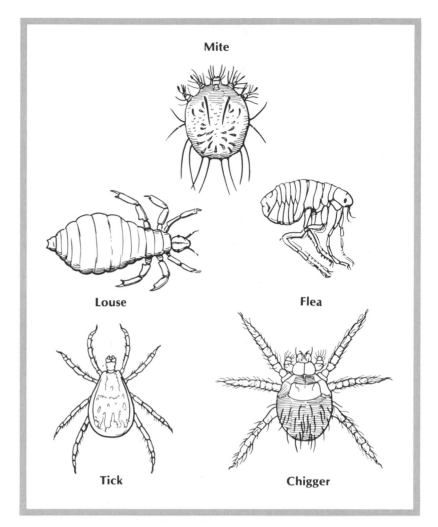

Mite

Louse

Flea

Tick

Chigger

fleas are not serious, and normally you do not need to see your physician if you have them. But they are very annoying and should be eliminated.

Treatment. Calamine lotion may help to relieve the itching, but the problem will continue until the fleas are eliminated. Persistent treatment of animals and their living areas is necessary. Once fleas are established, their elimination is difficult, and just putting a flea collar on your pet is not sufficient.

Various flea insecticides are available. Spray one of these on your pet's bedding, as well as on your own if you suspect that fleas have become established there. Furniture and carpeting also should be sprayed. Home foggers help eliminate the insects; however, be careful to remove other pets, such as birds and fish, because they are very sensitive to these insecticides. If you have a heavy infestation of fleas, or your own treatments are not effective, you may have to call in a professional exterminator.

CHIGGERS

Signs and Symptoms
• Intense itching;
• Pimple-like bumps or hives.

Chiggers, also known as red bugs or harvest mites, are the larvae of a type of mite. In the United States, they are found primarily in the South, although they can be found as far north as Canada. Chiggers live in areas of tall grass or brush and on the edges of woods. Farmers, hunters, hikers, and others who spend a lot of time in the woods are most likely to become infested.

The Diagnosis. The larvae prefer warm, moist places and usually take up residence around your waist, on your ankles, in the crooks of your elbows and armpits, in the groin area, and wherever clothing is tight. The small red insects attach themselves to the skin and insert a feeding tube to reach a source of blood, causing small red pimples and sometimes hives. Several hours after they have inserted their feeding tube there is intense itching at the site.

Chiggers remain in the same spot for 1 to 4 days and then drop off, full of blood. The best way to diagnose an infestation of chiggers is by identifying the mite itself. They can be found in the center of pimples that have not yet been scratched. In the United States, chiggers do not cause any diseases but are very annoying because of the intense itching. (See color photograph, page B-14.)

Treatment. *Medication.* Treatment is aimed at relieving the itching. Your physician may prescribe an antihistamine, and corticosteroid creams or lotions can be applied directly to the pimples.

TICKS

Signs and Symptoms
• Itching;
• Presence of ticks;
• Small hard lumps surrounded by a red circle.

Ticks are small, flat insects that feed on blood. They live in tall grasses, brush, and wooded areas and attach to animals or persons passing by. After walking through such areas, check for ticks. They often lodge in hair, around ankles, and in the genital area.

The Diagnosis. Ticks are most easily identified and removed before they attach themselves to the skin. Once embedded, they cause a small, hard, itchy lump surrounded by a red halo. Some ticks produce toxins that paralyze the nerves of the leg; the paralysis moves from the site of the tick up toward the trunk. (See color photograph, page B-14.)

How Serious Is a Tick Infestation? Tick infestation is the only insect infestation that can be serious because ticks may be carriers of Lyme disease (see page 854) or Rocky Mountain spotted fever (see page 855).

A condition called tick paralysis, which can resemble poliomyelitis, may occur after a tick has fed on the person for several days. It can be very serious but, if the tick is removed, the symptoms usually disappear.

Treatment. Do not scratch a tick bite. If you do, the body of the insect may break off, leaving the head embedded in your skin. Treatment consists of gently (slowly and steadily) removing the tick, preferably using tweezers.

Particularly in areas where Rocky Mountain spotted fever is known to be present, never detach a tick with your bare hands because infection may result.

To remove a tick, use tweezers to pull the tick firmly and steadily.

SEXUALLY TRANSMITTED DISEASES

Bacteria and viruses transmitted by sexual contact can cause various infections. Gonorrhea, chlamydia, and syphilis are bacterial infections. Herpes and venereal warts are viral infections. These infections will be discussed in the following pages. Many other diseases that often are sexually transmitted, such as hepatitis (see page 650) and AIDS (see page 848), are discussed elsewhere in this book.

GONORRHEA

Signs and Symptoms
- Thick, pus-like discharge from the urethra;
- Burning, frequent urination.

Gonorrhea is caused by the bacterium *Neisseria gonorrhoeae* and is a very common communicable disease. In the United States, almost 3 million cases are reported each year. It is most common in persons 15 to 29 years old and usually is contracted through sexual contact. It occurs in both men and women, but women are often carriers and have no symptoms, at least not for several weeks or months. Homosexual men also may have no symptoms, especially when the infection affects the pharynx or rectum.

The Diagnosis. In men, the first symptoms of gonorrhea generally appear between 2 days and 2 weeks after exposure to the bacteria. First, there is a tingling sensation in the urethra (the passageway that carries urine from the bladder to the outside of the body). A few hours later, urination becomes painful and a milky discharge is noted. As the infection progresses, urethral pain becomes more pronounced and large amounts of creamy, pus-like, discharge are produced.

In women, symptoms may not appear for 1 to 3 weeks. The infection usually affects the cervix and reproductive organs but can involve the urethra. In some women, gonorrhea causes frequent, urgent, and painful urination along with a pus-like discharge from the vagina or urethra. In most women, how-

ever, the only symptoms are a slight increase in vaginal discharge and some inflammation which may be evident only on physical examination. These symptoms are so mild that many women do not realize they have the infection. Often, the only suggestion that a woman may have gonorrhea is that men known to have had contacts have developed the disease.

In both sexes, rectal gonorrhea may result from anal intercourse with an infected person or from the infection spreading from the genital area. It may cause some discomfort in the anal area and rectal discharge, but in many cases no symptoms are present. Oral sex can produce pharyngeal gonorrhea with a sore throat, pain on swallowing, and redness of the throat and tonsils; again, many persons so affected have no symptoms. If the infection spreads to the eye, it can cause conjunctivitis.

To confirm a diagnosis of gonorrhea, your physician will take specimens of the discharge or infected tissue for culture. This must be done before antibiotic therapy is begun. The symptoms of gonorrhea are similar to those of a number of other sexually transmitted diseases including nongonococcal urethritis (see page 891) and cervicitis or vaginitis caused by *Chlamydia, Candida,* or other organisms (see page 1087). Often, several different infectious bacteria will be present; all must be treated. Blood tests for syphilis should be performed for all persons who have gonorrhea.

How Serious Is Gonorrhea? Gonorrhea is an acute infection that can become chronic if not treated. In men, chronic gonorrhea may develop into prostatitis or urethritis (see page 891). In women, it can spread to the uterus and fallopian tubes, causing pelvic inflammatory disease which may result in scarring of the tubes and infertility (see page 1104). Gonorrhea also can spread through the bloodstream to cause infection in other parts of the body. Fever, skin rash, and joint pain and stiffness are possible results. These complications can cause permanent damage. If treated adequately, gonorrheal infections usually can be cured. However, more and more strains of gonococci are appearing that are resistant to some types of antibiotic treatment.

Treatment. Because gonorrhea is quite contagious, it is important that you abstain from sexual contact until your infection is completely eliminated. General therapy for complications in men consists of hot sitz baths for prostatitis and bed rest, cold packs, and immobilization if the tubes at the back of the scrotum (epididymis) become infected. In women, infection of the fallopian tubes requires bed rest and possibly surgical treatment if this does not clear. Follow-up culture of infected sites is recommended.

Medication. It is important that all sexual partners be examined, that appropriate specimens be cultured, and that all infections be treated. Your physician will prescribe appropriate antibiotics. Analgesics also may be prescribed for relief of pain.

CHLAMYDIAL INFECTIONS

Signs and Symptoms
• Painful urination;
• Vaginal (women) or urethral (men) discharge.

Genital chlamydial infections in men and women are caused by the bacterium *Chlamydia trachomatis.* This organism is transmitted by either vaginal or anal sex.

Touching your eye with a hand that is moistened with infectious secretions can cause an eye infection, and a mother can pass the infection to her child during delivery. *Chlamydia trachomatis* is the most common cause of blindness worldwide; it causes serious eye infections in children in many developing areas including India, Africa, and the Middle East.

The Diagnosis. Diagnosis of a genital chlamydial infection can be difficult because in many cases, especially in women, there may be no symptoms. When symptoms are present, they are very similar to those of gonorrhea.

In men, chlamydial infection may cause a burning sensation during urination and a discharge from the urethra. The symptoms are milder than in gonorrhea and may appear 1

to 3 weeks after exposure to the bacteria. Women may experience burning urination, a thin vaginal discharge, or lower abdominal pain but many must rely on having their sexual partners inform them that they have the disease.

Tests for chlamydial infection involve identifying the bacteria in secretions from the cervix (women) or from urethral or seminal fluid (in men). Identification is either by culture of the bacteria or by a monoclonal antibody test.

How Serious Is Chlamydial Infection? It was once thought that chlamydial infections only affected men; women were simply carriers. However, it now is known that chlamydial infections can be serious both in men—causing inflammation of the urethra and epididymis—and in women—causing urethral infection and inflammation of the cervix and other pelvic organs. If you engage in anal sex, this organism may cause inflammation of the rectum. Conjunctivitis may occur during the first 2 weeks after birth, or chlamydial pneumonia may develop in the newborn.

Treatment. If the presence of a chlamydial infection is confirmed, or even highly suspected, both sexual partners must be treated, even though both may not have symptoms. Otherwise, they will pass the disease back and forth between them.

Medication. Antibiotics generally are prescribed for chlamydial infections. The infection should disappear within 1 to 2 weeks; if it does not, check again with your physician. He or she may use the results of cultures to monitor treatment response.

Prevention. Having only a monogamous sexual relationship is the surest way of avoiding the disease. Using a condom during sexual intercourse probably decreases the risk of chlamydial infection.

SYPHILIS

Signs and Symptoms

Primary:
• Painless sores on genitalia, rectum, tongue, or lips;
• Enlarged lymph nodes in the groin.

Secondary:

- Skin rash over any area of the body but especially on the palms of the hands and soles of the feet;
- Mouth sores;
- Fever;
- Headache;
- Soreness and aching in the bones and joints.

Syphilis is a complex disease caused by the spirochete (a type of bacterium) *Treponema pallidum.* Although once very prevalent, it became very uncommon among heterosexual persons compared with gonorrheal and chlamydial infections. However, recently the incidence has increased, especially in poor, urban areas of the United States. Usually transmitted by sexual contact, the organism gains entrance to the body through minor cuts or abrasions in the skin or mucous membranes. It also can be transmitted by infected blood and from a mother to her unborn child during pregnancy.

The Diagnosis. Syphilis has three stages. In the primary stage, painless sores appear on the genitalia, the genital area, the rectum (particularly in male homosexuals), or the mouth at 10 days to 6 weeks after exposure. Generally, these lesions are painless. Pain does occur if the sore becomes infected secondarily with bacteria. Your physician will also look for swollen lymph nodes in the groin area. Whenever possible, a rapid diagnosis can be made by microscopic examination of a discharge from open sores. A blood test is also available to test for the presence of the bacteria.

The second stage begins anywhere from a week to 6 months after the first stage. A red rash may appear on any surface of the body, including the palms of the hands and the soles of the feet. Lesions sometimes appear on the lips, mouth, throat, genitalia, and anus. During this stage, the lesions on the skin and mucous membranes are extremely infectious. You also may have flu-like symptoms—headache and aching in the bones and joints.

An intermediate period is called latent syphilis, during which no symptoms are present. During this time, syphilis is diagnosed by special blood tests. However, if the disease has not been treated adequately, the bacteria continue to spread throughout the body and there will be a relapse. The last

stage, known as tertiary syphilis, includes widespread infection which is often serious. By this time, the bacteria have spread throughout the body and may affect any of the internal organs including bones, heart, and brain. Examination of the spinal fluid may be necessary to determine whether the brain is involved.

How Serious Is Syphilis? Syphilis can be completely cured if the diagnosis is made early and the infection is treated appropriately. However, if it is not treated, the disease can lead to death. If a woman contracts the disease while she is pregnant, it can be transmitted to her unborn child, causing deformities or death of the child.

Treatment. In both the primary and secondary stages of syphilis, antibiotic therapy is the only treatment necessary. However, the disease is very contagious during these two stages, especially the secondary. Do not engage in sexual contact until at least two follow-up blood tests indicate that your infection has been eliminated. There is no vaccine against syphilis. Follow-up blood tests are required at regular intervals for at least 1 year to monitor treatment.

Medication. Penicillin is extremely effective in treating the early stages of syphilis and fairly effective in the late stages. For persons who are sensitive to penicillin, another antibiotic drug will be prescribed.

GENITAL HERPES

Signs and Symptoms

- Pain or itching in the genital area (women) or on the penis (men);
- Water blisters (vesicles) or open sores (ulcers).

Herpes is caused by the herpes simplex virus (HSV) and may affect the genital area (usually HSV-2) or the mouth and lips (usually HSV-1, see page 1175). Genital herpes is transmitted by vaginal or anal sex; the virus enters the body through tiny cuts in the skin or mucous membranes. It can infect the eyes by contact with a contaminated finger. It affects both men and women.

The Diagnosis. The initial symptom of HSV-2 is pain or itching of the skin around

SAFE SEX

Each year, the number of people in the United States who contract a sexually transmitted disease (STD) increases (this includes those—both heterosexual and homosexual—with the AIDS virus).

Some may be offended by open discussions of "safe sex," but it is important that you understand what behaviors put you and your family and friends at risk of contracting disease. All of us must take responsibility for protecting ourselves and our partners. Simply addressing these issues does not imply approval of the sexual practices discussed.

Most STDs are treatable, but AIDS has no cure and death is virtually certain. Therefore, education about this disease is especially vital.

Although AIDS can be spread through shared use of contaminated needles among drug abusers or, rarely, through blood transfusion, it usually is transmitted by sexual contact. The virus is present in semen and vaginal secretions and enters a person's body through the small tears in the vaginal or rectal tissues that can develop during sexual activity. AIDS is not considered to be a highly contagious disease; transmission of the virus occurs only after very intimate contact with infected blood or semen.

On the other hand, STDs such as chlamydiosis, gonorrhea, herpes, venereal warts, and syphilis are highly contagious, and many of them can be spread through even brief sexual contact. However, none of these infections is spread through casual contact such as handshaking, talking, sitting on toilet seats, or living in the same house with an infected person. The microorganisms that cause STDs, including AIDS, all die quickly once they are outside of the body.

The only sure way of preventing STDs and AIDS is through sexual abstinence or a relationship with only one uninfected person (straight or gay). If you have several sexual partners, either heterosexual or homosexual, you place yourself at high risk of contracting disease. And at present, no vaccine is available to prevent any of the STDs.

While condoms do not eliminate the risk, correct use of a condom and avoidance of certain sexual practices can decrease the risk of contracting AIDS as well as other STDs.

The condom, also known as a prophylactic, rubber, or safe, is a thin sheath, usually made of latex rubber, that covers the erect penis. When used correctly, a latex condom is effective both for preventing pregnancy and for decreasing the chance of contracting most STDs including AIDS. Condoms can be purchased over the counter at any drugstore and are available in various thicknesses, colors, and shapes. They may be lubricated or unlubricated, have a plain end or a reservoir end, and have a smooth (the most common), ribbed, or corrugated texture. They can cost as little as three for a dollar, but usually the cost ranges from 50 cents to a dollar each. Condoms sometimes are made of animal membrane; however, some experts believe that the pores in such natural "skin" condoms may allow the virus to pass through. To be effective, the condom must be undamaged, must be applied to the erect penis before any genital contact, and must remain intact and snugly in place until completion of the sexual activity.

About a third of the condoms now sold in the United States are bought by women. They can be kept in a pocket or purse until needed, and they provide protection against STDs. The condom can be placed on the erect penis of a woman's male partner as a part of the initial foreplay; a man who objects to a condom may be less opposed to wearing one if his partner puts it on for him. Most forms of female-directed contraception (i.e., the pill, the diaphragm) do not provide protection against STDs, although studies indicate that use of the spermicide nonoxynol 9, as with the vaginal sponge, does decrease the frequency of gonorrhea and chlamydiosis. Using spermicide in conjunction with a diaphragm also may help kill bacteria.

Different sexual practices carry different degrees of risk of contracting the AIDS virus. Receptive (passive) anal intercourse is the riskiest because this may damage the anal and rectal membranes and allow the AIDS virus to enter the bloodstream. The passive partner is at much higher risk of contracting the virus than is the active partner, although gonorrhea and syphilis can be transmitted from the passive partner's rectum. Most studies have focused on male homosexuals, but heterosexual anal sex probably carries the same risks.

Heterosexual vaginal intercourse, particularly with multiple partners, also carries a risk of contracting AIDS. The virus is believed to be transmitted more easily from the man to the woman than vice versa. This type of sex is how most other STDs are transmitted.

Oral/genital sex is a possible, but probably uncommon, means of transmission of the AIDS virus. However, inserting the penis in the mouth (fellatio) with ejaculation and swallowing of semen is the most common cause of throat gonorrhea; oral contact with the clitoris and vaginal opening (cunnilingus) is a frequent method of transmission of the herpes virus.

Herpes is probably the only disease that can be contracted by light (dry) kissing, but deep (French) kissing may transmit other STDs. Activities that involve only skin-to-skin contact such as hugging, massage, and mutual masturbation, with little or no exposure to body fluids, do not spread disease.

the genital area. This stage is known as the prodromal period and begins 2 to 20 days after exposure to the virus. Anywhere from a few hours to several days after the prodromal stage, sores begin to appear. In women they erupt in the vaginal area, external genitalia, buttocks, and anus; in men, they are on the penis, scrotum, buttocks, anus, and thighs. Sores may be present, but invisible, inside the cervix (women) or urethra (men). (See color photograph, page B-13.)

While the ulcers are present, it may be painful to urinate. The ulcers begin as small, tender, red bumps and become watery blisters within a few days. They then rupture, becoming ulcers that ooze or bleed. After 3 to 4 days, scabs form and the ulcers heal. You may experience pain and tenderness in the genital area until the infection clears. During the first outbreak, you may experience flu-like symptoms—headache and fever—as well as swollen lymph nodes in the groin.

Your physician can confirm the diagnosis by culturing the water blisters or early ulcers. A thorough examination for other sexually related diseases is important. Often at least one other sexually transmitted disease is present in addition to herpes.

How Serious Is Genital Herpes? There is no cure or vaccine for herpes at present. The virus remains dormant in the infected areas and periodically reactivates, causing symptoms. The disease is very contagious whenever sores are present.

Herpes generally does not cause any other serious permanent complications besides the sores. Newborn infants can become infected as they pass through the birth canal of mothers with open sores, with subsequent brain damage, blindness, and death. This infection is more common in infants of mothers who are having their first outbreak of active herpes infection at the time of delivery. The incidence of herpes infection in the newborn is increasing as the incidence of genital herpes in women increases.

Some studies suggest that previous genital herpes infections may be associated with a higher risk of cancer of the cervix and other genital areas, although the degree of risk is uncertain. Most evidence shows that human papillomavirus (HPV) (see Venereal Warts, below) accounts for most of the increased risk. All women should have Papanicolaou (Pap) smears on a regular basis (see page 1096). Those women who have had genital herpes should have a Pap smear every year.

Treatment. Topical treatment consists of keeping the sores clean and dry.

Medication. During the initial outbreak, the antiviral drug acyclovir in oral form helps speed up healing. This initial treatment does not prevent recurrences. However, if recurrences are frequent, oral acyclovir treatment can be used for a long time to suppress the herpes virus.

Prevention. Herpes is very contagious when the sores are present. Abstain from sexual contact until they are completely healed. Using a condom during sexual intercourse probably reduces the risk of acquiring the infection. A monogamous sexual relationship is the surest way of avoiding the disease.

VENEREAL WARTS

Signs and Symptoms
• Warty growths on the genitalia.

Venereal warts (also called genital warts) are caused by the human papillomavirus (HPV). This virus causes warts on the skin. Venereal warts affect both men and women and are easily transmitted through sexual contact. Persons with an impaired immune system and pregnant women are more susceptible.

The Diagnosis. Venereal warts are very similar to common skin warts in appearance. They may develop from 3 weeks to 3 months after exposure to the virus. In men, they usually appear near the tip of the penis and sometimes on the shaft or on the scrotum. In women, they may appear on the vaginal lips, inside the vagina, on the cervix, or around the anus. HPV can also cause cervical lesions. Your physician generally will be able to diagnose venereal warts by physical examination.

How Serious Are Venereal Warts? Venereal warts generally are not a serious condition, although they are contagious. However, women with cervical lesions caused by HPV have a higher risk of cervical cancer. Women with these lesions should have a Papanicolaou (Pap) smear each year (see page 1096).

Treatment. Treatment of both partners and removal of all the warts are important. Medications applied directly to the warts may be helpful. A surgical procedure involving freezing of tissues (cryosurgery) is often used.

Lasers are now used to remove large venereal warts as is electrodesiccation (drying the tissue by the use of electrical current) followed by removal of the wart at its base. These treatments may require local or general anesthesia.

CHAPTER 30

THE KIDNEYS AND URINARY TRACT

CHAPTER CONTENTS

YOUR KIDNEYS AND URINARY TRACT AT WORK

The kidneys and urinary tract form a complex system whose primary responsibility is removing excess fluid and waste material from the blood. In addition, the kidneys function as glands by producing hormones that are important in the production of red blood cells, in the regulation of blood pressure, and in the formation of bone.

The system has the following parts:

Kidneys. These are a pair of bean-shaped organs located against the back of the abdominal wall on either side of the spine at the level of the lowest ribs. Each kidney is generally about the size of your fist.

Ureters. These are muscular tubes, one from each kidney, that propel the urine to the bladder.

Bladder. This is a muscular bag that holds the urine.

Urethra. This is the narrow tube through which the urine leaves the bladder when it is being expelled from the body.

Most of us were born with two functioning kidneys. However, a single kidney is entirely capable of sustaining normal life.

The kidneys are able to vary their activities from day to day to adjust to the daily changes in kinds and amounts of food and fluids that are consumed. For example, suppose that one day you happen to drink large amounts of water or other beverages and on the next you drink almost none. Your kidneys are able to adapt accordingly, neither allowing your tissues to be flooded on the one day nor depleted on the next. They do this by carefully controlling the amounts of fluid and salts that are excreted in your urine. Although other organs such as skin, lungs, and intestine also excrete fluids, the kidneys are by far the most important organ for fluid excretion.

This is how the process works. Blood enters each kidney from the renal artery, a major branch of the aorta, the heart's main artery. Although together the kidneys account for less than 1 percent of the body's weight, 20 percent of the blood pumped from the heart at any given time is passing through them.

Once inside the kidney, the blood passes through a set of filtering systems called nephrons. These are the main functioning units of the kidney. Each kidney contains more than 1 million such units, each consisting of a tuft of small blood vessels, called a glomerulus, and some tubules.

First, the blood passes through the glomerulus. There, the blood cells, proteins,

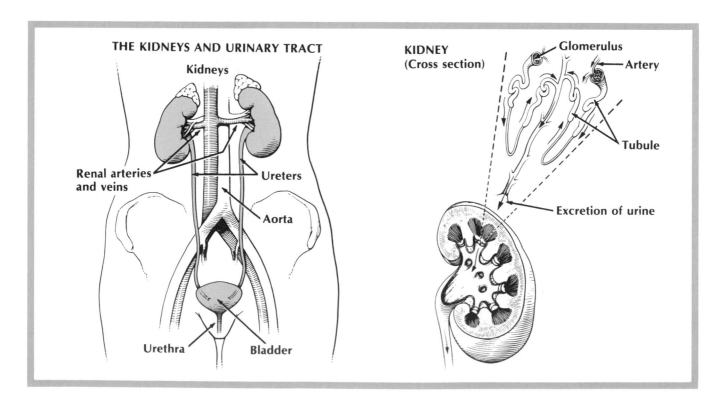

THE KIDNEYS AND URINARY TRACT

Kidneys

Renal arteries and veins

Ureters

Aorta

Urethra   Bladder

KIDNEY (Cross section)

Glomerulus

Artery

Tubule

Excretion of urine

large particles, and some of the water remain in the bloodstream and so pass through. Everything else, including a large volume of water, filters out and passes into the tubule.

In the tubule, an important process occurs to control what will be excreted in the urine and what will be reabsorbed back into the blood. Waste products (such as urea, creatinine, and uric acid) and excess salts, water, and calcium remain within the tubule. The other substances are absorbed, in precisely the amounts needed by the body, by the cells that make up the walls of the tubules. These absorbed substances are then returned to the bloodstream. Thus, the composition of the urine is determined by both the need to get rid of unwanted substances and the need to retain other substances.

The urine that has remained in the tubule emerges from the lower end of it, enters the ureter, and goes to the bladder where it will be stored. When the nerves of the bladder signal a feeling of fullness, the urine is voided through the urethra. On average, about 1.5 quarts (approximately 1.4 liters) of urine is excreted every day. But this is only a small fraction of the amount of fluid initially filtered through the glomerular capillaries into the tubules.

The blood that leaves the kidney contains salts, protein, sugar, calcium, and other substances vital to maintaining normal body function. This blood travels through the renal vein and circulates throughout the body.

Most of the time this cleaning process is performed flawlessly. Sometimes, however, problems occur in the kidney's ability to filter. For example, if the tubules are defective, valuable substances that ordinarily are returned to the bloodstream instead may be excreted in the urine. Or the glomeruli may leak protein into the urine, a condition called the nephrotic syndrome (see page 896). Injury, hypertension, exposure to toxins, kidney stones, tumors, and even infections in other parts of the body can cause kidney damage. Unfortunately, many kidney diseases often have no noticeable symptoms until they have done substantial and irreparable damage.

A good indication of whether the kidneys are functioning properly is obtained by a urinalysis, a simple test that is often performed during routine physical examinations. The urinalysis is the first step in determining the presence of kidney or related disease and in separating major problems from minor ones. Infection can be detected, and the bacteria causing it can be identified by growing a culture from the urine, so that the correct antibiotic can be prescribed (see page 1297).

Your primary physician is often the first to detect a kidney or urinary problem. He or she then may refer you to a nephrologist if the problem is in the function of your kidneys or to a urologist if the problem is with the urinary tract.

The remainder of this chapter will examine the diseases and disorders of the kidneys and urinary tract. Conditions specific for either females or males will be covered in the chapters Health Problems of Women (see page 1053) and Health Problems of Men (page 1111).

CONGENITAL KIDNEY DISORDERS

Because human beings need only one functioning kidney, many infants born with an abnormal or even a single kidney can lead normal lives.

Many of the following congenital defects cause no symptoms and often go undetected or are detected when tests are done for other purposes.

ANATOMIC ABNORMALITIES

Solitary Kidney. This term is used for the situation in which one kidney is missing. The other kidney performs the work of two, usually with no problems.

Horseshoe Kidney. The bottom ends of the two kidneys are connected, forming a horseshoe. This condition often goes undetected unless a kidney x-ray (intravenous pyelogram, or IVP; see page 885) is taken. Blood in the urine, kidney stones, urinary obstruction, and increased susceptibility to infection are complications of horseshoe kidney. These can be treated if and when they occur. The condition itself rarely leads to kidney failure.

Duplication of Kidney. The pelvis (the urine-collection portion) of the kidney is divided into separate compartments, each with its own ureter. This may occur in one or in both kidneys. There may not be any symptoms but this disorder carries with it an increased risk of infection or urinary obstruction.

Floating or Dropped Kidney. In this unusual condition the kidney moves up or down in the flank. In the past, various symptoms have been blamed on this condition, but it now is thought that a floating or dropped kidney usually is not a matter of concern and does not require any further testing or treatment.

Congenital Hydronephrosis. While the fetus is still in the uterus, its kidneys become distended with urine. It is a result of an obstruction to urine outflow. There are many causes of such urinary obstruction, the most common in males being narrowing of the urethral valves. Ultrasonography (examination with ultrasound) can detect the condition in the fetus. After birth, the cause of the condition can be determined by various special x-ray methods including retrograde and anterograde pyelography (see page 885). Infection may be the first indication of obstruction. An operation usually is necessary to relieve the obstruction and thus prevent kidney destruction.

MEDULLARY SPONGE KIDNEY

Signs and Symptoms
- Flank pain;
- Burning pain on urination or blood in the urine;
- Kidney stones.

Medullary sponge kidney is the result of an abnormality in the way the collecting ducts of the kidney drain the urine into the kidney's pelvis (the urine-collection portion of the kidney). If there are symptoms, they typically occur in adolescence or in the 20 years thereafter. Often there are no symptoms. Medullary sponge kidney is only rarely associated with serious kidney problems such as blood in the urine, kidney infection, or kidney stones. The diagnosis can be made by kidney x-ray (see page 885).

Treatment. The specific symptoms are treated. When there are no symptoms, physicians recommend drinking adequate quantities of water.

VESICOURETERAL REFLUX

Signs and Symptoms
- Recurrent urinary tract infections;
- Kidney x-ray may reveal scarring or stunted kidney growth;
- There may be protein in the urine.

Vesicoureteral reflux is the single most common urinary tract problem in children. It often occurs when there are anatomic abnormalities of the urinary tract. In a child with vesicoureteral reflux, the urine passes through the ureter from the bladder back to

X-ray of kidneys reveals duplication of the ureter on one side (arrow).

the kidney (refluxes) because the valve in the ureter does not function properly.

Reflux can be harmful to the kidney because it creates abnormal pressure and, most importantly, because it introduces bacteria from the bladder into the kidney. The kidney can become infected and, ultimately, damaged. Reflux is the most common cause of severe hypertension and end-stage kidney failure in children and young adults.

The Diagnosis. If your child is having recurrent urinary tract infections, your physician may suspect vesicoureteral reflux. Reflux can be detected during a kidney x-ray, or IVP (see below). However, the definitive test for this problem is the voiding cystourethrogram.

During this procedure, the child is catheterized (a thin flexible tube is passed through the urethra to the bladder [see page 882]) and x-rays are taken while the bladder is filled with fluid and then emptied. This shows whether the fluid stays in the bladder or flows back up (refluxes) to the kidney. It also allows an estimate of the severity of the

---

THE KIDNEY X-RAY

Intravenous pyelography, also known as IVP or as excretory urography, is an x-ray examination used to provide a detailed picture of the kidney and lower urinary tract. The IVP does not give the physician detailed information about kidney function.

If you are to undergo IVP, you will be instructed not to eat or drink for 6 hours prior to the test. You may be given a laxative to clean out your colon (this makes it easier to see your kidney).

The examination begins with the injection of contrast agent (a substance opaque to x-rays) into a vein in your arm. Your bloodstream will rapidly deliver it to your kidneys, where it is filtered through each glomerulus into the renal tubules. Later, it flows throughout the kidneys, down the ureters, and finally into the bladder. Throughout this approximately hour-long procedure, a series of x-rays are taken.

There is a related procedure called voiding cystourethrography. During this procedure, a catheter is inserted through the urethra into the bladder and x-rays are taken while the bladder is filled with fluid and subsequently emptied. This gives clear evidence of whether the fluid stays in the bladder or flows back up (refluxes) to the kidney.

If your physician suspects that you have an abnormality of your kidney or urinary tract, IVP is often one of the first radiologic tests done. One of its main uses is to determine if an abnormality of the kidney or its main artery is responsible for hypertension. It also is useful for determining the presence of congenital abnormalities, tumors, scarring of the kidneys, and stones in the urinary tract. An ultrasound or CT scan often is used to confirm the IVP findings.

IVP depends on the ability of each kidney to move the material throughout the urinary system. Thus, it is difficult to obtain a good IVP study when the kidneys do not filter properly.

Pregnant women should not have an IVP because the radiation can damage the fetus.

Most of the time there are no side effects after IVP, although some report nausea, vomiting, or pain in the arm where the injection was made. However, allergic reactions to substances injected into the body occasionally do occur, and so you should advise your physician of any allergies you may have. Of special concern are allergies to codeine, seafood, or radiologic contrast agents.

Intravenous pyelography (IVP) provides detailed view of the kidneys. Arrows show tumor.

problem, which is important in recommending treatment. A similar test, called a radionuclide cystogram, sometimes is used instead of the voiding cystourethrogram.

If your child does have reflux, a renal ultrasound examination or an IVP may be done to determine whether the kidneys have sustained any scarring or other damage.

How Serious Is Vesicoureteral Reflux?
The reflux may be mild, moderate, or severe. If the reflux in your child is mild, there is a good chance that the problem will disappear as the child grows. Moderate or severe reflux is less likely to disappear with time.

Reflux should never be ignored. Damage to the kidneys is a real danger with this problem. Kidney damage due to reflux is responsible for as many as 20 percent of the cases of end-stage renal failure in children and young adults.

Treatment. Treatment for vesicoureteral reflux depends on its severity.

Medication. Particularly when the reflux is mild to moderate, initially the child may be given low doses of antibiotics to keep the urine free of bacteria, thus preventing the refluxed urine from infecting the kidneys.

Typically, this involves a daily dose of an appropriate antibiotic.

Urine samples should be cultured at regular intervals to ensure that no bacteria are present.

Surgery. An operation may be considered for children who have severe reflux, who have moderate reflux that shows no sign of resolving as they grow older, who have urinary infections despite continuous antibiotic treatment, or who have other urinary abnormalities that make the resolution of reflux unlikely. Because of the increased risk of kidney scarring in young children with reflux, some infants and children under 5 years of age also may benefit from surgical treatment.

The operation for reflux involves reimplanting the ureter into the bladder. In 95 percent of cases, the reflux is abolished by this operation. However, urinary tract infections continue to occur in a small number of cases despite an apparently successful operation.

Children who undergo this operation should receive antibiotics for the first 3 months after the operation. At that time, another voiding cystourethrogram or radionuclide cystogram can be obtained to determine whether the problem has been corrected.

INHERITED KIDNEY DISORDERS

There are some kidney disorders that seem to run in families. If your physician finds one of these diseases in a member of your family, he or she may also do tests on other family members, even if they have no symptoms, to see if they also have the disease.

POLYCYSTIC KIDNEY DISEASE

Signs and Symptoms
- Flank pain;
- Blood in the urine;
- Excessive urination at night;
- Kidney stones;
- Anemia (in children);
- Hypertension.

In polycystic kidney disease, the kidneys contain clusters of cysts which interfere with

function and enlarge the kidneys. It occurs in both children and adults. The disease is much more common in adults and usually does not cause symptoms or problems until the second or third decade of life or later. It is estimated that 400,000 adult Americans have this disease; the number may be even greater because some persons with polycystic kidneys may never have symptoms.

The childhood form is often diagnosed shortly after birth. Problems associated with this disease include high blood pressure, anemia, kidney failure, and liver disease in early to middle childhood.

The Diagnosis. If the presence of polycystic kidneys is suspected, the examining physician probably will order an ultrasound examination (see page 1287) and perhaps a CT scan (see page 1286).

How Serious Is Polycystic Kidney Disease? With the adult form of the disease, hypertension and progressive loss of renal function often develop during adulthood. At times, bleeding into a cyst occurs and may be associated with flank pain. Renal stones occur more often in people who have polycystic kidney disease than in the general population. The majority of people with this disease reach end-stage renal disease by the time they are in their 40s or 50s, but some have end-stage renal disease earlier. Others may have only a mild to moderate loss of renal function throughout life. Once end-stage renal disease is reached, kidney dialysis or kidney transplantation is necessary to sustain life. Many of the adults with this disease also have liver problems, including liver cysts. The liver cysts can become infected, and this causes fevers and other symptoms.

The childhood form of the disease is very serious and may result in death in infancy or childhood.

Treatment. Currently, no treatment is available to prevent the cysts from forming and enlarging, but treatment is available for the symptoms and complications of polycystic kidney disease. Control of hypertension will help preserve what kidney function is remaining. Urinary infection must be treated promptly to prevent kidney damage. Puncture of cysts is sometimes necessary because of pain, bleeding, infection, or obstruction. Removal of a kidney is sometimes warranted. When end-stage renal disease ensues, kidney dialysis or transplantation has been successful.

The childhood form of the disease requires careful and consistent medical attention for the many complications. High blood pressure is common and usually requires medication. Most affected children will reach end-stage renal disease during childhood. Thus, dialysis or transplantation is used much earlier for this form of polycystic kidney disease. The associated liver disease is often severe.

CYSTINURIA

Signs and Symptoms
- Blood in the urine;
- Pain;
- Kidney stones.

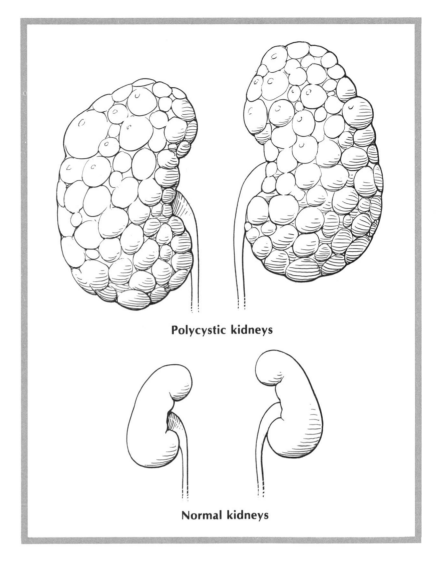

Polycystic kidneys

Normal kidneys

If you have cystinuria, your kidneys' tubules are not reabsorbing certain amino acids adequately. Excessive amounts of lysine, arginine, ornithine, and cystine are excreted in the urine. This inheritable disorder occurs in 1 of every 10,000 persons and is characterized by stones in the kidney, ureter, and bladder.

The Diagnosis. A special chemical analysis of the urine will reveal the presence of the substances found in cystinuria. If you pass a kidney stone, your physician will order a test to determine the exact composition of the stone. If the stone contains cystine, it is likely that you have cystinuria.

How Serious Is Cystinuria? Cystinuria is a serious disease. Many who have it require daily medication for the rest of their lives and may require numerous operations. People with cystinuria are likely to form cystine

Polycystic kidneys are enlarged from development of fluid-filled sacs. This condition can result in kidney failure.

stones that may damage the kidneys by causing ureteral obstruction or infection. Some will make many such stones. Fortunately, cystinuria rarely leads to kidney failure and does not affect other organs.

Treatment.   If you have cystinuria, a large fluid intake is recommended. Your best medicine is water. Because cystine is more soluble in alkaline solution, your physician may advise you to drink sodium bicarbonate or sodium citrate solutions in amounts needed to keep the urine alkaline. Those who do not respond to treatment with water and alkaline salts can be given other drugs that decrease cystine excretion. However, because of possible adverse side effects,

these should be used only if adequate fluid intake and alkalinizing solutions fail.

RENAL TUBULE DEFECTS

Renal Tubular Acidosis.   There are several inherited disorders in which the kidneys tend to excrete too much sodium and potassium in the urine. Chloride accumulates in the blood and it becomes acidic. In children, such tubular defects are often manifested by impaired growth. In adults, kidney stones may form and frequently lead to the diagnosis. Treatment generally consists of giving enough sodium biocarbonate or potassium bicarbonate to keep the blood in its normal range of alkalinity.

Vitamin D-Resistant Hypophosphatemic Rickets.   This is an inherited disorder in which the kidney is unable to retain phosphate normally. The result is impaired growth, rickets, and shortened adult stature (see Rickets, page 985).

ALPORT'S SYNDROME

Alport's syndrome is an inherited disease of the kidneys associated with blood in the urine and loss of hearing. It affects men more severely and more frequently than it affects women. The usual course of this syndrome in males is progression to loss of kidney function. Eventually dialysis or kidney transplantation is necessary, usually between adolescence and age 40. Females may have minimal or no symptoms but can pass the gene for the disease on to their children. Often, very similar inherited kidney disorders are not associated with hearing loss. These are referred to simply as hereditary nephritis.

CONGENITAL NEPHROTIC SYNDROME

Congenital nephrotic syndrome is evident shortly after birth and is most commonly found in families of Finnish origin. Its symptoms are low birth weight, very large placenta, and massive fluid retention. Infection, malnutrition, or renal failure may result in death during the first year of life. Early treat-

---

BLOOD IN THE URINE

Blood in the urine (hematuria) may be visible to the eye or, more commonly, may be apparent only when the urine is examined under a microscope. In the latter situation, hematuria is often diagnosed when a urinalysis is performed for some other reason, such as a screening test at the time of a routine or sports physical examination.

Hematuria may result from a wide variety of kidney or urinary tract problems such as infection, stones, glomerulonephritis, cysts, and tumors as well as others. However, many people with hematuria have no evidence of any of these problems, despite careful evaluation. The majority of such individuals have what is called benign hematuria.

Benign hematuria is not associated with any kidney damage or with any serious long-term effects. There are two forms of benign hematuria, a nonfamilial form and a familial or inherited form.

Nonfamilial benign hematuria (also called sporadic) typically is detected in childhood but may not become apparent until later. Aside from the presence of blood in the urine, all other findings related to the urine, blood, and kidneys are normal. Treatment is unnecessary. In many cases, the hematuria disappears gradually with time.

The familial form of benign hematuria is transmitted as an autosomal dominant trait. Therefore, several members of a family usually are affected, and screening of family members is helpful in establishing the diagnosis. Benign familial hematuria commonly is recognized in childhood. Typically, it persists throughout life but causes no kidney damage or other problems. No treatment is necessary.

In some children with isolated hematuria, a high concentration of calcium is found in the urine (hypercalciuria) and is believed to be the cause of the hematuria. These children may have an increased risk for having kidney stones.

ment, including transplantation, has been successful in some children.

SICKLE CELL DISEASE

Sickle cell disease occurs most frequently in blacks. People with this disorder may have an abnormal hemoglobin molecule, delay in growth, and, in infants, failure to thrive. Kidney problems include susceptibility to uri-nary tract infection, blood in the urine, and loss of the kidney's ability to concentrate the urine, which results in dehydration or loss of salt in the urine.

A progressive loss of kidney function can occur, more often in older people. Both dialysis and transplantation can be complicated by sickle cell disease but may be performed successfully. Those with only the sickle cell trait may notice blood in their urine but typically do not have serious kidney disease (see page 481.)

INJURY, INFECTION, AND INFLAMMATION OF THE KIDNEYS AND URINARY TRACT

There are many forms of injury of the kidneys and urinary tract. Because of their protected location within the body, traumatic injury is not common. However, the kidneys are quite susceptible to injury by toxic substances. Infection of the urinary tract is more common in women than in men. Inflammation of the kidney can be drug-induced, can be the result of an infection in the urinary tract or elsewhere in the body, or can be associated with disorders that also affect other organs.

This section is about problems common to both sexes. Problems affecting only males or only females are covered in the chapters Health Problems of Men (page 1111) or Health Problems of Women (page 1053).

INJURY OF THE KIDNEY AND URETERS

Signs and Symptoms
- History or evidence of physical injury;
- Blood in the urine;
- Severe pain in the flank;
- Nausea, vomiting, and swelling of the abdomen;
- Fever, sometimes;
- Internal bleeding;
- Shock.

Traumatic injury to the kidney and ureters is not common. It occurs mainly as a result of athletic activities or industrial or traffic accidents. Serious injury to the kidneys is relatively rare because they are protected by the rib cage and the heavy muscles of the back.

The Diagnosis. If you have been in an accident and have symptoms or signs that could indicate kidney damage, your blood and urine will be examined. A kidney x-ray (see page 885) or a CT scan (see page 1286) may be obtained. Another test that may be used is the renal scan to determine whether the blood flow to your kidneys has been jeopardized. If damage to or blockage of the renal arteries is suspected, a special x-ray study of the artery called arteriography or angiography probably will be done (see page 805).

How Serious Is Trauma to the Kidney and Ureters? Most often, injured kidneys are merely bruised, and the bleeding stops spontaneously. Sometimes, however, complications such as severe hemorrhage, infection, and shock may develop. After an injury to its blood vessels, the kidney's ability to function may be destroyed within a few hours.

Generally, kidney injuries require hospitalization.

Treatment. *Emergency.* As many as 20 percent of traumatic injuries to the kidneys require emergency operation because of massive hemorrhage.

Surgery. An injured kidney sometimes must be removed. Drainage of the space surrounding the kidney and repair of large kidney lacerations or a torn ureter may be necessary. Operation also is performed to remove clots or other obstructions.

Conservative Therapy. Often, treatment for kidney trauma consists of bed rest for 7

TOXIC INJURY OF THE KIDNEY

The kidneys are particularly vulnerable to toxic injury because of the vast quantity of blood circulating through them at any given time. Thus, if you have been exposed to a toxin, the effect may be greater on your kidneys than on other organs.

The four most common types of toxic injury to the kidney are as follows.

Analgesic Nephropathy

This condition occurs 3 to 5 times more often in women than in men and results from the long-term abuse of nonsteroidal anti-inflammatory drugs and analgesic drugs that contain phenacetin. It is one of the most common causes of chronic kidney failure. Its signs and symptoms include pus in the urine, anemia, and hypertension.

Lead Nephropathy

In children this usually results from ingestion of lead-based paint. Adults generally are poisoned from inhaling vapors produced when metal covered with lead-based paint is welded. Alcohol illegally distilled in an apparatus made from car radiators is another source of lead poisoning. If you have lead nephropathy, your symptoms may include gouty arthritis, hypertension, abdominal pain, and anemia (see Lead Poisoning, page 76).

Acute Uric Acid Nephropathy

Because it does not result from exposure to a toxin from outside of the body, this injury is unlike the previously mentioned toxic injuries. The cause is the body's overproduction of uric acid. It most often occurs in persons with bone marrow and lymph node disorders that have been treated with certain drugs. Its symptoms are diminished urine output and the presence of blood and uric acid crystals in the urine.

Nephropathy From Solvents and Fuels

Carbon tetrachloride and other solvents and fuels have the potential for causing damage to the kidneys. This is the reason for the warning on many commercial cleaners and sprays that they be used only in well-ventilated circumstances.

If your physician suspects that you have any of these toxic injuries, he or she will take a thorough medical history, paying particular attention to medications that you have taken and contacts that you have had with toxic substances. Blood and urine tests will be done. Toxic injury to the kidney may lead to chronic kidney failure if exposure to the toxic substance continues. Fortunately, most toxic injuries can be treated, and kidney function is restored simply by stopping exposure to the toxic substance at an early stage. Others, such as lead and urate nephropathy, require special treatment.

to 10 days with narcotics given for relief of pain. Within 6 months after the injury, an examination with IVP is generally done to make sure that the kidney has healed properly.

TRAUMATIC INJURY OF THE BLADDER AND URETHRA

Signs and Symptoms
- History of injury;
- Inability to urinate;
- Blood in the urine;
- Pain in the lower abdomen;
- Shock.

Traumatic injury to the bladder is not common because of the organ's location within the abdomen. When the bladder is injured, most often it happens during an operation such as hernia repair. The bladder also can be ruptured by bone fragments produced by a sharp blow to the pelvis.

Rupture of the urethra, the narrow tube that carries urine from the bladder, is more common but less dangerous. Most such injuries are limited cuts and bruises. In women, urethral damage is rare.

The Diagnosis. If your history and symptoms indicate a possible bladder or urethral injury, your physician will do a thorough examination of your abdomen and rectum. An x-ray will be obtained to determine if your pelvis is fractured. The physician also may do a cystoscopic examination which involves passing a special tube up the urethra into the bladder to permit visual inspection of this part of the lower urinary tract (see page 904).

How Serious Is Trauma to the Bladder or Urethra? These types of injuries usually require hospitalization. The most serious situation is a ruptured bladder that leaks urine into the abdominal cavity. This is a life-threatening situation because of the risk of infection, and it requires emergency surgery to repair the rupture and to remove the urine from the abdominal cavity.

The worst long-term complication of urethral injury is stricture, a severe narrowing of the urethra produced by stiffening of the scar that remains after the injured part of the urethra has healed.

Treatment. *Emergency.* The treatment of shock and hemorrhage takes priority (see page 304). These are treated by blood transfusions and fluid replacement given through a vein. Pulse rate and blood pressure are monitored constantly.

Medication. Antibiotics are given to prevent infection.

Surgery. An operation is necessary for a ruptured bladder. In the event of an injury to the urethra, a catheter (tube) may be passed through the urethra into the bladder to provide a route for the urine and left in place for several days.

URETHRITIS

Signs and Symptoms

- Frequent urination;
- Pain during urination;
- Pus in the urine;
- Discharge (in males).

Urethritis is an infection of the urethra, the tube that transports urine from the bladder during urination. The same organisms that infect the kidney and bladder can infect the urethra. In addition, because of the urethra's proximity to the vagina, sexually transmitted infections such as by herpes simplex virus and *Chlamydia* also are possible (see page 1088).

In men, urethritis often is the result of bacteria acquired through sexual contact; the vast majority of such infections are caused by the gonococci and *Chlamydia*. Reiter's syndrome is a combination of urethritis, arthritis, and an eye inflammation called conjunctivitis and is usually acquired through sexual contact (see page 1001).

The Diagnosis. It is difficult to differentiate between urethritis and cystitis in women because their symptoms are similar. One clue is provided by urinalysis. Approximately 30 percent of women who have painful and frequent urination do not have a significant amount of bacteria in their urine. This indicates that the inflammation is in the urethra and that it may not be the result of an infection.

Your physician will question you about your symptoms. If the illness began gradually more than 7 days prior to the examination and there is no blood in your urine, the symptoms are likely to be from infection with *Chlamydia,* particularly if there has been a recent change in sex partners. Bloody urine, a sudden onset of illness of short duration, and a history of previous infection suggest that a bacterial infection is the cause.

In men, the physician will attempt to squeeze a sample of the discharge from the urethra when the bladder has not been emptied for several hours. If no discharge can be obtained, a small swab can be inserted into the urethra to procure a sample for examination.

How Serious Is Urethritis? Never ignore urethritis. It is particularly dangerous because the symptoms may disappear without treatment. Because many cases are caused by sexual transmission, notify partners. When left untreated, conditions such as gonorrhea and *Chlamydia* infection can ultimately cause problems such as pelvic inflammatory disease, stricture of the urethra, sterility, arthritis, meningitis, and inflammation of the heart.

Treatment. Treatment depends on the cause. For *Chlamydia* infection, an antibiotic such as tetracycline is taken orally for 7 days. In most cases in which urethritis is caused by gonorrhea, penicillin is used. However, gonorrhea occasionally is resistant to penicillin, and a different medication may be chosen after appropriate laboratory tests. Antibiotics also are prescribed for other bacterial infections. In some situations, your physician will advise that your sexual partner also be treated.

CYSTITIS

Signs and Symptoms
- Frequent and urgent urination;
- Burning during urination;
- Pressure in lower abdomen;
- Blood in urine;
- Malodorous urine.

Often referred to as honeymoon cystitis, this infection commonly occurs as a result of sexual intercourse. During sexual activity, bacteria are introduced into the bladder through the urethra. Once inside the bladder, the bacteria begin to multiply. Usually, the body can rid itself of such bacteria by the process of urination, but when it cannot, cystitis or bladder infection may occur.

Although sexually active women between 20 and 50 years of age are the most likely to have cystitis, even young girls are susceptible to lower urinary tract infections because the anus, a constant source of bacteria, is so close to the female urethra. More than 90 percent of cystitis episodes are due to *Escherichia coli,* a species of bacteria commonly found in the rectal area. Males who are under age 50 and have normal urinary tracts rarely contract urinary tract infection.

The Diagnosis.   If you have the symptoms of cystitis, your physician will want a urinalysis on a urine sample collected in a special way. To do this, you wash the vaginal area or the tip of the penis with a disinfectant, pass a small amount of urine into the toilet to cleanse the urethra, and then collect the next portion of voided urine in a sterile cup for examination (this is midstream collection). If this urinalysis reveals an abnormal bacterial count, a culture to determine the kind of bacteria will be done so that appropriate treatment can be initiated.

(Note: Blood in the urine without pain or discomfort may not be the result of an infection, and the possibility of a kidney stone or a bladder or kidney tumor should be considered. See pages 898, 901, and 902 and consult your physician.)

How Serious Is Cystitis?   Although very uncomfortable and annoying, cystitis is not a serious disease. Some minor cases resolve without treatment. However, because of its proximity to the kidneys, your physician probably will treat your bladder if it is infected and will obtain a urine culture for testing (a week or two after treatment) to make sure that the infection is gone.

Treatment.   Cystitis is treated with antibiotics, typically for 7 to 10 days with a medication taken orally. Some physicians believe that shorter courses of treatment are adequate to cure the infection. The symptoms usually disappear within 24 to 48 hours after the first dose. Persons who have more than two infections within 6 months may need low-dose antibiotic therapy as a preventive measure indefinitely. Some women who are prone to bladder infection may benefit by taking a low dose of an antibiotic after sexual intercourse.

ACUTE PYELONEPHRITIS

Signs and Symptoms
- Flank pain;
- High fever;
- Shaking chills;
- Vomiting;
- Burning sensation during urination;
- Increased frequency of urination.

The majority of urinary tract infections affect the lower tract—the bladder and the urethra. Sometimes the bacteria travel up the ureters to the upper tract or kidneys, causing acute pyelonephritis (kidney infection).

Urinary tract infections are common, especially among females, and account for 6 million office visits annually in the United States. One to 3 percent of school-age girls have urinary tract infection; with the beginning of sexual activity, women have a marked increase in the frequency of infection.

Most bacteria gain access to the urinary tract via the urethra. Under normal circumstances, these bacteria are rinsed out of the body during urination (urine also has antibacterial properties that inhibit the growth of bacteria). However, certain factors increase the chances that these bacteria will take hold and multiply into a full-blown infection. Sexual intercourse, pregnancy, urinary obstruction, and the virulent nature of some bacteria all contribute to the likelihood of such an infection.

The Diagnosis. If your symptoms suggest a urinary infection, your physician will ask for a midstream sample of urine to determine the presence of bacteria. The combination of urinalysis followed by a urine culture if an abnormal bacterial count is found should reveal whether you have an infection. However, this is not an indication of whether or not the infection has invaded the kidney. There is no simple test to differentiate between kidney infection and lower urinary tract infection, although the presence of fever and flank pain suggests that infection has extended into the kidney itself.

How Serious Is Acute Pyelonephritis?
When properly treated, acute pyelonephritis rarely progresses to chronic renal disease, although it can be an immediate threat to life in an elderly or weakened person. It can also recur if the infection is not totally eradicated.

Treatment. Antibiotics are the first line of treatment. When recurrences are frequent or the kidney infection is chronic, there may be an underlying problem such as vesicoureteral reflux (a condition in which the urine flows backward from the bladder to the ureter) (see page 884). A kidney x-ray called an IVP (see page 885), a voiding cystourethrogram, renal ultrasound examination, or other diagnostic tests may be warranted.

ACUTE INTERSTITIAL NEPHRITIS

Signs and Symptoms
• Blood in the urine;
• Protein in the urine;
• Hypertension;
• Fever;
• Rash;
• Weight gain;
• Swelling.

Acute nephritis, an inflammation of the kidney, may affect the glomeruli, the tubules, or the spaces between. It is usually temporary and can be caused by a number of kidney diseases, allergic reactions to drugs, or the antibodies produced in response to a streptococcal infection. Some diseases that cause nephritis also cause kidney failure.

If you have interstitial nephritis, the inflammation is mainly confined to the spaces between the glomeruli and the tubules. This type of nephritis almost always is the result of an allergic reaction to a drug or to an infection elsewhere in the body.

Occasionally, some commonly prescribed drugs may cause acute interstitial nephritis. For this reason, your physician will question you about the medications you are taking. The most common such drugs are penicillin, ampicillin, and nonsteroidal anti-inflammatory drugs.

The Diagnosis. With acute interstitial nephritis or any other form of kidney inflammation, the kidneys are damaged and allow red blood cells and proteins to escape into the urine. Thus, a urinalysis is the first step toward making the diagnosis. Blood tests to assess kidney function also are needed. A kidney biopsy may be required to confirm the diagnosis and to evaluate the degree of damage.

How Serious Is Acute Interstitial Nephritis? Fortunately, kidney damage that results from acute interstitial nephritis usually is reversible. If the cause is related to the use of a drug, once that drug use is stopped the kidney begins to heal. Sometimes short-term dialysis is necessary (see page 908). Complete recovery is generally the rule, although progression to chronic renal failure may occur in rare cases.

Treatment. Avoidance of the drugs known to cause acute interstitial nephritis is essential. Fluid retention and swelling may be treated by restrictions on salt and fluid intakes. A drug is prescribed to treat the hypertension. Restriction of dietary protein intake may be appropriate.

Dialysis may be necessary for a short time if the kidneys are not functioning adequately. In some cases of acute interstitial nephritis, corticosteroid drugs such as prednisone are prescribed.

ACUTE GLOMERULONEPHRITIS

Signs and Symptoms
• Recent streptococcal or viral illness;
• Cola-colored or tea-colored urine;
• Hypertension;
• Fluid retention;
• Protein and red blood cells may be in the urine;

- Mild anemia possible;
- Headaches;
- Vision may be blurred;
- Generalized aches and pains.

Acute glomerulonephritis, an inflammation of the glomeruli, most often occurs after an infectious disease but sometimes it can be caused by other diseases or it can be a primary kidney disorder. If acute glomerulonephritis occurs after an infectious disease, it may be called acute post-infectious glomerulonephritis. The most common infection leading to acute glomerulonephritis is that caused by streptococci. Other infections that cause it are bacterial sepsis, pneumococcal pneumonia, typhoid fever, syphilis, and endocarditis (an inflammation of the lining of the heart). In addition, the kidney inflammation can be brought on by viruses such as those that cause mononucleosis, mumps, measles, or hepatitis or by echovirus or coxsackievirus. Acute glomerulonephritis is not actually a response to the infection or to the virus but is a result of the body's immune response elicited by the infection. Other causes are IgA (Berger) nephropathy, lupus erythematosus, vasculitis, Henoch-Schönlein purpura, and diseases of the glomeruli; these will be discussed in the following sections.

Acute glomerulonephritis rarely occurs after a streptococcal infection (strep throat or strep skin infection called impetigo) but when it does it happens in children ages 6 to 10. Typically, the glomerulonephritis develops some time after the person seems to be well again. In cases of strep throat, it takes anywhere from 6 to 10 days after the cessation of throat symptoms for acute glomerulonephritis to emerge; for strep skin infection, the latency period averages 2 weeks. In contrast, IgA (Berger) nephropathy may cause glomerulonephritis and blood in the urine immediately after an upper respiratory infection.

However, most strep infections do not cause glomerulonephritis. Only a few strains (types) of strep have this potential. Also, not everyone who gets acute glomerulonephritis has symptoms. In families who have experienced an outbreak of strep infection by a strain that can cause glomerulonephritis, there typically are three to four nonsymptomatic cases of acute glomerulonephritis for every one that produces symptoms.

The Diagnosis. If your recent health history and symptoms lead your physician to suspect acute glomerulonephritis, your throat or skin lesion will be cultured to determine if streptococcal organisms are still present. Blood studies will be done to identify your immune response, and a urinalysis will be obtained. If these tests suggest glomerulonephritis, a kidney biopsy may be used to determine the underlying cause.

How Serious Is Acute Glomerulonephritis? In most cases of acute glomerulonephritis, the fluid retention and hypertension resolve within a week. The abnormal urinary values may take several months to return to normal.

The prognosis appears to be better for children than for adults. Most children have a complete recovery and show no evidence of chronic renal disease later in life, although in a very small percentage of them a chronic form of glomerulonephritis may develop and slowly lead to renal failure. Adults do not do as well after acute glomerulonephritis, but no one understands the reasons for this. Adults who have had a particularly severe initial attack tend to be more prone to chronic kidney failure.

Those who have one attack of the disease generally do fine once the kidneys heal. Although recurrent attacks are unusual, a third to a half of those who have sporadic attacks have progressive renal deterioration.

Treatment. Your physician may advise you to stay in bed. Your salt and water intake may be restricted to minimize fluid retention and swelling. You will be given medication for your hypertension, and you may be placed on a special diet to restrict protein intake (if your serum creatinine or blood urea nitrogen value increases). If you have an active strep infection, your physician will prescribe medication such as penicillin. If the glomerulonephritis is caused by an organism other than strep, it will be treated with an appropriate antibiotic.

Henoch-Schönlein Purpura. This is an important cause of acute glomerulonephritis in children. The symptoms include a characteristic rash that is more prominent on the legs and buttocks, pain in joints with or without swelling or tenderness (especially in the ankles and knees), and abdominal pain.

Some children have blood in their stool. Not all children with Henoch-Schönlein purpura have abnormalities involving the kidney. When such involvement is present, there is blood and sometimes protein in the urine and these children have fluid retention and high blood pressure. Most patients with Henoch-Schönlein purpura recover without kidney damage. However, progressive renal damage does sometimes occur. Most children recover completely without specific treatment. In some cases, drugs such as corticosteroids may be prescribed.

Hemolytic-Uremic Syndrome. This disease occurs mainly in infants and young children; it occurs much less often in older children and only rarely in adults. In its typical form, an illness with diarrhea is followed abruptly by hemolytic anemia, a decrease in the blood platelet count, and rapid loss of kidney function. Other systems such as the central nervous system may be affected as well. Dialysis and blood transfusions often are required during the acute phase of the illness.

Most affected children have a complete recovery, but some are left with chronic kidney damage or damage to some other organs.

CHRONIC GLOMERULONEPHRITIS

Signs and Symptoms
* Protein in the urine;
* Blood in the urine;
* Hypertension;
* Gradual kidney failure.

Chronic glomerulonephritis is frequently associated with a slow, progressive loss of renal function. There are several diseases of the glomeruli that impair the kidney's ability to retain protein and red blood cells, and these diseases can and often do lead to chronic glomerulonephritis.

Membranous Glomerulonephritis. Irregular deposits of protein occur along the wall of the glomerulus. More than 80 percent of persons with this disease have nephrotic syndrome (abnormal loss of protein; symptoms include swelling and weight gain from fluid and sodium retention; see page

896). Males are more likely to have progression to chronic renal failure.

IgA Nephropathy. Also known as Berger's disease, this disease is characterized by recurrent episodes of blood in the urine. Young men are most often affected but it can occur at any age, even in children. In the majority of cases, renal function remains well preserved even after years of disease.

Focal and Segmental Glomerulosclerosis. This disease is characterized by scarring of some of the glomeruli. Persons with this disease may have nephrotic syndrome. Males are slightly more likely to have this ailment. Both children and adults are affected. The condition can be associated with vesicoureteral reflux (see page 884).

Mesangial Proliferative Glomerulonephritis. In this rare chronic disease, portions of the glomeruli are enlarged. Blood and protein are found in the urine. It occurs slightly more often in males than in females; older children and young adults are most commonly affected.

Diabetic Nephropathy. This may be the most common cause of end-stage renal disease in the United States. Approximately 50 percent of patients with insulin-requiring diabetes mellitus will have significant kidney disease within 12 to 20 years after the onset of their diabetes. This involvement of the kidney often is detected by routine urinalysis which shows protein in the urine; it also is detected if nephrotic syndrome (see page 896) or hypertension develops or the blood creatinine level (a measure of kidney function) increases. Once there is a significant amount of protein in the urine, end-stage renal disease usually follows within 5 to 10 years. Also, end-stage renal disease will usually result within 2 to 6 years after the creatinine value becomes high or hypertension develops. (For a more complete discussion of Diabetes, see page 707.)

Glomerulonephritis Secondary to Other Diseases. Several diseases that affect other organ systems can also damage the glomeruli. These include systemic lupus erythematosus (an immune disorder more common in women of childbearing age; see page 1006), amyloidosis, myelomas, and AIDS.

The Diagnosis. If you have chronic glomerulonephritis, it may be detected when your physician finds urine abnormalities, impaired renal function, or hypertension during a routine examination or an examination for an unrelated illness. Blood and urine tests and diagnostic studies to visualize the kidney (IVP, ultrasound examination, CT scan) may be done. Renal biopsy may be necessary to determine which disease is causing the chronic glomerulonephritis.

How Serious Is Chronic Glomerulonephritis? The outcome for chronic glomerulonephritis varies depending on its cause and the severity of the complications, particularly the high blood pressure and the protein loss in the urine.

Mesangial proliferative glomerulonephritis may or may not result in end-stage renal failure; if it does, this usually happens within 10 years after the diagnosis. If the leakage of protein into the urine can be controlled, there is a good chance of avoiding chronic renal damage. However, if there is no response to medication and the nephrotic syndrome persists, often the condition will progress to end-stage renal failure.

Children with focal and segmental glomerulosclerosis occasionally have spontaneous remission of their disease. In adults, however, spontaneous remission is not likely. Although the time for it to happen varies widely, most adults and children with this disease have a progressive decline in renal function. Those with large amounts of protein in their urine may progress to end-stage renal failure within months after the diagnosis. In at least 50 percent of those with focal and segmental glomerulosclerosis, end-stage renal failure develops.

Spontaneous remission of membranous glomerulonephritis is common among children but occurs in only 20 to 25 percent of adults with the disease. Those who have even a partial remission generally do not go on to end-stage renal disease. When it occurs, renal failure is most likely during the first few years after diagnosis. About 30 to 40 percent of those with membranous glomerulonephritis require dialysis or transplantation within 10 years after their diagnosis.

IgA nephropathy usually progresses slowly, if at all. Those with hypertension, large amounts of protein in their urine, and excess urea in their blood tend to have a worse outcome than do those with more moderate disease. In about a quarter of the persons who have this disease, end-stage renal failure develops within 25 years after diagnosis.

Good control of hypertension often will slow the progression of the renal failure of diabetic nephropathy, thus lengthening the time before dialysis or transplantation becomes necessary. Good control of the blood sugar concentration may be beneficial. Once renal failure begins, consultation with a nephrologist is important for advice and for planning for dialysis or kidney transplantation.

There are several glomerular lesions associated with lupus erythematosus. Some—such as minimal lupus glomerular lesion and mesangial lupus glomerulonephritis—generally do not cause substantial kidney damage. Others—such as diffuse proliferative lupus glomerulonephritis and membranous lupus glomerulonephritis—may produce end-stage renal failure, although this is becoming uncommon because of new treatment programs. About 85 percent of those with mild forms of the disease survive for at least 10 years.

Children with Henoch-Schönlein purpura usually do not have progressive kidney disease. However, when urinary abnormalities persist, kidney function may continue to deteriorate.

Treatment. If you have chronic glomerulonephritis, your treatment will be directed at your symptoms. You will be given medication for your hypertension and a diet low in protein and phosphate, adjusted to what your impaired kidneys can handle. In some people, glomerular lesions are treated with corticosteroids; others do not respond to this treatment.

When renal function deteriorates to the extent that maintenance of health or even life is not possible, dialysis or kidney transplantation must be considered (see page 911).

NEPHROTIC SYNDROME

Signs and Symptoms

- Large amounts of protein in the urine;
- Swelling around the eyes, feet, and abdomen;

- Increased weight from fluid retention;
- Poor appetite.

Nephrotic syndrome is the common feature of many diseases that affect the ability of the glomerulus to keep protein from being excreted in the urine. The most common causes of the nephrotic syndrome include diabetes mellitus, multiple myeloma, glomerulonephritis, and systemic lupus erythematosus (see pages 707, 493, 895, and 1006). Diseases of the glomeruli often result in this syndrome—for example, mesangial proliferative glomerulonephritis, focal and segmental glomerulosclerosis, and membranous glomerulonephritis (these are discussed in detail in the preceding section).

In children, the average age at detection is 3 to 4 years. The majority of these children have a form of nephrotic syndrome called minimal change disease (also known as lipoid nephrosis, nil lesion, or foot process disease). About 15 to 20 percent of the adults who have nephrotic syndrome that cannot be traced to infection, drug exposure, malignancy, a disease that affects multiple systems in the body, or hereditary disorders also have this form of the syndrome. The most common lesion that can result in nephrotic syndrome in adults is membranous glomerulonephritis; it accounts for up to 40 percent of adult idiopathic (no known cause) nephrotic syndrome (see page 895).

The Diagnosis. If you have the symptoms of nephrotic syndrome, your physician will do blood and urine studies. If these show large amounts of protein in the urine, he or she may recommend a renal biopsy for an accurate diagnosis and for formulating the best treatment plan. Children seldom require a renal biopsy for an accurate diagnosis.

How Serious Is Nephrotic Syndrome?
The seriousness of this syndrome depends on its cause and whether or not there are complications.

As a rule, if you have minimal change disease (a glomerular disease that often results in nephrotic syndrome), you can expect both remissions and relapses of the proteinuria (excessive protein in the urine). Prior to the development of antibiotics, infection was a leading cause of death. Now, however, the mortality rate is extremely low. The vast majority of children and adults with minimal change disease do not go on to progressive kidney failure.

When the syndrome is caused by infection or drugs, it often resolves after the infection is cured or the drug use is discontinued.

Some of the other lesions that can cause nephrotic syndrome do not have such a favorable outcome. Many people with focal and segmental glomerulosclerosis or membranous glomerulonephritis progress to end-stage renal disease. The more persistent the nephrotic syndrome, the worse the long-term outcome.

Treatment. Regardless of the underlying cause, treatment of nephrotic syndrome is aimed at alleviating symptoms and preventing complications. The most important predictor of outcome appears to be whether the proteinuria can be eliminated.

If you have one of the types of nephrotic syndrome that responds to corticosteroids, your physician will probably prescribe prednisone to decrease the urine's protein content. In minimal change disease, corticosteroid therapy enhances the body's tendency toward natural remission. The treatment usually consists of daily oral doses of prednisone for 2 months. Those who are going to respond generally do so within the first month.

Relapse after the medication is discontinued is not uncommon and usually occurs within the first year. If you have a relapse, your physician will most likely prescribe prednisone again, but the dosage will be reduced gradually over 3 to 6 months instead of being stopped abruptly.

Prednisone is a powerful drug and has significant side effects, the most common being increased appetite, weight gain, and facial puffiness (see Corticosteroid Drugs, page 1005). Some children require so much of the drug that their growth is slowed temporarily. Cyclophosphamide is another drug that can be given if there is no response to prednisone. However, this medication can cause bone marrow problems, bladder irritation, or, occasionally, problems with reproduction, so it is not the preferred drug.

Nephrotic syndrome caused by focal and segmental glomerulosclerosis or membranous glomerulonephritis does not always respond to treatment with prednisone. In these cases there have been encouraging results with the anti-inflammatory drug meclofenamate.

Other treatment measures used in nephrotic syndrome include a salt-restricted diet, medication for hypertension (if it is present), and diuretic drugs to control fluid retention. Some persons with nephrotic syndrome are especially susceptible to certain kinds of infections, and administration of pneumococcal vaccine is frequently recommended.

Recent experience with a class of drugs called ACE-inhibitors (a type of blood pressure drug) indicates that these drugs may be useful in some persons with nephrotic syndrome.

STONES, CYSTS, AND TUMORS

KIDNEY STONES

Signs and Symptoms
- Gradual development of pain, usually beginning in the flank and worsening until a narcotic drug may be needed to alleviate it;
- Pain moves downward to flank and groin, vulva, or testicle as the stone moves down the ureter;
- Persistent urge to urinate;
- Blood in the urine;
- Family or personal history of stones.

Few who have passed a kidney stone can forget the experience. Most people who have had this experience agree that it was one of the most excruciatingly painful episodes in their life. Occasionally, stones are passed with minimal or no symptoms.

Kidney stones (renal lithiasis) is a relatively common disorder. About 5 percent of women and 10 percent of men will have had at least one stone by the time they reach age 70. There is some tendency for kidney stones to recur: the annual recurrence rate is 3 percent after the first stone and 6 percent after the second stone. The tendency to have certain types of stones runs in families. Some types are associated with other conditions such as bowel disease, ileal bypass for obesity, or renal tubule defects.

A kidney stone is the result of a chemical reaction that occurs when the urine becomes too concentrated. Calcium salts, uric acid, cystine, and other substances in the urine crystallize to form a hard mineral deposit, often the size of a small pebble.

The following are the most common types of kidney stones in the Western hemisphere.

Calcium Stones. These account for 75 to 85 percent of all stones and are 2 to 3 times more common in men than in women. The first stone usually appears at age 20 to 30. Once you have had one calcium stone, you are likely to have another unless specific treatment is started. These stones usually are formed by calcium combining with oxalate, phosphate, or carbonate. The most common type is the calcium oxalate stone. The oxalate may be present as a result of the consumption of certain foods. In addition, some people with diseases of the small bowel may have an increased tendency to form oxalate stones.

Uric Acid Stones. Also formed mainly by men, uric acid stones account for up to 8

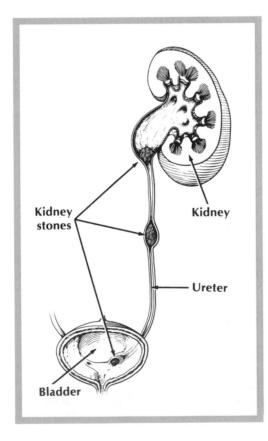

Kidney stones

Kidney

Kidney stones

Ureter

Bladder

Kidney stones can occur in the ureter, in the bladder, or in the kidney itself. Arrows depict common locations.

percent of all stones. Half of those with uric acid stones also have gout.

Cystine Stones. Persons who form cystine stones have the hereditary disorder cystinuria (see page 887). Men and women are equally likely to have cystine stones. These account for only 1 percent of stones.

Struvite Stones. Formed mainly in women, struvite stones are the result of urinary tract infection with bacteria that produce a specific enzyme. These stones can grow very large, producing the appearance of a stag's horn. They can obstruct the urinary tract and cause kidney damage.

Not all stones produce symptoms. It is not uncommon for stones to be discovered during x-ray studies made for an unrelated problem. Generally, the pain occurs when the stone breaks loose and begins to work its way down the ureter.

The Diagnosis. If your physician suspects that you have a kidney stone, he or she will request a chemical analysis of your blood and of a 24-hour collection of urine.

If you are having severe pain, you may be in the process of passing the stone, and your physician may prescribe a strong pain medication to help you through the episode. Often, a special kidney x-ray, an IVP, is made (see page 885). Hospitalization may be required.

Your physician will probably ask you to urinate through a strainer so that the stone can be recovered for analysis. Every effort should be made to determine the composition of your stone because this information suggests the cause and so allows the treatment to be planned accordingly.

How Serious Are Kidney Stones? Although the process is painful, the majority of kidney stones pass through the ureter and into the urine without causing any permanent damage. However, the underlying cause must be determined and treated to avoid further stone formation.

It is important to avoid complications such as urinary tract infection and obstruction, both of which can lead to extensive kidney damage.

Sometimes an operation is required to remove a stone, although new treatment methods such as kidney lithotripsy (see page 900) are replacing surgery in many instances.

Treatment. The selection of treatment depends on the type of stone and whether or not there are complications. However, there is one rule that applies to all kidney stone sufferers: Drink at least six to eight glasses of water every day and also drink at least one glass of water at bedtime and another at some time during the night. Adequate fluid intake dilutes the urine, thus making it less likely that crystals will form.

Medication. Whether or not you will need to take a medication that inhibits the growth of stones depends on the severity of your disease. With certain types of calcium stones (usually associated with excessive calcium excretion), a thiazide diuretic usually is successful in preventing the formation of new stones. A phosphate-containing preparation also may be prescribed to inhibit stone formation in the urine.

The calcium stone formation resulting from distal renal tubular acidosis, a defect in the ability of the renal tubules to filter acids, may be prevented by keeping the urine alkaline (see page 888).

If you have a uric acid stone, your physician may prescribe allopurinol and a medicine to keep the urine alkaline.

When a struvite stone is found, the first task is to suppress the infection that caused it. Several types of antibiotics may be prescribed.

Surgery. Obstruction, infection, or serious bleeding indicates that operation may be needed to remove a stone. In the past, stones were removed through an incision in the kidney, renal pelvis, or ureter or by passing an instrument up the ureter from the bladder. Now, a less-invasive treatment that uses shock waves (generated by sound) to fragment the stone is often successful (see Kidney Stone Lithotripsy, page 900).

Some calcium stones are caused by abnormally active parathyroid glands. The treatment for this condition is removal of parathyroid tissue to avoid future renal damage (see page 732).

Nutrition. Dietary excesses or deficiencies may contribute to stone formation. Be-

KIDNEY STONE LITHOTRIPSY

The majority of kidney stones pass without any intervention.

Until recently, anyone with a kidney stone that could not be passed and needed removal had to undergo a major operation and a 2-week hospital stay and was left with a large scar. Now, thousands of kidney stone operations are avoided every year because a relatively new technique, called kidney stone lithotripsy, is available. No incision is required, and the hospital stay may not exceed 2 or 3 days.

This procedure was developed in West Germany and was approved for use in the United States in late 1984. The lithotripter produces shock waves that pulverize the stones to small fragments which then are easily passed in the urine.

If you are to undergo lithotripsy, you will be given a general anesthetic agent (with newer machines, only a local anesthetic is needed). Then you will be lowered into a large tub of water so that your body is submerged up to your shoulders. Two x-ray devices within the lithotripter are used to locate your stone and to position you properly. Newer lithotripsy machines, now being developed, can be used without immersing you in a tub of water.

Because your body has the same acoustical properties as water, your body (neither soft tissues nor bones) is not hurt by the hundreds of shock waves that bombard you during the hour-long treatment. However, the kidney stone is so brittle that it crumbles. You will not feel the shock waves, but there is a loud noise that resounds throughout the treatment room every time a shock wave is generated by the machine, and you will be wearing earphones to protect your ears.

During the treatment, x-rays are made to determine the status of the stone. Typically, the stone begins to crumble after 200 to 400 shock waves; as many as 1,500 shock waves may be given during a treatment.

After the anesthetic wears off, you will be encouraged to walk about and to drink lots of water to wash out the small stone fragments.

This lithotripsy treatment is used for stones within the kidney itself or in the upper portion of the ureter. It does not appear to be helpful for stones in the lower part of the ureter. Stones that cannot be fragmented in the lithotripter often can be treated by lithotripsy in other ways. In one such procedure, percutaneous ultrasonic lithotripsy, a small incision is made in the skin and through it a cystoscope-like instrument is passed into the kidney. Then, a small ultrasound-producing unit is inserted to shoot sound waves at the stone; the physician removes the resulting fragments through the instrument.

In another variation of lithotripsy, a small instrument with an ultrasound-producing unit is passed up through the bladder and into the ureter (endoscopic lithotripsy). This works particularly well on ureteral stones that are inaccessible by the other methods.

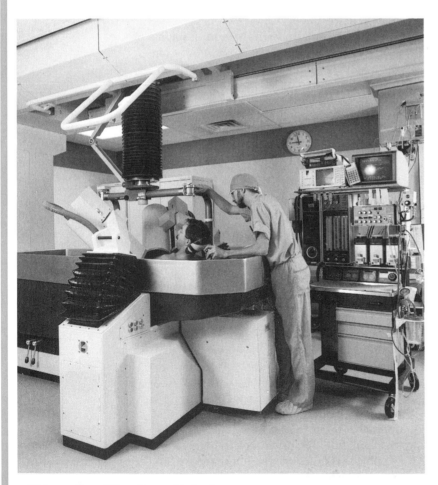

Kidney stone lithotripsy with bath.

cause specific factors vary, your physician may review your case and suggest appropriate dietary modifications.

BLADDER STONES

Signs and Symptoms
- Infection in some cases;
- Interruption of urine stream;
- Pain in penis;
- Unable to urinate except in certain positions;
- Blood in the urine.

Most bladder stones in Americans are the result of another urologic problem. Urinary infection and enlarged prostate are the most common causes. Ninety-five percent of all bladder stones occur in men.

The Diagnosis. If you have the symptoms that suggest a bladder stone is present, your physician will perform a thorough examination including a rectal examination. Urinalysis usually will reveal infection and blood in the urine (hematuria). Generally, bladder stones can be seen on an x-ray of the bladder.

How Serious Are Bladder Stones? Bladder stones usually pass without intervention. However, if they do not, they should be removed and the underlying cause should be identified and treated.

Treatment. Small stones can be removed with a cystoscope, a tube that is inserted into the bladder through the urethra. Larger stones may require a procedure called electrohydraulic lithotripsy. In this procedure, an instrument that dispenses an electric charge is placed in the bladder through the urethra. The electricity breaks up the stone.

Sometimes a medication is used to dissolve bladder stones.

KIDNEY CYSTS

Signs and Symptoms
- Often, none;
- Flank pain sometimes;
- Blood in the urine sometimes.

Kidney cysts are noncancerous lesions of the kidney. They usually are round and hollow and contain water-like fluid. They vary from very small to some that contain quarts of fluid. Unlike cancer, a cyst generally grows slowly and ceases to grow after it has attained a certain size.

Cysts in the kidney are very common. At least half of the population over age 50 probably has at least one kidney cyst. Some researchers have found a higher incidence of cysts in women than in men. The fact that infants and children rarely have these cysts suggests that the cysts are not inherited.

The Diagnosis. Usually, the cyst is found when an abdominal or kidney ultrasound examination (see page 1287) or CT scan (see page 1286) is done for some other reason. These methods usually can distinguish between benign cysts and cancer of the kidney.

How Serious Are Kidney Cysts? Most kidney cysts do not cause symptoms. Only when a cyst is extremely large will it impair renal function. However, cysts do sometimes rupture and collapse. Hemorrhage with the cyst can occur. Sometimes an infection or, rarely, a cancer will begin in a cyst.

Treatment. Generally, no treatment is required. In rare instances, however, operation or aspiration by a needle through the skin is required to collapse or decompress a cyst to relieve the pressure or pain and to prevent damage to the kidney.

CANCER OF THE KIDNEY OR URETER

Signs and Symptoms
- Blood in the urine;
- Flank pain;
- Abdominal mass may be felt during examination;
- Weight loss;
- Fatigue;
- Intermittent fever.

There are several varieties of cancer of the kidney and ureter, including the following.

Renal Cell Carcinoma. This is the most common cancer of the kidneys. It also is called renal adenocarcinoma or hypernephroma. It begins in one of the cells that form the lining of a renal tubule. About 18,000 new cases are diagnosed each year in the United States, and approximately 8,000 deaths annually are related to this malignancy. Renal cell carcinoma occurs twice as often in men as in women. The most common age at diagnosis is between 55 and 60.

Smokers, particularly those who smoke pipes or cigars, are at greater risk of renal cell carcinoma than are nonsmokers. In some instances, the disease appears to be hereditary. A large number of persons with von Hippel-Lindau disease, a condition affecting the capillaries of a part of the brain, also have renal cell carcinoma. People on dialysis for end-stage renal disease also have a higher incidence of this cancer.

Transitional Cell Cancer.   These tumors can occur in the kidney or ureter and account for 10 percent of all kidney cancers. They are associated with the abuse of analgesic drugs such as phenacetin. Transitional cell cancer typically affects middle-aged women.

Wilms' Tumor.   Children with cancer of the kidney usually have Wilms' tumor. It accounts for 95 percent of the renal cancers in children under age 14 and occurs in approximately 8 of every 1 million children under that age. The majority of the children with it are less than 7 years old at the time of diagnosis. The tumor usually is asymptomatic and is found when palpation of a child's abdomen detects a mass.

The Diagnosis.   When one of these cancers is suspected, a special kidney x-ray, an IVP (see page 885), a CT scan (see page 1286), or an ultrasound examination will be performed (see page 1287). Occasionally, additional tests are done, including a biopsy of the suspected mass (see page 1284).

Once the growth has been identified as a cancer, CT scanning often is used to determine its extent (see page 1286). Studies such as chest x-ray, bone scan, and liver tests also are done to ascertain whether the cancer has spread to other organs.

The presence of transitional cell cancer usually can be confirmed with an IVP (see page 885), followed by cystoscopy to determine the precise location of the tumor. A special examination of urine collected over a 24-hour period may also identify cancer cells.

How Serious Is Cancer of the Kidney?
The outcome with renal cell carcinoma depends on the extent to which the tumor has spread. If the tumor is in its earliest stage, 60 to 75 percent of these people will survive for at least 5 years. If the lymph nodes around the kidney have been infiltrated, the 5-year survival rate drops to 5 to 15 percent. When the cancer has spread to other organs, fewer than 5 percent survive for 5 years.

If a transitional cell cancer has not spread, the 5-year survival rates are very high. If the cancer has spread, the chance of surviving 5 years is 10 to 50 percent.

Children with Wilms' tumor generally have a good outlook if the disease has not spread. Overall, 85 to 90 percent survive for at least 5 years.

Treatment.   When it appears that a renal cell carcinoma has not spread beyond the kidney, the best treatment is removal of the entire kidney. Some surgeons advocate also removing the surrounding lymph nodes. Sometimes, radiation therapy may be used to prevent spread of the cancer.

If the disease has spread, there is no universally agreed upon method of treatment. Chemotherapy for kidney cancer is still in its infancy but has been effective in some cases.

In an early stage, a transitional cell cancer and the surrounding area are removed and an attempt is made to save the kidney itself. If the tumor is larger, the kidney and ureter are removed along with the portion of the bladder that is connected to the ureter (this is done to decrease the risk of bladder cancer).

A combination of treatments is used for Wilms' tumor. The mass is removed and the child is given chemotherapy. Sometimes, radiation therapy also is used.

BLADDER CANCER

Signs and Symptoms
- Blood in the urine;
- Pelvic pain;
- Difficulty in voiding urine.

Men are 3 times more likely to get bladder cancer than women are. Approximately 40,000 new cases of bladder cancer are diagnosed annually in the United States. The disease is responsible for more than 15,000 deaths each year.

Bladder cancer rarely occurs in those under age 40. It appears to be related at least partially to environmental factors. The disease is more prevalent among smokers and workers in the dye, chemical, and rubber industries.

The Diagnosis. The presence of blood in the urine without pain or discomfort is the most frequent early symptom. A common diagnostic error is to presume that blood in the urine means a bladder infection (see cystitis, page 892). If you have symptoms that suggest a possible bladder cancer, your physician may have a sample of urine examined for malignant cells. A special kidney x-ray called an IVP (see page 885) may be obtained and a cystoscopic examination (see page 904) that will enable the physician to see into the bladder will be performed. During the cystoscopic examination, a small sample of the bladder lining will be removed to be examined under a microscope for malignant cells.

If cancer is found, your physician may order a CT scan of the abdomen or pelvis as an aid in determining the stage of the cancer's growth (see page 1286). Tests to determine whether the cancer has spread beyond the bladder include a chest x-ray and blood studies.

How Serious Is Bladder Cancer? If the tumor is small and has not invaded deeply within the bladder (that is, it is superficial), the chances of recovery are good. About 50 to 70 percent of people with this type of bladder cancer will have a recurrence within 3 years but again the cancer will be superficial. About 12 percent of those whose initial disease is superficial eventually will have a more invasive cancer.

Approximately 45 percent of those whose cancer has invaded muscle or fat live at least 5 years, provided they have radiation therapy.

The vast majority of people whose bladder cancer has spread to other organs do not survive beyond 2 years despite treatment.

Treatment. For a superficial bladder cancer, treatment usually consists of removing the tumor itself. A major operation is not required because the surgeon is able to remove the tumor through a cystoscope.

After removal of a superficial tumor, cystoscopic evaluation with biopsy is repeated every 3 to 6 months to detect recurrence of the cancer. If superficial disease recurs, the tumor again will be removed cystoscopically. This time, the bladder may be infused with cancer-fighting drugs to decrease the chance of future bladder cancer.

If the disease has progressed to invade the bladder muscle and fat, the bladder probably will be removed. In men, the prostate gland also is removed, which frequently causes impotence. Women with advanced bladder cancer usually must also undergo removal of the ovaries, uterus, and a portion of the vagina.

Removal of the bladder makes it necessary to create an opening through which urine can pass. There are various ways to do this. In one of the more successful tech-

In an ileal conduit surgical procedure, the ureters are connected to an artificial bladder fashioned from a piece of intestine (ileum). An opening (stoma) is made in the abdominal wall. Urine drains into a pouch securely fastened to the skin.

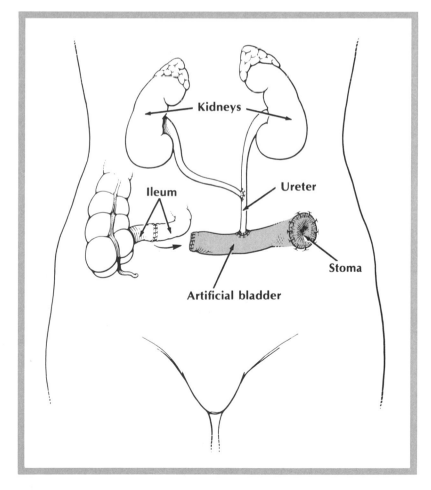

CYSTOSCOPY

Cystoscopy is an important technique for direct examination of the urethra and the inside of the bladder.

If you are to have a cystoscopic examination, you usually will be given a local anesthetic and will remain awake during the brief procedure. (Children generally are given a general anesthetic.) The cystoscope, a narrow tube, will be inserted through your urethra into your bladder. This tube carries a special lens and a fiberoptic lighting system, so that the examining physician can actually see the structures through which the cystoscope passes.

It may be necessary to remove a sample of bladder tissue for examination for cancer or other diseases or even to remove a small stone. All of this can be done through the cystoscope.

Cystoscopy is useful for evaluating various bladder problems—including recurring infection and pain during urination—for which no cause can be found. One of its most important uses is in the detection of bladder cancer. In women, cystoscopy is useful for detecting chronic inflammation of the urethra or bladder (see page 1108). In men, it sometimes is used to evaluate the degree of obstruction that an enlarged prostate may cause (see page 1124).

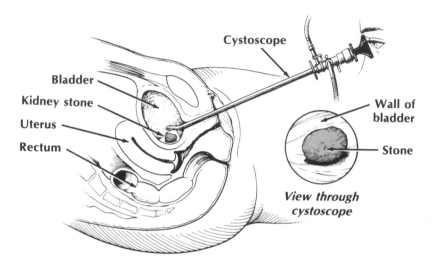

Cystoscope

Bladder
Kidney stone
Uterus
Rectum

Wall of bladder

Stone

View through cystoscope

Cystoscopic examination reveals a kidney stone in the bladder. This simple procedure usually is done under local anesthetic on an outpatient basis.

niques, the ureters are connected to an artificial bladder fashioned from a piece of intestine. The new bladder is attached inside the body near the navel. Then, an opening is created through the abdominal wall to drain the urine into a pouch worn against the body under the clothes. This is called the ileal conduit procedure.

Some physicians recommend radiation therapy and chemotherapy after this operation for invasive bladder cancer. When lymph nodes, bone, or other organs have been infiltrated by the tumor, chemotherapy can be administered. In 30 to 70 percent of people with metastatic disease (cancer that has spread to other organs), chemotherapy is helpful in arresting the spread of cancer and in alleviating pain. However, the benefit usually does not last more than 6 months, and then the cancer continues to progress.

A combination of chemotherapy followed by radiation therapy or surgical removal of the bladder prolongs life for some individuals with invasive disease.

BLOOD VESSEL PROBLEMS

Blood enters the kidneys from the renal artery, a major branch of the aorta (the main artery from the heart). Twenty percent of the volume of blood pumped from the heart at any given time passes through the kidneys. After the kidneys perform their filtering function, the blood returns by way of the renal vein to the inferior vena cava, the major vessel that carries blood from all parts of the body back to the heart.

Disorders of either the renal artery or the renal vein not only can affect the way the kidneys function but also can be a major cause of hypertension. In addition to the disorders described below, preeclampsia and eclampsia (rare but serious conditions that occur in pregnant women shortly before they give birth) (see page 207) and vasculitis (an inflammation of small arteries) (see page 1009) can result in blood vessel problems in the kidneys.

ACUTE ARTERIAL OCCLUSION

Signs and Symptoms
*   Abrupt onset of flank or abdominal pain;
*   Blood in the urine.

Acute blockage of the renal artery may occur after injury to the abdomen or side. It also occasionally occurs in people known to have heart disease (primarily mitral stenosis [see page 825] or atrial fibrillation [see page 817]). In such individuals, blood clots may travel out of the heart and through the aorta to lodge in the renal artery.

The Diagnosis. The diagnosis often is made by arteriography (a form of angiography [see page 805]). In this test, a catheter is inserted through the groin into the aorta and manipulated to reach the renal artery. Then, contrast agent is injected and x-rays are made. Occasionally, a renal scan is used to make the diagnosis.

Treatment. There is no specific therapy. The danger is that the affected kidney may cease to function. But, if this happens, the other kidney can take over the process of eliminating wastes. If arterial occlusion occurs in a person who has only one kidney (see Solitary Kidney, page 883), renal failure may occur (see page 906).

RENAL ARTERY STENOSIS

Signs and Symptoms
*   Usually none;
*   Hypertension.

Renal artery stenosis is a blockage of the renal artery before it enters the kidney. The result of this is development of hypertension which may be difficult to treat. Renal artery stenosis causes 1 to 2 percent of all cases of hypertension, but these are the most easily cured cases.

In the elderly, this condition most often results from atherosclerotic disease (see Atherosclerosis: What Is It? page 786). This disorder also occurs in women 20 to 40 years of age as a result of thickening of the artery wall (fibromuscular dysplasia).

The Diagnosis. This condition is suspected when your physician hears a bruit (loud noise) with a stethoscope over the kidneys. Particularly for young persons with this bruit, a special kidney x-ray called an

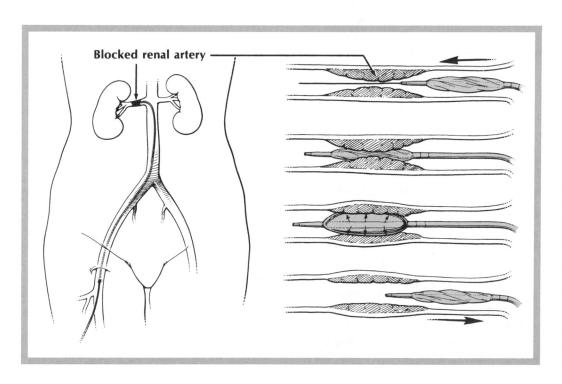

Blocked renal artery

Percutaneous transluminal angioplasty can be used to open a blocked renal artery. During the procedure, a catheter is threaded through an artery in the thigh up into the blocked renal artery. The artery is then dilated with a balloon situated at the tip of the catheter.

IVP (see page 885) is obtained. This may reveal decreased size of the affected kidney. A kidney ultrasound examination, which also measures arterial flow, may be helpful in identifying narrowing of the arteries. Then, an arteriogram is obtained to determine exactly where the blockage is located.

Treatment.   Sometimes this condition can be treated surgically. In the last several years, a new treatment has been successful, particularly in women with fibromuscular dysplasia. This consists of passing a special catheter into the renal artery and then inflating the balloon at the tip of the catheter in order to open the artery.

For some people, medication to control hypertension may be prescribed.

MALIGNANT HYPERTENSION

Emergency Symptoms
- Rapid increase in blood pressure;
- Blurred vision, severe headache;
- Shortness of breath;
- Chest pain;
- Seizures.

This is a potential medical emergency that generally occurs in individuals being treated for hypertension. For reasons that are not clearly understood, the blood pressure increases dramatically, and this causes such symptoms as blurring of vision, severe headache, distorted sensory perceptions, shortness of breath, and even seizures.

The Diagnosis.   Your physician will find a very high blood pressure and also may see worrisome changes on ophthalmoscopic examination of your eyes (see page 740). In addition, standard urinalysis may show an excessive amount of protein in your urine.

Treatment.   If this condition is treated promptly, the outcome is quite good. If it is not treated promptly, serious damage to the brain, eyes, heart, and kidneys may occur. The treatment may include hospitalization and intravenous administration of drugs to bring down the blood pressure. Then, the intravenous treatment is replaced by anti-hypertension drugs taken by mouth.

RENAL VEIN THROMBOSIS

Signs and Symptoms
- Severe pain in the lower back and flank;
- Large quantities of protein in the urine.

In this condition, a blood clot (thrombus) has developed in the vein leaving the kidney. It may occur shortly after significant trauma to the abdomen or back. It may be the result of a tumor blocking the blood flow in the renal vein. Or it may be associated with the nephrotic syndrome (see page 896). In rare cases, this occurs after severe dehydration, particularly in infants.

The Diagnosis.   Your physician may inject a dye through the groin into your vena cava (the blood vessel that returns blood from all parts of the body to your heart) and then into the renal vein. This dye will outline the blood clot in the renal vein.

Treatment.   Most often the treatment is anticoagulant medications (blood thinners). Over time, the renal vein reopens.

KIDNEY FAILURE

Kidney failure is defined as the situation when the kidneys are unable to perform their task of filtering waste out of the blood. It may be a result of infection, injury, exposure to toxins, various kidney diseases, diseases such as diabetes, systemic lupus erythematosus, or sickle cell anemia, or obstruction to the flow of urine from the kidney by a stricture, cancer, or chronic obstruction of the prostate.

There are two types of kidney failure. One is acute kidney failure, a sudden loss of kidney function. This often is related to the severe decrease in blood pressure that may occur with severe trauma or complicated surgery (states called traumatic shock or surgical shock) (see page 305), with severe infection (septic shock) (see page 306), or with a severe, complicated illness. Although acute kidney failure is a potentially life-threatening condition that requires hospitalization and round-the-clock care, the kidneys themselves generally are able to resume normal function over a period of several weeks to a few months after the crisis.

The other type, chronic kidney failure, is a slow, progressive destruction of kidney function, usually as a result of disease. End-stage renal disease is said to occur when the kidneys are functioning at only 5 to 10 percent of their capacity. At this point, kidney dialysis or transplantation is necessary to preserve life.

ACUTE KIDNEY FAILURE

Signs and Symptoms
- Fluid retention;
- Gastrointestinal tract bleeding;
- Seizures;
- Coma.

Acute renal failure is the term used to describe a rapid deterioration in the kidneys' ability to remove waste products from the blood. Thus, the wastes accumulate within the body. If something is not done to rid the body of these wastes, the person will die.

Sixty percent of all cases of acute renal failure are related to surgery or trauma with severe bleeding, severe dehydration, or shock. Exposure to certain toxins also may precipitate acute kidney failure. Another cause is obstruction to the flow of urine out of the kidney by a stricture, tumor, or chronic enlargement of the prostate (see page 1124).

There are many theories to explain how this kidney shutdown occurs. Some believe that cell debris obstructs the cavity of the tubule, thus interfering with its ability to filter out waste products. Others theorize that several factors combine to diminish blood flow through the glomeruli. We do know that many conditions can bring about acute renal failure, including the following.

Renal Ischemia.   This is the most common actual cause of acute renal failure. It is a deficiency of blood flow to the kidney as a result of obstruction or constriction of a blood vessel.

Nephrotoxic Agents.   Many common and uncommon substances can act as nephro-toxic substances. Contact with heavy metals or various solvents can induce acute renal failure.

Exposure to radiographic contrast agents such as those used during arteriography (see page 805) can precipitate acute failure. This is unlikely in a healthy person. But in 10 to 40 percent of those with an underlying kidney disease, especially diabetic kidney disease, this type of exposure can result in acute kidney failure.

Occasionally, a person with a life-threatening infection who is receiving an antibiotic such as streptomycin or gentamicin may go into acute kidney failure. The chance of kidney failure developing due to an antibiotic is greatly enhanced with age, underlying kidney disease, potassium depletion, liver disease, and the use of a diuretic or other nephrotoxic drug. In addition, the long-term use of a nonsteroidal anti-inflammatory drug occasionally can cause acute renal failure.

Extensive traumatic injuries can cause the release of the protein myoglobin, found in muscle, and this substance frequently causes acute kidney failure. Heat stroke, severe exercise, drug overdose, infection, or excessive alcohol intake also can activate the release of myoglobin and result in acute kidney failure.

Kidney Diseases.   Diseases such as interstitial nephritis (see page 893) and glomerulonephritis (see page 895) may result in acute renal failure.

The Diagnosis.   If you appear to have acute kidney failure and are not already in the hospital, you will be hospitalized. There, your physician will attempt to determine whether you have acute kidney failure or have some other kidney disease that affects kidney function.

How Serious Is Acute Renal Failure?
Acute renal failure is extremely dangerous. The mortality rates are highest among people whose acute renal failure developed after operation or traumatic accidents (50 to 70 percent) or who had coexisting heart or lung failure. The mortality rate is especially high (greater than 90 percent) in individuals who have had a recent stroke.

Other factors that can affect the outcome of acute renal failure poorly are old age,

KIDNEY DIALYSIS TREATMENTS

It has only been within the past 35 years that dialysis and kidney transplantation have given people with chronic and irreversible kidney failure the opportunity to live long after their kidneys have ceased to function. Dialysis is an artificial means of removing the waste products from the blood when the kidneys are unable to do so on their own.

Dialysis can be used as a temporary measure during acute kidney failure. This prevents the debilitating and ultimately fatal buildup of wastes in the blood and allows the kidneys time to heal so they can resume their work. It also can totally replace the kidneys when it is clear that chronic disease has rendered them useless.

When does a person with advanced kidney failure need dialysis? Every case is different. As a rule, however, most physicians try to manage chronic kidney failure for as long as possible with the conservative measures outlined in the previous section. Inevitably, however, there comes a time when the benefits of dialysis outweigh the risks.

For young and otherwise healthy people, transplantation is usually preferred over dialysis because it affords a better quality of life. Most of these individuals undergo dialysis until a suitable transplant donor is found. This will be discussed in detail in a later section (see page 911). However, transplantation is not an option for many people with kidney disorders because of their poor physical health and associated medical conditions.

In the United States, almost 100,000 persons are on dialysis, not counting those with acute kidney failure who are on dialysis only temporarily.

Dialysis machine artificially cleanses the blood of waste products in people whose kidneys no longer are able to do so on their own.

For acute situations, dialysis can be done in a hospital dialysis unit or in an intensive-care unit. Most persons with stable kidney problems have their dialysis in outpatient centers. Some forms of dialysis even can be done at home.

The complications associated with dialysis include infection, stroke, heart attack, obesity, peritonitis, and hernia.

Dialysis is not a panacea, but it can be credited with prolonging life in thousands of persons and saving lives in many others.

The several different types of dialysis are described in the following paragraphs.

Hemodialysis

This form of dialysis removes waste products directly from the blood. Before you can undergo hemodialysis, the most common

form of dialysis, an access to the bloodstream must be created surgically, usually in your arm or leg. One form of access is a fistula, a connection between an artery and a vein. After the initial wound heals, the limb appears normal, although the vein may bulge somewhat. Another type of access is a tube of synthetic material inserted between an artery and a vein.

As a rule, most persons on dialysis require 8 to 12 hours of dialysis per week, divided into several sessions. When you are connected to the dialysis machine, your blood is pumped from the vascular access into the artificial kidney which removes the waste products from the blood. This machine acts like the glomeruli because it makes the blood flow across membranes that let the waste compounds filter through. A solution in the machine helps to regulate the substances that are left in the blood and to remove excess fluid.

Peritoneal Dialysis

This form of dialysis utilizes your own peritoneal cavity (in the abdomen) to filter the blood. This cavity has a vast network of capillaries.

The first step is implantation of a catheter leading into the abdomen. Then, through this catheter, dialysis solution is repeatedly infused into and drained out of the abdominal cavity. The small blood vessels in the membrane that forms the inside surrounding lining of the abdomen filter waste products and water into the dialysis solution. This process is continued for as long as necessary.

Continuous Ambulatory Peritoneal Dialysis (CAPD)

Until the development of this method, peritoneal dialysis was not a viable option for those in need of ongoing dialysis. The procedure is similar to the peritoneal dialysis described above except that the abdominal cavity is infused only four or five times a day. This method can be performed by the person at home.

Continuous Cycling Peritoneal Dialysis

In this variation a machine automatically infuses dialysis solution into and out of your peritoneal cavity and drains several times over the course of the night while you sleep.

---

infection, gastrointestinal bleeding, and progression of an underlying kidney disease.

Treatment. If you have acute renal failure, your condition will be monitored closely for evidence of complications such as infection, heart or neurological problems, hypertension, or gastrointestinal bleeding. Should problems occur, they will be treated with the appropriate medication. Your physician also will alter your intake of fluid so that the intake is equal to the output.

Unlike chronic renal failure, acute renal failure can be reversible, and many people fully recover in 1 to 2 months. It may take as long as a year for full function to be regained, however. Occasionally, people progress to chronic renal failure.

Nutrition. You will probably be put on a high-carbohydrate low-protein diet. Essential amino acids and glucose may be given intravenously if your nutritional status is doubtful; this treatment sometimes provides a quicker recovery. Salt and potassium intake may be restricted.

Dialysis. More often now than previously, kidney dialysis is being used in the early stages of acute renal failure in an attempt to prevent complications (see page 907). The removal of excess waste by dialysis often makes the disease easier to control and makes the patient feel better. However, some people with acute renal failure can get through the crisis with minimal or no dialysis.

CHRONIC RENAL FAILURE

Signs and Symptoms
- Abnormal urinalysis;
- Hypertension;
- Loss of weight;
- Vomiting;
- Malaise;
- Headache;
- Decreased urine output;
- Fatigue;
- Decreased mental acuity;
- Muscle twitches and cramps;
- Gastrointestinal bleeding;
- Yellowish brown cast to the skin;
- Itching.

Unlike acute renal failure, chronic renal failure generally occurs over a number of years as the kidneys' nephrons are destroyed slowly and often imperceptibly.

Chronic renal failure is a particularly insidious disease because often there are no symptoms in its early stages. In many cases, *no* symptoms are apparent until kidney function has decreased to less than 25 percent of what is considered normal.

A number of diseases initiate the chronic kidney failure process, the most common being glomerulonephritis in any of its several forms (see page 895). Other causes include polycystic kidney disease, hypertension, pyelonephritis, vesicoureteral reflux, and use of analgesics (see pages 886, 906, 892, 884, and 436, respectively).

The single most common cause of end-stage renal disease in the United States is diabetes mellitus: nephropathy develops in approximately 50 to 60 percent of those with insulin-dependent diabetes (type I). Eventually, dialysis or kidney transplantation is necessary in these people.

If you have diabetes, the first signal of eventual kidney failure usually is an excessive amount of protein in your urine as detected by urinalysis. Normally, diabetics have albumin, a type of protein, in their urine 10 to 15 years after the onset of their diabetes. It is very important to control your blood pressure and to keep your blood sugar under good control. This will help to maintain kidney function. Transplantation, particularly if a related donor is found, may be an option for the younger diabetic person with chronic renal failure.

No matter what its cause, chronic kidney failure results in the buildup, in the blood, of wastes that a properly functioning kidney would excrete into the urine. A person with chronic kidney failure is said to have uremia, a term used to describe not only the wastes in the blood but also a host of metabolic and endocrine functions that also are impaired.

There are very few systems in the body that are not affected when chronic kidney failure occurs. The fluid retention that is common can cause congestive heart failure (see page 807). Other problems that could occur include: weakening of the bones so that they become susceptible to fracture; anemia; ulcers in the stomach; miscarriage in pregnant women; and changes in skin color. Even the central nervous system can be damaged—the affected person suddenly finds it difficult to concentrate or to remember and may have difficulty with the nerves and muscles in the arms and legs.

The Diagnosis. If your symptoms suggest chronic renal failure, your physician will want to establish that the condition is indeed chronic. X-ray studies can be used to determine if both kidneys are smaller than normal, a sign of chronic damage.

How Serious Is Chronic Renal Failure? This condition eventually may progress to

end-stage renal disease (see below). When this occurs, the kidneys simply are not capable of sustaining life. If the person is to live, either dialysis or kidney transplantation is needed.

Treatment. Treatment is begun immediately after chronic renal failure is diagnosed. Although there is no cure, there are things that can be done to control the symptoms, to minimize the complications, and to slow the disease's progression.

An important component of treatment is control of the underlying disease and its complications. Hypertension, congestive heart failure, urinary tract infections, kidney stones, abnormalities of the urinary tract, or the forms of glomerulonephritis that respond to therapy will be treated as appropriate. Severe anemia may require blood transfusion. A component of treatment not to be overlooked is education in preparation for when dialysis or kidney transplantation may be necessary.

Nutrition. A proper diet is extremely important. The problems of nausea, vomiting, and lack of appetite may be solved with use of a low-protein diet. Adequate calorie intake can be provided by carbohydrates and fat. Restricting salt intake may decrease an abnormally high blood pressure. Water intake may need to be regulated carefully. As the disease progresses, restriction of phosphate and potassium may become necessary.

END-STAGE RENAL DISEASE

Signs and Symptoms
- Kidneys permanently cease to function;
- Uremia and many resulting complications which may include hypertension, congestive heart failure, anemia, bone disease, gastrointestinal problems, urinary infection, and dementia.

When kidney function has deteriorated to between 5 and 10 percent of normal capacity, the condition is called end-stage renal disease. This means that the kidneys are incapable of sustaining life and that their function must be provided by either dialysis or a transplanted kidney.

KIDNEY TRANSPLANTATION

Transplantation and dialysis (see page 908) are the only two treatment options for persons with end-stage renal disease. In the past 15 years, more than 55,000 kidney transplantations have been performed in the United States.

Not everyone with end-stage renal disease is a suitable candidate for kidney transplantation. Those with infection, active glomerulonephritis, coronary artery disease, or other severe medical problems generally are considered not to be in good enough condition to undergo a major operation. People age 60 or over are more likely to have adverse reactions, including death, after transplantation than are younger individuals.

However, when successful, transplantation provides a healthier and better-quality life.

The actual operation itself is not a complicated procedure. What can be complicated is finding the right donor, which is important in order to lessen the chance of rejection of the new kidney. Compatibility is determined by blood tests that provide information about both the donor and the recipient, such as blood type and the nature of the antibodies present in each. A brother or sister of the recipient generally is the most likely to have compatible tissue. Unfortunately, a sibling donor is not always available, especially for a very young recipient, because donors have to be at least 18 years old to give their consent.

When a relative is not available as a donor, tissue-typing centers throughout the country are called on to help locate acceptable donors from among accident victims and others who have offered to donate their kidneys after their death (cadaver kidney). A kidney from a cadaver must be transplanted within 48 hours after the death of the donor. Thus, some people have to undergo long periods on dialysis until a compatible cadaver donor is available.

After the transplantation operation, the person receives immunosuppressant drugs to keep his or her body from rejecting the "foreign" kidney. Recently drugs such as cyclosporine have greatly increased the chances of acceptance. If the donor is a blood relative of the recipient, the chances are that by 1 year after the transplantation the kidney will still be well and functioning between 80 and 90 percent of normal. With a cadaver donor, about 80 percent of people have had no significant organ rejection by 1 year after operation.

In cases in which the transplanted kidney is rejected, a second or even third transplantation can be done. The rate of acceptance in these cases is significantly less than it is at the initial transplantation.

Improvements in preparing patients for transplantation and in monitoring their recovery have decreased mortality to as low as 5 percent in some medical centers.

Transplant recipients usually are hospitalized for 10 days to 6 weeks, depending on how well their body accepts the new kidney. The major hurdles are rejection and infection. Immunosuppressant drugs have greatly decreased rejection, but they make it harder for the body's immune system to fight infection. Because the transplant recipient must take an immunosuppressant medication for the rest of his or her life, he or she is prone to have infections.

Kidney transplant recipients need careful medical follow-up to enhance the success of the operation and to ensure good general health.

There are almost 100,000 persons in the United States on chronic dialysis and more than 20,000 persons are living with a functioning kidney transplant.

The largest group of persons with end-stage renal disease are those with type I (juvenile-onset) diabetes mellitus.

The Diagnosis. End-stage renal disease is never a surprise because it is the end of what generally is a long process of chronic kidney failure. Although chronic kidney failure may be silent initially, by the time the kidneys are functioning at only 20 to 25 percent of normal capacity the symptoms usually have become overt. The person usually has been under the care of a physician for 10, 15, or even 20 years when end-stage renal disease is diagnosed.

How Serious Is End-Stage Renal Disease?
End-stage renal disease is fatal unless dialysis is initiated or kidney transplantation is performed. Both of these methods have risks that can be life-threatening. Each individual is unique and should receive counseling from a nephrologist regarding the limitations of and expectations from these repeated treatments.

Treatment. Once a person has progressed to end-stage renal disease, the conservative measures used to manage chronic kidney failure—dietary restrictions, medications, and treating complications and underlying cause—are not enough. In some cases, kidney transplantation is not in the best interest of the individual because of poor general health. Dialysis then becomes the only option.

CHAPTER 31

THE LUNGS AND THE RESPIRATORY SYSTEM

CHAPTER CONTENTS

NORMAL VENTILATION

The primary function of your lungs is to provide oxygen to your blood and to remove carbon dioxide from it. Your lungs are suspended within your chest (thoracic cavity) which is enclosed on its sides, back, and front by your ribs and the cartilage and muscle between them. Your diaphragm, which consists of sheets of muscle, separates your thoracic cavity from your abdominal cavity.

Your lungs are soft and spongy. If you are healthy, your lungs probably are a mottled pinkish gray color, although even healthy lungs can become blackened from carbon particles in polluted air. Your right lung is divided into three sections (lobes); your left lung has two lobes. Your heart is between your lungs, nestled over one corner of your left lung.

To reach your lungs, air enters through your mouth and nose and then travels through the back of your throat (pharynx), through your voice box (larynx), and down your windpipe (trachea). The trachea branches into two main bronchial tubes, or air passageways. Each bronchial tube then branches into smaller passageways (bronchi) which divide several times more, finally forming much smaller tubes (bronchioles). The branching creates the appearance of an upside-down tree. The smallest bronchioles end in tiny closed elastic air sacs called alveoli. Your blood is carried to these air sacs by tiny blood vessels. These alveoli are where the actual exchange of oxygen and carbon dioxide with your blood occurs. Your lungs contain approximately 300 million such alveoli. If they could be stretched out on a flat surface, they would cover an area approximately the size of a tennis court.

The pleura, a double-layer membrane with a very thin lubricating layer of fluid between the two layers, covers the outside of your lungs and the adjacent chest wall. This membrane allows your lungs to move easily within the chest cavity as you breathe.

When you inhale, the muscles of your ribs contract, causing your ribs to move upward and outward. At the same time, your diaphragm contracts, pushing down toward your abdomen. These two actions increase the size of your chest cavity and thus cause your lungs to expand and air to be sucked into them. The individual alveoli also expand with air. During normal breathing, about a pint of air is pulled into your lungs in each breath. However, during heavy breathing, as much as 3 to 6 quarts of air may be sucked into the healthy lungs of an adult.

When you exhale, your diaphragm and rib muscles relax and they return to their original positions. This decreases the size of your chest cavity, compressing your lungs slightly and forcing the stale air, now carrying carbon dioxide, out of your body. The whole process of breathing in and out occurs automatically without your thinking about it.

Your respiratory system has several defense mechanisms that prevent foreign material from entering your lungs. Hairs in the nose filter out the larger particles. Special cells in your air passageways (the trachea and bronchial tubes) secrete mucus which helps keep the airways moist and lubricated and also catches bacteria, dust, and other foreign material. Tiny hair-like projections called cilia line your airways. These cilia continuously beat the mucus upward toward your throat to help keep the passageway to your lungs clean. Some substances may interfere with their function; for example, inhaling cigarette smoke causes the cilia to stop moving.

Lungs

Heart

Diaphragm

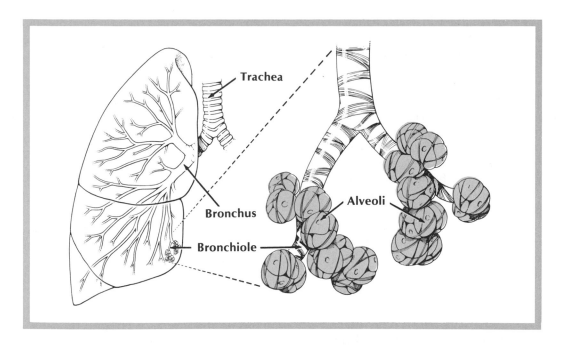

Enlargement of lung segment (right) shows bronchioles and alveoli. The alveoli exchange oxygen and carbon dioxide with your blood.

Your lungs are connected to your heart by the pulmonary veins and arteries (pulmonary comes from the Latin word *pulmo* for lung). Your blood travels throughout your body, returns to your heart, and is pumped by the right ventricle (the bottom right chamber of the heart) through the pulmonary artery to your lungs. The blood then passes through the arteries of the lungs into smaller and smaller vessels, similar to the branching of the bronchi. Finally, it flows into the smallest blood vessels, called capillaries, which are located in the membranes lining the alveoli. Capillaries are so tiny that often the cells of your blood have to pass through them single file. (For further discussion of these workings, see The Healthy Heart and Blood Vessels, page 782.)

After gases are exchanged in the alveoli, the blood, now carrying oxygen, passes into the smallest veins which merge to form larger and larger vessels until the pulmonary veins are formed. The pulmonary veins carry oxygenated blood from the lungs back to the heart, from which it is pumped out again to deliver oxygen to the cells of your body and to remove carbon dioxide.

RESPIRATORY INFECTIONS

If bacteria, viruses, or fungi enter the lungs and become established there, they can cause a number of diseases ranging from common and usually benign illnesses such as colds and flu to more serious illnesses such as pneumonia, bronchitis, and tuberculosis. (For a detailed discussion of the common viral colds, see page 860.)

BRONCHIOLITIS

Signs and Symptoms
- Wheezing;
- Exhaling heavily;
- Rapid breathing and rapid heartbeat;
- Sputum-producing cough.

A respiratory infection such as that caused by the influenza virus or a bacterium may cause your bronchioles (the small airways in the lungs) to become inflamed and to secrete an excessive amount of mucus. This usually is not serious in older children and adults, but in an infant the air passages are much narrower than in an adult and they may become partly or completely blocked. This makes it very difficult for the infant to inhale and exhale.

Bronchiolitis is fairly common, especially during the winter, primarily in children under 2 years of age, but it can occur in young adults under special circumstances. It usually is caused by a viral respiratory infection, often contracted from someone in the infant's household. In infants or families with a history of allergies or in infants with recurring bronchiolitis, an allergic reaction may be the cause.

The Diagnosis. Usually, bronchiolitis is preceded by mild nasal congestion for a day or two. Gradually, breathing becomes more and more difficult and may become more rapid with more vigorous exhalation. Wheezing, rapid heartbeat, and a cough are other symptoms. Fever may or may not be present.

In some cases, the infant may develop cyanosis (the lips and the beds of the fingernails become blue). Bronchiolitis can be serious if the airways become almost completely blocked and the individual has severe difficulty in breathing.

Treatment. Hospitalization might be needed, especially for an infant who is less than 2 months of age, has cyanosis, has had repeated attacks, or is breathing very rapidly and shallowly. Treatment consists of providing warm, moist air, perhaps with extra oxygen. Medications will depend on the nature and severity of the symptoms.

Most infants recover within 2 days to a week, although in rare cases an infant will not survive. About half of the children who contract bronchiolitis will have later episodes of wheezing and may be more susceptible to respiratory infections.

ACUTE BRONCHITIS

Signs and Symptoms
- Soreness and feeling of constriction in the chest;
- Cough;
- Chills;
- Overall malaise and slight fever.

The trachea and bronchi are the principal air passages of the lungs. When the mucous membranes that line the bronchi become inflamed, the condition is called bronchitis or tracheobronchitis. An occasional occurrence of acute bronchitis is to be expected; virtually everyone has bronchitis at some time, much as everyone has the common cold. However, a pattern of recurring bronchitis can represent a more serious health concern (see Chronic Bronchitis, page 927).

In most cases, this common ailment is the result of the same viral infections that cause the common cold (see Common Viral Colds, page 860). The infection spreads to the bronchi, producing the deep cough which, in turn, tends to bring up a yellowish gray sputum from your lungs.

The Diagnosis. The symptoms may include fever, a slight feeling of breathlessness, a sensation of tightness in the chest, and a wheezing sensation when you breathe.

If you have chronic lung or heart problems (including asthma, emphysema, or congestive heart failure), consult your physician if you think you have bronchitis. If you are otherwise healthy, the self-help treatments suggested below will probably be sufficient. In any case, because bronchitis most commonly is the result of a viral infection, your physician probably will be able to do relatively little to relieve your discomfort.

However, if you have fever, if your chest discomfort leaves you breathless, or if you cough up blood, call your physician. He or she will listen to your chest (using a stethoscope) and may obtain a chest x-ray, sputum culture, or other tests to rule out other causes.

In virtually all cases, acute bronchitis disappears in a matter of days and there are no lasting effects.

Treatment. *Self-Help.* Rest, aspirin for fever, drinking extra liquids, and a nonprescription cough medicine are the cornerstones of treatments for acute bronchitis.

Avoid other irritants to the airways, such as tobacco smoke. Remember that the act of coughing also is irritating to the trachea and bronchi, so make attempts to suppress your cough (see also Treating the Common Cough, page 918). You do not have to confine yourself to bed while suffering from acute bronchitis, but it is wise to remain in a warm environment in which the air is somewhat humid, perhaps from use of a vaporizer. Your physician may prescribe a bronchodilator drug to open narrowed passages in your lungs. If your sputum becomes yellow, gray, or green, your physician may prescribe an antibiotic.

Prevention. If you have repeated attacks of bronchitis, you may be able to trace their occurrence to the conditions in which you live. Cold, damp environments combined with excessive air pollution can make you more susceptible to acute bronchitis, so lifestyle changes may be advisable.

PNEUMONIA

Signs and Symptoms
- Cough which may bring up bloody sputum;
- Pain in the chest;
- Chills;
- High fever.

Pneumonia describes an inflammation of the tissues of your lungs. Rather than being an individual ailment, however, what your physician calls "pneumonia" actually can be any one of more than 50 different diseases. They range in seriousness from the mild discomfort that accompanies a cold to life-threatening conditions.

One key reason for this range of severity is that there are many causes of pneumonia. Among them are bacteria such as pneumococci, staphylococci, and streptococci; influenza and other viruses; and chemical irritants.

To make the subject of pneumonia more easily understood, the many varieties are classified into subtypes. For our purposes, three categories are useful: community-acquired, hospital-acquired, and aspiration pneumonia.

Community-Acquired Pneumonia.
Community-acquired pneumonia gets its name from the way it is acquired—that is, from the community at large rather than in the hospital (see Hospital-Acquired Pneumonia, below). Common causes of community-acquired pneumonia are pneumococci, mycoplasma, and the influenza virus.

Hospital-Acquired Pneumonia.
If you acquired your pneumonia while you were in the hospital, the kinds of possible infecting agents are much greater than if you were infected in the course of normal, everyday life.

Aspiration Pneumonia.
This type of pneumonia is the result of foreign matter

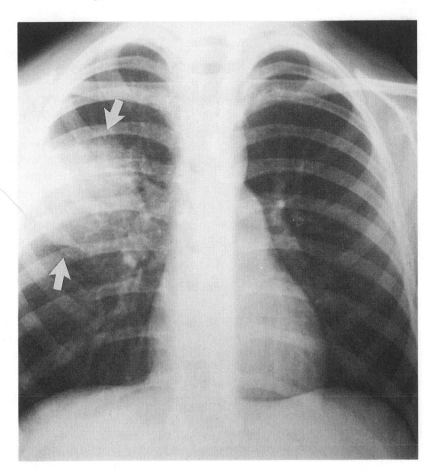

Chest x-ray reveals pneumonia in upper lobe of lung (arrows).

being aspirated into the lungs. Most commonly this occurs when the contents of your stomach enter your lungs after you have vomited.

Pneumonia is a common ailment, occurring in more than 1 in every 100 people annually. In fact, it is likely that everyone inhales certain causative agents with some frequency. However, the healthy person has sufficient defense mechanisms to be able to neutralize the infections. If your defense mechanisms are impaired by alcoholism, aging, injury, use of immunosuppressant drugs, or other causes, you may be more susceptible to pneumonia. In a person weakened by disease, pneumonia can be a deadly disease, which explains why long-term hospital patients with other chronic ailments often die of pneumonia.

The Diagnosis. The symptoms vary depending on the kind of pneumonia you have. A cough typically accompanies most kinds, as does a fever. Other symptoms include chills and breathlessness even when you have not exerted yourself. More serious symptoms include blood in the sputum pro-

TREATING THE COMMON COUGH

Most people think of the cough as just another disagreeable symptom of the common cold. In fact, the cough is a great deal more.

What Causes a Cough?

The cough is a protective reflex: it clears your breathing passages of secretions. As long as it accomplishes this task effectively, it is to be regarded as normal and even healthy.

However, a harsh or forceful cough can be an irritant to the lining of the airways, just as cigarette smoke can be irritating. The act of coughing causes the air passages to contract. When this happens over and over, it leads to inflamed membranes and helps to perpetuate the cough. Coughing is similar to scratching an itch on the skin: if overdone, it can do more harm than good.

Coughing is a symptom most often of viral upper respiratory infections—namely, colds and flu. Inflammation of the voice box (laryngitis) also may be associated with coughing.

Coughing occurs with a number of chronic disorders. Many smokers cough often and even violently; people with allergies and asthma also find themselves coughing involuntarily because of their ailments.

What Can Be Done?

A cough that accompanies the common viral respiratory infection may be treated by one or a combination of the therapies suggested below. However, if you have a persistent, unexplained cough or one that is dry and produces little or no secretion or interferes with your sleep—or your spouse's—consult your physician. He or she may want to find out if there is an underlying ailment that is producing your cough. For example, persistent coughing during the night may be due to regurgitation of the acidic content of your stomach and aspiration of this material into the bronchi (see Esophageal Reflux, page 593).

Throat Soothers

Honey, hard candy, or medicated throat lozenges may be effective in soothing simple throat irritation and preventing coughing if your throat is dry or sore.

Expectorants

If your cold or flu is accompanied by thick, sticky secretions in your throat, a cough medication called an expectorant may increase the flow of normal lubricants in your throat. The good news is that expectorants (the name comes from the verb "expectorate," meaning to spit) may help you to clear your throat of this material; the bad news is that these are not miracle drugs and in only a few cases do these medicines truly solve the problem. They may help but, in fact, drinking extra fluids is of primary importance. Breathing moist air also may help.

Cough Suppressants

A dry, irritating cough may be controlled by medications that act on the portion of your brain that controls your cough reflex. Termed antitussives (from the Latin word for cough), these include codeine and the related drug hydrocodone. They are available only with a physician's prescription and are to be used only as directed because they are narcotic drugs.

An over-the-counter drug that has similar effects is dextromethorphan. We recommend the cough-drop form of this medication, which spares you the extra cost of useless ingredients usually included in its syrup forms.

Antihistamines

One antihistamine drug, diphenhydramine, also has an antitussive effect. It is available as an over-the-counter drug.

Regardless of medications, however, remember this: harsh and prolonged coughing aggravates the situation, so cough as infrequently and as gently as possible. This is especially important when there is no secretion to raise from the lungs. Sipping liquids and breathing quietly sometimes can help you stifle a paroxysm of coughing.

If coughing persists at night, raising the head of your bed 6 to 8 inches may prevent the contents of your stomach from being aspirated. This is especially true for elderly people.

So, take care of your cough—and seek the guidance of your physician if it persists for more than 2 to 3 weeks.

duced by coughing, a bluish tinge to your skin (cyanosis), and even mental confusion. Pneumonia may appear to be a cold at first or may develop as a complication of a cold.

Your physician will listen to your chest to detect distortions in your breathing that suggest the presence of the infection. Chest x-rays also may be obtained to identify the location and extent of the infection.

A sample of your sputum may be tested to identify the infecting agent. Usually, the sample that you produce by coughing will be sufficient for this test but in some cases, other means, including the insertion of a catheter into the windpipe, may be necessary. Blood tests may also be conducted.

How Serious Is Pneumonia?   The seriousness of this disorder depends largely on your overall health. In young people, pneumonia typically is a passing discomfort that may remain undiagnosed and be regarded as simply a cold. However, in people weakened by disease (especially heart failure or lung ailments such as chronic bronchitis, asthma, or emphysema) and in the elderly, death can result—sometimes in 24 hours. Proper medical care, bed rest, and careful monitoring are essential.

Treatment.   Consult your physician because there is little you can do on your own and serious pneumonia can be life-threatening. The treatment your physician will provide depends on the cause (whether bacterium, virus, or other agent) and the severity of your symptoms.

Medication.   If the cause is bacterial, your physician will prescribe antibiotic drugs. Penicillin or erythromycin often is the drug of choice but your physician may consider other antibiotics, too, or even the nonantibiotic sulfadiazine.

Other Therapies.   Hospitalization may be necessary in serious cases; oxygen may also be administered.

Prevention.   Pneumococcal pneumonia may be prevented by injection of a pneumococcal vaccine (see also page 867). At present, it appears that this might give some degree of lifelong immunity to the disease, but the vaccine has not been in use for sufficient time to be certain. This type of pneumonia is common in certain groups of people—for example, those over age 65 and those at any age with heart or lung ailments. We recommend vaccination against the pneumococcus organism for healthy adults age 65 or older or for people with an immune deficiency disease or chronic illnesses such as heart disease, chronic lung disease, alcoholism, or if your spleen has been removed. If you are in one of these groups, ask your physician about this vaccine. You probably should have it.

TUBERCULOSIS

Signs and Symptoms

- Initially, symptoms are not apparent or are limited to a minor cough and mild fever;
- Later, fatigue;
- Weight loss;
- Cough which occasionally produces bloody sputum;
- Slight fever and night sweats.

Tuberculosis, often called "TB," is a chronic bacterial infection that can develop after you inhale droplets sprayed into the air (as from a cough or sneeze) by someone infected with *Mycobacterium tuberculosis.* This disease has been present since antiquity and, although its incidence has greatly decreased, TB continues to remain a health problem in the United States, particularly for infants and the very elderly. The disease has also been occurring more frequently in certain areas of the country and may be linked to the arrival of immigrants.

Your risk of contracting the disease varies directly with the frequency of your contacts with persons who have TB. The number of organisms released in a cough or sneeze is rather small, and the spread of infection to others is not as common as is the case with the common cold. Good ventilation and exposure to sunlight decrease the risk of exposure.

If you are exposed to the TB bacterium, the organism may gain entry to your lungs. Often, you are not aware of this exposure in that there are very few, if any, immediate symptoms. The spread of disease generally is limited or contained by your lymph nodes.

Usually within 2 to 3 months after the initial infection, a spot may be noticeable on an x-ray of your chest. This spot persists indefinitely and usually is no cause for concern.

In the United States, more than 95 percent of those acquiring an initial or primary TB infection have complete healing with no subsequent evidence of disease except the healed spots seen on a chest x-ray.

In some people tuberculosis can develop within weeks after the initial exposure. More often, the TB organism may lie dormant for many years before disease becomes apparent.

The disease may be reactivated under conditions in which the immune system is weakened, including old age, malnutrition, alcoholism, immunosuppressive therapy, or certain other illnesses such as AIDS or malignancies of the lymph or blood system. The disease also is common in the homeless and in refugees from Asia and Central America.

The Diagnosis. When you are infected, usually no symptoms are apparent initially, although there may be a mild cough and slight fever. Typical symptoms of later reactivation of the TB are fatigue, weight loss, lack of appetite, mild fever, night sweats, and coughing. Occasionally, the coughing may bring up blood from the lung. If the disease progresses, your physician may notice the development of cavities on your chest x-ray. More severe coughing may also result, occasionally along with discolored or bloody sputum.

The TB organism can spread through your lymph nodes and blood to almost any organ in your body. The areas commonly affected include the lining of the lungs (you may experience pain with breathing or coughing), the bones of the spine or large joints (pain is a major symptom), and kidneys (you may experience symptoms suggestive of a bladder infection; see Cystitis, page 892).

The preliminary diagnosis of TB often is based on review of your chest x-ray. In addition, your physician may obtain a sample of material from your sputum for staining and examination under the microscope. The diagnosis is confirmed by growing the organism in culture in the laboratory.

The easiest source of material for culture for the TB organism is sputum. Other common sources are urine and stomach secretions (obtained by placing a tube into the stomach). Your physician can obtain results from a staining test within 24 hours, but culture results may not be available for up to 6 weeks because the TB bacterium grows slowly. The culture results also will give information as to how well (or poorly) the bacterium will respond to treatment. Unusual forms of the TB organism are common and may require different or more intensive treatments.

A tuberculin skin test often is used to tell whether you previously have been infected with the TB organism. A common way of performing this test is to inject a small amount of tuberculin purified protein deriva-

tive (PPD) into your skin. If you have been infected by the TB organism, this injection will cause a reaction in your skin within 48 to 72 hours. The results of this test will be interpreted by your physician or a trained nurse 2 to 3 days after the injection.

When a very active infection is going on in your body or if your immune system is suppressed, the tuberculin test reaction may be falsely negative.

Treatment. In the past, sanatoriums often were used for persons who had active TB. This no longer is necessary unless you are unable to care for yourself. With modern therapies, hospitalization, enforced rest, or diet changes are seldom required to cure the disease.

Medication. If you have active TB, whether confined to your lungs or present in other areas of your body, your physician may prescribe at least two different medications to be used for prolonged periods. This is to prevent the development of resistance to the drug.

The drug regimens often include combined use of isoniazid and rifampin, although other combinations also can be used. Once these drug regimens are begun, symptoms often are relieved within 2 to 3 weeks, with improvement seen on the chest x-ray thereafter. In addition, generally after 2 to 3 weeks, you are no longer infectious. At times, the drug regimen needs to be changed or another drug added, depending upon your response to therapy.

All medications used for TB have some toxicity, and your physician will discuss this with you. Both rifampin and isoniazid may cause a noninfectious form of hepatitis (the key symptom is jaundice; see page 651). This generally is reversible if the medication is stopped. Rifampin may cause your urine, sweat, and tears to take on an orange or brownish color. If you are pregnant, your physician will discuss the potential effects of the medications on your pregnancy.

Prevention. If you have a positive tuberculin skin test, especially if you recently have been in close contact with a person with TB, your physician may consider giving you medication to decrease the risk of activation of the organism. Isoniazid often is prescribed to be used for up to a year.

In addition, your physician may consider giving isoniazid or a similar medication to others who live in your household or to persons who have been known to have been exposed in the past year.

Vaccines have been administered to millions of people worldwide and are known to be safe, although there is some question as to their value. Your physician may wish to consider these vaccines if you are a high-risk individual, but they are of no value in a person whose tuberculin skin test is positive.

LEGIONNAIRE'S DISEASE

Signs and Symptoms
- Malaise;
- Slight headache;
- Fever and shaking chills;
- Cough that produces mucus;
- Shortness of breath, chest pain.

Legionnaire's disease was first identified when a sudden, virulent outbreak of pneumonia occurred at a convention hotel in Philadelphia in July 1976, primarily among delegates to an American Legion Convention—hence its name. More than 200 people came down with a severe respiratory illness of unknown cause; 34 people died.

The cause eventually was identified as a previously unknown bacterium that subsequently was named *Legionella pneumophila*. The bacterium was then identified as being responsible for several other, smaller outbreaks of pneumonia, the earliest of which occurred in 1957. Children have come down with the disease, but most cases have occurred in middle-aged or older adults.

Legionella bacteria have been identified all over the world in all types of water-related environments. What is most important so far as disease is concerned is that the bacteria can thrive in warm, moist areas of the air-circulation systems of large buildings. They have been isolated from the evaporative coolers of large air-conditioning systems (the source of the outbreak in Philadelphia). The bacteria are spread through air ducts as aerosols and eventually are inhaled. Although these organisms have been found in a wide variety of places, the vast majority of similar sources are free of them and thus legionellosis is uncommon.

The Diagnosis. Legionnaire's disease usually begins with a slight headache and a feeling of malaise, followed in less than a day by a rapidly increasing temperature. Within 24 to 48 hours, the fever reaches 104°F in about half of the affected persons, and many have shaking chills.

A mild, dry cough usually begins early and gets worse over several days. The cough usually produces mucus. About 20 percent of these persons also cough up some blood in the mucus. Other common symptoms are shortness of breath, chest pain, and muscular pain. About a quarter of those with the disease have gastrointestinal symptoms including nausea and vomiting, diarrhea, and abdominal pain.

The disease usually gets progressively worse for the first 4 to 6 days; another 4 or 5 days may pass before recovery begins, although in some persons the illness is milder. The lungs usually continue to be congested for some days after the fever disappears.

To diagnose legionnaire's disease, your physician will take chest x-rays and obtain samples of your blood and mucus to identify the presence of the bacterium.

How Serious Is Legionnaire's Disease? Typically, legionnaire's disease is a very virulent disease, causing pneumonia severe enough to require hospitalization. Although most people recover, some hospitalized patients suffer from respiratory failure which is fatal in about 15 percent of the cases.

Treatment. Hospitalization may be required. You also may need intravenous administration of fluids, because of the fluid loss due to the high fever. You also may need supplementary oxygen.

Medication. Various antibiotics appear to be effective against legionnaire's disease. Erythromycin seems to be the safest and most effective antibiotic.

BRONCHIECTASIS

Signs and Symptoms
- Persistent cough that produces large amounts of sputum, usually gray-green;
- Appetite loss;

- Weight loss;
- Anemia;
- Recurring attacks of pneumonia.

Bronchiectasis is a chronic, abnormal expansion (dilation) of the walls of the bronchial tubes. The same condition occurs in

POSTURAL DRAINAGE AND CHEST PERCUSSION

With bronchiectasis (see page 921), cystic fibrosis (see page 933), lung abscess (see page 923), and certain other lung problems, a large volume of secretions may accumulate in the lungs. Especially if you have cystic fibrosis, your physician may recommend one or both of the strategies called postural drainage and chest percussion to help empty your lungs of the unwanted secretions.

Postural Drainage

This process uses gravity to clear the lungs. You position yourself so that the secretions are moved to your windpipe (trachea) so that you can then cough them out. Because the branches of your lungs point in various directions, it may be necessary for you to assume different positions to drain different areas of the lungs.

Some physicians recommend a time-consuming series of positional changes to raise secretions in cystic fibrosis, a childhood disease (see page 933). Others have found that compliance with these instructions decreases as the child with cystic fibrosis ages. Therefore, many physicians select certain of the positions in order to drain the areas of the lungs where most of the secretions are likely to lodge. (Usually these positions will be those that drain the lower portions of the lungs.)

Cystic Fibrosis

If you have cystic fibrosis, see your physician or a trained therapist at a cystic fibrosis center for specific instructions. Remember to cough during each position change to aid in raising the sputum.

Bronchiectasis

This condition is uncommon in upper lobes of the lungs because these lobes drain quite well when you are in an upright position. In these conditions, postural drainage may be simpler. You may drain lower portions of your lungs quite well by kneeling on a chair or couch and putting your hands on the floor. Stay in that position for about 10 minutes, and cough periodically.

Collect the expectorated sputum and note its color and approximate amount. If no sputum is produced, stop postural drainage until it becomes worthwhile. If you are taking antibiotics, remember that these work better and will be effective for a longer period if you keep your airways as free of secretions as possible.

Chest Percussion

Chest clapping (percussion) is another means of loosening secretions in the lungs.

Cup your hands and rapidly strike your chest wall with one hand and then with the other. You may wish to protect your skin with a bath towel. Be careful not to strike the heart area, breasts, floating ribs, shoulders, or kidneys.

Your physician may recommend a sequence that coordinates both chest percussion and postural drainage for maximum effect.

Parents and others concerned with a child's care should learn this technique. Adults also need help with this procedure when applying the procedure to the back which may be the most important area.

Postural drainage technique uses gravity to help clear lungs of unwanted secretions. Position shown here is designed to clear lower lungs.

persons who have chronic bronchitis, but in bronchiectasis the dilation of the bronchial tubes is more pronounced.

Some people are born with the condition but in most bronchiectasis develops as a complication of cystic fibrosis (see page 933) or diseases such as whooping cough, pneumonia, and tuberculosis. In about half of the cases, cystic fibrosis is the cause. Bronchiectasis occurs primarily in children and young adults; the illness usually is diagnosed within the first 20 years of life. It is much less common since the introduction of antibiotic treatment for pneumonia.

The Diagnosis. A chronic cough that produces large amounts of thick, often foul-smelling sputum is the primary symptom. The cough may be mild or severe. The sputum often contains streaks of blood and, if allowed to settle, will separate into three layers—a thick bottom layer containing pus, a middle layer of greenish fluid, and a top layer of froth.

As the disease progresses, symptoms such as fever, weight loss, general weakness, and anemia may develop. Your physician may use x-rays or a CT scan (see page 1286) to confirm the diagnosis. (A CT scan is a useful, noninvasive way of diagnosing bronchiectasis.) Bronchography (taking an x-ray of the lungs after injecting a material that appears opaque in the bronchial tubes on a chest x-ray) is not usually necessary unless surgical treatment is being considered and there is a need to define the extent of the disease precisely.

Treatment. Your physician may suggest chest physiotherapy which will include postural drainage and chest percussion (see Postural Drainage and Chest Percussion, page 922). You will be taught breathing exercises to help improve the functioning of your lungs. Avoid dust, smoke, and other respiratory irritants. Get plenty of exercise because deep breathing helps raise secretions. Eat a nutritious diet. Drinking lots of fluids helps to dilute the sputum in your lungs.

Medication. Because bacterial infections are associated with production of pus in bronchiectasis, antibiotics are usually prescribed. Unless a specific antibiotic is indicated by tests of your sputum, ampicillin,

tetracycline, or a similar drug is usually given. If you are allergic to penicillin-type drugs, your physician will prescribe a different medication. Your physician also may prescribe a bronchodilator to counteract the spasms in your bronchial tubes.

Antibiotics usually are prescribed for intermittent use. A common regimen would be to take the antibiotic for 7 to 10 consecutive days each month. Seldom should it be necessary to use an antibiotic continuously. At times it may be advisable to alternate among two or three kinds of antibiotics to prevent the development of a resistant bacterial strain.

Surgery. If you have no response to other treatments of if you are coughing up blood, surgical removal of the affected portion of the lung may be necessary. However, this is an option only if the disease is localized in one or two small areas of the lungs.

LUNG ABSCESS

Signs and Symptoms
- High and irregular fever;
- Sweats and chills;
- Shortness of breath;
- Cough that produces pus;
- Malaise and loss of appetite.

A lung abscess is a cavity in your lungs that is filled with pus. It usually occurs when infectious material from your mouth or throat is inhaled and an infection becomes established in your lungs. Dental disease often is the source of the infection.

Infectious organisms in the mouth usually are inhaled when a person is unconscious as a result of excessive alcohol consumption, general anesthesia, excessive sedation, or a disease of the central nervous system. In men over age 55 who smoke, lung cancer may cause a lung abscess by blocking a bronchial tube. Sometimes a lung abscess occurs as a complication of pneumonia. Other, rarer, causes of lung abscess are infections caused by tuberculosis or by fungal or parasitic organisms. In most cases, only a single abscess develops in the lung, although occasionally multiple abscesses appear.

The Diagnosis. Symptoms of a lung abscess develop slowly over several days or weeks. Initially, they are similar to those of pneumonia, including malaise, loss of appetite, fever, and chills. You may lose a considerable amount of weight.

A cough is present after the abscess ruptures into a bronchial tube. Large amounts of sputum that contains pus and sometimes blood may be expectorated. Depending on the type of organism causing the infection, the sputum may be foul-smelling. Chest pain is present in some cases.

In addition to a physical examination, your physician will have a series of chest x-rays taken if lung abscess is suspected and will take a sample of your sputum to check for bacteria or other organisms. Such information can lead to more effective treatment with specific antibiotics or other therapy.

How Serious Is a Lung Abscess?   Lung abscess is generally an acute disease although, if not treated adequately, it can become chronic. With correct treatment, most people with an acute abscess recover completely without surgery.

Treatment.   *Medication.*   Antibiotics are necessary. The particular antibiotic prescribed will depend on what bacterium your physician finds to be the cause of the infection. If the abscess is the result of other organisms, your physician will advise other specific treatment. (See also Tuberculosis, page 919, and Fungal Diseases of the Lungs, page 925.)

Other Therapies.   Postural drainage and chest percussion may be used to drain the lung abscess (see page 923). If your lung abscess does not respond to antibiotics or drainage and percussion, bronchoscopy (see page 940) may be appropriate. Surgery may be advisable if the abscess has been present for several weeks, if it has a thick wall, or if it has spread into the pleural space (see Empyema, below). Chest x-rays are often taken during the course of the disease to monitor progress.

EMPYEMA

Signs and Symptoms
* Dry cough;
* Fever and night sweats;
* Weight loss;
* Shortness of breath;
* Chest pain on deep breathing.

Normally, only a tiny amount of lubricating fluid is present in the pleural space, the space between the two layers of the pleural membrane that surrounds your lungs. Empyema (pus in the pleural space) occurs if infection is present in this space and there is an accumulation of pus.

This buildup of infected fluid—to a pint or more—puts pressure on your lungs, which may cause shortness of breath if the amount of fluid is large enough. You may experience chest pain on deep breathing due to pleurisy (inflammation of the pleural membrane; see page 925). This usually occurs early in the course of the disease but may disappear after more fluid is formed. A dry cough, fever and night sweats, and weight loss also may occur although, if the accumulation of fluid is small, you may have no symptoms at all.

Usually, empyema occurs as a complication of bacterial pneumonia, lung abscess, or certain other respiratory infections or after trauma to the chest or chest surgery. To confirm a diagnosis of empyema, your physician may perform thoracentesis; in this procedure, a needle is inserted through your chest wall to remove a sample of fluid from your pleural cavity.

Treatment.   Treatment consists of antibiotic therapy and draining of the infected fluid from the chest. Your physician will prescribe the antibiotic that is most effective based on the results of culture of the infected matter.

Surgery.   If the fluid in the pleural space flows easily, repeated thoracenteses may remove it. However, a thoracostomy—in which an incision is made in the chest wall under local anesthesia and a tube is inserted for drainage—is often necessary to ensure adequate removal of the fluid.

If this is unsuccessful, thoracotomy (opening the chest wall) may be performed under general anesthesia to permit thorough removal of the infection. When the lung has become trapped by marked thickening of the pleura (similar to a thick orange peel), surgery may be advisable to remove the thickening so that the lung can expand again.

PLEURISY AND PLEURAL EFFUSIONS

Signs and Symptoms
- Shortness of breath;
- Chest pain;
- Dry cough;
- Fever and chills.

Pleurisy is inflammation of the pleura, the double membrane that surrounds each of your lungs. Pleural effusions are accumulations of fluid in the pleural space. Pleurisy and pleural effusions occur as complications of an underlying disease such as tuberculosis, pneumonia, pulmonary embolism, pancreatitis, cancer, or congestive heart failure or of trauma to the chest or other serious conditions.

In pleurisy, the two inflamed layers of the membrane rub against each other when you inhale and exhale. This produces a sharp, fleeting pain in your chest that is made worse by coughing, sneezing, movement, and deep breathing. The pain is relieved when you hold your breath or, sometimes, when you apply pressure over the painful area.

When pleural effusions develop, the pain usually disappears because the fluid serves as a lubricant; however, if enough fluid accumulates, it puts pressure on the lungs and interferes with their normal function, caus-ing shortness of breath. A dry cough, fever, and chills sometimes occur as well, particularly if the fluid in the pleural space is infected (see Empyema, page 924). The outcome of pleurisy generally depends on the seriousness of the underlying disease.

The Diagnosis. Your physician may suspect the diagnosis on the basis of your symptoms, findings on examination of your chest with a stethoscope, and the results of a chest x-ray. Sometimes physicians inject a local anesthetic and insert a needle through the chest wall (between the ribs) and remove fluid for analysis.

At the same time, a sample of tissue for microscopic study may be obtained, particularly if your physician is concerned that the fluid collection may be caused by a cancer (see Lung Cancer, page 937), a chronic condition such as tuberculosis (see page 919), or sarcoidosis (see page 934).

Treatment. First, it is important to treat the underlying condition or illness that is causing the pleurisy or pleural effusion. However, in some cases the pleural effusion needs to be drained for several days by means of a chest tube.

Medication. Analgesics and anti-inflammatory drugs are generally prescribed. Sometimes codeine is prescribed to control the cough.

FUNGAL DISEASES OF THE LUNGS

Yeast and the spores of certain fungi, if inhaled, can become established in the lungs, causing disease. Most of these cause flu-like symptoms including fever, cough, and a general feeling of malaise.

HISTOPLASMOSIS

Signs and Symptoms
- Fever, cough, general malaise;
- Enlargement of liver, lymph nodes, spleen;
- Cough and difficulty breathing.
- No symptoms.

Histoplasmosis results from inhaling dust, particularly from chicken houses, bat-infested caves, and pigeon droppings, that contains the spores of the fungus *Histoplasma capsulatum*. Men are more likely than women to contract severe cases of the disease. In the United States, this disease is most common in the Mississippi and Ohio River valleys.

It is quite common to see one or more spots on the lung in chest x-rays in those who have had histoplasmosis in the past that went unrecognized or was symptomless.

The Diagnosis. There are four forms of histoplasmosis. The mildest form is almost indistinguishable from other diseases such as the common cold; it causes fever, cough, and a general feeling of malaise. If the fungus spreads from the lungs through the blood, it causes the second form with enlargement of the liver, lymph nodes, or spleen and, less often, oral or gastrointestinal ulcers. The third form, a chronic form, produces an illness similar to chronic tuberculosis; the symptoms are cough and difficulty breathing. The most serious form of histoplasmosis is the disseminated (widespread) form that can occur in persons with weakened immune systems.

To confirm histoplasmosis, your physician will obtain specimens of sputum, lymph nodes, bone marrow, liver, blood, urine, or oral ulcerations in order to check for the presence of the fungus.

How Serious Is Histoplasmosis?   In its mild form, histoplasmosis usually is benign and requires no treatment. The more serious forms of the disease can lead to death.

Treatment.   *Medication.*   If you have no symptoms, treatment usually is unnecessary. However, if symptomatic, amphotericin B, a fungicidal and fungistatic antibiotic, is effective in most cases of histoplasmosis; this drug must be given through a vein. At times, ketoconazole, which is taken orally, will suffice. If your lungs are affected, treatment will eliminate the fungus, but the lesions it produces in your lungs will remain.

ASPERGILLOSIS

Aspergillus is a genus of fungi that is found virtually everywhere. It may be present in nasal discharges and respiratory secretions of people who are exposed to them regularly (from the soil or farm dust), but they rarely cause problems in this group of people.

In persons with asthma (see Asthma, page 933), *Aspergillus* can produce a form of allergic response. In other susceptible persons, it can cause an unusual form of pneumonia. Both of these conditions, which are called aspergillosis, can be treated effectively with corticosteroids.

In persons whose lungs have been previously damaged, *Aspergillus* may collect within the lungs. The symptoms may include cough or coughing up blood, weight loss, and mild fever. Often, surgery is needed to control the bleeding.

If aspergillosis occurs in a person who has cancer of the blood (leukemia), the prognosis is poor, even with intravenous therapy with amphotericin B, an antifungal medication.

CRYPTOCOCCOSIS

Signs and Symptoms
* Low-grade fever;
* Chest pain;
* Cough.

Cryptococcosis is caused by a yeast, *Cryptococcus neoformans,* that lives in soil and on dried pigeon droppings. Disease results when a person inhales the organism. Most susceptible are those with weakened immune systems, such as persons with leukemia or Hodgkin's disease, those taking corticosteroids, and those with AIDS.

The Diagnosis.   In some cases, only mild symptoms, such as a low-grade fever, chest pain, and a cough, possibly producing sputum, occur. More serious cases resemble bronchitis and lesions develop in the lungs. The yeast may remain in the lungs, or it may spread, especially to the central nervous system where it causes increasingly severe headaches, followed by nausea, vertigo, loss of appetite, vision disorders, and mental deterioration.

Your physician may take an x-ray to detect changes in the lungs, and samples of sputum, pus, or spinal fluid may be taken to check for the presence of the yeast.

How Serious Is Cryptococcosis?   Some mild cases clear without treatment but, because this condition usually affects people whose immune systems are already greatly weakened, cryptococcosis can lead to death, especially if it spreads from the lungs.

Treatment. *Medication.*   Amphotericin B and flucytosine usually clear up the infection in about 6 weeks. Surgical removal of the nodules that form in the lungs may be advisable.

COCCIDIOIDOMYCOSIS

Signs and Symptoms
- No symptoms;
- Fever, chills, backache, headache;
- Chest pain;
- Red spotty rash;
- Swelling of knees and ankles;
- Cough, nasal congestion.

Coccidioidomycosis is caused by breathing in spores from the fungus *Coccidioides immitis* which exists in the soil in certain arid parts of the southwestern United States, Mexico, and Central and South America. In the United States, it was first discovered and is very prevalent in California's San Joaquin Valley and hence its more popular name, San Joaquin or valley fever. It may affect anyone, but if you are pregnant or if your immune system is weak, you are especially vulnerable. The disease tends to be more serious in dark-skinned people.

The Diagnosis. Most commonly there are no symptoms with coccidioidomycosis. Nine of every 10 people who have moved into the desert areas of the southwestern United States test positive for this fungus within 4 or 5 years after their move. In approximately 10 percent of these, chest pain will develop. This, along with fever, chills,

and other flu-like symptoms, usually begins 10 to 30 days after exposure to the mold. Nasal congestion and a mild cough may be followed by bronchitis. One to 2 days after the fever begins, a red spotty rash, similar to that of measles, appears, and your knees and ankles may swell.

How Serious Is Coccidioidomycosis?
Usually the disease clears up without complications, although in some cases the lesions formed in the lungs may be difficult to cure and, in rare cases, this disease may recur after weeks or months. Occasionally the infection spreads throughout the body, causing lesions in the lungs, bones, and other organs.

Treatment. You will need bed rest and treatment of the flu-like symptoms until the fever disappears.

Medication. If you have no symptoms, treatment usually is unnecessary. If you have symptoms, your physician may prescribe amphotericin B. This is given through a vein, and it helps in most cases. Ketoconazole taken by mouth is less effective but may be used between courses of amphotericin B in treating a recurrence of the disease.

Surgery. In severe cases, surgical drainage of lung abscesses or pleural fluids may help.

CHRONIC LUNG CONDITIONS

There are three chronic lung disorders in which obstruction to the flow of air out of the bronchial passages is a prominent symptom. In one, chronic bronchitis, there is a persistent inflammation of the lining of the bronchial passages commonly, but not always, associated with obstruction to the outflow of air. Another, emphysema, is characterized by swelling of the air sacs (alveoli) and destruction of the walls between them; there almost always is some degree of bronchitis associated with emphysema, and chronic obstruction to the outflow of air is prominent. Physicians often refer to emphysema and chronic bronchitis as chronic obstructive lung disease (COLD) and chronic obstructive pulmonary disease (COPD).

In the third disorder, asthma, allergic factors are mainly responsible. Obstruction to the outflow of air is intermittent, occurring in "attacks," and is a consequence of spasm of muscles encircling the bronchial tubes. *(For a detailed discussion of Asthma, see page 466.)*

CHRONIC BRONCHITIS

Signs and Symptoms
- Chronic cough that produces mucus;
- Shortness of breath.

This disorder consists of chronic inflammation and thickening of the lining of your bronchial tubes. There may be enough narrowing of these air passages to interfere with breathing and often to induce spells of coughing. In addition, the inflammation causes the glands of your bronchial tubes to produce excessive amounts of mucus, increasing the congestion in your lungs and further hampering your ability to breathe. It is a persistent disease, lasting for long periods and recurring often, and it may become permanent.

Most people with chronic obstructive pulmonary disease (COPD) have a combination of chronic bronchitis and emphysema, but one of these diseases is usually dominant. Those with chronic bronchitis tend to be over age 35 and often are overweight or obese.

Smoking is the major cause of chronic bronchitis; however, air pollution and dusts or toxic gases in the workplace also can cause bronchial irritation and chronic inflammation. The disease is more prevalent in men than in women. About 20 percent of adult men have chronic bronchitis; however, because more women are smoking, the number of women with the disease is increasing.

In bronchitis, the main branches leading from the airway to the lungs (the bronchi) become inflamed and thickened, narrowing the passageway for air to travel to the lungs.

The Diagnosis.   The primary symptom of chronic bronchitis (as distinct from emphysema) is a chronic cough that produces large amounts of mucus. The diagnosis of chronic bronchitis is based on the presence of a persistent (for at least 3 months of the year for more than 2 consecutive years) cough that produces mucus. Initially, the cough usually appears during the winter months; then, over the years, it becomes almost continuous. As the disease worsens, relapses of the cough become more frequent and more severe and you may experience shortness of breath.

In diagnosing chronic bronchitis, your physician will take your medical history, perform a physical examination, obtain lung function tests, and take a chest x-ray.

How Serious Is Chronic Bronchitis?
Chronic bronchitis is a serious disease. In people with severe disease, the likelihood of long survival is poor. However, if the disease is detected early and the affected person does not smoke, the outcome is more optimistic.

Treatment.   If you smoke cigarettes, stop smoking. Other primary goals of therapy are relief of symptoms and avoidance of respiratory infections. Also, your physician will teach you how to deal with the disease.

One of the things you can do to prevent aggravation of your cough is to avoid fumes such as paint odors, exhaust fumes, and even certain cooking odors and perfumes. Avoid dust, extremely humid or dry air, and cold air. During the winter, use a humidifier in your home, particularly in the bedroom.

If at all possible, avoid exposure to anyone who has a cold because such an infection may severely aggravate your bronchitis. Make sure you dress appropriately for the temperature, and stay away from large groups of people during the winter when colds and flu are common. If you do come down with a respiratory infection (typical symptoms include cough, a change in color or amount of sputum, and fever), call your physician promptly and get treatment.

Unless your physician advises against it, get a flu shot (see Influenza Shots, page 854) yearly and be vaccinated against pneumococcal pneumonia (see Immunizations, page 867). Note, however, that the pneumonia

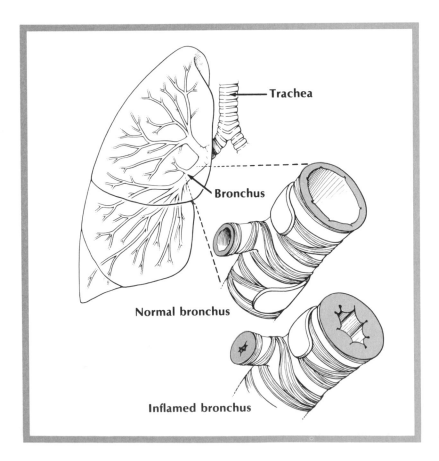

Trachea

Bronchus

Normal bronchus

Inflamed bronchus

vaccine (Pneumovax) provides lifelong immunity against common strains of *Pneumococcus.* Seldom is a second vaccination necessary.

Drinking large quantities of fluid helps to dilute the thick mucus in your lungs and so may make removal by coughing easier. Keep in mind, however, that beverages containing caffeine and alcohol tend to remove fluid from your body, so limit the amounts you consume.

Medication. Your physician may prescribe a 7- to 10-day course of broad-spectrum antibiotics (antibiotics that are effective against many kinds of bacteria; examples are ampicillin, erythromycin, and tetracycline). These will be used if your sputum changes in color, volume, or thickness, changes that may indicate the onset of a respiratory infection. Your physician also may prescribe a bronchodilator if lung tests indicate the presence of spasm of your airways.

If your body's ability to get oxygen from your lungs into your blood is significantly impaired, your physician may prescribe oxygen therapy, on either a continuous or a supplemental basis. Devices are now available that permit oxygen delivery both in the home and in portable containers to allow maximum mobility.

EMPHYSEMA

Signs and Symptoms
- Shortness of breath;
- Chronic, mild cough.

The term emphysema is used as a synonym for chronic obstructive pulmonary disease (COPD). Emphysema is quite common and in most cases is caused by smoking over a long period, although heredity and preexisting asthma may have some effect. Emphysema is most likely to develop in cigarette smokers, but cigar and pipe smokers also are at risk. (Most of the latter group smoked cigarettes initially.) Emphysema is more common in men than in women, but this difference is changing because more women are smoking.

Normally, your lungs contain 300 million elastic air sacs, called alveoli, in which oxygen is added to your blood and carbon dioxide is removed from it. Emphysema occurs when the alveoli lose their natural elasticity, become overstretched, and rupture. Several adjacent alveoli may rupture, forming one large space instead of many small ones. This process occurs slowly and does not affect all of the alveoli to the same extent, but it does prevent the lungs from functioning efficiently. Smoking may cause the elastic fibers that make up the walls of the alveoli to dissolve, damaging cells that produce a substance necessary for maintaining healthy elasticity.

Emphysema is characterized by a narrowing of the smaller breathing passages of the lungs. Smoking tends to cause spasm and narrowing of these small passages through direct irritation. As a result, it takes much longer for air to flow into or out of your lungs, and the exchange of oxygen and carbon dioxide in your lungs is greatly slowed. This leads to shortness of breath.

In some persons, emphysema is caused by an inherited deficiency of an enzyme,

In emphysema, the air sacs of the lungs (the alveoli) lose their natural elasticity, becoming enlarged, and may rupture, thus preventing the normal exchange of oxygen and carbon dioxide with your blood.

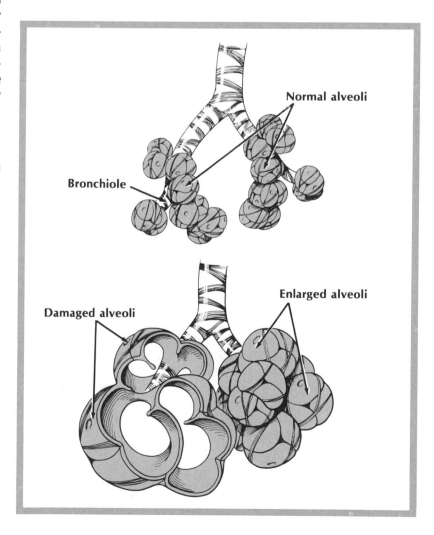

Normal alveoli

Bronchiole

Damaged alveoli

Enlarged alveoli

BREATHING TECHNIQUES

If you have emphysema or another chronic lung disorder, you may be helped by practicing some simple breathing exercises. You can develop a new breathing pattern by learning to control the emptying of your lungs (expiration) by the use of your abdominal muscles. You can also increase the efficiency of your lungs and your inspiratory (inhaling) muscles.

Diaphragmatic Breathing

Lie on your back with your head and knees supported by pillows.

Begin the exercise by breathing in and out slowly and smoothly in a rhythmic pattern. Relax.

Now, place the fingertips of one hand on your abdomen, just below the base of your rib cage at the center of your chest. As you inhale slowly, you should feel your diaphragm lifting your hand.

Practice pushing your abdomen against your hand as your chest becomes filled with air. Make sure your chest remains motionless while you do this. Try this while inhaling through your nose and counting slowly to 3; then exhale while counting slowly to 6.

Practice diaphragmatic breathing on your back until you can take 10 to 15 consecutive breaths in one session without tiring. Then practice it on one side and then on the other. Progress to doing the exercise while sitting erect in a chair, while standing up, walking, and, finally, while climbing stairs.

Pursed-Lip Breathing

Try the diaphragmatic breathing exercises with your lips pursed. That is, with your lips puckered (the flow of air should make a ''sssssss'' sound) inhale deeply through your mouth and exhale. Repeat 10 times at each session.

Deep-Breathing Exercise

This exercise is simple but is a good discipline. While sitting or standing, pull your elbows firmly backward as you inhale deeply. Hold the breath in, with your chest arched, for a count to 5 and then force the air out by contracting your abdominal muscles. Repeat this deep breathing 10 times.

The Regimen

With your physician's guidance, develop a regimen of breathing exercises. Do them daily, perhaps twice or even four times every day.

Inhale . . .   . . . Exhale

DIAPHRAGMATIC BREATHING

THE CONTROLLED COUGH

If you have a chronic lung disorder that causes an accumulation of secretions in your lungs, you must clear them out in order to prevent infection. There are several simple ways to accomplish this, including postural drainage (see Postural Drainage and Chest Percussion, page 922) and the controlled cough.

Sit on the edge of a bed or chair. Lean slightly forward. Your feet should be on the floor, and you should be confident of your balance.

Inhale a deep breath through your nose, hold it for a moment, and then cough twice. Try two short and sharp coughs—do not try to do it all at once with explosive, uncontrolled coughs because they tend to collapse your air-

ways, trapping mucus and air. This, in turn, may lead to shortness of breath.

Relax for a moment, then repeat this procedure. Keep a box of tissues close at hand in case your cough produces sputum.

By starting with gentle coughing and working up to harder coughs, you will develop a skill at clearing your lungs of secretions.

called alpha-1-antitrypsin, which normally protects the integrity of the elastic fibers in the walls of the alveoli. On testing of their blood, such persons will be found to have low levels of this enzyme and likely will have severe emphysema in the third or fourth decade of their lives. Although unproven, smoking may block the action of this enzyme and thereby produce emphysema in persons without the inherited trait.

The Diagnosis.   The primary symptom of emphysema is shortness of breath that can slowly worsen over time, becoming severe, especially after respiratory infections. As emphysema develops, you will become less and less able to tolerate exercise or even mild exertion. A mild cough that produces small amounts of sputum may be present as well. In severe cases, weight loss results. Your physician will make a diagnosis of emphysema on the basis of your symptoms, medical history, lung function test results, and chest x-ray findings. He or she often will notice an increase in the size of your chest.

How Serious Is Emphysema?   Emphysema is a serious, chronic disease. The outcome can be poor if the involvement is

An enlarged chest can be one characteristic sign of emphysema.

extensive. There is no specific treatment for reversing the changes of emphysema.

On the other hand, if detected early, emphysema is largely a preventable disease—so stop smoking. If you stop before symptoms are present, you may prevent further progression of disease.

YOUR HOME SUPPLY OF OXYGEN

If you have a chronic lung disease, your physician may prescribe the use of oxygen at home. This has become routine and, when proper procedures are followed, it is safe and may make you more comfortable.

Taking Proper Precautions
Fire burns faster in an oxygen-rich environment, so take special care when using oxygen in your home. Keep objects that produce sparks, flames, or intense heat well away from the area where the oxygen is located. These include smoking materials, matches, lighters, electric radiant heaters, and electrical

appliances such as heating pads, radios, and hair dryers. Keep flammable materials away from the area too. These include alcohol, aerosol sprays, combustible liquids, and any petroleum-based household substances including Vaseline and perfumes.

Never expose the oxygen tank and its attachments to temperatures above 125°F.

Handling the Equipment
Be sure that the oxygen cylinders are well secured to prevent them from tipping over. They are heavy and hazardous. When not in use, seal the tanks properly with protective caps.

When installing the regulator, follow the technician's instruc-

tions precisely. Before the regulator is attached, open the valve slightly and then close it immediately. This clears out dust or combustible material.

The Traveling Tank
If you require oxygen 24 hours a day, your physician may also recommend use of a portable oxygen tank that allows you to travel beyond the reach of the large tank and its hose. The rules and regulations cited above apply equally to portable tanks. Portable containers carry only a limited amount of oxygen. Longer trips (more than several hours) require more preparation to ensure a continuous oxygen supply.

SMOKING AND CHRONIC OBSTRUCTIVE PULMONARY DISEASE

Smoking is the primary cause of chronic obstructive pulmonary disease (COPD) such as emphysema and chronic bronchitis. Compared with nonsmokers, deaths caused by chronic bronchitis and emphysema are significantly more frequent in people who smoke heavily.

By the time symptoms of COPD appear—typically, cough, shortness of breath, and difficulty tolerating exercise—damage has already occurred to your lungs. If you do not stop smoking, your disease will get worse.

Tobacco Smoke

Tobacco smoke contains a mixture of chemicals, gases, and tiny droplets of tar. Thousands of substances have been identified in tobacco smoke; the toxic effects of many of them remain unknown. Some components are filtered off when you draw the smoke through the remaining unburned tobacco; however, as the cigarette burns, these chemicals are vaporized again and each puff of smoke thus contains more of the components. Most smokers inhale the cigarette smoke, which makes it even more dangerous.

Cigarette smoke contains 2 to 6 percent carbon monoxide. Carbon monoxide is a toxic gas that combines with hemoglobin (carboxyhemoglobin). When this occurs the hemoglobin molecule cannot transport oxygen to the tissues. Many smokers have carboxyhemoglobin levels of 8 to 10 percent in their blood whereas a nonsmoker commonly has only up to 1.5 percent. (A person dying from acute carbon monoxide poisoning has blood carboxyhemoglobin levels of 30 to 40 percent.) Thus, your tissues are deprived of needed oxygen.

The tar found in cigarettes contains substances that cause cancer. Irritants in tobacco smoke cause your air passages to constrict and your bronchial tubes to produce excess mucus, and they cause you to cough. These irritants also may impair the function of the immune system cells in your lungs and may upset the normal balance of pulmonary enzymes, which makes you more susceptible to respiratory disease. Finally, inhaled tobacco smoke stops the action of the cilia in your airway. Cilia are the tiny hair-like projections in your windpipe and bronchial tubes. They help expel foreign material from your lungs.

Cigar and Pipe Smoke

Cigarette smoking is not the only cause of chronic respiratory disease. Although less dangerous than cigarette smoking, cigar smoking and pipe smoking are not innocuous; because this smoke is more irritating, you are less likely to inhale it.

Marijuana Smoke

Marijuana smoking also can lead to chronic respiratory disease. It contains many of the same irritants found in tobacco smoke. It also contains substances that are not present in tobacco smoke, such as delta-9-tetrahydrocannabinol. Some of them are respiratory irritants.

Marijuana usually is smoked in ways that make it more dangerous than cigarette smoking. Marijuana smokers usually inhale deeply and hold the smoke in their lungs, or they use a specially constructed pipe that concentrates the smoke and sends it into the lungs under pressure. Studies show that this inflames the airways and causes carcinogenic (cancer-prone) changes in the respiratory cells. In addition, it makes the lungs more susceptible to infection by any fungi or bacteria that might be present in the marijuana. Researchers have found significant decreases in the lung capacity of people who smoke marijuana daily. These smokers are at risk for COPD as well as laryngitis and chronic rhinitis.

Quit Smoking

If you are a smoker, our recommendation is clear—stop smoking. Unfortunately, however, many people do not quit until they have symptoms of respiratory disease.

If you need help in kicking the tobacco habit, see Tobacco, page 407.

Treatment. Treatment cannot restore your lungs to normal, but therapy can keep your disease from getting worse and can teach you how to use your damaged lungs most efficiently.

The most important step is to stop smoking (for help, see the chapter on Tobacco, page 407). If you do not stop, your disease almost certainly will get worse. Also, avoid other respiratory irritants that may cause shortness of breath or tightness in your chest. These include fumes from paint and automobile exhaust, some cooking odors, certain perfumes, dust, cold air, and extremely humid air.

During cold weather, wear a soft scarf or

a cold air mask (obtainable from any pharmacy) over your mouth and nose to warm the air that is entering your lungs. For the same reason, breathe through your nose because cold air can cause spasm of the bronchial passages. Using a humidifier in your home also may help. Finally, avoid exposure to persons with respiratory infections such as a cold or flu.

People with emphysema are particularly prone to pneumonia, acute bronchitis, and other serious respiratory diseases. A change in the color, volume, or thickness of your sputum may signal the onset of a respiratory infection. Your physician may prescribe a 7- to 10-day course of broad-spectrum antibiotics (antibiotics such as ampicillin, tetracycline, and erythromycin that are effective against many bacteria). Bronchodilators may be useful if you experience bronchial spasms as well.

Emphysema causes shortness of breath because your alveoli are less efficient in exchanging oxygen and carbon dioxide. Also, airways can be narrowed and thus respiratory muscles must work harder. But there are several things you can do to increase the efficiency of your lungs.

First, take the medications your physician prescribes. Second, exercise regularly. Less-strenuous exercise such as walking or cycling can increase your exercise tolerance; thus, we strongly recommend them. Third, practice breathing techniques prescribed by your physician. Some people are able to improve their tolerance of exercise through this special training of the muscles that control inhalation and exhalation. The training can improve the strength and endurance of these muscles. Your physician will teach you how to do it correctly (see Breathing Techniques, page 930). Finally, see your physician promptly if your condition worsens or if a respiratory infection develops.

Sometimes physicians prescribe home oxygen therapy on either a continuous or supplemental basis (see Your Home Supply of Oxygen, page 832).

ASTHMA

Signs and Symptoms
- Shortness of breath;
- Cough;
- Tightness of the chest;
- Wheezing.

Asthma is characterized by spasms of the muscles in the walls of the bronchial tubes of your lungs. Normally, the muscles surrounding your bronchial tubes contract only as a protective reaction to prevent harmful substances from entering your lungs. With asthma, the muscles of the bronchial tubes react at inappropriate times, often through allergic mechanisms and against substances that would not damage the lungs.

For a detailed discussion of Asthma, see page 466.

CYSTIC FIBROSIS

Signs and Symptoms
- Cough;
- Exercise intolerance;
- Recurring pneumonia;
- Chronic diarrhea.

Cystic fibrosis is an inherited disease that affects both the respiratory and digestive systems. It is the most common fatal hereditary disease in white children in the United States, affecting approximately 1 in every 2,000 infants. It also is one of the more common causes of chronic lung disease in children.

The disease seldom affects black, Asian, or Jewish children. It occurs in boys and girls equally. It is inherited on a recessive basis, which means that a child can have cystic fibrosis if both parents are carriers of the disease. (In this case the parents will have no symptoms themselves.)

Cystic fibrosis affects the mucus and sweat glands of the body. The first symptom in a newborn infant may be blockage of the intestine due to thick, clay-like meconium (the dark-green material present in an infant's intestine that makes up its first stool).

As the infant grows older, chronic respiratory disease may develop, including bronchitis, bronchiectasis (chronic, abnormal dilation of the bronchial tubes), collapsed lung due to blockage of the airways, pneumonia, or fibrosis of the lung.

These problems occur because the mucus in the child's lungs is very thick and sticky. Instead of serving as a lubricant, it clogs the respiratory system and allows bacteria and other microorganisms to grow within it, impairing the body's natural defenses. General symptoms are chronic cough, shortness of breath, exercise intolerance, poor appetite, and decreased energy. The pancreas may not provide the enzymes needed to digest fats and proteins completely, resulting in chronic diarrhea and malnutrition. The child's sweat glands also are affected, causing the sweat to be extremely salty. As a result, the child may suffer salt depletion and heat exhaustion when he or she sweats in hot weather.

The Diagnosis. If your child has chronic respiratory or pancreatic disease, your physician may perform lung function or stool tests or may also order a sweat test to measure the amount of salt in your child's perspiration. This test is often performed on 2 consecutive days for an accurate diagnosis. If the test is positive and your child has siblings, test them also.

How Serious Is Cystic Fibrosis? Cystic fibrosis is very serious and ultimately fatal. About half of the individuals with this disease live beyond age 26, although as techniques to treat cystic fibrosis have improved, some people have survived beyond their 30s. Mild forms of the disease may not produce symptoms until adulthood.

Treatment. Treatment is a long-term process, and frequent checkups are important.

If bowel symptoms are present, your child should receive a high-protein, low-fat diet. For instance, give skim milk instead of whole milk. Other than that, no special diet is required so long as the child is given a pancreatic enzyme preparation to supply the missing digestive enzymes; this comes as a capsule or powder to be taken with solid food. If your child is deficient in sodium or perspires heavily because of fever or hot weather, salt supplements may be given.

There are special exercises that parents can help their child perform to loosen and promote drainage of the mucus (see Postural Drainage and Chest Percussion, page 922). Your child should do these exercises one or more times daily. A health practitioner can provide instruction on how to do them correctly. Inhaling an aerosol may help as well. Finally, because your child's immune defenses against respiratory disease are weakened, it is important that vaccines be given against all respiratory diseases including whooping cough (pertussis), measles, and influenza.

Medication. Respiratory infections require prompt treatment with the antibiotic appropriate for the bacteria causing the illness. Children with cystic fibrosis may require breathing treatments along with medications to help relieve wheezing. Occasionally, oxygen supplementation is needed. Treatments with corticosteroids, aerosolized antibiotics, or amiloride, or with a substance that can dissolve mucus, are being tested.

Prevention. If you have a child with cystic fibrosis, each additional child will have a 25 percent chance of having the disease, a 50 percent chance of being a carrier, and a 25 percent chance of having normal genes.

Since the recent description of the cystic fibrosis gene, our understanding of the cause, diagnosis, and treatment of this disease is rapidly changing. Specialists in cystic fibrosis can advise you on the latest developments.

SARCOIDOSIS

Signs and Symptoms
- There may be none;
- Malaise;
- Fever;
- Shortness of breath, especially with exercise;
- Weight loss.

The cause of sarcoidosis is unknown. It can affect nearly any part of your body, including your skin, eyes, peripheral nerves, liver, lymph nodes, and heart, but in 90 percent of cases, it affects the lungs.

Sarcoidosis appears to involve the immune system. The helper T lymphocytes, one of the types of white blood cells that protect your body from disease, seem to overrespond, causing a buildup of inflammatory cells in your tissue. In the lungs, this accumulation of cells distorts the walls of the alveoli (the small air sacs of your lungs), the bronchial tubes, and blood vessels, altering the normal diffusion of oxygen into blood in your lungs.

Sarcoidosis occurs in a higher percentage of blacks than whites in the United States, although all races are affected. Women are affected more often than men. It occurs primarily in individuals between the ages of 20 and 40, although in rare cases it can develop in children and elderly people.

The Diagnosis. Sarcoidosis may cause a general feeling of malaise, fever, and shortness of breath, especially during and after exercise. Usually, however, there are no symptoms, especially early in the disease. Many times, sarcoidosis is first suspected on a routine chest x-ray. To confirm the diagnosis, your physician may perform a lung biopsy using a fiberoptic bronchoscope to obtain tissue for examination (see Bronchoscopy, page 940). Sometimes, biopsy of skin, lymph node, or sclera of the eye is simpler if these structures are involved. Occasionally, the blood calcium level is higher than normal, and this may be a clue to the eventual diagnosis.

How Serious Is Sarcoidosis? Sarcoidosis usually is a slow or chronic disease. About half of the affected persons recover completely or with only minor lasting effects, even without treatment. About 10 to 15 percent, however, have chronic disease that stays active or comes and goes intermittently for many years. In 5 to 10 percent, sarcoidosis leads to death, usually after many years.

Treatment. *Medication.* If you have pronounced symptoms or if the disease does not resolve spontaneously after 4 to 6 months, your physician may prescribe corticosteroids which are then tapered off over several months or even years as the condition improves as judged by chest x-rays or other tests. If the disease reappears, another course of corticosteroids may be required. However, this course of corticosteroids is likely to continue for a longer time than in the initial treatment cycle because results generally are not as good with a second course of treatment.

INTERSTITIAL LUNG DISEASE

Signs and Symptoms

- Shortness of breath;
- General fatigue and weakness;
- Loss of appetite and weight;
- Cough.

Interstitial lung disease refers to a group of more than 180 diseases that are chronic, nonmalignant, and noninfectious. These diseases are characterized by infiltration of inflammatory cells into the walls of alveoli (the air sacs of your lungs), which causes abnormal formation of scar tissue in the connective tissue that supports the alveoli. If the disease progresses, scarring develops to the point such that the lungs may be destroyed. In most interstitial lung disorders, the causes are not known. These ailments generally affect people over 50 years of age.

A major consequence of the formation of abnormal scar tissue is impairment of the transfer of oxygen from the air to the blood. Thus, if you are affected, you may notice fatigue, malaise, and a shortness of breath, particularly upon exercising. In addition, a cough that produces no sputum, along with a sensation of chest discomfort, occasionally is present.

The Diagnosis. Your physician may suspect an interstitial lung disease based on your symptoms and the sounds he or she hears on examination of your chest with the stethoscope. He or she will probably order chest x-rays and lung function tests, both of which generally reveal significant abnormalities. Bronchoscopy with biopsy may be performed for confirmation of the diagnosis (see Bronchoscopy, page 940) or to rule out an infectious or malignant condition that may mimic the disease on chest x-ray.

An open biopsy of the lung may be necessary to confirm the diagnosis. This is a surgical procedure, performed under general anesthesia, in which the chest wall is opened and a small sample of lung tissue is removed for examination under the microscope.

How Serious Is Interstitial Lung Disease? These diseases have variable courses, depending on their cause. Some are progressive and ultimately fatal; others become stable or have a fluctuating course.

A common type of interstitial lung disease is sarcoidosis (see page 934). Other types of interstitial lung diseases are idiopathic pulmonary fibrosis, pulmonary alveolar proteinosis, and Goodpasture's syndrome.

Idiopathic Pulmonary Fibrosis. This is a chronic noninfectious, nonmalignant disorder that causes progressive shortness of breath. Average duration of life after the onset of symptoms is 4 to 5 years, but many affected persons live much longer. Males and females are equally affected; the disorder commonly develops in the middle years of life but it can occur at any age.

The diagnosis can be strongly suspected when certain typical sounds are heard through the stethoscope and certain characteristic patterns are seen on the chest x-ray and in results of lung function tests. However, lung biopsy, either by bronchoscopy or surgery, also may be required. If there is a history of occupational exposure to asbestos (see Asbestosis, page 942), there could be a coexisting lung cancer. Treatment may consist of corticosteroids, but only a small percentage of affected persons are helped. Lung transplantation has occasionally been used for this disorder.

Pulmonary Alveolar Proteinosis. This rare disorder occurs when material builds up within the alveoli (air sacs of the lungs). It occurs primarily in men, usually between the ages of 20 and 50. The cause is unknown.

In pulmonary alveolar proteinosis, the shortness of breath is minimal compared with the extent of involvement seen on the chest x-ray. (In contrast, in idiopathic pulmonary fibrosis the shortness of breath is greater than would appear likely from the relative lack of disease evident on the chest x-ray.) The problem may worsen over time or may disappear spontaneously.

Sometimes material from within the alveoli can be removed from the lung under general anesthesia. In this procedure (whole lung lavage), the material is literally rinsed from the lung—first from one lung and then from the other at a later date. Persons with this disease usually recover, although occasionally the disorder may recur.

Goodpasture's Syndrome. The cause of Goodpasture's syndrome is unknown. It occurs most often in young men. It causes hemorrhage of the lungs and glomerulonephritis (a type of inflammation of the kidneys) (see page 893).

Although the hemorrhage itself can be life-threatening, the lung symptoms can range from mild to severe. The diagnosis is made by biopsy of either lung or kidney. The

course of the disease varies widely. Your physician may prescribe corticosteroids or cyclophosphamide to control the disorder. In addition, your physician may elect to "filter" your blood to remove antibodies which may play a role in causing this disease.

ATELECTASIS

Signs and Symptoms
- Shortness of breath;
- Fever;
- Decreased blood pressure and rapid heartbeat;
- Severe, hacking cough.

Atelectasis consists of a collapse of portions of a lung or sometimes of an entire lung. It is caused by obstruction of bronchial passages in the lungs (commonly, by a plug of mucus), by accidental inhalation of a foreign object, or by outside pressure from a tumor, aneurysm, or enlarged lymph node. Sometimes it occurs as a complication after abdominal surgery when breathing may be shallow and portions of the lung are not expanded. It also may be associated with a bacterial infection. When obstruction occurs, the air beyond the obstruction is absorbed by the blood and that part of the lung collapses.

Atelectasis can come on slowly (as with a growing tumor) and produce only mild respiratory symptoms. If a massive, sudden collapse of the lung occurs, there is pain on the affected side, sudden shortness of breath, decreased blood pressure, rapid heartbeat, fever, and shock (see Shock, page 303). Atelectasis may cause a severe, hacking, unproductive cough. In making a diagnosis, your physician will look for an airless area on your chest x-ray.

Treatment. The first goal is to remove the cause of the obstruction. If coughing, suctioning, or other therapeutic measures do not work, fiberoptic bronchoscopy (see also page 940) may be performed. Ampicillin or other medication may be prescribed to eliminate infection.

Prevention. Atelectasis is much less likely to occur after you have had an operation if, during postoperative recovery, you are encouraged to take deep breaths frequently and are up and walking as soon as possible. Commonly, an apparatus to teach you rapid, forceful inspiration is prescribed.

If you smoke or have chronic bronchitis or emphysema, you are less likely to have atelectasis after your operation if you discontinue smoking at least 3 to 4 days before your surgery. For several days before surgery you also can use bronchodilator medications (administered by an inhaler) and you can inhale an aerosol moisture periodically. Your physician may prescribe prophylactic use of an antibiotic that is effective against various organisms.

PNEUMOTHORAX

Signs and Symptoms
• Often, none;
• Breathlessness.

Pneumothorax is the presence of air in the pleural space outside the lung but inside the chest. It also is referred to as collapsed lung.

When it occurs spontaneously, pneumothorax usually is thought to be due to rupture of a bleb (a blister containing air) on the surface of the lung. This spontaneous pneumothorax is most frequent in people under age 35 or 40.

Air also can enter the pleural space by other means. Air can enter the mediastinum (the space in the center of the chest between the lungs), especially during an asthmatic attack, and then rupture into the pleural space, causing a pneumothorax. When a lung biopsy specimen is taken at the time of bronchoscopy (see also page 940) or during thoracentesis (removal of fluid from the pleural space), the pleura lining the lung may be penetrated, causing a leak of air which then may cause a pneumothorax.

How Serious Is Pneumothorax? There may be no symptoms if the pneumothorax is small (a small amount of air in the pleural space), or there may be shortness of breath if a large amount of air is in that space.

The Diagnosis. If your physician suspects a pneumothorax, a chest x-ray may be taken to confirm the diagnosis and to determine the amount of air present.

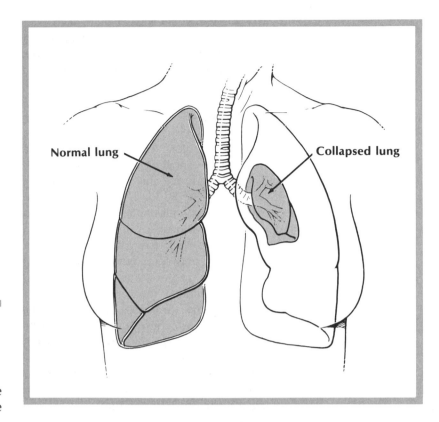

Normal lung   Collapsed lung

Treatment. If your lung is less than 20 to 25 percent collapsed, your physician may choose to watch the progress by a series of chest x-rays until the air is completely absorbed or the lung completely reexpanded.

If collapse of the lung exceeds 25 percent or if you are short of breath at rest, your physician may recommend removing the air through your chest wall. This can be done with a needle, but it is better performed by inserting a tube and applying constant suction for 24 hours or more. The latter procedure also helps to prevent recurrence of pneumothorax.

LUNG CANCER

Signs and Symptoms
• None;
• Cough that brings up sputum, sometimes blood-streaked;
• Shortness of breath;
• Chest pain;
• Hoarseness;
• Loss of appetite and weight.

Lung cancer is the leading cause of cancer death in the United States in both men and women. More than 100,000 men and

A collapsed lung (pneumothorax) results if air escapes from the lungs but is retained in the chest cavity.

50,000 women have lung cancer each year, and the number is increasing. The number of women with lung cancer is increasing because of increased smoking in this group over the last 30 years.

Lung cancer occurs mainly in people between ages 45 and 70. Cigarette smoking accounts for 85 percent of all lung cancers. Other risk factors for lung cancer include industrial carcinogens and, according to preliminary evidence, high concentrations of radon (see The Radon Risk, page 335). Primary lung cancer is uncommon in nonsmokers, but a cancer of the breast, colon, prostate, testis, kidney, thyroid, bone, or other organ may spread (metastasize) to the lungs.

Nonmalignant tumors such as carcinoid or hamartoma are occasionally seen in the lungs. At times, these tumors have to be removed surgically if they are causing symptoms or if the diagnosis is uncertain.

More than 20 types of malignant and benign tumors have been identified as originating in the lungs. A benign tumor is a mass of abnormal tissue that does not spread and can be completely removed surgically. It is not life-threatening and is not likely to recur. A malignant tumor, however, is an abnormal growth of cells that can invade and destroy nearby tissue or organs and can spread (metastasize) to other parts of the body.

Almost all primary malignant cancers of the lung are one of four types: squamous cell carcinoma, adenocarcinoma, large cell carcinoma, and small cell carcinoma. Squamous cell carcinoma (also called epidermoid carcinoma) usually arises from the cells lining the central bronchi (the largest air passages of the lungs), making it one of the easier cancers to identify early through examination of your sputum. Squamous cell lung cancer accounts for about 25 to 30 percent of primary lung cancers.

Adenocarcinoma usually arises in the lining of the smaller bronchi (air passages). It is now the most common type of primary lung cancer, causing about 35 percent of cases. It is named for the glandular structures that the tumor cells form (*adeno* means gland). It may spread to the lymph glands in that particular area of the lung and then, through the bloodstream, to other organs. Because it arises on the periphery of the lung it is more difficult to identify early than is squamous cell carcinoma.

Bronchioloalveolar cell carcinoma, a subtype of adenocarcinoma, accounts for less than 5 percent of cases. It seldom spreads beyond the lungs; it affects the alveoli (air sacs) of your lungs.

Undifferentiated large cell carcinoma also appears in the periphery of the lung and spreads through the bloodstream. It accounts for approximately 15 to 20 percent of lung cancers.

Finally, small (oat) cell carcinoma also develops in the central areas of the lung, making it easier to identify. Named for the small, round or oval shape of the cancer cells as seen under the microscope, it is one of the more aggressive cancers. It tends to cause narrowing of the bronchi by compressing them. Small cell carcinoma accounts for about 20 to 25 percent of lung cancers.

The Diagnosis. Five to 10 percent of lung cancers are detected on routine chest x-rays, prior to the development of symptoms. If you are between ages 50 and 70 and you smoke one pack of cigarettes or more daily, have an annual chest x-ray and sputum examination for malignant cells. If symptoms are apparent, the location of the tumor may determine the nature of the symptoms you experience. Routine sputum examinations

Chest x-ray reveals an abnormal mass in lung (arrow). Subsequent biopsy confirmed this to be lung cancer.

for malignant cells also may detect lung cancers before symptoms occur.

In many cases, a new cough develops because an enlarging cancer is beginning to block an air passageway. Often, the cough will produce moderate amounts of sputum that may contain pus and may be streaked with rust-colored or even bright red blood. Coughing up large amounts of blood is rare

but, when it does happen, it indicates that the cancer has invaded a large blood vessel.

Persistent chest pain suggests that the tumor has invaded the chest wall. Infection in a lung because of blockage of an airway may cause fever, chest pain, and loss of weight. If the main bronchi are blocked by a tumor, that portion of the lung may lose volume (see Atelectasis, page 936). Later in

SMOKING AND LUNG CANCER

Approximately 85 percent of the cases of lung cancer that occur each year can be traced to smoking. People who smoke more than one pack a day have a 20 times greater risk of lung cancer than do those who have never smoked. A person who has smoked two packs of cigarettes or more daily for 20 years has a 60- to 70-fold increased risk of cancer than a nonsmoker has.

Your risk of lung cancer decreases if you quit smoking, but it does not return to the risk level of persons who have never smoked.

Currently, lung cancer is more common in men than in women; however, because more women are smoking, their incidence of cancer is increasing rapidly. Lung cancer now surpasses breast cancer as the most common cause of cancer death in women. The American Cancer Society estimates that, by the year 2000, equal numbers of women and men will die from lung cancer.

Your risk of lung cancer increases with the number of cigarettes you smoke each day, the number of years you smoke, the amount of smoke you inhale, and the amount of tar and nicotine in the cigarettes you smoke.

Cigarette smoke contains a number of toxic gases plus tiny

**Normal
lung tissue**

**Lung tissue
with severe emphysema**

Cigarette smoking is a leading cause of lung cancer and emphysema as depicted above.

droplets of tar. Tar contains numerous carcinogens (substances that cause cancer) as well as cocarcinogens (substances that accelerate the production of cancer cells). Small (oat) cell carcinoma and squamous cell cancer are most strongly associated with cigarette smoking. Small cell cancer is a particularly aggressive cancer that spreads rapidly. It is most common in men who are heavy smokers. It seldom occurs in nonsmokers.

Cigarette smoke contains 2 to 6 percent carbon monoxide, a toxic gas that interferes with the ability of your body to transport and use oxygen. Irritants in cigarette smoke impair the function of the tiny microscopic hairs (cilia) that remove

unwanted substances in your lungs and upset the normal balance of pulmonary enzymes, making you more susceptible to respiratory disease.

By 10 years after they quit smoking, the death rate of those who smoked more than 20 cigarettes a day decreases by two-thirds, but still does not reach the level of those who have never smoked. Unfortunately, however, many people do not quit until they already have symptoms of respiratory disease or have developed cancer.

The most effective way to quit smoking is just to stop—go "cold turkey." But this generally is not easy. For tips on quitting, see Tobacco, page 407.

BRONCHOSCOPY

Bronchoscopy is a procedure in which a flexible tube is passed down your airway to allow your physician to see the inside of your air passages. Your doctor can look for tumors, foreign objects, areas of internal bleeding, and abnormalities of your lungs and air pas-

Rigid bronchoscope

Flexible bronchoscope

sageways. The bronchoscope also has an open central channel through which your physician can remove excess secretions, obtain biopsy specimens, and introduce saline to rinse your lungs (lavage).

There are two types of bronchoscopes: the rigid bronchoscope which is larger, rigid, and requires a high degree of skill to use; and the fiberoptic bronchoscope which is flexible and only 3 to 7 mm in diameter. Most bronchoscopic examinations in children require use of the rigid instrument. The rigid bronchoscope is often used in adults if a foreign body is present, dilation is required, or a laser is to be used in the tracheobronchial passages. Otherwise, the flexible fiberoptic instrument is used. It contains glass fibers that transmit light and return a magnified picture of the passageways of your lungs. Your physician can watch the progress of the bronchoscope on a small television-like screen.

You will not be permitted to eat for at least 6 to 12 hours before bronchoscopy is performed. Fiberoptic bronchoscopy usually is performed under local anesthesia, but may be done under general anesthesia. The anesthetic agent, which depresses your cough and swallowing reflexes, usually is administered through your nostrils or mouth. Your physician also may give you a sedative to help you relax. The bronchoscope is then inserted through either your mouth or your nose. The procedure may be performed while you are sitting or lying down. Lidocaine jelly is used as an oral anesthetic and as a lubricant to protect your air passages.

When the flexible fiberoptic bronchoscope is used, the procedure is painless and there seldom are complications. After the procedure, you should not eat or drink anything for about an hour because your swallowing and cough reflexes still are depressed.

LUNG REMOVAL

Surgical removal (resection) of the tumor is the preferred treatment for people who have lung cancer that has not spread (metastasized) to other parts of the body. Depending on the extent of the cancer, people with squamous cell carcinoma, large cell cancer, or adenocarcinoma are candidates for surgical treatment. Surgery seldom is performed for small cell carcinoma because this type of cancer spreads too rapidly and too extensively to be totally removed surgically.

The Outlook
In those whose cancer is detected

early enough so that surgical removal can be done, approximately 80 percent survive 1 year, and 50 percent are alive at 5 years after the operation. If the cancer recurs, however, the outlook generally is quite poor, although chemotherapy or radiation therapy may decrease the size of the tumor, prolong life, and relieve pain and other symptoms.

The Procedure
The tumor and the tissue immediately surrounding it, such as a lobe or even an entire lung, are removed. Usually, the lymph nodes draining the involved lung are removed as well. Radiation therapy sometimes is used in conjunction

with removal. Normally you will be hospitalized for a week to 10 days after the operation, although it will take much longer before you recover completely. Many people are able to resume their normal activities in 4 to 6 weeks. However, the rate and degree of recovery depend on the general condition of your lungs and the amount of lung tissue removed as well as your overall health.

The Risk of Recurrence
After resection, be sure to have regular medical checkups to detect recurrence of the cancer, either within your lung or in other parts of your body.

the progression of the cancer, weakness and weight loss develop. Various other symptoms may develop as the cancer spreads to the liver, brain, bone, heart, and adrenal glands.

Generally, lung cancer is first suspected either because of your physical symptoms or because an abnormal mass appears on a routine chest x-ray. Loss of appetite and weight may be the first signs of a lung cancer. In this case, the first step is to determine with certainty whether or not cancer is present. In addition to a regular chest x-ray, tomograms (special chest x-rays that give a highly localized view of the lung) or other special studies such as a CT scan (see page 1286) may be obtained.

Your physician may compare old and new chest x-rays to help determine if an abnormal finding on the new chest x-ray was present previously and if it has changed in size. Examination of your sputum may reveal the presence of cancer cells, particularly if the tumor is centrally located. A CT scan is useful for revealing very small lesions and determining if the cancer has spread to other sites. Your physician also may perform a complete blood cell count and liver function tests.

Fiberoptic bronchoscopy, or possibly rigid bronchoscopy (see page 940), may be performed in order to view the air passages and to obtain a biopsy (sample of tissue for examination of the tumor).

How Serious Is Lung Cancer? Lung cancer is a very serious disease and has a very poor outlook. Overall, about 10 percent of patients survive for 5 years; however, the outcome depends upon the stage of the disease when it is discovered, your general health and age, the type of cancer, how rapidly it grows, and what type of therapy is given. Only 20 to 25 percent of all lung cancers can be removed surgically at the time of initial diagnosis. Once symptoms of lung cancer appear, the disease may be fairly well advanced and not treatable by operation.

Small cell cancer is very serious because of its tendency to spread early, often before symptoms are apparent. The 5-year survival after diagnosis is approximately 5 percent. After surgery, approximately one-third of those with squamous cell carcinoma and one-fourth of those with adenocarcinoma or large cell carcinoma survive 5 years.

Treatment. Basically there are three treatment options for lung cancer: surgery (removal), chemotherapy, and radiation therapy. Laser surgery can be used to restore breathing when tumors obstruct central air passageways. Usually, this is done only when surgical removal of the cancer is not possible.

Surgery is the preferred treatment for those who do not have small cell cancer (see Lung Removal, page 940). Small cell cancer usually cannot be removed surgically, so other forms of treatment are used. Approximately 20 to 25 percent of the persons with primary lung cancer can have their tumor surgically removed. Because lung cancer commonly occurs in people who have smoked heavily for many years, the lung not involved with cancer may be severely damaged by emphysema. Therefore, the surgeon cannot always remove the cancerous lung safely because the other lung may not be able to meet the person's oxygen needs. This situation can be clarified by breathing tests before the operation.

Radiation therapy, in which a beam of radiation is focused on the cancer cells at doses that destroy the cancer but do not harm surrounding tissue, is used in some patients. Combination chemotherapy is the preferred treatment for patients with small cell carcinoma. Frequently, radiation treatment is added to the treatment program.

OCCUPATIONALLY RELATED LUNG DISEASE

Hazardous materials in the workplace can cause lung disease if inhaled in quantity over time. Perhaps the best known of these diseases is asbestosis, which has numerous manifestations. Coal miner's disease and silicosis (caused by inhaling silica) also are well known. In addition, various industrial and agricultural dusts and some fungi cause diseases, usually named after an occupation or the type of dust inhaled.

ASBESTOSIS

Signs and Symptoms
- Chest pain;
- Shortness of breath;
- Decreased exercise tolerance;
- Cough (sometimes).

Asbestos was used extensively as an insulation in building construction for many years until 1975 when it was replaced by other materials such as fiberglass and slag wool. There are four types of asbestos fibers—chrysotile, amosite, anthophyllite, and crocidolite—and all can cause respiratory disease. Disease may result when large amounts of the fine asbestos fibers accumulate in your lungs and you are unable to expel them.

More than 9 million workers are estimated to be at risk of this respiratory dis-

ASBESTOS REMOVAL FROM BUILDINGS

Up to the early 1970s, asbestos commonly was installed in buildings as an all-purpose low-cost insulation and fire-resistant fiber. It was sprayed onto beams, used as insulation for floors and ceilings, mixed into cement and floor tiles, and placed around pipes and boilers in schools, office buildings, and shopping malls. It is expensive to remove.

Asbestos in the Air
The problem is friable asbestos—asbestos that is flaking off. When disturbed during routine maintenance work, the tiny fibers can easily be released from the surface. These loose fibers may stay in the air for weeks. The vast majority of the people who work in or go into buildings containing friable asbestos have a very small risk of contracting respiratory illness from the fibers, but what level of asbestos exposure is safe has not yet been determined.

Various federal, state, and local government regulations now require asbestos control or removal, particularly in schools. Many insurance companies will not finance buildings containing asbestos.

The Removal Process
The first step in removing asbestos

Asbestos, like the pipe covering shown here, can be hazardous to your health. Removal is a job for experts.

from a building is to determine the extent of the problem by obtaining counts of the asbestos fiber in air within the building. Owners of the building can hire an environmental consultant who specializes in asbestos to survey the building. The consultant should not be involved with anyone in the business of removing asbestos.

Asbestos removal is safest, easiest, and cheapest when the building is empty, although this is not always possible. In a building with tenants, the ideal removal plan consists of removing the material from those areas that are exposed because of maintenance work or renovations and then cleaning out the rest when the building is empty before complete renovation or demolition. Until complete removal is possible, teach maintenance workers how to recognize and avoid the hazardous material. Also, monitor the air continuously if the asbestos is disturbed.

Removal of asbestos is a job for experts. Buildings should be demolished only after the portion to be torn down on a given day is dampened with water to prevent formation of dust clouds containing asbestos.

ease. People exposed to asbestos include workers in mining, milling, manufacturing, and installation of asbestos products. Trades that install asbestos products include pipe fitters, boiler makers, ship builders, and construction workers. Asbestos was sprayed on steel girders of buildings to prevent buckling in a fire. Asbestos also was used in fire-smothering blankets and safety clothing, as filler for plastic materials, in brakes and clutch linings, and in cement and floor tiles. Demolition workers and do-it-yourself home renovators working on older buildings are at risk.

You do not need to handle the material yourself in order to be exposed to the fibers. Electricians, painters, and others who worked next to the person installing asbestos insulation are at risk, as is the person who shook out and washed the clothes of someone who worked with it. Occasionally, groups of cases have occurred in neighborhoods and communities near asbestos plants and mines.

The Diagnosis. Asbestos exposure may cause asbestosis (a form of interstitial fibrosis or pneumoconiosis), mesothelioma (a cancer of the lining of the lung or abdomen), or lung cancer. Pulmonary asbestosis may result when the fibers accumulate around your bronchioles, the smallest air passageways. Your lungs react to the fibers by covering them, forming small masses of scar tissue. Symptoms appear when the scar tissue causes your lungs to lose their elasticity. The first symptom of asbestosis is the gradual appearance of shortness of breath upon exertion.

The severity of disease is directly related to the duration of your exposure and to the amount of fiber inhaled. Usually, at least 10 years of moderate to severe exposure must occur before symptoms of asbestosis appear. On your chest x-ray, the scar tissue will appear as small, scattered, opaque areas. They are first evident in the lower parts of your lung but gradually spread upward as the disease gets worse. Eventually, your entire lung may be affected, producing a honeycombed appearance.

Provide your physician with a detailed history of your work activities and any other sources of possible exposure to toxic dusts. Tell your doctor about the availability and use of dust masks and other respiratory protection devices. An abnormal chest x-ray may suggest that you have been exposed to asbestos but does not necessarily mean you have asbestosis. The disease itself is diagnosed only if you have a history of exposure, suggestive chest x-ray and physical findings, and symptoms of debilitating pulmonary fibrosis (the abnormal development of scar tissue). This becomes important if you wish to seek compensation.

Another result of prolonged exposure to asbestos may be the development of pleural plaques around your lungs. These areas of thickening of the pleura, the double membrane that surrounds your lungs, usually occur along the lower part of the chest wall or near the diaphragm. The presence of pleural plaques confirms that you have been exposed to asbestos but does not mean that your lungs are impaired unless you have other symptoms or signs.

Mesotheliomas, malignant tumors arising from the pleura, are a relatively rare type of cancer. Mesotheliomas may develop 20 to 40 years after the exposure to asbestos fibers and can occur even if the exposure was for only a year or two, or even less. Many persons with mesothelioma have no history of exposure to asbestos. The symptoms include chest pain, gradual appearance of shortness of breath, and weight loss. In about half of those with mesothelioma, the disease spreads, producing tumors in other parts of the body. In other cases, the tumors are limited to the chest. Pleural effusion, the buildup of fluid between the two layers of the pleural membrane, often contributes to shortness of breath and chest pain. The disease usually is fatal within 8 to 14 months; 75 percent of the affected persons die within a year after diagnosis.

Finally, if you smoke and have been exposed to asbestos, you have a much greater chance of developing lung cancer than does someone who smokes but has not been exposed. If you do not smoke, your chance of getting lung cancer from exposure to asbestos is much less. If you still smoke, quitting will help decrease your chance of getting cancer.

Treatment. There is no effective treatment for asbestosis. If you are a young or middle-aged worker who is exposed to asbestos, avoid further exposure. If you have been exposed to low levels of the fiber and you discover this late in life, you may acquire the disease. It probably will progress slowly and further risk from working with asbestos is probably low, assuming that you do not smoke and the asbestos control program at your worksite is satisfactory.

PNEUMOCONIOSIS AND SILICOSIS

Signs and Symptoms
* Shortness of breath;
* Cough that produces sputum (sometimes).

We will describe two types of pneumoconiosis here: coal worker's pneumoconiosis, and silicosis. Both are caused by inhaled industrial particles that become permanently deposited in the lungs.

Coal worker's pneumoconiosis, also known as black lung disease or anthracosis, is caused by inhaling coal dust for prolonged periods, usually at least 10 years. Coal worker's pneumoconiosis is much more common in miners of anthracite coal (located primarily in the eastern United States) than in miners of bituminous coal (located primarily in the western United States).

Silicosis is caused by the inhalation of free silica (crystalline quartz); it is a severe disease caused by inhalation of industrial dust particles. Mining, stone cutting, quarrying (especially of granite), blasting, road and building construction, industries that manufacture abrasives, and farming are occupations that produce exposure to free silica. It usually takes 15 to 20 years of exposure before symptoms develop; however, unprotected workers in occupations with intense exposure to silica, such as sandblasting in confined spaces, tunneling through rock with a high quartz content, and manufacture of abrasive soaps, may develop silicosis in less than a year.

The Diagnosis. In most cases, both coal worker's pneumoconiosis and silicosis cause no respiratory symptoms unless you are a cigarette smoker. These diseases are diagnosed when small, irregular, opaque areas are seen on your chest x-ray and you have a history of exposure to coal dust or silica. With long-term exposure, these irregular areas become larger and combine into more regular, small, rounded nodules.

However, both coal worker's pneumoconiosis and silicosis may develop into progressive massive fibrosis, also called complicated pneumoconiosis. The symptoms may be severe shortness of breath and cough. Only a small percentage of those with coal worker's pneumoconiosis develop massive fibrosis; the mechanism that causes it is unknown. Those with silicosis, however, are likely to develop progressive massive fibrosis.

Fibrosis is diagnosed when an opaque area with a diameter larger than ½ inch is seen over the smaller opaque spots on your chest x-ray. The opaque areas combine so that they may cover the entire lobe of the lung. At this stage, the disease has progressed to cause shortness of breath and a cough that produces mucus. The symptoms are often more severe than the chest x-ray appearance suggests.

How Serious Are Coal Worker's Pneumoconiosis and Silicosis? In their early stages, coal worker's pneumoconiosis and silicosis do not cause respiratory impairment. However, if massive fibrosis develops, which it ultimately does in silicosis, respiratory impairment occurs and, despite avoidance of further exposure, death results. Survival may be less than 2 years. In addition, persons with silicosis have a 3 times greater risk of tuberculosis than does the average person.

Treatment. There is no specific treatment for either of these diseases. If you have one, avoid additional exposure to dust. If you smoke, by all means stop. Limit your exposure to all respiratory irritants—cold air, dry air, extremely humid air, and irritating fumes.

If you have silicosis and your tuberculin skin test is positive, you will need treatment to prevent tuberculosis, even if symptoms are not present.

Prevention is the best course of action. Wear a dust mask and take other steps to prevent exposure to the dust if you are working in an occupation that puts you at risk of developing one of these diseases. In addition, do not smoke.

OCCUPATIONAL ASTHMA

In about 2 percent of those with asthma, the cause is related to occupation or environment. Some agents that are known to cause asthma are wood dust, grain dust, tobacco, pollens, synthetic dyes, gum arabic, and rosin (soldering flux). Inhalation of one of these agents does not mean you will develop asthma, however. A small percentage of the population seems to be genetically disposed to allergies which may be provoked by exposure to one of these agents.

The symptoms are the same as those of acute asthma: shortness of breath, cough, tightness of the chest, and wheezing. The diagnosis of occupational asthma depends primarily on your medical history and the results of pulmonary function tests, possibly including a bronchial provocation test in which you are exposed to the allergic substance in a laboratory and your reaction is measured.

Treatment consists of bronchodilators and avoiding the substance that causes your asthma. Sometimes, you may have symptoms of asthma for years afterward even though you are no longer coming into contact with the offending agent (see also Asthma, page 933).

ALLERGIC ALVEOLITIS

This lung disease is caused by exposure to organic dusts. It goes by many names, usually relating to the occupation in which it is acquired. The best known are farmer's lung and byssinosis (see page 947). Grain dust can cause illness in farmers and in those who work in grain elevators.

Other illnesses include humidifier lung, which is caused by humidifiers, heating systems, and air conditioners that are contaminated by a fungus. Bagassosis results from fungi in moldy sugarcane fiber (called bagasse), and suberosis is caused by inhaling moldy cork dust. Sequoiosis is caused by moldy redwood sawdust; maple bark stripper's disease is caused by rotting maple tree logs and bark. Finally, mushroom picker's disease is caused by moldy compost, and detergent worker's lung is caused by dust containing spores from enzyme additives.

All of these dusts generally cause the same symptoms in those who are sensitive. These symptoms include a persistent cough that produces large amounts of sputum (which is the lung's way of trying to get rid of an irritant), wheezing, and shortness of breath. Tests reveal decreased pulmonary function. In all cases, those who smoke are more susceptible and have more serious symptoms than nonsmokers.

Generally, avoiding the irritating dust relieves the symptoms. Drinking plenty of liquids, using a non-contaminated humidifier, and, if necessary, using a bronchodilator prescribed by your physician also help.

BYSSINOSIS

This asthma-like disease sometimes is found in workers who produce cotton or, to a lesser extent, flax, jute, and hemp yarn and rope. Also known as brown lung and Monday fever (although it does not cause a fever), it is caused by inhaling dust from the raw plant bales. Those who work with cotton and other fibers during the cleaning processes that precede spinning—blowing, mixing, and carding (straightening)—are at greatest risk.

The disease may develop soon after first exposure or after years of working in the industry. You may feel a tightness in your chest toward the end of the day on Monday, the first day after the weekend. At first, the symptoms do not appear during the rest of the week, but in about 10 to 25 percent of affected persons the chest tightness gradually begins to persist for several days and eventually throughout the week and into weekend and vacation periods.

Byssinosis generally is not serious, and bronchodilators and antihistamines help clear up the symptoms. If the disease persists or gets worse, however, it can lead to chronic illness such as emphysema and chronic bronchitis. Thus, you probably should stop working in the industry. When exposure to the fibers stops, the illness will clear up.

INDUSTRIAL BRONCHITIS

Bronchitis in coal miners and workers exposed to cotton, flax, or hemp dust is called

FUMES SMOKE, AND GASES

Exposure to high concentrations of toxic fumes and gases and to smoke can cause various respiratory symptoms.

Industrial Fumes and Gases

Long-term low-level exposure or accidental exposure to high levels of industrial toxic chemicals can cause various temporary and sometimes chronic respiratory symptoms. Usually, the lower respiratory tract is affected, causing symptoms such as shortness of breath, cough, and chronic bronchitis (see page 927). A sampling of toxic chemicals includes: ammonia, cyanides, formaldehyde, acid fumes, hydrogen sulfide, diazomethane, halides, nitrogen dioxide, isocyanates, ozone, phosgene, phthalic anhydride, and sulfur dioxide.

The industrial process of heating certain metals, such as cadmium, chromium, nickel, and beryllium, to high temperatures and then cooling them quickly releases fumes that can cause various respiratory diseases if inhaled. These include bronchitis, inflammation of the lungs, lung cancer, and metal fume fever. Metal fume fever is a flu-like illness that can result from exposure to fumes from copper, magnesium, zinc, and certain other metals. The symptoms usually appear several hours after work and then clear up within 24 hours. However, they return when the worker is exposed to the fumes again.

If you work in an industrial trade that uses high heat, such as welding, brazing, smelting, pottery making, and furnace work, you are most at risk. Using nonhazard-ous compounds, ensuring that ventilation is adequate, and using safe machinery and work practices can help prevent exposure to toxic fumes.

In all cases, workers who are exposed to these fumes and gases and who also smoke have a greatly increased risk of lung cancer.

Air Pollution

Given the right atmospheric conditions, air pollution caused by automobiles, power plants, and factories can result in increased levels of ozone and sulfer dioxide in the air. This often causes wheezing in people who have asthma and may cause shortness of breath in elderly people, young children, and persons with chronic cardiopulmonary disease. On days when the ozone level is high, usually after a long stretch of hot, humid weather, it is best that those at risk stay indoors.

Indoor air pollution also can be a problem, especially because concerns about energy efficiency have resulted in construction of houses that are more tightly sealed. Therefore, fumes that once were of little concern tend to build up in the house instead of escaping to the outside. One example is cigarette smoke which, besides having major health effects on the smoker, also affects nonsmokers who are exposed to it. For instance, passive cigarette smoking has been shown to cause increased respiratory infections and decreased lung function in children whose parents smoke. When ventilation is poor, wood smoke and fumes from kerosene floor heaters can aggravate asthma.

Another potentially hazardous agent is formaldehyde. It is present in urethane foam insulation and in some types of flooring used in con-struction of new houses, mobile homes, and furniture. When the products are new there may be a pungent odor due to formaldehyde fumes which may irritate the eyes, nose, throat, and airways (trachea and bronchi). The formaldehyde gradually evaporates so that within a few months it should cause no problem. People with asthma may note worsening of the problem during these weeks or months.

Smoke

More fire fighters and fire victims die from smoke inhalation than from burns. Smoke inhalation has several effects on the lungs. It usually causes some degree of inflammation of the lower respiratory tract, which can develop into pulmonary edema if the exposure is severe enough.

Whenever anything burns, carbon monoxide is produced and, when inhaled, interferes with transportation of oxygen by the blood. All smoke contains this odorless gas. Be careful, therefore, when you have any fire indoors that produces smoke (such as indoor barbecuing). The effects of inhaling carbon monoxide are so subtle as to be unnoticeable, and you can become unconscious without realizing anything is happening.

Smoke that contains a heavy concentration of floating particles also irritates the lungs.

Many plastics, polyurethanes, and other synthetic materials used in home furnishings give off various toxic gases when they burn. They are particularly dangerous to the lungs and may cause a severe, although temporary, illness. Long-term exposure, as in fire fighters, may increase the risk of chronic illness, although this is difficult to measure.

industrial bronchitis. Fumes from ammonia, strong acids, certain organic solvents, chlorine, hydrogen sulfide, sulfur dioxide, and bromine also may cause bronchitis. It remains unclear whether the bronchitis in these workers is caused by the dusts to which they are exposed or whether the exposure aggravates bronchitis from other causes, such as smoking.

Industrial bronchitis, like acute bronchitis, generally causes shortness of breath and a chronic cough that produces sputum. This is an acute disease. It clears up with rest, plenty of liquids, and elimination of exposure to the irritant. Sometimes use of a humidifier or vaporizer also helps.

FARMER'S LUNG

Farmer's lung is a type of lung disease that results from repeated inhalation of dust from moldy hay containing the spores of a fungus. Only a small percentage of people exposed to the spores actually develop the disease, and then only after considerable exposure. Asthma does not predispose you to being susceptible. In fact, people with asthma or hay fever are unable to tolerate exposure to the quantity of dust required to cause farmer's lung.

In acute cases, the symptoms are fever, chills, cough, and shortness of breath. You also may experience loss of appetite, nausea, and vomiting. If you avoid exposure to moldy hay, your symptoms will usually decrease in severity within hours, although it may take weeks before you recover completely. Your physician will review your medical history and may perform a physical examination, chest x-ray, and pulmonary function tests to confirm the diagnosis.

The disease can be chronic—particularly if you are continuously exposed to low levels of the fungus over long periods. A cough that produces sputum, progressively worsening shortness of breath during exertion, fatigue, and weight loss are symptoms of chronic disease.

If you avoid exposure to the fungus, the acute disease does not develop. If you cannot avoid moldly hay, be sure to use a protective dust mask. Also, it may be possible to prevent the growth of the fungus by using chemicals. In severe cases, corticosteroids may be prescribed.

SILO-FILLER'S DISEASE

Silo-filler's disease is an acute illness that results from inhalation of fumes given off by moist silage. The gas given off is nitrogen dioxide. When inhaled, it is irritating to the bronchi and lungs.

The severity of the illness depends on the length of time the farmer is in the silo. Farmers sometimes die in silos filled with the yellowish gas and acrid odor of oxides and nitrogen. With less exposure, there may be only irritation of the respiratory tract, such as a runny nose and mild cough.

If mild breathlessness occurs, see your physician soon. Often, irritation of the lungs leads to pulmonary edema (a collection of fluid in the lungs) which can be serious and result in permanent damage to the lungs. There may be an associated bronchiolitis (inflammation of the tiny airways near the alveoli) which also may cause permanent damage to your lungs. For this reason, many physicians give corticosteroids to try to avoid this permanent problem.

THE LUNGS AND THE CARDIOVASCULAR SYSTEM

The workings of your heart and lungs are interrelated. Blood travels through your lungs to be oxygenated each time it passes through your heart. Thus, if a blood clot forms in your blood vessel system and then travels through your bloodstream, the clot eventually may block an artery in your lungs, resulting in pulmonary embolism or death of tissue (infarction). Chronic lung disease can lead to heart failure (cor pulmonale).

PULMONARY EMBOLISM

Signs and Symptoms
- Sudden shortness of breath;

- Chest pain;
- Anxiety;
- Cough that produces blood-streaked sputum;
- Excessive perspiration.

Emergency Symptom

- Sudden loss of consciousness.

An embolus is a small clot of foreign material—usually a blood clot but sometimes a globule of fat, an air bubble, tissue from a tumor, or a clump of bacteria—that blocks an artery.

Most emboli come from blood clots (called thrombi) in the veins of the lower extremities or pelvis. They are carried by the bloodstream through the right side of the heart to the lungs. They also may arise from the walls of the heart. If a clot arises in the left side of the heart, the embolus will not go to the lungs but instead will go to the brain or some other part of the body. Tissue death (infarction) occurs when the blood supply to the tissue is blocked.

An embolism (sudden blockage caused by an embolus) can occur in any small artery, but the lungs are particularly vulnerable because all of the blood in your body passes through your lungs every time it circulates.

Pulmonary emboli affect as many as 500,000 persons in the United States yearly and may cause as many as 50,000 deaths each year. In persons under age 45, it occurs more often in women than in men; after that age it occurs equally in both sexes. Surgery, prolonged bed rest or inactivity (such as prolonged sitting when on an automobile or airplane trip), stroke, heart attack, obesity, and hip or leg fracture increase your risk of having a pulmonary embolism. Also, anything that increases the tendency of your blood to clot may make you more susceptible.

The Diagnosis. The symptoms depend on the size of the embolus and how healthy your cardiopulmonary system is. They include sudden chest pain, shortness of breath, a feeling of anxiety, sweating, and cough that sometimes produces blood-streaked sputum. Massive embolism or embolism occurring in a person with serious preexisting heart or lung disease may cause sudden loss of consciousness and even death.

Pulmonary thromboembolism may be difficult to diagnose, particularly if you have underlying cardiopulmonary disease. Your physician may need a chest x-ray, a lung scan, or a pulmonary angiogram (dye is injected into an artery of the arm or leg and then flows into the arteries of the lung so that they are highlighted on the x-ray). Pulmonary angiography is the most accurate test for detecting emboli; however, it requires a high degree of experience to perform and interpret correctly. Your physician may recommend other tests as well.

How Serious Is Pulmonary Embolism?

Pulmonary embolism can be very serious; about 10 percent of affected persons die within the first hour. However, if you survive

---

LUNG AND HEART TRANSPLANTATION

Lung transplantations were first performed in the early 1960s; however, after 10 years of poor success, lung transplantation was abandoned. Then, in the late 1970s, a new immunosuppressant drug called cyclosporine was introduced. This revived the possibility of performing lung transplantation. However, studies in animals found that the supply of blood to the new lungs was insufficient, and that the transplants did not heal adequately.

In the 1980s, a solution was found: transplant the lungs and heart together. In 1981 the first successful heart-lung transplantation was performed. Transplanting both organs together helps ensure that the new lungs and trachea receive enough blood to be able to heal.

The list of problems and limitations is long. Finding donor lungs and hearts can be very difficult because the lungs of brain-dead accident victims often are damaged. To be usable, lungs must match the recipient's body size, blood type, and tissue compatibility. Recently, by using new immunosuppressant drugs and new procedures, many double-lung and single-lung transplantations have been successfully performed, opening up the possibility that a donated heart and lungs can help save the lives of up to three people instead of only one. If a lung transplantation recipient's heart is healthy, it often can be donated to someone in need, in a double transplantation.

Lung transplantation is a risky, expensive, and very complicated procedure that is performed only on patients whose only hope for survival is transplantation and in cases that have a high possibility of success.

Most recipients of successful lung transplants seem to recover to carry on relatively normal lives in the short term. The long-term outcome is not yet known.

the initial attack and have appropriate diagnosis and treatment, the outlook is good. You should return to normal in a few weeks unless other serious disease is present.

Treatment. *Medication.* Your physician may prescribe anticoagulant therapy to prevent further blood clots from forming or clots already present from enlarging. Heparin usually is the drug that is given, often in conjunction with warfarin. Other medications may be given in order to dissolve existing clots. All of these medications do have side effects. Their use must be closely monitored.

Surgery. Surgery is rarely necessary, but it may be helpful in persons with recurring emboli for whom other treatments have not been effective or with a sudden, massive embolus.

Prevention. After an operation, you will be encouraged to get up and move around as soon as possible or to perform active and passive leg exercises. When on a trip, walk periodically or at least wiggle your toes and move your feet while sitting. If you are immobilized, keep your legs elevated and perhaps wear support stockings. All of these can help prevent pooling and clotting of blood in your legs, a frequent cause of emboli.

In some cases, if you are at risk for recurrent pulmonary embolism, you may be helped by taking low doses of heparin, warfarin (Coumadin), or antiplatelet drugs such as aspirin.

COR PULMONALE

Signs and Symptoms
- Chronic cough that produces sputum;
- Shortness of breath with exercise;
- Wheezing;
- Weakness and easy tiring;
- Bulging of the veins in the neck;
- Swelling of the lower extremities;
- Enlargement of and tenderness in the liver.

"Cor pulmonale" means enlargement and eventual failure of the right ventricle (the lower right chamber) of the heart due to pulmonary disease. Because the heart and lungs are closely associated in function and physical location, diseases of the lungs often affect the heart as well.

Blood goes from the right side of the heart into the lungs where carbon dioxide is removed from and oxygen is added to the blood. Normally, it does not take a great deal of pressure to push the blood into the lungs, so the muscular walls of the right ventricle are not as strong as those on the left side which pumps blood out to the rest of the body. However, when the lungs are impaired by emphysema, fibrosis, or other severe chronic lung disease, it takes more effort to pump blood into them. Although the heart is able to compensate for a while, eventually it fails, making this a very serious disease.

To diagnose cor pulmonale, your physician will probably do a physical examination and take your medical history, perform a pulmonary function test, take a chest x-ray, and record an electrocardiogram.

Life expectancy with cor pulmonale is generally the same as that with the underlying pulmonary disease. Once symptoms appear, on average the survival is for 2 to 5 years. If the underlying cause is uncomplicated emphysema, survival may be considerably longer.

Treatment. Your physician may arrange specific treatment for the underlying respiratory disease. In addition, he or she may advise the use of oxygen, restriction of salt and fluid intake, and diuretics.

CHAPTER 32

THE MUSCLES AND BONES

CHAPTER CONTENTS

JOINT DISORDERS
Osteoarthritis
Rheumatoid Arthritis
Joint Replacement
Juvenile Rheumatoid Arthritis
Joint Disorders of Childhood
Inflammatory Arthritis
Infectious Arthritis
Rheumatic Fever Arthritis
Gout

Acute Painful Shoulder
Bursitis
Corticosteroid Drugs
CONNECTIVE TISSUE DISEASES
Systemic Lupus Erythematosus
Scleroderma
Sjögren's Syndrome
Polymyositis and Dermatomyositis
Polymyalgia Rheumatica
Vasculitis

A
Your bones are alive and always changing, providing support for your body and functioning as your body's depository for important minerals.

B
Many of your skeletal muscles are paired, enabling your body to move. These muscles are connected to your bones by tendons.

A

B

THE MUSCULOSKELETAL SYSTEM AT WORK

As its name suggests, the musculoskeletal system consists of muscles (from the Latin word *musculus*) and bones (from the Greek word *skeletos,* which means dried-up body). The bones in the human body are interconnected at junctions called joints. Most joints are essentially hinges that allow the bones to move within certain prescribed limits. Others move in a different way, such as the hip and shoulder, which are ball-and-socket joints, and the backbone (vertebral column), which has limited movement.

The musculoskeletal system provides mobility and also provides protection for our internal organs, with the ribs surrounding the fragile lungs and the heart and the skull protecting the brain. Until the system breaks down, whether due to accident, disease, or simply wear and tear over time, most of us take this miracle of mechanics for granted.

Breakdowns can occur at any time and for various causes. This chapter discusses a range of potential problems, beginning with injuries sustained as we go about our daily activities, such as an ankle sprain. Amputations, whether congenital or surgical, make physical and psychological demands on the body, and the rehabilitation efforts needed to deal with these demands are presented. Common ailments of the foot and back, problems that are widespread in our population, are discussed at length. Diseases of the bones, muscles, and joints, from the arthritis and osteoporosis so common in our elderly population to more unusual ailments such as lupus and gout, also are considered.

To understand how these events or ailments affect our muscles and bones, we need first to know the constituent parts and the basic workings of the musculoskeletal system. Essential to such an understanding is a familiarity with not only the muscles and bones but also the joints.

THE BONES

There are 206 bones in the human body. These rigid parts are composed of osseous tissue (from the Latin word for bony, *osseus*). Osseous tissue, in turn, consists of various substances, among them proteins, minerals, and bone cells.

The proteins form a framework to which the minerals, in particular a compound of calcium and phosphate, are attached. The bone cells monitor the ongoing process whereby the calcium phosphate mineral is deposited or withdrawn. The bones are alive and always changing, providing support for the body and also functioning as the body's depository for these important minerals. Inside certain bones is the marrow, a soft core that manufactures blood cells (see page 476).

Problems with the bones vary. Some are the result of trauma in which a bone is broken or bruised, such as fractures (see page 955) or dislocations (see page 957). Others, such as osteoporosis (see page 982) or osteomalacia (see page 985), result from a malfunction of the complex balance of the chemistry of bone.

THE JOINTS

The ends of the bones that meet in a joint are cushioned with a layer of cartilage, which absorbs some of the shock or weight involved in movement. Among the other elements of a joint are a liquid called synovial fluid, a membrane, a protective casing called the capsule, and bands of fibrous tissue called ligaments, which bind the parts of a joint together.

As with bone problems, joint ailments are many and varied. Osteoarthritis, perhaps the most common, is mainly the result of wear and tear on the joints (especially the cartilage) and usually affects a single joint at a time (see page 995). Others, such as rheumatoid arthritis, occur for reasons that are not well understood, but they produce pain and discomfort in many or even all joints, with inflammation in the synovial membrane and the cartilage (see page 997). Joints may also sustain injuries from trauma (certain knee injuries, for example; see page 966).

THE MUSCLES

There are some 650 muscles in the body. The muscles are fibers with an elasticity that sets them apart from other body parts. This key characteristic allows the muscles to expand and contract and thus produce movement at the joints.

Virtually all the muscles are paired. In your arm, for example, the contraction of your biceps muscle will cause your arm to flex, whereas a contraction of the opposing triceps muscle causes your arm to extend. The muscles are connected to the bones by tendons.

Not all muscles produce movement of the skeleton. In addition to the skeletal (or striated) muscles, there are smooth (or nonstriated) muscles. These muscles are found in such internal organs as the stomach and bladder and in the walls of blood vessels. They usually are arranged in sheets and also are called involuntary muscles because they are not under conscious control. Heart (or myocardium) muscles are another type of muscle. They are also beyond the mechanism of voluntary control. The smooth muscles and the heart muscles are not considered a part of the musculoskeletal system.

Most muscle problems occur because of strain or overexertion. The back pain that occurs in the usually sedentary person who elects to rearrange the furniture is the result of the sudden or unusual demands put on poorly conditioned muscles (see page 992). The muscle soreness experienced by the rookie jogger who overdoes it at the start of an exercise program is a similar problem. Common sports injuries include sprains or pulled muscles (see pages 960 and 959).

This chapter discusses each of the injuries mentioned above and also numerous others. However, regardless of whether or not you have an injury, you will find valuable guidance about exercise (see page 959). Exercise is a critical component of good health, but exercise can be detrimental, especially when proper care is not given to the muscles and bones. Proper care can involve a simple program of loosening exercises or the avoidance of certain kinds of activities if you

already have certain joint or other musculoskeletal problems. Being careful now may save you pain, time, and money later.

Several medical professionals are largely concerned with problems of the musculoskeletal system. If you or your primary-care physician believe that a specialist is necessary to treat your ailment, you may see a rheumatologist, orthopedic surgeon, physiatrist, or physical or occupational therapist.

A rheumatologist is a physician who has special training in diseases of the musculoskeletal system (such as arthritis and other joint diseases). If you have rheumatoid arthritis, lupus, or a less common joint ailment or if your arthritis is not responding to treatment, you may want to seek the care of a rheumatologist.

If your bone disorder requires a surgical procedure, you should consult an orthopedic surgeon. Orthopedics is the surgical discipline concerned with preventing or correcting disorders of the body's moving parts, including the skeleton, joints, muscles, ligaments, and cartilage. An orthopedic surgeon is a physician with additional training in this specialty.

A physiatrist is a specialist in physical medicine and rehabilitation. Also a physician, the physiatrist is specially trained to help restore the useful function of injured or damaged joints or limbs. The program the physiatrist offers for rehabilitation may include special clothing or equipment, exercise, pain control treatments, or other approaches.

A physical therapist is a licensed professional, but not a physician, who helps you recover by using various means including such physical agents as heat, water, light, massage, and exercise. An occupational therapist is also a licensed professional. Often, occupational therapists work with physical therapists. These specialists in occupational rehabilitation can help you to accomplish tasks that your ailment or injury prevents you from doing.

COMMON INJURIES

Although the body's mechanical system is extremely durable, muscle and bone injuries are commonplace. Excessive stress can cause the rigid bones to break and, when

extended beyond their usual range, the flexible muscles or joints can be strained or damaged. Whether the event is a fall from an apple tree at 8 years of age or a tennis tumble at 65 years, most of us experience a wide variety of musculoskeletal injuries in our lifetimes. The most common of these are discussed below.

FRACTURES

Signs and Symptoms

- A swelling or bruising over a bone;
- Deformity of a limb;
- Localized pain that is intensified when the affected area is moved or pressure is put on it;
- Loss of function in the area of the injury;
- In a compound fracture, the broken bone breaks through adjacent tissues and protrudes from the skin.

Fractures occur as a result of a physical force being exerted on the bone that is greater than it can withstand. Thus, quite simply, a fracture is a broken bone. Fractures are common injuries, so common that in the course of their lives most people sustain one or more fractures.

Bone breaks are classified into several categories. A simple fracture is one in which the bone has been broken but does not come through the nearby soft tissues. A comminuted fracture is one in which the bone splinters into several pieces. When the bone does protrude from the skin, it is termed a compound fracture.

Fractures are also classified according to the way the bone itself is broken. If the bone actually snaps into two or more parts, it is called a simple or complete fracture. When the break is limited to a crack and the bone is not separated into two parts, the fracture is termed incomplete. An impacted fracture occurs when one fragment of bone is embedded into another fragment of bone.

Yet another variety of bone break occurs in people with bones weakened by disease. Bone cancer (see page 988) or a bone disorder such as osteoporosis (see page 982) can result in weakened bones that fracture spontaneously or with only minor stresses exerted on them. Such breaks are termed pathologic fractures because the principal cause is an underlying disease.

Compound fractures break through the skin. Simple fractures, of which there are several varieties, do not. Simple fractures are classified according to the way the bone is broken. Examples include: greenstick, transverse, oblique, comminuted.

Compound   **Simple**   **Greenstick**   **Transverse**   **Oblique**   **Comminuted**

The risk of fracture varies with age. The skeleton is flexible in children, so their bones are more likely to bend than to break. As a result, when a child experiences a fracture, it is often a type of incomplete fracture called a green-stick fracture. The bone doesn't snap neatly like a dried twig but cracks more like a green stick. In the elderly, bones are likely to be brittle, and falls or other events that would have no effect on younger bones can cause fractures.

Still another variety is the stress fracture. The stress fracture is really a hairline crack and often is invisible on an x-ray for up to 6 weeks after injury. The recommended treatment for stress fracture is likely to be rest rather than operation or the therapies discussed below.

The Diagnosis.   Your physician will begin with a physical examination. In the event of a compound fracture, the bone protruding from the flesh makes the diagnosis obvious. In some instances of simple and incomplete fractures, however, identifying the fracture isn't always easy. Severe sprains and incomplete fractures sometimes closely resemble one another.

An x-ray is the means of confirming the diagnosis, and often x-rays will be taken from two different angles. In the case of suspected skull or vertebral fractures, the physician may also order a computed tomographic (CT) scan (see page 1286).

How Serious Is a Fracture?   The seriousness of bone fractures depends on the location of the break and the damage sustained by the bone and adjacent tissues.

When certain minor bones of the hands or feet are broken, your physician will recommend only that you avoid using the affected area. For more serious fractures, dangerous complications can occur if proper treatment is not provided. In any fracture, the adjacent area must be examined carefully to establish whether blood vessel or nerve damage occurred. In cases of injury to the skull or the back, the danger of brain injury (see page 535) or spinal damage (see page 552) must also be considered. Compound fractures must be treated to ensure that the bone and adjacent tissues don't become infected (see Osteomyelitis, page 987).

The time required for recuperation from a broken bone varies with the age and health of the patient and the nature of the fracture.

In children, a minor break may be entirely healed within a few weeks. In the elderly, a serious fracture may require months to repair. In some instances, a fracture that is healing particularly slowly may require a second operation in which bone tissue taken from another bone is grafted onto the fracture. The source of bone for a graft is often the thigh bone.

With prompt and proper treatment and a sound rehabilitation program, the outlook most often is for a complete recovery.

Treatment.   All suspected fractures should be treated with proper first aid (see page 308) and examined by a physician, and an x-ray should be taken. (See also Sprains, page 310.) If the bone has been displaced, it must be set in its proper position if it is to heal properly. The setting of the bone is called reduction. For cases in which it can be done without an operative procedure, it is termed closed reduction. A local anesthetic will be used, and your physician will reposition the bone using x-rays as a guide.

Surgery.   If surgery is required, the procedure is termed open reduction. Usually, a general anesthetic is administered, and an incision is made to gain access to the broken bone so it can be set in its proper position.

A fracture that is immediately adjacent to or extends into a joint may require a device such as a pin, plate, or screw—or even a special kind of glue—to hold it in place. During a surgical procedure, the device is fastened to the bone to maintain the proper position of the broken parts with respect to one another. One advantage of this approach is that use of the injured limb can often be resumed in a matter of weeks rather than a longer time—even months—because the device can carry some of the weight or stress on the bone.

In some instances, especially in elderly persons with osteoporosis or another disorder that has led to a deterioration of the bone or joint, an artificial joint may be inserted (see Joint Replacement, page 998).

Immobilization.   After the bone has been set, it is usually necessary to immobilize it and, in some cases, also the adjacent joints. Preventing motion between the two ends of the bone lessens pain and facilitates healing. Means of accomplishing this include casts, splints, and occasionally traction. In some cases, however, no such artificial means are necessary. A broken rib, for example, will be held in place by the mass of chest muscles that surround it. If a finger or toe is broken, it may simply be taped to an adjacent digit.

1. Casts and Splints. A cast may be applied to, for example, a broken arm to immobilize it. First the arm is covered with a soft material to protect the skin from irritation. Then, bandages saturated with plaster are wrapped around the limb. When the plaster dries over a period of a day or two, the cast will be rigid. However, to avoid changing the shape of the cast during the drying process, the cast should not be handled with the fingertips (the palm of the hand can be used to maneuver it) or rested on a flat surface. Rest it on pillows to avoid flattening, which can put pressure on the skin beneath the plaster. Casts made of fiberglass or plastic dry more quickly, usually within 30 minutes, than those made of plaster of Paris.

Occasionally, a splint may be applied. This is a device used to immobilize, support, and correct injured, displaced, or deformed structures. It is often used instead of a full cast to prevent motion of a dislocated joint or of the ends of a fractured joint.

2. Traction. For instances in which a broken bone is difficult to immobilize by other means (as with the thigh bone, which is protected by a dense layer of muscles), a mechanical system of weights is sometimes used to hold broken parts of the bones in the proper position. Traction, the force created by this system, is especially useful for fractures in which ends of the broken bone tend to override one another because of the surrounding musculature.

Rehabilitation. After the bone has been set in its proper position and immobilized, the next most important part of any treatment program is rehabilitation. This process begins as soon as possible, even if the broken bone is still within a cast. Movement of adjacent tissues is important to blood flow, which enhances the healing process and prevents the formation of blood clots. Movement also helps maintain muscle tone, and it may limit wasting (atrophy) of the muscles and withering of the bones due to prolonged immobilization. It also helps prevent the stiffness in joints that occurs when they are not used.

Medication. In most cases, medication is limited to analgesics to reduce pain and antibiotics to reduce the risk of infection.

DISLOCATIONS

Signs and Symptoms
- An injured joint that becomes misshapen and immovable, usually after having been subjected to a blow, fall, or other trauma;
- Swelling and intense pain.

A dislocation is, at its simplest, a joint that is out of place. It is an injury in which the joint ends of bones are forced from their normal positions. The joint will no longer function properly, and the unnatural movement of the bones may have caused damage to the structure of the joint and perhaps to its muscles, ligaments, nerves, and blood vessels.

In some cases, the cause of the dislocation is an underlying disease (such as rheumatoid arthritis; see page 997) or a congenital weakness. In persons who have sustained dislocations previously, the joint may become weakened and will dislocate spontaneously.

The Diagnosis. After sustaining a dislocation, the joint will become difficult or impossible to move. The pain is likely to be intense and to become more severe at any attempt to move the joint. There usually will be a visible change in the configuration of the joint, sometimes with swelling.

If your physician suspects that you have a dislocation, an x-ray will be taken to confirm the diagnosis and to determine whether an accompanying fracture (see page 955) is present. A CT scan also may be taken if spinal damage is suspected.

Nursemaid's Dislocation. This common and often misdiagnosed dislocation of the elbow is found in children younger than 5 years. It usually occurs when a child's arm is suddenly pulled or jerked by an adult. The immature elbow cannot withstand this stress and a dislocation occurs. The child typically experiences pain and limited motion in the elbow. Generally, x-rays are taken to rule out any other problems. When the bones are returned to their proper position, the pain ceases. The usual treatment approach also involves several days of immobilization, often with a splint or cast.

How Serious Is a Dislocation?

If a vertebra is dislocated, there is a risk of spinal cord damage and, potentially, paralysis. Similarly, nerve damage is a risk when a shoulder or hip is dislocated.

In most cases, however, a simple dislocation without substantial nerve or tissue damage can be corrected by a physician. The joint then will be immobilized for a short time (typically, 2 weeks). After a period of recuperation, the joint is likely to be nearly or fully normal.

For cases in which the joint has been weakened and spontaneous dislocations occur, a surgical procedure, in which the ligaments of the joint are tightened to prevent such recurrences, may be needed.

Treatment. Any suspected dislocation should be treated with proper first aid (see page 312) and examined by a physician, and an x-ray should be taken. In the case of a suspected vertebral dislocation, however, don't move the injured person: wait for professional care (see Spinal Injuries, page 309). The displaced bones in the joint must be returned to their proper position. This setting of the bones is called reduction.

The dislocation should be treated as quickly as possible. If it is not treated within half an hour, the swelling and pain are usually such that treatment without an anesthetic is not feasible. It is also crucial, however, that any treatment be provided by a person with proper training. Further damage can result from improper attempts at reduction.

Immobilization. After the joint has been returned to its normal position, it is usually necessary to immobilize the joint, usually with a splint.

Rehabilitation. After the joints have been set in their proper positions and immobilized, rehabilitation begins. This may start even if the joint is in a cast. Movement stimulates blood flow in adjacent tissue, which enhances the healing process. Movement also maintains muscle tone and limits the wasting of the muscles and withering of the bones due to prolonged immobilization. It also helps prevent the stiffness in joints that results from extended disuse.

Be sure to follow your physician's advice about limiting the physical activity of the affected joint. Too rapid a return to normal activity puts you at risk of reinjuring the joint.

Medication. In most cases, the medication used to treat a dislocation is limited to analgesics to reduce the pain and an anesthetic if operation is needed. Antibiotics are needed only rarely.

SEVERED TENDONS

Signs and Symptoms
- A deep cut accompanied by an inability to move a finger, toe, or other joint.

A severe cut of the tissues of the hand, foot, forearm, or calf may damage the tendons, the fibrous tissues that connect muscle to bone. Severing a tendon will result in an inability to move the affected joint.

A severed tendon requires attention of two kinds. First, the wound must be closed immediately to aid healing and prevent infection. Second, the tendon must be repaired surgically. Sometimes both can be done in one procedure when the wound is initially treated, but in some cases the cut must be allowed to heal before the operation is performed. In general, however, reattachment is usually done within a week of the injury.

The Diagnosis. The key symptom, an inability to move a finger, toe, or other joint, suggests that the tendon has been severed, and so the musculature is no longer linked to the bone it usually maneuvers. This injury must be distinguished from a severed nerve, which may have the same effect by preventing muscle contraction.

If your physician suspects that a fracture may accompany the injury, an x-ray may be taken of the affected area.

How Serious Is a Severed Tendon?

In most cases, prompt repair of a severed tendon allows the affected area to return to nearly normal. However, some stiffness and a decrease in the range of movement often result.

Treatment. If you suspect a severed tendon, seek immediate medical help.

SPORTS INJURIES

Most injuries that occur during athletic activity result from unusual demands put on bones, muscles, or other tissues. The novice runner who struggles to complete 5 miles the first day on the track will have undreamed of aches and pains; the over-40 ex-jock who comes out of retirement for the company softball game is an excellent candidate for sprain and pain.

An injury-free life is an unrealistic goal. However, a few sensible rules will help you avoid inconvenient, painful, expensive, and, at times, disabling injuries.

Consult Your Physician

If you are older than 40 years, obese, or a heavy smoker, if you have had unexplained chest pains, heart problems such as a previous heart attack, irregular heart rhythms, or other serious health problem, or if you lead a largely sedentary life, consult your physician before starting a vigorous exercise regimen. Your physician may suggest a stress test (see page 804) to evaluate the condition of your heart and lungs and offer valuable do's and don't's specific to your physical condition.

Warm Up Before Exercising

To avoid injury, invest a minimum of 5 to 10 minutes in stretching and loosening your muscles. The increased blood flow of such a warm-up will reduce tension in the muscles, improve their range of motion, and may even increase your level of performance. Simultaneously, you are reducing significantly the chance of muscle pulls, strains, and other injuries.

Cool Down After Exercising

After your workout, it is just as important to allow your muscles to cool down. Muscles used during a workout have contracted, and most repetitive activities also can cause them to become permanently shortened. To restore balance to the muscles, a session of stretching after the workout is critical. Muscles that aren't treated by this staged return to normal are more likely to sustain pulls, strains, and spasms (see page 959).

Pace Yourself

Sudden and unfamiliar exertions are most likely to cause injuries. If you are bent on improving your performance, do so—but at a sensible pace. Don't double your distance or duration overnight. Develop a program that allows your body to become conditioned to the activity so that over time it adjusts to the challenges you offer it.

Select the Sport That Is Right for You

If you have a painful back or perpetually sore knees, the pounding of jogging is not for you; perhaps a daily swim or a ride on a stationary bicycle more nearly suits your needs. *See page 382 for guidance in selecting the exercise most suitable to you.*

Make It a Habit

Working out only once a week, no matter how vigorous the activity, puts you at risk of injury (and fails to provide you with maximal aerobic and conditioning benefits; see page 794). Try to establish a schedule of a minimum of three 20-minute workouts a week.

Take Care of That Injury

When you sprain an ankle or twist a knee, make sure you get medical advice and then follow it. A key element is almost sure to be what physicians commonly refer to as the tincture of time. Allow the injury to heal before testing it too vigorously (see page 969).

Surgery. Tendons are stretched taut like elastic. When severed, the two pieces may snap back from the tear and be difficult to retrieve. As a result, an incision may be required to enlarge the cut. In some instances, tissue from another tendon may have to be used to repair the damaged tendon.

Rehabilitation. After operation, the area of injury usually is immobilized. Upon instructing you to resume physical activity, your physician also may recommend an exercise program. Recently, advances have been made in the use of passive exercise (principally flexing movements involving no stress on the injured area) that help decrease the long-term stiffness.

PULLED MUSCLE (MUSCLE STRAIN)

Signs and Symptoms

- Localized pain when an injury occurs, followed by tenderness and, in some cases, swelling;

- Stiffness or tenderness that occurs during the 24 hours immediately after sustaining a pulled muscle (or muscle strain);
- If the muscle seems to have no function whatsoever, the muscle may have been ruptured.

A so-called pulled muscle (or muscle strain) is the result of too great a demand being put on a muscle. A minor muscle pull results from overstretching or overworking the area. There is no loss of strength, but soreness results.

A more serious muscle pull occurs when some of the fibers of a muscle actually tear, causing the muscle to contract and to bleed internally. In rare cases, the entire muscle may be torn apart, either partially or, less frequently, entirely. When this occurs, the muscle is ruptured.

One of the most common muscle strains occurs to the hamstrings. A group of muscles at the back of the thigh, the hamstrings enable you to flex your knee and extend your thigh, motions that occur when you run. A muscle pain or weakness at the back of the thigh may well indicate an injury to your hamstring muscles.

A second common muscle injury is the so-called groin pull (or strain). No one specific muscle is injured when you sustain a groin pull; rather, the tendons and muscles of the groin (including abdominal, leg, and pelvic areas) may be strained or torn. The pain or muscle spasms in the groin area can result from repetitive overuse or a single traumatic event.

The Diagnosis. The discomfort in the area (which may include tenderness, muscle spasms, and swelling) is the key to diagnosis. An x-ray may be taken to rule out bone injury as a cause of the problem.

How Serious Is a Muscle Pull? A complete and rapid recovery can be expected from most muscle pulls when they are treated with the simple measures described below and given proper rest during recuperation.

However, if you suspect that a muscle has been ruptured or that a bone may have been fractured (see page 955), or if the pain persists for more than a few days, seek professional medical help. An operation may be required to repair the damage.

Treatment. Apply ice or cold packs to the injured area for the first 24 hours after injury, then use a heating pad or hot baths thereafter. At times, particularly if swelling is extensive, cold packs can be used throughout the entire recovery of a muscle injury. Elevating the injured muscle and the use of a compression wrap such as an elastic (Ace) bandage may help reduce and prevent swelling, although you should not bind it tightly. Try not to use the injured muscle while it is painful, usually a period of no more than several days.

Medication. For minor muscle pulls, aspirin or another over-the-counter drug may be taken to reduce the pain. For moderate or more severe muscle strains, consult your physician before taking medication because he or she may prescribe an anti-inflammatory drug to reduce the swelling, a muscle relaxant, or an analgesic for pain, depending on the injury.

Surgery. If the muscle is ruptured, operation may be the best option.

Prevention. The key to avoiding muscle pulls is appropriate conditioning and a routine of muscle stretching and loosening exercises before exercising (see page 959). In some cases, a program of muscle development for chronically weak muscles may help avoid recurrent muscle pulls.

SPRAINS

Signs and Symptoms
- Rapid swelling, sometimes accompanied by discoloration of the skin;
- Impaired joint function;
- Pain and tenderness in the affected area.

Emergency Symptoms
- If an audible popping sound and immediate difficulty in using the joint accompany the injury, apply ice and seek emergency medical care.

Although the term is often used loosely to identify a wide range of injuries, a true sprain involves damage to the ligaments that connect the bones. A sprain occurs when a traumatic event such as a violent twist or stretch causes the joint to move outside its normal range of movement and tissues of the ligaments are torn.

The most common sprains occur in the joints of the ankles, knees, and arches of the foot. In all three cases, a fall or stumble can cause the weight of the body to be placed on the joint in an unnatural position, resulting in a sprain.

The Diagnosis.   Any joint can be sprained. If the joint ceases to function, the injury is more likely to be a fracture (see page 955) or a dislocation (see page 957) than a sprain. If you suspect bone or serious ligament damage in the joint or if the pain and difficulty in moving the joint do not go away within 2 or 3 days, seek professional medical care. Your physician may order an x-ray to rule out a fracture.

How Serious Is a Sprain?   In general, the greater the pain, the more serious the injury, but sprains vary in severity from minor to those requiring operation. Repeated minor sprains can also lead to a weakening of the joint. In most cases, a sprained joint will be able to bear weight within 24 hours and be fully healed within 2 weeks.

Treatment.   For a simple sprain, apply ice to reduce swelling during the first 24 hours after injury. Support the joint with a supportive wrap such as an Ace bandage, and rest it in an elevated position. Resume normal activity slowly, testing the injured joint gradually after a day or more has passed.

Medication.   If you seek medical help, your physician may prescribe an anti-inflammatory drug. You may want to take aspirin or some other analgesic for pain.

Surgery.   If your sprain is serious enough that the joint is unstable, operation may be required to repair ligaments that have been torn or detached from the bone. Your physician also may elect to immobilize the area of the sprained joint in a cast or splint. If such measures are required, carefully follow your physician's advice on rehabilitation, which may involve a supervised physical therapy program and an exercise program to strengthen the muscle surrounding the sprained joint.

An ankle sprain involves damage to ligaments that connect muscles to bones.

Wearing a simple elastic ankle support may be of value when exercising if you often experience ankle sprains.

Prevention.   Taping, bracing, or wrapping knees, ankles, wrists, or elbows can be a convenient and efficient means of preventing recurrent sprains. The ankle devices that are laced and have supports on the inner and outer sides of the ankle seem to be as effective as taping of the chronically sprained ankle. Exercises can also be of value for strengthening the muscles of a joint weakened by recurrent injury.

SHIN SPLINTS

Signs and Symptoms
- Pain on the shin (the front part of the leg above the ankle and beneath the knee).

When pain occurs on the front, inside portion of the large bone of the lower leg, the tibia, it may be the result of shin splints. The fibers of the membrane that ties the muscles to the front and side of the tibia are irritated and inflamed, producing pain and occasional swelling.

Most often, shin splints are the result of the repeated pounding on hard surfaces that is characteristic of certain athletic activities, typically running or playing sports such as basketball or tennis or long marches (by army recruits, for example).

The Diagnosis. In addition to examining your leg, your physician may order an x-ray of the area to rule out a hairline crack or stress fracture of the tibia (see Fractures, page 955).

Treatment. As with other minor musculoskeletal injuries, rest, ice, and protection (wrapping with Ace bandages or tape) are effective treatments of shin splints. Sometimes heat is used in hot soaks or a whirlpool bath to reduce discomfort.

Medication. Your physician may prescribe aspirin or another over-the-counter anti-inflammatory medication.

Other Therapies. In some cases, a soft insert in the shoe also can reduce some of the shock sustained in vigorous physical activity. A similar but specially fabricated device (orthotic) may be prescribed if a structural abnormality of the foot is found.

Avoiding exercise such as running or basketball, which involves a persistent pounding of the legs, for 2 weeks to 2 months in favor of bicycling or swimming may eliminate the problem.

MUSCLE CRAMPS

Signs and Symptoms
- Sudden and sharp muscle pain, often in the legs;
- A distorted lump of muscle tissue visible beneath the skin.

A cramp, sometimes called a charley horse, is actually a muscle spasm in which the tissue contracts, producing sudden and intense pain. One especially common variety of muscle cramp occurs in the calf muscles of the leg during sleep. But overuse, injury, muscle strain, or simply remaining in the same position may result in muscle cramps. They commonly occur in an athlete who is overfatigued and dehydrated during sports that are played in warm weather.

Certain activities characteristically result in so-called professional cramps. Writer's cramp is the classic example—the thumb and first two fingers of the writing hand experience a cramping sensation as a result of long periods spent gripping a pen or pencil. In the past, watchmaker's and seamstress's cramps were common afflictions.

How Serious Are Muscle Cramps? Almost everyone experiences muscle cramps at some time, although for most people they are only an occasional inconvenience. For some, however, muscle cramps, especially at night, are a nagging problem. If you experience frequent and severe cramps that interfere with sleep, consult your physician.

Intermittent claudication, a distinct form of cramps in the legs that is associated with exercise, is caused by an inadequate blood supply to the calves (see Antherosclerosis of the Extremities, page 834). Another form of exercise-related cramps in the legs is caused by nerve compression in the spine (see Lumbar Stenosis, page 994). See your physician if you repeatedly have cramping in the legs with exercise. Potassium loss in the urine from the use of diuretics (medication used for hypertension to accelerate fluid loss) or from excessive sweating is often blamed for muscle cramps, but it is an uncommon cause.

Treatment. When a cramp occurs, try to extend the affected muscle. Gently straighten the limb because stretching the contracted muscle usually will provide immediate relief. Try compressing and massaging the affected muscle. Immersion in a hot bath or the use of a heating pad also may provide relief. Cold packs also may reduce muscle spasm or relax a tense muscle. At times, voluntarily contracting the muscles that are opposite to those that are cramped may reduce the intensity of pain. For example, if you are experiencing a leg cramp, force the front of your foot upward toward your knee and hold it there until the cramp lessens.

Prevention. Avoid dehydration, do stretching exercises before and after your workouts, and don't overfatigue your muscles.

Medication. If recurrent cramps disturb your sleep, your physician may prescribe diazepam or diphenhydramine.

THIGH BRUISE

Signs and Symptoms
• Pain and tenderness in the muscles at the front of the thigh that occur suddenly and are aggravated by movement.

The set of four muscles on the front of your thigh that allow you to extend your leg is called the quadriceps femoris. When these muscles are torn or strained, especially from physical contact, the resulting injury is termed a thigh bruise or contusion.

The Diagnosis. Pain and swelling of the front part of the thigh along with an inability to bend (flex) the knee as much as the opposite knee without pain usually indicate a thigh bruise or contusion. Often there is discoloration under the skin, beginning with a redness and progressing to the characteristic black-and-blue bruise. This injury can take anywhere from a week to months to heal. X-rays are often required to exclude a fracture.

Treatment. Relief from the discomfort of the injury may be obtained from some combination of rest and the use of ice immediately after the injury. A supportive wrap (Ace bandage) and leg elevation are useful for reducing swelling. Short-term use of crutches may be advisable to keep weight off the injured leg. Supportive wraps (or tape) will provide some protection when activity is resumed, as will properly fitted pads if contact sports are involved.

TENNIS ELBOW

Signs and Symptoms
• Recurrent pain on the outside of the upper forearm below the crease of the elbow;
• In some cases, pain extending down the forearm toward the wrist.

The name tennis elbow is a misnomer in that many persons who experience it have never played tennis. Both tennis elbow and a related ailment called Little League elbow are elbow pains that are thought to result from repeated, tiny tears in the tendons that attach the musculature of the lower arm at the elbow.

So-called tennis elbow produces pain on the outside of your forearm near your elbow when you exercise the joint. Tiny tears in tendon tissue cause the discomfort. In some cases, a forearm support band (see inset) worn just below the elbow can provide relief.

The tears can result from a wide variety of activities that involve a repeated, rotary motion of the forearm. Hitting a backhand in tennis, painting a house, or wielding a screwdriver all have been known to precipitate tennis elbow. Little League elbow usually occurs in a youngster, and often the cause is the strain of pitching a baseball.

The Diagnosis. A physical examination will probably be sufficient for your physician to reach a diagnosis, but to rule out other complications, an x-ray of the painful area may be taken. If you have tennis elbow, the x-ray will be normal.

How Serious Is Tennis Elbow? In most cases, the discomfort will fade over time, perhaps 6 to 12 months. In youngsters with Little League elbow, continued use of the arm despite the pain can lead to fracture.

Treatment. The application of ice to the elbow, massage, use of a splint at night, and rest are suitable treatment approaches.

Prevention. In order to avoid recurring episodes of tennis elbow, you may want to use a forearm support band. Worn just below the elbow, it can relieve stress placed on the inflamed tendons. Strengthening exercises can be done with a hand weight (with your elbow cocked and the palm down, repeatedly bend your wrist).

Medication. Aspirin or another over-the-counter anti-inflammatory medication is effective for reducing the pain of tennis elbow. In certain instances, a steroidal medication may be injected. However, because these are powerful drugs, their use is recommended only in extreme cases (see Corticosteroid Drugs, page 1005).

RUNNER'S KNEE

Signs and Symptoms
• Pain at the front of the knee, often accompanied by swelling.

With the continuing popularity of jogging, many people have experienced runner's knee. The pain in one or both knees is caused by small sprains of the ligaments of the knee. The sprains usually are the result of overuse or misuse rather than a single traumatic event (see also Knee Injuries, page 966). The pain usually isn't constant but is felt when you move your knee.

The Diagnosis. As a rule, the diagnosis is made on the basis of the degree of discomfort: if the knee is severely sprained, the cartilage may be damaged and movement is limited or impossible. However, no abnormality will be found on an x-ray, and a surgical procedure is rarely necessary.

How Serious Is Runner's Knee? Given proper rest and treatment, the pain of runner's knee will disappear over time, usually within a matter of weeks. However, if the cause of the problem is not addressed, the problem may recur.

Treatment. Apply ice to the sore knee and avoid the activity that caused the discomfort. Also avoid deep knee bends because they will strain the sore tissues.

Prevention. The most common reason for runner's knee is an improper training program. Proper review and instruction by a person knowledgeable in sports medicine may prevent recurrences. It may be necessary, however, to change your exercise program.

Some people switch from jogging to swimming or bicycling, activities that put much less stress on the knees. In some cases, orthotic devices may be used to correct flatfeet or other alignment problems in the legs. If these are the cause of the symptoms, you may be referred to a physiatrist or physical therapist.

Support for the kneecap in the form of a light brace can also help. Another important strategy is a stretching and exercise program to maintain the balance and flexibility of the muscles (see Exercise and Fitness, page 377).

Medication. Aspirin and other anti-inflammatory drugs can be effective for reducing the pain and discomfort associated with runner's knee. Injection of an anti-inflammatory steroidal medication also may be recommended. However, steroids are used only in extreme cases (see Corticosteroid Drugs, page 1005).

ACHILLES TENDINITIS

Signs and Symptoms
- A dull ache or pain in the Achilles tendon, especially when running or jumping;
- A mild swelling or tenderness may accompany the discomfort.

Emergency Symptoms
- Pain and inability to move the foot may require emergency treatment, usually a surgical procedure.

Achilles tendinitis is an inflammation of the tendon that links the leg muscles to the bone at the back of the heel, commonly called the heel cord. The pain is the result of tiny tears in the tissue. Most often, they occur during strenuous exercise.

The Diagnosis. An x-ray taken of the area will be normal if you have Achilles tendinitis.

How Serious Is Achilles Tendinitis? Unless the Achilles tendon has been severed, conservative treatments such as rest, ice, and perhaps a change in exercise program should be sufficient to allow the tendon to repair itself over a period of weeks.

Treatment. Resting the affected area is often the best treatment. It may be advisable to switch to another form of exercise, at least temporarily. Applying ice to the Achilles tendon can also provide relief. An orthotic device may be used to elevate the heel within the shoe, relieving the strain on the stretched tendon.

Operation usually is required only when the tendon has been torn completely (ruptured).

Medication. Aspirin and other anti-inflammatory drugs can help reduce the pain and discomfort associated with Achilles tendinitis.

BASEBALL FINGER

Signs and Symptoms
- Swelling and pain in the last joint of the finger;
- Inability to straighten the finger.

Also known as mallet finger or jammed finger, this injury occurs when the tendon that connects the muscles at the end of the finger is forcibly separated from the bone. It often results when the end of the finger is struck by a thrown or batted ball.

The Diagnosis. The injury is usually the result of a traumatic event, so an x-ray will be taken of the injured joint. If the finger appears normal on the x-ray, the possibility of fracture will be ruled out (see page 955).

How Serious Is Baseball Finger? Given proper treatment, the injured finger can be used normally within approximately 8 weeks, although a permanent deformity of the finger often persists.

Treatment. *Immobilization.* A baseball finger usually is treated by immobilizing the end of the affected finger with a splint. The last joint will be splinted in an extended position for approximately 6 weeks to allow the tendon to repair. After the splint has been removed, the finger should be returned to normal use gradually. Gentle, range-of-motion exercises will be recommended by your physician.

A surgical procedure is usually necessary only when a fracture accompanies the injury.

Medication. Aspirin or another anti-inflammatory drug may relieve the discomfort of the injury.

HEEL PAIN

Signs and Symptoms
- Pain in the heel of the foot when weight is placed on it;
- If the pain does not cease when the heel is relieved from weight-bearing, there is the risk of a stress fracture, and medical help should be sought.

The heel pad consists of fibrous tissue that cushions the underlying structure of your foot when you put weight on it. Pain in the heel is thought to result from tears or inflammation of the heel pad where it attaches to the heel bone. Also called painful heel syndrome, this common ailment may cause mild to intense pain.

The Diagnosis. Your physician will determine whether the pain is constant or whether it occurs only when you step down on your heel. An x-ray may be taken to rule out a stress fracture. However, stress fractures are often not apparent on an x-ray for up to 6 weeks after injury.

Sometimes the x-ray shows a spur of bone projecting forward from the heel bone (the calcaneus). Although in the past these bone spurs have been blamed for heel pain (and then surgically removed), they are not ordinarily a cause of pain. Therefore, surgery is rarely appropriate.

Another type of x-ray called a bone scan (see page 1287) may also be used to confirm the diagnosis.

How Serious Is Heel Pain? In most cases, the pain will fade or disappear in a matter of weeks. It can recur, however, especially if you wear improper footwear (poorly fitted athletic shoes or those that lack cushioning of the heel) when performing weight-bearing exercise. Wearing a different pair of well-fitted shoes each day may be helpful. Some people find that the only way to avoid a recurrence of the problem is to modify their activity, switching from jogging or tennis to swimming or bicycling. In most patients, however, the prognosis is complete recovery.

Treatment. Apply ice to your sore heel. Massage and gentle stretching also may provide some relief. Soft-soled running shoes may help, as can inserting a rubber sponge pad into the shoe with the portion of the pad under the painful area removed. If the heel pain proves especially persistent, your physician may prescribe an orthotic device—a heel cup that is custom-made of molded polyethylene foam.

Medication. Try aspirin and other over-the-counter anti-inflammatory drugs first. If they do not help, consult your physician. Your physician may inject your heel with an anti-inflammatory steroid drug such as cortisone, but the use of such drugs is recommended only when conservative measures are ineffective (see Corticosteroid Drugs, page 1005).

KNEE INJURIES

Signs and Symptoms
- Pain and swelling in the knee;
- Instability of the knee;
- A popping sound, a snapping sensation, or a physical locking of the joint.

Emergency Symptoms
- When the knee locks rigidly in one position or a traumatic event produces intense pain and the knee ceases to function properly, seek emergency medical help.

Knee injuries result from a wide variety of causes. Acute knee injuries can occur during contact sports such as football, and the wear and tear of time can result in chronic knee problems.

Two key factors make the knee joint susceptible to injury. First, its location leaves it exposed, both to unexpected trauma and to practically nonstop use. The second factor is the complexity of the knee. It is more than a hinge. Its range of motion is unique among

Heel pain may result from tears or inflammation of your heel pad where it attaches to your heel bone. This pain rarely results from bone spurs.

your body's joints: it must slide and glide and swivel as well as bend.

The Diagnosis.   If you sustain a knee injury, your physician may administer an anesthetic before the examination because the knee may be painful to touch and it will need to be examined in a variety of positions.

The external examination is often followed by one or more tests that provide a look at the joint's internal structure and the damage it has sustained. Traditional x-rays are one means of looking within the knee. Others include arthrography, in which the knee is x-rayed after a dye is injected into the joint space (see page 1291), and magnetic resonance imaging (MRI), in which a computerized image of the structure of the knee is assembled by a machine on the basis of the tissue's response to a magnetic field. Arthroscopy also may be done, in which the physician examines the interior of the knee by inserting a tube and fiberoptic equipment through a small incision (see Arthroscopy, page 968).

How Serious Is a Knee Injury?   The severity of a knee injury varies, depending on the type of damage the joint sustains. There are several major categories into which most knee injuries are classified. All can produce pain and instability of the joint.

Meniscal Tears.   The meniscus is the crescent-shaped cartilage in the knee between the ends of the bones of the thigh and lower leg. Certain impact and twisting injuries can produce tears in this meniscus, causing pain in the joint. A popping sound sometimes occurs at the moment of injury.

Often the injury will cause you to collapse. In some cases, you will be able to get up and even resume activity, but more likely a cartilage tear in the knee will produce immediate swelling and continuing pain. Even if it heals over a period of weeks, it may recur.

Loose Bodies.   Some knee injuries involve pieces shredded from the inner surface of the kneecap (the patella) or cartilage (meniscus) that are torn from their proper positions and float about in the joint cavity. The effect is similar to a pencil being caught in a door hinge. Even a small piece of loose cartilage

This torn ligament is a common form of knee injury. Swelling occurs and the joint becomes unstable.

can become pinched in the knee joint and "lock" the joint or cause pain.

Treatment.   The treatment required for a knee injury varies with each injury. For relatively minor knee injuries, the proper treatment approach is summarized by the acronym P.R.I.C.E.: protection, rest, ice, compression, and elevation (see page 969). Stop using the knee when you injure it. Use ice and compression to limit swelling. Keep your leg elevated to help reduce pain and swelling.

If your joint has sustained major damage, a reconstructive surgical procedure will be required, perhaps to reset the bones if they are dislocated or fractured or to reattach torn or ruptured ligaments. Often, minor damage can be repaired by arthroscopy, which involves a small incision rather than a large opening and much greater tissue repair (see Arthroscopy, page 968).

Rehabilitation.   After surgery, a splint, brace, or cast may be applied for the initial recuperation period. After you are allowed to move the knee, you will be given a program of exercises to follow to restore range of motion and strength to the joint. A physical therapist or rehabilitation specialist may oversee your recuperation.

ARTHROSCOPY

Until the development of a device called the arthroscope in 1972, injuries of the knee and other joints often required operation, an extended hospital stay, and a long and painful recuperation. Although some problems still require large incisions to open the knee or shoulder for reconstructive surgical procedures, many less serious injuries can now be corrected with the arthroscope.

The Instrument

The arthroscope (*arthro* for joint and *scope,* meaning to view) consists of a tube, an optical system of magnifying lenses, and a fiberoptic light source.

The Procedure

After an anesthetic is administered (either local or general), a small incision is made on one side of the kneecap (or shoulder or other joint to be examined). The incision is often so small that stitches are not required to close it after completion of the procedure.

The tube of the arthroscope is then inserted. Through the eyepiece or on a screen, the physician is provided a look at the inside of the joint. A sterile fluid may be injected into the joint space to enlarge it and enhance visibility.

The Options

Once inside the joint, the arthroscope offers an opportunity not only to examine the tissues but also, through the use of attach-

ments, to take a biopsy specimen or even to perform minor surgery. Floating bits of cartilage can be removed, and minor tears and other knee disorders can be treated in this way. The arthroscope is also of value in diagnosing various joint diseases.

The Recuperation

Unlike traditional procedures in which the joint itself is opened, little time is needed for the joint to heal after arthroscopy. The procedure rarely takes more than an hour, and the individual usually can return home shortly thereafter. Although the joint should not be subjected to vigorous physical activity for several days, most normal activities can be resumed immediately.

The arthroscope allows your physician to visualize the interior of your knee or other joints, as well as to perform various tests and repairs without resorting to major surgery. Right: arthroscopic views of normal meniscus (top), torn meniscus (middle, see arrow), and normal anterior cruciate ligament.

P.R.I.C.E.

If you sustain a minor injury, protection, rest, ice, compression, and elevation are the words to remember—P.R.I.C.E. This self-help treatment can help speed your recovery.

Protection

Immobilize the affected area to encourage healing and to protect it from further injury. The use of elastic wraps, slings, splints, crutches, or canes may be necessary.

Rest

Avoid activities that cause pain or swelling; rest is essential to tissue healing.

Ice

To decrease pain, muscle spasm, and swelling, apply ice to the injured area. Ice packs, ice massage, or slush baths all can help.

Compression

Swelling can result in loss of motion in an injured joint, so compress the joint until the swelling has ceased. Wraps or compressive (Ace) bandages are best.

Elevation

To reduce swelling, raise the swollen arm or leg above the level of your heart. This is especially important at night.

PRINCIPLES OF SPORTS REHABILITATION

At its simplest, the task of sports rehabilitation is to enable the injured athlete to return to normal physical activity, good health, and full function. The approach to, speed of, and eventual result after any rehabilitation are influenced by various factors, including your age, level of normal physical activity, body structure, and conditioning at the time of injury.

The rehabilitation process consists of four principal stages.

Stage 1

Stage 1 is concerned with controlling the inflammation and pain of the injury. A P.R.I.C.E. treatment approach is usual (protection, rest, ice, compression, and elevation; see above).

Stage 2

The second step endeavors to restore the full range of motion in the injured joint. Exercises, done by yourself and, at times, an assistant moving the muscles surrounding a joint, may be advised by a physical therapist. Muscle strengthening exercises will follow, usually with isometrics (in which the extremity is not moved but the muscles are flexed). Light weight training, perhaps with a rubber or elastic tube, may follow. When substantial strength and normal range of motion have been restored, additional exercises, perhaps using a stationary bicycle (for lower extremity injuries) or swimming (for upper body injuries), can be very helpful.

Stage 3

Only in stage 3 of rehabilitation do you return to biomechanical skill patterns related to specific sports. For example, a baseball pitcher recovering from an operation on the arm would resume throwing a baseball at this stage. Accompanying the gradual resumption of specific skill activities is a general cardiovascular endurance program, perhaps involving long-distance biking, swimming, or running.

Stage 4

Upon your return to normal activity and condition, your physician may prescribe a maintenance program, stage 4 of rehabilitation, to enable you to maintain flexibility, strength, and endurance. Skipping any of the steps in this process may put you at risk of reinjury or a prolonged recovery.

ABSENCE OR LOSS OF A LIMB

Some people are born without one of their limbs. Such congenital absences occur as the result of a developmental defect. The cause also may be a drug or other substance, but more often the cause is unknown.

The loss of a limb after birth is a significant medical event. A major operation usually is involved in such an amputation, whether it is precipitated by a traumatic event such as an automobile accident or by a considered medical decision to remove the limb because of complications of a disease.

In addition to drawing upon the body's healing capacity, an amputation also makes psychological demands on the patient to adjust to the change. The adjustment involves not only learning to live with altered physical capacities but also accepting the change in body image.

Your doctor and other health-care professionals can help you make the necessary adjustments. An artificial limb may be fitted to help you live as normally as possible (see below); if you become depressed or have difficulty adjusting to an amputation, seek psychiatric help also.

Surgical amputations that are performed after birth are done for a wide variety of reasons. Some people with advanced diabetes (see page 707) develop poor circulation in the extremities (because of narrowing of the channels in the arteries), and the ulcers and gangrene that can result lead to the need to amputate a foot or leg. Circulatory problems due to other causes also can produce gangrene (see page 835). Certain bone cancers (see page 988) are best treated by removing the tumor, which may require amputation of an arm or leg.

Sometimes an amputation is the result of an accident. When a finger or toe or larger body part is severed, it is an emergency requiring immediate medical attention.

How Serious Is an Amputation?   Amputation that results from an accident has various attendant risks, including blood loss and shock. As with any invasive procedure, there is also the risk of infection. The risk is greater if the amputation is accidental as opposed to surgical. In either case, your physician or surgeon will take all possible precautions to avoid infection.

In most cases, the amputation procedure itself isn't life-threatening. The problem, therefore, is dealing with the consequences of the amputation. These range from living with the immediate pain of the amputation to adjusting your lifestyle. The loss of a leg, for example, will have a significant impact on your mobility and balance, changes to which you must adjust.

The surgical removal of a body part also can be an emotionally demanding event. There may be pain in the stump or the sensation, sometimes painful, that the limb or part of the limb is still present (so-called phantom limb sensations). Your self-image, self-confidence, and self-worth also may be affected. If an artificial limb is required, it will be tailored to your needs in regard to both its function and its appearance.

When a severed body part is reattached surgically, the usefulness of the part varies from case to case. In some instances, the reattached part regains most or all of its usefulness, whereas in others sensitivity, flexibility, and strength are impaired.

ARTIFICIAL LIMBS

When cancer surgery, gangrene, an accident, or another illness or event results in the loss of a limb, a replacement part (prosthesis) may be substituted.

An artificial limb can never replicate the movement, flexibility, strength, and sensitivity of your original arm or leg. Yet, once you adjust to it, the prosthesis allows you to live a nearly normal life.

A physiatrist or physical therapist can help you recover. Exercises are prescribed to keep your remaining muscles in condition, and a temporary prosthesis is provided. At first, it is worn for short periods. Gradually, day-long use is achieved. After the tissues have healed fully and you have adjusted to the temporary prosthesis, a specially designed artificial arm or leg can be fabricated.

The permanent limb must be tailored to meet your specific needs. A balance must be struck between the physical demands for mobility and strength and concern with appearance of the limb.

Treatment.   In the event of a medical emergency involving a severed body part, proper precautions must be taken to ensure that both the patient and the part be properly cared for in advance of reattachment (see page 312).

Surgery.   Remarkable advances have been made in recent years in reattaching severed fingers, hands, and even limbs. Through the help of a microscope, fine surgical repairs and reattachments of tiny tissues are possible. The results depend on many factors, but if the severed body part has had proper care and a trained surgeon is available, the chances for a successful reattachment are good.

Rehabilitation.   A physician or a physical therapist will propose a program of rehabilitation; in some cases, a team approach is used, involving physical and occupational therapists under the guidance of a physiatrist (a physician who specializes in physical medicine).

At its simplest, the program will consist of a plan for achieving as normal a life as possible, and it will include exercises to help maintain the strength of the muscles that remain. When an artificial limb or other equipment is required, the program may involve other exercises, instruction on the use of crutches, counseling, and other aspects to allow a return to normal activity. The artificial limb usually is fitted after the pain and swelling that follow the operation have abated, and then a training process will help in mastering the different movements involved in using the prosthesis or artificial limb (see Artificial Limbs, page 970).

Medication. Treatment may involve analgesics to reduce pain and antibiotics to fight infection.

MUSCLE, TENDON, AND SOFT TISSUE DISORDERS

The tissues of your muscles are elongated and elastic, a function that allows muscles to extend and contract. When you move a limb, one muscle contracts to produce the movement; when you return the limb to its original position, contraction of the opposite muscle is required.

Equally important to movement are the tendons, the tissues that connect the muscles to the bones. In most parts of the body, the tendons are interwoven with the muscles or are simply short connectors between the ends of the muscles and the bones. In the hands and feet the tendons are long and cord-like, but throughout your body the fibrous tendons convey the movement of the muscles to the bones. Thus, a muscular contraction causes the attached bones and tendons to move.

As with the rest of the musculoskeletal system, we tend to take our muscles and tendons for granted—until pain or stiffness or immobility alerts us to their malfunctions. In the following pages, a number of common muscle, tendon, and soft tissue disorders are considered, from the transient discomforts of the muscle cramp to the paralyzing disorder muscular dystrophy.

TENOSYNOVITIS

Signs and Symptoms
* Difficulty in straightening a finger or thumb: the finger seems to hesitate when you try to point it and straightens in a sudden, jerking motion;

* Tenderness and pain in the finger;
* Movements are accompanied by a crackling sound;
* Pain on movement of the wrist or shoulder.

Emergency Symptoms
* A joint that becomes heated and inflamed may be infected, and you should seek immediate medical help (see also Infectious Arthritis, page 1002).

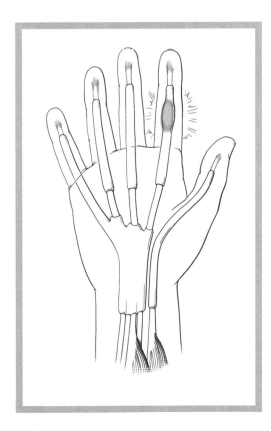

Each of the cable-like tendons in your hand is sheathed in a protective membrane called a synovium. When inflamed or infected, tenosynovitis can result. Treatment varies from rest to medication to surgery.

One form of tenosynovitis is called trigger finger. The sheath that protects the tendon of a finger becomes inflamed, making it difficult to straighten the finger.

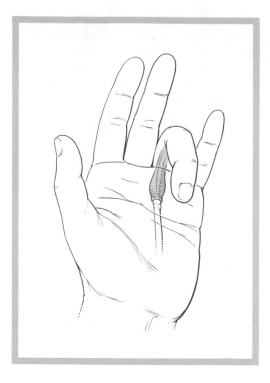

Long, cable-like tendons run through your hand and into each finger. Each is protected by an individual membrane called synovium, the same tissue that shields the joint cavity in your knee or other large joints (see page 953). In tenosynovitis, the membranous sheath becomes inflamed or infected.

The cause can be overuse, as may occur in factory workers or typists whose work involves countless repetitions of the same hand movements (see Carpal Tunnel Syndrome, page 974).

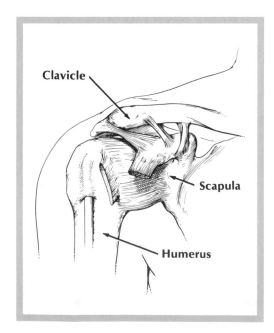

The shoulder joint is a complex structure. Tough tendons attach muscle to bone. Ligaments help hold the joint together.

Tenosynovitis also can be caused by an infection, often one resulting from a puncture wound. It also can occur in the wrist or, even more commonly, in the bicipital tendon in the shoulder.

One type of tenosynovitis is called trigger finger. The characteristic symptom of trigger finger is an inability to straighten a finger. In a typical case, you decide to straighten your finger but it doesn't respond; then you glance down and suddenly it jerks into position.

This problem is most common in women at or beyond middle age. An x-ray may be needed to rule out any bone involvement.

How Serious Is Tenosynovitis?   If the cause is a bacterial infection, tenosynovitis must be treated immediately because the infection may cause permanent functional damage to the affected tissues.

When the tenosynovitis is the result of overuse, time and rest may produce a full recovery. If the activity that led to the tenosynovitis is resumed, symptoms will likely recur; thus, a change in habits may be required.

Treatment.   *Medication.*   If the cause of the discomfort is an infection, an antibiotic will be prescribed.

An analgesic or anti-inflammatory drug such as aspirin may reduce the pain of non-infectious tenosynovitis. In some cases, injection of a steroid drug such as cortisone may relieve the symptoms. However, steroid drugs are recommended only when more conservative measures fail (see Corticosteroid Drugs, page 1005).

Surgery.   If the diagnosis is infectious tenosynovitis, an immediate operation may be required. The operation will release the buildup of pus and limit spread of the infection. When the cause is mechanical rather than an infection, persistent tenosynovitis may be relieved by a surgical incision in the membrane; this procedure may restore full movement.

TENDINITIS

Signs and Symptoms
- Pain and tenderness just outside a joint, especially your elbow or shoulder.

A minor injury or excessive use can produce soreness in the shoulder or elbow. The cause is usually a small tear or inflammation of the tendon that links the muscles to the bone.

Tendinitis is most common in the elbow (see Tennis Elbow, page 963) and the shoulder. An x-ray may be taken of the area of soreness to rule out any bone involvement.

How Serious Is Tendinitis?   Tendinitis can cause permanent damage to the tendons. The natural tendency to favor the painful area also can lead to stiffness. A vague discomfort at age 30 can, if the overuse is continued for years, lead to a loss of flexibility due to scarring of the tissues.

Sometimes the discomfort of tendinitis disappears within a matter of weeks, especially if you rest your elbow or shoulder. In elderly people and those who continue to use the affected area, tendinitis often heals more slowly and usually progresses to a chronic condition. The ligaments and tendons about the shoulder may gradually stiffen, a condition leading to a loss of movement; this is termed frozen shoulder (see Acute Painful Shoulder, page 1004).

Treatment.   Rest is essential. Do not use the affected area for several days. A sling is sometimes helpful, as is an Ace or other bandage that compresses the affected area. Also, elevate and apply ice to the area. This may help reduce discomfort and swelling.

Medication.   An analgesic such as aspirin will help reduce the discomfort.

If tendinitis persists, your physician may inject the area with a steroid drug such as cortisone (see Corticosteroid Drugs, page 1005).

Surgery.   When a tendon is torn, a reconstructive operation may be necessary.

Exercise.   Although rest is a key part of treating tendinitis, prolonged inactivity can cause stiffness in the joints. Flexibility of the joint should be maintained by doing gentle, range-of-motion exercises after a few days of resting the area. This can help prevent frozen shoulder.

Prevention.   A recurrence of tendinitis can be avoided by warming up before exercising and cooling down after exercise (see page 959). Strengthening exercises also may help avoid further episodes of tendinitis.

FIBROSITIS

Signs and Symptoms
* Generalized aches and pains accompanied by stiffness;
* Overall fatigue, often exaggerated by an inability to sleep;
* Headaches and a vague tingling sensation in the muscles may accompany the other symptoms.

Fibrositis is an ailment characterized by aches, pain, and stiffness in the joints and muscles. Its name literally identifies the key symptom—inflammation *(itis)* of the body's fibrous connective tissues.

The discomfort resembles the muscular aches of a persistent flu, but without attendant fever. The discomfort of fibrositis tends to be present most of the time, although to varying degrees. The stiffness generally worsens with inactivity and may be relieved with activity.

Fibrositis is not the result of infection, but it may be the result of a specific injury or emotional tension. The symptoms—vague and nagging irritations that interfere but little in most activities—are likely to persist for years.

The pain is felt in the muscles and at the points where the muscles are attached to the bones by the ligaments. Common tender points are the front of the elbow and hip joint, the rear of the knee or shoulder, the base of the neck, and along the vertebrae. The pain and soreness may result from muscle fatigue or prolonged tension, and it may be aggravated by motion.

Fibromyalgia and fibromyositis are other terms that are used interchangeably with fibrositis. Although anyone can have fibrositis, more women than men have it, usually in middle age.

The Diagnosis.   Diagnosing fibrositis is largely a matter of excluding other ailments with similar symptoms, because no one test confirms or excludes the presence of fibrositis. Your physician may order laboratory tests to rule out other ailments such as rheumatoid arthritis, but the test results all will be normal if fibrositis is present. Such results may make you even more anxious: the pain of fibrositis is so generalized and its diagnosis is so generalized that many people begin to believe that their problem is largely psychological. Yet the pain of fibrositis is very real indeed. That isn't to say, however, that psychological factors such as stress don't contribute to the discomfort. Strategies to reduce stress may help reduce the aches and pains of fibrositis (see page 399).

How Serious Is Fibrositis?   Although chronic, this disorder is not crippling and will not lead to disability. It will not require operation, and long-term treatment is likely to consist of physical conditioning and strategies to improve sleeping habits. The minor discomfort may not go away; however, it also won't get progressively worse.

Treatment.   Your physician will offer reassurance that rheumatoid arthritis or other serious underlying disease is not present. Sometimes, small changes in life-style can reduce the discomfort. Try a firmer mattress. Take more care to maintain proper posture (see The Importance of Posture, page 989). A ritual of daily relaxation exercises or a change in daily routine to avoid certain known physical and emotional stresses also may help.

Other Therapies.   Hot baths and massages have some value for short-term relief. Aerobic training (see page 378) has proved to be of value in some cases. Although claims have been made that food allergies can cause this disorder, there is no evidence to support them.

Medication.   Fibrositis in most cases is relieved by aspirin or other anti-inflammatory drugs, although physicians occasionally prescribe other medications.

COSTOCHONDRITIS

Signs and Symptoms
* Pain in the chest, usually at the front of the rib cage;
* Swelling of the tissues around the sternum may also occur.

The name comes from the Latin word *costa* for rib and the Greek word *chondros* for cartilage. Logically, then, this disorder is of the cartilage of the rib cage.

The pain and soreness are the result of an inflammation of the cartilage. The inflammation may be caused by a blow or trauma sustained by the rib cage, but often the cause is unknown. The pain is exaggerated by movement of the ribs and by pressure exerted directly on the affected area (see Chest Wall Pain, page 296).

When it first strikes, the pain of costochondritis can be a source of anxiety because it is often confused with that of a heart attack. Costochondritis itself is not a medical emergency, but the sudden onset of especially severe and intense chest pains should prompt you to seek immediate medical help because of the dangers of a heart attack.

Costochondritis is also known as Tietze's syndrome, after the German surgeon who identified it.

The Diagnosis.   Tenderness, with or without swelling, at the junction of the ribs is the key symptom, but a chest x-ray, electrocardiogram (see page 802), and blood tests may be needed to exclude heart disease or underlying lung ailments.

Treatment.   Given time and proper rest, the symptoms may disappear. Exercise may aggravate the symptoms, so avoid activities that worsen the discomfort.

Medication.   Aspirin and other anti-inflammatory drugs may reduce the discomfort. A steroid drug such as cortisone also may be injected into the affected area (see Corticosteroid Drugs, page 1005).

CARPAL TUNNEL SYNDROME

Signs and Symptoms
* A numbness or tingling sensation in your fingers and hand;
* Pain from your wrist, which may seem to shoot up into the forearm or down into the palm of the hand or surface of the fingers;
* The numbness or pain may be worse at night, and it may awaken you. Often the discomfort will occur after a day in which you have used your hand or wrist forcefully, and it may be relieved by shaking the hand or getting up and walking about.

The carpal tunnel is a passageway through the wrist (carpal is from the Greek word *kar-*

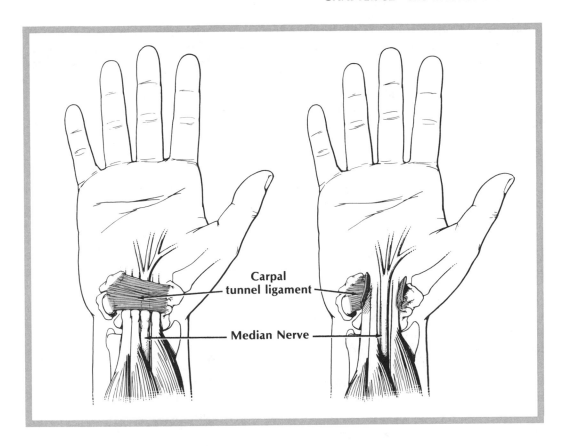

Carpal
tunnel ligament

Median Nerve

A narrow tunnel through your wrist—the carpal tunnel—protects your median nerve, which provides sensation to your thumb, index and middle fingers, and the thumb side of your ring finger. When swelling or inflammation occurs at the tunnel, the median nerve can be compressed, producing pain and numbness. If conservative treatment is not effective, the carpal tunnel ligament may be severed (right) to relieve the compression.

palis, which means wrist). Bounded by bones and ligaments, the carpal tunnel protects the nerves and tendons that extend into the hand.

When the tissues that constitute the tunnel become swollen or inflamed, the median nerve is compressed. Because this key nerve provides sensation to your thumb, index, middle, and ring fingers, pressure on it produces the numbness and pain that characterize carpal tunnel syndrome. Often both wrists are affected in this ailment.

This syndrome is common to certain professions in which the wrist is subject to repetitive stresses and strains, especially those involving pinching or gripping with the wrist held flexed. Thus, blacksmiths have traditionally had a high incidence of carpal tunnel syndrome. Typists, carpenters, grocery clerks, factory workers, meat cutters, violinists, mechanics, and, uncommonly, hobbyists such as golfers or canoers also may be subject to the discomfort of carpal tunnel syndrome.

The problem isn't always an independent medical problem, however; it often accompanies other diseases or events. Some pregnant women find that their tendency to retain water and gain weight leads to carpal tunnel syndrome, but the symptoms disap-

pear after childbirth. Some endocrine disorders such as diabetes and, rarely, hypothyroidism (see page 730) and acromegaly (see page 723) also are accompanied by the syndrome, as is rheumatoid arthritis (see page 997). In general, women approaching middle age are most likely to suffer from carpal tunnel syndrome.

The Diagnosis. A diagnostic key is that the numbness in the fingers does not include the little finger. An electromyogram may be needed (see page 1294), which will indicate whether the electrical impulses traveling along the median nerve are slowed in the carpal tunnel; slowed impulses indicate that the nerve is being compressed. A Tinel sign test also may be done: after the physician taps on the front of your wrist, a shooting pain into your hand or forearm is a positive sign, which usually is a reliable indication that the syndrome is present. Atrophy or loss of bulk in the muscles of your thumb may be present.

How Serious Is Carpal Tunnel Syndrome?
With proper treatment, the pain can be relieved and no permanent damage is sustained by the hand or wrist.

Treatment. Conservative treatments include simply resting the joint and wearing a splint, which immobilizes the wrist but allows the hand to function almost normally so usual activity can be conducted. A splint often helps, especially in relieving the nighttime symptoms.

Medication. The affected area may be injected with a steroid drug such as cortisone. But this treatment usually is used only when more conservative strategies have failed (see Corticosteroid Drugs, page 1005). If the problem recurs after two injections of cortisone, your physician may recommend an operation.

Surgery. When the pain of carpal tunnel syndrome is persistent, an operation may be the best option. This involves division of the ligament that is pressing on the nerve. After recuperation, normal use of the wrist and hand usually returns within a few weeks to months.

ARTHRITIS AT THE BASE OF THE THUMB

Signs and Symptoms
- Pain at the base of your thumb, especially when performing simple activities such as opening a jar or turning a key in a door;
- Clumsiness or pain in the area when holding a small object.

This common problem may affect anyone, but it most frequently occurs in middle-aged women. Often the cause is unknown, but previous thumb fractures and certain varieties of arthritis, including rheumatoid arthritis (see page 997) and gout (see page 1003), are thought to be the cause in some cases. A physical examination and x-rays will reveal the extent of the problem.

Treatment. Initial treatment generally is limited to resting your thumb and taking aspirin or other over-the-counter analgesics for the discomfort. A brace also may be used to limit the movement of the sore area.

Surgery may be necessary if more conservative means do not relieve the discomfort. Ligament or bone positions may be changed, and a cast and physical therapy of several months' duration may be required.

GANGLION

Signs and Symptoms
- A lump on your wrist;
- Accompanying pain, especially when your wrist is extended or flexed, may be present, but usually the lump is painless.

A ganglion is a swelling that appears beneath the skin, usually on the back of the wrist but in some instances on the top of the foot, on the front of the wrist, or in the fingers. It results from an accumulation of a jelly-like substance that has leaked from a joint or tendon sheath. Usually rubbery to the touch, a ganglion may vary in size.

The Diagnosis. A physical examination will be done and, in some cases, other tests or an x-ray will be needed to exclude other problems. An ultrasound examination (see page 1287) is sometimes useful to confirm the diagnosis.

How Serious Is a Ganglion? A ganglion is essentially harmless. However, if you observe a bump on your wrist or foot, seek your physician's counsel in order to rule out other causes such as a malignancy. If the ganglion is painful, your physician may be able to relieve the discomfort through surgical or other means, but in most cases the harmless, small lump requires no treatment and has no effect on your activities.

Treatment. *Surgery.* Your physician may burst the ganglion simply by putting

A swelling that appears beneath the skin, usually on the back of the wrist, is called a ganglion. This is a harmless condition, but consult your physician to rule out a malignancy.

pressure on it after puncturing it in several places with a needle or may drain the jelly-like contents with a needle. A surgical procedure is regarded as unnecessary in most cases, but if the ganglion is painful and does not respond to drainage, it can be removed surgically.

DUPUYTREN'S CONTRACTURE

Signs and Symptoms
- An inability to straighten one or several fingers;
- A small lump or area of tightness in the palm of your hand.

This disorder is named after the early 19th-century French surgeon, Baron Dupuytren, who described it. It is characterized by a hardening of the lining of tissue beneath the skin (the palmar fascia).

Dupuytren's contracture usually isn't painful, but a progressive deformity of the hand may result. A similar hardening and shrinkage of tissue also may occur on the soles of the feet. Dupuytren's contracture is most common in the ring and little fingers, but it can affect any finger, the thumb, the soles of the feet, and even the penis (see Peyronie's disease, page 1143).

The cause of Dupuytren's contracture is unknown, but there appears to be a strong genetic component because the ailment tends to run in families. Another common trait is that many persons with Dupuytren's contracture are middle-aged men, and some are alcoholic or have epilepsy. The reason for such linkage is unknown. The condition probably is not related to a single traumatic event.

The Diagnosis. A physical examination is usually reliable for diagnosing Dupuytren's contracture. Dimpling of the skin over the affected area is fairly characteristic. A cord of immobile tissue may also be beneath the skin. A change in the position of the wrist does not affect a contracture.

After the condition has been diagnosed, it is important to monitor its progression. To do so, your physician may ask you to place your hand palm down on a tabletop or other flat surface. If you are unable to hold your fingers and hand flat, treatment may be necessary. Even if the test is negative, you should repeat it periodically. If the result in-

dicates that the condition has worsened, surgical treatment may be in order.

How Serious Is Dupuytren's Contracture? Although this common disorder is rarely painful, the decreasing flexibility of the fingers can be debilitating over time. In many cases, however, treatment is not required.

When an operation is necessary, most or all normal movement often can be restored, although in some people the problem may recur.

Treatment. *Surgery.* Surgical treatment will involve removing the shrunken tissue and, in extreme cases, skin grafting or other surgical intervention. The hand will be bandaged with the fingers in a straightened position for a few days or weeks, after which a course of physical therapy involving finger and hand exercises will be begun.

REFLEX SYMPATHETIC DYSTROPHY SYNDROME

Signs and Symptoms
- Pain and tenderness in a hand or foot that develop in the weeks or months after an injury, heart attack, or stroke;
- Thin or shiny skin in the affected area, accompanied by increased sweating and hair growth.

Reflex sympathetic dystrophy syndrome usually affects a hand or foot, but it also may strike the kneecap or hip. The pain is usually a burning sensation, and accompanying

A thickening and hardening of tissue beneath the skin on the palm of your hand can lead to an involuntary contraction of one or more fingers. Called Dupuytren's contracture, this progressive deformity can be corrected surgically.

symptoms will likely include a swelling due to water retention and a tenderness in the joints. The syndrome usually advances over a period of months to a second phase in which the skin becomes cool and shiny. In some cases, contracture may follow (see Dupuytren's Contracture, page 977).

In two-thirds of the cases, an accident, heart attack, stroke, or injury precipitates reflex sympathetic dystrophy syndrome. Most often, it occurs in people older than 50 years, and men and women are equally likely to be affected.

The Diagnosis.   X-rays may be needed if your physician suspects reflex sympathetic dystrophy syndrome. Typically, they will reveal that the bones have been weakened by a loss of minerals. The syndrome can lead to irreversible damage to the affected area if it is not treated promptly.

Treatment. *Medication.* An analgesic may be used to reduce the pain. A program of heat and cold and exercise also may be added to the treatment to relieve the pain and tenderness. In some cases, corticosteroid drugs may be prescribed (see page 1005).

MUSCLE TUMORS

Signs and Symptoms
* A lump in muscle tissue perceptible on the surface of the skin;
* Pain in the affected area;
* A rapid increase in the size of the lump.

Muscle tumors are rare, and when they do occur they are usually benign. However, a malignant muscle tumor (rhabdomyosarcoma) can be life-threatening and requires immediate treatment.

The Diagnosis.   If you observe any sort of lump under your skin, see your physician. Most lumps under the skin are lipomas. They consist of fat and are located between the skin and the muscle layer. Often they are identified easily with slight finger pressure and move readily. It is not unusual to have several such collections. These lumps are rarely a cause for worry.

Your physician will examine the lump and, if concerned, may order a traditional x-ray, a magnetic resonance imaging scan, or a computed tomography scan of the area (see pages 1286 and 1287). A biopsy of the tissue also may be required, in which a sample of tissue is removed for laboratory analysis.

Treatment.   If the tumor is benign, it may require no treatment or will simply be excised. If it is malignant, however, surgical removal, radiation treatments, or chemotherapy may be necessary.

MUSCULAR DYSTROPHY

Signs and Symptoms
* Muscle weakness, characterized by an apparent lack of coordination, clumsy gait, and an inability to elevate your arms over your head;
* Progressive crippling, resulting in loss of mobility.

Muscular dystrophy is a progressive disease in which the muscle tissues decrease in size and grow weaker (the word dystrophy comes from the Greek prefix *dys,* which means bad or painful, and the word *trephein,* which means nourishment; literally, dystrophy means insufficient nourishment). The most common variety of this rare ailment is called Duchenne's muscular dystrophy. Pseudohypertrophic muscular dystrophy is a common synonym for it.

For reasons not yet understood, the muscles in persons with Duchenne's muscular dystrophy lack a key protein essential to muscle function. In the absence of this protein, the muscles grow progressively weaker, yet they may appear larger than normal because fat tissue replaces the lost muscle.

The tendency to have this rare disease is inherited. Duchenne's muscular dystrophy usually strikes at an early age (often before the age of 5 years), and it affects only males.

The Diagnosis.   In the toddler, a decrease in mobility skills—walking, climbing stairs, and difficulty in lifting the arms over the head—may indicate Duchenne's muscular dystrophy. The physician is likely to order a biopsy of the muscle tissue (a small sample of tissue is removed for laboratory examination).

How Serious Is Muscular Dystrophy?

Muscular dystrophy is a crippling disease. In most cases the arms, legs, and spine become progressively deformed; by the teenage years, most patients need a wheelchair. Because of their susceptibility to chest infection, most patients with muscular dystrophy die before adulthood, usually of pneumonia or other chest infection.

Treatment. There is no cure for muscular dystrophy. The best treatment regimen involves trying to minimize the deformities through physical therapies.

Prevention. Although little is known about treating Duchenne's muscular dystrophy, it is clear that the disorder is inherited in more than half the cases. Because the affected genes are carried by females, any woman with a family history of muscular dystrophy should seek counseling before pregnancy. The odds are 1 in 2 that a male child of a carrier will have the disorder.

PROBLEMS OF THE FEET

Our feet carry us where we want to go. They also complain about excesses of heat or cold, and they alert us when they are injured or mistreated. But, if we are lucky—and sensible enough to wear properly fitted footwear—most of us spend almost no time worrying about them.

When the feet are sore, mobility is painful. If foot problems occur, you may want to seek the guidance of your physician or a podiatrist. The latter, although not a medical doctor, is a licensed professional whose area of expertise is the examination of the human foot and the diagnosis, prevention, and treatment of foot disorders.

In the following pages, we discuss some of the most common foot problems.

CORNS AND CALLUSES

Signs and Symptoms

- A thickened layer of skin, often between the toes.

Corns and calluses are the result of constant pressure or repeated friction on the skin, producing a thickening and hardening of the skin. Corns are smaller (less than a quarter-inch long) than calluses.

Shoes that fit poorly are often the cause of corns or calluses on the feet (see also Bunions, below). Calluses on the hands usually result from the pressure or friction of repetitive labor: if you wield a shovel or other hand tool daily you will find your hand lined with calluses over time.

How Serious Are Corns and Calluses?

Corns and calluses are common and are rarely more than minor discomforts. However, in the diabetic, infection and other complications can occur, so special care should be taken (see Foot Problems and Diabetes, page 981). If a corn or callus becomes painful or ulcerated, consult your physician.

Treatment. In most people, curing a corn or callus is a matter of eliminating the cause. If improperly fitted footwear is the cause, wear shoes of soft leather and the proper shape. In a few weeks, the corn or callus should disappear. If the problem persists, your physician may refer you to a foot specialist (a podiatrist) who may remove the tissue surgically.

BUNIONS

Signs and Symptoms

- A bony protrusion at the base of your big toe;
- Accompanying pain and limitation of motion.

TREATING YOUR CALLUSES

You can gradually thin some of the thickened skin of corns and calluses by rubbing the skin with a towel whenever it has been softened by a shower or bath. The alkalinity of the soap along with the soaking in water soften your skin so you can rub off the upper layers.

Use a pumice stone as a mild abrasive during or after bathing to reduce the thickness of callus tissue. This is not recommended, however, if you have diabetes or poor circulation.

When the base of your big toe extends beyond the normal profile of your foot, the bump that results is called a bunion. To prevent a bunion, avoid shoes with narrow toes or high heels.

Bunion

To avoid an ingrown toenail (A), don't clip your toenails too short. Clip them straight across.

When a toe takes on a claw-like, clenched appearance, it is termed hammer toe (B). Most often, the second toe is affected. An orthotic appliance inserted into the shoe may be sufficient to relieve discomfort. To help avoid hammer toe, wear shoes that fit properly.

A bunion occurs when the big toe overlaps another toe. The condition is the result of an inherited trait called hallux valgus (from the Latin *valgus* which means bowlegged and *hallux* which means big toe) and results in a minor deformity of the foot.

The base of the big toe is thrust out beyond the normal profile of the foot, producing the bump known as the bunion. The bunion often is subjected to constant rubbing that, in turn, results in a thickening of the skin (see Corns and Calluses, page 979).

This common but minor problem is several times as likely to occur in women as

men. Although some people are genetically predisposed to develop the condition, more often the ailment results from forcing the foot into a tight shoe with a pointed toe and a high heel.

The Diagnosis.   Your physician may request x-rays from several angles to confirm the visual diagnosis.

How Serious Is a Bunion?   A bunion usually causes minor discomfort. However, accompanying bursitis or osteoarthritis can develop, causing pain and stiffness (see pages 1006 and 995, respectively). A bunion can make finding suitable shoes difficult, and often the shoes are unsatisfactory in appearance. If your bunion becomes very painful and annoying, consult your physician.

Treatment.   Shoes that fit properly are often the best remedy and preventive for the discomfort of a bunion. The shoes should provide ample room for your toes. If bursitis develops, you may find that a hole cut in the upper surface of an old shoe in the area of the bunion will provide relief. Commercially available felt pads may be helpful. In rare and extreme cases, an operation may be performed to realign the bones and remove excess bone tissue.

HAMMER TOE AND MALLET TOE

Signs and Symptoms
- A claw-like or mallet-like clenched appearance to a toe;
- Accompanying pain and difficulty in movement.

Unlike a bunion, which affects the big toe (see page 979), hammer toe may affect any toe (although most commonly the second toe is affected). The toe becomes bent and painful. Generally, both joints in a toe are affected, giving it a claw-like appearance. Hammer toe can result from wearing shoes that are too short, but the deformity also occurs in persons with long-term diabetes who have muscle and nerve damage as a result of the disease (see Foot Problems and Diabetes, page 981).

A

B

A mallet toe has a deformity of the end of the toe that gives it a malletlike appearance.

How Serious Are Hammer Toe and Mallet Toe? Both hammer toe and mallet toe can be painful and make walking and other movements uncomfortable and more difficult.

Treatment. Your physician or a podiatrist may prescribe an orthotic appliance to position your toe properly and relieve the pressure and pain in the toe. Make sure you wear shoes that fit properly. A corrective surgical procedure is another possibility in some cases.

INGROWN TOENAIL

Signs and Symptoms

- Pain, swelling, and redness around a toenail.

An ingrown toenail is a condition in which the sharp end of a toenail grows into the flesh of the toe, often the big toe. It can result from unusually curved toenails, poorly fitted shoes, or toenails that are cut improperly. The tissue around the nail may become infected.

Treatment. If the tissue around the nail has become infected, your doctor will pre-

---

FOOT PROBLEMS AND DIABETES

If you have diabetes, you are at special risk for foot problems. Cuts, blisters, corns, calluses, and other conditions that are rarely more than minor irritations to non-diabetics can rapidly become serious medical problems. Gangrene or infection can result and, in severe cases, amputation of your foot or leg may be required (see Diabetes Mellitus, page 707).

Be alert for symptoms of the potential complications outlined below and seek proper care if you observe them. However, if you have insulin-dependent diabetes, the risk of foot problems is low in the first 10 years or so that you have the disease.

Blood Vessel Disease

Circulatory problems in the small blood vessels of the legs often occur in persons with long-term diabetes. This tendency helps explain why the incidence of gangrene among men and women older than 40 years is many times greater in diabetics than in the general population.

Decreased circulation may result in cold, dusky red feet. This renders the feet more vulnerable both to burns and to injury from cold.

Diabetic Neuropathy

Accompanying the decrease in circulation is a loss of nerve tissue and sensitivity in the feet. The loss of sensitivity in the feet (and, in some patients, the hands) results in a decrease in sense of touch and ability to experience pain, heat, and cold. Your legs and feet may feel numbed, as if they've "gone to sleep."

This insensitivity also increases the risk from cuts, abrasions, bruises, and burns. Small injuries can go unnoticed and become infected or even ulcerous (see Foot Ulcers, page 982). Burns or frostbite can occur without your being aware of it. To prevent such injuries, take steps to avoid exposure to extremes of heat or cold.

Charcot's Joint

Another serious long-term complication of diabetic neuropathy is Charcot's joint. This uncommon problem occurs with long-stand-

ing nerve deterioration. The small bones of the arch of the foot gradually disintegrate, and the feet rather quickly become swollen and very flat. Charcot's joint can have crippling results, although there is little pain.

Foot Infections

Research has not yet established whether the diabetic is more susceptible to infection, but it is known that an infection is usually more severe in the diabetic and responds more slowly to treatment than in the nondiabetic. Markedly increased blood sugar concentration probably accelerates or worsens infections, and keeping the blood sugar value within satisfactory limits likely will have a favorable effect on the infection. Abscesses on the sole of the foot, on ulcer sites, in the vicinity of nails, and between the toes are common problems.

Many of these problems can be prevented or their complications minimized by proper foot care. For advice on day-to-day foot care, see Proper Care of the Feet in Diabetes (page 983).

scribe an antibiotic and may also trim the portion of the nail that has grown into the toe (a minor procedure that is done in the office). Warm soaks, a topical antibiotic, and rest also may be advised.

Prevention.   To avoid chronic recurrence of ingrown toenails, don't clip your nails too short; also, cut them straight across rather than curving them to match the shape of your toes. Wear socks and shoes that fit properly, and avoid excessive pressure on your feet and toes.

FOOT ULCERS

Signs and Symptoms
* An open sore on the skin surrounded by inflamed tissue;
* If the tissue is infected, pus is discharged from the ulcer.

The diabetic, in particular, is at risk for foot ulcers. A foot ulcer can be the result of long-term blood vessel or nerve deterioration or even of bedsores from prolonged immobilization.

The Diagnosis.   If the ulcer is thought to be the result of arterial problems, the physician will check for the presence or absence of pulsation in the arteries of the foot. If necessary, a special ultrasound test will be done to check for blockage of the arteries to the leg. Particularly if there appears to be a need for operation, arteriography also may be done to examine the blood vessels themselves and identify abnormalities (see page 805).

Ulcers from an inadequate arterial blood supply are ordinarily found at or near the toes, whereas ulcers produced from poor veins tend to be located near the ankle. Ulcers resulting from a nerve deficit are often on the soles, frequently at the site of a callus.

See your physician if a foot ulcer develops.

Treatment.   *Surgery.*   Many foot ulcers heal without surgery, but sometimes an operation on the arteries or even amputation is needed.

Prevention.   Your physician may recommend use of special stockings or support hose to help circulation and prevent future ulceration. In the case of an ulcer from poor veins, foot elevation may be recommended. This means that, as much as possible, the foot should be elevated above the heart to assist in drainage and to lessen the associated swelling.

BONE DISEASES

At left is normal bone; illustration at right shows osteoporotic bone, which is more porous and thus weaker and subject to fracture.

The 206 bones in the human body consist of hard, rigid tissue. The bones are the skeletal framework to which the muscles are attached and within which the organs are located.

Our bones are made up of proteins, sugars, minerals, and other materials. They are living, changing tissues that produce blood cells and act as a storehouse for the minerals calcium and phosphate. Given the range of activities that take place within the bones, a range of problems and malfunctions can occur.

Some of the diseases that may affect bone, such as osteoporosis, are common whereas others, such as fibrous dysplasia or Paget's disease, are uncommon or rare. However, they all result in failure of the function of the remarkable structural system we know as the skeleton.

OSTEOPOROSIS

Signs and Symptoms
* Low back pain;

- Loss of height over time, with an accompanying stooped posture;
- Fractures of the vertebrae, wrists, or hips.

Most cases of osteoporosis are the result of an acceleration of the normal changes our bodies undergo as we age. Unfortunately, varying degrees of osteoporosis are found in 1 of every 4 women older than 45 years and in 9 of 10 women older than 75 years. These women have primary osteoporosis, in which the store of calcium in the bones is gradually depleted; this form usually is more evident after the onset of menopause. Men start with a larger reserve of bone minerals, and so their loss of bone density due to osteoporosis becomes evident later in life and to a lesser degree. A calcium-poor diet, smoking, a sedentary lifestyle, early menopause, and being underweight all heighten the risk of osteoporosis.

The term osteoporosis is from the Greek *osteon* for bone and *porus* for pore or passage. The disorder results in the bones literally becoming more porous. The percentage of calcium stored in the bones decreases over time, causing the skeleton to weaken and leading, in some cases, to fractures. This demineralization has various causes.

Osteoporosis also can accompany endocrine disorders such as acromegaly and Cushing's syndrome (see pages 723 and 719) or can result from excessive use of drugs such as corticosteroids. In such cases, the problem is termed secondary osteoporosis. The treatment must be directed at curing the principal ailment or not using the offending drug.

The Diagnosis. Your physician may observe osteoporotic bone in a routine x-ray of the chest or spine before you even know you have the disease. In many cases, however, the first symptom of osteoporosis is a fracture. A hip or wrist may break with a minor fall or accident (although in some cases spontaneous hip fractures precipitate the fall). When an x-ray is taken of an osteoporotic bone, its shape is the same as that of normal bone (unless a fracture is found) but its density is less. The image is less distinct, and this finding suggests weaker bone.

If your physician suspects you have osteoporosis, appropriate blood or urine tests must be done to exclude other causes for a loss of bone density. One or several x-ray-like tests also need to be done, including CT

PROPER CARE OF THE FEET IN DIABETES

If you have diabetes, you should spend a few minutes of each day caring for your feet. By doing so, you may minimize future foot complications. A few commonsense guidelines follow.

Keep Your Feet Clean

Wash your feet carefully every day. Use warm water and mild hand soap or a cleanser recommended by your doctor. Dry them thoroughly with a soft, clean towel. To prevent dry skin, apply a moisturizing lotion (*not* between the toes). Wear only soft, absorbent, clean socks or hose, and avoid shoes and socks that are tight enough to restrict circulation or cause your feet to perspire excessively. Avoid socks made from synthetic material because they do not allow evaporation of moisture and thus keep the skin soggy.

Examine Your Feet Daily

Examine your feet carefully, including tops, bottoms, areas between the toes, and the toenails. You can use a small mirror if you have difficulty seeing the bottom of your feet. Look for cuts and scrapes, cracks, calluses, bruises, corns, or signs of infection such as swelling or redness. Consult your doctor if you notice any areas of soreness or infection. In any case, your physician should inspect your feet routinely at your regularly scheduled visits.

Take Proper Care of Your Toenails

Do not use nail scissors or clippers because they can cause injury. With an emery board, file the nails straight across rather than curving them to match the shape of the toes. Don't keep them too short, a precaution that will help avoid ingrown nails; this is a common ailment but, for the diabetic, a potentially serious one.

Avoid Injury

Exercise increases circulation and helps maintain the health of the feet. However, in selecting your physical activities consider the risk of injury. Also avoid extremes of hot and cold. When your feet or legs become tired, sit down and elevate your feet for a few minutes before continuing with your activities.

(see page 1286) or photon absorptiometry, to define the degree of bone density loss.

How Serious Is Osteoporosis? Fractures are the key consequence of osteoporosis. Although the fractures tend to heal normally, they often occur with very little or no unusual stress, and further fractures may occur once healing has taken place.

Osteoporosis also affects lifestyle: you must learn to live with it. For many people, this means adopting more sensible dietary and exercise programs to minimize future bone loss and taking a commonsense approach to daily activities to avoid putting the bones at risk.

The vertebral fractures characteristic of osteoporosis rarely require surgical treatment. Called compression fractures, they may cause minimal discomfort if they are minor; if they are more extensive, a painful episode of backache may result. Commonly, the pain begins abruptly, centers in the back (but may radiate around the trunk), is aggravated by movement and relieved by heat, and gradually subsides over the next 1 to 2 months. Over a period of years, however, a sequence of spinal compression fractures can lead to dowager's hump or widow's hump, resulting in an increasingly bent-over posture.

Osteoporosis can be crippling when the bones are weakened severely. The disorder also is associated with perhaps 40,000 deaths annually, largely from complications of surgery or immobilization after hip fractures.

One of the long-term effects of osteoporosis can be a series of vertebral compression fractures that, over time, can produce the stooped posture commonly called dowager's hump.

Treatment. *Exercise.* A regular, reasonable exercise program is a crucial part of the battle against osteoporosis. Research suggests that weight-bearing exercise (that is, exercise such as walking rather than swimming) may help the bones to regain calcium. In addition, exercise can improve your musculature, which may help avoid future falls and fractures.

Select your exercise carefully. Appropriate exercises for an elderly woman include walking, riding a stationary bicycle, and working out on a rowing machine. Paradoxically, the serious female competitive runner is often vulnerable to osteoporosis because of a decrease in estrogen production and scanty or absent menstrual periods that may accompany extreme leanness.

Prevention. Although there is little agreement among researchers as to whether osteoporosis can be fully prevented, there is an emerging consensus that the more calcium a woman has stored in her skeleton before menopause, the less her risk of developing significant osteoporosis. To that end, a young woman should adopt dietary and exercise programs that foster deposition of calcium in her bones.

Eat foods high in calcium, including dairy products, leafy green vegetables, beans, nuts, and whole-grain cereals. One often advocated precaution is to take a calcium supplement if your dietary calcium intake is deficient. The value of this advice has yet to be proved adequately, but a calcium intake of approximately 1,000 milligrams per day from diet or supplements may help you maintain maximal calcium status. For the elderly woman with osteoporosis, the same strategies apply.

Weight-bearing exercise is important to women younger than 40 years who are concerned about the risk of developing osteoporosis. Good preventive exercises include jogging, walking, tennis, bicycling, dancing, rope-jumping, cross-country skiing, and almost any activity that combines movement with stress on the limbs, including weight training. In general, adopting an exercise program that serves the basic goals for cardiovascular fitness (see page 793) will help avoid bone loss.

Medication. At the time of menopause, estrogen replacement therapy may be recommended. This course of medication will replace the supply of estrogen as the ovaries cease to supply it, enabling the skeleton to slow its rate of absorption and retain calcium stores. The use of estrogen supplements has a danger of endometrial cancer and is recommended only for women at high risk of osteoporosis. A combined hormone program of estrogen and progesterone will help decrease the risk of developing this cancer. Supplemental calcium, taken in the form of calcium carbonate, and vitamin D often are prescribed. Fluoride therapy is still considered experimental and must be used only under close medical supervision.

Surgery. In the event of fractures, an emergency operation may be required to set a broken wrist, hip, or other bone. In some cases, a replacement hip joint may be required if the affected bones are badly eroded by osteoporosis (see Joint Replacement, page 998). Physical therapy is a key part of the recovery from any fracture.

OSTEOMALACIA AND RICKETS

Signs and Symptoms
- Pain in the bones of your arms, legs, spine, and pelvis, with actual tenderness of the bones;
- Progressive weakness.

In Children
- In addition to the above symptoms, a child with rickets may have bowlegs and develop a pigeon breast (projection of the chest) and a protruding stomach;
- A slight fever and restlessness at night.

Osteomalacia means softening *(malakia)* of the bones. This softening occurs from a loss of the mineral calcium from the skeleton. The bones become flexible and gradually are molded by forces, such as bearing weight, that are exerted on them. Deformities can then result. When osteomalacia occurs in children, it is termed rickets.

One of the two most common causes of osteomalacia is a problem of fat malabsorption called steatorrhea. In this condition, the body is unable to absorb fats, and they are passed directly out of the body in the stool. The result of this problem is that vitamin D, which is usually absorbed with fat, and calcium are poorly absorbed. This poor absorption can be a result of digestive disorders

such as nontropical sprue and short-bowel syndrome (see pages 621 and 623).

The other common cause of osteomalacia is an increased amount of acid in the body fluids because kidney function is faulty. Called tubular acidosis, this problem occurs in persons with congenital or acquired kidney disorders (see page 888). In simple terms, this increased acid gradually dissolves the skeleton (just as vinegar will soften an eggshell).

A less common cause of osteomalacia is a dietary shortage of vitamin D, a key component in the body's process of calcium absorption. Because milk is supplemented with vitamin D and because even small exposures to sunlight result in the manufacture of vitamin D in the skin, osteomalacia and rickets rarely result from a lack of vitamin D in our society. However, if you or your child has trouble digesting milk products, your physician may advise taking vitamin D supplements to be sure that no deficiency occurs (see Lactose Intolerance, page 623). A long-term deficiency of calcium in the diet also can result in osteomalacia, but it usually causes osteoporosis. There is also a hereditary form of rickets with shortened adult stature, often called vitamin D-resistant rickets (see page 888).

The Diagnosis. If your physician suspects osteomalacia or rickets, a blood test may be done to measure the amounts of the minerals calcium and phosphorus. X-rays of the affected bones must be obtained. Infrequently, a bone biopsy, in which a small sample of bone tissue is removed for analysis, also may be needed to confirm the diagnosis.

Once osteomalacia is diagnosed, the next and most essential step is to find out whether the cause is an intestinal problem (malabsorption) or a kidney defect.

How Serious Is Osteomalacia? In most cases, when the mineral deficiency is eliminated, so are the symptoms. In children and adults, most of the mineral depletion in the bones can be corrected with appropriate treatment, and the skeletal deformities will disappear in time.

Treatment. *Medication.* Treatment is usually directed toward correcting the underlying problem. Calcium and vitamin D supplements may be necessary.

Surgery. In extreme cases, particularly in vitamin D-resistant rickets, skeletal deformities may require surgical correction.

PAGET'S DISEASE OF THE BONE

Signs and Symptoms
- Pain and a sensation of warmth over the involved bones;
- Headache;
- Bowing of a lower limb;
- Hearing loss.

The disorder called Paget's disease (also known by the technical name osteitis deformans), named after a mid-19th century English surgeon, is the reverse of osteoporosis (see page 982). Paget's disease of bone initially occurs when too much bone tissue is broken down. In response, the body increases the rate at which new bone is formed. However, the new bone is laid down in a disordered pattern and may be softer and weaker than normal bone. The result of Paget's disease is somewhat like that of osteoporosis, however, in that the bones grow weak and may become deformed and even fracture.

Most cases of Paget's disease of bone are diagnosed in patients between the ages of 50 and 70 years, although in rare instances it has been found in young adults. Occasionally, it runs in families.

The Diagnosis. If your physician suspects that you have Paget's disease of bone, blood and urine tests may be done to determine whether the amounts of by-products from the bone breakdown process are higher than normal. Traditional x-rays and bone scans (see page 1287) may also be needed. In rare instances, a bone biopsy is done to obtain a sample of affected bone tissue to help decide on appropriate treatment.

How Serious Is Paget's Disease of Bone? In many people, the disease is without symptoms. In fact, it may be discovered by accident when a routine x-ray or blood test is done.

In patients with symptoms, usually only one area of the body is affected, most likely the spine, skull, pelvis, thighs, or lower legs. However, multiple sites can be involved. The affected bones can become deformed and subject to fracture. In most cases, the disease tends to progress very slowly.

In rare cases, serious, long-term complications range from deafness to congestive heart failure. Rarely, a malignancy of the bone may develop.

Treatment. Patients who don't have symptoms usually require no treatment.

Medication. In its early stages, treatment to reduce pain and inflammation is all that is required. Aspirin and other mild analgesic and anti-inflammatory drugs are sufficient. If the disease progresses, however, stronger medications such as the hormone calcitonin may be needed. When the usual treatments are ineffective, the cell-destroying agent mithramycin also may be used.

Surgery. When deformities occur, an operation may be required. This, however, is uncommon.

FIBROUS DYSPLASIA

Signs and Symptoms
- Bone pain, especially in the lower part of your leg;
- Difficulty in walking;
- Rarely, fractures and multiple bone deformities;
- Often, fibrous dysplasia will cause no symptoms.

This disorder bears some resemblance to Paget's disease (see above) in that it is characterized by abnormal cystic growth of bone tissue. In the case of fibrous dysplasia, however, the bone tissue is fibrous rather than bony. Typically, it first appears in childhood. The cause of fibrous dysplasia is unknown. This disorder may affect one bone or several bones. One form of fibrous dysplasia is associated with premature sexual maturation in girls (Albright's syndrome; see Sexual Precocity, page 139).

The Diagnosis. The presence of fibrous dysplasia is confirmed with x-rays of the bone or with a bone biopsy, in which samples of bone tissue are removed for laboratory examination (see page 1284).

Treatment. Although fibrous dysplasia is not curable, excess fibrous growths may be removed surgically from affected bones. Bone grafts also may be necessary.

OSTEOGENESIS IMPERFECTA

Signs and Symptoms
- Fragile bones resulting in fractures;
- The white part of the eyes (sclera) is deep blue or black;
- Limb deformities, particularly bowing;
- Flatfeet;
- Short stature.

Osteogenesis imperfecta is a rare inherited disease in which the bones are abnormally brittle and fragile. Fractures may occur at birth or later when the child begins to walk.

Hearing impairment is common during adolescence and later in life.

There are various forms of the disease. In the less severe forms there is often a marked reduction in the number of fractures once a child reaches adolescence

The Diagnosis. The diagnosis is made with x-ray studies of the bones

How Serious Is Osteogenesis Imperfecta?
The most severe forms of osteogenesis imperfecta are often fatal. Many children with severe disease die of cardiorespiratory complications during infancy or childhood.

Treatment. The treatment for less severe types of this disease involves trying to reduce the risk of fractures. It is important that all fractures be set promptly and skeletal deformities corrected. Genetic counseling should be considered before another pregnancy.

OSTEOMYELITIS

Signs and Symptoms
- Intense pain and a sensation of heat at the site of the affected bone;
- Tenderness and swelling;
- Fever;
- Fatigue.

Osteomyelitis is an inflammation of the bone marrow (from the Greek words *osteo* for bone, *myelos* for marrow, and *itis* for inflammation). It usually occurs as the result of a bacterial infection, often one introduced at the time a wound, fracture, or other injury is sustained. It also may be carried to the bone via the blood.

Osteomyelitis is more common in children than adults, but it is now rare in the United States. It usually can be treated successfully with antibiotic drugs, but it can recur.

The Diagnosis. If osteomyelitis is suspected, a blood test, traditional x-ray, a bone scan (see page 1287), or needle biopsy (see page 1284) may be used for diagnosis. A surgical biopsy of the bone also may be necessary, in which a sample of the bone, pus, or other tissue from the deep abscess is removed for laboratory examination.

Treatment. An extended course (3 weeks or more) of penicillin or other antibiotic drug is the usual treatment. Bed rest and immobilization of the affected bones are also recommended. In some instances, surgical removal of infected tissues may be necessary.

ENDOCRINE DISORDERS AND THE BONES

Your endocrine system controls various functions in the body. Consisting of glands that secrete hormones, the endocrine system affects virtually all body functions and parts. Your bones are no exception. Each of the following disorders affects the bone.

Acromegaly
This condition is the result of too much growth hormone being secreted by the pituitary gland. It occurs in adulthood. Persons with acromegaly have characteristically large hands, feet, jawbone, and skull (see Pituitary Tumors, page 723).

Gigantism
Gigantism is a rare ailment that also is caused by too much growth hormone. It occurs in children and results in accelerated growth and excessive adult height (see Pituitary Tumors, page 723).

Hypopituitarism
Children whose pituitary glands produce too little growth hormone suffer from hypopituitarism. This disorder results in dwarfism (see Hypopituitarism, page 725).

Hyperparathyroidism
In this condition, too much parathyroid hormone is produced. One result is that too much calcium is released from the bones, sometimes resulting in a weakening of the skeleton with cystic changes (see Hyperparathyroidism, page 732).

BONE TUMORS

Signs and Symptoms
- A hard lump on the surface of a bone;
- Accompanying pain;
- Fractures of the bone.

Tumors that begin in bone are rare. If cancerous, the malignant cells often have traveled (metastasized) from a cancer elsewhere in the body. The exceptions are a blood cancer called multiple myeloma that begins in the bone marrow (see Multiple Myeloma, page 493) and osteosarcoma, which is the most common primary bone malignancy. Both of these are much less common than metastatic bone cancers. More often, bone tumors are benign.

The Diagnosis. X-rays are helpful, but they may not yield a firm diagnosis. In order to rule out a malignancy, a biopsy, in which a small sample of the tissue is removed for laboratory examination, may be done.

How Serious Is a Bone Tumor? A benign growth rarely presents any health risk. If the tumor is the result of a cancer that has metastasized from another site or is a bone malignancy, the survival rate varies.

Treatment. Benign tumors occasionally require surgical removal.

The cancerous bone tissue of osteosarcoma is removed surgically and anticancer drugs are prescribed. Sometimes the limb can be preserved by removing the diseased portion of the bone and reconstructing the arm or leg. This is followed by a program of rehabilitation.

THE BACK AND BACK PROBLEMS

More than 30 separate bones form the backbone, the flexible assembly that runs from the base of the skull to the tailbone. These bones, the vertebrae, are stacked on top of one another. In the spaces between these bones are spongy cushions, the discs, which

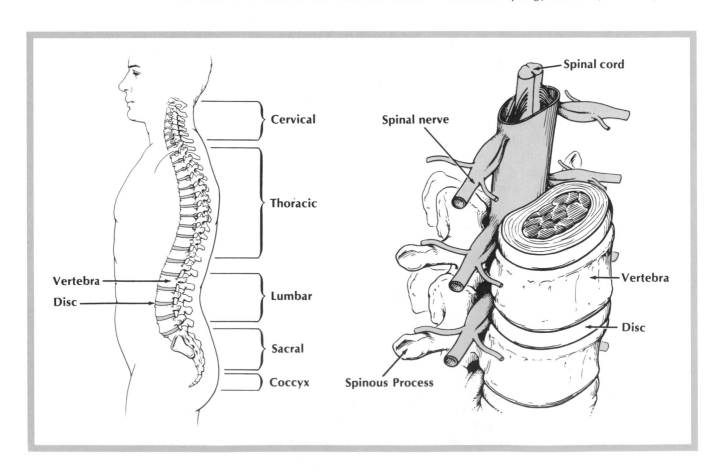

THE IMPORTANCE OF POSTURE

Parents, teachers, and drill sergeants alike are famous for ordering their wards to stand up or to sit up straight. Like it or not, it's excellent advice. People who both stand up and sit up straight all day, every day, are at less risk for backache because poor posture is one of the more common causes of backache.

What Is Proper Posture?

Imagine that strings connect your ears to the bones that protrude from your ankles. Now, starting with your knees bent and shoulders hunched, pull those theoretical strings taut by standing up. When you stand as straight as possible, the string should extend up your leg just behind the kneecap and across the meat of your thigh and pass by the tip of your shoulder.

What Is Poor Posture?

One extreme is the slouch, in which the shoulders are rolled forward (called kyphosis). In people who perpetually slouch, the muscles of the chest are shortened and flexibility is reduced. In the opposite postural extreme, the swayback (also known as lordosis), the

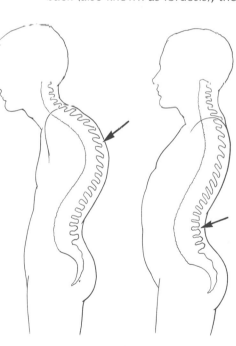

stomach sticks out too far in front and the buttocks too far in the rear—and the backbone takes on an exaggerated curve between the pelvis and ribs (the lumbar region). Such a swaybacked posture puts much pressure on the lower back and contributes to back problems.

Attention!

The military stance may seem a bit exaggerated, but you should apply some of its rules to your upright posture. Keeping your backbone straight is an obvious one; holding your shoulders back helps too. Don't forget to pull in your stomach and buttocks, trimming your profile, and pull in your chin.

Sit Up Straight!

A slouched posture when seated can only aggravate back discomfort: in general, sitting puts more stress on your back than standing does.

Sit in chairs with either straight backs or low-back (lumbar) support. The seat should be high enough that your thighs rest horizontally on the seat. That way, your weight is more evenly distributed and your back isn't forced to assume a disproportionate amount of your weight.

Wear Proper Footwear

Wear shoes that provide your feet with good support. High heels, in particular, put stress on your back. So, to help avoid backache, wear shoes with low or flat heels.

Practice Makes Perfect

Knowing what good posture is isn't enough. You have to practice it. Of course, it isn't easy to change years of bad habits, but you must concentrate on maintaining a proper upright posture at all times.

Common forms of improper posture are kyphosis, left, in which shoulders roll forward, and lordosis, swaybacked posture.

◄ **For proper posture, stand straight and imagine that a string extends from your earlobe to your instep.**

have a strong, fibrous outer skin that protects a gel on the inside. The entire assembly for the vertebrae and discs is held together by a network of ligaments and muscles.

The intricate structure of the back is a remarkable piece of engineering: it bends and twists and bears the weight of our bodies and the loads we carry. The backbone also protects the spinal cord, the main pathway for the central nervous system.

The complexity of the structure contributes to the potential for problems. Seemingly minor changes in the alignment or balance of any part—whether a disc, a vertebra, or muscles—can make any movement painful. When the nerves that travel through the backbone are affected, there is a risk of pain in any part of the body because virtually the entire skeleton is served by these nerve tissues. If the back suffers serious trauma, there is a risk of permanent damage to the spinal cord and resulting paralysis (see Spinal Cord Trauma, page 552).

The following pages consider back problems from the simple backache nearly everyone experiences occasionally to rarer ailments such as spondylosis. In addition, strategies are given to help you avoid back pain and injuries—and to deal with them if they occur.

PROLAPSED DISC

Signs and Symptoms
- Mild to severe pain in your back or neck;
- If the prolapsed disc is in your neck, numbness or weakness of an arm or hand

may occur; often, serious neck and upper extremity pain is present;
- If the damaged disc is in the middle or lower part of your back, numbness or weakness may occur in the buttocks, legs, or feet;
- A shooting pain that occurs if you cough, sneeze, or strain;
- Usually one arm or one leg is affected significantly more than the other arm or leg.

The discs are the cushioning pads located between the bones (vertebrae) of the back. When one of the discs ruptures, the resulting condition is called a prolapsed disc. This disorder is also known as herniated disc (and also as a slipped disc, although there is no actual slippage).

The discs are composed of a fibrous outer skin that contains a soft, jelly-like substance. Age or strain may cause the disc to develop a bulge (herniate). The result can be a loss of the cushioning effect, allowing pressure on nearby nerves, which causes pain.

A prolapsed disc is most likely to occur in the lower back, although any disc can be affected. The condition does occur in children, but it is more likely to develop in adults.

The Diagnosis.   A careful physical examination and probably a series of x-rays, some CT scans (see page 1286), or MRI scans (see page 1287) are used to determine the extent of the injury and also to rule out other conditions that cause similar symptoms, such as a spinal tumor or a circulatory problem (see pages 554 and 834, respectively). The material protruding from the disc is not visible on routine x-rays, but sometimes it can be seen on an MRI or CT scan. If surgery is necessary, another x-ray test called myelography, which requires injection of a dye into the spinal column, may be required (see page 1292).

How Serious Is a Prolapsed Disc?   In most people, a prolapsed disc will repair itself if given time (usually 2 to 6 weeks) and proper rest (sometimes complete bed rest). In some instances, an operation may be necessary.

Treatment.   The most common prescription for a prolapsed disc is decreased activity and, in some cases, bed rest. Two weeks

If one of the discs that cushion vertebrae in your back ruptures, a portion of the disc's jelly-like interior can be displaced, putting pressure on a spinal nerve (as shown here) or on the spinal cord. This condition is variously known as a prolapsed, ruptured, herniated, or, more commonly, a slipped disc.

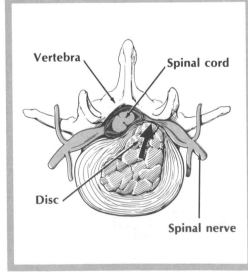

Vertebra   Spinal cord

Disc

Spinal nerve

of such a regimen is often the recommended duration (see also Treatment for Your Backache, page 993). After 1 or 2 weeks of markedly decreased activity, activity usually can be resumed, although slowly and progressively. Conservative physical therapy measures such as the use of heat or ice, massage, gentle exercises, and sometimes traction are often helpful.

Surgery. Sometimes compressed nerves from disc protrusion do not heal with rest. In such cases, a surgical procedure called a laminectomy may be necessary to remove the disc or the part of the disc that is compressing the nerve.

In the lower back, this procedure usually is done by making an incision in the back, removing a small amount of bone covering the disc, and then removing part of the disc material. All of the disc cannot be removed when the approach is from the back. Although a similar procedure is sometimes done in the neck or upper back, it is occasionally desirable to remove the disc by approaching it from the front. In this case, it is not necessary to remove any bone, and a larger amount of disc can be removed. Often, fusing together the vertebrae on either side of the damaged disc is considered when this approach is used.

These two operative procedures require an incision, leave a surgical scar, and, of course, require a period of wound healing. Nevertheless, they allow the surgeon to see directly the nerve that is being compressed and to remove the disc, ligament, bone, or other material that is compressing the nerve.

Other Therapies. In an effort to avoid the surgical incision and decrease the recovery time, two other options have been tried for a carefully selected group of patients with nerve compression from disc protrusion.

Chymopapain, an enzyme derived from the tropical papaya tree, can be injected into the disc. It causes the disc to shrink, reducing the pressure on the nearby nerve and, in many cases, eliminating the pain.

Another procedure, called percutaneous discectomy, allows the disc to be removed from between the vertebrae with a mechanical device that fits into a large needle. This large needle is inserted through the skin into the disc, much like the needle used to inject chymopapain into the disc.

Unfortunately, sometimes the nerve compression cannot be relieved with the chymopapain or the percutaneous technique. In other patients, the nerve compression is not necessarily due to disc material. In these situations, the more conventional surgical procedure may be the only solution.

BACK MUSCLE STRAINS AND SPASMS

Signs and Symptoms
- Back pain and stiffness.

Back pain can result from a movement: lifting a barbell or other heavy object can strain a muscle, as can a sneeze or other everyday movement. Back pain also often occurs for no obvious reason; in some people, the stresses of life seem to produce backaches. Most often, though, the pain results from a muscle pull or strain.

Back pain can occur at any point on the spine, but the most common point is in the lower back. Back problems are among the most common ailments of humankind. Young or old, male or female, short or tall, most Americans experience some back discomfort in their lifetimes.

The Diagnosis. When you complain of backache, your physician will first review your medical history, perform a physical examination, and obtain diagnostic studies such as an x-ray of your spine to try to eliminate serious spinal problems (see Prolapsed Disc, page 990, and Spondylosis, page 992).

You might feel pain at the very moment you strain the muscle. In some cases, a gradual soreness develops at night and you awaken to a discomfort. Regardless of how the pain develops, it is often difficult for your physician to pinpoint the cause. Whether or not you have a history of back problems also will be important for diagnosis.

How Serious Are Back Strains and Spasms? There is no denying the discomfort that accompanies a sore back. Every movement can be painful, and simply going about daily life can seem like agony. In some people, low-back pain can be so intense that they virtually are immobilized.

Usually, the problem will subside given time and rest, although recurring episodes of back discomfort are the rule rather than the exception. Every case is different, but by using a combination of simple treatments, practicing good posture (see page 989), and using sensible strategies for protecting your back (see below), you may avoid or minimize future back problems.

Treatment.   Most back spasms or simple strains require rest, and in a few days you will be able to return to normal activities. In the meantime, there are various possible treatments. Operation is rarely the preferred treatment for backache, but if more conservative treatments such as rest or heat or ice

fail (see Treatment for Your Backache, page 993), your physician may refer you to a neurologist, neurosurgeon, physiatrist, or orthopedic surgeon for an evaluation of your condition.

SPONDYLOSIS

Signs and Symptoms
* Back pain;
* Tenderness and difficulty in moving your back;

HOW TO PROTECT YOUR BACK

Certain everyday activities put your back at risk for injury. Lifting is one obvious example, but have you considered that how you sleep and sit are critical to the health of your back? Here are some simple strategies to consider.

Lifting
Bend your knees, not your back. Whether the object to be picked up weighs a fraction of an ounce or a hundred pounds, squat with your back straight and let your legs do the lifting. Bring tension on your muscles gradually: don't jerk or lunge to lift the load.

Sleeping
Lying down provides relief for backache—and also an opportunity for backache prevention. Don't sleep on your stomach unless your abdomen is cushioned by a pillow; sleep on your side with your legs drawn up slightly toward your chest. Make sure your mattress provides your back with proper support (use a bed board of ½-inch plywood if the mattress is too soft or sags).

Avoiding Stiffness
If you find yourself seated at a desk, standing in one position, or behind the wheel of a car for hours everyday, you are at risk for stiffness and muscle fatigue. Make

it a point to break the routine at frequent intervals. When standing, shift your weight from one foot to the other periodically; when sitting, get up—even for a few seconds—as often as possible. Take frequent breaks when driving and get out and stretch. A small pillow at the base of the back can also help you support the spine.

Weight Loss
One important cause of backache in the United States is being overweight: extra pounds at the midriff put strains and stresses on your back. If you are overweight, try to reduce and to establish an appropriate exercise program (see page 377).

The golden rule is simple: use your knees, not your back, when lifting.

To avoid aggravating your backache when you sleep or lie down, sleep on your stomach only if your abdomen is cushioned by a pillow (top). If you sleep on your back, support your knees and neck with pillows (middle). Best option: sleep on your side with your legs drawn up slightly toward your chest.

- Pain in the back of your thighs;
- Mild cases of spondylosis are usually symptomless.

Spondylosis is a disorder in which the spine, over time, becomes stiff and loses flexibility. The name is derived from the Greek words for vertebra, *spondylos,* and condition, *osis.*

The cause can be excessive use, injury, or simply the aging process. Whatever the cause, the discs between the vertebrae become worn, and the spaces between the vertebrae narrow. Bony spurs also can develop. The result is the pain and stiffness of spondylosis.

Spondylosis is sometimes referred to as degenerative joint disease or osteoarthritis of the spine. However, it is not to be con-

fused with ankylosing spondylitis (see page 1001).

The Diagnosis.   An x-ray of your spine will be taken to determine the condition of the discs and vertebrae. If you have had problems with prolapsed discs, you may be more susceptible to spondylosis.

How Serious Is Spondylosis?   For most people, living with spondylosis is a matter of developing strategies for dealing with the discomfort, although in rare cases, spondylosis in the lower back can lead to difficulty in urinating, defecating, and walking (see Lumbar Stenosis, page 994.)

Treatment.   Your physician is unlikely to be able to offer a simple solution. A combi-

---

TREATMENT FOR YOUR BACKACHE

The causes of back pain are numerous, ranging from minor strains and sprains (see page 992) to a slipped disc (see Prolapsed Disc, page 990) and various chronic problems of the spine. Although diagnosing the precise cause isn't easy, it is important that certain potential underlying causes be ruled out, so see your physician when you have back pain.

Medication
Analgesics such as aspirin can help ease the pain. Depending on the diagnosis, stronger pain killers or muscle relaxants also may be prescribed. A corticosteroid drug may be injected if the pain is localized in one definable area (see Corticosteroid Drugs, page 1005).

Physical Therapy
Your physician or physical therapist can design specific treatment and exercise programs for you. An exercise that might help one person could harm another. So be sure to follow instructions.

Basic therapy includes application of alternating heat and cold and gentle massage to your back. For some disorders, braces, corsets, or mechanical traction can help. These measures may take some of the pressure off the affected area. In addition, exercises to stretch and strengthen the muscles of your back can reduce the risk of future back problems. Again, because needs vary, see your physician or physical therapist for specific instructions.

Lie Flat on Your Back
Always sleep on a firm surface or mattress or insert a board beneath your mattress. During an episode of back pain, try to remain flat on your back with your legs drawn up for long periods. For a strain or sprain, 3 or 4 days of such rest should bring relief (if not, consult your physician). If you have a prolapsed disc, you will be instructed in the proper care.

Surgery
If none of the other approaches provide relief, you may be re-

ferred to a neurologist, neurosurgeon, or orthopedic surgeon. In some cases, surgical alternatives can resolve back problems, but spinal surgery is not to be taken lightly. Try the more conservative approaches first because an operation is required in less than 1 percent of all cases of backache.

Self-Help
A physician's advice is important, but it's far from the whole story. Follow medical advice carefully, but also use common sense in going about everyday activities. If you are overweight, lose those extra pounds. Be careful when lifting. A reasonable approach to exercise will help your general condition. In addition, your physician can recommend specific exercises to strengthen the muscles that support the vertebrae.

Also, maintain proper posture (see page 989), protect your back when lifting or doing any exercises that put your back at risk (see page 992), and simply think ahead as you pursue your normal activities. A little prevention may save you a lot of pain.

nation of an analgesic drug such as aspirin, physical therapy, and other self-help approaches will likely be recommended (see Treatment for Your Backache, page 993).

LUMBAR STENOSIS

Signs and Symptoms
- Pain in the buttock, thigh, and calf associated with walking and standing;
- Pain stops with sitting or bending forward.

Lumbar stenosis can result from either arthritic changes or a congenital narrowing of the spine that produces a compression of the lower end of the spinal canal. Symptoms can be similar to those caused by blockage of the arteries to the lower extremities (see Arteriosclerosis of the Extremities, page 834).

The Diagnosis.   Your physician will examine the arteries of your lower legs and may order special tests to make sure the arteries are functioning properly. If these vascular studies are normal, a CT scan of the spine may be needed to determine whether the spinal canal is narrowed.

Treatment.   If symptoms persist, a specialist may be needed to consider whether an operation (called a laminectomy) is needed to relieve pressure on the spinal nerves.

SCOLIOSIS

Signs and Symptoms
- A sideways curvature of the spine;
- Asymmetrical rib cage with one shoulder blade protruding.

Scoliosis is an abnormal curvature of the spine (from the Greek word *skoliosis,* meaning curvature). Usually a curve to one side develops, followed by a compensating bend in the opposite direction.

Poor posture and congenital defects of the spine are the causes of scoliosis in only a small percentage of cases. Most cases are of unknown origin, probably traceable to genetic factors. The deformity may begin during infancy (more often in boys) or in the preschool years and immediately after. Often, however, the signs go undetected until adolescence. Adolescent girls are more likely to have scoliosis than boys.

The Diagnosis.   A visual examination is usually sufficient to recognize the condition, although x-rays of the spine may be needed to determine the extent of the curvature.

How Serious Is Scoliosis?   Scoliosis may be a chronic and progressive disorder. If left unchecked, the vertebrae at the scoliotic curve will rotate, resulting in widely separated ribs on one side of the body and narrowed spaces on the other. In severe cases, heart and lung problems may develop over a period of many years.

Treatment.   Once scoliosis is diagnosed, a program of exercises may be recommended to strengthen the muscles of the spine and

A sideways curvature of the spine is called scoliosis. Exercises and a brace may be the only treatment required.

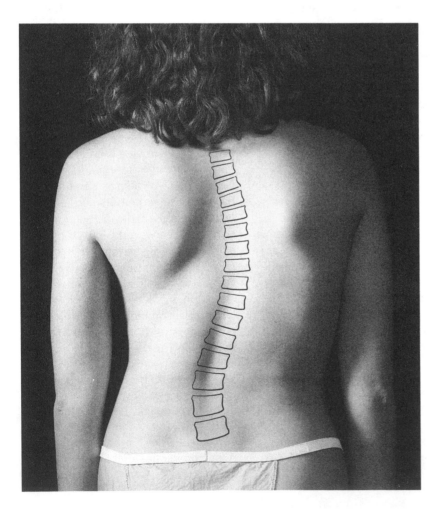

improve posture. A spinal brace also is commonly used to prevent further curvature of the spine. The brace is molded to fit the pelvic region and pads are fitted to the frame to apply correct pressure at the apex of the curve. If conservative measures are ineffective, surgical procedures can be used to correct the problem (see page 993).

JOINT DISORDERS

The ends of the bones that meet in a joint are cushioned with a layer of resilient tissue called cartilage. The cartilage has a very smooth surface. Surrounding the joint space is a membrane called the synovial membrane which produces synovial fluid to lubricate the joint. Surrounding this membrane is a fibrous, protective casing called the capsule; binding all the parts of a joint together are bands of fibrous tissue called ligaments.

Problems that occur in the joints may be the result of mechanical failure of the parts (as with osteoarthritis, the so-called wear-and-tear arthritis). Often, however, the cause of joint disorders is an inflammation produced by infection, disease, or some unknown cause. Most joint ailments caused by inflammation are termed arthritis, from the Greek words *arthron,* for joint, and *itis,* for inflammation. The following pages outline the common and some of the more unusual varieties of arthritis.

fingers are affected, often multiple joints become arthritic.

Although the precise mechanisms are unknown, it is clear that wear and tear is a principal cause of osteoarthritis. This explains the alternative names for osteoarthritis: degenerative joint disease and wear-and-tear arthritis (osteoarthrosis, another term, is used interchangeably with osteoarthritis). Thus, the athlete who sustains joint injuries and the laborer whose joints are challenged every day by demanding physical activity are at heightened risk of developing arthritic joints later in life.

Here's what occurs in the joint of a person with osteoarthritis. The cartilage that cushions the impact on the joint gradually deteriorates. Its smooth surface roughens, and it loses its cushioning effect. Over time, the ends of the bones also are affected, with bone growing along the sides to produce lumps. Each of the steps in this process produces pain.

OSTEOARTHRITIS

Signs and Symptoms
- Pain in a joint during or after use;
- Discomfort in a joint before or during a change in the weather;
- Swelling and a loss of flexibility in a joint;
- Bony lumps on the end joint of the finger (called Heberden's nodes) may develop. Similar lumps on the middle joint of the finger (called Bouchard's nodes) also may develop.

Osteoarthritis is one of the most common disorders known to humankind. It has been recognized for centuries and affects tens of millions of Americans. Many elderly people have osteoarthritis but don't realize it until their physician recognizes it on a routine x-ray.

Osteoarthritis initially strikes only one joint if the knee or hip is involved; if the

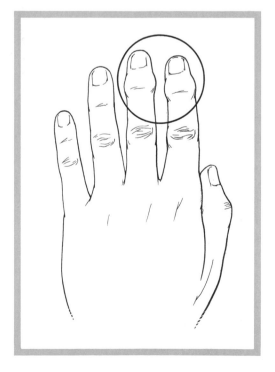

In people with osteoarthritis, a bony lump at the end joint of the fingers may occur. These lumps, called Heberden's nodes, most often occur in women. Although initially painful, they are of little more than cosmetic concern.

Osteoarthritis commonly occurs in the neck or back. The usual progression involves the development of bone spurs on the sides of a damaged vertebra, as seen on x-rays of the bone. The knee and hip also are commonly affected. In young people, osteoarthritis is relatively rare, although osteoarthritis of the knee is not uncommon in young adults.

The Diagnosis.   The presence of pain in either one or a few joints is a key to the diagnosis of osteoarthritis; the sheer prevalence of the disorder is another. If an x-ray is taken of the affected joint, bone spurs (called osteophytes) may be evident, indicating the presence of osteoarthritis. Blood tests may be done to exclude rheumatoid or other forms of arthritis.

Another clue may be the presence of Heberden's or Bouchard's nodes, bony lumps that appear over a period of years in the end and middle joints of the fingers. Your physician may inquire whether your parents also had them because there apparently is a genetic tendency for Heberden's nodes. Women have them about 10 times as often as men.

How Serious Is Osteoarthritis?   Osteoarthritis doesn't go away, although the pain tends to fade within a year of its appearance. Over time, the ends of the bones that rub together (after the breakdown of the cartilage) become polished in a process called eburnation. Still, the effects of osteoarthritis are crippling in only rare cases.

Age is a significant factor in the disorder: it is more likely in elderly people than in the young, and some joints tend to be more affected over time.

Treatment.   *Exercise.*   Although osteoarthritis is the wear-and-tear disease, appropriate exercise can be a valuable treatment approach. A physician or a physical therapist (if your doctor refers you to one) should advise you on an exercise program, but range-of-motion and muscle strengthening exercises can help prevent future problems and avoid stiffness.

Other Therapies.   Consult your doctor about the use of heating pads, hot water bottles, and hot baths. If your neck is affected by osteoarthritis, a cervical collar may be prescribed during acute episodes.

Weight control can be an invaluable adjunct to other treatments: excessive weight puts unnecessary pressures on the joints and can exacerbate the condition. Good posture also can be an aid, especially for osteoarthritis of the spine (see The Importance of Posture, page 989).

Medication.   Aspirin is one of the most effective drugs for treating arthritis. If aspirin is not well tolerated, many other anti-inflammatory drugs can be used to reduce the pain and discomfort.

If inflammation is severe, your physician may recommend an injection of a corticosteroid drug. This is most likely for cases in which a weight-bearing joint, such as a knee or ankle, is affected (see Corticosteroid Drugs, page 1005).

Surgery.   When long-term deterioration has occurred, a hip or knee replacement operation may create a useful joint (see Joint Replacement, page 998). When the joints in the hands have deteriorated significantly, an operation also may be appropriate.

Illustration below shows a common deformity characteristic of rheumatoid arthritis. Joints in the hand may lose strength and be painful during flare-ups of the disease.

RHEUMATOID ARTHRITIS

Signs and Symptoms
- Pain and swelling in the smaller joints of your hands and feet;
- Overall aching or stiffness, especially after sleeping or periods of motionlessness;
- Affected joints are swollen, painful, and warm to the touch during the initial attack and ensuing flare-ups.

Rheumatoid arthritis, unlike the more common osteoarthritis (see page 995), is not the natural result of time and the wear and tear of normal use. Rather, it is thought to be an autoimmune disease in which the body's immune system attacks itself. The ailment is not yet well understood, but researchers suspect that an unidentified virus stimulates the immune system, but the disease-fighting cells inflame the joints.

Unlike osteoarthritis, which affects only the musculoskeletal system, rheumatoid arthritis is a systemic disease that, in some patients, affects such organs as the heart, lungs, and eyes. It also tends to affect more than one joint at a time, resulting in an overall stiffness and aching. By the same token, it is generally symmetrical in its assaults, affecting both feet or both hands. It also may result in small lumps, called rheumatoid nodules, under the skin near the elbow, the ears or nose, the back of the scalp, over the knee, or under the toes. They range in size from that of a pea to perhaps that of a walnut. Usually the lumps are not painful and present no physical problem.

The disease can strike at any time, but most often it develops between ages 20 and 50 years. (A variant of rheumatoid arthritis called juvenile rheumatoid arthritis is discussed on page 1000.) Roughly 3 times as many women as men have rheumatoid arthritis. An estimated 7 million Americans have the ailment.

The Diagnosis. The principal area of attack of rheumatoid arthritis is the synovium, the membrane that lines your joints (for discussion of the configuration of a joint and its parts, see page 953). This smooth membrane becomes inflamed when affected by rheumatoid arthritis, and swells and reddens. Researchers have discovered that the disease-fighting cells of the immune system are especially active in the synovial tissues of patients with rheumatoid arthritis.

Accompanying the inflammation of the synovium are other changes in the joint. Tissue in the cartilage tends to proliferate, which also produces an erosion of surrounding tissues, including ligaments, muscles, and bones. In addition to contributing to the discomforts of rheumatoid arthritis, these changes also produce a looseness in the joints.

If your physician suspects you have rheumatoid arthritis, a thorough physical examination will be conducted. Your doctor will try to establish whether your discomforts are found on both sides of your body. If they are, a diagnosis of rheumatoid arthritis is likely, but laboratory tests will be done to confirm it.

A special blood test that determines the erythrocyte sedimentation rate (see page 1282) helps confirm the presence of rheumatoid arthritis, as does another blood test for an antibody called rheumatoid factor. Four of five patients with rheumatoid arthritis have this abnormal antibody. As the disease advances, x-rays may be useful for following its progression. In particular, an x-ray method in which an opaque fluid is injected into the joint, called arthrography, may be used.

How Serious Is Rheumatoid Arthritis?
Rheumatoid arthritis is the most debilitating form of arthritis. People with this disease often have deformed joints, which lead to loss of mobility. Also, some people experience sweats and fevers along with loss of strength in muscles attached to affected joints. Yet, even when stricken with severe forms, the individual with rheumatoid arthritis usually retains flexibility in the joints and has less pain than the appearance of the deformed joints would suggest.

Often, the disorder is chronic, although it tends to come and go. Periods of increased disease activity, called flare-ups or flares, alternate with periods of relative remission, during which the swelling, pain, difficulty in sleeping, and weakness fade or disappear. It is difficult to predict how severe the disease will be in any one person. Persons who have more or less continuous symptoms for 4 or 5 years are more likely to have a lifetime of problems with the disease. Some of them

JOINT REPLACEMENT

When a joint disorder such as osteoarthritis or rheumatoid arthritis has crippled a hip or knee joint, a surgical procedure called arthroplasty may be the best treatment.

Arthroplasty is a re-forming of the joint. The operation may simply smooth the damaged lining of a joint, but a replacement arthroplasty involves an actual replacement of certain parts of the joint itself with a plastic or steel device.

The most common joint replacement is done on the hip. In a hip arthroplasty, a steel ball on a stem replaces the top of the thigh bone (femur). The cup of the pelvis is also re-placed with a polyethylene cup. Both implants are fastened with a special glue. Recent developments include artificial joints covered with a material that allows bone tissue to grow into it and a short-stem hip replacement.

Knees, finger joints, and other joints can be replaced with prostheses. The results are generally remarkable: people who were unable to walk before their hip arthroplasty frequently walk out of the hospital a few weeks later—under their own power and free of pain. Although the durability of these prostheses is not yet clear, evidence to date suggests that replacement parts are durable with moderate use.

Normal hip socket

Metal prosthesis

Acrylic cement

At left is a normal hip. When the hip is broken or deteriorated from arthritis or osteoporosis, the joint may be replaced with a prosthesis like that shown at right.

will have "burned-out" or remission rheumatoid arthritis after 10 to 20 years. Results of the sedimentation rate test will be more normal, but joint deformities will remain, as will some pain and impaired joint function.

The cyclic nature of rheumatoid arthritis presents researchers with one of the most confusing aspects of the puzzle. There is no cure, but with proper treatment, a strategy of joint protection, and changes in lifestyle, most patients are able to live long, productive, and nearly normal lives after the disease develops. However, proper medical care is essential for dealing with this chronic disorder.

Treatment. *Rest and Exercise.* The key strategy is to establish a proper balance of rest and exercise. The preservation and restoration of function to affected joints involve muscle-building, range-of-motion, and other exercise; yet, a suitable balance of exertion and rest must be maintained. At times, the use of a splint at night is useful.

Because of the ebb and flow of the disease, strategies used during flares and periods of remission differ. The intense disease activity of a flare-up puts you at risk of joint damage, so a combination of rest, pain reduction strategies, and even immobilization of the involved joint is usual. During flares, keep exercise of the affected joints to a minimum to avoid damaging your joints. During periods of remission, exercise and normal activities are encouraged. Still, it is equally important to recognize your limits and avoid undue fatigue. Follow the advice of your physician or physical therapist carefully. No specific diet is useful, but observe general principles of good nutrition and avoid obesity.

Medication. Anti-inflammatory drugs, in particular aspirin, are basic to treating the pain and inflammation of rheumatoid arthritis. Corticosteroid drugs such as prednisone may be very effective for relieving pain and inflammation, but they provide no lasting benefit and they should be used with great caution because of their numerous side effects. In fact, they relieve the pain so effectively that often patients are tempted to use their joints freely and may suffer lasting joint deformities. Prednisone is also an ingredient in some nonapproved arthritis cures, and although such cures may give momentary relief, they also may lead to long-term harm. (See also Corticosteroid Drugs, page 1005.)

In some cases, a wide variety of other drugs are used, including nonsteroidal anti-inflammatory agents, antimalarial drugs, gold salts, and experimental medications used in an attempt to suppress the overactive immune system.

JOINT DISORDERS OF CHILDHOOD

There are numerous rare skeletal problems peculiar to children. Among them are the following.

Legg-Calvé-Perthes Disease

This disorder (also called Perthes' disease) occurs more often in boys than in girls and may be discovered between the ages of 5 and 9 years.

The result of Perthes' disease is a deterioration of the top portion of the thighbone (femoral head) due to defective circulation to that part. This is called avascular necrosis. The cause is unknown.

The child generally complains of pain in the hip and may walk with a limp. At other times, pain may be noticed in the knee. The diagnosis is made with an x-ray. In the early stages of the disease, however, conventional x-rays may be normal. At times, a radionuclide study is helpful (see page 1287).

Healing usually requires a period of 2 to 3 years. In years past, bed rest and later a sling to keep weight off the leg and hips were advocated. More recently, because the outcome seems unrelated to these rather extreme measures, crutches have been advocated or, at times, no treatment. Your physician may instruct you in physical therapy measures to keep the head of the thighbone (femur) in the hip socket.

The vast majority of children with this disorder completely heal without deformity. Some, however, are left with a deformed head of the thighbone that, in later adult life, may cause hip pain and dysfunction. In these few individuals, surgery may be needed.

Slipped Capital Femoral Epiphysis

During the growth spurt just before puberty, the thighbone's (femur's) insertion into the hip can slip out of position, rotate sideways, and slide upward. This unusual condition is called a slipped capital femoral epiphysis. The major symptoms are pain in the knee, thigh, or hip and a limp that involves lurching to the side and outward turning of the foot. Symptoms usually evolve gradually over weeks or months, but they can also appear suddenly in association with an injury.

The capital epiphysis slips most commonly in boys between the ages of 11 and 14 years, particularly those who are tall and overweight. It happens more often in blacks than whites. In one-fourth to one-half of cases, it affects both the left and the right sides.

A slipped capital epiphysis is considered an emergency that requires hospitalization. If x-rays confirm the diagnosis, the child is put in traction in a hospital bed and prepared for surgery. If a slip is detected early, while it is still mild, it can be fixed with an operation in which metal pins are inserted to prevent further displacement. However, if the slip progresses until it is severe, it can deform the hip and interfere with normal walking. Even after extensive bone-cutting surgery to correct an advanced case, the child risks developing arthritis prematurely.

Osgood-Schlatter Disease

Children between 11 and 15 years, boys more frequently than girls, may have pain and swelling at the bony protuberance just below the kneecap, on the shinbone (tibia). This is the point at which tendons from the kneecap are inserted into the tibia. (It is also the point at which irritation from kneeling on hard surfaces can cause bursitis, known as housemaid's knee.)

Osgood-Schlatter disease is usually treated with rest and will resolve over time as the skeleton matures.

Congenital Dislocation of the Hip

In this condition, the hip socket into which the head of the femur fits is too shallow at birth, making the joint especially susceptible to dislocation. The problem can lead to an altered shape of the bones of the joint, which may require extensive surgery later in life.

Even if a baby appears to be entirely healthy, the pediatrician should be on the alert for this condition during the first year of life of the child. Early recognition can permit simple treatment with splinting, which is usually successful. Congenital dislocation of the hip tends to recur in families, so alert your pediatrician if you or your spouse had the condition.

Clubfoot

Technically known as talipes equinovarus, this sometimes hereditary deformity of the foot is present at birth. It can be treated with casts or splints during the first few years of life, usually with good results (see page 48).

Surgery. When a joint has become badly damaged or deformed, an operation may restore usefulness. Occasionally, joint replacement (see page 998) may be necessary for severely eroded joints.

JUVENILE RHEUMATOID ARTHRITIS

Signs and Symptoms
- Swelling and stiffness in the joints;
- Fever and skin rash;
- Fatigue and irritability;
- Associated inflammation of the eye.

Juvenile rheumatoid arthritis resembles rheumatoid arthritis (see page 997) but also differs in significant ways. Among the differences are the age of the typical patients (juvenile rheumatoid arthritis affects children, and rheumatoid arthritis affects adults) and the long-term nature of the ailment. In most cases, juvenile rheumatoid arthritis is not a lifelong disorder and its symptoms fade with adulthood.

There are several subcategories of the disorder, each with its own distinguishing characteristics. When four or fewer joints are affected, it is termed pauciarticular juvenile rheumatoid arthritis; children with this type tend to have little or no disability after several years of disease. The form called polyarticular juvenile rheumatoid arthritis is more virulent and the prognosis is frequently chronic joint problems. About two of every three children with acute febrile juvenile rheumatoid arthritis, another form, have no signs of active disease by adulthood. No causes of juvenile rheumatoid arthritis have been established.

The Diagnosis. The disorder is diagnosed on the basis of observed symptoms because there is no one test that confirms it. However, various blood tests may be conducted.

How Serious Is Juvenile Rheumatoid Arthritis? As with rheumatoid arthritis, there is a risk of permanent joint damage from juvenile rheumatoid arthritis. In addition, however, the growing child also may be in danger of experiencing abnormal bone growth. For example, the disease may accelerate growth in one leg bone but not in the other, producing one leg that is longer than the other.

Another risk is that a child will often instinctively keep an affected joint motionless to avoid pain. This can result in weakened and contracted muscles and even a deformity over time.

Treatment. In general, treatment resembles that for the adult form of rheumatoid arthritis (see page 997).

Medication. Aspirin is generally the preferred drug treatment; if aspirin is not well tolerated, other anti-inflammatory drugs may be prescribed.

Other Therapies. Range-of-motion exercises and splints to prevent loss of motion and deformity are used on affected joints.

A balance must be struck in order to maintain some semblance of normal activity and yet provide sufficient rest to avoid fatigue and excessive stress on affected joints. During periods of severe disease activity, bed rest or tutoring at home may be necessary, but it is important, for psychological and physical reasons, to avoid isolating a child from his or her normal routine.

Surgery. If severe joint damage is sustained, reconstructive procedures or joint replacement (see page 998) may be required, but in general it is advisable to wait until the affected joints have reached maturity.

INFLAMMATORY ARTHRITIS

Signs and Symptoms

Psoriatic Arthritis
- In the patient with psoriasis (see page 1160), an accompanying form of arthritis may occur, especially in the knee and elbow joints.

Reiter's Syndrome
- A form of arthritis transmitted by sexual contact, which is characterized not only by pain in the joints but also by a penile discharge (urethritis), a painful inflammation of the eye (conjunctivitis), and a skin rash.

Ankylosing Spondylitis
- A form of arthritis that affects the joints of the body's trunk, including the hips,

shoulders, and ribs, but especially the back and neck. Pain and stiffness are early signs, but in advanced cases a poker spine—a very stiff, inflexible backbone—is common.

Arthritis of Inflammatory Bowel Disease

• In patients with inflammatory bowel disease, a characteristic form of arthritis also may occur. Peripheral joints—those of the hands and feet, in particular—are affected most often, and the pain and stiffness are most noticeable in the morning.

All four of these forms of arthritis have a genetic factor. Each of them has characteristic gene markers that indicate a genetic predisposition to the disease. The presence of the marker can be established by a tissue-typing test, although the presence of a certain gene doesn't mean you will get these ailments. Rather, the gene confirms a tendency to the ailment and reinforces the observation that these disorders tend to recur within families. What makes one individual develop one of these disorders and another not remains a mystery.

Psoriatic Arthritis. Psoriasis is a common skin disease in which areas of the skin assume an inflamed, reddish color (see page 1160). The surface of the skin of the elbows and knees may become scaly. The fingernails may become pitted and discolored. In about 1 in 10 people with psoriasis, the skin problem is accompanied by psoriatic arthritis. More women than men suffer from these ailments, and typically they strike persons in their 20s and 30s.

In most people, the effects of psoriatic arthritis are minor, resulting in some pain and discomfort in affected joints but having little effect on overall health.

Treatment. In most cases, simple anti-inflammatory drugs such as aspirin and range-of-motion exercises are the basic treatments. In more difficult cases, stronger drugs also may be prescribed.

Reiter's Syndrome. Although not well understood, Reiter's syndrome usually appears in stages. The penile discharge occurs first, generally after sexual exposure to the infection. Some time later (a few days or weeks), joint pain occurs, often in the knee, heel, or fingers. Skin lesions such as those of psoria-

sis may also appear, as may an eye inflammation called conjunctivitis (see page 759).

Reiter's syndrome may appear once or episodically. Attacks tend to last a few weeks or months. It occurs only in persons with a genetic predisposition to it and primarily in whites (blacks rarely get it). Reiter's syndrome rarely leads to permanent damage to the joints, although the inflammation of an acute attack can produce tenderness and pain. Reiter's syndrome is the most common cause of arthritis in young men.

Treatment. Anti-inflammatory drugs such as aspirin usually are prescribed to treat Reiter's syndrome, but stronger drugs also may be prescribed.

Ankylosing Spondylitis. Individuals with this disorder have the same gene marker that is found in persons with Reiter's syndrome. It tends to be an inherited disorder—more than half of those who have ankylosing spondylitis have relatives who also have it.

Over time, the affected vertebrae in the person with ankylosing spondylitis will fuse, producing this characteristically stooped-over posture.

Males are affected more often than females, generally during the third decade of life. Occasionally, the patient already has inflammatory bowel disease (see Crohn's Disease, page 626, and Ulcerative Colitis, page 628).

The name is derived from Greek words that identify the characteristic symptoms: rigid *(ankylosing)* spine *(spondyl)* with accompanying inflammation *(itis)*. The usual disease course involves a soreness in the spine and other joints of the trunk. As the disease progresses, the affected bones begin to grow together, rendering the joints immovable. In addition, some people develop a peripheral arthritis resembling rheumatoid arthritis.

In most cases, ankylosing spondylitis is a mild condition, often going undiagnosed for decades; in rare cases, it can be crippling. In serious cases, eye, heart, and other complications may result.

Treatment.   The chronic pain and stiffness may be relieved with anti-inflammatory drugs. However, essential to treatment is a program of physical exercise. In part, this means proceeding with regular activity as much as possible, but it also means habitually performing range-of-motion and stretching exercises to combat the tendency of ankylosing spondylitis to reduce flexibility. Good posture is important (see The Importance of Posture, page 989), and smoking is discouraged because of the long-term potential for the disorder to limit air exchange because of its effects on the rib cage. A surgical procedure may be an option in advanced cases.

Arthritis of Inflammatory Bowel Disease.
In about 1 of 10 patients with ulcerative colitis (see page 628) and 1 of 5 with Crohn's disease (see page 626), one or more sore joints accompany the digestive disorder.

Treatment.   In the short-term, the joint pain, often in the hands or feet, usually is treated with aspirin or other anti-inflammatory drug. Control or cure of the inflammatory bowel disorder is the long-term solution.

INFECTIOUS ARTHRITIS

Signs and Symptoms
- Pain and stiffness in one joint, typically a knee, shoulder, hip, ankle, elbow, finger, or wrist;
- The surrounding tissues are warm and red;
- Chills, fever, and weakness.

Emergency Symptoms
- If you have all three of the above-described signs and symptoms, immediate medical attention is required.

A joint infection can be caused by bacteria, virus, or fungus. Typically, the infecting agent enters the body and spreads to the joint via the bloodstream. In some instances, an open wound or puncture provides the infection direct access to the joint.

Infectious arthritis, unlike other joint disorders, can occur in anyone at any time: the infecting agents are not limited by a person's age, sex, or race.

What Are the Types of Infectious Arthritis?

Lyme Disease.   Lyme disease is named for the town on the Connecticut coast where it was first observed. It is contracted from a tick bite. Usually, a disc-shaped rash will develop around the bite, and other symptoms may follow, including fever, chills, sore throat, fatigue, and nausea. Some weeks later, stiffness and pain may occur in the joints. Because of the time lapse between symptoms, Lyme arthritis, as it is also known, is not always diagnosed correctly (see page 854).

Gonococcal.   Roughly a third of those who contract gonorrhea, a sexually transmitted bacterial disease (see page 875), also experience pain in several joints. A rash also may result. This type of infectious arthritis is reported 10 times more frequently in women than in men.

Staphylococcal.   When a boil or other infection releases the staphylococcal bacterium into the bloodstream, it can spread to a knee or other joint. The pain is usually intense and sudden.

Tuberculous.   A small number of people with tuberculosis have an accompanying arthritis. The symptoms are usually few, so it may go undiagnosed. If you have tuberculosis and experience slight joint pain, consult your physician.

Viral. Arthritis symptoms may occur in persons who have hepatitis B, rubella (German measles), mumps, and other diseases caused by viruses. In general, however, the arthritis requires no specific treatment but resolves with the treatment of and recovery from the underlying disease.

The Diagnosis. If your physician suspects a form of infectious arthritis, he or she may remove fluid from the joint with a needle in order to conduct laboratory tests. Blood tests may also be done.

How Serious Is Infectious Arthritis? In most cases, prompt diagnosis and treatment of a joint infection result in a rapid and complete recovery.

Treatment. Because of the risk of permanent damage to the bone or cartilage, a joint infection needs to be treated immediately. Unless the cause of the infection is viral, an antibiotic drug will be prescribed. Hospitalization may be necessary, and a needle may be used to drain the infected joint or the joint may be opened surgically and damaged tissues removed. If serious damage has been sustained, surgical reconstruction of the joint may be necessary.

During recuperation from an infection, the joint may be immobilized with a splint. After the infection has been eliminated, physical therapy may be necessary to regain strength and mobility in the affected joint.

GOUT

Signs and Symptoms
- Severe pain that strikes suddenly in a single joint, often at the base of your big toe;
- Accompanying swelling and redness.

Also called crystal-induced arthritis, gout occurs when uric acid crystals accumulate in the affected joint. Some uric acid is derived from a food substance in the diet known as purines, but the greater part is produced by our bodies daily. If you have gout, the normal balance is lost: too much uric acid is produced by your body or too little is excreted. When the amount of uric acid in your blood and body fluids increases, uric acid in the

---

RHEUMATIC FEVER ARTHRITIS

The management of rheumatic fever is one of modern medicine's success stories. Once it caused serious heart problems in many children. With the advent of antibiotic drugs, however, its risks have been reduced greatly, especially with prompt treatment.

However, a form of arthritis is a common side effect of the illness. This form of arthritis characteristically occurs several weeks after a streptococcal infection, usually of the throat. Your joints become swollen, reddened, and painful to move. Typically, your joints are affected in a manner often described as migratory: first, one joint is painful for a time and then the pain seems to migrate to another joint.

Rheumatic fever arthritis is not strictly an infectious arthritis but rather is a hypersensitivity reaction in the joints. In general, the treatment of rheumatic fever arthritis is the same as that for rheumatic fever, although your physician may remove fluids from swollen joints with a needle in order to reduce the discomfort (see Rheumatic Fever, page 823).

---

fluid around the joints (synovial fluid) forms crystals and gout results, typically in the joint at the base of the big toe.

Ninety percent of gout sufferers are men older than 40; 1 in 4 has a family history of the ailment. Gout has long had a reputation for being an illness that results from the excessive consumption of food and drink, but gout can strike at any time and for no apparent reason. People who are obese or who suffer from hypertension may be at greater risk for crystal-induced arthritis. An attack may be provoked by the stress of an injury such as a fracture or a surgical procedure. Thiazide diuretics, a common treatment of high blood pressure that reduces the water content of the body, may raise uric acid levels in the blood and provoke gout in the susceptible person.

The Diagnosis. An episode of gout begins within a matter of hours. A joint that seemed entirely normal will become intensely painful, red, and swollen. The joint will remain very painful for several days, although the discomfort will subside gradually over the next 1 to 2 weeks, and the joint will be left apparently normal and pain-free. Even though the joint at the base of the great toe is involved most frequently, other joints in the feet, ankles, knees, hands, and wrists may be affected.

To confirm the diagnosis, your physician may withdraw some fluid from the affected joint to look for crystals of uric acid within the white blood cells. Blood tests for levels of uric acid also may be done, but they can be misleading because the levels may be nearly normal during an acute attack of gout. In addition, many people with high levels of uric acid never experience an attack of crystal-induced arthritis.

Sometimes, a long-term accumulation of uric acid may produce lumps, called tophi, just beneath the skin. The most common site is the cartilage of the ear.

What Is Pseudogout?   Pseudogout is a related ailment that involves the deposit of crystals of a calcium salt rather than uric acid in the joints. The affected joints are more likely to be knees, wrists, and ankles than those of the foot. Pseudogout strikes women and men with roughly equal frequency, but the age at onset is late, typically 70 years. The ailment is also known as calcium pyrophosphate dihydrate crystal deposition disease.

How Serious Is Gout?   Acute attacks can be treated effectively and future attacks can be prevented with maintenance medication. After an attack has run its course (usually a matter of days and no more than a few weeks), the affected joint usually returns to normal. When the ailment is not properly treated, however, permanent joint damage and kidney problems caused by uric acid deposits or even stones may result.

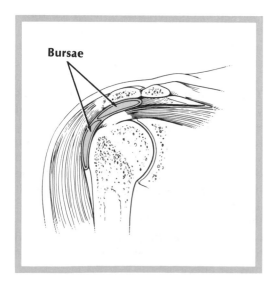

Treatment.   *Medication.*   Colchicine, in use for centuries, is still valuable for acute attacks of gout. Indomethacin also can be used for acute attacks. Other drugs, including probenecid and allopurinol, may be used between attacks to control the levels of uric acid in the body.

Pseudogout is usually treated with anti-inflammatory drugs, although colchicine is effective in some cases.

Nutrition.   Although food and drink are no longer thought to be the main factors causing gout, if you have gout, avoid excessive consumption of alcohol, maintain your weight within reasonable limits, and avoid foods that contain purines. Purine-rich foods include sardines, anchovies, sweetbreads, liver, and kidney. Remember, attempts at rapid weight reduction may provoke an acute attack.

ACUTE PAINFUL SHOULDER

Signs and Symptoms
- Pain in your shoulder;
- Limited range of motion;
- Pain in your upper arm or neck.

Also known as frozen shoulder, bicipital tendinitis, and periarthritis of the shoulder, acute painful shoulder occurs at the point where the tendon of the biceps muscle passes, like a rope through a pulley, over the head of the humerus (upper arm bone). Inflammation can develop easily in this area, often for no particular reason, although excessive use of the shoulder may be the cause.

An acute attack may occur suddenly and remain painful for several weeks or more than a month. Pain may extend well into the biceps area.

Motion, particularly extending your arm to the side or putting on a coat, may produce pain. Some people may hold the affected arm close to the body and avoid moving it. However, if the joint is not extended through its range of motion with some frequency, even during the acute phase when it is painful to do so, ligaments and other tissues about the joint will stiffen and the shoulder will freeze. Movement of the joint will then be very limited, even after the inflammation subsides.

Bursae

Overuse of a joint can lead to bursitis, an inflammation of the bursa, which serves as a cushion between bone and fibrous tissue (see page 1006).

Episodes of acute painful shoulder tend to recur. In some instances, the biceps will actually tear, requiring surgical repair. In such cases, there will be a visible distortion or bulge near the shoulder and accompanying pain.

In other cases, the ligaments that surround the shoulder joint (the rotator cuff) also may be torn. The symptoms may resemble those of acute painful shoulder, but a shoulder cuff tear can be distinguished by the finding that the shoulder can be moved readily to the side and overhead by someone else, whereas the injured person is unable to accomplish these motions. Again, surgical repair of the tear may be needed.

Treatment. *Medication.* During the acute phase of frozen shoulder, your physician probably will prescribe anti-inflammatory drugs in generous amounts. In very severe instances, prednisone may be given by mouth for limited periods. If pain and inflammation persist, a prednisone injection into the joint may be helpful (see Corticosteroid Drugs, below).

Other Therapies. Your physician will determine the amount of motion to be performed each day. If, despite exercise, your shoulder remains too limited in its range of motion, the joint may be forcibly put

---

CORTICOSTEROID DRUGS

Corticosteroid drugs are modified forms of the human hormones cortisone and hydrocortisone made in the adrenal gland. This family of drugs has an important place in the treatment program of today's physician.

The Uses

The corticosteroid drugs have a strong anti-inflammatory effect that will reduce the swelling, pain, redness, and heat of sore joints. In addition to their obvious value in treating disorders of the adrenal glands, corticosteroids can be invaluable remedies for a wide range of other ailments, including skin diseases, allergies, certain tumors, and numerous types of arthritis and other musculoskeletal problems. These drugs can be taken in tablet form for a sustained period (sometimes for years), applied topically to the skin, dropped into the eye, or injected directly into a localized area. They also are used for long periods to prevent rejection of the transplanted organ in persons who have had transplantation.

The Risks

With sustained, long-term use of corticosteroid drugs, the risk of side effects is great. The adrenal glands tend to atrophy. Weight gain, a loss of bone mineral akin to that in osteoporosis (see page 982), muscle weakness, water retention, hypertension, a rounding of the facial features (commonly called moonface), thinning of the skin, and other problems also can result. No individual suffers all of these side effects, of course, and with short-term use the chances of having none are good. The risks with topically applied corticosteroid medications are regarded as so small that they are now available without a prescription.

For persons who take prednisone daily for 3 to 6 months or longer, particularly if side effects such as rounding of the face and thinning of the skin have occurred, the adrenal glands may have atrophied and the related function of the pituitary gland may have decreased. In such cases, the adrenal glands no longer can produce the needed amounts of hydrocortisone when the body is faced with the stress of surgery, severe infection, or injury, and the person may die for lack of the hormone. When such persons have a

surgical procedure or sustain injury, physicians prescribe generous amounts of prednisone or other corticosteroid drugs, which are given intravenously or by muscle injection to provide for the increased hormonal needs.

If you take prednisone daily, have this information readily available in case of an emergency.

Cortisone by Injection

Cortisone injections have remarkable effects for the treatment of such acute conditions as bursitis and tendinitis. Also, they are invaluable for relieving the pain and swelling in individual joints affected by chronic osteoarthritis or rheumatoid arthritis. Often, a single injection will relieve an acute condition permanently, but more injections can be given if necessary. However, as few as six injections within a 12-month period can damage bone and joint structure, so your physician is unlikely to administer more than three or four within a calendar year.

Corticosteroid drugs differ from anabolic steroid preparations (male sex hormones), which sometimes are inappropriately used by athletes to increase muscle bulk (see page 439).

through its normal range of motion while you are under a general anesthetic.

BURSITIS

Signs and Symptoms
- Pain and swelling in the area of your elbow, hip, knee, shoulder, big toe, or other joint.

A bursa is a sac-like membrane found in many joints (there are actually 78 on each side of the body). The bursa acts as a cushion between the bone and the fibrous tissues of the muscles and tendons, facilitating movement by limiting the friction. When a bursa becomes inflamed, the resultant disorder is termed bursitis (see page 1004).

Repeated physical activity often leads to bursitis: throwing a baseball and swinging a tennis racket are common causes. Job-related tasks also can lead to bursitis, as typified by housemaid's knee (in which the bursa at the front of the knee becomes inflamed). Bursitis usually can be traced to events of overuse or pressure, but there may be no such obvious cause.

The Diagnosis. Your physician will conduct a physical examination and inquire about recent activities. By palpation, he or she may also identify tenderness in a localized area. If another cause of the discomfort is suspected, an x-ray may be taken of the affected area; if bursitis is the cause, the x-ray images will be normal.

Treatment. Bursitis usually disappears within 2 weeks, given reasonable care of the painful joint. Anti-inflammatory drugs such as aspirin may help relieve the discomfort. A local injection of a corticosteroid drug also may be given (see Corticosteroid Drugs, page 1005).

When bursitis occurs repeatedly in the same joint, the affected bursa may be removed surgically.

CONNECTIVE TISSUE DISEASES

Collagen is a fibrous protein found in your skin, bone, ligaments, and cartilage—in fact, the connective tissue collagen is an essential element of every part of your body. It normally functions as a network or frame for many tissues, including the liver, muscles, and heart. Some disorders (for example, systemic lupus erythematosus, scleroderma, and polymyositis) involve inflammation of the collagen.

The characteristic common to all these disorders is inflammation of the connective tissue, an inflammation that is of unknown cause. Many physicians believe that the body's own defense mechanism, the autoimmune system, malfunctions and begins to attack itself, damaging the skin, muscles, and other body parts.

SYSTEMIC LUPUS ERYTHEMATOSUS

Signs and Symptoms
- Joint pain, swelling, and redness that come and go from day to day, most often in your fingers and wrists;
- Rashes, especially across the nose and cheeks;
- Localized chest pain accompanied by coughing;
- Sunlight sensitivity that produces rash and fever reactions;
- Inexplicable fatigue.

Systemic lupus erythematosus is a chronic disease of unknown origin. It typically affects the synovial membrane in the joints, producing pain and inflammation. Both the joint discomforts and the rash tend to be episodic, with alternating periods of remission and flares.

The typical person with lupus is a female between the ages of 15 and 35 years. Ten times as many women as men have systemic lupus erythematosus. Lupus sometimes appears for the first time during pregnancy, usually with little or no effect on the unborn child.

The Diagnosis. The condition can be diagnosed with an antinuclear antibody test to determine whether a particular protein, typically found in the blood of lupus patients, is present. A blood test for rheumatoid factor may be done; a creatinine test also may be used because lupus can have effects on kidney function.

How Serious Is Lupus?   For many people with lupus, the disease is not a major illness. For some, however, it is a serious disease that must be managed carefully in order to avoid serious complications that can result in internal bleeding, reduced resistance to infection, depression, kidney disease, and serious joint damage. Typically, lupus is a lifelong ailment that comes and goes. As its name implies, it may affect virtually every organ system in the body.

Treatment.   *Medication.*   The approach to systemic lupus erythematosus depends on its severity, but the major treatments involve medications. Corticosteroids (see page 1005), anti-inflammatory agents, and other drugs often are used.

Other Therapies.   Avoidance of excessive exposure to the ultraviolet rays in sunlight is often recommended, but discuss this and other strategies with your physician. Because of long-term risks associated with lupus, your physician will want to monitor the changing status of the disease.

SCLERODERMA

Signs and Symptoms
- A thickening and tightening of the skin, especially on your arms, face, or hands, resulting in a loss of flexibility;
- Puffy hands and feet, particularly in the morning;
- Joint pain and stiffness.

Scleroderma, also known as progressive systemic sclerosis, means hard *(sclero)* skin *(derma)*. This disorder leads not only to a hardening of the skin but also to a permanent shine and tightness of the affected tissues.

As with other connective tissue disorders, the protein collagen is affected by scleroderma. The exact cause is unknown, but the disease course involves the development of excessive collagen in the skin, producing the hardened effect. Two theories about the cause of scleroderma are a malfunction of the body's immune system and the gradual failure of tiny blood vessels in the skin. The latter theory may help explain the thickening and hardening of the collagen.

Most people with scleroderma contract it between the ages of 20 and 40 years, although it is not unheard of in children and the elderly. Women are about 4 times as likely to get scleroderma as men.

The Diagnosis.   Your physician will conduct a thorough physical examination if scleroderma is suspected, and special attention will be given to the skin of your hands, face, feet, and arms (see color photograph, page B-16). The physician may inquire about the presence of Raynaud's phenomenon, a tendency for the skin color of the fingers to change from a dead white pallor to a blue and finally a pinkish hue. This may occur with emotional stress or exposure to cold.

A biopsy, in which a tissue sample is removed for laboratory study, also may be done on affected skin.

How Serious Is Scleroderma?   The usual course of the disease involves an initial phase of approximately 2 years during which the affected tissues harden and stiffen. After that time, the skin effects of the disorder are unlikely to progress and may even lessen somewhat, although in rare instances the hands may be crippled permanently.

In a minority of people, organ involvement can occur, producing hypertension, lung problems, kidney failure, and intestinal tract problems that can lead to malnutrition. In rare cases, these long-term effects can be life-threatening.

Treatment.   *Medication.*   The approach depends on the severity of the case, but there is no known treatment for this condition. Your physician may prescribe a blood vessel dilator if Raynaud's phenomenon is present; hypertensive drugs to treat high blood pressure; analgesics like aspirin for joint pain; antibiotics for intestinal problems.

Other Therapies.   Exercise is essential for cases in which the skin is affected. Movement can limit the stiffening effects and help maintain blood flow.

Because nicotine causes the blood vessels to contract, cessation of smoking is recommended.

When hands are to be subjected to cold (such as by reaching into a freezer), gloves should be worn for protection.

If heartburn occurs, antireflux measures (see page 593) can be used and eating should be avoided in the 3 to 4 hours before bedtime. An antacid medication also may be recommended to protect the esophagus (see page 594).

SJÖGREN'S SYNDROME

Signs and Symptoms
- Dryness about the eye, characterized by a feeling of sandiness or grittiness in the eye;
- Dry mouth.

This disorder often accompanies rheumatoid arthritis (see page 997) or other ailments such as lupus (see page 1006), scleroderma (see page 1007), or polymyositis (see below). Most people who suffer from Sjögren's syndrome are middle-aged women.

The eyes become red, dry, and painful. They may feel as if a foreign body has become lodged in the eye but, on examination, none is found.

Treatment. ***Medication.***   Eye drops may be useful for treating the discomfort in the eyes; dry mouth may be relieved by stimulating the production of saliva. Corticosteroids or other drugs may be prescribed in severe cases.

POLYMYOSITIS AND DERMATOMYOSITIS

Signs and Symptoms
- Weakness in the hip or shoulder muscles;
- Pain, swelling, heat, and redness in the small joints;
- Reddish patches of skin on the face, knuckles, elbows, knees, or ankles.

Polymyositis is a rare disorder in which the muscles *(myo)* become inflamed *(itis)*; when a skin inflammation accompanies the muscle weakness, the disorder is termed "dermatomyositis" (from the Greek word *derma* for skin).

Adults between 30 and 60 years of age and children between 5 and 15 years old are most likely to have these disorders, but they can strike at any age. Women are about twice as likely to have polymyositis or dermatomyositis.

The Diagnosis.   Your physician will perform a physical examination and inquire about the symptoms. The accompanying weakness may make it difficult to climb stairs or even comb your hair.

Blood tests may be done to determine the presence of certain muscle enzymes and rheumatoid factor (see page 1283). A test called electromyography, which measures the electrical patterns of your muscles, may also be done (see page 1294). In addition, a biopsy, in which a tissue sample is removed for laboratory study, may be conducted on affected muscles.

How Serious Are Dermatomyositis and Polymyositis?   Dermatomyositis and polymyositis can disappear within a few months after they develop; however, they also can be fatal. A particular danger is the potential effect on the muscles of the throat, making swallowing difficult. Lung problems also may occur.

Treatment. ***Medication.***   The primary treatment of polymyositis or dermatomyositis is medication. Prednisone (see Corticosteroid Drugs, page 1005) is the key drug, although other medications may be used if prednisone does not relieve the symptoms.

Other Therapies.   Once the medication begins to take effect, your physician will recommend an exercise program.

POLYMYALGIA RHEUMATICA

Signs and Symptoms
- Pain and stiffness in the muscles of your

VASCULITIS

Vasculitis is a term used to describe conditions caused by inflammation and damage to the blood vessels, especially the arteries. Inflamed arteries may cause various general symptoms such as fever, weakness, and malaise or, if a particular organ is involved, may cause more specific symptoms such as abdominal pain if the arteries to the gut are involved.

In general, no specific blood tests can be used to diagnose the various forms of vasculitis, including polyarteritis, allergic angiitis and granulomatosis, hypersensitivity vasculitis, and cranial arteritis. With these ailments, the erythrocyte sedimentation rate is often elevated (see page 1283). The diagnosis is confirmed by removing a segment of an artery for laboratory examination (see Biopsies, page 1284).

Corticosteroids, at the lowest dose that prevents symptoms, are most often used for treatment. Occasionally, aspirin is also effective for treating the following conditions.

Polyarteritis

This serious disorder involves an inflammation *(itis)* of many *(poly)* arteries. Inflammation can result in obstruction of the vessels, reducing the supply of blood reaching the affected area. The skin, intestines, kidney, and heart are at greatest risk; typical symptoms include weight loss, fever, weakness, and fatigue. Occasionally, if the lung is affected, asthma symptoms may occur or, if the gut is involved, abdominal pain and bloody diarrhea may occur.

Middle-aged men are the most likely to suffer from polyarteritis, although there is a juvenile form of the illness. In the past, this disease was often fatal; but with proper treatment many persons with polyarteritis can lead normal lives.

Allergic Angiitis and Granulomatosis

Also called Churg-Strauss disease, this ailment closely resembles polyarteritis nodosa, but the lungs usually are involved in allergic angiitis. Asthmatic attacks are common. Blood and erythrocyte sedimentation rate tests (see page 1283) may be done to confirm the diagnosis.

Hypersensitivity Vasculitis

This form of vasculitis is the result of exposure to a drug or foreign agent. Occasionally, the skin is involved.

Cranial Arteritis

This disorder occurs almost exclusively in people older than 50 years and affects women more often than men. Also termed temporal or giant cell arteritis, this condition is characterized by headache and a tender, thickened artery that can be felt at the side of the head. Malaise, fatigue, loss of appetite, weight loss, and sweating are common accompanying symptoms. Occasionally, pain on chewing and vision problems also are experienced.

The diagnosis is suspected from the medical history, and it will be confirmed by biopsy of a piece of the affected artery. Recovery is the general rule, although in some cases it requires 1 to 2 years of treatment with corticosteroid drugs or aspirin.

---

lower back, thighs, and hips or neck, shoulders, and upper arms;
• Slight fever, fatigue, and weight loss.

The name of this ailment is from the Greek words that mean many *(poly)* muscles *(myo)* in pain *(algia)*. Rheumatica (or its equivalent, rheumatism) is an ancient word for muscle and joint soreness.

Polymyalgia rheumatica is thought to be the result of an inflammation of the blood vessels that serve the muscles. It affects elderly people, usually those older than 50 years, and is more common in whites than in other races. Women are affected more often than men.

The Diagnosis. Information about the onset of the pain is important for diagnosis. In polymyalgia rheumatica, the pain usually strikes suddenly and may involve most muscles, although the neck and shoulders are often the most painful. The discomfort is likely to be worse in the morning, but it may occur at night also. There are no specific tests to confirm the diagnosis, but certain x-ray or laboratory tests may be used to eliminate other possible causes for the discomfort.

How Serious Is It? Left untreated, polymyalgia rheumatica may lead to eye problems and weight loss. However, the typical disease course is about 5 years, after which it usually disappears. It may be associated with inflammation and tenderness in arteries just under the scalp (see Cranial Arteritis, page 1009) or other major arteries in the body. A biopsy of an artery may be appropriate.

Treatment. Corticosteroids (see page 1005) usually will produce improvement within a few days. These drugs usually are used in the smallest dose that will control the symptoms until the disease runs its course. Aspirin and other anti-inflammatory drugs also may be prescribed.

CHAPTER 33

MENTAL HEALTH

CHAPTER CONTENTS

THOUGHT DISORDERS
   Schizophrenia
   Brief Reactive Psychosis
   Alcohol- or Drug-Induced
      Psychosis

ADDICTIVE BEHAVIOR
   Alcohol Dependency
   Compulsive Gambling
   Caffeine Addiction

DRUG DEPENDENCY
   Central Nervous System
      Depressants
   Central Nervous System Stimulants

   Opioids
      Detoxification
      Hallucinogens
   Marijuana and Cannabis
      Compounds

PSYCHOSOMATIC ILLNESS
Conversion Disorder
Somatization Disorder
Hypochondriasis
   Minnesota Multiphasic Personality
      Inventory (MMPI)
Chronic Pain Disorders
   Chronic Pain Centers

WHAT IS MENTAL HEALTH?

Defining mental health is difficult—professionals have debated this for generations. Mental health does not imply an absence of emotion or conflict but rather an ability to cope with life's transitions, traumatic experiences, and losses in a way that allows your personality to remain intact and even contributes to emotional growth.

Instead of attempting to repress all conflicts and distress, the mentally healthy person learns to accept them, to understand them, and to cope with his or her reactions to them so that life can go on.

Thus, a definition of mental health to some degree is bound by culture and circumstances. Different cultures have different ways of coping with stress. For example, in one country the death of a close relative may be received with wailing while in another the ability to carry on without a display of emotion is considered healthy. Behavior that is considered highly erratic in one culture may be perfectly acceptable in another.

Within the bounds of everyday life, however, there are certain traits that are characteristic of mental health. The ability to function may be the most obvious. A mentally healthy person is able to sustain relationships with family and friends and to carry out his or her responsibilities in the workplace and at home. Such responsibilities may vary—holding down a steady job, caring for children, or some other activity—but the common denominator for the mentally healthy is the ability to meet these responsibilities with some semblance of harmony with loved ones and society (see Controlling Stress, page 399).

The healthy person also has a realistic perception of the motivations of others. Although not always accurate, these perceptions do not involve bizarre delusions such as imagining that the mailman is planning to hurl a Molotov cocktail at one's front door. Unlike a psychotic, the theoretically "healthy person" has normal thought processes that are essentially logical and reasonable. The process of conversing with others is similarly reasoned and rational. Ideas proceed in a rational manner from one to the next, rather than jumping helter-skelter.

DEFINITIONS

In our society, anxiety and lack of self-esteem may be the two biggest obstacles to achieving mental health. Anxiety may be a symptom of unresolved or stressful conflict. At times, anxiety may be made evident by actual physical symptoms. A person's lack of self-esteem may be the result of failing to live up to expectations. In addition, complaints of fatigue, insomnia, and poor concentration are common and may be clues to an underlying depressive disorder.

The term "personality" suggests characteristic ways of thinking, behaving, and reacting to one's surroundings. When an individual habitually uses inappropriate or stereotyped ways of coping with his or her environment, he or she is said to have a personality disorder.

If a person's thinking processes are disordered by delusions, hallucinations, or both, the condition is known as psychosis. Schizophrenia is an example.

The state called dementia is a progressive and incapacitating deterioration of mental capability as a result of organic brain disease. Brain tissue function is impaired to such a degree that there is a decrease in or loss of intellectual abilities that affects social interactions or occupational performance. Probably the most striking feature of dementia is memory loss, although depression or anxiety also can occur. Alzheimer's disease is one familiar and much discussed example. Dementia usually is irreversible.

Because dementia generally is the result of organic brain disorders, it is discussed in the chapter titled The Brain and Nervous System (see page 503).

Even when your physician suspects a psychiatric disorder, he or she should give due consideration to the possibility that medical diseases are producing the symptoms and signs. The possibility of an underlying medical condition should be eliminated by appropriate laboratory and radiological tests; only then is a psychiatric diagnosis appropriate.

Many common psychiatric disorders can be treated by your family physician. In some situations, referral to a mental health specialist such as a psychiatrist or psychologist will be needed.

A psychiatrist is a medical doctor (M.D.) who completed a 4-year course of study in a recognized medical school and 4 years of postgraduate training (residency) in the specialty of psychiatry. Most psychiatrists are certified as specialists in psychiatry by the American Board of Psychiatry and Neurology. Some psychiatrists subspecialize in subjects such as child and adolescent psychiatry, geriatric psychiatry, or forensic psychiatry. Because psychiatrists are physicians and trained in the use of drugs, they may use medications and write prescriptions.

A psychologist is a person trained in the specialized area of dealing with emotional issues in people. Most psychologists have an advanced degree (Ph.D.) and additional clinical internship training in dealing with patients. Psychologists perform psychometric evaluations of patients, use psychotherapy, and sometimes carry out biofeedback relaxation techniques. Psychologists do not prescribe medications or do physical examinations on their patients. Many psychologists are involved in psychological research and some specialize in helping certain types of patients such as those with physical or sexual impairments.

A psychoanalyst is a psychiatrist or psychologist who has had special training in the practice of psychoanalysis, which is a form of psychotherapy. Psychoanalysis is a highly specialized type of therapy and usually is available only in the larger cities for a limited number of problems.

When a person suspected to have a psychiatric disorder is referred to a psychiatrist or psychologist, this mental health professional will conduct a mental status examination to test thinking patterns. Orientation, level of awareness, thought, attention, and judgment will be evaluated in an attempt to gain some insight into the person's illness. The psychiatrist or psychologist will evaluate emotional state and behavior and determine whether there is any evidence of disorders of perception such as hallucinations or disorders of memory.

We will introduce the term "nervous breakdown" only to discard it. At times the term is used to describe a serious mental illness in a person who is unable to deal with the stresses and strains of ordinary life. However, the term is not very specific and thus is not helpful in diagnosing a mental health problem and making recommendations for treatment.

This chapter discusses a host of common psychiatric problems. Some of the ailments are true diseases or disorders; others may be matters of personal adjustment to a life-change or specific event.

DEVELOPMENTAL PROBLEMS

Mental health is not the absence of conflict—it is the ability to cope with it. As we progress through life, most of us encounter certain predictable patterns of conflict. Being able to recognize these as such, rather than assuming that our difficulties are unique, can be very reassuring.

For centuries, as far back as the ancient Hindus, mankind has recognized various stages of life. For example, Shakespeare referred to the "seven ages of man." Contemporary psychologists speak of a predictable pattern of adjustments that people make as they pass from infancy and childhood through the teenage years on to adulthood and into old age.

ADJUSTING TO ADOLESCENCE

Interest in sexuality is a hallmark of the teenage years, a period when puberty turns the child's body into that of an adult. But, contrary to popular belief, the teenager is rapidly maturing in many other aspects of life.

The adolescent's most important question is "Who am I?" and the effort to answer it usually points away from parents and toward the peer group. His or her quest for personal identity and separation from family may involve acting "cool," experimenting with smoking, drinking, or sex, and wearing unusual or sexually suggestive clothing. This process of breaking away can be frustrating to parents. But rebellion is an essential part of the adolescent's attempt to take responsibility for his or her own behavior and direction.

The adjustment to adolescence can be viewed as a three-stage process. During early adolescence (ages 12 to 15), the theme is separation. The intense ties to parents and siblings characteristic of childhood are dissolving, and the adolescent is likely to be increasingly anxious and emotionally fragile. He or she may express the emotional upheaval by a behavior that is often termed "acting out"—dressing like a rock star, writing graffiti, or losing interest in school achievement.

Middle adolescence (ages 16 to 18) is a time of coming to terms with sexual identity and relationships with the opposite sex. For many teenagers this means being recognized as a "real man" or a "real woman," often through provocative dress and behavior. By late adolescence (ages 18 to 20), the young person is resolving the separation problem and is preoccupied with establishing his or her adult identity, particularly in terms of career. Although adolescence is a time of turmoil and rebellion for many, the majority of teenagers pass through this phase of life relatively smoothly (see The Teenage Years, page 141).

ADJUSTING TO ADULTHOOD

During young adulthood—from the early 20s to the early or middle 40s—men and women are faced with critical decisions and choices. Most enter into a career, select a mate, and establish a family. This means giving up the free time enjoyed as children and adolescents in order to get on with the business of life.

For most young adults, this is a period when intimacy and isolation are the major emotional issues. The emotional disorders of this time typically reflect anguish or protest against failures at intimacy.

The onset of middle adulthood—mid-life or middle age—begins in the fifth decade of life and, psychologically speaking, tends to occur somewhat earlier in women than in men. In mid-life, it is normal to look back at the road not taken, to review past successes and failures, satisfactions and disappointments, and to evaluate them in the context of youthful dreams and aspirations. The childless individual may have to come to terms with the family that he or she might have had. Parents whose children are leaving home face the "empty nest." Men see consolidation of their career and may become concerned about decreasing sexual desire and performance. By mid-life we begin to recognize our own limitations as well as our own mortality.

At this stage it is also not uncommon to feel trapped—by financial burdens, by social and professional roles, and even by chronology, as the generation caught between the responsibilities for aging parents and those for children. To cope, the person at mid-life may try to escape or repress negative feelings or may begin to turn outward toward the rest of society and feel ready to "make a contribution" to others (see Young Adulthood, page 167, and The Middle Years, page 223).

ADJUSTING TO AGING

Emotional adjustment during old age is greatly affected by the decline most people experience in physical health. At least 3 of every 4 people past age 65 have at least one chronic physical disorder; 1 of 10 finds it difficult to move about away from home. By this age less than 20 percent of men—and even fewer women—are still in the work force. Major losses, such as the death of a spouse, have occurred, and one quarter of people over 65 live alone. Fifteen percent suffer from either a functional or an organic brain disorder, such as Alzheimer's disease, and 5 percent are in nursing homes.

As a result of such limitations, older people often feel isolated, lack social contacts, and lose out on intellectual stimulation, all of which tend to contribute to a decrease in mental capacities (see The Later Years, page 235).

PROBLEMS IN CHILDHOOD

Despite its image as a carefree time of life, childhood is far from easy. Many children experience emotional difficulties of one sort or another as they deal with a wide range of issues including self-control, learning to socialize with peers, and separation from parents.

As a result, it is not uncommon for parents to become easily alarmed, wondering whether every nightmare is an indication of phobia or every hectic day is a sure sign of hyperactivity. For the most part, however, serious emotional problems are diagnosed on the basis of a long-term pattern of symptoms and not the occasional wet bed or playground fight.

In the pages that follow are some of the more common childhood problems that have mental or psychiatric origins (see also School Phobias, page 137).

ENURESIS

Signs and Symptoms
- Involuntary voiding of urine at least twice a month by a child at least 5 years old.

"Mommy, I wet my bed." Virtually every parent hears those words at one time or another, and many young children do have "accidents" during the night now and then.

However, true enuresis is the involuntary voiding of urine at least twice a month in a child age 5 or older. Usually it does not indicate an emotional problem. Children vary markedly in the age at which they are physiologically ready to stop wetting.

If the child has never been totally dry for a year, the condition is known as primary enuresis. Eighty percent of children who wet their bed suffer from primary enuresis. Secondary enuresis is when the child has had a dry period of at least a year before the appearance of the problem. It often develops temporarily in conjunction with a stressful change in the child's environment. Common examples are the birth of a sibling, the first week of school, or a parent's going away on a trip.

Enuresis is much more common in boys than in girls. The child invariably urinates during the first third of the night and remembers nothing of the occurrence. Although in 1 percent of the cases enuresis continues into adulthood, most children are continent by adolescence. Aside from wet pajamas, enuresis itself causes no direct impairment of the child's life, but social ostracism by peers (at sleep-overs and camp, for example) and anger and rejection by parents can damage self-esteem.

Treatment. Limiting the child's intake of liquids before bedtime is one way to make it easier for him or her to stay dry. Getting the child up to go to the bathroom at night also may help. Behavior modification techniques often are effective in eliminating enuresis. For example, many parents use wall charts with gold stars awarded for dry nights to inspire the child to work toward token rewards and favorite treats.

Behavior modification devices with an alarm to awaken the child have been useful for children who are motivated to stop wetting. When prescribed and supervised by a physician, a medication, such as imipramine, may help when the problem persists.

In the case of secondary enuresis, the child should be examined to rule out any organic problems—for example, infection, seizure disorder, or diabetes. Should the problem appear to be a reaction to stress, psychotherapy or family therapy may be helpful.

Although having to change bed linens repeatedly because of the bedwetting can be exasperating, it is important to express support rather than anger to the child, in order to enlist cooperation and avoid further loss of self-esteem.

ENCOPRESIS

Signs and Symptoms
• Repeated passage of feces (stool) into inappropriate places (other than toilet or potty) by a child at least 4 years old.

Encopresis is repeated defecation in inappropriate places, such as underwear or the floor. By definition, the diagnosis of encopresis is made only after the age of 4 and does not include instances of stool incontinence with an organic cause. Encopresis is 5 times more common in boys than in girls.

Twenty-five percent of children with encopresis also have enuresis (see page 1015). Usually, the stools are hard and painful because the child holds back for long periods of time. Because the constipation makes defecation painful, the child may resist having a bowel movement. Use of stool softeners and suppositories can help the dilated rectum resume its normal size.

How Serious Is Encopresis? Sometimes the condition develops in association with psychosocial stress, such as entering school or the birth of a sibling. But the condition may be part of a passive-aggressive relationship with the parents, especially if deliberate smearing is evident. If the child feels ashamed, he or she may try to avoid potentially embarrassing situations such as attending camp.

Treatment. Establishing regular routines for sitting on the toilet, use of a high-fiber diet and stool softeners, and treatment by behavior modification techniques—such as

a system of rewards for stools successfully passed in the toilet—are often helpful. Never shame or punish your child. While suppositories and enemas may be necessary to relieve severe retention and impaction, do not use them repeatedly.

Family therapy also can be a way of examining an overall pattern of oppositional behavior. Parents may learn greater respect for the child's autonomy, and the child can learn more direct ways to express anger.

LEARNING DISABILITIES

A child with a learning disability is one who shows inadequate development of a specific academic skill. This is not the result of a demonstrable physical or neurological disorder, mental retardation, or insufficient educational opportunities. Usually there is an impairment in one particular cognitive area of maturation—reading, arithmetic, language, or speech. (For a comprehensive discussion of learning disabilities, see page 133.)

OBESITY

Signs and Symptoms
• Weight greater than normal by 20 percent or more.

Obesity, which is defined as overweight by 20 percent of normal body weight or more, is caused by the consumption of more calories than the body can use. The excess calories are stored as fat, producing the excess body weight.

There is evidence that early feeding patterns may play a major role in a cultural rather than genetic transmission of obesity from one generation to the next. Today's American children are said to be notably less physically fit than their counterparts in previous generations. They are less active and engage in considerably less exercise, which markedly decreases their caloric needs. Another cause may be the nature of foods eaten—fast foods, snack foods, and sweets, those perennial children's favorites, are extremely high in calories.

How Serious Is Obesity? The frequency of obesity in children ranges from 16 to 33 percent; the estimates vary. Of those who are obese when they are 10 and 13 years old, 80 percent will be obese when they are adults. These children tend to be less popular with peers and do less well at sports, which causes them to have a poorer self-image.

Treatment. If your child is obese, you may find it helpful to keep a diary of everything he or she eats for a week and of all physical activities. An examination by a physician who knows the child's history can help determine the child's appropriate weight.

If weight gain can be kept to a minimum while growth in height continues, the obesity gradually will be corrected. This is most likely to be achieved by changes in eating and activity patterns, and such changes are more likely to produce a healthier and longer-lasting result than might be achieved by a drastic or rigidly planned diet (see also page 126).

MENTAL RETARDATION

Signs and Symptoms
- Score of 70 or below on an individually administered intelligence test;
- Slow acquisition of developmental milestones (motor, language) and social and emotional immaturity;
- Poor school performance in most or all subjects.

Persons with mental retardation have limited mental capacity. The disorder is most evident during the school years. Mild mental retardation may not be recognized until the child is exposed to demands of school learning. Although some affected persons may be dull in appearance and have physical problems, many others are normal in appearance and have a pleasant, appealing personality. As adults they may be productively employed in routine jobs.

A person who scores 70 or below on one of the individually administered intelligence tests (for example, the Wechsler, the Stanford-Binet, or the Kaufman test) may be diagnosed as mentally retarded. These persons have difficulty interacting with others as demonstrated by poor social skills, difficulty in communicating, and an inability to function from day to day.

About 3 percent of school-age children are believed to be mentally retarded. The disorder is more common among boys, with a boy-to-girl ratio of approximately 3-to-2. Mental retardation has many causes. About 25 percent of cases are due to inborn chromosomal or metabolic abnormalities such as Down syndrome (see page 57) or phenylketonuria (PKU; see page 8). Mental retardation may be caused by prenatal rubella or toxoplasmosis or by heavy maternal alcohol consumption. Children have also been found to become mildly retarded in certain economically or socially deprived situations in which they lack adequate language models, they are chronically understimulated, or their environment is unstructured and unpredictable.

Treatment. The evaluation of a retarded child is done by a pediatrician, a child psychiatrist, a clinical psychologist, an audiologist, and a speech pathologist. Their education requires special classes for slow learners conducted by special education teachers. These classes provide an atmosphere in which the child can learn academic skills at his or her own level of ability. The child may be able to attend "mainstream" classes for subjects such as art and physical education. Help for speech and hearing problems may also be necessary.

Depending on the child's intelligence level, parents and teachers can be effective in helping him or her learn to manage personal needs. Many mentally retarded persons can profit from special occupational or vocational training. As adults, they can perform competently in supervised work situations. When mental retardation appears to have environmental causes, preschool training (in programs such as Head Start) may offset some of the cultural deprivation (see also Mental Retardation in the Preschool Child, page 113).

INFANTILE AUTISM

Signs and Symptoms
- Appears to live in his or her own world;
- Exhibits bizarre reactions to people and details in the environment;
- Poor communication;
- Lack of cuddling, and even abhorrence of physical contact;
- Virtually total lack of social interaction.

Infantile autism (now often called pervasive developmental disorder) is one of the most severe mental illnesses of childhood. The autistic child is extremely unresponsive to other people. He or she communicates very poorly, does not cuddle, and may even seem to be repulsed by physical contact. He or she fails to seek comfort when distressed, does not imitate adults normally (for example, doesn't "wave bye-bye"), and has virtually no social interaction.

The autistic child may exhibit stereotyped body movements (hand-flicking or -twisting, spinning, head-banging); is fascinated by parts of objects (say, spinning the wheels on a toy car); gets very upset over even the slightest change in his or her environment (movement of furniture or bric-a-brac, for example); and is unreasonably insistent on routines.

Autism usually appears before the child is 30 months old. The autistic child often does not speak or may only mimic sounds made by others, has difficulty naming objects, and makes bizarre facial expressions and gestures. Occasionally, an autistic child will have an extraordinary talent, similar to the case of the adult "idiot savant."

We do not know how the disorder develops, although maternal rubella (see page 862), PKU (see Phenylketonuria, page 8), encephalitis (see page 529), or meningitis (see page 527) may predispose a child to it. It is 50 times more common in siblings of autistic children than it is in the general population. It occurs 3 to 4 times more frequently in boys than in girls.

Treatment. It is very difficult to treat this disorder. The most effective treatments use a combination of special education, behavioral therapy, and medication. Many autistic children function at a subnormal intellectual level. Others are intellectually bright and perform well in school subjects but have severe social adjustment problems. Not all children with autism are severely incapacitated. Some have a mild form of autism that produces social awkwardness, but they function in school and eventually may become gainfully employed.

PROBLEMS IN ADOLESCENCE

Adolescence is a time of tumultuous changes in a child's physical and emotional makeup. Many observers have called the adolescent "a child in an adult's body."

A classic situation is that in which the adolescent is unreasonably critical of his or her appearance. "I hate my nose!" "Don't I look fat in these pants?" Nearly every adolescent finds something disagreeable about the way he or she looks. These comments often reflect concerns about self-image. Sometimes, such statements are obvious bids for reassurance; the child wants to hear that he or she is worthy of love.

In some cases, however, there is a hidden message. For example, the child whose parents have recently divorced may be saying that he or she believes the divorce happened because there is something wrong with him or her. The most constructive course of action is to ask why he or she feels that way. Often, it is not necessary to do any more than provide a willing ear.

The adolescent's difficulties center not only on his or her intense self-awareness and sexuality but also on the often traumatic and uneven journey from being a dependent child to a young adult who is beginning to separate from parents. In the following pages, we will discuss problems faced by adolescents.

ADOLESCENT DEPRESSION

Signs and Symptoms
- Depressed or irritable mood most of the day, nearly every day;
- Marked loss of interest in nearly all activities;
- Changes in appetite and weight (usually a loss of appetite leading to weight loss; sometimes increased eating);
- Trouble sleeping at night or excessive daytime sleeping;
- Daily fatigue or energy loss;
- Continued feelings of worthlessness or inappropriate guilt;
- Trouble concentrating or indecisiveness, nearly every day;
- Recurrent thoughts of death or suicide.

It is a rare teenager who looks cheerful most of the time. Many of them sleep for hours on end when offered the opportunity. But if many of the previously listed signs and symptoms appear, the teenager may be depressed.

It is important for parents to be alert and to take steps to be sure the adolescent is evaluated by a physician to rule out physical illness; if untreated, depression may last for months. A child psychiatrist may be consulted to confirm that the adolescent is depressed. Teenage depression is serious because suicide is the second leading cause of death among adolescents.

Depression sometimes is an obvious reaction to a disturbing event such as the death of a relative, the break-up with a close friend, failure at school, or a move to a new environment. Often there is no apparent cause. Such depressions tend to run in families (see also page 1038).

Treatment. Adolescent depression is treated with a combination of antidepressant medications and psychotherapy (see page 1026). Psychotherapy alone is used for milder forms of depression; medication is necessary for severe depression. Where there is a risk of suicide, treatment in a hospital psychiatric unit is often necessary.

TEENAGE PREGNANCY

Signs and Symptoms
- Adolescent is sexually active;
- Late or missed menstrual period;
- Swelling or tenderness of the breasts;
- Nausea, particularly on awakening;
- Weight gain, particularly around the middle;
- Sudden distaste for certain foods.

Because teenagers sometimes are sexually active, it is important to be sure that each teenager fully understands how pregnancy occurs and is informed about methods of contraception. A young woman may become pregnant even before her first period because the first egg may be released before menstruation begins.

Pregnancy may be the result of ignorance, denial ("it can't happen to me"), or seeking to be loved. A teenage girl may become pregnant intentionally in order to have a baby to love or to avoid losing her boyfriend.

TEENAGE SUICIDE

Tragically, each day 18 American adolescents take their own lives. Although for most of the 20th century, suicide rates increased with increasing age, reaching a plateau at mid-life, by the 1960s the pattern had begun to change, and suicide is now the second leading cause of death among people between the ages of 15 and 24 years. In fact, the incidence of suicide in this age group has tripled over the past 20 years and seems to be still increasing.

Why this trend has occurred is complex. One factor is that we live in a society in which the family structure is radically changing, and teenagers have enormous difficulties coping with the highly emotional issues of separation and identity. They may also feel unwanted by their families or have trouble in school which leads to feelings of failure. Pregnancy and trouble with the law can be overwhelming to a teenager.

Teenagers who attempt suicide may be looking for help to escape a life that seems intolerable or attempting to "punish" their parents whom they perceive as uncaring or unfair. The suicidal teenager may not know how to deal with pain and a feeling of failure. Family losses—a divorce, or a parent's death, for example—are often associated with teenage suicide, and depression and psychosis may be involved. Finally, there are the cases of accidental suicide, either from drug abuse or from deviant sexual practices.

If a teenager threatens suicide, take him or her seriously. (For further information, see Warning Signs of Potential Suicide, page 1040.) Psychotherapy can be helpful to the suicidal teenager, especially by focusing on how to deal with loss or anger (see also page 1026).

Treatment. Should pregnancy occur, it is essential to see a family physician or obstetrician without delay. If the pregnant girl plans to continue the pregnancy (either to keep the baby or to arrange for subsequent adoption), prenatal care is essential to ensure the health of mother and baby (see page 184). Should she decide to terminate the pregnancy, doing so early in the pregnancy is safer; however, the abortion must be performed only by a licensed physician in an established hospital or clinic (see also page 199).

ANOREXIA NERVOSA

Signs and Symptoms
- Unrealistic fear of becoming fat;
- Excessive dieting and exercise;

- Significant weight loss or failure to gain weight during a period of growth;
- Refusal to maintain a normal body weight;
- Absence of menstrual periods;
- Preoccupation with food, calories, and food preparation.

Many teenagers go on a diet but give it up after a few days or weeks. Those who go on to develop anorexia nervosa persist to the point of emaciation despite warnings from their family and friends.

This disorder occurs almost exclusively in adolescent girls and young adult women, although a few cases (less than 10 percent) are in males. Typically, an adolescent girl who is normal in weight, or somewhat overweight, begins to eliminate snack foods and high-calorie foods from her diet. She begins to skip meals, and her food restriction becomes increasingly stringent. Often, the dieting is accompanied by frantic exercise.

She may take great interest in reading recipes, counting calories, preparing food, and baking for her family. She may encourage others to eat but avoid eating herself. This food restriction results in progressive loss of body fat. Even more serious physical changes result when self-induced vomiting and inappropriate use of laxatives and diuretics are begun in order to speed the weight loss.

The specific cause of anorexia nervosa is not known. Multiple factors play a role. Some individuals seem to have a biological predisposition that becomes apparent at the time of puberty. Individual psychological factors, such as a fear of sexuality, may play a role, as may family pressures and conflicts. Social influences that emphasize the desirability of extreme thinness encourage the dieting process.

When the problem is identified early, treatment can prevent progression of the illness, and complete recovery is possible. However, the illness can be severe and last for several years. In extreme cases, death may result.

Treatment.   In most instances, psychotherapy, diet counseling, and counseling for the parents are recommended while the adolescent with anorexia nervosa remains at home. When weight loss is out of control and dangerous practices such as vomiting and abuse of laxatives and diuretics have caused physical harm, hospitalization becomes necessary for more intensive treatment.

BULIMIA NERVOSA

Signs and Symptoms
- Recurrent episodes of binge eating;
- Self-induced vomiting or laxative abuse;
- Weight within fairly normal range;
- Fear of becoming fat.

Often called the "gorge and purge" disorder, bulimia nervosa involves the consumption of enormous amounts of food—usually high-calorie sweets—in a short time. The gorging may continue until interrupted by a feeling of fullness or a stomachache. Self-induction of vomiting (the most common form of purging) and abuse of laxatives occur because the individual fears gaining weight.

The disorder occurs chiefly in late adolescent and young adult women. Men also binge eat but rarely are concerned about it.

Unlike persons with anorexia nervosa, women who binge and purge usually realize that their eating is abnormal and they often become depressed after binges. Bulimia nervosa is serious because the habit is disruptive to work and social life. Purging can have very serious health consequences by depleting the body of water and potassium and can even result in death.

Treatment.   Bulimia is usually treated with behavior modification techniques and psychotherapy, sometimes in conjunction with antidepressant medication. When binging and purging are out of control and there are physical complications, hospitalization may be necessary (see page 159).

DRUG AND ALCOHOL ABUSE

The abuse of drugs, both legal and illegal, is alarmingly common among adolescents. Depending on the drug and on the teenager, it may be merely experimentation or a serious addiction.

For information on the symptoms and treatment of drug abuse, see Medications and Drug Abuse, page 431, and Drug Dependency, page 1046.

VICTIM OF VIOLENCE

Signs and Symptoms
- Multiple bruises;
- Multiple old fractures;
- Unexplained injuries;
- Pain in the genital area;
- Sudden changes in behavior;
- Loss of appetite;
- Problems in school;
- Abdominal pain.

It often is harder for teenagers to tolerate violence than it is for adults because they are far more emotionally intense and responsive, have a tenuous sense of self, and often lack supportive adults to whom they can turn.

This is especially true in cases of physical or sexual abuse by a relative, friend, or other trusted figure. Often, the victim is afraid to report the problem, fearing adult retaliation and also fearing the loss of the adult's love. When an adolescent has unexplained injuries or pain or exhibits sudden changes in behavior, it is wise to seek professional help.

Treatment. Sometimes an adolescent will confide in a trusted adult, such as a teacher, a relative, or a member of the clergy. If the adolescent has suffered a major trauma such as violence, sexual or physical abuse, or rape, psychotherapy and, in the case of incest, family therapy can help this young person cope with the reality of the situation and restore his or her self-esteem.

PROBLEMS IN THE ELDERLY

Just as children and young people experience difficulties in adjusting to the changes that are occurring in their bodies and in their lives, so do the elderly. The changes in the elderly are physical, which may result in a loss of mobility, in sexual problems, or in a general feeling of being unable to cope. Changes in circumstances may produce isolation or loneliness. As one ages, often one experiences greater difficulty in facing and dealing with changes. Some of the following problems are often found in the elderly.

DEPRESSION IN THE ELDERLY

Signs and Symptoms
- Loss of interest or pleasure in usual activities;
- Feeling sad or "blue";
- Poor appetite and weight loss;
- Sleep disturbance;
- Loss of energy and fatigue;
- Difficulty in concentrating, or memory loss.

In an older person, depression can be difficult to recognize. Often, a depressed elderly person does not present what we have come to regard as the typical profile of the depressed person, a person who is supposed to be generally sad and tearful. Depression in the elderly occasionally may be manifested in various complaints such as fatigue, weakness, insomnia, poor appetite, restless anxiety, poor concentration, or lack of interest in sex. In rare cases, however, a depressed older person may become so withdrawn that he or she appears to have difficulty understanding even simple requests (see Dementia, page 518). A more common presentation is a person with mild to moderate dementia (such as Alzheimer's disease, see page 516) with a coexisting major depression. At times, physicians find it difficult to diagnose depression in the elderly. Many of the typical symptoms are part of normal aging.

There are various causes of depression among the aging. These include loneliness (especially after loss of a spouse); chronic illness and pain; difficulties in getting around or even performing simple tasks; frustration over memory loss; and lack of a sense of purpose in the absence of a job or a family to worry about. Sometimes depression may actually be a sign of a medical illness (such as hypothyroidism; see page 730). Your physician will need to rule out medical disorders with symptoms that mimic depression. Many medications can contribute to depression in the elderly. Often, no cause for depression is found (see page 1038). There may be a biochemical explanation for the frequency of this disorder, but the research is not yet conclusive.

Treatment. If a medication is causing or contributing to the depression, it may be gradually withdrawn under careful supervision. Depression among the elderly can often be alleviated through nonmedical means: participation in group activities that provide companionship and regular outings; regular visits from young people ("adoptive grandparent" programs); and, in the case of relatively healthy retirees, performing volunteer work in the community.

For more serious forms of depression, further evaluation and treatment including the use of antidepressant drugs and electroconvulsive therapy may be required (see page 1039) under the careful supervision of a physician.

PARANOID REACTIONS IN THE ELDERLY

Signs and Symptoms
- Delusions that last for months or longer and involve real-life situations such as being followed, being poisoned, having a disease, or being deceived by a spouse.

Paranoid symptoms and delusions occur occasionally in the elderly, at times in those who are hard of hearing. When paranoid symptoms occur, the first typically will be that the older person is highly suspicious of a member of the family or a friend. These symptoms may be a sign of depression or early dementia (see page 519). The correct diagnosis must be made before therapy can begin.

Treatment. Antipsychotic drugs such as haloperidol (Haldol) or trifluoperazine (Stelazine) often can be helpful, although these medications must be used with caution in a person who is not under a doctor's supervision.

SLEEP DISORDERS IN THE ELDERLY

Signs and Symptoms
- Confusing days and nights (day/night reversal);
- Prolonged delay in falling asleep;
- Frequent nocturnal awakening.

Sleep disturbance is a common problem among the elderly and is worse in those with psychiatric disorders. At best, sleep in old age is "not what it used to be"; falling asleep takes longer than for younger people, the elderly have less deep sleep, and they frequently wake up during the night. In general, elderly people also need less sleep.

There are two potential causes of sleep disturbance in the elderly. First, they may be in pain, often from such common ailments as arthritis. Second, the elderly person may not be getting enough activity during the day. Especially in institutions, where bedtime may be scheduled for as early as 7 p.m., sleeping through until morning may not be likely.

Other possible causes include medical problems such as congestive heart failure (see page 807), esophageal reflux (see page 593), frequent urination (see page 1109), anxiety, depression, pain, excessive use of stimulants (coffee in the evening, for example), or alcohol or drug use. An aging person with frequent sleep disturbances not only exhausts his or her caretakers and family but tires himself or herself out.

Treatment. When a person is not sleeping well because of pain, aspirin or acetaminophen may help when sleeping pills do not. A moderate exercise program, a quiet, comfortable bed, and a drink of warm milk at bedtime can improve the sleeping pattern. When there are no identifiable physical or psychological causes, occasional use of a short-acting benzodiazepine or a sedating tricyclic antidepressant can be helpful, but not on a regular basis. Because these drugs can be habit-forming, they should not be freely administered without a search for possible causes for the sleeplessness. (For a general discussion of sleep disorders, see page 1028.)

CHAPTER 33 Mental Health

PERSONALITY PROBLEMS

Although there are many types of personality disorders, they all reflect an inability to accept the demands and limitations of the outside world. These disorders may regularly interfere with a person's behavior and with his or her interactions with family or persons at work or play.

Before the diagnosis of a personality disorder can be accepted, physicians must rule out medical and neurological changes that can mimic personality disorders. Often, persons with personality disorders have had emotional problems during childhood.

Only about one-fifth of those with personality disorders seek psychiatric help and treatment. The majority experience long-standing difficulties in marriage, in maintaining stable employment, and in friendships.

Persons with personality disorders often do not recognize the reasons for their problems. They tend to blame others for their own actions or thoughts. Treatment generally consists of psychotherapy (see page 1026), although occasionally a drug is used. The key to therapy is establishing a trusting relationship. Treatment may be long and frustrating.

PASSIVE-AGGRESSIVE PERSONALITY DISORDER

Signs and Symptoms (at least *five* of the following)
- Procrastinates;
- Sulky, irritable, or argumentative behavior;
- Tends to work slowly or deliberately do a bad job on tasks that he or she does not really want to do;
- Protests (unrealistically) that everyone is making unreasonable demands;
- "Forgets" obligations;
- Believes that he or she is doing a much better job than others think he or she is;
- Resents useful suggestions from others on how to be more productive;
- Fails to do his or her share of the work, thereby obstructing others' efforts;
- Unreasonably criticizes or scorns people in positions of authority.

Passive-aggressive personality disorder is a pervasive pattern of passive resistance to demands for adequate performance, both in social circumstances and in the workplace. It begins in early adulthood and occurs in various contexts.

Persons with this disorder have a resentment of responsibility in both work and social spheres. They show this resentment through the signs and symptoms listed above rather than openly expressed anger, by using procrastination, inefficiency, and "forgetfulness" to avoid fulfilling their obligations. Rather than take responsibility for their own actions, they tend to blame and manipulate others.

Treatment.   Professional counselling may be of value in identifying and changing the destructive patterns of passive-aggressive behavior.

ANTISOCIAL PERSONALITY DISORDER

Signs and Symptoms
- Lack of concern regarding society's rules and expectations;
- Repeated violation of the rights of others;
- Unlawful behavior;
- Lack of regard for truth;
- In parents, neglect or abuse of child or children;
- Physical aggression, including spouse abuse;
- Lack of steady job;
- No regular address.

A person with antisocial personality disorder shows a lack of concern in regard to the expectations and rules of the society in which he or she lives and repeatedly violates the rights of others. The popular term for an individual with this disorder is sociopath.

Although the diagnosis is limited to persons over age 18, it requires a history of antisocial behavior. Before age 15, the individual often has displayed a pattern of lying, trouble with the law, truancy, delinquency, and substance abuse and may have run away from home. As an adult, the person often commits acts that are against the law, fails to live up to the requirements of a job or financial or parenting responsibilities, and is reckless in personal behavior (driving while intoxicated, for example). He or she is unable to sustain a long-term relationship with one sexual partner, frequently abuses alcohol or drugs, and is aggressive and irritable.

Antisocial personality disorder is not just a medical term for criminality; it describes a long-standing disorder that usually lands those who have it not in a psychiatrist's office but in court or prison.

Suicide, alcoholism, vagrancy, and social isolation are common among those commonly called sociopaths, but what is remarkable is their apparent lack of anxiety or depression in situations in which such emotions might be expected. Despite all their run-ins with the law, they can present a charming and strikingly normal facade.

Treatment.   There is no simple or widely effective method of treating the sociopath.

HISTRIONIC PERSONALITY DISORDER

Signs and Symptoms
- Relationships that appear very intense but are in fact superficial;
- Highly dramatic and engaging manner, emotions expressed in exaggerated way;
- Self-centered;
- Constantly seeking attention and praise;
- Sexualization of relationships;
- Low tolerance of frustration.

This problem usually makes for stormy and ungratifying interpersonal relationships. It is diagnosed much more frequently in women than in men, and it seems to run in families. The behavior might be a combination of learned and inherited characteristics.

Treatment.   There is no widely effective method of treating histrionic personality disorder. In some cases, however, psychotherapy (see page 1026) can have a beneficial effect.

PARANOID PERSONALITY DISORDER

Signs and Symptoms
- Suspicious of and overly sensitive to perceived injuries, slights, and tricks by others;

- Frequent blaming of others;
- Secretive;
- Lack of humor or insight;
- Exaggerated sense of own importance.

Individuals with this disorder are overly worried that others are "out to get them." Because they spend a great deal of energy looking for hidden, sinister meanings behind the behavior of others, they are easily offended. They show a limited range of emotions and may appear cold and humorless. They easily become hostile.

Treatment.   Treatment is difficult, although psychotherapy (see page 1026) may be of help.

SCHIZOID PERSONALITY DISORDER

Signs and Symptoms
- Aloofness and emotional coldness;
- Lack of close friendships;
- Isolation;
- Lacking in energy;
- Indifferent to praise from or criticism by others.

The person with schizoid personality disorder appears to have little need for other people and usually is a loner. He or she may live in nearly total social isolation, lacking any close friendships and remaining aloof from everyone he or she encounters.

Treatment.   Treatment of schizoid personality disorder is difficult. In some cases, however, psychotherapy (see page 1026) may be beneficial.

SCHIZOTYPAL PERSONALITY DISORDER

Signs and Symptoms
- Disordered or magical thinking;
- Odd speech (vague or metaphoric);
- Inappropriate ideas of reference (attributing unusual significance to neutral events);
- Suspiciousness.

Persons with schizotypal personality disorder show many similarities to schizophrenics (see Schizophrenia, page 1042) in their odd ways of thinking, perceiving the world, and speaking, but their symptoms are not sufficiently pervasive or strong to warrant a diagnosis of schizophrenia. Although they are often socially isolated, the difficulties these persons have are primarily in understanding (cognition) and not interpersonal (as with the schizoid personality).

Treatment. There is no known cure for schizotypal personality disorder. Psychotherapy (see page 1026) may be beneficial in certain cases.

BORDERLINE PERSONALITY DISORDER

Signs and Symptoms
- Chronic difficulty in maintaining a positive self-image;
- Moodiness;
- Interpersonal problems;
- Impulsive, often damaging behavior (such as suicide attempts).

People with borderline personality disorder can be thought of as having "stable instability." They have chronic problems such as moodiness, sudden angry, sad, or fearful periods, or feeling empty inside. Despite the fact that they do not get along well with others, they usually do not like to be alone. They tend to characterize others as either "all good" or "all bad" as a defense mechanism.

Treatment. Treatment of borderline personality disorder is difficult and often unsuccessful. In certain cases, psychotherapy (see page 1026) may be helpful.

NARCISSISTIC PERSONALITY DISORDER

Signs and Symptoms
- Exaggerated sense of own importance, power, and talents;
- Seeks admiration;
- Indifferent to emotions and needs of others;
- Difficulty in coping with rejection.

The narcissistic person has an inflated sense of his or her own uniqueness, importance, and gifts. When rejected, he or she displays excessive anger or shame and has trouble viewing others realistically, characterizing them as "perfect" or "worthless," with very little in between.

Treatment. There is no known cure for narcissistic personality disorder, although psychotherapy (see page 1026) may be effective for certain people.

AVOIDANT PERSONALITY DISORDER

Signs and Symptoms
- Exaggerated worry over being rejected or humiliated, resulting in avoidance of close ties with other people;
- Low self-esteem.

Avoidant persons are called this because their preoccupation with their own shortcomings, and consequent fear of rejection, causes them to withdraw from other people. They often do seem to wish for intimacy, however, despite their lack of close ties.

Treatment. Treating avoidant personality disorder is difficult, and there is no known cure. In certain cases, however, psychotherapy (see page 1026) may be beneficial.

DEPENDENT PERSONALITY DISORDER

Signs and Symptoms
- Views self as inept or helpless;
- Avoids personal responsibility and allows others to assume it for important life decisions and aspects;
- Chronically unable to meet the ordinary demands of life, but is not mentally retarded.

People who are dependent permit others to take over the important aspects of their lives and to make major decisions for them. They see themselves as inadequate and, in order to avoid taking responsibility, willingly subordinate their own desires and needs to those of other people.

Treatment. There is no known cure for dependent personality disorder, but psychotherapy (see page 1026) may be appropriate.

OBSESSIVE-COMPULSIVE PERSONALITY DISORDER

Signs and Symptoms

- Pervasive pattern of perfectionism and inflexibility;
- Symptoms begin by early childhood;
- At least five of the following are present:
  1. So bent on perfection that he or she has great difficulty in completing a task;
  2. Preoccupied with details—rules, regulations, lists, and schedules—and often loses sight of the point of the activity;
  3. Displays a strong need to control situations, unreasonably insistent that everyone "do it my way," and is unwilling to delegate tasks because of the belief that no one else can do them correctly;
  4. Overzealous devotion to work in preference to leisure activities and friendships (workaholism) without apparent financial necessity for this;
  5. Markedly indecisive because of worry about priorities;
  6. Highly moralistic and inflexible about moral and ethical questions, without a basis in cultural or religious identification;
  7. Displays affection only in restricted ways;
  8. Is stingy with time, money, or gifts, even when the stinginess offers no personal gain;
  9. Is a "pack rat," unable to throw anything away, no matter how worthless the object may be.

PSYCHOTHERAPY

Psychotherapy is a method of treating emotional problems by means of a supportive working relationship between the therapist and the patient. In the sanctuary of the therapist's office, the patient is encouraged to feel comfortable while discussing his or her problems and conflicts and optimistic that he or she can be helped. The therapist may interpret the problems and suggest different ways to cope with them.

There are dozens of different kinds of therapy. Basically, however, there are two categories.

In one category are the psychodynamic therapies. These are designed to help you understand better the psychological forces that motivate your actions, with the goal that these insights reveal possibilities for change. Psychoanalysis is a well-known example of this kind of therapy, although in recent years it has been used only rarely.

In the second category are the behavior therapies which, as the name implies, deal not with inner feelings and motivations but instead use specific techniques to change specific behavioral symptoms. Therapy to create a dislike for smoking is an example of behavior therapy.

Psychotherapy cannot change the world around you. Therapy sessions will not eliminate job stress or financial problems or change the personality of a difficult spouse. What it can do, however, is help you learn to cope more effectively with your environment, to evaluate your priorities and responses to stress, and to understand and accept yourself as you are.

In practice, most therapies involve a mixture of self-exploration by the patient and supportive-directive work from the therapist. Psychodynamic therapy may be one-on-one between therapist and patient, or it may be in a group setting. Psychodrama is a unique form of group therapy. It may last for only a few sessions dealing with a specific problem, or it may be long-term and open-ended. Psychodynamic therapy usually is a combination of discussion, explanation, relaxation, exploration, and support. It attempts to make connections between the patient's internal experiences and his or her responses to life events.

Broadly speaking, behavior therapy covers a group of related methods and techniques all based on learning theory. Rather than assuming that the problem that brings you to the therapist's office is symptomatic of an underlying psychological disorder, behavior therapists work on the problem behavior itself. They concentrate on helping you learn to change your response to a particular problem situation. In order to achieve this, they most frequently use classical conditioning principles—the basis for Pavlov's famous experiment with dogs. Through systematic desensitization, for example, which is repeated exposure to a situation or stimulus that frightens or upsets you, you can learn to conquer a phobia or an anxiety state.

Other methods of behavior therapy include anxiety management training, social skills training, and assertiveness training.

The term obsessive-compulsive personality disorder (sometimes shortened to compulsive personality disorder) describes individuals who tend to be preoccupied with detail, rules, and procedures. Often these individuals insist on a procedure being done a specific way. Sometimes they are ineffective because of their indecisiveness. Obsessive-compulsive individuals place a higher value on work and possessions than on interpersonal relationships. They often have difficulty expressing warm, emotional feelings toward others and are sometimes perceived as being aloof, cold, or indifferent.

Treatment. There is no specific treatment for this personality disorder.

GRIEF RESPONSES

The word "grief" refers to our subjective feelings and emotions after the loss of a loved one (usually through death, but also after the dissolution of a relationship). The collective processes by which grief is resolved are known as mourning.

GRIEVING

Signs and Symptoms
- Shock;
- Disbelief;
- Protest;
- Fear;
- Anger;
- Despair.

Many researchers have studied the process of mourning in an attempt to find a predictable pattern. Generally, on learning of the loss you are likely to feel shocked, fearful, and disbelieving. It is not at all uncommon to feel angry at the departed person. As the reality of the loss begins to sink in, you may go through a period of missing the person so much that you find yourself searching for him or her. Coming to terms with the futility of the search then may lead to despair.

A healthy process of mourning goes from recognition of the loss to eventual acceptance of it. No two people experience grief in exactly the same way, but this overall pattern is a guideline.

Your responses will depend on many factors. For example, if the deceased suffered from a chronic disease, his or her death may seem like a blessing; and the time spent in what is known as anticipatory grief, or mourning before the actual loss, can diminish the impact of death. The death of a young child, on the other hand, is likely to leave a parent grief-stricken no matter how much anticipatory grief has taken place. The public behavior of a grieving person is greatly affected by family style and cultural influences. In some cultures, weeping and wailing is the norm; in others, a "stiff upper lip" is required.

Treatment. There is no single treatment for grief. But time and counseling can help soften the hard edge of loss. In fact, grief has traditionally been assumed to expend itself over a year (or more), as you pass through the events of a full calendar year without the presence of the loved one.

Signs and symptoms persist much longer. Even though you never get over the loss entirely, after healthy grieving you can return to a normal life.

It may be helpful to talk with a psychiatrist or psychologist, or a member of the clergy,

---

ABSENT GRIEF REACTION

Although our culture tends to praise people who appear serene in the face of great pain, refusing to deal with the reality of a loss—or being unable to face it—can be unhealthy in the long run.

Grief that is not expressed openly comes out in other ways. Often, signs of an absent grief reaction only show up over time. The bereaved may seem oddly euphoric. He or she may begin to experience persisting physical symptoms similar to those the deceased had. Or his or her behavior may become unaccountably erratic on the anniversary of the loss or on occasions of significance to the departed, such as a birthday or favorite holiday.

The absent grief reaction may be displaced onto another loss that seems trifling by comparison or onto the problems of another person.

Dealing with grief is essential. If your loved one is avoiding it, encourage that person to seek counseling.

who may focus on both the positive and negative aspects of your relationship with the person for whom you grieve. If your relationship was one of excessive dependency, resolving your grief may be more difficult. Often, such dependent relationships also have a negative or hostile side, as is often the case for the loving but covertly angry spouse of an alcoholic.

Tranquilizing or antidepressant drugs usually are not appropriate in the treatment of uncompleted grief response.

SLEEP DISORDERS

Sleep disorders are among the most commonly reported life problems. It is important to realize that our sleep patterns change as we go through life.

All sleep is not the same. By measuring brain waves, sleep researchers have identified several different stages of sleep which recur at fairly regular cycles throughout a night's sleep. We progress from wakefulness to drowsiness to moderate sleep to deep restorative sleep. The duration of deep sleep decreases with age. Dream sleep, or rapid-eye-movement (REM) sleep, occurs 1 to 2 hours after you fall asleep. The first REM sleep period is the longest. You may experience several shorter REM sleep periods as the night progresses. During REM sleep, our eyes move rapidly behind our closed lids.

REM sleep cannot be truly called light or deep sleep; it is a different kind of sleep. It is the stage when most dreaming occurs and it is characterized by faster breathing and heart rates than in the other sleep stages. REM sleep also is characterized by penile erections in males.

During REM sleep, your brain waves, as displayed by an electroencephalograph (EEG; see page 1294), suggest faster electrical activity at lower amplitude than at other stages of sleep, which makes the waves superficially similar to those of wakefulness. REM sleep is not absolutely vital for life.

The brain undergoes a number of changes during sleep. The brain consumes increased amounts of oxygen and has increased blood flow. People awakened during REM sleep may recall vivid dreams. During a normal night's sleep there are four or five REM-sleep periods; they occur about once every 90 minutes as part of the sleep cycle and total about 1½ hours.

Sleep disorders are of various kinds and may be the result of physical conditions, stress, or other factors.

INSOMNIA

Signs and Symptoms
- Inability to sleep enough at night;
- Difficulty falling asleep;
- Night awakening in an adult.

Insomnia is defined simply as too little sleep. A person with insomnia may complain that he or she "didn't sleep a wink," although in fact there usually was some sleep.

An occasional individual claims to hardly sleep at all and yet actually does sleep for 4 or more hours a night. What may be happening is frequent awakenings, leading to the perception of no sleep. In older people, sleeping less and awakening more often at night seems to be common and is not insomnia.

The causes of insomnia are many and varied. A change in your environment, such as a new work schedule or jet lag, can cause difficulty in sleeping. Drinking excessive amounts of coffee, tea, or cola drinks can cause insomnia. If you are especially sensitive to caffeine, even a cup or two during the day can keep you awake at night. The use of other stimulants (amphetamines, methylphenidate) also contributes to insomnia.

Although a drink or two of an alcoholic beverage seems to help some people relax enough to fall asleep, even moderate amounts of alcohol can distort normal sleeping patterns. The ability to fall asleep may be increased but sleep is poor later during the night as the blood alcohol level decreases. The use of certain medications can cause insomnia. Most of the psychoactive drugs—such as the barbiturates and benzodiazepines—actively interfere with the sleep cycle, particularly with prolonged use.

Insomnia may be secondary to another medical condition such as sleep apnea (see page 1030), restless legs syndrome (see page 1031), drug abuse or withdrawal, or endocrine abnormalities like Cushing's syndrome (see page 719) and hyperthyroidism (see page 727). Long-term use of sleeping medications is a common cause of distorted sleep cycles and consequent insomnia.

In regard to psychological factors, insomnia may be a symptom of a transient problem or of a long-term underlying disorder. Sometimes people go through periods of sleeplessness because of temporary anxiety—over an upcoming job interview or examination, for example. In middle-aged and older people, depression may result in insomnia, particularly during the early morning hours. Chronic anxiety, reflecting fears, can cause insomnia. People who tend to have nightmares may find themselves awakening suddenly while in REM sleep.

Treatment. The first thing to consider when you are suffering from insomnia is how to make simple changes in your bedtime routine that will help you sleep. Examples of changes that may help you feel sleepy include restricting your bedtime reading and television viewing to light topics that are not emotionally upsetting—for example, no horror stories. Avoid strenuous exercise or emotional upset in the period immediately preceding bedtime. Taking a warm bath or drinking a cup of warm milk may help you relax. Exercise during the day may help your body feel fatigued enough to need rest at bedtime. Even though you may be tired from your sleepless nights, avoid napping during the day so that you can reestablish a pattern of sleeping at night. Habitual daytime naps may be a cause of insomnia. If you do not have time for physical exertion during the day, take a walk before bedtime, but do not do anything too strenuous or you probably will have trouble dropping off to sleep.

Finally, if you are tossing and turning, do not try to force sleep; get up and stay up until you are too tired to stay awake and then go to bed and try to sleep.

If you are unable to reestablish a sleeping pattern by using a home remedy, it is a good idea to have a careful medical evaluation because there are many potential causes of insomnia. If the problem is sensitivity to caffeine or medications, excessive alcohol intake, or the use of stimulants, eliminate these, if possible, from your daily routine. If an underlying psychological problem is contributing to insomnia, psychotherapy may be helpful.

Be cautious about the use of sleeping pills. If you are awake at night because of pain from a medical or surgical condition, a sleeping medication may be advised for a short time along with use of an analgesic such as aspirin or acetaminophen. Sleeping pills (also

WHAT IS NORMAL SLEEP?

"Sleep" is the word we use to define both a biological state and a behavioral state in which we are quiet and relatively unresponsive to external stimuli. Sleep is regular and recurring, and easily reversible (unlike a coma, for example). Most people spend about one-third of their life in the state of unconsciousness that is sleep, about 7½ hours a night for a middle-aged adult.

When we do not get enough sleep, we may feel less alert and vigorous—or confused and fatigued. Lack of sleep affects not only energy level but also mental and social functioning. Sleep deprivation over prolonged periods has been found to cause hallucinations, delusions, and psychosis in normal persons. In fact, going long periods without adequate sleep is so well-recognized as disorienting and demoralizing that forced sleep deprivation is a widely used brainwashing technique.

Sleep patterns vary considerably according to age. The newborn infant may spend as much as half of its total sleeping time in REM sleep and may sleep five or six times a day. Infants fall into REM sleep immediately, whereas adults must pass through other stages of sleep first.

Some researchers have suggested that the frequency of REM sleep in newborns may reflect a need for stimulation from within, to allow the central nervous system to mature in an orderly fashion. Others suggest that REM sleep has a role in processing new information, which is acquired at a very high rate in childhood. As the child grows, the sleeping habits become more organized: frequent, unpredictable periods of sleep give way to two naps in the daytime, gradually decreasing to one and then to the adult pattern of one long nocturnal period with no daytime nap.

In later years, however, many people seem to return to frequent daytime naps and sleep less at night. These patterns vary with individuals, depending on neurological development and other factors but the overall progression has been identified as the norm through the human life span.

known as sedatives or hypnotics) not only lose their effectiveness after 4 to 6 weeks but they also may disturb your sleeping pattern and thus contribute to the insomnia.

SLEEP APNEA

Signs and Symptoms
- Excessive daytime sleepiness;
- Extremely loud snoring;
- Observed episodes of breathing stoppage during sleep;
- Morning headache;
- In children, enuresis (bedwetting).

Sleep apnea (from the Greek *a pnein,* "without breathing") is a disorder in which there are recurrent episodes of breathing stoppage during sleep. It is caused by an obstruction to the movement of air in the upper respiratory passages.

At night, people with sleep apnea tend to snore very loudly, and in the daytime they often are very sleepy. They may wake up with a headache. They may black out or feel disoriented during the day but be unable to remember the episode.

In sleep apnea, the muscles in the walls of the throat (pharynx) relax so that the walls collapse on themselves as the sleeper approaches the deeper levels of sleep. The flow of air is thus obstructed. After 20 to 30 seconds or more of no exchange of air, the person awakes toward a lighter level of sleep, the muscles regain their normal tone (tenseness), the obstruction is relieved, and the cycle begins anew.

The obstruction to breathing prevents the person from ever reaching the deeper levels of restorative sleep, so this person feels as if he or she had been without sleep even though he or she may have been asleep all night.

In adults, obesity is a contributing factor, and weight reduction often gives relief. Some persons who are of normal weight or moderately overweight may experience sleep apnea. This diagnosis can be suspected from their excessive daytime sleepiness and their pattern of snoring—periods during which breathing ceases followed by deep gasps and then the resumption of breathing. The diagnosis can be confirmed by studies in a sleep laboratory (see page 1031).

More than half of all cases of sleep apnea are diagnosed in people age 40 years or older. Sleep apnea is a major contributor to daytime drowsiness; 20 to 60 percent of people with severe daytime sleepiness have sleep apnea.

Treatment. Weight reduction is of great importance and often gives substantial relief—but many obese persons find it difficult to adhere to a low-calorie eating schedule, even with the promise of some relief from distressing symptoms.

Sleep disorder specialists sometimes will help the affected person learn to use a machine that delivers air through a mask at a pressure somewhat greater than that of the surrounding air. This may be of considerable benefit.

Surgical procedures to increase the size of the throat have not been effective.

NARCOLEPSY

Signs and Symptoms
- Abnormal tendency to sleep during the day;
- Desire to sleep longer than the usual 7 to 8 hours;
- Episodic attacks of REM sleep during the day that may cause attacks of muscle paralysis;
- Memory loss;
- Dream-like hallucinations.

Narcolepsy (from the Greek *narke* meaning stupor) is popularly known as the sleeping sickness. It is the abnormal tendency to sleep during the day. The person with narcolepsy experiences episodes of uncontrollable sleepiness. He or she then sleeps briefly and awakens refreshed, only to become sleepy again within an hour or so. Although these sleep attacks usually occur after meals, they may also occur during active times—for example, while the person is driving a car, having a conversation, or making love.

Possible aggravating factors include environmental causes, such as alternating work weeks (i.e., working nights one week and days the next). It is likely that narcolepsy represents a neurological problem of sleep-wake mechanisms in the brain.

The Diagnosis. Although daytime sleepiness is a symptom of both sleep apnea and narcolepsy, there is an important observable difference. Unlike the person with sleep apnea, the person with narcolepsy has brief sleep attacks and feels refreshed upon awakening. Many cases of narcolepsy are associated with cataplexy. This consists of attacks of paralysis of various muscles, at times even provoked by laughter. When such an attack occurs, the person will experience weakening of the knees, the jaw will drop, and the person even may fall to the floor. During awakening after a night's sleep, the person with cataplexy may be unable to move for a few minutes, a condition called sleep paralysis. Many also have hallucinations that seem like dreams.

Narcolepsy is usually diagnosed between the ages of 15 and 25. Often, the clue is difficulty in staying awake in class. Men and women are affected in equal numbers.

Treatment. To prevent sudden sleep attacks, plan naps so that your body will feel rested when you need to be awake. Allow plenty of time for sleep at night. Forced naps—say, one to four of them for 10 minutes or so each—when you are really feeling drowsy can enable you to function normally without medication. Because you may be especially sleepy after a meal, eat light or vegetarian meals during the day and avoid a heavy meal just before an important activity. Caffeine—especially coffee, tea, or cola drinks—used in moderation may help you stay awake.

Learning to adjust to living with narcolepsy and to cope with the emotional problems your illness may be causing in your workplace and relationships may help enormously.

Medication. Medical treatment of narcolepsy includes stimulant pills such as dextroamphetamine and methylphenidate. If you have cataplexy, your physician may prescribe an antidepressant to suppress the attacks of REM sleep.

RESTLESS LEGS (NOCTURNAL JERKING MOVEMENTS)

Signs and Symptoms

- Unpleasant creeping sensations deep inside the calves and occasionally in the feet, thighs, or arms while awake, especially while lying down;
- Irresistible urge to move the legs;
- Possible worsening of symptoms during times of stress.

Restless legs syndrome is a condition in which your legs feel extremely uncomfortable unless you move them. This discomfort commonly begins shortly after you go to bed. Often, you feel as if you want to get out of bed and walk or move your legs. Such activity briefly relieves the symptoms, but they return. These symptoms usually last for an hour or more. Myoclonus (from the Greek *myo-,* for muscle, and *klonos,* for violent motion) is the name given to these contractions. They should not be confused with leg cramps (see page 962).

With restless legs syndrome, you may feel creeping sensations deep inside your calves while you are awake (especially when lying down). Occasionally, your feet, thighs, or arms are similarly affected. They feel unpleasant but not painful.

These disorders are not dangerous, although they can be uncomfortable and disruptive to sleep.

Treatment. These related disorders are seen mostly in middle-aged and older people and seem to get worse during times of stress. Muscle relaxation techniques can be helpful, as can a warm bath before bed. In some cases, your physician may prescribe a medication such as clonazepam or some

---

SLEEP CLINICS

Many hospitals and medical centers have sleep clinics for the purpose of diagnosing sleep disorders. The person enters the unit during the early evening hours and spends the night in a comfortable bed. Electrocardiographic (ECG, or heart monitor, see page 1293) and electroencephalographic (EEG, brain monitor, see page 1294) recordings are often used throughout the night. In addition, breathing is monitored.

In men who have problems with impotence, the occurrence and duration of nocturnal erections also can be monitored.

The results of these studies often allow the specialist in sleep disorders to identify the problem and offer appropriate treatment.

other benzodiazepam. These tranquilizers help in some persons but cause unacceptable sleepiness in others.

NIGHTMARES AND NIGHT TERRORS

Signs and Symptoms
- Nightmares: Unpleasant or frightening dreams that usually take place during the second half of a night's sleep;
- Night terrors: screaming and arousal from sleep, with no memory of a frightening dream except perhaps a frightening image.

A nightmare is a dream from which you may awaken in fright. Especially when they recur, nightmares may suggest a psychological disturbance or stress brought on by a difficult situation. However, perfectly normal persons have nightmares from time to time.

Night terrors are usually disorders of childhood. They are common between ages 3 and 5 years and happen much less often after that. During deep sleep the child wakes up screaming, apparently is terrified, and is unable to explain what happened or to be comforted or fully awakened. Although the terror may last for 10 or 20 minutes, the child generally will be unable to remember the episode the next morning.

Night terrors can be distinguished from regular nightmares because they usually happen during the first third of the night but nightmares are more usual near morning. Night terrors are far more terrifying than nightmares, and the affected person will not be able to remember what happened, aside from a frightening image. On the other hand, a nightmare may be remembered as a long, movie-like dream.

Night terrors seem to run in families. In adults they can get worse with the use of alcohol, and emotional tension can make them more likely to occur. Usually, persons who frequently have nightmares or night terrors are experiencing considerable conflict and stress in their waking lives.

Treatment. Children usually outgrow night terrors. In adults often there is no specific treatment for nightmares, but psychotherapy (see page 1026) can help.

SLEEPWALKING

Signs and Symptoms
- Walking or other activities (opening closet doors, going to the bathroom, driving) during sleep;
- Activity usually occurs during the first third of the night;
- Duration is typically a few minutes to half an hour;
- Confusion or disorientation on awakening is characteristic.

Sleepwalking describes not only walking but other activities performed during sleep—rearranging furniture, dressing or undressing, and even getting into a car and driving. It usually occurs during the first third of the night and can be very brief or can go on as long as half an hour.

The sleepwalker's eyes are open, the facial expression is blank or dazed, and he or she will be confused or disoriented if awakened. It is commonly believed that sleepwalkers do not get hurt during their "travels," but this is a misconception; it is not unusual for a sleepwalker to be injured by tripping or loss of balance.

Sleepwalking occurs at various ages although young children, who often sit up in bed and appear to be awake, rarely leave the bed and actually walk. Sleepwalking occurs most frequently between the ages of 6 and 12. In children, sleepwalking is believed to be caused by psychological factors including fatigue and prior sleep loss. With adults, there may be personality disturbance as well as anxiety or conflict. Sleepwalking also seems to run in families.

Treatment. There is no specific treatment for sleepwalking. To prevent injury, however, it is a good idea to make the room and

---

SHIFT DISORDERS

Some persons have a sleep disorder caused by rotations in their work shifts. They may be chronically tired and have insomnia (see page 1028). In general, if a person routinely works at night, the bedroom should be as quiet as possible for sleep during the day. It is better to remain "shifted" on the days not working. However, for many people, this is not possible. Avoid use of sleeping pills.

house safe for the sleepwalker: avoid leaving objects, electrical cords, or small furniture in the middle of the bedroom where it can be tripped on, and block the top of a staircase with a gate. Avoiding use of alcohol and other central nervous system depressants can be helpful.

Medication.   When medication is considered necessary, short-acting tranquilizers such as benzodiazepines have been helpful in some cases.

BRUXISM

Signs and Symptoms
- Grinding, gnashing, or clenching of the teeth during sleep.

Bruxism is grinding or clenching of teeth during sleep. About 15 percent of normal people report this. Sometimes it can be so violent that the teeth are damaged. Often, it is so loud that the person is unable to duplicate it while awake. Bruxism usually seems to occur in the early part of the night.

Treatment.   Sometimes bruxism is caused by a problem in occlusion (the way the upper and lower teeth fit together when the jaws are closed). However, psychological factors usually are involved. People with bruxism seem to be especially anxious, and they are often tense and appear to be suppressing anger. Bruxism often gets worse after alcohol intake. Psychotherapy, alcohol abstinence, and adjustment of the bite may help. A dentist can create a plastic guard to wear during sleep to prevent further damage to the teeth if this is warranted.

ANXIETY DISORDERS

Ours has been called the age of anxiety. Anxiety is a common emotion and, in its mild form, may be helpful in adapting to stressful situations. It is widespread but often hard to explain.

Although in popular speech the word "anxiety" may mean no more than worry or concern, in medicine it is defined specifically as a painful or apprehensive uneasiness of mind about some impending or anticipated ill fortune. It is an emotional reaction that manifests itself in various physical symptoms of different degrees of intensity.

PROBLEMS OF ANXIETY

Signs and Symptoms
- Tension over or terror about a danger whose source is often unrecognized;
- Rapid heartbeat or respiration;
- Tremor;
- Gastrointestinal distress;
- Motor tension (trembling, muscle aches, restlessness, inability to relax);
- Perspiring;
- Dry mouth;
- Dizziness;
- Impatience and irritability, insomnia, or difficulty in concentrating;

- With generalized anxiety disorder or anxiety neurosis, persistent anxiety for at least a month without any specific phobia or panic attack;
- Possible drug abuse to avoid symptoms.

Anxiety involves tension over or terror about a danger whose source is unrecognized.

Anxiety and fear are normal emotions: the fight-or-flight response is natural in the face of danger or stress. The symptoms—quickened heart rate, increased blood pressure and muscle tension, and increased awareness—represent an almost involuntary response marked by several physical reactions that are the result of an increased flow of catecholamines (chemicals in the blood that include epinephrine and that stimulate the sympathetic nervous system).

The fight-or-flight reaction gives a person the extra strength needed to overcome or to escape from a dangerous situation. An important characteristic of anxiety, however, is that you cannot always determine exactly what that dangerous situation is.

The Diagnosis.   The signs of anxiety are similar to those of fear—your heart begins to pound faster, you breathe rapidly, you may tremble, and your stomach becomes upset. Unlike ordinary fear, however, with anxiety you may not know exactly what it is that has you so distressed, or the apparent source of anxiety may seem minor compared with the intensity of your emotional reaction.

Fear is a reaction to an understandable, identifiable, current danger; anxiety is a conscious reaction to an unconscious stimulus. Anxiety also can be the first noticeable sign of depression or full-blown psychosis. Anxiety may be a response to a specific stress, in which case it may be termed situational anxiety; it also can be a generalized feeling of uneasiness called free-floating anxiety.

The generalized anxiety disorder, or anxiety neurosis, features persistent anxiety for at least a month, without any specific phobia or panic attack. The symptoms may include muscle tension, trembling, muscle aches, inability to relax, restlessness, sweating, palpitations, rapid breathing and pulse, dry mouth, dizziness, nausea, stomach pain, apprehension, impatience, irritability, insomnia, difficulty concentrating, and fatigue on awakening.

Anxiety can be associated with physical illness. Sometimes people try to avoid anxiety by abusing drugs such as alcohol, barbiturates, and anti-anxiety agents and even may become dependent on a medication. Occasionally, these drugs contribute to the anxiety state. Anxiety disorders sometimes can be traced back to childhood fears, stresses, or losses that are reactivated later in life.

Treatment. Treatment may include anti-anxiety medications (such as benzodiazepines), psychotherapy (see page 1026) to help you understand the conflicts that are producing the anxiety, and behavior therapy (see page 1036) to teach relaxation techniques. Do not try to resolve your anxiety by using anti-anxiety medications for a long time because there is a risk of dependency and addiction. Short-term use with the smallest dose that is effective is safer (see Controlling Stress, page 399).

PANIC ATTACKS

Signs and Symptoms
- Feelings of fear or extreme tension and a sense of impending doom;
- Shortness of breath;
- Palpitations, chest pain or discomfort, or feelings of choking or smothering;
- Dizziness or unsteadiness;
- Sense of unreality;
- Tingling in the extremities (hands or feet); hot and cold flashes; inexplicable perspiration;
- Trembling;
- Fear of losing one's mind, dying, or losing control;
- Nausea, vomiting, or diarrhea.

A panic attack is an unexplained and unprovoked fight-or-flight response. Your body displays the normal physiological response to a life-threatening situation or extreme physical exertion, but there is no apparent stimulus. All of a sudden you are panting, your heart is pounding, your head is swimming, and your palms are damp.

Panic disorders tend to run in families, and many researchers believe that biochemical factors may play a crucial role in this condition. It is a fairly common disorder, found in 1 to 2 percent of the population. But, because so many of the symptoms of a panic attack resemble those of an organic disorder, people often fail to recognize them and end up visiting physicians in the mis-

HYPERVENTILATION

Hyperventilation (from the Greek *hyper* meaning over or above and the Latin *ventus* for wind) is breathing too heavily with, paradoxically, a sensation of not being able to get enough air. A common occurrence during anxiety, it causes various symptoms including faintness and a tingling sensation in various parts of the body. This is why a person may feel faint upon hearing very bad news or at other traumatic life moments.

When you breathe quickly, an imbalance of gases is created in your blood, and this causes the symptoms. Because you are anxious, you often are not even aware that you are breathing too quickly.

Because hyperventilation is so often associated with or provoked by anxiety, it is occasionally treated with tranquilizers. However, such medication is unnecessary in most cases.

Hyperventilation can be relieved by a homespun remedy you might recognize as the traditional cure for hiccups. Simply hold your breath or try breathing into and out of a paper bag so that the exhaled carbon dioxide is reinhaled. This will help to restore the proper balance of blood gases and thus relieve the accompanying sensation.

taken belief that they have cardiac or respiratory problems.

Treatment. *Medication.* In the majority of cases, one of the family of drugs called the tricyclic antidepressants will relieve the problem of panic attacks. Many victims of this disorder also live in a constant state of fear of the attacks themselves, and brief treatment with anti-anxiety drugs may be helpful.

Other Therapies. Psychotherapy (see page 1026) can help uncover the underlying causes, but behavior therapy, and relaxation therapy in particular (see page 1036), may be useful in eliminating the symptoms.

PHOBIAS

Signs and Symptoms
* Persistent, irrational fear of a specific object, activity, or situation;
* Compelling desire to avoid what is feared;
* Fear may be recognized as excessive or unrealistic but you still want to avoid it;
* Impaired ability to function at normal tasks.

A phobia (from the Greek *phobos,* fear or flight) is a persistent, irrational fear of something—either an object, such as an insect, or a situation, such as being in crowds. This produces a compelling desire to avoid the feared object or situation.

Even though the person with the phobia may understand that the fear is excessive or unrealistic, he or she is unable to control the emotional response and will try to avoid the object at virtually all cost.

The Diagnosis. If the phobia causes no major disturbance in your life it is not considered to be a disorder. When the fear impairs your ability to function at normal tasks, however, then it needs to be diagnosed and treated.

One example is agoraphobia, fear of being in public places. Nearly a million people in this country, 85 percent of them women, suffer from agoraphobia which usually begins between the ages of 18 and 35. Another common example is claustrophobia (from the Latin *claustrum,* an enclosed place), the irrational fear of being in a con-

fined or crowded place. Morbid fear of heights is acrophobia (from the Greek *akros,* high).

Some degree of discomfort in any of these situations may be perfectly normal under certain circumstances, but when the fear becomes irrational and uncontrollable to the extent that normal social interactions and daily life are affected, it is considered to be a phobia. The fear is usually experienced not only at the time the person faces the object of the phobia but also when he or she anticipates encountering it (anticipatory anxiety). Phobias may be a part of anxiety or panic attacks.

ANTI-ANXIETY MEDICATIONS

Treating anxiety with drugs has come a long way since barbiturates were widely used for this purpose. Today, a family of drugs called anxiolytics are used to relieve the symptoms of anxiety. Most of these anxiety-fighting drugs are from a family called the benzodiazepines. Examples include lorazepam (Ativan), diazepam (Valium), alprazolam (Xanax), and chlordiazepoxide (Librium).

Like barbiturates, anxiolytics are sedatives and central muscle relaxants. And, also like the barbiturates, they are addictive. What makes them an improvement over barbiturates, however, is that they depress the respiratory system less and therefore are less risky with suicidal patients.

Anxiolytics are widely prescribed for various disorders including anxiety disorders and phobias. If you have an anxiety disorder or a related syndrome (such as hypochondriasis), you may have sudden attacks of intense fear as well as shortness of breath, pain and pressure in the head and chest, sweating, and numbness of the fingers and toes. You may also experience insomnia, depression, phobias, obsessions, compulsions, and other problems and may be likely to abuse alcohol and sleeping pills.

Anxiolytics usually are administered orally. Potential side effects of these medications include drowsiness, ataxia (inability to coordinate voluntary muscle movements), and confusion. It is important not to drive or attempt to operate heavy machinery while using them. Using alcohol while being treated with anxiolytics is especially dangerous. In older or extremely agitated people, low doses of anxiolytics may cause transient states of excitement, in which case the drug should be discontinued. When the therapy is no longer needed, it is important to withdraw the anxiolytic drug gradually because otherwise restlessness, insomnia, nightmares, and even seizures can occur. Anxiolytic drugs must be used cautiously by people who have or have had alcohol dependency.

Treatment. According to psychotherapy theory, phobias do not represent a reaction to real danger but are an underlying fear or hidden conflict within the affected person. His or her fears of forbidden sexual or aggressive impulses—of danger from within—are transposed onto some external object—for example, snakes. This is a defense mechanism known as displacement.

For this reason, psychotherapy (see page 1026) to uncover the original meanings of the fears and to help the person learn to cope with them can be helpful. But behavior therapy (see page 1026) also can be quite successful for phobias. One widely used approach is systematic desensitization in which the person is repeatedly exposed to the frightening stimulus until the fear diminishes. For example, he or she may begin by thinking about snakes and then go on to looking at pictures of them and, finally, to seeing some live ones. Antidepressant drug therapy may help some patients who have a phobic disorder.

OBSESSIVE-COMPULSIVE DISORDER

Signs and Symptoms
- Recurrent persistent ideas, thoughts, or impulses that are experienced involuntarily and appear to be senseless;
- Repetitive behavior that is performed regularly, even though it appears senseless.

Individuals with an obsessive-compulsive disorder experience recurrent obsessions (persistent thoughts) or compulsions (persistent behaviors) or both that are perceived as being senseless and repugnant. Obsessions include thoughts of violence, fears of contamination, fears of becoming infected, and doubt. Examples of compulsions include repeated checking of the doors to make sure they are locked, repeated handwashing, and counting steps while walking. The obsessions and compulsions do not always occur at the same time in the same person. The disorder seems to be slightly more common in females than males. This disorder generally begins in late adolescence or young adulthood; it rarely is seen in children. At times, the disorder is accompanied by depression or anxiety.

A person with an obsessive-compulsive disorder may do virtually everything in a meticulous, precise, orderly fashion. When the compulsive need is not fulfilled, the person may experience overwhelming anxiety.

Treatment. Behavior psychotherapy is helpful at times. Your physician may advise antidepressants or other drug therapy.

RELAXATION TECHNIQUES

Although relaxation techniques resemble meditative and contemplative methods that have been part of Eastern and Western religious practices for centuries, they were introduced as psychotherapeutic relaxation training in the 1920s by Edmund Jacobson who used them to teach hypertensive people to relax.

There are many different approaches to relaxation therapy. In progressive muscle relaxation, you learn to focus on each muscle. First, you tense a muscle and hold that tension for 5 or 10 seconds until you can easily identify the muscle or muscle group involved by slight discomfort. Then, you slowly release the muscle, repeating the procedure with various muscle groups so that you become familiar with the sensation of relaxing your entire body. The muscle tension levels may be monitored on a biofeedback machine during the training sessions.

In other relaxation therapies the approach differs. In autogenic training, you concentrate on self-suggestions of warmth and heaviness in the limbs. Hypnosis involves having suggestions of relaxation and mental calm provided by the hypnotist. Biofeedback is a method of relieving symptoms of distress by relaxing the muscles. It is used to reduce stress and, as a part of systematic desensitization, to treat phobic anxiety. It involves the monitoring of one of the physiological systems—heart, respiration, or skin resistance—so that you can become more aware of your own body's stress and thus control it.

The various methods of meditation—such as Zen, yoga, or transcendental meditation—are based on using mental repetition of a neutral word or symbol in a quiet, comfortable environment.

The ideal setting for relaxation training is a quiet room where you can rest comfortably on the floor or in a reclining chair or bed. You need to feel relatively quiet but not tired. An instructor can be a great help in directing your attention toward your inner self so that you will learn to concentrate and to relax at the same time and be able to do it yourself at home. Listening to a tape can be used, although live training may be more effective. Eventually, you learn to relax without verbal cues from another person.

POST-TRAUMATIC STRESS DISORDER

Signs and Symptoms

- Persistent reexperiencing of a traumatic event in intrusive recollections, distressing dreams, hallucinations, distress at anniversaries of the trauma, and avoidance of thoughts, feelings, and activities associated with the trauma;
- Feeling of detachment or estrangement from others, inability to have loving feelings;
- Markedly diminished interest in significant activities;
- In young children, developmental regression in such areas as toilet training and language;
- Sense of a foreshortened future, no hope of family life, career, or living to old age;
- Increased arousal (not present before the trauma), with at least two of the following: trouble sleeping, anger, difficulty concentrating, exaggerated startle response, and physiological reaction to situations that remind the person of the traumatic event.

Post-traumatic stress disorder occurs among survivors of events that are generally acknowledged as traumatic—rape, war, torture, earthquake, or death camps. A physical trauma is often involved, but there is always a characteristic psychological component: the person has lived through a period in which he or she was faced with intense fear, helplessness, loss of control, and the threat of annihilation.

Very young and very old people who experience major traumas seem to be especially susceptible to post-traumatic stress, presumably because young children have inadequately developed coping mechanisms and the elderly may be overly rigid and have fewer social supports.

The symptoms may appear immediately after the event or be delayed by 6 months or more. There may be a sense of estrangement from other people and of difficulty enjoying activities that were previously pleasurable—particularly those associated with intimacy, such as sexual contact.

Flashbacks are one aspect of post-traumatic stress disorder in victims of major life traumas—an automobile accident, an airplane crash, a wartime experience, kidnapping or hostage situation, or physical assault—in which the original experience was one of intense fear and utter loss of control. The flashback is a vivid sense of reliving the experience, and the person may perceive it as real.

"Survivor guilt" is also a common problem in the case of those who survive traumatic episodes in which other people have died or who survived only through means incompatible with conventional morality.

Treatment. *Medication.* Minor tranquilizers such as diazepam (Valium) and chlordiazepoxide (Librium) can decrease the symptoms of anxiety.

Other Therapies. Behavioral techniques, especially relaxation therapy and progressive desensitization, may be used to decrease the symptoms such as anxiety and phobia. Psychotherapy (see page 1026) can provide support and, in severe cases, the insight and catharsis needed for the person to cope with the reaction to the original trauma.

DEPRESSION AND MOOD DISORDERS

There are various kinds of depression, and they may have some symptoms in common. These symptoms may include withdrawal from usual activities, disturbed sleep, loss of appetite, inability to concentrate or to make decisions, decreased energy level, feelings of worthlessness and guilt, and even thoughts of suicide and death. When the depression is mild, changes in the environment may lead to some improvement, but not when the depression is severe.

There also are age-associated features. In early childhood, separation anxiety is a common factor. In early adolescence in boys, negative and antisocial behavior may occur. Sexual acting out, truancy, and running away are seen in older boys and girls. In the elderly, pseudodementia—depression that is evident primarily as a loss of intellectual functioning—must be carefully differentiated from the true dementia caused by organic mental disorder.

This section deals with various kinds of depression and the treatment options that are available to you. In addition, it discusses the warning signs of potential suicide, a complication of any serious depression.

SITUATIONAL DEPRESSION

Signs and Symptoms
- Sense of helplessness and gloom;
- Grief;
- Loss of self-esteem;
- Feeling that life is meaningless;
- Anxiety or worry;
- Irritability;
- Retreat from relationships with others.

Also known as a depressive reaction, situational depression is a prolonged episode of "the blues" that may occur after a disappointment or loss or during mid-life.

Situational depression is not the same as normal grieving after the death of a loved one, illness, or other misfortune, although it may be triggered by such an event.

Depression also may be a side effect of certain medications, particularly in a person who tends toward depression.

Treatment.   Situational depression may be relieved when the problem that triggered it fades. On the other hand, the person may become so depressed that there is a risk of suicide. Consequently, it is important to provide emotional support.

At first, when the person is acutely depressed, psychotherapy can provide that support while antidepressant medication helps to relieve the symptoms. Then, when the symptoms are relieved, psychotherapy can help the person understand why the depression occurred: Are there solutions to their external life problems that might prove less stressful? Did the episode that triggered the depression recall a childhood conflict long buried in the unconscious? Does he or she have low self-esteem, view the situation as hopeless, or feel uncomfortable expressing negative feelings such as hostility or anger? Would a change of scenery or routine be helpful?

One of several different types of therapy may be suggested in the case of depression. Cognitive therapy can help the person view his or her situation differently by identifying and testing self-defeating ways of thinking about it (negative cognitions). For example, a person who tends to be pessimistic is likely to suffer from feelings of hopelessness. Someone who expects failure may be apathetic and unwilling to exert himself or herself. Once the therapist has helped the person to identify these thinking patterns, new approaches to the situation can be developed.

Family therapy can help the person improve his or her marriage or family life or both, so that the depression does not adversely affect other family members and the family members do not contribute further to the depression.

MAJOR DEPRESSIVE DISORDER

Signs and Symptoms
- Change in physical demeanor—either a noticeable slowing down or "dragging," or a discernible speeding up or agitation;
- Distinct quality to the depressed mood (different from the feeling one has after the death of a loved one);
- Lack of response to environment changes (day/night, sun/rain, leisure/work);
- Loss of interest in activities usually enjoyed, including sex;
- Poor appetite and attendant weight loss;
- Early morning awakening;
- Self-reproach or inappropriate guilt;
- Suicidal behavior;
- Sometimes, hallucinations or delusions;
- No apparent "trigger" (precipitating event).

A major depressive disorder, sometimes called endogenous depression, is not merely sadness or grief but is a genuine psychiatric illness that affects both the mind and the body. Depressed people tend to retreat from human relationships, to have trouble functioning in society and using their talents, to be unable to enjoy life, and even to feel suicidal.

Stricken with much more desperate feelings than merely the "blues" or being "down in the dumps," these people are incapacitated, are unable to hold a steady job, derive no pleasure from their lives, and have difficulty interacting with others. Sometimes, although not always, they may have psychotic symptoms such as hallucinations or delusions. By and large, however, the physical symptoms of depression—a characteristic hollowness around the eyes, uninflected speech, and a gait resembling sleepwalking—are the signs of depression.

Depression is more common among women than among men. Because it is both debilitating and associated with suicidal tendencies, a major depressive disorder is considered serious. But this type of depression, even in its most severe form, generally is self-limited. It will run its course and terminate without treatment within 6 months to a year. Meanwhile, however, the person's existence may be almost intolerable, and suicide is a great temptation.

Treatment. Because depression is so common, many therapies have been developed to treat it. At first, treatment of a major depression often includes hospitalization, especially if the person is threatening suicide or displays suicidal behavior.

The various types of therapy have some characteristics in common. Virtually all therapeutic situations operate on the assumption that people can change, that they can learn to cope better with life traumas and inner struggles. The depressed person usually visits the psychiatrist because he or she believes that there is light at the end of the tunnel.

Psychotherapy. Psychotherapy is used, often in conjunction with medication, to help the depressed person understand the sources of his or her depression and to find other ways of coping with inner conflicts.

Cognitive therapy is a short-term psychotherapy developed to treat both depression and anxiety. The idea is that self-defeating patterns of thinking make us feel depressed because our negative thoughts influence our feelings. In cognitive therapy, you may be asked to write down your negative thoughts. The therapist then helps you identify the distortions in them and suggests constructive alternatives.

Antidepressive Medications. Medications to treat depression come in two main types, the tricyclic antidepressants (TCAs) and the monoamine oxidase inhibitors (MAOIs).

Antidepressants are more helpful when the depression has discrete episodes that seem to have a life of their own rather than in chronic or situational depression. Imipramine (Tofranil) and amitriptyline (Elavil) are the most frequently used tricyclic antidepressants, the most common type of antidepressant medication. However, these medications do not deal with the intrapsychic and interpersonal issues that may have contributed to the depression. For this reason, the most effective treatment may be to combine both medication and psychotherapy.

Electroconvulsive (Shock) Therapy. In the movies, electroconvulsive therapy (ECT) has been depicted as repressive and cruel, but actually it is considered by many psychiatrists to be one of the most effective and humane treatments for depression. It is used primarily for major depressive episodes.

Unlike antidepressants, ECT works quickly (often within a few days) and is more likely to be decisively helpful when the problem is serious. Physicians do not know exactly how it works, but it may alter the rate at which brain chemicals, called catecholamines, affect the central nervous system cells.

Before undergoing ECT, the patient is anesthetized with a barbiturate and a muscle relaxant. Side effects commonly include temporary memory loss, headaches, and muscle aches. Nonetheless, ECT remains the most effective treatment available for major depression. Its risks are significantly lower than the risks of untreated severe depression (which include suicide).

MANIC-DEPRESSIVE ILLNESS

Signs and Symptoms
- Alternating pattern of emotional highs (characterized by high-spirited behavior) and emotional lows or depressions;
- The manic and major depression episodes may alternate rapidly every few days;
- Symptoms of depression are prominent and last for a full day or more.

Manic-depressive illness is known to mental health professionals as bipolar disorder. It is characterized by recurring periods of mental illness in which episodes of excitement and hyperactivity (mania) either

WARNING SIGNS OF POTENTIAL SUICIDE

Too often, family and associates are shocked at a suicide, saying things like, "I had no idea; he seemed so happy." In fact, the person's behavior may not match descriptions of these warning signs precisely but, related to the person's normal personality, changes may be evident. When a person displays warning signs of potential suicide, it is important to keep a close watch on him or her (to see that the opportunity for suicide does not arise), and to seek professional help as soon as possible. Begin by calling your local suicide hotline or a local psychiatrist or psychologist.

A person who is contemplating taking his or her own life may show one or more symptoms (see below), but it is important to keep in mind that these warning signs are only guidelines. There is no one type of suicidal person.

The Signs

Withdrawal
The person is unwilling to communicate and appears to have an overwhelming urge to be alone. He or she is withdrawing into a shell. Trouble at work can be a symptom of a withdrawal from the workplace, just as poor grades can signal a retreat from school. Rejection of forms of recreation the person usually considers pleasurable may also be a warning sign.

Moodiness
Although we all have our ups and downs, when the shifts are drastic—an emotional "high" one day followed by being "down in the dumps" the next—there is cause for alarm. Sudden, inexplicable calm after a spell of gloom is a danger sign; it may indicate that the person has decided on suicide as the solution to the problem.

Life Crisis or Trauma
In a deeply depressed person, divorce, death, or an accident can trigger a suicide attempt. The loss of self-esteem that may occur after loss of a job or a financial setback may produce suicidal thinking.

Personality Change
The wallflower turns into the life of the party, or vice versa. Or there might be a change in attitude toward personal appearance or a change in energy level.

Threat
The person may state outright that he or she wants to commit suicide, saying things like "I wish I'd never been born," or "You're going to be better off when I'm gone." The popular assumption that people who threaten suicide never really do it is not true.

Gift-Giving
The person begins to "bequeath" his most cherished belongings to friends and loved ones.

Depression
The person appears to be physically depressed and is unable to function socially or in the workplace.

Aggression
The suicidal urge may be manifested in the person's sudden participation in dangerous activities such as high-speed driving or unsafe sex.

The risk that the suicide actually will be completed is increased in older men, in people who have lost a spouse (by divorce or death), in alcoholics, in those with a history of previous suicide attempts, or in those with a family history of suicide.

---

occur alone or alternate with periods of depression.

Everyone has moods, but bipolar disorder is characterized by extreme and unpredictable mood swings from highly excited euphoria to the darkest depths of despair and depression. In a normal person, mood changes are a response to events in the environment but, when elation or depression occurs without relation to the circumstances, this is manic-depressive illness.

The person's feelings are so intense that they take over completely, and contact with the real world is lost. The manic phase usually is the episode that may require the person to be hospitalized. During the manic episode, the person may feel very "high" or irritable. His or her euphoria may not be obvious to those who do not know the person well, but friends and loved ones will come to recognize it as unusual or as typical of the manic phase. His or her speech and thoughts seem to run at high speed, so fast that it is difficult to understand them. The speech may become so laden with puns, jokes, and plays on words that, after a while, it makes little sense.

The self-esteem of the individual with manic-depressive illness may soar, often to the point of delusions of grandeur. In fact, he or she is likely to be hyperactive, eager to take on far more activities than reasonably can be handled. Should such activities be thwarted, however, irritability may result. There may be an inability to judge the consequences of actions, manifested in shopping sprees, self-destructive sexual activity, unwise business decisions, or reckless driving. The person may change moods frequently, alternately laughing and crying, and there may be fleeting delusions or hallucinations.

If untreated, the manic episode may last for weeks, during which the person is physically restless, highly talkative, likely to sleep less, and easily distracted.

During the depressed phase (which is the more frequent form of the illness), the person appears depressed for most of the day, nearly every day. He or she loses interest and pleasure in nearly all activities, may lose or gain a great deal of weight, and usually has a change in sleeping patterns. He or she may be fatigued, suffer from feelings of worthlessness, and have trouble concentrating. The person may withdraw completely, speaking only rarely. Often, there are recurrent thoughts of death and suicide. If untreated, the depressive phase may last for months.

Often, two or more complete cycles (a manic episode and a major depression that follow each other with no period of remission) will occur within a year. This situation may be called rapid cycling and seems to be more chronic than other types of bipolar disorder. Although major depression is more common in women, bipolar disorder is equally common in men and women. It is estimated that about 1 percent of the adult population have had this disease.

The disorder usually appears between the ages of 15 and 25. It occurs much more often in immediate relatives of people with bipolar disorder than in the general population.

Treatment. *Medication.* Tranquilizing drugs are helpful in controlling the manic phase. Antidepressant drugs can be used to treat the depression episodes. Lithium carbonate is the standard treatment for manic episodes, and the regular use of this drug may prevent uncontrolled mood swings.

Other Therapies. In severe cases, electroconvulsive therapy may be necessary

(see page 1039). It is always important to be aware that the danger of suicide is present. When the person appears to have suicidal tendencies, it is important for those closest to him or her to express a caring attitude (see Warning Signs of Potential Suicide, page 1040). In these cases, however, the person will probably need to be hospitalized.

Hospitalization also is needed if the person is in a depressed phase and regresses so much that he or she is unable to take care of personal needs at home. Likewise, if electroconvulsive therapy is prescribed or if the antidepressant medication is expected to have severe side effects, admission to the hospital may be appropriate. On the other hand, considering how severe the depressed phase often is in bipolar disorder, it is surprising how many people are treated successfully as outpatients.

During the depressed phase, psychotherapy usually serves only as a means of emotional support. The therapist will explain the illness to those closest to the patient, establish a rapport with the patient, and foster a sense of hope and planning for the future. A structured daily program for the person may be provided, and the therapist will be sure to determine the risk of suicide and intervene when necessary.

SEASONAL AFFECTIVE DISORDER

Signs and Symptoms
- Depression caused by a specific season of the year, most often winter;
- Headaches, irritability, low energy level;
- Crying spells.

Seasonal affective disorder (SAD) is an extreme form of the "winter blahs." True forms of this disorder are unusual; most people with "cabin fever" do not have SAD.

People who do have it tend to sleep a great deal in the winter. They may gain a great deal of weight because they gorge on carbohydrates. Low on energy and highly irritable, they get many headaches, feel very stressed, and may have crying spells. The cause of SAD is not yet known, but it may be linked to the body's biological clock that controls temperature and hormone production. It usually begins in adolescents or young adults and is more common among women than men. Some people outgrow it, but it may last a lifetime.

Treatment. A recent innovation in the treatment of SAD uses fluorescent bulbs for light therapy. Patients are allowed to read, but not sleep, for several hours a day in front of specially designed, bright lights. The symptoms usually subside within a few days but reappear if therapy is stopped. The use of full-spectrum light bulbs to extend the hours of sunlight artificially is being investigated.

THOUGHT DISORDERS

A psychosis is an impairment of thinking or mood in which a person's interpretation of reality and of daily events is severely abnormal. Psychosis is actually a symptom of a disordered brain; there is substantial evidence that chemical abnormalities cause the problem.

SCHIZOPHRENIA

Signs and Symptoms
- Two or more of the following for at least 1 week: delusions, prominent hallucinations for much of the day, incoherence, lack of or inappropriate display of emotions, bizarre delusions (such as talking with Martians);
- Problems or decreased ability to function in work, social life, and hygiene;
- Continuous signs for at least 6 months;
- No evidence of an organic cause or of mood disturbance with psychotic features.

Schizophrenia is the most common and destructive of the psychoses. It may be difficult to treat, and it is the most likely to be permanent. The affected person withdraws from the people and activities in the world around him or her and retreats into a world of delusions and fantasies.

The schizophrenic is unable to sustain self-initiated, goal-directed activity and has delusions that are often multiple, fragmented, or bizarre—that he or she is being persecuted, or that the FBI wants to kill him or her.

There may be a loosening of associations, with the affected person's conversation jumping from one idea to a completely unrelated one. Or the schizophrenic may chatter away and yet fail to convey any information. Speech is vague, very abstract, or repetitive. The schizophrenic may play with language, making up new words that seem highly important but make no sense to anyone else.

Hallucinations are common, and the person is especially likely to hear voices, although schizophrenia is not to be confused with cases of multiple personality. The schizophrenic's face tends to be expressionless and the voice is a monotone. The normal sense of self has been lost. The schizophrenic is likely to be socially withdrawn. Conversely, the schizophrenic may be clingy and intrusive with strangers. There is a marked lack of response to the surrounding environment. The schizophrenic may appear very rigid or in a stupor or may display inappropriate excitement through odd mannerisms and grimacing. Pacing and rocking are common. The schizophrenic may have a disheveled, bewildered appearance and may dress or groom eccentrically.

Schizophrenia usually appears during adolescence or early adulthood, although it may begin in middle or late adult life. The cause is not known, although many believe it is an inherited disorder. There is some evidence that genetic influences combine with environmental ones.

Schizophrenia seems to be equally common in both sexes. Once the signs appear, it is uncommon for the person to return to the level of functioning achieved before the disorder began. Usually, there are acute periods of schizophrenic behavior with residual impairment between episodes.

There are different types of schizophrenia: the catatonic type (which may involve stupor or mutism, or rapid alternation between the extremes of excitement and stupor); disorganized schizophrenia (when the person is incoherent and either expressionless or displays inappropriate emotions); and paranoid schizophrenia (characterized by a preoccupation with one or more systematized delusions such as the belief that the person is a famous individual or with frequent auditory hallucinations related to a single theme).

Treatment. Because there are more theories about schizophrenia than about virtually any other mental disorder, there also are many treatments. Generally, individuals with acute or severe episodes of schizophrenia are treated in the hospital.

Electroconvulsive therapy in the hospital may be used in acute cases. Antipsychotic drugs, such as one of the phenothiazines, usually are prescribed to decrease excitement and agitated depression and to improve the person's thought processes. Frontal lobotomy—the surgical cutting of the frontal lobes of the brain in order to decrease aggression—has fallen out of favor because its results are both unpredictable and irreversible. Antipsychotic drugs usually produce an improvement and allow the schizophrenic to be released from the hospital. However, if the person fails to continue to take the medication, the symptoms invariably return.

Supportive psychotherapy (see page 1026) may help the person with schizophrenia to return to a more normal, less-withdrawn life.

BRIEF REACTIVE PSYCHOSIS

Signs and Symptoms
- Disordered thinking or delusions (false beliefs)—anything from thinking that a dead grandmother is alive to believing that all restaurant food is poisoned—that the person will not give up even in the face of logical argument;
- Disorders of perception (especially hallucinations);
- Language disorders (conversation that makes no sense, wanders, or is literal to an extreme);
- Disturbance of affect (the emotion the affected person appears to express is either not consistent with what he or she is thinking or shifts much more rapidly than normal);
- Symptoms last at least a few hours but no more than a month.

When a person suddenly displays psychotic symptoms for at least a few hours but not more than a month and eventually returns to his or her previous level of functioning, the diagnosis is brief reactive psychosis.

The symptoms often appear after an extremely stressful event such as the loss of a loved one or combat duty. The person goes through turmoil, experiencing a rapid fluctuation of emotions or overwhelming confusion. He or she may be aware of it, or the symptoms may be obvious from his or her conversation.

Behavior and dress may be bizarre, and the psychotic may adopt peculiar postures. He or she may frequently scream or, on the other hand, become mute. Speech may be foolish, often involving the repetition of nonsense phrases. There may be passing hallucinations or delusions, and the person is disoriented and has trouble remembering things.

This disorder usually appears during adolescence or in the early adult years. Often, the symptoms will subside in a day or two. Afterward, the person may continue to feel a loss of self-esteem or be mildly depressed for a while.

Treatment. *Medication.* Treatment involves use of drugs often referred to as major tranquilizers, such as chlorpromazine (Thorazine) or haloperidol (Haldol), which are antipsychotics. They do not really induce tranquility but instead decrease or completely eliminate psychotic symptoms and behavior.

These antipsychotic drugs appear to act by blocking the chemical receptors in the brain that normally link via dopamine, a chemical nerve messenger. Although they are very effective, they do cause a range of side effects: dry mouth, sensitization of skin to sunlight, constipation, loss of bladder control, blurred vision, orthostatic hypotension (feeling of faintness on rising quickly from chair or bed), or a tremor.

Other Therapies. Psychotherapy (see page 1026) is also helpful in providing support and helping the person to cope with the emotional trauma from which the psychosis originated.

ALCOHOL- OR DRUG-INDUCED PSYCHOSIS

Signs and Symptoms
- Delirium;

- Aggression, hostility, or violent behavior;
- "Bad trip" or fearful mental disorientation (panic, delusions, hallucinations) after use of hallucinogenic drug;
- Behavior resembling schizophrenia after use of certain combinations (such as alcohol and barbiturates) or overdoses of drugs (such as sleeping pills or antidepressants).

This disorder is known technically as psychoactive substance-induced organic mental disorder. It is a psychosis caused by the use of certain drugs (particularly hallucinogens or amphetamines), by overdose of common drugs, or by alcohol abuse or untreated withdrawal.

The affected person displays all or many of the symptoms of acute psychosis or schizophrenia—disorientation, violence, visual hallucinations (see pages 1042 and 1043). Often, the delirium is so similar to psychosis that the only way to be certain that it has been caused by chemical means is through laboratory tests. Overdoses of cocaine or amphetamines are two major causes.

Even in people who are usually calm and controlled, aggression and violent hostility may be produced. Untreated withdrawal from these drugs or from alcohol may cause delirium, seizures, or terrifying hallucinations. Even some drugs used for medical reasons may cause psychosis-like behavior after a person takes an overdose of them. These include over-the-counter sleeping pills and antihistamines as well as antidepressants and drugs used for Parkinson's disease.

A psychotic reaction to hallucinogenic drugs such as LSD or PCP (angel dust) and occasionally marijuana or hashish, popularly known as a "bad trip," is a frightening, disorienting mental reaction. The person experiences panic, anxiety, and a feeling of disorientation. The fear is of "losing one's mind" and is often accompanied by delusions and hallucinations.

Treatment.   For his or her own safety, a person who is on a "bad trip" needs to be isolated in a safe, quiet environment and accompanied by someone who will provide reassurance. Treatment with an antipsychotic drug such as haloperidol may be necessary to bring the person back to reality.

ADDICTIVE BEHAVIOR

Although the word "addiction" tends to bring drugs to mind, people can be addicted to a wide variety of substances and practices, from coffee or tobacco to compulsive gambling. However, the term "addictive behavior" also refers to psychological dependencies such as overeating.

The main characteristic of addictive behavior is that the person feels a compelling need to engage in the particular activity or to use the addictive substance without deriving pleasure or gain from it.

"The main point," wrote Dostoevsky, a compulsive gambler, "is the game itself. I swear it is not greed for money, although I am sorely in need of money."

In this section we discuss the addictive behavior that accompanies the use of alcohol and other addictive behaviors. We also consider the use and misuse of substances such as alcohol and tobacco. Drug dependency is discussed in a later section (see page 1046).

ALCOHOL DEPENDENCY

Signs and Symptoms
- Feeling of guilt about drinking;
- Tendency to drink too much;
- Desire to continue drinking after friends say the person has had enough;
- Irritation when family or friends comment on the person's drinking;
- Arguments with loved one about drinking;
- Inability to remember previous evening's activities upon awakening, with assurance from companions that person did not pass out (black out);
- Regret over things done or said while drinking;
- Efforts to avoid family or friends while drinking;
- Financial problems;
- Inability to meet the demands of a steady job;

- Eating irregularly while drinking;
- Arrest for driving while under the influence of alcohol, or car accident after drinking;
- "The shakes" upon awakening, which disappear after "a little drink";
- Steady drinking for several days at a time;
- Delusions or hallucinations after periods of drinking;
- Loss of memory and concentration;
- Repeated declarations that the person has resolved to give up drinking altogether, with denials that he or she has a drinking problem.

Alcoholism is a chronic and often progressive disease characterized by periods of preoccupation with alcohol, impaired control over alcohol intake, and repetitive use of alcohol despite the known risk of adverse consequences related to drinking. In this context, alcoholism is alcohol dependence.

Often, a person begins to become dependent on alcohol after discovering that having a few drinks helps to relieve stress from family problems, difficulties at work, or social isolation. Despite occasional hangovers and the fact that this relief is only temporary, he or she gradually falls into the pattern of drinking whenever he or she feels tense. Unfortunately, the more an alcohol-dependent person drinks, the less tension he or she can tolerate without alcohol.

The actual number of drinks is not the critical issue, because some people can easily become intoxicated after very little. The diagnosis of alcohol dependency is made when the person has difficulty getting through the day without regular alcohol consumption. We are not yet certain of the cause of alcoholism, although it does seem to run in families and there is some evidence pointing to a genetic predisposition. It tends to be underdiagnosed because one classic trait of alcoholics is that they deny their dependency.

About 5 percent of the adult population in the United States is said to have alcoholism. It is more common among men than women (although the prevalence among women is increasing) and among the urban poor and minority groups.

Treatment. In treating alcoholism, a fundamental principle is "Once an alcoholic, always an alcoholic." Most research indicates that an alcoholic is unable to become a normal social drinker. Consequently, treatment is designed to eliminate alcohol totally from that person's routine. He or she must never take another drink. Alcoholics Anonymous (AA) is the most effective treatment known. It provides group support, a 12-step abstinence program with a spiritual base, and gentle confrontation of the various ways in which alcoholics deny their illness. In conjunction with AA, aversive therapy may be used to discourage drinking: the drug disulfiram (Antabuse) blocks the normal oxidation of alcohol so that acetaldehyde accumulates in the bloodstream and causes unpleasant symptoms such as rapid pulse and vomiting.

Psychotherapy (see page 1026) may be suggested to help restore the person's self-esteem and establish new patterns of healthy behavior (see Alcohol Abuse, page 417).

COMPULSIVE GAMBLING

Signs and Symptoms
- Gambling gradually proceeds from occasional to habitual, with higher and higher stakes risked and other interests—family, and sometimes work—neglected;
- Most important reason to gamble is craving for the painful but pleasurable tension derived from risk;
- When money is lost, feels guilty and tries to keep it a secret;
- Once started, continues, whether winning or losing, until the place closes or has no money left;
- In order to afford the habit and pay debts, may resort to unlawful activities (larceny, fraud, embezzlement).

Gambling tends to be a compulsion more frequently among men than among women. It often goes hand-in-hand with excessive drinking. It is serious to the extent that it disrupts personal life and may cause financial ruin.

Treatment. Treatment includes psychotherapy (individual and group) (see page 1026) and support groups such as Gamblers Anonymous.

CAFFEINE ADDICTION

Signs and Symptoms
- Anxiety manifestations;
- Muscle twitching and sensory disturbances such as ringing in ears or flashing of light;
- Heart palpitations;
- Gastrointestinal pain or diarrhea;
- Periods of inexhaustability;
- Insomnia;
- Withdrawal symptoms if daily intake is interrupted: headache, drowsiness and lethargy, irritability, nervousness, vague depression, or occasional yawning;
- Depression;
- In women, fibrocystic breast syndrome (benign lumps in breast tissue).

People who are addicted to coffee easily recognize a "caffeine high": their heart pounds, they are jumpy, and they may have gastric distress. When they try to give up coffee, they get a headache and often feel drowsy. Caffeine is found not only in coffee but also in chocolate and cola drinks.

Treatment. Caffeine addiction can be cured by discontinuing or decreasing intake. When you are thirsty, drink decaffeinated beverages or water. Symptoms should begin clearing up in 4 to 10 days.

DRUG DEPENDENCY

Dependence on drugs, whether prescription or illegal, is dangerous because of its long-term physical effects, its disruptive effect on family and work, and the risks associated with sudden withdrawal. Frequently, a person is able to maintain a dependence on a prescription drug by collecting prescriptions from various unsuspecting physicians. Illegal drugs are hazardous not only by their nature but also because of the risk of contamination with other dangerous substances. In most cases, help is essential, whether in the form of support groups, drug-free residential communities, or day-care centers.

CENTRAL NERVOUS SYSTEM DEPRESSANTS

Signs and Symptoms
- Drowsiness or coma;
- Slurred speech;
- Lack of coordination;
- Memory impairment;
- Confusion;
- Tremor or decreased muscle tone;
- Agitation;
- Paranoia;
- Inappropriate display of emotions.

Central nervous system depressants, also known as downers, include prescription drugs such as sedatives, hypnotics, and anti-anxiety agents. The effects of their use resemble those of drunkenness but without alcohol consumption. Aside from the difficulties usually caused in the person's family and work lives, there is also a danger of death from an overdose.

Glue. Young children may sniff glue, which is a central nervous system depressant, when they are as young as age 6 or 7 years. The glue is sniffed directly from the tube or in plastic bags or from smears on pieces of cloth. At first a few sniffs may give a "high," but the child develops a tolerance in a matter of weeks or months. Chronic users may have to use several tubes before achieving the desired effect. The initial symptoms are similar to those of alcoholic inebriation, including slurred speech, dizziness, breakdown of inhibitions, drowsiness, and amnesia. The child may have hallucinations, may lose weight, and occasionally may lose consciousness.

Barbiturates. Most people begin taking barbiturates for relief from unbearable tension, anxiety, or inadequacy. Middle-aged people may obtain the drug from their physicians in response to complaints of nervousness or trouble sleeping, and they may be chronically intoxicated for years without anyone around them realizing it, until their ability to work becomes impaired or they begin to exhibit signs such as slurred speech. Teenagers or young adults may ingest barbiturates to "get high."

Barbiturates, especially the short-acting kind such as secobarbital, produce psychological dependence as well as physical dependence after 1 or 2 months of taking doses above the recommended therapeutic level. The most commonly available on the black market are secobarbital (reds, red devils), phenobarbital (yellows), and a combination of secobarbital and amobarbital (reds and blues, rainbows). Some young adults take barbiturates intravenously.

Benzodiazepines.   Two drugs of the benzodiazepine group, chlordiazepoxide (Librium) and diazepam (Valium), are often prescribed to control anxiety as well as to control the symptoms of alcohol withdrawal. These are frequently abused, particularly by persons who obtain prescriptions from multiple physicians, and can cause marked central nervous system effects.

Treatment.   A child with a glue-sniffing habit should be seen by a child psychologist.

Treatment of addiction to barbiturates or benzodiazepines includes getting the person to withdraw from the drug safely—withdrawal symptoms can range from mild (such as anxiety, weakness, profuse sweating, and insomnia) to seizures—and preventing him or her from starting again. The latter usually is achieved with the help of drug support groups (see also Detoxification, page 1048).

CENTRAL NERVOUS SYSTEM STIMULANTS

Signs and Symptoms
- Agitation;
- Rapid speech;
- Irritability;
- Difficulty concentrating;
- Debilitating cycle of "runs" (heavy use for several days a week) and "crashes" (letdowns when the user is forced to stop using the drug because of agitation, paranoia, and malnutrition);
- Nasal congestion (with cocaine).

The most widely used central nervous system stimulants are amphetamines and cocaine. Amphetamines (also known as uppers) produce an extraordinarily high degree of psychological dependence that amounts to a compulsion. A high degree of tolerance to the euphoric effects develops in abusers. The effects last for several hours. There is less physical dependence in the sense of a biochemical or physiological need and, therefore, less of a withdrawal syndrome of the kind found in alcohol or heroin addiction.

Some people view cocaine as a safe "recreational" drug. In reality, cocaine is far more dangerous than once thought. Cocaine generally is taken by sniffing (snorting), although it is being smoked in a crystalline form (crack) with increasing frequency. Occasionally, cocaine is taken by injection through a vein. The drug is rapidly absorbed, and its effects begin quickly with initial stimulation and enhancement of mood.

Cocaine triggers a release of the hormones epinephrine and norepinephrine from your sympathetic nervous system. These hormones stimulate your heart to pump faster and more powerfully. Also, your blood pressure and body temperature increase, you become more alert, and your appetite diminishes. These reactions result in the rush of euphoria, the illusion of control and heightened sexual drive commonly associated with using cocaine.

Even a single modest dose of cocaine can kill you. Injecting or smoking crack can be more dangerous because a greater amount of the drug is absorbed into your bloodstream. Cocaine can overwork your heart, forcing it to beat too fast and too powerfully. As your heart tires, it becomes susceptible to irregularities in its rhythm, which can cause your heart to stop. Cocaine also can induce coronary artery spasm, a sudden narrowing of the arteries leading to your heart. Such spasms can cause a blood clot to form, even in otherwise normal arteries. If the spasm or clot completely blocks the flow of blood to your heart, it can cause a heart attack, dangerous heartbeat irregularities, or sudden death.

Thus, cocaine can kill you quickly, even if your heart is perfectly healthy. The size of the dose is not important. Superbly conditioned athletes have succumbed to the potent and variable effects of cocaine after a single modest dose.

The chronic use of cocaine can disrupt eating and sleeping habits and can produce psychological disturbances such as irritability and disturbed concentration. After the euphoria of cocaine subsides, the user often feels irritable or may have an acute anxiety reaction along with occasional hallucinations. The craving for cocaine can become overwhelming. When smoked as crack, cocaine is almost instantly addictive.

Treatment. A person who withdraws from amphetamines may experience a depression so severe that he or she becomes suicidal. Withdrawal also commonly produces extreme lethargy, fatigue, anxiety, and terrifying nightmares. The amphetamine psychosis is generally self-limiting, however, and treatment usually requires little more than supportive measures. Psychotherapy (see page 1026) can be used, but the person's dependence on the drug often interferes with its effectiveness. Drug support groups with multi-step abstinence programs are helpful.

Treatment of a cocaine overdose is a medical emergency. It may require hospitalization in an intensive-care unit for monitoring of blood pressure and heart rhythm and for treatment of seizures if they occur.

Treatment of chronic cocaine abuse often requires the combined efforts of the family physician and mental health professionals. Individual and group psychotherapy (see page 1026) are often useful.

OPIOIDS

Signs and Symptoms
- Depression, often of an agitated type;
- Anxiety symptoms;
- Impulsiveness;
- Fear of failure;
- Low self-esteem, hopelessness, and aggression;
- Limited coping strategies and low frustration tolerance;
- Need for immediate gratification;
- Friends who are drug users.

Opium (Greek for juice) is produced from the milky discharge from the unripe seed capsules of the poppy plant. Opioids include opiates (substances naturally produced from opium), such as heroin and morphine, and synthetic substances that have morphine-like action and are prescribed as pain-relievers, anesthetics, or cough suppressants (such as codeine and methadone).

Heroin, an illegal drug, usually is taken by injection. Because addicts tend to be indifferent in regard to hygiene when using syringes, infections of the skin and systemic organs are common, especially tuberculosis and low-level chronic hepatitis without jaundice. Hepatitis B, like the AIDS virus, is transmitted by shared use of needles, and both are common among intravenous drug users. In recent years there has been a steady increase in the number of opiate addicts from middle-class homes.

Treatment. Although it was once believed that addiction to these narcotic drugs is easily acquired and hard to break, a follow-up study of drug users among Vietnam veterans found that most of the men who used narcotics extensively in Vietnam stopped when they came home and had not begun again. Treatment involves safe withdrawal from the addiction (often with the use of methadone) and supportive psychotherapy (see page 1026) to help in the return to a productive life.

MARIJUANA AND CANNABIS COMPOUNDS

Signs and Symptoms
- Introversion;
- Lack of drive;

DETOXIFICATION

When a person is intoxicated with alcohol or any other drug, it may be necessary to carry out a process called detoxification. The chronic alcoholic is in danger of seizures or delirium tremens (DTs) or even death if detoxification is not carried out in a systematic manner. Similarly, the person who has been using drugs such as benzodiazepam or barbiturates is in danger of seizures. Whether the intoxicating drug agent is alcohol, an opioid such as heroin, a barbiturate, or a tranquilizer, the person is likely to be very uncomfortable for a number of days after the withdrawal from the addictive substance is begun.

Detoxification includes supportive measures—for example, sometimes the amount of intoxicant used is decreased slowly. When the addiction is to a drug of the benzodiazepam family, the use of decreasing amounts is important to avoid the risk of seizures. Detoxification often requires a week or more of treatment, ideally in a hospital. Once detoxification has been safely accomplished, the person should enter a program of re-education about drug use. These programs often last several weeks and can be in a hospital or on an outpatient basis or both.

HALLUCINOGENS

In the 1960s, various "experiments" were conducted, largely by young people, regarding the effects of hallucinogenic drugs on their consciousness. Recreational use of such powerful chemicals as LSD and PCP has waxed and waned in recent years, but the hazardous practice is still commonplace.

The Drugs

LSD (lysergic acid diethylamide) is not addictive. However, it does produce profound changes in mood and thought processes that may result in hallucinations and a state resembling acute psychosis. Unusually brilliant and intense perceptions may accompany the other effects. With a "bad trip," acute panic reaction or psychotic symptoms may occur; suicide attempts also have been known to occur. In addition, rapid heart rates, hypertension, and tremors are often noted.

PCP (phencyclidine) sometimes is described as a dissociative anesthetic. It is used widely by veterinarians to immobilize large animals briefly. It also is either smoked or injected and is used to adulterate LSD, amphetamines, or cocaine sold on the street. The most common street preparation is angel dust, a white granular powder containing the drug at 50 to 100 percent strength.

In low doses (5 mg), PCP produces excitement, incoordination, and absence of sensation (analgesia). In high doses it can cause drooling (hypersalivation), vomiting, stupor, or coma. PCP overdose symptoms often resemble those of an acute schizophrenic reaction. Chronic use of PCP causes insomnia, anorexia, and severe changes in behavior including chronic schizophrenia. When there is acute psychosis associated with PCP, the person is at high risk for suicide or violence toward others.

Dealing With the Effects

Usually, the psychotic effects of LSD wear off in 12 to 18 hours, and psychiatric help is unnecessary. Protection so that the person cannot physically harm himself or herself (or others) and companionship and reassurance are essential. Disturbing recurrences of symptoms may appear even months later. Abrupt abstinence from LSD does not produce withdrawal symptoms although mental health professionals are often needed for supportive reassurance after a panic episode that may follow the use of LSD.

When a person takes an overdose of PCP, prompt use of life-support measures in a hospital intensive-care unit is needed to treat coma, convulsions, and breathing difficulties. Death has been known to occur from PCP overdose.

- Poor judgment;
- Disorientation;
- Agitation;
- Delirium.

Marijuana, which is smoked, is not highly addictive. Marijuana cigarettes are made from the leaves and flowers of the plant. Hashish is made from the concentrated resin of the same plant, *Cannabis sativa*, and is also smoked. The psychoactive substance in them, delta-9-tetrahydrocannabinol (THC), is absorbed more rapidly from marijuana smoke than after oral ingestion of cannabis compounds.

A person who is acutely intoxicated with marijuana or hashish feels relaxed and euphoric, an effect similar to mild or moderate drunkenness. Thinking usually is impaired, and concentration and perceptual and psychomotor functions are affected. The effects of marijuana are relatively benign, but the drug can bring on severe emotional disorders in persons with psychotic or neurotic problems.

Chronic marijuana abusers may lose interest in the everyday events of life and socially desirable goals. They devote more and more of their time to buying and using the drug.

Increased heart rate, redness of eyes (conjunctival injection), and decrease in lung function have been found in chronic users. Chronic users develop tolerance and need to smoke more frequently to obtain the euphoria.

Treatment. When habitual abuse of these substances is suspected, psychotherapy may be of help in developing self-esteem, providing support, and pointing the way toward a more productive and satisfying pattern of living.

Withdrawal from chronic use of marijuana includes sweating, tremors, nausea, vomiting, diarrhea, irritability, and difficulty in sleeping (see also page 440).

PSYCHOSOMATIC ILLNESS

Only in the 20th century has there been a comprehensive scientific attempt to understand the complex relationship between psychiatric health and physical health. In the past, such links were usually superstitious ones: for example, a person who contracted a crippling illness was said to have incurred the anger of the gods. The term psychosomatic (from the Greek *psyche,* soul, and *soma,* body) was coined in the 19th century.

Psychosomatic illnesses are those that may begin at a time of crisis in a person's life, show a time relationship with stressful situations, and clear up when the situation changes for the better or the person learns to adapt.

The psychosomatic disorders are characterized by physical symptoms that are caused by emotional factors. Only one organ system, such as the skin or gastrointestinal tract, is usually affected. The symptoms often resemble those that normally accompany emotional upset, but in psychosomatic disorders they are more intense and last for a sustained period.

Somatoform disorders are those in which the physical symptoms suggest a physical disorder, but no organic cause can be found and there is a strong suggestion that the symptoms are caused by psychological factors or conflicts. In these disorders, the person does not intentionally produce the symptoms. In somatoform pain disorder, the person is preoccupied with pain, although there are no adequate physical findings to account for the pain or its intensity.

CONVERSION DISORDER

Signs and Symptoms
- Physical problem suggesting a physical disorder;
- Link between the appearance of the symptom and a psychosocial stress;
- No awareness of intentionally producing the symptom;
- Although pain or sexual dysfunction may exist, the symptom is not limited to these problems.

Conversion disorder, also known as hysterical neurosis, is the appearance of a physical problem that appears to have an organic cause but really is an expression of a psychological conflict or need. The classic examples are paralysis, seizure, and blindness, but vomiting and false pregnancy also can be conversion symptoms. Usually, the disorder enables the person to keep the internal conflict out of conscious awareness, to avoid a particularly disliked activity, or to receive support from others that might not otherwise be forthcoming. This disorder usually appears in adolescence or early adulthood.

Treatment. Because there generally is a correlation between the appearance of a conversion disorder and a stressful situation, the problem usually will clear up when the situation improves or the person adapts. Psychotherapy (see page 1026) and hypnosis have been successful in the treatment of this disorder.

SOMATIZATION DISORDER

Signs and Symptoms
- History of many physical complaints or the person believes that he or she is sickly, beginning before age 30 and lasting for several years;
- Various symptoms for which no organic cause is found and which have been the reason the person takes prescription medicine, visits a physician, or makes lifestyle changes (these symptoms include gastrointestinal symptoms, pain, cardiopulmonary problems, conversion symptoms, sexual dysfunction, and female reproductive abnormalities).

In somatization disorder the person has many physical complaints that last for several years and have no physical basis found by a physician. The affected person often is vague or highly dramatic about the complaints. The problems usually are gastrointestinal, sexual, pain-related, cardiopulmonary, and neurological (such as paralysis).

The symptoms usually begin in adolescence and the disorder is more common among females.

Treatment. Through psychotherapy (see page 1026), it may be possible to determine the psychological motivation for the disorder.

In stressful situations, people tend to suppress their emotions, particularly aggressive ones, and this may lead to the formation of psychosomatic symptoms. As a result, although the physical symptoms need to be treated, supportive psychotherapy may be of enormous help.

HYPOCHONDRIASIS

Signs and Symptoms
- Obsessive preoccupation with fear of illness or supposed illness;
- No apparent physical disorder that can account for the physical signs or sensations;
- Disturbance lasts at least 6 months;
- Belief of illness is not of delusional intensity—that is, the person can accept the possibility that he or she may not in fact have a serious disease.

Hypochondriasis is an obsessive preoccupation with supposed ill health in which the patient interprets physical signs or sensations as evidence of physical illness. No physical disorder can be found on thorough physical evaluation, but the unwarranted fear of disease persists.

Change in heart rate, perspiration, or gastrointestinal pain may be interpreted as evidence of a serious disease. Or the person may become preoccupied with a specific organ—for example, worrying that he or she has heart disease. There usually is a considerable amount of "doctor-shopping," during which the hypochondriac visits a series of physicians and is disappointed at being told that all is well.

Often, the person gives the impression of relishing the misery of the imagined ailment while bemoaning its consequences; the hypochondriac usually is overdemanding of physicians and unappreciative of their help. The symptoms rarely fit any pattern known to medicine.

Unlike Münchausen's syndrome, in which the person fabricates a physical illness or self-inflicts injury in order to gratify an inordinate need for attention, hypochondriacs genuinely believe that they are physically ill.

MINNESOTA MULTIPHASIC PERSONALITY INVENTORY (MMPI)

This is an objective personality test consisting of more than 500 standard true-or-false questions that can provide a description of the overall personality profile of an individual. When used correctly, it reveals a great deal about a person's grasp of reality, impulse control, depression, guilt, major defenses, and symptoms due to psychological problems. Fairly sophisticated interpretations of the MMPI are offered by commercial computer services.

Treatment. As with all somatoform disorders, once a diagnosis is made (which includes eliminating genuine organic causes for the person's complaint), psychotherapy (see page 1026) can often be helpful in aiding the person to work through the conflicts that underlie the disorder.

CHRONIC PAIN DISORDERS

Signs and Symptoms
- Preoccupation with pain for at least 6 months;
- No physical disorder or effects of injury to account for the pain, or a complaint of pain or resulting social or occupational impairment grossly in excess of what would be expected from the physical findings.

Chronic pain disorder (somatoform pain disorder) is preoccupation with pain without physical findings adequate to explain the pain or its intensity. The person's pain may be inconsistent with the anatomy of the nervous system or may mimic a known disease entity (as in angina or sciatica) without any apparent organic cause being revealed by extensive diagnostic evaluation.

There may be evidence that psychological factors are contributing to the pain, especially if the pain is clearly associated with an environmental stimulus that seems to be related to a psychological conflict or need. Sometimes the pain seems to enable the person to avoid some disagreeable activity or to get support from family, friends, or professionals that otherwise might not be available. But there do not always seem to be psychological factors. In somatoform pain

CHRONIC PAIN CENTERS

In 1976, a survey found 17 pain clinics in the United States. At present, there are between 500 and 1,000.

In these centers, physicians and therapists representing various specialties work with the patient toward the goal of pain control. This team approach is essential because with chronic pain it is unlikely that any one technique will work. The professionals in an interdisciplinary center treat not only the pain itself but also the disruption it usually causes within a marriage and family as a result of the person's disability, loss of income, depression, and anxiety. A chronic pain center may treat people as inpatients or outpatients.

Because there is no licensing procedure, it is important to investigate carefully before enrolling at a pain clinic. In most cases, an interdisciplinary pain-treatment program is the most likely to produce results.

disorder there is no physical explanation to account for the pain—for example, the tension headaches caused by muscle spasm.

This disorder is serious because of its effect on the person's daily life. Typically, he or she becomes incapacitated, quits working, goes from physician to physician, uses too many pain-killers without relief, and, basically, assumes the role of an invalid. As a result, he or she is likely to be depressed.

In this disorder, which usually begins between ages 30 and 50, the pain typically appears suddenly and worsens severely over a few weeks or months. There is some evidence that people with this disorder tend to be close biologic relatives of people with more painful injuries and illnesses, depression, or alcohol dependence. Somatoform pain disorder is diagnosed almost twice as frequently in females as in males. The problem is especially difficult when pain without apparent cause occurs after an industrial accident and there is a claim for compensation.

Treatment. As with other somatoform disorders, organic causes need to be eliminated. In compensation cases, quick resolution yields the best chance for relief.

Pain management centers have been developed to help people with chronic pain cope with their problem. Such centers usually provide drug withdrawal, learning better living habits, biofeedback, relaxation and physical therapy, and group psychotherapy (see Chronic Pain Centers, above).

CHAPTER 34

HEALTH PROBLEMS OF WOMEN

CHAPTER CONTENTS

THE FEMALE ORGANS

GYNECOLOGICAL ORGANS

Gynecological organs are those associated with childbearing, including the ovaries, fallopian tubes, and uterus. The term gynecology means the study of women—from the Greek words *gyne,* meaning woman, and *logos,* meaning study.

The two ovaries are located about 4 or 5 inches below the waist, midway in the pelvic cavity. Each is only about the size of an almond. At birth, the ovaries are already stocked with a lifetime supply of roughly 1 million ova, or eggs. Between puberty and menopause, the ovaries generally release one egg each month, at the midpoint of the menstrual cycle. They also produce the female sex hormones estrogen and progesterone.

Between each ovary and the uterus lies one of the fallopian tubes. Each of these tubes is the thickness of a lead pencil and contains a passageway no wider than a needle. Each is approximately 4 inches long and is connected to the uterus. The uterus itself is hollow and shaped like an upside-down pear. In a nonpregnant woman, it is about 2.5 inches long.

The walls of the uterus are thick and lined with powerful muscles that contract during childbirth to push the fetus out. The narrow

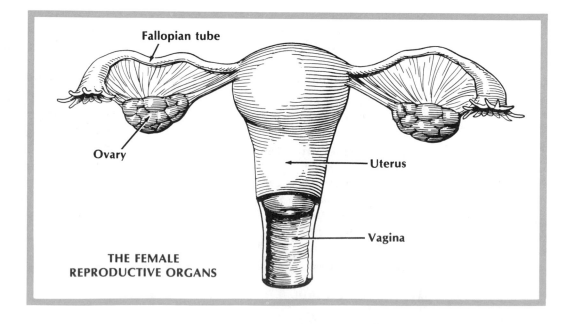

Fallopian tube

Ovary

Uterus

Vagina

THE FEMALE
REPRODUCTIVE ORGANS

neck of the uterus is called the cervix, and it also has thick walls. Ordinarily, the opening of the cervix is exceedingly small: big enough for menstrual fluids to pass through but not large enough that a tampon, for example, could accidentally be thrust up into it. During childbirth, the cervical opening expands enormously.

The cervix extends out into the vagina, which is a muscular canal about 5 inches long. Most of the time the walls of the vagina touch, but they can expand to accommodate something as small as a tampon or as large as a fetus. Cells in the vaginal walls secrete lubricants. In girls, the hymen—a thin membrane—partly blocks the opening of the vaginal canal. It is eventually stretched or broken by first intercourse or by an activity such as horseback riding or some other sport. In rare cases, a physician has to make an incision in the hymen before a girl can menstruate.

The opening to the vagina is shielded by the external genitalia. The whole area is called the vulva. It consists of the mons pubis, the labia, the clitoris, and the opening (vestibule) of the vagina. The mons pubis is the pad of fatty tissue at the base of the abdomen that becomes covered with hair at puberty. The labia are double folds of tissue that extend downward on either side of the vagina; the outer folds are the labia majora and the inner folds are the labia minora (*labium* is the Latin word for lip). Where the labia meet, near the front of the body, they cover a small protrusion, which is the tip of the clitoris. During sexual arousal, the clitoris, like the male penis, becomes erect. Important glands, called Bartholin's glands, are located in the vestibule of the vagina; the substances they secrete lubricate the vaginal opening.

Between the clitoris and the vagina is another, smaller opening, the entrance to the urethra. The urethra is a passageway, about 1.5 inches long, that leads to the bladder, where urine is stored. The bladder is located between the pubic bone and the uterus. Both males and females have a bladder and urethra; however, men and women develop different urinary problems, or sometimes the same problem affects them differently. Consequently, this chapter will also cover women's urinary disorders (see page 1108).

The Pelvic Examination.   A pelvic examination is a simple procedure that can be

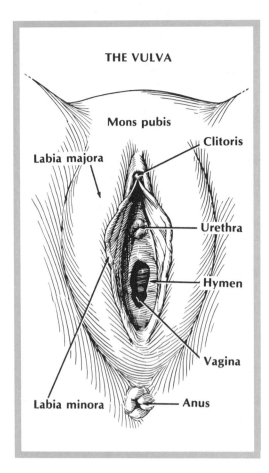

THE VULVA

Mons pubis

Labia majora

Clitoris

Urethra

Hymen

Vagina

Labia minora

Anus

As part of the pelvic examination, your physician will insert two gloved fingers inside your vagina. While simultaneously pressing down on your abdomen, he or she can examine your uterus, ovaries, and other organs. ▼

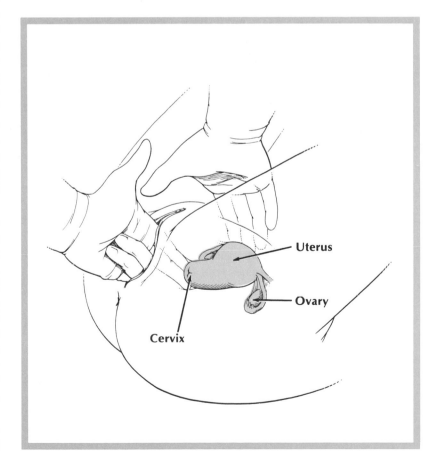

Uterus

Ovary

Cervix

SELECTING A GYNECOLOGIST

Gynecologists are physicians who are trained to treat disorders that affect a woman's reproductive system. You would consult a gynecologist for menstrual problems (problems with your periods) and problems affecting your breasts; for cancer that develops in any of your reproductive organs; for treatment of infertility or of sexually transmitted diseases; for difficulties during menopause (change of life); and for advice on birth control, abortion, or sexual problems. Because gynecologists also are trained as obstetricians, many of them handle pregnancy and childbirth. Many women choose to use a gynecologist as their primary-care physician.

In some areas of the country, gynecologists are not available. In these areas, general practitioners, family practitioners, and internists can provide routine gynecological care. Another alternative is the certified nurse-midwife (CNM), a nurse who has had specialized training. CNMs deliver babies under some circumstances and provide well-woman care, including routine breast examinations and pelvic examinations with Papanicolaou (Pap) smears (see pages 1055 and 1096). They always work with one or more physicians who are available for consultations and in emergencies.

You may not need a gynecologist for routine care, but you should consult one for serious conditions. To select a gynecologist, you can ask another physician to recommend someone, or you can call a local hospital for suggestions.

During your first visit to the gynecologist, you will be looking for answers to important questions. Is the physician willing to take the time to explain things in language you can understand? Will he or she readily answer questions over the telephone? Most of all, are you comfortable with this person? If you are not, you will want to consult other gynecologists before making a final choice.

cervix. This is done, with the speculum in place, by rubbing the cervix gently with a small spatula, brush, or cotton swab. The sample is sent to a laboratory for a Pap test (see page 1096), which is used to screen for cancer of the cervix, or for other tests.

Internal organs such as the uterus and ovaries cannot be seen, but your physician can examine them by touch (palpation). To do this, the physician inserts two lubricated, gloved fingers into your vagina. By pressing down on your abdomen with the other hand while maneuvering the fingers inside the vagina, he or she can locate the uterus, ovaries, and other organs, judge their size, and confirm that they are in the proper position and have normal muscle tone. By exploring the contours of these organs, your physician sometimes can detect tumors or cysts.

To palpate the same organs from a different angle, and to examine your rectum, the physician also may insert a finger into the rectum and manipulate that finger, together with one or more fingers in the vagina.

As the physician palpates your internal organs, you may feel somewhat uncomfortable. However, the experience should not be painful; if you do experience pain or tenderness, say so immediately. There will be less discomfort if you can relax the muscles in your pelvic area. It often helps to take slow, deep breaths.

A routine gynecological checkup generally also includes an examination of your breasts. In addition, the physician takes a medical history. He or she will want to know the date of your last menstrual period, unless you are too young to menstruate. You will generally be asked about past pregnancies, childbirths, and abortions and about what form of birth control you are using, if any. You usually will be weighed and have your blood pressure measured, and you may be asked for urine and blood samples for laboratory analysis.

The American College of Obstetricians and Gynecologists recommends that you have a pelvic examination once a year, beginning when you are in your early to middle 20s, or even earlier if you are sexually active. If you have never had a pelvic examination, you may approach the first one with a certain amount of anxiety; many women do. You may have to go through the procedure a couple of times before the examination begins to seem routine and nonthreatening.

done by your gynecologist or family physician. You will be asked to lie flat on your back on an examining table with your knees bent. Usually, your heels rest in metal supports called stirrups. The physician first examines your external genitalia to make sure they look normal—no sores, discolorations, or swellings, for example. The internal examination is next. To see the inner walls of the vagina and the cervix, the physician inserts an instrument called a speculum to hold the vaginal walls apart and then shines a light inside, looking for lesions, inflammation, signs of abnormal discharge, or anything else that is unusual. Generally, the next step is to take a sample of cells from the

The Breasts.   For the most part, the breasts consist of fat and connective tissue that protect a network of milk-producing glands and blood vessels. During lactation, these glands secrete milk and empty it into a system of ducts that eventually come together just behind the nipple. The breasts are attached to the muscles of the chest wall (the pectoral muscles) by connective tissue.

The nipples are made of erectile tissue. Some are constantly erect and protruding, some are inverted (turn inward), and others are normally flat but become erect when it is cold, when something brushes against them, or during sexual arousal. All three types of nipple are perfectly normal.

Encircling the nipple is the areola, a ring of tissue the same color as the nipple. Oil glands in the areola lubricate the nipple during breast-feeding; in some women, these glands are visible as small bumps. Many normal women have hairs growing at the edges of the areola. There is no reason to remove them. In some women who take birth control pills, the number of hairs increases.

Some women are self-conscious about their breasts: they think that their breasts are too small or too large, or they are concerned because one is larger than the other. Actually, size makes no difference either in sexual responsiveness or in ability to nurse a baby. Women who have small breasts are as

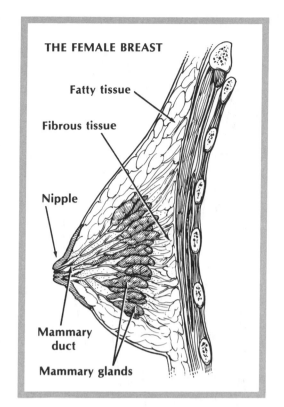

THE FEMALE BREAST

Fatty tissue

Fibrous tissue

Nipple

Mammary duct

Mammary glands

responsive as women with large breasts and they can feed an infant just as successfully. Furthermore, it is normal and usual for the two breasts to be somewhat different in size and shape. For some reason, it is common for the right breast to be smaller than the left.

MENSES AND MENSTRUAL DISORDERS

PUBERTY AND MENARCHE

Puberty begins when a girl is about 8 years old. Her pituitary gland begins to secrete two key hormones in increasing amounts: follicle-stimulating hormone and luteinizing hormone. These hormones travel via the bloodstream to the ovaries, where they trigger growth and change.

The ovaries at birth actually contain all the ova (eggs) they will ever have. However, the eggs remain almost dormant until stimulated by a surge of pituitary hormones. Then the ova begin to enlarge and to develop additional layers of outer cells, and these cells start to produce another hormone called estrogen. During childhood, a girl's body produces estrogen in very small quantities, but

at puberty her estrogen level increases about 20-fold. Meanwhile, the ovaries themselves grow in size as the ova develop, and other internal reproductive organs also grow and mature.

Soon there are external signs of change. The girl's breasts begin to bud as estrogen induces the development of milk ducts. One breast may start to grow before the other does, and the two may develop at different rates; usually, they become approximately equal in size. Next, the girl develops pubic hair and, later, underarm hair. She experiences a growth spurt, and as her hips and breasts become more rounded, she begins to look more like a woman.

Approximately 2 years after a girl's breasts begin to bud, she generally reaches menarche and menstruates for the first time.

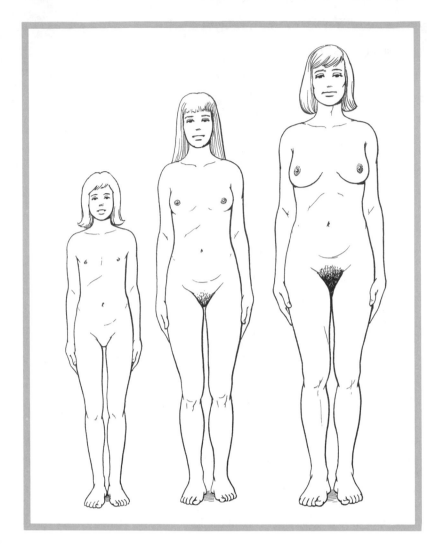

The female body, before, during, and after puberty.

nourished. Apparently, before hormonal changes can begin, a girl either must have reached a critical body weight, around 106 pounds, or perhaps must have reached that weight and also must have the right amount of body fat and body water. At any rate, girls who are overweight usually have their first menstrual period earlier than those who are not. However, girls who are very athletic, are malnourished, or have a chronic, debilitating disease generally begin menstruating later.

If a girl's breasts begin to bud before she is 8 years old or if she has her first period before age 9 years, it is advisable to consult a physician. This rare condition is called precocious puberty. It has several possible causes. Premature sexual development can be a symptom of something serious (see Sexual Precocity, page 139), but it is usually treatable.

It is also a good idea to consult a physician if a girl has no breast development by the age of 14 years or has not begun to menstruate by the time she is 16 years old—especially if she is concerned about it.

For the first few years after menarche, it is normal for a girl's menstrual cycle to be irregular and for her to skip a cycle altogether at times. Her ovaries probably are not releasing an ovum every single month. However, it is wise to assume that once she has begun to menstruate, she can become pregnant.

In medical terms, puberty ends only after menstruation is established and regular.

Menarche marks the beginning of her reproductive life, and menopause (the cessation of ovarian functioning) will mark the end of it. The term menarche is derived from the ancient words for month—*men*—and beginning—*arche*.) Males have no counterpart for menarche, which marks a dramatic change in a female's biological status. A girl's attitude toward menstruation, and her feelings about what it means to be a woman, may be influenced by the way her family and friends respond to her first menses.

Menarche is considered to have occurred in the normal fashion when it happens after age 9 years and before 16 years. On the average, American girls begin menstruating at 13 years, and that is earlier in life than previous generations of American women did. For the past 100 years, the average age at menarche in the United States has been dropping at the rate of 3 or 4 months every decade. Medical experts believe the change has happened because girls today are better

THE NORMAL MENSTRUAL CYCLE

The menstrual cycle begins on the first day of flow of one menstrual period and ends on the first day of flow of the next. The release of an egg (ovum), a single cell barely visible to the naked eye, occurs approximately in the middle of the normal menstrual cycle.

Even before birth, the ovaries are completely stocked with all the eggs a woman will ever have. Three or four months before birth, a female fetus has approximately 7 million eggs; at birth, only 1 million remain—the rest have been absorbed by the body. By the time of menarche, the number is down to a mere 400,000, and by menopause, only a few are left. Normally, only one ovary releases an egg each month, in random order.

Each month, even as you menstruate, several follicles have begun to develop in one of your ovaries, and your next cycle is under way. These follicles are tiny sacs, each containing a single, immature egg. After a week or so, one follicle begins to outgrow the others, which then shrink to normal size. Meanwhile, the ovaries secrete more and more estrogen, much of it produced by the outer cells of that single, dominant follicle. The estrogen acts on the endometrium (the lining of the uterus), causing it to grow and thicken. A day or two before ovulation, estrogen levels peak; they then start to fall, and the dominant follicle begins to produce tiny amounts of the hormone progesterone. The follicle swells, ruptures, and releases the egg. Other events include a slight increase in body temperature and a change in secretions from the glands in the cervix.

After it is released from the follicle, the egg floats into the fallopian tube and begins a journey to the uterus that generally takes about 6 days. While it is in transit, it can be fertilized if sperm are present. Fertilization generally takes place within 24 hours after ovulation, before the egg has traveled more than a third of the way down the tube.

Even as the egg drifts toward the uterus, its empty follicle in the ovary is being transformed. Once again, the follicle enlarges rapidly—at this stage, it is called the corpus luteum—and it begins to secrete large quantities of progesterone and estrogen. Under the impact of these hormones, the endometrium continues to develop. Its glands secrete substances and release nutrients; its blood supply increases, as do the number of tiny blood vessels in the tissue. By the end of the menstrual cycle, the uterine lining has doubled in thickness, and large amounts of nutrients have been stored there, ready to nourish a fetus.

If pregnancy occurs and a fertilized egg implants itself in the endometrium, hormones secreted by the corpus luteum will help to sustain it. If that does not happen, the egg disintegrates or leaves the body in vaginal secretions, usually even before menstruation begins. Meanwhile, within about 2 weeks after ovulation, the corpus luteum begins to shrink, and levels of both estrogen and progesterone decrease. The uterus starts to shed its lining, and menstrual bleeding, known as menses, begins.

Menstrual flow actually consists not only of blood but also of vaginal and cervical secretions and tissue sloughed from the lining of the uterus. By the fourth or fifth day of your period, the endometrium has become thin, but the process of rebuilding it has already begun. Menstruation ends when the outer surface of the endometrium has been restored.

On the average, a menstrual cycle is 28 days long, although cycles that are anywhere from 23 to 35 days long are considered normal. If your cycle does not fall within this range, it may still be completely normal, although extremely long or extremely short cycles are sometimes associated with infertility. On the average, the menstrual period itself lasts 4 days; periods

MENSTRUAL CARE

In the past, menstruating women used cloths to catch their menstrual flow, rinsing them out and reusing them. Today, commercially made sanitary napkins are available, as are tampons and menstrual sponges that can be inserted into the vagina to absorb menstrual fluids.

Boxes of napkins and tampons are often labeled "regular" or "super." These terms refer to the product's ability to absorb, rather than to its physical size. Because there are no common standards, and one brand's "regular" may be as absorbent as another brand's "super," you will have to find out by trial and error what works for you. Because of the risk of toxic shock syndrome (see page 1061), many physicians now advise women to alternate tampons with napkins, not to leave tampons in place for very long, and to use napkins at night.

An inexpensive alternative to napkins and tampons is the menstrual sponge. It is a natural sponge that is worn internally and can be rinsed out and reused. Menstrual sponges have not been sterilized, nor have tampons. The same precautions apply to sponges as to tampons: do not leave them in place for too long, and use a pad at night.

If, during your period, your vagina or vulva begins to itch or becomes irritated, you may have been using a napkin or tampon that is scented or deodorized. Some women are allergic to the chemicals used in these products. Menstrual fluid is actually odorless until it comes into contact with bacteria and air. In general, a woman who bathes often and changes napkins, tampons, or sponges often should have no problem with odor.

From a health point of view, it is not harmful to have intercourse while you are menstruating. Some women use a diaphragm, lubricated with contraceptive jelly, to block menstrual flow temporarily.

as short as 2 days or as long as 7 are not unusual.

At some point in your life, your period will likely become temporarily irregular for no obvious reason. You may skip a period or have one that is much longer, shorter, or heavier than normal. Sometimes this change simply reflects your age: menstrual periods are apt to last longer both at menarche and as you approach menopause. However, at

ORAL CONTRACEPTIVES

Oral contraceptives are highly effective: their failure rate is less than 1 percent. Today's birth control pills are very different from the original formulation in that manufacturers have reduced the dose of female hormones. When oral contraceptives contained high levels of estrogen, they caused heart and circulatory disorders in some women. With the newer, low-dose pills, although there *are* still risks involved in taking them, the danger is now slight, especially for anyone younger than 30 years. Smoking may increase these risks.

Two types of oral contraceptives are available. The combination pill, which contains both estrogen and progesterone, has only one-tenth as much estrogen as the original birth control pill did and half as much progesterone. The so-called mini-pill, which has only progesterone, is also low-dose. The result of these changes is that it is now statistically safer to take the pill than it is not to use birth control at all because the death rate associated with normal pregnancy or elective abortion is higher than that associated with taking the pill.

The Pill Is Not for Everyone
Some women should not use oral contraceptives. You should not be taking the combination pill if you have a history of strokes, blood clots, high blood pressure, severe diabetes, or breast or uterine cancer; if you have active liver disease or sickle cell disease; if you may already be pregnant; or if you are breast-feeding. Some physicians

also will advise you to avoid the pill if you are depressed, have migraines, or are a heavy smoker; if your menstrual periods are infrequent (see page 1065); or if you have stopped menstruating altogether (see page 1063). In addition, because studies show that the risks associated with oral contraceptives increase with age, physicians generally recommend that all women who smoke should stop taking the pill once they are older than 35 years and that every woman should stop taking it after age 40 years.

Side Effects
Because there is still some small risk that the pill will cause a stroke, there are danger signs to watch for if you are taking it. If you are having more headaches than usual or if you feel faint or begin to have speech difficulties, call a physician. If you know you are going to have an operation and you are taking high-dose pills, stop using the oral contraceptive about a month before the procedure because the pill increases your risk of developing a blood clot after the operation. These effects are not a cause for concern with the low-dose pills.

Oral contraceptives also have other, less serious, side effects. Especially when you first start to take the pill, you may sometimes bleed slightly between menstrual periods, or you may not menstruate at all. There are dozens of birth control pills on the market, and usually your physician can eliminate these problems by prescribing a different brand. Some women menstruate regularly while they are taking the pill but stop having periods after

they discontinue using it. This effect is almost always temporary. Roughly 5 percent of women who use oral contraceptives develop some increase in blood pressure after about 5 years. In most cases, their blood pressure returns to normal if they stop taking the pill.

Other possible side effects include nausea, breast tenderness, fluid retention, depression, and nervousness. In addition, you may gain a little weight, either because of water retention or because the pill has increased your appetite and you are eating more.

Drug Interactions
If you are getting a new prescription of any kind, remember to tell the physician that you are taking the pill because it can interact with other drugs.

The Good News
Not all side effects are harmful, and oral contraceptives have some beneficial effects that are a welcome bonus. While you are taking the pill, you are less likely to have heavy menstrual bleeding or severe cramps or to develop breast lumps, iron-deficiency anemia, ovarian cysts, endometrial or ovarian cancer, or rheumatoid arthritis. Your periods should be regular, light, and predictable. Young women taking the pill also seem to have lower rates of uterine cancer than other women. Furthermore, there is no convincing evidence that women who take the pill develop breast cancer or any other type of malignancy more often than women who don't. (For information on other birth control methods, see page 175.)

other times, stress may play a role. A woman's monthly cycle is regulated by hormones ultimately controlled by the hypothalamus, an area at the base of the brain that acts as a kind of thermostat for the whole system. Given the complexity of the system and the fact that both physical and mental stress can affect the hypothalamus, it is remarkable that women's cycles are as regular as they are.

The sections that follow suggest specific guidelines to help you distinguish ordinary menstrual irregularity from times when you need to consult a physician. Many of the disorders, such as amenorrhea and dysmenorrhea, have similar names. They incorporate two Greek words, *men,* meaning month, because menses are a monthly occurrence, and *rhoia,* meaning flow.

TOXIC SHOCK SYNDROME

Signs and Symptoms
- Sudden fever of 102°F or higher;
- Vomiting or diarrhea;
- Dizziness, a feeling of weakness, fainting, disorientation;
- A rash resembling a sunburn, particularly on your palms and the soles of your feet.

Toxic shock syndrome (TSS) is a rare but potentially dangerous disorder that has been associated most often with the use of tampons and occasionally with the use of contraceptive sponges, especially by women younger than 30.

In the early 1980s, there was a small epidemic of TSS, for the most part involving young, menstruating women who had been using a particular brand of super-absorbent tampons. Researchers reported that TSS seemed to be caused by toxins, or poisons, produced by a type of bacteria called *Staphylococcus aureus.* These bacteria often are present in the body and cause no problems. Some researchers theorized that when super-absorbent tampons were left in place for a long time, they could become a breeding ground for these bacteria. Others suggested that the super-absorbent fibers in the tampons scratched the surface of the vagina and thus made it possible for the bacteria or their toxins to enter the bloodstream.

The brand of tampons associated with the original TSS epidemic was taken off the market. Since then, the number of cases of TSS has declined, despite the fact that today most tampons contain some super-absorbent fiber. In recent years, there have been a few cases of TSS in women who had been wearing a diaphragm or a contraceptive sponge. However, 25 to 30 percent of those who develop TSS today are *not* young, menstruating women, but are older women, men, or even children; often, it strikes soon after an operation.

The Diagnosis.   Call your physician immediately if you experience the above symptoms, especially if you are menstruating or have just finished menstruating and have been using tampons. (Even before you call, remove the tampon.) Tell the physician what your symptoms are, how long you have had them, and when your period started.

Other possible symptoms include a headache, sore throat, aching muscles, and bloodshot eyes. The rash may appear on various parts of your body, including the palms of your hands and the soles of your feet; after a week or so, the skin on the hands and feet generally begins to peel.

How Serious Is TSS?   TSS symptoms develop suddenly, and the disease is actually fatal in about 3 percent of all cases. It can cause blood pressure to plummet, and if that happens, you may go into shock. Kidney failure also results in some cases.

Treatment.   If you develop a serious case of TSS, you will need antibiotics. Because *Staphylococcus aureus* organisms can be resistant to penicillin and ampicillin, some other type of medication may have to be used. If your blood pressure begins to drop, you will have to be hospitalized and given medication to stabilize it and fluids to prevent dehydration.

Prevention.   You can reduce your chances of getting TSS by wearing tampons less often or by giving them up altogether. Women who are known to have problems with *Staphylococcus aureus* infections should not wear tampons at all. Physicians often suggest that women who prefer tampons should alternate them with sanitary napkins, they advise against wearing tampons overnight or between menstrual periods, and they suggest choosing brands that are low in absorbency. Unfortunately, current labeling does not accurately reflect how absorbent a product is. One brand's "regular" is sometimes more absorbent than another brand's "super." However, if a tampon leaves your vagina dry or is hard to pull out, it is more absorbent than you need.

TSS tends to recur—up to 30 percent of persons who have had it once get it again, although subsequent attacks are not usually as serious. Women who have had TSS are advised not to use tampons at all.

PREMENSTRUAL SYNDROME

Signs and Symptoms
• A predictable pattern of physical and emotional changes that occur just before menstruation.

Physical changes may include bloating, fluid retention, weight gain, breast soreness, abdominal swelling, clumsiness, aching, swollen hands and feet, fatigue, nausea, vomiting, diarrhea, constipation, headaches, skin problems, or respiratory problems.

Emotional changes may include depression, irritability, anxiety, tension, mood swings, difficulty in concentrating, or lethargy.

For 2 to 5 percent of women, premenstrual syndrome (PMS) is a severe problem. Many others experience it to a moderate or mild degree. The symptoms can develop any time after the midpoint in your menstrual cycle, and they disappear soon after your period starts. They tend to wax and wane from month to month, and they are more apt to trouble women in their 20s and 30s.

No one really knows what causes PMS. It is undoubtedly related to cyclic changes in hormone levels because symptoms disappear during pregnancy and after menopause. Stress can aggravate the problem, but it is not the sole cause. PMS has been unfairly blamed at times for symptoms arising out of emotional states.

The Diagnosis. A physician will attribute a particular symptom to PMS only if it is part of a predictable premenstrual pattern. Hence, your physician may ask you to keep a record for several menstrual cycles before you come in for a consultation. On a calendar or in a diary, you record all symptoms, along with the day you first noticed them and the day they disappeared. Note, too, the day your period began.

How Serious Is PMS? PMS can be hard to tolerate but, because it does not reflect any harmful underlying disorder, it is not considered serious. There is no cure for it except menopause—although it usually disappears of its own accord before that. However, some of the symptoms of PMS can be treated by a physician.

Treatment. *Medication.* Each of the medications currently used to treat PMS actually fails to help most women; yet, because individual reactions differ, each does help some women.

To reduce water retention and bloating, a physician can prescribe a diuretic. It is easy to become dependent on diuretics and to search for ever stronger agents because of the perceived distress from swelling. You can try oral contraceptives (see page 1060), although they aggravate symptoms about as often as they relieve them. For severe irritability, tranquilizers may help, although they pose their own risk. Progesterone also is being prescribed on an experimental basis. Low-dose progesterone begun 10 days before the menstrual flow begins does not affect fertility, nor does it act as a contraceptive. However, large doses of progesterone administered for 15 to 20 days a month can prevent conception and may cause infertility. Vitamin B_6 supplements have been used widely, but there is no evidence that they are effective, and large doses of this vitamin are dangerous.

Nutrition and Exercise. By avoiding salt in the last few days before your period, you can reduce bloating and fluid retention. If you also avoid caffeine, you may feel less irritable and tense and have less of a problem with breast soreness. Many women say that vigorous exercise helps because it provides an emotional lift at a time when they need one.

Women who have only mild PMS sometimes find that just recording their symptoms for a few months is all the help they need. Once it is clear that their problems are predictable and short-lived, PMS is easier to tolerate.

MITTELSCHMERZ

Signs and Symptoms
- Pain in the lower abdomen at the time of ovulation;
- Sometimes slight vaginal bleeding accompanying the pain.

Mittelschmerz (a German word meaning middle pain) occurs at the midpoint in the menstrual cycle, at the time of ovulation. Typically, the pain is a dull ache that lasts anywhere from a few minutes to a few hours; it may or may not be accompanied by minimal bleeding.

The cause is unknown. According to one theory, when an ovarian follicle ruptures and releases an egg, fluid from the follicle may escape into the abdominal cavity and cause irritation. The bleeding may be caused by the rapid drop in estrogen that occurs at the time of ovulation.

The timing and location of the pain usually serve to identify mittelschmerz. On rare occasions, the pain is severe enough to be confused with appendicitis (see page 624). It does not seem to indicate any underlying disorder.

Treatment. *Medication.* You can take a mild analgesic to ease the pain.

PAINFUL MENSES

Signs and Symptoms
- Pain in the lower abdomen during menstruation, possibly extending to the hips, lower back, or thighs;
- Nausea, vomiting, diarrhea, or general aching during menstruation.

It is normal to have mild abdominal cramps on the first day or two of your period—more than half of all women do. However, 10 percent experience such severe pain that they cannot manage their normal routine unless they take medication.

The problem is called primary dysmenorrhea if the pain is *not* a symptom of some underlying gynecological disorder but is an exaggeration of normal processes. (The prefix *dys* means difficult, *men* signifies month, and *rhoia* means a flow.) Medical experts believe that primary dysmenorrhea is caused by excessive levels of prostaglan-dins, substances that make the uterus contract.

Painful menstruation is known as secondary dysmenorrhea when it is caused by a gynecological disorder. In general, a secondary cause is suspected when the pain lasts longer than the first 1 to 3 days of the menstrual period, occurs between periods with or without bleeding, occurs a few days before your period begins, and is accompanied by spotting or by gushing of blood. The underlying cause could be fibroids (see page 1097), adenomyosis (see page 1104), a sexually transmitted disease (see page 875), endometriosis (see page 1101), pelvic inflammatory disease (see page 1104), or an ovarian cyst or tumor (see page 1105).

The Diagnosis. Your physician's first concern is to check for the underlying disorders that cause secondary dysmenorrhea. You will have a pelvic examination (see page 1055) and perhaps blood tests and a urinalysis. The physician may use ultrasound to get a picture of your internal organs (see page 1287) or laparoscopy (see page 1297) for a direct look.

How Serious Is Dysmenorrhea? Primary dysmenorrhea is painful but not harmful. It is more common during adolescence, and it is apt to ease or disappear altogether by the time you are in your mid-20s or once you have had a baby. Secondary dysmenorrhea is more serious, but most of the underlying disorders that produce it are treatable.

Treatment. *Medication.* For primary dysmenorrhea, your physician may prescribe an analgesic drug. Medications such as ibuprofen, mefenamic acid, naproxen, and indomethacin work for about 80 percent of the women who take them. Oral contraceptives and aspirin also may relieve the discomfort.

For secondary dysmenorrhea, the treatment varies with the underlying cause.

ABSENCE OF PERIODS

Signs and Symptoms
- In young girls: menstruation has not yet begun at age 16 (primary amenorrhea);
- In adult women who are not pregnant: absence of menstruation for 6 months or longer (secondary amenorrhea).

If you reach the age of 16 years without ever menstruating, the chances are that you are developing normally but a little later than most girls. If you are very athletic or if you are quite thin, menarche could be delayed (see below). However, because there is a small possibility that you have a hormonal abnormality, consult a physician, especially if other sexual changes also have been delayed—if your breasts and pubic hair have not yet begun to grow, for example. Failure to menstruate also is called amenorrhea, a word that combines the Greek negative prefix *a-* (the equivalent of the English *un-*) with *men,* for month, and *rhoia,* meaning flow. If you have never menstruated, the condition is called primary amenorrhea.

If you have been menstruating for years and suddenly you miss one or several periods, you have secondary amenorrhea. There are several possible explanations for this. You might be pregnant, perhaps you lost a lot of weight rather quickly or have been exercising a lot (see below), or you may have been under stress. Very obese women sometimes fail to menstruate. You also could be taking a medication that suppresses menses as a side effect. If you just quit taking oral contraceptives, you may not have a period for several months. In addition, breast-feeding can delay menstruation, and if you are reaching the age of menopause (see page 1067), it would be normal to begin skipping periods.

Secondary amenorrhea due to such causes is quite common. More serious problems, such as tumors or disorders of the pituitary gland, also can cause amenorrhea, but they are rare (see Pituitary Gland Disorders, page 723). Failure to resume menstruation after childbirth, particularly if lactation does not take place either, may mean that the pituitary gland failed either partly or completely at the time of delivery, a condition called postpartum pituitary necrosis.

If you have been menstruating regularly and your period is more than 2 weeks late, you may want to see a physician to find out whether you are pregnant. However, if you are sure you could not be pregnant and you have no other symptoms, there is no harm in waiting for 6 to 9 months before consulting a physician. Keep in mind, though, that even though you are not menstruating, you could still become pregnant if you do not take precautions.

The Diagnosis. Whether you have primary or secondary amenorrhea, your physician may do a pelvic examination (see page 1055). He or she will check to see whether your vaginal walls seem moist and otherwise normal and will examine cervical mucus, looking for signs that your ovaries are producing normal amounts of estrogen. Another way to determine your estrogen status is to have you take progesterone for a few days, and then wait to see whether you bleed from the vagina. Bleeding indicates that estrogen is not the problem, and the physician may want to check whether you have polycystic ovaries (see page 1107). If you do not bleed despite taking progesterone, the general indication is that your ovaries are secreting little or no estrogen and that you are not ovulating. Several disorders can suppress ovulation; blood tests and x-rays can help your physician determine the cause.

SPORTS AND MENSES

Female ballet dancers, female joggers, and women who are involved in vigorous sports frequently find that they skip menstrual periods or stop menstruating altogether. This is more likely to happen if you are young, especially if your cycle is generally irregular. In fact, teenagers who train heavily are often in their late teens before they actually have their first menstrual period.

Medical experts believe that several factors are involved, including stress and perhaps the ratio of fat cells in your body to other cells (going on a crash diet and losing a lot of weight very rapidly also can interfere with menstruation). In both cases, you stop menstruating because your ovaries do not produce estrogen in the cyclic manner that causes the uterine lining to thicken and then shed (see page 1058).

If you reduce your exercise schedule or gain weight, you probably will begin to menstruate again. If that does not work—or if you do not want to exercise less or gain weight—your physician may suggest that you take estrogen in low doses. There is a good reason for this recommendation. If you are not producing normal amounts of estrogen you may be susceptible to osteoporosis (see page 982), a thinning of the bones that can make fractures more likely in later years.

Be aware, however, that you cannot simply forget about birth control just because your reproductive system seems to have shut down. You could ovulate at any time and be at risk for pregnancy.

How Serious Is Amenorrhea?   Amenorrhea is seldom a sign that anything is seriously wrong. However, if you are not menstruating, you may find it difficult to become pregnant. If that happens, your physician will probably refer you to a specialist in infertility.

Treatment.   *Medication.*   Your physician may prescribe various types of hormones to see whether your ovaries are functioning normally.

Provided no underlying disorder is causing your amenorrhea, treatment is generally unnecessary. However, because women who are not menstruating seem susceptible to osteoporosis (see page 982), your physician may suggest that you take estrogen and a calcium supplement.

If an underlying disorder *is* to blame for either primary or secondary amenorrhea, the treatment will depend on what the disorder is.

INFREQUENT PERIODS

Signs and Symptoms
- Fewer menstrual periods than the usual 11 to 13 per year.

Some women ovulate and menstruate normally but less often than most. This is called oligomenorrhea, a term that combines three Greek words: *oligo,* which means few, *men,* for month, and *rhoia,* for flow.

It is normal to menstruate less frequently as you approach menopause. However, some women have infrequent menses all their adult lives—no one knows exactly why. Occasionally, a woman not nearing menopause begins to menstruate infrequently and at the same time develops acne and an unusual amount of hair on her face and body; the problem may be an excess of androgen, produced either by her adrenal gland or by a tumor of the ovary (see Adrenal Gland Disorders, page 718, and Idiopathic Hirsutism, page 722).

The Diagnosis.   Your physician will take a careful history, do a pelvic examination (see page 1055), and is likely to order blood and urine tests to measure levels of various hormones.

How Serious Is Oligomenorrhea?   In most cases oligomenorrhea presents no danger to your health and requires no treatment. However, if you menstruate infrequently and find you cannot become pregnant, you may need to see a specialist in infertility.

Treatment.   *Medication.*   If the cause of your oligomenorrhea is that your ovaries are producing too little estrogen, your physician may prescribe estrogens to compensate. This treatment will restore normal menstruation and help prevent osteoporosis (see page 982).

If the cause of your problem is too much androgen, treatment will be dictated by findings concerning the underlying causes (see Adrenal Gland Disorders, page 718).

HEAVY PERIODS

Signs and Symptoms
- Menstrual periods that last longer than 7 days;
- Periods in which bleeding is unusually heavy.

Heavy periods are common, especially in young women who are not yet ovulating regularly and in older women approaching menopause. However, any woman at any time in her reproductive life may experience heavy menstrual bleeding; some women have heavy periods almost every cycle. Menorrhagia, the medical term for heavy periods, is derived from the Greek words *men,* meaning month, and *rhegnynai,* meaning to burst forth. The disorder also is known as hypermenorrhea.

Often, heavy periods reflect some spontaneous disturbance of the hormone cycle. However, they also can be caused by fibroids (see page 1097), pelvic infection (see page 1104) or, rarely, endometriosis (see page 1101). An intrauterine device (IUD) used for birth control also can cause menorrhagia; when that happens, the IUD often has to be removed.

If your heavy period is a one-time occurrence and your period arrives late, you could be having a miscarriage. Call a physician immediately because, if the miscarriage is incomplete, you may need to have dilation and curettage (D and C)—a minor operation in which the physician gently scrapes out the uterus (see below)—or perhaps a simple suction procedure.

You probably do not need medical help if you have a single heavy period that is not late and you have no reason to think you were pregnant. In that case, simply reduce your activity until the bleeding eases. If it does not stop within 24 hours, call your physician.

If you have several heavy periods, see a physician to make sure that you are not developing iron-deficiency anemia from the loss of blood and that you have no underlying disorder.

DILATION AND CURETTAGE

Dilation and curettage—generally referred to as a D and C—is a minor surgical procedure in which a physician first dilates the cervix and then inserts a thin, spoon-shaped instrument and uses it to scrape the lining of the uterus.

The opening to the cervix is normally tiny and tight. To dilate it during a D and C, a physician may insert a series of tapering rods, each thicker than the previous one, or stretch it with other types of instruments.

The traditional D and C involves scraping the uterine lining with a curette, a long, thin, spoon-shaped instrument. However, today physicians sometimes use vacuum aspiration—low-pressure suction— to remove endometrial tissue.

Often, a D and C is used to diagnose a problem. If you have been menstruating too often or very heavily, the physician may be able to determine the cause by examining uterine scrapings under a microscope (see Heavy Periods, page 1065, and Dysfunctional Uterine Bleeding, page 1067). Sometimes the D and C itself cures the problem, temporarily or permanently. In addition, a D and C is useful for diagnosing uterine fibroids (see page 1066), endometrial polyps (see page 1098), uterine cancer (see page 1099), and cervical cancer (see page 1095).

D and C also can be used for treatment of certain problems rather than for diagnosis. Endometrial polyps that protrude through the cervix may be removed during a D and C, and, very occasionally, fibroids can be scraped away, although usually a major operation is required. D and C sometimes also is done to remedy a condition called endometrial hyperplasia (see page 1098) in which the uterine lining has become too thick.

In addition, if you have a miscarriage or an incomplete abortion, you may need to have the remaining uterine lining or products of conception scraped or suctioned away to prevent infection. Although the D and C used to be the standard method for early abortion, it largely has been replaced by vacuum aspiration (see page 199).

D and C can be done in a physician's office with a local anesthetic. However, sometimes physicians prefer to do the procedure in a hospital and use a general anesthetic; then the pelvic muscles relax completely and a more thorough examination is possible.

If you have a D and C done in a hospital, you generally can go home the same day or the next day. You may experience some vaginal bleeding for a few days afterward and may have some cramps or back pain, but you usually can resume normal activities almost immediately. However, you should not have sex or use tampons for a few weeks, until the cervix is once again normal and the endometrium is healed completely.

Although a D and C is a minor procedure, no operation is entirely without risk. In rare cases, infection or hemorrhage develops, the uterus or surrounding organs are perforated during the procedure, or complications due to the anesthesia develop.

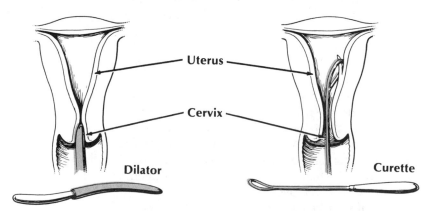

To perform a dilation and curettage (D & C), your physician will start by using a series of surgical instruments called dilators. These tapering rods are used to open (dilate) the cervix. After dilation, your physician inserts another instrument, called a curette, which is used to scrape a small amount of tissue from the wall of the uterus.

The Diagnosis. Your physician will do a pelvic examination (see page 1055) to check for abnormalities of the uterus. The physician may also do a Pap test (see page 1096) and a biopsy of the cervix (see page 1094) or the endometrium. In addition, you might have a blood test to make sure you are not anemic and to check for signs of other problems that could be causing the heavy bleeding. If you are anemic, other sources of blood loss should be evaluated.

How Serious Is Menorrhagia? Menorrhagia is inconvenient, and it can be distressing. However, there is rarely any serious underlying disorder, although you do have to be careful not to become anemic.

Treatment. *Medication.* If you are young and your uterus is in normal condition, the physician will probably prescribe estrogen or progesterone or both, often in the form of birth control pills, to reduce the bleeding. If you are already taking the pill and are still having heavy periods, or you cannot take the pill for some reason, other medications can be used. If you are anemic, you may need iron tablets.

Surgery. If you are older or if you are a young woman but after a few months on medication you are still having heavy periods, your physician may schedule a dilation and curettage to try to identify the underlying disorder that is causing the problem. Even if the dilation and curettage (see page 1066) does not establish the cause, it often stops the heavy bleeding.

DYSFUNCTIONAL UTERINE BLEEDING

Signs and Symptoms
- Vaginal bleeding that occurs at irregular intervals and is unpredictable in amount or duration.

Dysfunctional uterine bleeding is usually painless. It happens most often in girls who have just begun to menstruate, in women approaching menopause, or as a consequence of stress or illness. In most cases, the uterine lining has overdeveloped because the ovaries are not producing hormones in the normal way.

When dysfunctional uterine bleeding is not due to life stage or stress, the underlying cause may be polycystic ovarian disease (see page 1107). Less frequently, the problem is an estrogen-producing ovarian tumor or abnormal estrogen metabolism due to liver disease. However, if you have been taking a medication that contains estrogen, that could be to blame.

The Diagnosis. Your physician will want to take a careful menstrual history and do a pelvic examination (see page 1055) to make sure the source of the bleeding is actually the uterus and not the bladder, vagina, or cervix. Your physician also will try to determine whether an ectopic pregnancy or an early miscarriage could cause the bleeding.

How Serious Is Dysfunctional Uterine Bleeding? If the bleeding continues, and it is not due to menarche or menopause, it should be treated. Dysfunctional bleeding usually can be controlled by medication; if not, a dilation and curettage (see page 1066) generally is effective. Women with chronic bleeding are apt to be infertile.

Treatment. *Medication.* If the bleeding is moderately severe, your physician may prescribe a short course of oral contraceptives containing a relatively high dose of estrogen. If the problem is severe, hospitalization, bed rest, and injections of estrogen or progesterone may be required. After this treatment, iron replacement may be needed if you have become anemic, and you may take oral contraceptives for several months to prevent a recurrence.

Surgery. If hormone therapy fails to control the bleeding, your physician may do an endometrial biopsy or a dilation and curettage to determine the cause of bleeding. In fact, the dilation and curettage sometimes solves the problem.

MENOPAUSE

Signs and Symptoms
- Hot flashes: a sudden reddening of the face associated with a feeling of warmth;
- Painful intercourse, due to a gradual thinning of vaginal tissues and lessening of lubrication;

- Emotional problems such as nervousness, depression, irritability, insomnia;
- Much later, back pain and brittle bones due to osteoporosis;
- No signs or symptoms.

Menopause is a natural stage of life (see page 1058). In the simplest terms, it is a transition from the time when you menstruated and could have children to the time when you no longer experience the monthly menstrual flow and can no longer become pregnant. In technical terms, it happens when the ovaries no longer produce enough estrogen to stimulate the lining of the uterus and vagina properly.

A generation ago, women were expected to be unstable and unhappy during menopause. Today, the pendulum has swung the other way, and people tend to assume that a woman should have no problems at all—and many women do not. About 25 percent of all women notice no changes during menopause, except the gradual cessation of menstruation. Fifty percent notice slight changes, and the remaining 25 percent report some or all of the symptoms listed above.

Menopause comes naturally to most women at some time between ages 40 and 55 years. Once you are in midlife, you will suspect you are approaching menopause when your periods become irregular and unpredictable. You may menstruate more often or less often; you may skip some periods altogether; you may have shorter periods or longer and heavier ones. Perhaps one-third of all women experience no such irregularities—one day they simply stop menstruating. However, for most women, menopause is a gradual process that takes anywhere from several months to several years as the ovaries produce less and less estrogen. Estrogen is still being produced elsewhere in the body, but the total amount available decreases dramatically around the time of menopause. Finally, the amount of estrogen is so low that it can no longer stimulate the endometrium to proliferate and grow, at which point menopause has been reached.

Medically, the word menopause simply means the permanent end of menstruation. It is derived from the Greek words for month *(men)* and cessation *(pausis).* Literally, menopause occurs when you menstruate for the last time, though in popular use the word generally refers to a period of several years, from the first menstrual irregularities to the time when the body has adjusted completely to hormonal changes.

Although girls in this country have been reaching menarche at younger ages than previous generations did, women have been experiencing the onset of menopause somewhat later in life. It is not unusual now for a woman to be menstruating in her mid-50s. However, the median age at the last menstruation is 50 to 51 years. Because a woman's life expectancy may be almost 80 years, about a third of her life is likely to occur after menopause.

The dramatic decrease in estrogen levels that leads to menopause is responsible for hot flashes and vaginal changes. Hot flashes happen when blood vessels dilate. Some women experience very mild flashes (or flushes, as they are also called), but others are extremely uncomfortable during flashes. If you are in the latter group, you may wake up drenched with perspiration many times in the course of a night. During the day, you may feel conspicuous and embarrassed when flashes strike, because you feel your face heat up and you begin to perspire. It helps to remember that most of the time the flashes produce only a slight change in skin color and go unnoticed by others.

To some degree, all women experience gradual changes in the vagina during menopause: a thinning of vaginal tissues and a lessening of lubrication may mean that intercourse becomes painful. If sex does become uncomfortable, a water-soluble lubricating jelly should solve the problem. Another result of vaginal changes and a parallel thinning of tissues in the urinary tract is that you may become more susceptible to both vaginal and urinary infections.

Osteoporosis can be a more serious problem. It is a disorder common in old age in which the bones become porous and brittle (see Bone Diseases, page 982).

A small percentage of women develop emotional problems during menopause that seem to be linked to hormonal changes. However, the connection is difficult to prove or disprove because midlife can be a difficult time for both women and men—children leave home; a spouse may die; parents may be in poor health or may die; it becomes harder to find a job. Any of these changes could trigger the kind of depression and anxiety that sometimes are associated with menopause.

On the other hand, menopause also can affect your physical and mental health in positive ways. For instance, if you have endometriosis, the symptoms may disappear after menopause, and fibroids usually shrink (see pages 1101 and 1097). In addition, you no longer need to worry about becoming pregnant.

The Diagnosis. During the premenopausal years, see a physician if you begin bleeding between periods, if you have prolonged or excessive menstrual bleeding, or if you go for 6 months without menstruating and then suddenly have a period. All of these changes can be perfectly normal at that stage of life. However, because they could also be symptoms of a malignant growth such as cancer of the uterus, it is better to have them checked. Your physician will want to take a history and do a pelvic examination (see page 1055). If the physician has any suspicion that you might have uterine cancer, he or she will do an endometrial biopsy, an office procedure in which a sample of tissue is excised from the lining of the uterus (see page 1099). At times, dilation and curettage may have to be done (see page 1066).

You may also want to see a physician to get relief from hot flashes and other problems of menopause or because you have skipped a period and want to be sure you are not pregnant. In these cases, the physician will also probably take a history, do a pelvic examination, and—if appropriate—do a pregnancy test.

Because you may still be ovulating, your physician undoubtedly will advise you to continue to use birth control for a time even after you seem to have stopped menstruating. One rule of thumb: if you had your last period while you were younger than 50 years, you should continue to use contraceptives (other than birth control pills) for 2 years after that; if you were older than 50 years, use contraceptives other than birth control pills for 12 months.

How Serious Are the Problems Associated With Menopause? Most menopausal problems are not considered serious because they do no harm and they are self-limiting: if you do nothing about them, they will go away of their own accord within a couple of months or a couple of years. However, osteoporosis is debilitating, particularly if it results in numerous fractures.

Treatment. *Medication.* Estrogen replacement therapy can relieve hot flashes and halt the thinning of vaginal tissue temporarily; it also may delay the progression of osteoporosis.

Estrogen replacement therapy was popular during the 1970s, until researchers linked it to an increased risk of cancer of the lining of the uterus (endometrial cancer). Today, the treatment has changed: it generally involves the lowest effective dose of estrogen (for example, 0.625 milligrams of premarin daily) combined with a progesterone, because studies show that adding progesterone reduces the risk of endometrial cancer. Typically, estrogen replacement therapy involves taking tablets of estrogen for the first 11 to 15 days of every month and then taking estrogen and progesterone together for about 10 days; then you stop taking both medications, at which point you will have vaginal bleeding for several days. Women who are taking this therapy to relieve hot flashes and vaginal problems generally continue to do so for many years.

Some medical experts would like to see estrogen therapy more widely used to prevent osteoporosis, arguing that the disease has reached almost epidemic proportions; others urge caution because of the potential dangers involved. Many physicians think that you should seriously consider estrogen replacement therapy if you are especially at risk. You are at risk if you are small-boned or thin, smoke, drink alcohol, or come from northern European stock, especially if someone in your immediate family, such as your mother or an aunt, has had osteoporosis.

Most physicians definitely recommend estrogen replacement therapy for women who went through menopause prematurely. Menopause is considered premature if you stopped menstruating before the age of 40 years, either naturally or because your ovaries were surgically removed (see Hysterectomy, page 1100).

While you are taking estrogen, be sure to have a yearly mammogram (see page 1180). You should also be checked regularly for cancer of the endometrium. Endometrial cancer (see page 1099) can often be detected while it is still at an early stage by an endometrial biopsy.

For the emotional problems that sometimes occur during midlife, treatment depends on the specific symptoms. Possible treatments include antidepressants for severe depression, mild sleeping pills for temporary insomnia, and psychotherapy when it is appropriate. Estrogen replacement is usually ineffective for relieving emotional problems.

Nutrition and Exercise.   To prevent osteoporosis, you need a diet rich in sources of calcium, such as milk and some green vegetables. Before menopause, according to most medical experts, a woman should have at least 1,000 milligrams of calcium a day; after menopause, she should have 1,500 milligrams. Most physicians who prescribe estrogen replacement therapy to prevent osteoporosis also advise their patients to take calcium pills. In addition, they suggest regular exercise because there is evidence that weight-bearing exercise, such as walking and jogging, can slow the loss of bone. Exercise also may yield a feeling of well-being (see page 984).

POSTMENOPAUSAL BLEEDING

Signs and Symptoms
- Vaginal bleeding that occurs a year or more after your final menstrual period.

If you suddenly begin to bleed from the vagina after menopause, there are many possible explanations. You may have developed a vaginal infection, or you might occasionally bleed a bit after intercourse or from douching just because the walls of your vagina are thinner and more fragile (see page 1068). Estrogen, taken as a medication, also can cause bleeding. Because cancer of the endometrium (see page 1099) also can be a cause of bleeding, see a physician as soon as possible.

The Diagnosis.   Your physician will do a pelvic examination (see page 1055). His or her first concern will be to establish where the blood is coming from because the source could be almost anywhere in your reproductive tract, including your uterus and its lower part, the cervix, or the vagina. It

could even be coming from your urinary tract or rectum.

If it appears that you are bleeding from the vagina, your physician will probably want to do a cervical biopsy to determine the possible causes (see Biopsies, page 1284) and a dilation and curettage to be sure the vagina is the only source of bleeding. Both are minor surgical procedures. During a cervical biopsy, a small piece of tissue is cut from the cervix; in dilation and curettage, the inner walls of the uterus are scraped (see page 1066). Your physician also may order blood and urine tests.

Sometimes even after exhaustive study, a physician cannot find any explanation for an episode of postmenopausal bleeding. If the bleeding never recurs, there is no reason for concern, but if it happens again, you will have to be reexamined until the cause is finally found.

How Serious Is Postmenopausal Bleeding?   It can be trivial, or extremely serious, or anything in between, depending on what is causing the bleeding.

Treatment.   Treatment depends on the underlying disorder. For example, if the tissue lining your vagina has become fragile, your physician may prescribe a vaginal cream or suppository that contains estrogen. Vaginal infections generally are treated with antibiotics. If you have cancer, you will need an operation, radiation, chemotherapy, or some combination of these treatments.

PRIMARY OVARIAN FAILURE

Signs and Symptoms
- First menstrual period has not occurred by age 16 years;
- Breasts and pubic hair may not have developed;
- Genitals may not look normal.

Because of chromosome abnormalities, some girls are born without all the usual internal or external organs of their sex. Sometimes this is noticeable at birth, but often the first clue is that the girl does not begin menstruating at puberty. She may or may not develop breasts and pubic hair, depending on the nature of her genetic problem.

One third of the girls who fail to menstruate have a disorder called gonadal dysgenesis (abnormal ovaries). There are several different types of gonadal dysgenesis, but the most common—it occurs in 1 out of every 2,500 female newborn babies—is Turner's syndrome. A teenage girl with Turner's syndrome is very short, her body is childlike in appearance, her breasts have not developed, and she has little or no pubic or underarm hair. Her internal reproductive organs are also childlike, and her ovaries are simply streaks of fiber with no follicles or ova; these are known as streak gonads.

Complete testicular feminization is another congenital problem that may result in a failure to menstruate. At puberty, the girl develops breasts but little or no pubic or underarm hair. Her genitals appear to be normal, but the vagina is short and she has no cervix; some girls have no vagina at all. She has no uterus, ovaries, or fallopian tubes; instead, somewhere in her abdominal cavity, she has undescended testes. She is generally feminine in her behavior and outlook. The undescended testes are slightly at risk as a site for cancer.

The Diagnosis. When girls reach their late teens without menstruating, most often they are simply late in developing (see page 1057). However, if a physician has reason to think congenital problems might be involved, these problems will be checked because hormone treatment can make a great difference in many such cases. The physician will do a pelvic examination (see page 1055) and may order a chromosome study and blood tests to measure circulating hormones. Because the physician will want to know exactly which chromosomes are abnormal, chromosome studies are often helpful.

A physician also can learn more about the status of the ovaries by prescribing a course of the female sex hormone progesterone. If the ovaries are producing estrogen, a course of progesterone will induce bleeding from the uterus; this is called withdrawal bleeding. This bleeding also implies that the uterus has an endometrium (lining) that can be stimulated.

How Serious Is Primary Ovarian Failure? It can be serious because of the risk of cancer. In some cases of primary ovarian failure, enough of the ovary is normal for the girl to menstruate occasionally and eventually to conceive, but most often she never menstruates and is infertile. However, if she is treated at puberty with female sex hormones she will develop breasts and all the usual secondary sex characteristics and will be protected to a considerable extent from developing osteoporosis.

Treatment. *Medication.* Physicians generally prescribe estrogen and progesterone to develop and maintain secondary sex characteristics.

Surgery. Specialists advise removal of streak gonads if the chromosome abnormality that produced them is the sort (testicular feminization) that predisposes them to cancer. Surgery also can correct the look of genitals that are sexually ambiguous or even create a vagina that will be functional for purposes of intercourse but not reproduction.

ABNORMALITIES OF THE HYPOTHALAMUS, THYROID, PITUITARY, ADRENAL GLANDS, AND OVARIES

Signs and Symptoms
- Disruption of menstrual periods.

The menstrual cycle is governed by a complex cascade of hormones. The hypothalamus, which is a part of the brain, sends chemicals called releasing factors directly to the pituitary gland; the pituitary then releases pituitary hormones (called gonadotropins), which travel through the bloodstream to the ovaries where they cause ovarian follicles to produce estrogen and progesterone (for more details, see Pituitary Gland Disorders, page 723). Estrogen and progesterone prepare the uterus for a possible pregnancy. Things can go wrong at any stage in this process.

As a result, menstrual irregularity is sometimes caused by problems in the distant hypothalamus, a part of the brain that can be affected by illness, drug abuse, a drastic loss of weight, or stress. More rarely, the hypothalamus develops a disorder such as a tumor or infection, and that affects menstruation.

If the pituitary gland stops producing its hormones, the ovaries are the first organs to be affected. When a young girl fails to develop sexually, it may be either because her pituitary is not producing enough gonadotropins or because of ovarian failure (see page 1070). Sometimes the pituitary produces too much of the hormone prolactin, either in reaction to certain drugs, such as tranquilizers and oral contraceptives, or—very rarely—because of a pituitary tumor. Prolactin helps prevent pregnancy while a woman is breast-feeding; released in excess at other times, it can prevent ovulation and menstruation (see Galactorrhea, page 1078).

Sometimes, the ovaries themselves develop cysts or tumors and fail to release their hormones in normal amounts (see page 1105). The menstrual cycle also can be disrupted by disorders of the thyroid gland (see Thyroid Disorders, page 727). If your thyroid is overactive, you may stop menstruating or have scanty periods; if it is underactive, menstruation can be prolonged and heavy and you also may lose interest in sex. Changes in the adrenal glands also can cause changes in menstrual patterns, which can be corrected with medication.

The Diagnosis. Blood tests can be done to measure the levels of various hormones circulating in the blood. If pituitary hormones seem to be present in normal amounts, for example, but you show signs of estrogen deprivation, such as a thinning of the vaginal walls, the problem may be with the ovaries. Blood tests can be done to identify adrenal problems, or x-rays can be taken to check for tumors. A laparoscope, a thin, tube-like instrument equipped with a light (see page 1297), can be used to look for ovarian cysts. And, of course, the physician will want to do a general physical examination and a pelvic examination (see page 1055).

How Serious Are These Abnormalities? Some abnormalities, such as malignant tumors, are serious. Others are not—for example, menstrual irregularity that is simply a reaction to stress or to tranquilizers that you have been taking.

Treatment. *Medication.* The treatment used depends on the underlying problem. If a hormone is not being produced in the normal way, it often can be given as a medication—estrogen, for example, or a thyroid hormone for hypothyroidism.

Surgery. If the basic disorder is a tumor, surgery or radiation generally is needed.

PROBLEMS OF THE BREAST

During puberty, the normal breast rapidly develops fibrous tissue (stroma). The adult breast has more fatty tissue. The breast changes in response to monthly variations in hormone levels.

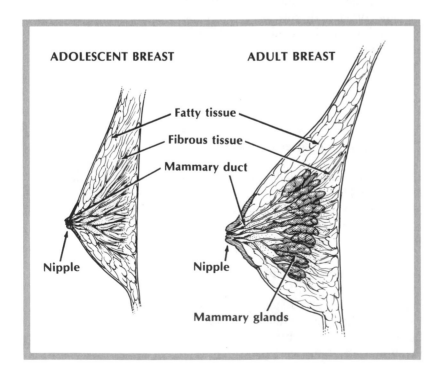

ADOLESCENT BREAST **ADULT BREAST**

Fatty tissue
Fibrous tissue
Mammary duct
Nipple
Nipple
Mammary glands

THE NORMAL BREAST

From the time a woman reaches puberty until after menopause, her breasts change continually as her hormones fluctuate. At puberty, when the body begins to produce estrogen in quantity, the breasts rapidly develop both stroma—a framework of connective tissue—and a system of glands and ducts. However, it is the fat cells that are deposited at the same time that provide the bulk of the breast tissue.

From puberty on, your breasts change every month, growing larger over the course of the menstrual cycle. During the first half of the cycle, your ovaries release estrogen, which causes new cells to grow in glands, ducts, and other breast tissue, and more blood flows to the breasts. During the second half of the cycle, glands in the breasts are bombarded with progesterone as well as estrogen, and they begin to secrete substances that are the precursors of breast milk. If you do not become pregnant, your hormone levels decrease, your body absorbs both the secretions and the new cells, and the blood supply to the breasts diminishes. In some women, the breasts become so engorged toward the end of the menstrual cycle that they are painful (see Premenstrual Tenderness and Swelling, page 1074). Others have cysts in their breasts that enlarge at that time (see page 1074). Birth

BREAST-FEEDING

Many women prefer to breast-feed their babies. Although infants also thrive on formula, breast milk is easier to digest and contains antibodies that protect the baby from infections. In addition, many women find it very pleasant.

Once you have given birth to a baby, your pituitary gland begins to produce increased amounts of a hormone called prolactin, which stimulates cells in your breasts. These cells begin to absorb nutrients from your bloodstream and use these to produce milk. Because this process takes a little time, for a few days after birth the breasts produce a thin white fluid, called colostrum, rather than milk. Like milk, colostrum is nourishing and has antibodies. After 3 to 5 days, the milk is produced. Prolactin controls the quantity; up to a point, the more the baby takes, the more prolactin your pituitary produces, and the more milk you will have. Once the child stops nursing, milk production ceases within a week or two.

The flow of breast milk is controlled by the let-down reflex—otherwise milk would continually leak from your breasts. When the baby suckles, your nipples respond by sending sensory impulses to the hypothalamus in the brain. The hypothalamus immediately signals the pituitary gland to release hormones (principally, oxytocin) that travel via the bloodstream. When they reach the breasts, they cause the cells surrounding the alveoli—the cavities where the milk is stored—to contract, expressing milk out into the ducts. All of this takes only 30 to 60 seconds. Once breast milk is established, the let-down reflex is easily triggered; often, just the sound of the baby crying stimulates it. However, stress can interfere with the reflex; thus, you need supportive people around you, especially when you are just starting to breast-feed.

If you feel a sharp pain in your nipple while the baby is suckling, the nipple may have developed a thin crack. Your physician can recommend a cream to apply that will help it heal. If you feel a small, hard lump in one breast, you may have a blocked milk duct. Try massaging the area and bathing it with hot water. If the lump does not go away, call the physician because it may be an infection (see Breast Infections, page 1076). If so, you will need antibiotics. You usually can continue to breast-feed the baby despite the infection.

To some extent, the prolactin protects you from becoming pregnant. However, it is wiser not to rely on it because you occasionally may ovulate while breast-feeding, even if you do not menstruate.

When you stop breast-feeding, unless you taper off gradually, your breasts may become engorged and painful for a few days until the milk dries up. Women who bottle-feed from birth have the same problem. Your physician can prescribe a drug to suppress lactation. If that does not work, ice bags and a tight breast binder may help.

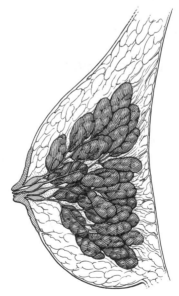

NORMAL BREAST   **LACTATING BREAST**

If you breast-feed, the system of ducts and glands within your breast expands as milk is produced (lactation).

control pills also can cause breast tenderness and swelling as a side effect, although this is not a problem for most women who take them.

During pregnancy, the breasts enlarge considerably—together, they may gain as much as a pound. The duct system, stimulated by hormones produced by the placenta and the pituitary gland, grows and branches. More cells are laid down in the stroma, and fat cells are added. The nipple and the areola are apt to grow larger and, in light-skinned women, to become darker; these changes are often permanent.

Once a baby is born, other hormones affect the breasts. Milk production is regulated by prolactin, which is produced by the pituitary gland. When the baby is weaned and breast stimulation ends, prolactin production eases off, the flow of breast milk ceases, and eventually the breasts return to their normal size and condition.

At menopause, the breast changes that accompanied the menstrual cycle cease. Some problems, such as cystic breast lumps, diminish or disappear. However, the likelihood of breast cancer rises. It is a particularly deadly form of cancer, but diagnosing it early makes a big difference. For that reason, examine your breasts once a month at every age, but especially after menopause (see Breast Self-Examination, page 1076). At age 40 years, begin having mammography (see page 1080), and after age 50 years, have mammography annually.

PREMENSTRUAL TENDERNESS AND SWELLING

Signs and Symptoms
- Breasts that are swollen and painful just before menstrual periods.

Just as your uterine lining thickens each month in preparation for a possible pregnancy, over the course of the month your breasts develop new cells in their glands and ducts to prepare for breast-feeding (see page 217). Thus, in the week or so before you menstruate, your breasts enlarge. For some women the change is extreme and uncomfortable.

Breast engorgement is one of the symptoms of premenstrual syndrome (see page 1062). No one knows exactly what causes this syndrome, but it may be related to hormonal changes that take place toward the end of the menstrual cycle.

The Diagnosis. Your physician may ask you to keep a record of all your premenstrual symptoms for a few months, noting particularly the day on which your breasts become uncomfortable, the day the discomfort ends, and the day your period starts. Although it can be painful, premenstrual breast tenderness is not considered serious.

Treatment. *Medication.* Your physician may prescribe a diuretic. It can be taken for the last 10 days before the onset of your period or for 1 or 2 days before your symptoms usually appear.

Self-Help. You may feel more comfortable if you cut down on salt intake at the end of your cycle, because salt causes tissues to retain more fluid, which makes engorgement worse. Some women find that it also helps to avoid caffeine, sugar, and alcohol. A comfortable brassiere, worn 24 hours a day, may help too.

LUMPS IN THE BREAST

Signs and Symptoms
- One or more lumps in the breasts, which may or may not be painful;
- A greenish or straw-colored discharge may be expressed from the nipples.

The vast majority of breast lumps are not malignant. Nevertheless, some are, so if you find a lump call your physician. If it is late in your menstrual cycle, you may prefer to wait a few days because the lump may disappear after menstruation, which would indicate that it is a harmless cyst.

Cysts are produced by a benign condition called fibrocystic changes. (It is also sometimes called chronic cystic mastitis, mammary dysplasia, or benign breast disease.) A cyst is a fluid-filled sac that tends to get bigger toward the end of the menstrual cycle, when your body is retaining more fluid. Some cysts are very tiny, but others can be as large as a hen's egg. If pressed, the large ones may change shape slightly, and they can be moved about a bit under the skin.

No one knows what causes cysts. Because they generally disappear after menopause, ovarian hormones are probably involved. You are most likely to develop fibrocystic changes between the ages of 25 and 50 years, with one lump or several located in both breasts.

Breast lumps that are not cysts and are not cancer are most likely to be fibroadenomas (or adenofibromas), benign tumors that most often are found in young women. A fibroadenoma has a firm, smooth, rubbery feeling and a well-defined shape. It can be moved about under the skin.

There are also other types of lumps. An infection can produce a lump (see page 1074), as can severe injury. A lump could also be a lipoma—a tumor of the fatty tissues. It may be an intraductal papilloma (see page 1078), especially if it is blocking a duct, which would cause a cyst. None of these conditions are malignant.

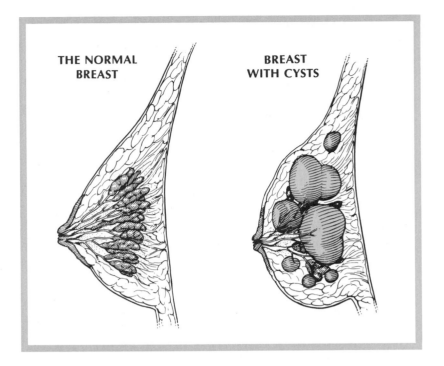

THE NORMAL BREAST

BREAST WITH CYSTS

The Diagnosis. Your physician's chief concern will be to make sure the lumps in your breast are not cancer. If you have a single lump that feels like a cyst, your physician may try to aspirate its fluid contents by using a thin needle. This can be done in the physician's office, and you may not even need a local anesthetic. If the fluid can be aspirated, the lump will disappear, an indication that it was a cyst. The fluid can be sent to a laboratory to be analyzed for signs of malignancy. If you have a family history of breast cancer, you will want to be sure this is done.

If a lump does not feel like a cyst, or if it does feel like one but the physician is unable to draw out any fluid, your physician may recommend a mammogram, a special breast x-ray (see page 1080). If the lump is large enough, ultrasonography is sometimes useful (see page 1287). A lump that refuses to yield fluid may still be a cyst.

If mammography or ultrasonography shows a solid area rather than a hollow cyst, the next step is a biopsy to remove some or all of the lump and examine it under a microscope. A needle biopsy, which removes a very small core of tissue, can be done in a physician's office with local anesthesia. A surgical biopsy, removing the whole lump, is another way to determine that the lump is not malignant—mammography and ultrasonography can be misleading and a needle biopsy might remove a nonmalignant area of an otherwise malignant tumor. A sur-

gical biopsy is done in a hospital, with either local or general anesthesia.

How Serious Are Breast Lumps? If they are not malignant, they are not harmful beyond occasional discomfort. According to some recent studies, if you have fibrocystic changes you are not more likely to develop breast cancer than anyone else. (Older studies suggested a slightly increased risk.) However, women with lumpy breasts may have more trouble detecting a malignant tumor, should one develop.

Treatment. *Medication.* Many women prefer to take mild analgesics, such as aspirin, and otherwise tolerate the discomfort. Good breast support, worn even at night, is also effective. Danazol and bromocriptine relieve breast pain for many women, but both can have unpleasant side effects and both are expensive. Vitamin E is sometimes used, but there is no solid evidence that it works.

Surgery. Cysts are aspirated to ensure that they are simply cysts; otherwise, they need not be removed or treated unless they are painful or recur after aspiration. Fibroadenomas and other benign tumors may be left, or they can be removed if they are large or uncomfortable. Lumpectomies (removal of lumps) are done in a hospital, often on an outpatient basis.

BREAST SELF-EXAMINATION

Although 75 percent of all breast lumps are benign, some are not. Thus, regular self-examination can save your life because breast cancer is curable if it is caught early.

Examine your breasts once a month. If you have not yet reached menopause, the best time is a few days after your period ends because your breasts are less likely to be tender or swollen. If you are no longer menstruating, pick a day of the month and do the examination regularly on that day.

Stand in front of a mirror. With your arms at your sides, look at the skin on your breasts for any sign of puckering, for dimples, or for changes in the size or shape of the breasts. If your nipples are not normally inverted, look to see whether they are now pushed in. Rest your hands on your hips, then place them behind your head; in each position, check for the same signs.

Next, step into the shower and, once your breasts are wet and soapy, place your left hand behind your head and examine your left breast with your right hand. Think of your breast as the face of a clock, and place your right hand at 12 o'clock, at the top of the breast. Hold your hand flat, fingertips pressed together, and make a tiny circling motion, feeling for lumps. Move the hand to 1 o'clock, to 2 o'clock, and so on. Once you return to 12, slide the fingertips closer to the nipple and repeat the motions you just went through, going around the clock in a circle within the first circle; then make an even smaller circle. Continue until you have checked the

tissue under the nipple; look for discharge from the nipple at that time. Finish by examining the area adjacent to your breast, below your armpit, because it also contains breast tissue. Repeat the

Use your eyes and hands to search for lumps, thickened areas, or swelling in your breasts. While lying and standing, a circular massaging motion is appropriate (see top and bottom illustrations). Both are necessary for a complete exam. Soap and water during a shower can facilitate the procedure. At center: A mirror also can be helpful. Elevate your arms and look for changes in the natural symmetry of both breasts. Also look for any unusual discharge from your nipples.

whole procedure using your left hand on your right breast.

In addition, examine your breasts while you are lying on your back. Again look for nipple discharge. To examine your right breast, put a pillow under your right shoulder and place your right hand under your head. To examine the left breast, place the pillow under the left shoulder and your left hand under your head.

If your breasts are normally lumpy because of fibrocystic changes (see Lumps in the Breast, page 1074), you will want to make a note of how many lumps you have, where they are located, and their approximate size. Then, with each self-examination, you can check for changes.

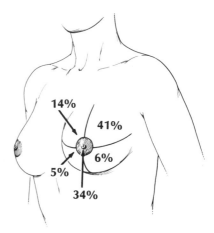

Seventy-five percent of all breast cancers occur under the nipple-areola region or in the upper, outer portion of the breast.

Forty-one percent of all breast cancers are found in the upper outer quadrant of the breast; 34 percent, in the central portion; 14 percent, in the upper inner quadrant; 5 percent, in the lower inner quadrant; and 6 percent, in the lower outer quadrant.

Nutrition. If you smoke or if you drink caffeinated substances, you may want to cut down or quit altogether. Although the evidence is inconclusive, some women have reported that their lumps subsided after they stopped smoking or gave up caffeine.

BREAST INFECTIONS

Signs and Symptoms
- A red, tender, painful swelling or lump in the breast;
- Swelling of the nearby glands in the armpit;
- Fever.

Breast infections, sometimes called mastitis, are not uncommon in women who are nursing a baby or who recently have stopped breast-feeding. Such infections generally are caused by bacteria that enter the breast through a cracked nipple. If the infection is severe, it can become an abscess. Surrounding tissues protect themselves by secreting a substance that hardens into a kind of wall around the infection, and pus collects inside it.

The Diagnosis. In a woman who is breast-feeding, the symptoms listed above strongly suggest an infection. However, breast infections occasionally do develop in women who have not been breast-feeding. Because the symptoms are similar to those of a rare form of cancer, in such cases the physician will want to test carefully to rule out malignancy. This testing may include a mammogram, a needle biopsy, or a surgical biopsy (see pages 1080 and 1079).

How Serious Are Breast Infections? Breast infections usually respond quickly to antibiotics. If they do not and an abscess forms, it can be drained.

Treatment. *Prevention.* If you are breast-feeding, keep your nipples clean and dry between feedings and do not wear clothing that irritates them. Do not allow the baby to chew on your nipples.

Medication. Your physician will prescribe an antibiotic and perhaps an analgesic for pain and fever. If you are breastfeeding, these drugs should have no harmful effects on either your milk supply or the baby, although you probably will be advised to give the baby the other breast until the infection clears up. Meanwhile, you can massage the infected breast gently to expel milk and prevent painful engorgement.

Surgery. Usually, the antibiotic is sufficient. If it is not, the abscess can be drained:

the physician may aspirate it with a needle or make a small incision at the edge of the areola to let the pus out. The incision leaves a minimal scar.

NIPPLE PROBLEMS

Signs and Symptoms
- Discharge from the nipple;
- Nipple that is indented, as if pulled in from below;
- Lumps in the areola (the area surrounding the nipple);
- Scaling of the nipple.

It is always wise to pay attention to changes in your nipples. Although most often the cause is benign, it could be cancer.

If whitish or greenish fluid leaks from your nipples, it is probably breast milk, especially if it comes from both nipples (see Breast-feeding, page 217, and Galactorrhea, page 1078). If the fluid is greenish or straw-colored, it may be due to fibrocystic changes (see page 1074). A discharge that is dark red or black contains blood; you may have a tiny, benign tumor growing in a milk duct (see page 1075), although breast cancer is a remote possibility.

Indented or retracted nipples are normal if you have had them since puberty. Later in life, if a previously normal nipple develops an indentation, it can be a sign of cancer.

Lumps in the areola are generally cysts, formed because oil glands have become blocked. If an infection develops, a cyst may become a boil.

Scaling of the nipple is usually due to benign changes. If it persists, a biopsy may be necessary to exclude an underlying cancer.

The Diagnosis. If you have nipple discharge, your physician will want to examine your breasts and get a sample of the discharge for laboratory analysis. To be sure no malignancy is involved, he or she may do other tests. For a newly retracted nipple or a bloody discharge, tests for cancer are definitely in order (see page 1078). Your physician's physical examination will likely identify a cyst or boil.

How Serious Are Nipple Problems? Nipple discharge and retracted nipples are serious only when they are symptoms of cancer. Cysts can be ignored unless they become infected, in which case antibiotics usually will solve the problem. If nipple scaling persists, see your physician.

Treatment.   For boils, antibiotics generally are prescribed. Whether or not surgery is necessary depends on the underlying problem.

GALACTORRHEA

Signs and Symptoms
* Whitish or greenish discharge from the nipples, usually from both breasts;
* May be accompanied by amenorrhea (missed menstrual period, see page 1063).

Normally, you produce breast milk only after giving birth and perhaps for a few days before. If your nipples leak milk at other times, you have an unusual condition called galactorrhea (from the Greek words *gala,* for milk, and *rhoia,* for flow).

Galactorrhea is something of a mystery. Researchers report that in about 50 percent of the cases a cause cannot be found, and in 25 percent of the cases it is due to a type of pituitary tumor called a prolactinoma, which is usually benign but secretes prolactin, the hormone that regulates the production of breast milk (see Pituitary Tumors, page 723). In the remaining 25 percent of the cases, galactorrhea has various causes—for instance, it can be a symptom of hypothyroidism or a side effect of a medication. Drugs that can cause galactorrhea include methyldopa (a medicine used for high blood pressure), phenothiazines (a category of tranquilizers), several types of antidepressants, and dextroamphetamine.

The Diagnosis.   The physician will examine your breasts and the fluid they are producing to make sure it is not the bloody discharge that occasionally is associated with breast cancer (see below). Your medical history will reveal whether the galactorrhea could be a side effect of some drug. If it is not, the physician will probably test for hypothyroidism (see page 730). Blood tests may be done to check your prolactin level, and a CT scan (a type of x-ray, see page 1286) of the hypothalamus and pituitary can be taken.

How Serious Is Galactorrhea?   Galactorrhea is no threat to your health unless it is

caused by a pituitary tumor. Such tumors grow slowly and some eventually stabilize. They often can be treated successfully with medication; if that fails, operation or radiation can be used.

Treatment.   *Medication.*   For hypothyroidism, thyroxine is prescribed. If you have a pituitary tumor or tests find no explanation for your galactorrhea, the physician probably will prescribe bromocriptine, which can shrink a tumor and reduce prolactin levels. Bromocriptine often cures galactorrhea even when it is of unknown origin.

Surgery.   For a large pituitary tumor, surgery may be necessary. Because such tumors tend to recur, you may need long-term treatment with bromocriptine or radiation.

INTRADUCTAL PAPILLOMA

Signs and Symptoms
* Watery or bloody discharge from the nipple;
* A very small lump beneath the nipple.

Intraductal papillomas are tiny, benign tumors that grow within the milk ducts of the breast at the point where they reach the nipple. Relatively uncommon, these tumors are often too small to feel.

The Diagnosis.   Your physician will go through the usual diagnostic procedure for breast lumps (see page 1074) to make sure you do not have breast cancer. He or she will apply gentle pressure in the areolar area to try to identify the duct containing the papilloma so that the duct can be excised with the tumor. Intraductal papillomas are benign but should be removed because that is the only way to be sure the lump is a papilloma rather than a cancer.

Treatment.   *Surgery.*   If there is a palpable lump, a surgeon can remove it. When no lump can be found, careful follow-up is necessary, including regular mammograms.

CANCERS OF THE BREAST

Signs and Symptoms
* A lump or thickening in the breast, which may not be painful or even tender;

- Clear or bloody discharge from a nipple;
- Retracted nipple;
- A change in the contours of the breasts—one may be higher than the other, for example;
- Any flattening or indentation of the skin of the breast;
- Redness or pitting, like the skin of an orange.

One of every 10 women will develop breast cancer at some point in her life. Although the disease often can be treated successfully if it is caught early, breast cancer still kills more women than any other cancer except lung cancer.

Scientists do not know what causes breast cancer. However, studies have identified certain factors that make it more likely for a woman to develop the disease. You run a higher risk than most women if your mother, her mother, an aunt, or a sister had breast cancer, especially if she developed it while young or if she had it in both breasts. Your risk is increased if you have never had children or if you were older than 35 years when you had your first child. If you already have had cancer in one breast, your chances of developing it in the other one are increased. The risk of breast cancer also rises with age.

There is very little you can do about most of these risk factors. However, you can be alert for the symptoms listed above so a malignant tumor can be caught in its early stages. All women older than 20 years should examine their breasts once a month (see Breast Self-Examination, page 1076). If you are between 20 and 40 years old, have a physician examine you at least once every 3 years; if you are older than 40 years, have an examination once a year. Many cancer experts believe that women should have mammography every year or two (see page 1080), beginning in their 40s. Women older than 50 years should have mammography annually.

The Diagnosis.   Your physician will examine your breasts carefully. He or she may squeeze the nipple area gently to see whether there is any discharge and will feel your armpits for signs that the lymph nodes might be involved because breast cancer can spread through the lymph system. A mammogram is the next step.

If you have a breast lump that is identified on ultrasonography as a cyst, the physician may use a thin needle to try to draw fluid from it. The fluid can be analyzed for malignant cells. In addition, if the lump disappears after the fluid is withdrawn, the chances are that it is simply a cyst (see Lumps in the Breast, page 1074).

A surgical biopsy, usually removing the entire lump, is the only way to be absolutely certain whether a lump is malignant. Your physician probably will advise such a biopsy if fluid cannot be drawn from the lump, if the lump does not collapse after the fluid has been drawn out, if the lump recurs, or if the fluid contains blood or malignant cells.

A needle biopsy of a particularly accessible lump may be done in a physician's office with local anesthesia. Surgical biopsies are generally done in a hospital with local or general anesthesia. The surgeon removes the entire lump for microscopic and biochemical examination by the pathologist. If the results are positive, the lump is malignant; if not, you will be told that it is benign. In more than 80 percent of biopsies, the lump is benign.

How Serious Is Breast Cancer?   A breast tumor itself is not lethal. The disease kills by metastasizing—that is, by spreading through the lymph system or the bloodstream to other parts of the body. Thus, if breast cancer is caught early, while the tumor is small and before malignant cells have spread to

Breast cancer spreads (metastasizes) through the lymph system (shown here) and through the bloodstream.

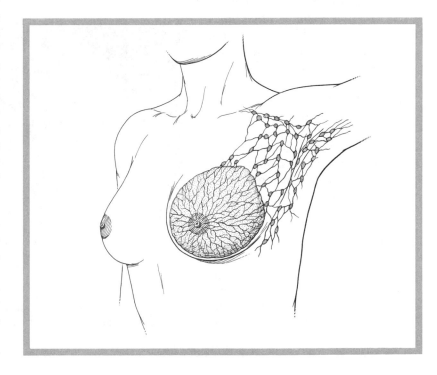

neighboring lymph nodes, there is about a 90 percent chance of a cure. However, in half of cases the cancer already has spread to other parts of the body before it is discovered. Nevertheless, the disease often can be controlled for years by drugs, radiation, or surgery.

Treatment. *Surgery.* Surgery is the primary treatment for breast cancer, although there is considerable controversy about how much of the breast needs to be removed (see Surgery for Breast Cancer, page 1081). Today, surgery is often combined with radiation therapy, hormone therapy, or chemotherapy.

As part of virtually every operation for breast cancer, the surgeon removes some lymph nodes from the armpit so they can be tested for signs of malignancy. The presence or absence of a malignant tumor in the lymph glands of the armpit is most important for planning treatment after the operation.

Radiation. If the surgeon finds that the cancer has reached your lymph nodes, he or she may recommend using radiation in the chest area to kill any cancer cells that may have escaped surgical removal. If the cancer eventually metastasizes and as a result you develop bone cancer, radiation may be used to ease the pain.

Hormone Therapy. If your breast cancer recurs, if tumors develop at distant sites, or if the cancer is too far advanced for surgery to make much of a difference, you still may be able to prolong life and relieve symptoms by taking hormones. Some tumors respond to treatment with hormones, either to drugs that counteract estrogen or sometimes to an added dose of estrogen. Among the anti-

---

MAMMOGRAMS

A mammogram is a special breast x-ray that can detect tumors so small that your physician cannot feel them. Mammography saves lives by identifying breast cancer at a stage when it is potentially still curable. However, the test is not infallible. Occasionally it fails to show a tumor, and at other times it indicates a problem when there is none. Screening by mammography is best combined with regular breast examinations done by a physician and with self-examination (see page 1076).

There is controversy within the medical profession about the age at which women should begin to have regular mammograms. Young women rarely develop breast cancer, and, in any case, their breasts are often so dense that they do not x-ray well.

Most medical experts agree that women younger than 35 years who are not in a high-risk category need not have mammograms and that those older than 50 years

Arrow reveals breast cancer on a mammogram, produced by a special x-ray device (top) that can detect tumors before they can be felt.

should have them annually. Controversy has centered on whether screening is necessary for women in their 40s and on whether a woman should have a baseline mammogram (to establish a norm for her breasts) at age 35 years. Recent studies indicate that regular mammograms do save lives among women in their 40s, but the value of the baseline x-ray remains questionable.

Today, this seems to be the best advice:

If you are younger than 40 years, you do not need mammography unless you develop a problem or are in a high-risk category (for instance, if you have a family history of breast cancer).

If you are between 40 and 49 years and have a family history of breast cancer, have a mammogram once a year.

If you are between 40 and 49 years, have no symptoms or self-found lumps, and have no family history of breast cancer, have a mammogram once every 2 years.

After the age of 50 years, have a mammogram annually.

SURGERY FOR BREAST CANCER

Caught early, breast cancer can sometimes be treated with radiation alone. However, in most cases a malignant tumor must be surgically removed.

During the operation, the surgeon also removes lymph nodes from the nearby armpit because the only way to tell whether the cancer has begun to spread (metastasize) is to examine those nodes under a microscope. If malignant cells are present, you will need additional treatment, either radiation or drugs. If only a few of the nodes test positive for cancer, that is a much better sign than if many of them do.

In operating for breast cancer, surgeons can remove a variable amount of tissue, and there is controversy about which procedures have the best long-term results. Every case is different. Your physician will consider the size of the tumor, its location, the type of cancer and its rate of growth, and whether the malignancy seems to have spread. The surgical possibilities are listed below.

Radical Mastectomy

Until 10 years ago, this was considered the only option. Now it is seldom done, except when a tumor has invaded muscle underlying the breast. Because a radical mastectomy removes a layer of chest muscles (the pectorals) along with the breasts and lymph nodes, it leaves the patient with less tissue covering the chest, which makes it hard to fit a prosthesis, and with an arm that has a tendency to swell and has some loss of mobility.

Modified Radical Mastectomy

The surgeon removes the entire breast along with lymph nodes from the armpit. However, be-

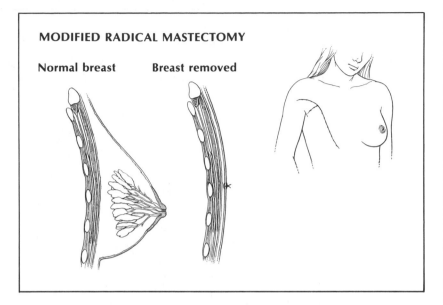

MODIFIED RADICAL MASTECTOMY

Normal breast   Breast removed

In a modified radical mastectomy the entire breast, along with lymph nodes from the adjacent armpit, is removed. Chest muscles remain intact.

cause the chest muscles are spared, problems are less likely to develop in the adjoining arm, the cosmetic result is better, and it is easier to do prosthetic reconstruction. The cure rate with the modified radical procedure seems to be about the same as that with the traditional radical mastectomy.

Simple Mastectomy

The surgeon removes only the breast and takes sample lymph nodes from the armpit.

Subcutaneous Mastectomy

The breast tissue is removed, but the skin and some superficial tissue are left in place. An artificial breast made of synthetic material (silicon) can then be inserted under the skin. Some nodes from the armpit also are excised.

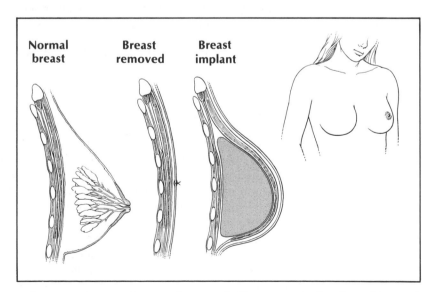

Normal breast   Breast removed   Breast implant

In breast reconstruction, a soft cone of silicone can be implanted beneath the skin.

Lumpectomy

The surgeon removes only the lump itself or else makes a wedge-shaped incision to remove surrounding tissue also. In either case, nodes are taken from the armpit. Lumpectomies generally are done only if the tumor is small, and they ordinarily are followed by radiation treatments to kill any cancer cells left in the area. Further treatment is always necessary if the lymph nodes in the armpit test positive for cancer; even when the nodes test negative, radiation, hormone therapy, or chemotherapy are sometimes used as a precaution. Recent studies indicate that if the cancer is caught early and the lumpectomy is followed by radiation, your chance of surviving is as good as with a modified radical mastectomy. (The lumpectomy is also sometimes called tylectomy, wide excision, segmental resection, or a partial mastectomy.)

Breast Reconstruction

Today, many women who have had a mastectomy have breast reconstruction done. Usually, a soft cone of silicon is implanted either under the skin or under the chest muscle. However, a plastic surgeon also can construct a whole

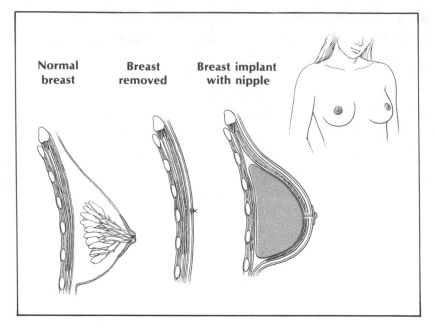

Normal breast   **Breast removed**   **Breast implant with nipple**

For cosmetic reasons, your surgeon can save the nipple of your reconstructed breast.

new breast from muscle or fatty tissue transferred from the abdomen or elsewhere in the body and covered with skin taken from the other breast or from somewhere else. Breast reconstruction does not make it any more or less likely that cancer will recur.

It is important that you and your physician discuss thoroughly the various options that are available for the removal of the cancer and for reconstruction of the breast.

To help you make the best decision, have a family member or a trusted friend sit in on the discussion.

Several self-help groups are available to help women who have had a mastectomy. You can ask your physician to contact Reach to Recovery, a program offered by the American Cancer Society. Volunteers will call on you in the hospital to give you practical advice and moral support.

estrogens that often are used are tamoxifen, androgens (the male hormone), and progesterones.

Hormone therapy can stop a tumor from growing or actually cause it to shrink; it can give you a partial or complete remission. If one hormone stops working, another may help. In this way, physicians can stall the disease for years. When hormones are no longer effective, your physician may try corticosteroids, such as prednisone, alone or combined with drugs used in chemotherapy.

Chemotherapy. The anti-tumor drugs given in chemotherapy are more toxic than

hormones, and all of them suppress the immune system to some degree, which can leave you vulnerable to infections. They also have many of the same unpleasant side effects as radiation: nausea, diarrhea, and fatigue. In addition, you may temporarily lose some or all of your hair. However, chemotherapy can often slow metastasis. It can sometimes bring about a complete remission, although the reprieve is usually temporary.

Chemotherapy seems to work better for women who have not yet gone through menopause. Physicians use various drugs in different combinations, sometimes also adding a corticosteroid or tamoxifen.

VAGINAL AND VULVAR DISORDERS

The vagina is the passageway that connects the uterus to the external genitals. It is about 5 inches long and its walls are lined with strong muscles. Most of the time the vagina is so narrow that the walls touch, but it can expand dramatically. The neck of the uterus, the cervix, extends into the vagina at the upper end. In young girls, the other (outer) end is partially blocked by a thin membrane called the hymen. It is rare for a hymen to close off the vagina altogether. The membrane is sometimes semicircular and covers just part of the vaginal opening, or if it is circular it generally has at least one hole in it.

A woman's external genitals are called the vulva (see page 1055). They include the mons pubis, a pad of fatty tissue at the base of the abdomen that is covered with hair after puberty, and the lip-like folds of tissue—the labia majora and, inside them, the labia minora—that shield the vagina and urethra. Just behind the mons pubis, where the labia come together, is the clitoris, a small protrusion that becomes distended during sexual arousal. The urethra, the tiny opening just behind the clitoris, leads to the bladder, where urine is stored. Behind the urethra is the vagina. Various glands located in the vulva and the vagina lubricate the area.

DEVELOPMENTAL DISORDERS

Signs and Symptoms

- Little or no vagina, or a very short vagina and no cervix;
- Genitals in a female that somewhat resemble male genitals.

At the moment of conception, the embryo acquires either male (XY) or female (XX) chromosomes. For the next 40 days, males and females are indistinguishable. Then, if the fetus has a Y chromosome, testes will develop. If a Y chromosome is not present and two X chromosomes are present, ovaries will develop. These organs secrete male or female hormones, respectively, and, in response, the fetus develops either a female or a male urogenital tract.

Something can go wrong at any stage. For instance, in a female fetus, an internal duct called the mullerian duct develops into fal-lopian tubes, a uterus, and the upper portion of the vagina. If something interferes with this process, the baby may be born without a vagina, with one that is very short, or perhaps without a uterus or ovaries. This condition is known as mullerian agenesis. Because most of the abnormalities are internal, and as long as the child has a vaginal opening, there may be no sign of the problem until she reaches puberty and fails to menstruate.

A girl born with little or no vagina also could have the condition called complete testicular feminization (also called androgen resistance syndrome). She has no cervix, uterus, or ovaries but instead has testes—often internally. She was genetically programmed to be a male but has abnormal androgen receptors; thus, before birth, male hormones were not able to connect with those receptors in the usual way to produce male genitals. At puberty, she develops breasts but little or no pubic or underarm hair. However, she is apt to be completely feminine in her attitudes and identity.

Sometimes a female is born with genitals that seem sexually ambiguous. She may have an unusually large clitoris, almost like a tiny penis, or the labia majora may be partially fused together and look a bit like a male scrotum. The commonest cause for ambiguous genitals is congenital adrenal hyperplasia (see page 722), sometimes called pseudohermaphroditism. In such cases, the body does not produce enough of certain enzymes at a crucial time in fetal life. A female born with this condition is usually normal internally.

When a baby is born with ambiguous genitals, a specialist should be consulted immediately. The child will be "assigned" a sex, depending on the chromosomes and what the genitals and internal organs are like; early operation can then alter the genitals, if necessary. If the genital ambiguity is due to congenital adrenal hyperplasia, fetal shock (addisonian crisis) might develop unless the physician is on the alert to prevent it (see page 720).

The Diagnosis. The physician will do a physical examination and take a family history because developmental disorders often (but not always) run in families. Laboratory tests done on blood or skin cells can establish which chromosomes caused the condition, and this information can have a bearing on how the problem is treated. Laboratory tests also can identify abnormality of androgen receptors.

How Serious Are Developmental Disorders? Most girls who have mullerian agenesis are infertile, but some have a normal or near-normal uterus and ovaries and can conceive and give birth if a surgeon creates an artificial vagina. Girls with congenital adrenal hyperplasia actually have normal internal organs; if the abnormalities in the vulva are surgically corrected and they get proper medication, they, too, can have children. Girls with testicular feminization are invariably infertile, but they have a normal appearance except for female hair distribution.

Treatment. *Medication.* For congenital adrenal hyperplasia, physicians usually prescribe glucocorticoids (cortisone-related steroids) to allow breasts to develop and menstruation to occur. For testicular feminization, ordinarily the testes are removed because of the risk of malignancy, and estrogens are given at puberty to create and sustain secondary sex characteristics such as breasts.

Surgery. For girls born without a normal vagina, surgeons can create an artificial one. This is generally done if there is a chance that the girl can have children, but it also allows sexual activity. In cases of testicular feminization, the testes usually are removed because there is a risk that they will become cancerous.

VULVITIS

Signs and Symptoms
* Swelling of the vulva, with redness and itching;
* Blisters that may ooze or crust over;
* Skin of the vulva may thicken and turn whitish when the condition is chronic.

Vulvitis is an inflammation of the external genitalia, or vulva. (The Greek suffix *itis* means inflammation.) It can be caused by an allergic reaction to a vaginal spray, to the detergent with which you wash your underwear, or to a medication, or it could be simply from poor hygiene. The inflammation also may be caused by a bacterial, viral, or fungal infection (see page 846) or be cancer (page 1086).

The Diagnosis. Your physician will do a pelvic examination (see page 1055) and may also order blood tests, a urinalysis, and other laboratory tests. If a venereal disease could be involved, you may be tested for that. If the inflammation persists, you may need to have a biopsy to make sure there is no malignancy; this is apt to be an office procedure done with a local anesthetic. Except when it is caused by cancer, vulvitis is seldom serious.

Treatment. *Medication.* The medication used depends on what is causing the problem. Whatever the cause, a cortisone cream usually will relieve the itching.

Self-Help. Keep the area clean and dry; wear loose, absorbent clothing and cotton underpants. If the vulvitis consistently occurs after the use of a spray or deodorant, contact your physician. The cause of the vulvitis may be an allergy. Bear in mind that an allergic reaction usually takes several days to develop (see Skin Allergies, page 457).

ATROPHIC VULVAR DYSTROPHY

Signs and Symptoms
* Dry, itchy, reddened areas in the vulva;
* Later, these areas may turn white or develop blisters;
* Some areas turn white and thicken;
* Skin becomes papery or shiny; clitoris and vaginal opening may shrink.

Dystrophy is a kind of degeneration of tissue; the word is derived from the Greek words for bad *(dys)* and nourishment *(trophe)*. It is more likely to occur in women who are past menopause. The term lichen sclerosus et atrophicus is sometimes used for this condition. This term implies that the skin around the rectum, as well as the vulva, is involved. Malignancy may develop in the affected skin. Leukoplakia (whitish areas) may require biopsy.

The Diagnosis.   To make sure you do not have cancer, your physician may do a vulvar biopsy (cut out a small piece of tissue to be analyzed). For this procedure, your physician usually will use either a local or general anesthetic. During a physical examination, the physician also will check for signs of an underlying infection. A urinalysis, blood tests, and perhaps other laboratory tests probably will be done. Except when cancerous, vulvar dystrophy is not serious.

Treatment.   *Medication.*   Treatment depends on the source of the problem; however, a cortisone cream generally will relieve symptoms.

It is important to have periodic examinations to identify potentially malignant changes, if they should develop.

PRURITUS VULVAE

Signs and Symptoms

- Intense itching, burning, or irritation in the genital area.

Pruritus means itching (the Latin word for "to itch" is *prurire*). When the vulva itches, possible explanations include seborrheic dermatitis (see page 1157), an allergy (see page 457), an infection (see page 1177), or occasionally some systemic disease. Before puberty and after menopause, the vulva sometimes itches and is irritated for no discernible reason; the problem may be an inadequate amount of estrogen.

The Diagnosis.   Infections generally are identified by laboratory tests done on samples of vaginal discharge or vaginal tissue or by colposcopy (examination with an instrument that magnifies the surface of the vagina). The source of an allergy may be obvious; if not, tests can be done. Pruritus vulvae is not serious. However, if you develop patches of whitened skin in the vulva, see your physician.

Treatment.   *Self-Help.*   If the itching is not accompanied by discharge or other symptoms, you can wait a couple of weeks before calling a physician while you try to solve the problem yourself. Stop using feminine hygiene sprays or other products that could be irritating your vulva. Wear cotton underpants, avoid panty hose, and bathe the area once a day with unscented soap.

Medication.   A physician can prescribe a corticosteroid cream to help relieve the symptoms. Otherwise, medication depends on the underlying cause of the problem. If an infection called condyloma, caused by human papillomavirus, is identified, a minor operation may be needed.

Surgery.   If whitened skin (leukoplakia) develops in the vulva, your physician may suggest a minor surgical procedure to remove it. If an infection caused by the human papillomavirus is identified, removal with a laser procedure (see page 1095) may be indicated.

GENITAL WARTS

Signs and Symptoms

- Tiny pink or red swellings in the genital area that grow quickly;
- Several warts close together can take on a cauliflower shape.

Genital warts (also known as venereal warts or condyloma acuminata) are common. They are caused by the papillomavirus, and usually you get them from direct sexual contact with someone who has them. The incubation period is 1 to 6 months. These warts can grow on the vulva, the walls of the vagina, the cervix, or the perineum (the area between the external genitalia and anus). Because they thrive on moisture, they often appear with a disorder that produces a vaginal discharge or during pregnancy, when the vagina is unusually moist.

The Diagnosis.   Your physician usually can diagnose genital warts by their appearance. However, because other sexually transmitted infections, such as gonorrhea or syphilis (see page 875), also can occur as a result of the sexual exposure that caused the warts, you may need other tests to rule these out and perhaps a biopsy to rule out cancer (see page 1086).

How Serious Are Genital Warts?   By themselves, genital warts are mainly a nuisance because they have a tendency to recur. However, they also have been associated with cancer of the cervix and of the rectum. If you have had genital warts, be sure to have a Pap smear annually (see page 1096).

Treatment. *Medication.* If you have an ongoing infection, your physician will treat that because the warts may disappear when the infection does. Otherwise, the physician may paint the warts a few times with a chemical that often clears them up (do not use over-the-counter wart paints).

Surgery. If medication does not work or if the warts recur, your physician can try cryosurgery—freezing the wart with liquid nitrogen—which is quick and painless. Some physicians prefer to start with cryosurgery. Other possibilities are electrical cauterization and laser surgery (see page 1095). Your sexual partner also must be treated or you may become reinfected.

BARTHOLIN'S GLAND ABSCESS

Signs and Symptoms
- A hot, tender, swollen lump just inside the vagina.

Bartholin's glands—named for Danish anatomist Casper Bartholin—are located at the entrance to the vagina, one on each side. They can become infected, sometimes as a result of gonorrhea. At first, the infection may ooze pus, but if the opening to the gland becomes blocked, an abscess results.

The Diagnosis. Your physician will look for symptoms of a vaginal infection (see page 1087) and will have laboratory tests done.

How Serious Is Bartholin's Gland Abscess? The abscess itself generally responds to treatment, although sometimes a benign Bartholin's cyst forms afterward and may need to be removed surgically. Gonorrhea is dangerous and can leave you sterile unless it is treated.

Treatment. Your physician will prescribe antibiotics for the infection. If the abscess does not respond to antibiotics, the physician may lance and drain it.

SEBACEOUS CYSTS

Signs and Symptoms
- A soft, smooth lump in the skin of the vulva, sometimes with a tiny dark dot in the center.

Sebaceous glands, just beneath the surface of the skin, produce an oily substance that keeps skin supple. If the opening of a sebaceous gland is obstructed, a fluid-filled cyst may develop. Such cysts are painless and common, but they are prone to infection. An infected cyst may burst and drain, only to recur, because the sac of the cyst remains.

Physicians identify sebaceous cysts by the way they look. They are harmless and most people simply ignore them.

Treatment. If a cyst becomes infected, your physician can prescribe an antibiotic. A cyst that is bothersome can be removed surgically as an outpatient operation with a local anesthetic.

CANCER OF THE VULVA

Signs and Symptoms
- A small, hard, itchy lump in the skin of the vulva;
- Vulvar ulcer with raised edges; may bleed or seep fluid.

Cancer of the vulva is rare. It occasionally occurs in atrophic (vulvar) dystrophy (see page 1084). It accounts for just 3 to 4 percent of all tumors of the female reproductive organs. It is more common after menopause.

To diagnose a suspicious lump in the vulva, the physician removes a tiny piece of tissue for laboratory analysis. Cancer of the vulva generally grows very slowly, and early treatment means a complete cure.

Treatment. *Surgery.* Usually, a vulvectomy is necessary: the surgeon removes the tumor, surrounding skin, and perhaps lymph glands in the groin and the skin between the lymph glands and tumor. The type of cancer and size of the tumor determine how much tissue must be removed. Sometimes radiation therapy also is needed.

PUBIC LICE

Signs and Symptoms

- Grayish insects the size of a pinhead in pubic hair;
- Tiny white particles clinging to the hair (the eggs of the lice);
- Severe itching.

You can catch pubic lice by having intercourse with someone who has them or, rarely, from clothing or bedding. Sometimes the lice—which also may be found in hair on other parts of the body—produce no symptoms. Then again, you may have itching and a slight, bluish rash. Pubic lice often are called crabs because they hang on with crab-like claws. The problem is also known as pediculosis pubis (the Greek word for louse is *pediculus*).

Treatment. *Medication.* Your physician may suggest an over-the-counter medication such as RID (pyrethrins with piperonyl butoxide) or may prescribe lindane (Kwell; gamma benzene hexachloride). Lindane is more potent and sometimes causes allergic reactions. It should not be used by pregnant women or infants. These medications may have to be applied again a week later, and your sexual partner also will need to be treated. If you have crabs in your eyelashes or eyebrows, do not use RID or Kwell because they can damage your eyes; use an ophthalmic ointment (physostigmine) instead.

To keep from becoming reinfested, dry clean your clothing, sheets, blankets, and towels or wash them in very hot water. Wash enough for day-to-day living and set everything else aside for 2 weeks where it will not come into contact with human beings. This interval is time for the louse eggs to hatch and the lice to die of starvation. Treat infested mattresses the same way.

VAGINITIS

Signs and Symptoms

- Unusual discharge from the vagina;
- Itching, irritation;
- Pain during intercourse;
- Pain in the lower abdomen;
- Vaginal bleeding.

If you have some of the symptoms listed above, you may have a vaginal infection (vaginitis), which is common and treatable, or a sexually transmitted disease, which is more serious but is also treatable. It is possible to have either disorder and have no symptoms. Sexually transmitted diseases are discussed on pages 162 and 875.

Vaginitis is an inflammation of the vagina, usually caused by an infection. A vaginal infection can be sexually transmitted, but you may catch it in other ways. However, as with a sexually transmitted disease, you should tell your sexual partner that you have an infection and that he may need treatment. Do not have intercourse until your symptoms have disappeared.

There are three common kinds of vaginitis: trichomoniasis, yeast infections, and nonspecific vaginitis.

Trichomoniasis. This is caused by a parasite. You may have no symptom at all, or you may develop a smelly, greenish yellow, sometimes frothy, discharge. Trichomoniasis is most often acquired through intercourse, but you can also pick it up from toilet seats or from a damp towel or bathing suit used by someone who has the infection.

Yeast Infections. A fungus causes yeast infections. The main symptom is itchiness, but you also may have a white discharge that resembles cottage cheese. You are more likely to develop a yeast infection if you are pregnant or diabetic, if you are taking antibiotics, corticosteroid medications, or the pill, or if you have an iron deficiency.

Nonspecific Vaginitis. This type is now more often called bacterial vaginosis. It is thought to be caused by several different organisms, including *Gardnerella vaginalis*. Many women have no symptoms at all, but others develop a white or grayish, fishy-smelling discharge that coats the vaginal walls.

The Diagnosis. Your physician makes a diagnosis by taking a history, doing a pelvic examination (see page 1055), and identifying the organisms responsible through laboratory analysis of samples of discharge or tissue scrapings. Sometimes blood tests are also helpful.

How Serious Is Vaginitis?   Vaginitis is common and, because it tends to recur, annoying.

Treatment.   *Medication.*   Trichomonal vaginitis usually is treated with metronidazole tablets, and yeast infections are treated with miconazole or clotrimazole, often as suppositories. For nonspecific vaginitis (bacterial vaginosis), metronidazole, ampicillin, or doxycycline may be prescribed.

NONSPECIFIC URETHRITIS

Signs and Symptoms
* Frequent urination accompanied by a stinging or burning sensation;
* Lower abdominal pain;
* Occasional thin vaginal discharge.

Nonspecific urethritis is an inflammation of the urethra (see page 891) that is sometimes caused by *Chlamydia.* It also may be caused by a bacteria called *Ureaplasma urealyticum.* The symptoms occur within 10 to 20 days after exposure. However, most women have no symptoms at all, and if the disease is untreated, complications such as pelvic inflammatory disease (an infection of the fallopian tubes, ovaries, uterus, or cervix) can develop later. Men are more likely to have symptoms. Therefore, if your sex partner develops urethritis you should be checked; his infection could be due to *Ureaplasma, Chlamydia,* or some other sexually transmitted disease.

The Diagnosis.   Your physician makes a diagnosis by taking a history and doing a pelvic examination (see page 1055) to rule out any other contributing cause and then identifies the responsible organisms through a urine culture.

How Serious Is Nonspecific Urethritis? Generally, this disease is more annoying than serious, particularly if it is recognized and treated early.

Treatment.   Antibiotics are the standard treatment for nonspecific urethritis.

ATROPHIC VAGINITIS

Signs and Symptoms
* Soreness, burning, or itching in the vagina;
* Slight bleeding after intercourse;
* Painful intercourse.

Atrophic vaginitis is an inflammation of the vagina caused by degeneration of the vaginal tissue. (Atrophic combines the Greek word *trophe,* for nourishment, with the negative prefix *a.*) The problem is most likely to develop after menopause, although it can occur during breastfeeding. In both situations, your estrogen production decreases, and the walls of the vagina may become drier, thinner, and less elastic and may bleed easily.

A pelvic examination (see page 1055) may be all that is necessary to diagnose the problem, although your physician may order laboratory tests if a vaginal infection is

---

VAGINAL PAIN

When vaginal pain occurs during intercourse, it is called dyspareunia (from the Greek prefix *dys,* meaning something bad or difficult, and *pareunos,* meaning lying beside). It is often caused by a vaginal infection (see page 1087) or by herpes. The symptoms are vaginal soreness or persistent or recurrent pain during intercourse. Sometimes the vagina is simply irritated by a douche, feminine hygiene spray, or contraceptive cream or jelly.

Dyspareunia also can result from bladder problems such as cystitis or urethritis (see pages 892 and 891). If intercourse causes deep internal pain, you may have endometriosis (see page 1101) or tears in the ligaments that support your uterus (see Loss of Pelvic Support, page 1090), or you could have some other disorder of the cervix, uterus, fallopian tubes, or ovaries.

If you are breast-feeding or are past menopause, the vaginal tissues may have thinned because you are producing less estrogen (see page 1068). If you recently had a baby, the vagina may have been scarred by an episiotomy (see page 212). Sometimes a woman is tense during intercourse and her vagina does not become sufficiently lubricated. Some women also have a problem called vaginismus—involuntary contractions of muscles at the opening to the vagina. Vaginal cancer is very rare, but it, too, could be the source of the pain (see page 1091).

To determine the causes of vaginal pain, your physician will do a pelvic examination (see page 1055) and may order blood tests, a urinalysis, or other laboratory tests. Treatment depends on what is causing the pain.

suspected. Atrophic vaginitis is likely to be little more than a discomfort, but it can interfere with your sex life.

Treatment. *Medication.* In breast-feeding women, the problem is temporary. If you have passed menopause, your physician may recommend estrogen replacement therapy (see page 1069); or you can apply estrogen directly to the vagina as a cream or suppository. These are not cures but provide a kind of daily maintenance.

If the primary problem is painful intercourse, use of a water-soluble lubricant may help. Regular sexual activity actually improves circulation in the vagina and helps keep the tissues supple.

POSTMENOPAUSAL VAGINITIS

Signs and Symptoms
- Vaginal soreness, burning, or itching after menopause;
- Unusual, thin, watery vaginal discharge;
- Painful intercourse;
- Swelling or redness of the vulva.

Because your overall estrogen level is decreased after menopause, vaginal tissue becomes more fragile. You may develop tiny sores or cracks. These can produce the symptoms listed above and make you more vulnerable to vaginal infections (see page 1087). To reach a diagnosis, your physician will take a history and do a pelvic examination (see page 1055). The physician also may send samples of the discharge to a laboratory to be analyzed.

Treatment. *Medication.* If you have developed an infection, your physician will probably prescribe antibiotics. Estrogens applied to the vagina (diethylstilbestrol cream or suppositories, for example) may thicken and help lubricate the tissue. However, they also can cause renewed bleeding from your uterus.

VAGINAL CYSTS

Signs and Symptoms
- Small swellings in the walls of the vagina;
- A lump that bulges out of the vaginal opening.

VAGINAL HYGIENE

Washing your genitals once a day with a mild soap and water is sufficient. In a normal woman, douches and feminine hygiene sprays are unnecessary, and at times they can be harmful.

Normally, the vagina is self-cleansing. The vaginal walls produce their own fluid, and it carries dead cells and other organisms away with it as it flows downward. This healthy discharge is either clear or milky, although it is yellowish when it dries. It is somewhat slippery and has a mild, not unpleasant odor. It increases in amount at about the time of ovulation and during sexual arousal. If you have a copious vaginal discharge that is a different color or that has a strong smell, you probably have a vaginal infection (see page 1087) and should see a physician.

If you use a vaginal hygiene spray, never spray it directly into the vagina because it can irritate vaginal tissues. If you have been using a spray and the skin of your vulva becomes red and irritated, stop using the spray—you may be allergic to chemicals in the spray.

Some commercial douches also contain irritating chemicals. In addition, they can change the normal acidic vaginal environment, a condition that discourages the growth of yeasts and other organisms that can cause infections. In fact, dilute vinegar douches may be prescribed to help maintain normal acidity as well as for their cleaning action. Douching also can wash away the plug of mucus that normally covers the cervix and prevents infectious organisms from getting into the uterus.

Despite all these negative effects, there *are* some problems for which your physician may advise douching. If so, be sure to hang the douche bag no more than 2 feet above your hips to reduce the fluid pressure; otherwise, vaginal organisms may be forced up into your uterus, where they can cause an infection.

The bacteria and yeasts that cause vaginal infections tend to thrive in hot, moist conditions. For that reason, it is a good idea to wear cotton underpants or synthetic underpants with a cotton crotch and to avoid tight panty hose. Tight, nylon underpants and hose trap heat and moisture in the genital area. One last point: always wipe your anus from front to back to avoid contaminating the vagina with bacteria from a bowel movement.

Several types of benign cysts can develop in the vagina. The most common are inclusion cysts and Gartner duct cysts. Inclusion cysts are caused by trauma—after operation or childbirth, for example, the vaginal walls may not heal to perfect smoothness. Gartner duct cysts are vestiges of a duct that serves a purpose before birth and then disappears.

Sometimes, a Gartner cyst enlarges enough to poke through the vaginal opening.

If a physician has reason to suspect cancer, the cyst may be biopsied. However, most cysts are identifiable during a pelvic examination.

Treatment. *Surgery.* You may elect to ignore a vaginal cyst. If it causes discomfort, however, a cyst can be removed surgically. If it is small enough, it can be removed in a physician's office with local anesthesia.

LOSS OF PELVIC SUPPORT

Signs and Symptoms
- A bulge in the walls of the vagina;
- A feeling of fullness and discomfort when you bear down internally, sometimes with backache;
- Stress incontinence (when you laugh or cough, you leak a little urine);
- Difficulty in passing urine or defecating;
- A sensation of bearing down or of pelvic pressure when lifting or when you are on your feet for a long time.

The organs that fill the lower abdomen—such as the bladder, uterus, and small intestine—are supported by the pelvic floor, a sheet of muscles and ligaments. These muscles also help close off the urethra where it leaves the bladder. They can become stretched or slack as a result of childbirth or aging or because of a hereditary weakness. When that happens, some of your internal organs may prolapse—that is, they may sink lower in your body. As a result, you may have any of the symptoms listed above or none at all. Prolapse is more likely to happen to elderly women and to those who have given birth to several children.

Sometimes the uterus droops downward into the vagina. In extreme cases, the cervix may actually protrude from the vaginal opening. When either the bladder or the urethra prolapse, they produce a bulge in the front wall of the vagina. A bulge in the back wall may mean that either the small intestine or the lower rectum has prolapsed. When that happens, bowel movements may become difficult.

The Diagnosis. The telltale bulges in the vaginal wall usually make prolapses easy to diagnose during a pelvic examination (see page 1055). However, your physician may want to analyze a urine specimen just to be sure you do not have a urinary tract infection (see page 1108), which could be aggravating your symptoms.

How Serious Is Loss of Pelvic Support?
Minor prolapses are common, especially in elderly women. As long as yours is minor and you are not feeling too uncomfortable, there is no rush to treat the problem. Exer-

If muscles that form the pelvic floor weaken, the uterus may sink lower (prolapse) into the vagina (see arrow).

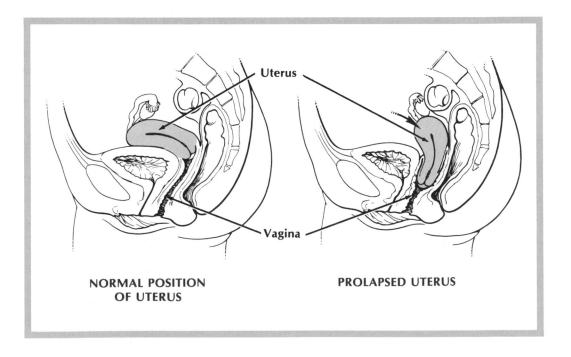

NORMAL POSITION
OF UTERUS

PROLAPSED UTERUS

cise and diet may resolve it. However, when the bladder or urethra slips, sometimes urine is trapped in the bladder for long periods, and a breeding ground for bacteria is created. Thus, you may have repeated urinary tract infections, and a surgical repair may be the best solution. A prolapsed lower rectum does not generally require operation unless the bulge is large.

Treatment. *Self-Help.* Simple exercises (called Kegel exercises) are sometimes the only treatment that is necessary (see Exercises for Incontinence, this page). Other possible remedies include going on a diet if you are overweight and eating high-fiber foods (they will help you move your bowels without straining).

If these measures are not enough, your physician can fit you with a vaginal pessary, a rubber device that fits around the cervix and helps to prop up prolapsed organs. You will have to remove it regularly to clean it.

Surgery. If an operation is necessary, you can have a procedure called a vaginal repair. The surgeon elevates the prolapsed organ, or organs, back into place and tightens the muscles and ligaments of the pelvic floor. For a symptomatic prolapsed uterus, sometimes a vaginal hysterectomy (see page 1100) is done at the same time, although that should be a last resort.

VAGINAL TUMORS

Signs and Symptoms
- Watery discharge from the vagina;
- Bleeding after intercourse or a pelvic examination;
- Pain during intercourse;
- A frequent or urgent need to urinate or painful bowel movements.

Vaginal tumors are extremely rare. Of all the different types of cancer that can develop in a woman's reproductive organs, only about 1 percent are cancers of the vagina. They are most likely to occur between the ages of 45 and 65 years, and 95 percent of them are slow-growing squamous cell tumors. They often extend to the bladder or rectum, causing painful defecation or a frequent, urgent need to urinate.

In recent years, a different type of vaginal

EXERCISES FOR INCONTINENCE

If you urinate involuntarily at times (stress incontinence), the muscles of your pelvic floor may have become weakened as you grew older. By investing 20 minutes a day in simple exercises that can be done anywhere, you may be able to regain bladder control.

The muscles that control the bladder are those surrounding the anus and vagina; they are called the pubococcygeal muscles. In the 1950s, Dr. A.M. Kegel developed an exercise regimen to strengthen them.

Begin by contracting your anal sphincter, as you would to prevent a bowel movement. Relax, and then repeat the contraction. Do this 20 or 30 times. Repeat the whole set of contractions several times over the course of the day. As the tone in your pubococcygeal muscles gradually improves, you should have better bladder control; as a bonus, many women find that they also are more sexually responsive.

---

tumor, called clear cell adenocarcinoma, has been diagnosed in very young women born to mothers who took diethylstilbestrol (DES) during pregnancy. Beginning in the 1940s, DES, a synthetic estrogen, often was prescribed for women who seemed in danger of miscarrying. By 1971, it had become clear that DES produced a birth defect in which a type of glandular tissue normally found in the cervical canal was incorporated into the vaginal walls. The condition is called vaginal adenosis, and many so-called DES daughters have it. It does not need treatment, but it must be watched because it can lead to clear cell adenocarcinoma. The worst-case estimate is that 1 in 700 DES daughters will get this cancer; some experts predict it will be only 1 in 7,000. The peak years for vulnerability are between the ages of 15 and 22 years. DES daughters also may have a higher than normal chance of developing cervical cancer (see page 1095).

If you are a DES daughter, contact a gynecologist, both because of the risk of vaginal cancer and because DES can cause other, less serious problems. You should see your gynecologist as soon as you begin menstruating or, at any rate, by age 14 whether or not you are menstruating. Afterward, you should have regular checkups. Clear cell adenocarcinomas are fast-growing and in the early stages sometimes produce no symptoms. However, with regular checkups, your physician can spot the problem early, and it can be treated.

The Diagnosis. Sometimes a Pap test (see page 1096) is the first clue to the existence of a vaginal cancer: its results are positive because the specimen contains cancerous cells from the vagina, not from the cervix. When a vaginal tumor is in such an early stage that the physician cannot see or feel it, Schiller's test can be performed. For this test, the cervix and walls of the vagina are painted with an iodine solution; normal tissue stains dark brown, but malignant cells do not stain. Because adenosis tissue and some other benign conditions also fail to stain, Schiller's is not a definitive test for cancer, but it does show the physician which area to biopsy. Colposcopy also may be performed to identify the source of abnormal cells (see page 1296).

For a DES daughter, pelvic examinations may include a careful inspection of the cervix and the vagina, a Pap smear not only of the cervix but of the vaginal walls, and Schiller's test.

How Serious Are Vaginal Tumors? They are rare but can be deadly: overall, the 5-year survival rate without recurrence is about 30 percent. The statistics are somewhat more encouraging for clear cell adenocarcinoma: the survival rate is 80 to 85 percent.

Treatment. *Surgery.* The extent of the operation depends on where the tumor is located, how far it extends, and your age and condition. If the malignancy is localized and in the upper third of the vagina, the surgeon probably will remove the uterus and that part of the vagina and also some pelvic lymph nodes to find out whether the cancer has spread via the lymph system, or you might have less extensive operation with radiation therapy afterward. Plastic surgery can often reconstruct the missing section of the vagina.

CERVIX, UTERUS, AND FALLOPIAN TUBE DISORDERS

Your uterus, or womb, is the organ that shelters the fetus when you are pregnant. It is hollow and, except during pregnancy, about 2.5 inches long. Powerful muscles, buried in the thick walls of the uterus, contract during childbirth in order to expel the baby. The uterus is shaped like an upside-down pear. The narrower end, the cervix, extends down into the vagina, and the cervix, too, has thick walls. Its opening is ordinarily very tiny.

Two thin tubes, called the fallopian tubes, are connected to the uterus, one on each side of its broad top. Each tube is about 4 inches long and about the thickness of a lead pencil, with an inner channel that is needle-thin. Each tube extends from the interior of the uterus to a place close to the ovary. Once a month, one of the ovaries releases an egg which travels down the fallopian tube to the uterus.

DEVELOPMENTAL DISORDERS

Signs and Symptoms
• Failure to begin menstruating at puberty;
• Inability to conceive or carry a pregnancy to term.

Because of genetic problems or because something goes wrong during prenatal life, some women are born with abnormalities of the cervix, uterus, or fallopian tubes. These can range from an almost total absence of female reproductive organs (see page 1083) to minor discrepancies that nevertheless make it difficult to conceive or carry a pregnancy to term.

Some women born to mothers who took a synthetic estrogen called diethylstilbestrol (DES) during their pregnancies have an abnormal cervix or a uterus that is T-shaped rather than the usual pear shape. During pregnancy, the cervix may be too weak to support the fetus, or the uterus may not expand enough. DES daughters are more likely to miscarry than most women. Although these congenital abnormalities are not life-threatening, they are distressing to women who want children.

The Diagnosis. If a physician suspects a developmental disorder in the uterus or fallopian tubes, he or she may order a type of x-ray called a hysterosalpingogram (also known as a uterotubogram). Because soft tissues cannot be seen on an x-ray, this procedure uses a special dye that does register on the film. The dye is injected into the uterus and travels up the fallopian tubes and into the abdominal cavity where it is absorbed by the body. While the dye is spreading, a radiologist takes a series of x-rays. The procedure can be somewhat uncomfortable, especially if pressure is used to force the dye through the tubes; you may be given a local anesthetic, injected into the cervix, or an oral medication to help you relax. A hysterosalpingogram is usually made during the first half of the menstrual cycle, before ovulation, to avoid any risk that a fertilized egg might be exposed to radiation, which could lead to birth defects.

Two other procedures allow a physician to look directly at the ovaries, fallopian tubes, and the outside of the uterus. For culdoscopy, which is rarely done now, a small incision is made in the back wall of the vagina and an instrument with a built-in light is inserted through the incision. For laparoscopy (see page 1297), a similar instrument is inserted through an incision made near the navel. Both procedures are done under general or spinal anesthesia in a hospital.

Treatment. *Surgery.* Surgeons sometimes can correct a cervix that is unable to sustain a pregnancy to term and fix certain structural problems of the uterus. However, infertility specialists usually try to rule out every other possible cause before they consider operation, even if the uterus does not look completely normal.

CERVICAL EROSION

Signs and Symptoms
• Reddish patch on cervix, visible during pelvic examination;
• Occasionally, whitish or slightly bloody vaginal discharge;
• Bleeding with or after intercourse.

If you develop a reddish patch on your cervix, it could be cervical erosion, a condition that occurs when the cervix has been scraped, perhaps by an intrauterine device or during intercourse. A related disorder, cervical eversion (also called cervical ectopy) looks very similar, but it develops because a type of cell that normally lines the cervical canal is growing on the outside of the cervix. Cervical eversion is normal dur-

ing the early teens, and it often occurs during pregnancy and in women who are taking the pill; the reason is unclear. Many women with erosion or eversion have no symptoms. Some medical researchers think these disorders can lead to cancer; most disagree. There is evidence, however, that they may make you more susceptible to infection.

The Diagnosis. Your physician's chief concern will be to rule out more serious problems. Thus, a Pap smear (see page 1096) will be used to check for cancerous cells, and samples of discharge or tissue scrapings may be sent to a laboratory to check for infection (see page 1095). Colposcopy may be performed (see page 1094).

Treatment. *Surgery.* As a precaution, your physician may recommend cauterizing the cervix with heat or cryosurgery (application of extreme cold) to facilitate healing of the eroded area.

CERVICAL POLYPS

Signs and Symptoms
• Bleeding after intercourse, between periods, or after menopause;
• Unusually heavy periods;
• Heavy, watery, bloody discharge from the vagina;
• Crampy pelvic pain.

If you have these symptoms, see a physician immediately because they could be due either to harmless cervical polyps or to cervical cancer (see page 1095). Polyps sometimes cause no symptoms at all and may be found during a routine pelvic examination.

Cervical polyps are growths, rather like grapes, that generally protrude from the mouth of the cervix. You may have a single polyp or a cluster. They are common and often occur during pregnancy because of hormonal changes. They also may appear after the cervix has been injured.

They are rarely cancerous, and a small one may not even produce symptoms. However, large polyps can cause bleeding or make it difficult for you to become pregnant, so you may want to have them removed.

The Diagnosis. Because polyps are very occasionally malignant, your physician will probably do a Pap test (see page 1096) and perhaps a biopsy (see page 1094) in which a sample of tissue is removed for laboratory analysis.

Treatment. *Surgery.* A single polyp can be removed in a brief office procedure with local anesthesia. If you have many large polyps, you may have to be hospitalized for the operation. If the polyps recur—which rarely happens—you may need dilation and curettage (see page 1066) to remove them permanently; in this minor surgical procedure, the surgeon gently scrapes the lining of the uterus.

CERVICITIS

Signs and Symptoms
- Vaginal discharge that is clear, grayish, or yellow;
- Pain during intercourse;
- Frequent, urgent need to urinate; painful urination;
- Burning or itching in the genital area;
- Bleeding after intercourse.

Cervicitis is an inflammation of the cervix (the Greek suffix *itis* means inflammation). It can be caused by a local infection, especially if the cervix is damaged during childbirth. However, cervicitis is also a symptom of vaginal infections, of various sexually transmitted diseases (see page 875), and of pelvic inflammatory disease (see page 1104).

The Diagnosis. During a pelvic examination (see page 1055), the physician swabs the cervix to get a tissue sample; this sample is sent to a laboratory to identify the organism responsible. Your physician also may do a Pap test (see page 1096) to rule out cervical cancer. On occasion, colposcopy (see this page) is performed.

Treatment. Your physician will prescribe the antibiotic or sulfa drug that is most effective against the organisms involved. In severe cases, the cervix sometimes is cauterized with cryosurgery (application of extreme cold) or with an electrically heated instrument in an office procedure.

NABOTHIAN CYST

Signs and Symptoms
- A fluid-filled lump on the cervix, noted during a pelvic examination.

A nabothian cyst (named for Martin Naboth, a German anatomist) occurs when a mucus gland on the cervix is obstructed, either because new tissue grows over it, usually after childbirth, or—in an elderly woman—because thinning cervical tissue has trapped natural secretions.

It is diagnosed generally by inspection during a pelvic examination (see page 1055). A nabothian cyst rarely requires treatment.

Treatment. *Surgery.* If necessary, the cyst can be removed by cauterizing it or through cryosurgery (application of extreme cold). This is an office procedure and seldom requires even local anesthesia.

CERVICAL DYSPLASIA

Signs and Symptoms
- Abnormal cervical cells found as a result of a Pap smear.

Sometimes a Pap test (see page 1096) shows a type of cell that is considered to be precancerous. The condition is called dysplasia (*dys* is the Greek prefix meaning bad, and *plasis* means molding). Mild dysplasia often disappears of its own accord. However, if it does not, it can be the first step in a process that will lead to cancer some years later.

Dysplasia is found most often in women between the ages of 25 and 35 years, but it can occur at any age from the teen years on. It has been linked to sexually transmitted diseases caused by viruses, and it is more apt to occur in women who have many sex partners or who began to have intercourse before they were 18 years old.

The Diagnosis. If your Pap smear reveals dysplasia, your physician may want to have a second smear done. When abnormal cells are found, you will need to have a colposcopy and biopsy. This is generally done in the physician's office. A colposcope is an instrument equipped with a magnifying lens and a light. The physician uses it to examine the cervix while doing a biopsy—removing a bit of the cervix to send for laboratory analysis. You may or may not need a local anesthetic for this. If the biopsy result is negative, you will be asked to come back for another Pap test in 4 to 6 months.

How Serious Is Cervical Dysplasia? It may simply disappear. If it does not, it can be treated successfully.

Treatment.   *Surgery.*   Mild forms of dysplasia usually are treated by cauterization, cryosurgery, or laser surgery.

Cauterization destroys the abnormal tissue with heat, electricity, or chemicals. It can be done in a physician's office or in a hospital on an outpatient basis. Usually, no anesthesia is necessary. Cautery occasionally causes scarring that makes Pap smears difficult to interpret afterward.

In cryosurgery, the tissue is destroyed by application of extreme cold in the form of liquid nitrogen. The procedure can be done in the physician's office.

For laser surgery, a high-energy beam of light is used to burn away the dysplasia. There is little or no damage to surrounding tissue, and the area heals quickly. This is usually an outpatient hospital or office procedure.

For advanced dysplasia, sometimes a cone biopsy is done: a cone-shaped slice of the cervix is removed and analyzed. This is a major surgical procedure that is done with general anesthesia in a hospital. You will have to rest at home for a few days afterward. If the analysis shows that the surgeon excised all the abnormal tissue, no further treatment may be required. Conization can sometimes make it difficult for a woman to become pregnant because it decreases cervical mucus, and in rare cases it leaves her with a tendency to miscarry. If you become pregnant and you have had a cone biopsy, tell your physician about it.

After being treated for dysplasia, your doctor may recommend a Pap smear twice a year for the next 2 years and once a year after that to make sure there is no recurrence. For severe dysplasia or actual surface cancer, the usual treatment is a hysterectomy (see page 1100).

CANCER OF THE CERVIX

Signs and Symptoms
- Bleeding from the vagina after intercourse, between periods, or after menopause;
- Watery, bloody discharge from the vagina; it may be heavy and smelly;
- In later stages, a dull backache and general poor health.

Cervical cancer is one of the more common cancers that affect the female reproductive organs. It is most likely to occur between the ages of 30 and 55 years. Fortunately, it is slow-growing and almost 100 percent curable when it is caught at the precancerous stage, called cervical dysplasia (see page 1094), or while it is still carcinoma in situ—meaning that it is located on the surface of the cervix in the top layers of cervical tissue.

You are more likely than most women to develop cervical cancer if you have had a sexually transmitted viral infection, such as genital warts or herpes; if you began having sex before you were 18 years old; if you have had many sex partners; or if you have had many pregnancies, starting at a young age.

The Diagnosis.   Your physician will do a Pap test (see page 1096) and probably a colposcopy and biopsy (see pages 1094 and 1095). A colposcope is an instrument with a magnifying lens that permits a close look at the cervix. For a biopsy, the physician removes a fragment of tissue from the cervix for a laboratory analysis; this is the only way to determine whether tissue is malignant.

If the biopsy shows that you do have cancer, the physician may do a conization and a dilation and curettage, gently scraping the uterine lining for tissue samples (see page 1066) to find out whether the cancer has spread to the uterus. Then he or she will determine the stage of the disease on the basis of the extent of the tumor. This "staging" of the cancer is the key to determining how extensive the treatment must be. Treatment can be much more conservative for carcinoma in situ (cancer located on the surface) than for an invasive malignancy that extends deep into cervical tissue or has spread to other organs.

How Serious Is Cancer of the Cervix?

Almost every woman treated when the cancer is in an early stage is cured. Cervical cancer is less deadly than most malignancies as long as it has not spread beyond the uterus. Even then, invasive cancer of the cervix is the cause of death in only 3 percent of American women who die of cancer.

Treatment. *Surgery.* Carcinoma in situ (surface cancer) can be destroyed by laser surgery, freezing, or cauterization. A cone

biopsy is another possibility: the surgeon removes a cone-shaped piece of the cervix for analysis. If all the border areas have normal cells, the physician can assume that the biopsy removed all the cancerous tissue, although sometimes radiation therapy is advised afterward as a precaution. If the borders of the cone contain cancer cells, a second conization may be necessary, or perhaps a hysterectomy. A cone biopsy is a major operation done in a hospital with general anesthesia. The 5-year cure rate for can-

---

THE PAP SMEAR

Since the early 1940s, the death rate of women with cervical cancer has decreased by 70 percent, largely because so many women have been screened by the Pap smear. Although it is not infallible, this test detects 95 percent of cervical cancers and—what is more important—detects them at a stage when they cannot yet be seen with the naked eye but can be treated and almost invariably

cured. Occasionally, the Pap smear will identify an endometrial or ovarian cancer.

The Pap smear, which is named for G.N. Papanicolaou, its developer, is done during a pelvic examination (see page 1055). At most, it causes slight discomfort. Using a wooden spatula, brush, or cotton swab, your physician gently scrapes the entire surface of the cervix to gather cells and also takes a cell sample from inside the cervical canal by inserting a cotton swab. The cells are sent to a laboratory for microscopic analysis.

A negative result means that your cervix is normal; a positive result indicates some abnormal cells. A positive result does not prove that you have cancer or even dysplasia (see page 1094), a precancerous condition, but it usually does mean you should have further evaluation, such as colposcopic examination and biopsy.

You should have your first Pap smear soon after you start having intercourse, and a year later you should have a second one. If both have normal results, you can have Pap smears done thereafter at intervals agreed on by you and your physician, unless you are in a high-risk group, in which case you should be tested once a year. Women most at risk are those who began having intercourse before they were 18 years, who have had many sex partners, who have had herpes or venereal warts, or who have had multiple sex partners. You can stop having Pap smears once you are older than 60 years and have had two normal smears since your 60th birthday.

If your mother took a synthetic estrogen called DES while she was pregnant with you, you are in a high-risk category. You should have a Pap smear done at least once a year, beginning at age 14 years, or earlier if you began menstruating earlier.

Uterus

Vagina

Cervix

The Pap smear is a simple procedure. With a speculum in place (1) a cell sample is obtained. The sample is removed by use of a cotton-tipped swab or by using a tiny wooden spatula (2). The sample then is smeared onto a glass slide (3) for examination under a microscope.

cer in situ (surface cancer) is almost 100 percent. For cancer that involves more tissue than cancer in situ but has not spread beyond the cervix, the 5-year cure rate is 90 percent.

For an invasive cancer that involves a large part of the cervix and extends into the uterus, a radical hysterectomy generally is done: the surgeon removes your uterus (including the cervix), upper vagina, some surrounding tissue and lymph nodes, and the fallopian tubes, but one or both ovaries may be left in place in a young woman. You may have radiation therapy afterward. If a biopsy of the nodes indicates that the cancer has already spread through your system, you also may have chemotherapy.

Radiation. For cervical cancer, the cure rates for operation and radiation are nearly identical: among women with localized cancer (confined to the cervix) treated with radiation, 75 to 90 percent survive for at least 5 years; among those with cancer that has spread beyond the cervix, the 5-year survival rate is about 45 to 55 percent. Radiation treatments often involve both radiation delivered by a machine and internal radiation from radioactive material implanted in the uterus or in the upper part of the vagina and left there for several days while you remain in the hospital. The implanting is done under general anesthesia.

Radiation has some distressing side effects, although not everyone experiences them. They can include diarrhea, rectal bleeding, and fatigue. For a few months afterward, you may have trouble retaining urine. If you did not have a hysterectomy, the radiation treatments probably will disrupt your menstrual cycle and they may give you symptoms of menopause, such as hot flashes, if you have not yet passed menopause. Radiation therapy also can cause some narrowing and shortening of the vagina. However, use of a lubricating jelly just before having intercourse generally solves the problem.

You will need regular checkups and tests for at least 5 years after treatment for cervical cancer.

FIBROIDS

Signs and Symptoms
• Heavy or prolonged menstrual periods;

• Pain or pressure in lower abdomen or lower back.

Emergency Symptoms
• Sudden, sharp pain low in the abdomen.

A fibroid is a benign tumor that develops within the uterine wall or is attached to it. Although you may have a single fibroid, you are more likely to have several of them. They can be as small as a pea or as large as a grapefruit. Most women who have them have no symptoms. (Fibroids also are called leiomyomas, myomas, or fibromyomas.)

Normally, fibroids grow slowly. However, they respond to increased levels of estrogen and so may expand rapidly during pregnancy or if you take oral contraceptives or estrogen replacement therapy. After menopause, these tumors usually shrink and often disappear completely as long as you are not taking estrogen replacement therapy.

Fibroids are rarely malignant, and most cause few problems. They also are extremely common: about 20 percent of women older than 35 years have them. Nevertheless, if you have fibroids, have regular checkups to make sure they do not grow too large. If your periods become very heavy, you could develop iron-deficiency anemia. Fibroids can make conception difficult, and if you are pregnant, they could cause a miscarriage or interfere with delivery. Sometimes, a fibroid attached to the uterine wall becomes twisted and starved for blood and oxygen. If that happens, you may suddenly feel a sharp pain low in your abdomen, and you will need an emergency operation to remove the tumor.

The Diagnosis. Fibroids usually are identified because the physician can feel them during a pelvic examination (see page 1055). If there is any question about what they are, your physician will order CT or ultrasonography (see page 1287) or do a dilation and curettage (see page 1066), a minor surgical procedure in which tissue is scraped from the lining of the uterus.

Treatment. If you have no symptoms, treatment may be unnecessary. If you have symptoms and are not planning to have children, your physician probably will recommend a hysterectomy (see page 1100)— removal of the uterus. As an alternative, a surgeon can simply remove the fibroids. However, this procedure, called a myomectomy, is also a major operation and has a higher rate of complications than a hysterectomy. In about 10 percent of cases, the fibroids return.

RETROVERSION OF THE UTERUS

Signs and Symptoms
• Occasional backaches during menstruation.

In most women, the uterus is tipped forward, its closed end higher than the cervix and closer to the front of the body. About one woman in five has a tipped (retroverted) uterus—it tilts backward and down. Most affected women have no symptoms and no problems. However, a tipped uterus can cause occasional backaches, especially during menstruation. In very rare cases, intercourse is painful when the penis penetrates deeply.

A physician can tell during a pelvic examination (see page 1055) whether your uterus is tipped. Retroversion of the uterus is not a disease, and treatment is rarely necessary. If you have retroversion of the uterus and you become pregnant, the uterus generally will right itself. The condition does not interfere with a normal delivery.

Unfortunately, pregnancy is no cure. The uterus generally returns to its original position after a term pregnancy.

Treatment.   Surgery. If intercourse is painful, your physician can fit you with a pessary, a rubber cap that covers the cervix and props up the uterus. If that does not eliminate the pain, the physician may suggest a ventro-suspension, an operation that will fasten the uterus permanently in its new position.

ENDOMETRIAL POLYPS

Signs and Symptoms
• Spotting between menstrual periods, especially after intercourse or douching;
• Pelvic cramps;
• Heavy or prolonged periods.

Endometrial polyps are small, soft growths in the lining of the uterus (the endo-

metrium). They are almost never malignant, and they occur most often at about the time of menopause. You may have one or a cluster of them.

Usually, endometrial polyps will have no symptoms. However, sometimes polyps protrude into the vagina, causing cramps as they expand the opening of the cervix. If protruding polyps become twisted and lose their blood supply, they can become infected. Polyps often occur together with endometrial hyperplasia (see page 1098) or solid growths called fibroids (see page 1097).

Protruding polyps are visible during a pelvic examination (see page 1055). When you have polyps that do not protrude and do produce symptoms, your physician will generally do a dilation and curettage (see page 1066), a minor operation in which the lining of the uterus is scraped. This procedure may diagnose and cure the problem simultaneously. Endometrial polyps are almost always harmless.

Treatment.   Surgery. Polyps can be removed during dilation and curettage, which is usually done in a hospital on an outpatient basis with local anesthesia. Once removed, they are analyzed to be sure they are not malignant. On occasion, they may recur.

ENDOMETRIAL HYPERPLASIA

Signs and Symptoms
• Bleeding between menstrual periods;
• Heavy or prolonged menstrual periods.

Endometrial hyperplasia occurs when the uterine lining—the endometrium—grows too thick. Teenagers and women approaching menopause are most apt to have this problem.

It is easy to treat, but it must be distinguished from a precancerous condition called adenomatous hyperplasia.

The Diagnosis. If your physician suspects endometrial hyperplasia, an endometrial biopsy will be done, in which a small sample of the endometrium is removed for laboratory analysis. This office procedure is somewhat uncomfortable.

Treatment. If you are young, taking birth control pills for a few months often will solve the problem. If oral contraceptives fail or if you are an older woman, you should have a dilation and curettage (see page 1066), a procedure in which tissue samples are scraped from the uterine lining. If laboratory analysis of the tissue shows precancerous cells, you probably will have to have a hysterectomy (see page 1100). Although you could try hormone therapy instead, you run the risk that cancer will develop later.

CANCER OF THE UTERUS

Signs and Symptoms
- Vaginal bleeding after menopause;
- Before menopause, heavy periods or bleeding between periods;
- A pink, watery discharge from the vagina.

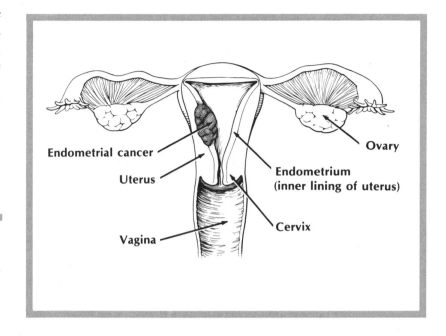

Cancer of the uterus also is called endometrial cancer because it starts in the endometrium, the lining of the uterus. One of the most common of the cancers that afflict American women, it is almost always curable if caught early. It most often occurs after menopause, between the ages of 50 and 70 years. Although researchers do not know the precise cause, excess estrogen replacement after menopause seems to be involved.

Obesity does predispose one to endometrial cancer. Furthermore, it makes treatment (operation and irradiation) difficult.

Today, estrogen replacement therapy uses lower doses of estrogen, combined for part of the month with progesterone. Thus, if you are taking appropriate estrogen replacement therapy, you have no greater risk of uterine cancer than the population at large. However, estrogen taken alone for menopausal symptoms may cause bleeding. Thus, bleeding caused by endometrial cancer may be mistakenly attributed to the estrogen, and diagnosis is delayed.

Women who are at high risk for uterine cancer include those who have never given birth to a child, those who were still menstruating at age 52, and those with a history of infertility or irregular periods. Women who have been taking birth control pills actually may have a decreased risk of endometrial cancer.

The Diagnosis.   In its earliest stage, uterine cancer produces no symptoms. Pap smears (see page 1096) detect it in less than half the cases, and it is not noticeable during a pelvic examination (see page 1055). The first clue is apt to be vaginal bleeding.

If you develop symptoms, your physician can do an endometrial biopsy. In this office procedure, the physician removes a small piece of tissue from the uterine lining for laboratory analysis; usually, you do not need anesthesia. If you do have uterine cancer, the biopsy detects it most of the time.

For a more accurate diagnosis, dilation and curettage (see page 1066) is necessary: the surgeon dilates the cervix and gently scrapes tissue samples from the uterine lining for analysis. It usually requires some form of anesthesia, and it is often done in a hospital or in an outpatient clinic.

If you have cancer and there is reason to think it may have spread beyond the uterus, your physician will want to do a series of tests to locate any secondary tumors.

How Serious Is Uterine Cancer?   It is usually slow-growing and is apt to be still localized when it is discovered. Thus, most women who have it can be cured. When it is diagnosed early, the 5-year survival rate is 88 percent; even when it has already spread to adjacent tissue, the rate is 75 percent. Rarely, the tumor is a faster-growing, deadlier type, and results are not as good.

Treatment. *Surgery.* Most physicians will recommend a hysterectomy (see page 1100), the removal of your uterus. Your fal-

Endometrial cancer is a common disorder that develops in the lining of the uterus (endometrium). It usually is curable if diagnosed early.

lopian tubes and ovaries also will be removed because the cancer tends to spread to those organs also.

Radiation. If the cancer already has extended beyond the uterus, radiation therapy may be given after the operation. Sometimes, radiation is used instead of operation. It may be deep x-ray therapy delivered by a machine or a radium implant inserted in the uterus or vagina while you are under general anesthesia. The radium implant is left in place for a few days, and you will be hospitalized for the duration. A combination of these methods also may be required.

Medication. If the cancer has metastasized (spread) to other parts of your body, progesterone can often stop it from growing, sometimes for 2 to 3 years or even longer.

HYSTERECTOMY

A hysterectomy is the removal of the uterus. (The Greek word *hystera* means womb; *ektome* means incision.) You may have to have a hysterectomy if you develop cancer of the uterus; if you have severe endometriosis (see page 1101), fibroids (see page 1097), or pelvic adhesions which bind the uterus to neighboring organs; if you have severe and uncontrollable bleeding; or if the uterus has dropped down and is protruding from the vagina. There are also other reasons hysterectomies are performed.

Hysterectomies are not all alike. A partial hysterectomy leaves the cervix and the base of the uterus intact. In a total hysterectomy, the entire uterus, including the cervix, is removed. A total hysterectomy with bilateral salpingo-oophorectomy is removal of your uterus, cervix, fallopian tubes *(salpingo),* and both ovaries *(oophor),* whereas a radical hysterectomy extends even further and also includes removal of the upper part of the vagina and some lymph nodes. The extent of the problem that made the hysterectomy necessary determines how much is removed.

In doing a hysterectomy, the surgeon most often makes an incision in your lower abdomen, either horizontally just above the pubic hair or vertically from the navel to the hairline. However, sometimes a vaginal hysterectomy is indicated. This is accomplished through an incision made at the top of the vagina. Either operation takes 1 to 2 hours under general anesthesia. If you have a large ovarian or uterine tumor or cancer, the abdominal approach is necessary. Many surgeons prefer it, in any case, because it gives them a better look at various pelvic organs. Hysterectomy by the vaginal approach usually is selected for the management of uterine prolapse.

Although some surgeons routinely remove the ovaries to prevent ovarian cancer in women older than 40 years, this is a controversial tactic. On the one hand, ovarian cancer is deadly—it has a cure rate of only 10 to 20 percent. On the other hand, cancer of the ovaries is uncommon.

If you have a hysterectomy, you probably will remain in the hospital for 5 to 7 days. Possible complications include pelvic infections, kidney and bladder infections, and hemorrhage. After you get home, for a time you will have to forgo tub baths and douches, driving the car, and lifting heavy objects, and for 6 to 8 weeks you must forgo sex and active sports.

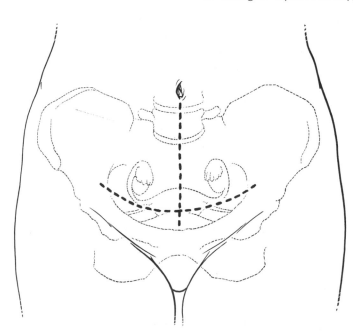

In performing an abdominal hysterectomy, your surgeon may elect either a horizontal or a vertical incision.

Other anticancer medications also can be used.

HYDATIDIFORM MOLE

Signs and Symptoms
- During pregnancy, the uterus grows much faster than it should;
- Vaginal bleeding, severe nausea and vomiting, no fetal movement;
- Passage of grape-like tissue from the vagina;
- High blood pressure.

A rare benign growth called hydatidiform mole sometimes develops at the beginning of pregnancy from tissue surrounding the fertilized egg that would normally produce a placenta. In such cases, the fetus dies. (If placental tissue is left in the uterus after childbirth or a miscarriage, a mole also can develop, sometimes years later.)

If you have the symptoms listed above, see a physician as soon as possible. It is essential that the tumor be removed. It grows quickly and can become large. In addition, although more than 80 percent of such moles are benign, 15 percent develop into a condition called invasive mole. This mole—still benign—reaches so deeply into the uterine wall that it can cause a hemorrhage and other serious problems. Two to 3 percent of hydatidiform moles are followed by a choriocarcinoma, a fast-growing malignant tumor that soon spreads to other parts of the body.

Hydatidiform moles are more common in older women. One occurs in about every 2,000 gestations in the United States and more often in some other parts of the world.

The Diagnosis.   To make sure you are not experiencing some other complication of pregnancy in which the fetus is normal, your physician probably will use ultrasonography. Because hydatidiform moles produce quantities of human chorionic gonadotropin, a hormone that can be detected in urine or blood, your physician may order a urine or blood test.

How Serious Are Hydatidiform Moles?
A noninvasive mole can be removed easily, and invasive moles and malignant tumors also are treatable. In fact, for choriocar-

cinoma, the overall cure rate is 75 to 85 percent.

Treatment. *Surgery.*   The mole can be removed, usually by suction, in a procedure similar to dilation and curettage (see page 1066). Afterward, the physician will monitor your levels of human chorionic gonadotropin, which should return to normal. If they do not, you may have developed either an invasive mole or choriocarcinoma. Your physician may recommend that your uterus be removed (see Hysterectomy, page 1100), but he or she is more likely to suggest chemotherapy.

Chemotherapy.   For both invasive moles and choriocarcinoma, chemotherapy provides good results. Furthermore, you can still have a child afterward, and you avoid a major operation.

ENDOMETRIOSIS

Signs and Symptoms
- Painful menstruation—pain may begin before and extend several days after a period;
- Occasional heavy periods;
- Sharp pain deep in the pelvis during intercourse;
- Infertility;
- Pain when straining at stool.

Endometriosis occurs when bits of the endometrium (the tissue that lines the uterus) somehow escape the uterus and become implanted on other pelvic organs. Most often, the implants develop on the outside of the ovaries, the fallopian tubes, or the uterus or its supporting ligaments.

These mislocated cells imitate the menstrual cycle (see page 1058), first thickening and then bleeding as menstruation begins. Because the implants are embedded within other tissue, there is nowhere for the blood to go. They form blood blisters, irritating the surrounding tissue, which may create a cyst to encapsulate the blister. The cyst, in turn, may become a scar or an adhesion (abnormal tissue that binds organs together). Scars and adhesions on the ovaries or fallopian tubes can prevent pregnancy.

Experts estimate that 10 to 15 percent of American women of childbearing age have endometriosis. Most have no symptoms and require no treatment, but for some this is a progressive disease that becomes more painful and debilitating over time. Endometriosis, which may occasionally run in families, is most likely to occur between the ages of 25 and 40 years in women who have not had children. The cause is uncertain, but some experts believe the implants occur when menstrual flow backs up into the fallopian tubes and spills into the pelvic cavity.

Menopause usually cures mild or moderate endometriosis. However, if you have estrogen replacement therapy, it may be reactivated.

The Diagnosis. Although a physician often can feel patches of endometriosis during a pelvic examination, laparoscopy is the only way to confirm the finding. It is important to be certain because ovarian cancer produces similar symptoms, and the hormones usually prescribed to treat endometriosis can make cancer grow faster. A laparoscope is a slim instrument equipped with a light. It is inserted into the abdomen through a small incision, and the physician looks through it to see your pelvic organs. Laparoscopy is a minor procedure done with local or general anesthesia, often on an outpatient basis (see page 1297).

How Serious Is Endometriosis? Endometrial implants are rarely malignant, but they frequently prevent pregnancy. Although the symptoms may wax and wane, they generally get worse with time. There is often no real cure short of menopause.

Treatment. *Pregnancy.* If you have endometriosis in an early stage, your physician may suggest that you become pregnant soon if you want to have children because it may become more difficult to conceive later on. During pregnancy, endometriosis implants generally shrink and the symptoms may disappear. However, women with endometrio-

PELVIC PAIN

Any time you have a pain in the pelvic region that lasts more than a few hours, that recurs, or that is accompanied by other symptoms such as fever or vaginal bleeding, see a physician. Your physician will ask a great many questions about what the pain is like. Such information is important for diagnosis. Some of the most significant distinctions involve whether it is acute (like the onslaught of pain and fever that sometimes marks the beginning of pelvic inflammatory disease) or chronic (meaning that it has been with you for a while) and, if it is chronic, whether it is episodic (it comes and goes) or continuous. You also will be asked whether the pain is associated with your menstrual periods, bowel or bladder habits, intercourse, or physical activity.

Acute Pain

Pelvic Infection
If you develop severe pain in the lower abdomen a few days after a menstrual period, perhaps accompanied by fever or vomiting, you may have acute pelvic inflammatory disease (see page 1055). The pain often starts in the middle of the abdomen and gradually moves lower down and to both sides, a sign that the infection has spread from the uterus into the fallopian tubes.

Your abdomen will be tender when pressed. You may have a smelly discharge from the vagina or vaginal bleeding. If you suddenly develop signs of shock, such as cold, clammy skin, rapid breathing, or an irregular heartbeat, get medical help immediately: an abscess, caused by the infection, has perforated and you are hemorrhaging internally.

Complications of Early Pregnancy
During the first trimester of pregnancy, pain in the lower abdomen or back may mean you are having a miscarriage (see page 209). The pain may be dull and constant, or sharp and intermittent. You may have spotting or heavy bleeding from the vagina. Call a physician immediately. If the pain is severe enough and the bleeding heavy enough, the fetus may be dead. You may need dilation and curettage to prevent infection.

Ectopic Pregnancy
If you develop a sudden, constant, severe pain in the lower abdomen, especially if it is located only on one side and is followed by vaginal bleeding, you may have an ectopic pregnancy. That means a fertilized egg is developing in one of your ovaries or fallopian tubes rather than in the uterus. If you faint soon after the pain strikes, you are probably in shock because the tube has ruptured. You will need emergency treatment (see Ectopic Pregnancy, page 202).

Nongynecological Causes
Acute abdominal pain is not al-

ways caused by the reproductive organs. Appendicitis, for example, often begins as a sudden, intense pain in the general vicinity of the navel, then changes to pain in the lower right side of the abdomen (see page 624). Diverticulitis and bladder infections cause pain in the lower abdomen. With diverticulitis, when the pain is very intense it sometimes feels like a belt around the body (see page 631). Gallstones can cause attacks of severe, spasmodic pain, starting in the upper abdomen and streaking toward the right shoulder blade (see page 661).

Episodic Pain

Dyspareunia
Pain that occurs only, or primarily, during intercourse is called dyspareunia. It has several possible causes. If you are breast-feeding or are past menopause, your body is no longer producing estrogen in the same quantities, and the vaginal tissue may have become thinner and more fragile (see page 1068). Also, the walls of your vagina may be irritated because of an allergic reaction; you may have vaginal cysts (see page 1089), a vaginal infection, or a sexually transmitted disease such as herpes or genital warts (see page 1085). If you recently had a baby, the discomfort could be due to scars from an episiotomy (see page 212).

The problem also could be a bladder infection (see page 1108). It also could be loss of pelvic support (see page 1090). If pain occurs only when your partner thrusts deeply, the cause probably lies in the uterus or beyond: it could be pelvic inflammatory disease (see page 1104), an ectopic pregnancy (see page 202), endometriosis (see page 1101), or cysts or a tumor in the ovaries (see page

1105). Finally, if none of the above conditions explain the pain, you may have vaginismus: for psychological reasons, during intercourse your vagina produces little lubrication and the vaginal muscles go into spasms.

Midcycle Pelvic Pain
Some women experience pain in the lower abdomen at midcycle, when they ovulate. Called mittelschmerz (see page 1063), the pain is typically a dull ache that can last a few minutes or a few hours.

Dysmenorrhea
Severe pain during menstruation may be due to excess prostaglandins produced by the endometrium (see page 1063). Or the problem may be temporary, a result of giving up oral contraceptives or of using an intrauterine device. However, if you also have a fever and have had a heavy, unpleasant discharge between menstrual periods, you may have a vaginal or pelvic infection (see page 1104).

Chronic Pain

Endometriosis or Adenomyosis
Pain in the lower abdomen that begins a little before a menstrual period starts, continues throughout the period, and actually gets worse right afterward is apt to be caused by endometriosis (see page 1101) or by adenomyosis (see page 1104). In either case, the pain often accompanies heavy menstrual flow. In endometriosis, the kind of tissue that normally lines the uterus is found implanted on other pelvic organs such as the ovaries and the fallopian tubes. In adenomyosis, that same tissue be-

gins to grow inside the walls of the uterus.

Chronic Salpingitis
If you have had pelvic inflammatory disease (see page 1104), especially if you have had recurring bouts of it, you may develop chronic pain in the pelvis. It generally gets worse during menstruation and during intercourse.

Pelvic Pain Syndrome
Some women experience considerable pelvic discomfort every month during the 7 to 10 days before they menstruate. The pain is worse when they sit or stand and better when they lie down; the lower back and legs also may ache. Intercourse may be painful, and normal vaginal discharge is sometimes increased. Symptoms associated with premenstrual syndrome (see page 1062), such as headaches, insomnia, and fatigue, also may be present. This problem may be caused by congestion due to the increase in blood flow to the uterus just before menstruation.

Nongynecological Causes
Chronic pelvic pain also can originate with nonreproductive organs in the urinary and intestinal tracts. A bladder infection (see page 1108) sometimes causes a gnawing pain just above the pubic bone while you are urinating; you also may have a burning sensation in the urethra. Other symptoms are a frequent, urgent need to urinate and occasionally blood in the urine. Irritable or spastic colon produces a crampy abdominal pain often accompanied by nausea, vomiting, diarrhea, or constipation. If abdominal pain accompanies a distended abdomen and follows several days of constipation, you may have a blockage of the intestine.

sis are more likely than most to have a pregnancy outside of the uterus (ectopic pregnancy) (see page 202).

Medication.   Birth control pills may relieve the symptoms. If that treatment is not sufficient, various hormones can be used to stop menstruation completely for a time. Danazol (a testosterone derivative with the brand name Danocrine) often is given. It sometimes actually shrinks implants; after 6 months on danazol and then withdrawal of the drug, some women do conceive.

Surgery.   If drugs fail, the implants can be removed surgically or destroyed with electrocautery, although some surgeons believe that laser surgery, done during laparoscopy, is less likely to produce scars and adhesions. Unfortunately, recurrences are common. If nothing else works and the pain is severe, removal of your uterus and ovaries may be necessary (see Hysterectomy, page 1100).

ADENOMYOSIS

Signs and Symptoms
* Menstrual cramps that last throughout a period; they get worse as you grow older;
* Prolonged and excessive menstrual bleeding.

In adenomyosis, some of the endometrial tissue that lines the uterus begins to grow *within* its muscular walls. This is most likely to happen late in the childbearing years and after you have had children. Many women who have adenomyosis have no symptoms.

During a pelvic examination (see page 1055), the physician generally finds that the uterus is enlarged and tender. That fact, and the symptoms listed above, indicate adenomyosis, which is generally harmless but can be painful.

Treatment.   If you are nearing menopause, your physician may prescribe painkillers and suggest no other treatment because the problem generally disappears when menstruation ends. If the pain is severe or menopause is years away, the physician may suggest that your uterus be removed (see Hysterectomy, page 1100).

PELVIC INFLAMMATORY DISEASE

Signs and Symptoms
* Severe pain and tenderness in lower abdomen, perhaps with fever and vomiting (acute disease);
* Mild, recurrent pain in lower abdomen, perhaps with backache, irregular menstrual periods, infertility (chronic disease);
* Pain during intercourse;
* Periods that start early or are heavy;
* Copious, foul-smelling vaginal discharge.

Emergency Symptoms
* Severe pain low in abdomen; nausea, vomiting, and signs of shock, such as faintness.

Strictly speaking, pelvic inflammatory disease (PID) is an infection of the fallopian tubes; it is also known as salpingitis. However, infections of the ovaries, uterus, and cervix also have come to be called PID.

The bacteria responsible for PID are usually sexually transmitted. Salpingitis develops in almost 15 percent of women with gonorrhea. However, other bacteria also can cause PID, and the infection can sometimes be traced to childbirth or to procedures such as an endometrial biopsy or dilation and curettage. Every year, about 1 million American women develop PID. Some have no symptoms and are never diagnosed; some develop a low-level, chronic infection; and others have an acute attack.

If you use a diaphragm or if your partner uses a condom, you are somewhat protected from PID. If you use an intrauterine device (IUD), you are more likely to develop the disorder. You are most vulnerable to infection during menstruation. If you have PID, your sexual partner should be treated, too, even if he has no symptoms. If he has the infection, he may reinfect you.

The Diagnosis.   During a pelvic examination (see page 1055), your physician will use a cotton swab to take samples from your vagina and cervix. They will be sent to a laboratory for analysis to determine what organism is causing the infection. If there is any question about the diagnosis, or about how widespread the infection is, the physician can do a laparoscopy: he or she will insert a thin, lighted instrument through a small incision in your abdomen in order to see your pelvic organs. This hospital procedure is usually done on an outpatient basis with local or general anesthesia.

How Serious Is PID? If it is not treated, PID can be serious. An abscess may develop on the fallopian tubes or the ovaries, creating a surgical emergency if it perforates. If the tubes or ovaries become damaged or scarred, you may be unable to conceive. PID also can lead to peritonitis, an inflammation of the membrane that lines the abdominal cavity. Peritonitis is always serious and needs intensive treatment with antibiotics. In rare cases, if bacteria invade the bloodstream, PID can lead to blood poisoning (septicemia) and inflammation of the joints.

The long-term consequences of PID can be severe; they include chronic pelvic pain due to adhesions, lingering infection, and ectopic pregnancy in which the fetus grows outside the uterus, usually in one of the fallopian tubes.

Treatment. *Medication.* A physician rarely waits for the results of laboratory tests before giving medication. Thus, to begin with, you may be given a combination of antibiotics; the physician may give you a different medication once the laboratory results are known. You also may be given a painkiller. Bed rest will be advised. You may even be hospitalized for a short time if you have a severe case or if it fails to respond quickly to medication. PID recurs in about 15 to 25 percent of cases.

Surgery. Operation is rarely necessary. However, if an abscess ruptures or threatens to rupture, it may have to be drained or removed.

OVARIAN DISORDERS

Each of the two ovaries is about the size of an almond. They are located in the abdomen, above and to the side of the uterus and about 4 to 5 inches below your waist. At birth, a female has roughly 1 million undeveloped eggs, or ova, already stored in her ovaries, each housed in its own follicle. From the time of puberty until menopause, every month one ovum grows until rupture of its follicle releases it; the ovum then floats downward to the uterus via the fallopian tube. Normally, this ovulation process takes place in only one ovary, and the ovaries release an egg in random order.

The ovaries also produce the female sex hormones estrogen and progesterone, which regulate the menstrual cycle. During the first half of the cycle, your ovaries secrete estrogen. Most of it is manufactured by the outer cells of the single follicle where the ovum is growing. Estrogen causes the uterine lining to thicken so that it will be ready to receive a fertilized egg.

Just before ovulation, the same follicle begins to produce tiny amounts of progesterone. After the egg has been released, the follicle expands rapidly—at this stage it is called the corpus luteum—and steps up production of both progesterone and estrogen.

These hormones act together to complete the development of the uterine lining. If pregnancy occurs, hormones secreted by the corpus luteum will help to sustain the pregnancy. If it does not occur, the corpus luteum will begin to shrink, and levels of estrogen and progesterone will decrease. As a result, the uterus will shed its lining during menstruation.

OVARIAN CYSTS AND BENIGN TUMORS

Signs and Symptoms
- Usually no symptoms;
- Dull ache in the abdomen or a sense of pressure or fullness;
- Pain during intercourse;
- Delayed, irregular, or painful menstrual periods;
- Firm, painless swelling of the lower abdomen;
- Abrupt onset of sharp pain in the lower abdomen.

Emergency Symptoms
- Sudden, severe abdominal pain with fever and perhaps vomiting.

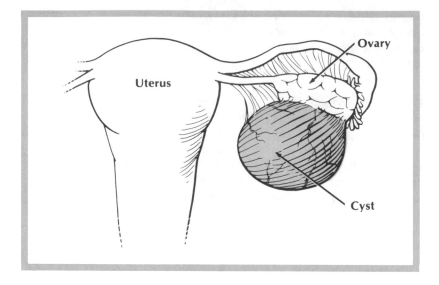

Ovary

Uterus

Cyst

An ovarian cyst is a growth on an ovary. The growth may be detected during a routine pelvic examination.

Most ovarian cysts are harmless and disappear of their own accord. Other types of cysts should be taken as a warning. Often, they are benign themselves and do not even cause symptoms—they are found during a routine pelvic examination. However, women who develop such cysts between the ages of 50 and 70 years have a higher risk of ovarian cancer than most and should have regular pelvic examinations.

A cyst is a sac and often is filled with fluid; a tumor is a solid lump. Benign tumors do not invade neighboring tissue or spread to other parts of the body the way malignant tumors do. However, if a benign tumor or ovarian cyst is large, it can cause abdominal discomfort. In some cases, it may interfere with the production of ovarian hormones and result in irregular bleeding from the vagina or an increase in body hair. If a large

An ovarian cyst that becomes twisted may produce pain and other symptoms and may require immediate treatment.

tumor or cyst presses on the bladder, you may need to empty your bladder more frequently because its capacity has been diminished.

If a tumor or cyst becomes twisted, you may experience spasmodic pain. Sudden or sharp pain may mean a cyst has ruptured. The twisting or rupture of a cyst occasionally predisposes to an infection. If you have severe abdominal pain, fever, and vomiting, or if you have symptoms of shock such as cold, clammy skin and rapid breathing, get help immediately.

The Diagnosis. If your physician finds something that feels like an ovarian cyst or tumor during a pelvic examination (see page 1055), he or she may order an ultrasound examination and perhaps a laparoscopy to confirm the diagnosis. For laparoscopy, a minor surgical procedure, a slim, lighted instrument is inserted into the abdomen through a small incision so that the physician can see your ovaries (see page 1297).

Treatment. If you have a cyst and no symptoms and are younger than 40 years, you can wait through two or three menstrual cycles to see if it goes away. If it does not, your physician may prescribe hormones or consider removing it surgically.

Surgery. An operation or other procedure is necessary if a cyst causes problems or does not regress or disappear in two or three menstrual cycles. Sometimes, the cyst can be drained through a laparoscope, but more often it is surgically removed in a hospital. If you are older than 40 years and the cyst is larger than 2 inches in diameter or if you are postmenopausal, the cyst should be removed surgically. Tumors also are removed. If a cyst or tumor is not too large, the ovary can be left intact. At other times, one or both ovaries and their fallopian tubes may have to be removed, and sometimes the uterus also is removed.

CANCER OF THE OVARY

Signs and Symptoms
- Usually, no symptoms initially;
- Vague abdominal discomfort and mild indigestion;
- Swollen abdomen and pain in the lower abdomen (late stage of the disease).

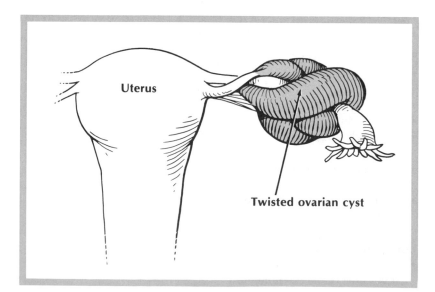

Uterus

Twisted ovarian cyst

In the United States, ovarian cancer affects 1 woman in 70. It can be deadly. In its early stages, it produces few noticeable symptoms, and it most often is discovered in the course of a routine pelvic examination. If it is not found early, it eventually becomes painful, and the tumor may produce fluid that causes the abdomen to swell. Seventy to 80 percent of the time, the disease is already in this advanced stage when it is diagnosed.

Ovarian cancer generally develops after menopause. If you have never been pregnant or have had trouble conceiving, you are somewhat more likely to get cancer of the ovaries. Conversely, you are less likely to get it if you have had several children or have taken birth control pills. However, in either case, an annual pelvic examination still is important because early diagnosis and treatment give you the best chance for a cure.

The Diagnosis. If a pelvic examination (see page 1055) reveals a growth on the ovary, your physician will order a series of tests. They may include ultrasonography to get a picture of the inside of your abdomen; x-ray studies of the colon, kidney, and ureters (tubes connecting the kidneys to the bladder) because an ovarian tumor can distort the shapes of these organs; and laparoscopy in which a surgeon makes a small incision in your abdomen to get a direct look at the ovaries. During laparoscopy, the physician may remove a tiny piece of the tumor for laboratory analysis—the only way to be sure whether it is malignant. Three out of four ovarian tumors are not malignant.

How Serious Is Cancer of the Ovary? When ovarian cancer is caught early, the 5-year survival rate is 60 to 80 percent. Overall, the survival rate is only 30 to 40 percent because this type of malignancy is seldom found soon enough. Nevertheless, with aggressive surgery and chemotherapy, women with advanced ovarian cancer are now surviving longer.

Treatment. *Surgery.* If a tumor is found early and you are a young woman and want to have children, the surgeon may remove only one ovary and its fallopian tube. However, the most common type of tumor often occurs in both ovaries. When that is the case or when the disease already has begun to spread, the surgeon removes both ovaries

and also the uterus, fallopian tubes, nearby lymph glands, and a fold of tissue known as the omentum because ovarian cancer often spreads to the omentum. In addition, the surgeon takes many samples of tissue within the abdomen and fluid from the abdomen to be examined for cancer cells.

Radiation. Operation often is followed by radiation or chemotherapy. If the surgeon was unable to remove the whole tumor, radiation therapy generally can shrink it, giving chemotherapy a better chance.

Chemotherapy. The oncologist (cancer specialist) will probably treat you with a combination of several drugs. After chemotherapy, a tumor usually shrinks. However, 12 to 18 months later, it often begins to grow again. Because it is then resistant to the original drugs, a different combination of drugs will be used in the second course of chemotherapy.

POLYCYSTIC OVARIES

Signs and Symptoms
- Unpredictable menstrual periods, or failure to menstruate;
- Infertility;
- An unusual amount of facial hair.

This is a disease of young women. Most who get it never had a normal menstrual rhythm in their teens and eventually may

Polycystic ovary is a rare disorder involving irregular menstrual periods and an excess of facial hair. The ovaries develop cysts and fail to release eggs.

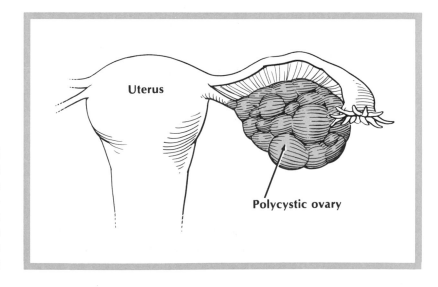

Uterus

Polycystic ovary

stop menstruating altogether (some never start). Their faces are rather hairy and they are apt to be overweight; if they do menstruate, they may have severe cramps. Most of the time, they do not ovulate. For reasons that are not yet understood, their ovarian follicles develop but form cysts instead of releasing an egg; eventually, each ovary is a mass of small cysts.

This rare disorder is also known as the Stein-Leventhal syndrome. It causes infertility, but that is often treatable.

The Diagnosis.   During a pelvic examination (see page 1055), your physician generally can feel that the ovaries are enlarged. Blood tests will reveal a typical pattern of hormones present in abnormal amounts.

Treatment. *Medication.* If you do not want to become pregnant, your physician may prescribe birth control pills or long-acting progestins such as medroxyprogesterone to suppress ovulation and forestall any possible precancerous changes in the lining of the uterus. If you want to conceive, you will be given a fertility drug. Clomiphene induces ovulation about 75 percent of the time, and 35 percent of those who take it eventually become pregnant. If clomiphene does not work, your physician can give you gonadotropins.

Surgery.   If, despite medication, you fail to conceive, you can have an operation called an ovarian wedge resection, in which the surgeon removes a wedge-shaped section of the ovary.

BLADDER AND URETHRAL DISORDERS

The bladder lies between your pubic bone and your uterus. It is the sac where urine is stored after it has been produced by your kidneys. The bladder has stretchable, muscular walls that expand as it fills with urine. When those walls contract, the urine is squeezed out into the urethra, a thin tube about 1.5 inches long. The opening to the urethra is located between the clitoris and the vagina (see page 1055).

Both males and females have a bladder and urethra, but these organs are constructed somewhat differently in the two sexes. For that reason, different problems can develop, and some disorders are more likely to develop in women than in men. For example, because in women the urethra is close to both the vagina and the anus, which often harbor bacteria, and is shorter than in the male, infections of the bladder (cystitis) and urethra are more common in women. In addition, some older women experience urinary problems, such as incontinence, when the muscles of the pelvic floor, which support the bladder and other internal organs, become weakened and allow those organs to sag lower in the body.

This section covers urinary tract problems common to women. For other urinary disorders, see page 889.

CHRONIC URETHRITIS

Signs and Symptoms
- Discomfort on urination, which persists or recurs;
- Frequent urination.

Sometimes irritation and inflammation of the urethra persist over weeks or months, with or without evidence of a bacterial infection. When this happens, you feel the need to urinate frequently, and urinating is uncomfortable. As the chronically inflamed urethra has undergone periods of healing, it has gradually narrowed.

Inflammation that extends into the bottom of the bladder is called trigonitis. A lighted, tubular instrument (see Cystoscopy, page 904) that can be inserted into the bladder is used to diagnose trigonitis.

Treatment. *Medication.* Antibiotics or sulfa drugs may be prescribed if there is evidence of actual infection. Other treatments—for instance, stretching (dilating) the urethra with an instrument—also are often helpful.

URINE INCONTINENCE AND OTHER URINE LOSS PROBLEMS

Signs and Symptoms
- Involuntary urination;
- Small amounts of urine escape under pressure—for instance when you cough or sneeze.

If you find that you need to urinate so suddenly and urgently that you cannot hold back, you have urgency incontinence. A low-grade urinary infection is often to blame. If you lose control only a little bit, and only when you cough, sneeze, laugh, or lift something, it is stress incontinence. It generally is due to weakening of the muscles of the pelvic floor that support the bladder and close off the top of the urethra. Those muscles can deteriorate because of childbirth, being overweight, or aging (see page 1090). Incontinence also can be caused by disorders such as Alzheimer's disease (see page 516).

If the physician suspects an infection, he or she will want a urine sample for laboratory analysis. If not, you may have a bladder x-ray. The condition is annoying but not dangerous.

Treatment. *Medication.* Bladder infections are treated with antibiotics (see page 847). Sometimes use of an estrogen cream in the vagina will strengthen the muscles of the pelvic wall and lessen or eliminate urinary incontinence.

Surgery. For stress incontinence, pelvic floor muscles can be tightened surgically, or you can be fitted with a pessary (a device that encircles the cervix) to wear in your vagina during the day to support the pelvic organs.

Self-Help. You can strengthen pelvic muscles with simple exercise (see Exercises for Incontinence, page 1091).

IRRITABLE BLADDER

Signs and Symptoms
- Sudden and sometimes uncontrollable urge to urinate;
- Frequent need to urinate during the night.

HONEYMOON CYSTITIS

Some women develop symptoms of cystitis (see page 892), such as frequent, painful urination, almost every time they have intercourse. The symptoms generally last for a day or two and then disappear, only to recur the next time the woman has sex. The problem is sometimes called honeymoon cystitis, although it is actually a form of chronic urethritis—it is generally the urethra, not the bladder, that is inflamed. (The Greek suffix *itis* means an inflammation.)

In most cases, the symptoms are caused by an infection, often by *Chlamydia* (see page 891). However, if you have been soaking in bath oils or using feminine hygiene sprays or douches, these could be irritating your urethra. Another possibility is that the urethra is being bruised by sexual activity, thus the term honeymoon cystitis.

If bath oils, sprays, or douches are the problem, you can simply quit using them, and the symptoms should disappear. Otherwise, see a physician. Your physician will ask for a urine sample and have it tested for bacteria. If you do have an infection, it generally can be cleared up with antibiotics. However, sometimes laboratory tests fail to find any microorganisms that could be responsible; and some women, even after treatment with an antibiotic, continue to have symptoms whenever they have intercourse. In such cases, your physician may suggest preventive measures. An antibiotic, such as a low dose of nitrofurantoin or trimethoprim-sulfamethoxazole (Bactrim or Septra) may be taken every time you have sex.

There are other things you can do to make honeymoon cystitis less likely. Wash your genital and anal areas daily with mild soap and water. Before you have sex, be sure your partner's hands and penis are clean. After intercourse, empty your bladder immediately to flush bacteria out of the urethra. Use a water-soluble lubricant during intercourse to make penetration easier and bruising less likely; do not use petroleum jelly because it is not water-soluble.

You may have an irritable bladder—one that contracts uncontrollably at times—if you often need to urinate so suddenly and urgently that you do not always make it to the bathroom. The problem is fairly common. Sometimes an infection is to blame, but often the cause is unclear, although the bladder seems to be chronically inflamed. This disorder can be distressing, but it is not dangerous. It should be distinguished from an inflamed bladder.

The Diagnosis. The physician will want a urine specimen for laboratory analysis. You may have a special kind of x-ray taken while you are urinating (a voiding cystogram). Cystoscopy is another possibility (see page 904); this is a procedure in which a lighted instrument is inserted through the urethra into the bladder.

Treatment. *Medication.* Antibiotics are used to treat infections. Drugs such as imipramine or calcium channel blockers can relax the muscles that make the bladder contract. Other medications can reduce the activity of the nerves that control the contraction.

Self-Help. When irritable bladder is not due to an infection, it often is treated by exercising and strengthening the bladder muscles: when you urinate, practice holding back the urine for as long as possible (see Exercises for Incontinence, page 1091).

CHAPTER 35

HEALTH PROBLEMS OF MEN

CHAPTER CONTENTS

MALE GENITAL ORGANS

In terms of function, the main purpose of the male genital organs is to produce sperm cells and transport them to the female reproductive system. As with the female genital organs (See Health Problems of Women, page 1053), there is some overlap between the genital system and the urinary system, with some of the same organs being used in each. The link is so close that a genital system disorder frequently causes symptoms in the urinary system, and vice versa. The urologist is the physician who deals with both the genital and urinary organs in men; urologists also deal with urinary tract problems in women.

The main male genital organs are the penis, the testicles, the vas deferens (duct through which the semen passes), the seminal vesicles, and the prostate gland.

The penis is a sexual organ and also transports urine. The urethra, which runs the length of the penis through its center, carries the urine and the semen. There are many blood vessels in the penis and these are involved in producing an erection. During sexual arousal, these vessels supply blood to three cylindrical, sponge-like structures that run parallel to the urethra along the length of the penis. As these structures fill with blood, the penis expands, straightens, and stiffens.

The testicles (or testes) are two oval organs about 2 inches long. They are contained in a pouch of skin, called the scrotum, which hangs below the abdomen and behind the penis. In each testicle there is a tightly packed mass of coiled tubes surrounded by a protective capsule. The testicles begin to produce the sperm cells that are used in reproduction at about the time of puberty, and this process continues throughout life. In addition to producing sperm cells, the testicles secrete the male hormone testosterone which enters the bloodstream and plays an important role in the development and maintenance of the typical masculine physical characteristics (such as facial hair, greater muscle mass and strength, and deeper voice).

Sperm production must take place at a temperature that is lower than the temperature within the body. This is made possible by the testicles' location outside of the body. The cords that suspend the testicles within the scrotum help to maintain the correct temperature for sperm production. When the outside temperature is lowered, the cords draw the testicles upward, nearer to the body and thus in a warmer place. When the outside temperature is increased, the cords lower the testicles, decreasing their warmth.

The sperm cells that are constantly being produced within each testicle are transported to the epididymis (the cord-like structure near the top of the testes) and then stored in the seminal vesicles. The mixture of the sperm cells with the fluids formed by the seminal vesicles and the prostate gland forms the semen that is ejaculated during sexual activity. Although sperm cells make up only a small portion of the semen, a single ejaculation contains as many as 500 million sperm. After sexual intercourse, one of these cells may survive to reach and fertilize an egg in the female (see also page 181).

The prostate gland contributes fluids to the semen which, among other things, appear to increase the ability of the ejaculated sperm to survive within the acidic environment of the vagina. As a man ages, the prostate gland frequently enlarges. Sometimes

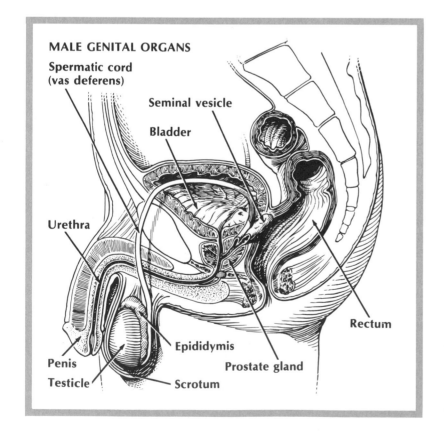

MALE GENITAL ORGANS

Spermatic cord (vas deferens)

Seminal vesicle

Bladder

Urethra

Penis

Testicle

Epididymis

Prostate gland

Scrotum

Rectum

this causes the gland to press against the urethra. This pressure makes urination more difficult and may require surgical correction (described later in this chapter).

PROBLEMS RELATED TO TESTICLES AND SCROTUM

The testicles (testes) play two important roles: they produce the sperm cells used in reproduction, and they secrete hormones (for example, testosterone) that play a key role in male body development. Their location in the scrotum, a pouch outside of the pelvic area, keeps them at a temperature lower than that within the body, which is required for sperm production.

The relatively exposed location of the testicles and scrotum does make them prone to injuries. But it also makes it easy to examine them for potentially life-threatening problems, such as cancer.

This section covers the main problems that can be encountered in the testicles themselves, in the epididymis (the cord-like structure near the top of the testes) and vas deferens (sperm transport tubes), and in the spermatic cords (which suspend the testicles) within the scrotum. Self-examination of the testicles also is described.

TESTICULAR TORSION

Signs and Symptoms
- Sudden, generally severe, pain in one testicle;
- Elevation of one testicle within the scrotum;
- Nausea and vomiting;
- Sensation of faintness;
- Swelling;
- Fever.

Emergency Symptoms
- Sudden, severe testicular pain that arises spontaneously or after strenuous physical activity.

Each testicle is suspended within the scrotum on a spermatic cord which contains the blood vessels that supply that testicle. In testicular torsion, the testicle twists on its spermatic cord, cutting off the blood supply to the testicle. Testicular torsion sometimes occurs without any apparent cause, even during sleep. At other times, it happens after strenuous physical activity.

Testicular torsion is uncommon. When it does occur, it is usually in young children, although it also may occur around the time of puberty. However, testicular torsion can happen at any age.

The Diagnosis.   Severe local pain, often accompanied by nausea, faintness, and vomiting, with no precipitating physical injury suggests testicular torsion. However, these same symptoms can also be caused by inflammation within the scrotum and by a tumor. The symptoms of testicular torsion and epididymitis (see page 1115) are similar. One way to distinguish between the two ailments is to lift the painful testicle while standing; with torsion, the testicle will probably hurt more as a result; with epididymitis, it will probably hurt less.

In some cases, a surgical procedure may be necessary to establish the diagnosis and to correct the testicular torsion.

How Serious Is Testicular Torsion?   If you experience severe pain in a testicle, seek immediate medical help. If the torsion is not

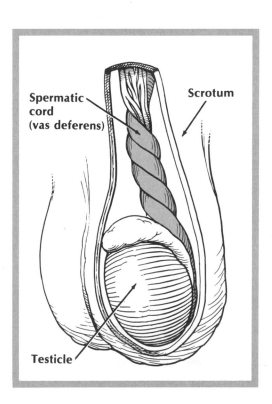

Spermatic cord (vas deferens)

Scrotum

Testicle

In testicular torsion, the testicle twists on its spermatic cord, cutting off the blood supply and producing sudden, severe pain.

corrected within a few hours—often by an operation—the testicle will atrophy due to lack of a blood supply and will have to be removed from the scrotum.

It is uncommon for the twisted cord to untwist spontaneously, without medical intervention.

Treatment. *Surgery.* If you have testicular torsion, your physician may arrange for a prompt corrective operation to return the testicle to its normal position and to anchor it in place. In addition, the testicle on the other side usually also is anchored in place as a precaution to prevent possible torsion of that testicle in the future.

Other Therapies. Sometimes it is possible for the physician to manipulate the twisted testicle carefully and to return it to its normal position. In this case, an operation later probably will be desirable anyway, to secure the testicles in their normal position and thus prevent a recurrence.

TESTICULAR FAILURE

Signs and Symptoms
- Infertility;
- Possible lack of sexual drive;
- Delay of puberty or of development of male characteristics, in some cases.

The term "testicular failure" refers to the inability of the testicles to produce sperm or, in some cases, to produce male hormones. The causes of such failure include chromosomal abnormalities present before birth, problems affecting sexual maturation, and damage to mature, normally developed testicles caused by disease, drugs, or injury. Testicular failure is uncommon.

The Diagnosis.
Testicular failure is one of many possible causes of infertility. To diagnose infertility, the physician must interview and examine both sexual partners and also perform blood, urine, and semen tests (see Chapter 36, Health Problems of Partners, page 1129). The diagnosis will depend on the results of such tests.

In cases of slowed or absence of sexual maturation, the diagnosis will be by interview, physical examination, and related tests as appropriate.

How Serious Is Testicular Failure? Testicular failure is neither life-threatening nor the first stage in some degenerative process. Instead, its seriousness relates to the symptoms themselves—infertility, possible lack of sex drive, or delayed sexual maturation. Restoration of a normal sex drive or continuity of normal sexual development often can be achieved by the administration of male hormones. However, fertility rarely can be restored.

Treatment. *Medication.* Male hormones are administered for some types of testicular

---

INJURY TO THE TESTICLES

Because the male genital organs are not protected by being inside the abdomen, like the female's, they are more prone to injury. Suspended at a variable (and temperature-dependent) distance from the abdomen, the testicles can come into contact with objects that can hurt them.

The severity of the pain caused by a blow to the testicles is something that every male is familiar with from an early age. There can be no doubt about what happened when your testicles have been struck. Fortunately, however, lasting injury to the testicles is rare. The sponginess of their tissues and the flexibility of their location enable them to absorb considerable shock without permanent harm.

If your testicles have been struck by a blunt object or in a fall and the pain and any swelling of the scrotum go away within about an hour, there probably is no serious damage. If the scrotum remains swollen or is bruised, however, or if the pain persists, seek medical care promptly.

If your scrotum has been struck and penetrated by a sharp object, visit an emergency room immediately.

The same precautions apply in the case of babies and children. Persistent pain, swelling, or bruises signal the need to see a doctor promptly. A young male can become infertile from an untreated testicular injury even though he has not reached the age of sexual maturity at the time of the injury.

There are many causes of pain in the testicles other than injury. Most of these causes are described in this chapter. The important thing to remember is this: if severe pain persists, see a doctor or go to an emergency room. Untreated testicular injury or other conditions affecting the testicles can have serious complications such as blood clots, infertility, or even loss of a testicle. (Loss of a single testicle does not cause impotence, infertility, or loss of sex drive or other male characteristics.)

failure. These are often effective in cases of delayed puberty or lack of sex drive.

EPIDIDYMITIS

Signs and Symptoms
- Pain in the scrotum, generally severe, which develops gradually over several hours or days;
- Fever;
- Swelling.

At the rear of each testicle is a coiled tube that transports sperm to the vas deferens. This tube is the epididymis. Epididymitis is inflammation of this tube. The swollen area will feel hot and sausage-shaped to the touch. Epididymitis usually is caused by bacteria. Sometimes it also can arise from nonbacterial unknown causes.

The Diagnosis. Pain about the testicles that develops over several hours and is accompanied by fever suggests epididymitis. Usually, only one testicle is affected. The physician may take a urine sample and a sample of prostate gland secretions to identify the infecting organism.

How Serious Is Epididymitis? Epididymitis usually is an acute ailment that can be corrected with medication without any damage to the genital organs. Occasionally, chronic epididymitis develops, and this requires surgical treatment for relief of symptoms.

Treatment. *Medication.* Antibiotics generally are prescribed to combat epididymitis that is of bacterial origin. Because your sex partner may be infected with the same bacteria, similar treatment of your partner will probably be necessary.

Other Therapies. Treatment for epididymitis also includes bed rest, application of ice packs to the scrotum, elevating the scrotum, and use of analgesic agents to relieve pain.

SCROTAL MASSES

Signs and Symptoms
- Lump or swelling in the scrotum;
- Possible local pain or tenderness.

Scrotal masses have various causes. These include tumors, cysts and other inflammations, physical injury, and inguinal hernia.

The tumors may be either benign or malignant. Tumors growing within the testicles themselves most often are malignant (cancerous); those located elsewhere within the scrotum are usually benign (noncancerous). Cancer of the testicles is discussed later in this chapter.

A common type of painless, benign cyst is the spermatic cyst or spermatocele. It grows adjacent to the epididymis near the top of a testicle. Hydrocele and varicocele, described later in this chapter (see pages 1116 and 1117, respectively), also are painless, benign sources of scrotal swelling. Hematocele is a scrotal mass caused by physical injury, and it consists of an accumulation of blood. With an inguinal hernia, a portion of the intestine may drop into the scrotum and cause it to bulge.

The Diagnosis. Every scrotal mass should be evaluated by a physician. If the mass is a tumor, it could be malignant. The tumor must be removed surgically before an accurate diagnosis can be made. Blood tests and a painless ultrasound examination (see page 1287) help to distinguish the many harmless causes of scrotal masses from tumors.

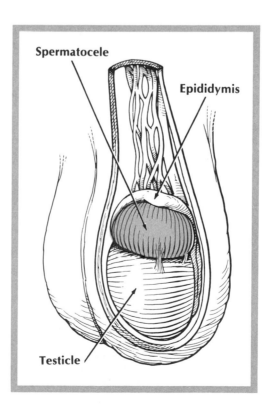

A common, painless and benign growth, called a spermatocele, may occur atop the testicle.

How Serious Are Scrotal Masses? Malignant tumors are serious. If detected before the cancer spreads (see Self-Examination of the Testicles, below), they usually can be treated effectively. The various other causes of scrotal masses are generally not serious and, apart from inguinal hernia, do not require treatment.

Treatment. *Surgery.* If you have a testicular tumor, surgical removal of the tumor is necessary. Testicular cancer requires surgical removal of the entire testicle and possibly additional treatment as well.

Inguinal hernias generally require surgery (see Inguinal Hernias, page 671). Other causes of scrotal masses usually do not require any treatment.

HYDROCELE

Signs and Symptoms

• Soft, usually painless, swelling in the scrotum.

The term hydrocele comes from the Greek *hydro* for water and *cele* for tumor. A testicular hydrocele is a collection of watery fluid in the sheath that holds the testicle. Normally, this sheath contains just enough fluid to lubricate the testicle. The larger amount, which makes the hydrocele, develops either because the body produces too much fluid or because it does not absorb enough fluid. Hydroceles are a common cause of scrotal swelling and may occur with one or both testicles. Hydroceles may occur at any age but are most common in older men.

The Diagnosis. To help differentiate a hydrocele from a tumor or other source of swelling, the physician will carefully feel the swollen area and probably will shine a light at the scrotum. If the swelling is a hydrocele, the light will shine through it. A painless ultrasound examination also may be performed.

How Serious Is a Hydrocele? A hydrocele is not serious. Treatment is usually not

---

SELF-EXAMINATION OF THE TESTICLES

Cancer of the testicles is a potential killer—but, if detected early, it can usually be cured.

A simple examination that takes only a minute or two can detect a growth in the testicles in its early stages. Like the breast self-examination for women, self-examination of the testicles is easy and important, and it may turn out to be life-saving. Because cancer of the testicles occurs more often in younger men than in older men, monthly self-examination of the testicles should begin at high-school age.

Perform the examination after a shower or warm bath, when the skin of the scrotum is loose and relaxed. Examine one testicle at a time. Grasp the testicle and roll it gently between your thumb and forefinger. As you do so, feel for any lump on the surface of the testicle. Also, notice if the testicle is enlarged, hardened, or otherwise different from what it was at the last examination. (A small firm area near the rear of the testicle is a normal part of the testicle; the cord leading upward from the top of the testicle is also a normal part of the scrotum and is not a growth.)

If you feel a lump on a testicle or any change in the testicle, this does not necessarily mean that you have cancer. But visit your physician soon to find out.

A regular self-examination of the testicles can identify dangerous growths early—in time for a cure. Grasp and roll the testicle between your thumb and forefinger, feeling for lumps, swelling, hardness, or other changes.

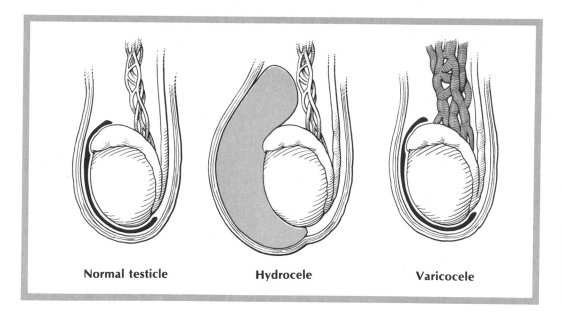

| Normal testicle | Hydrocele | Varicocele |

A hydrocele is a generally harmless but abnormal accumulation of watery fluid within the scrotum; the condition usually requires no treatment. A varicocele is a swelling within the scrotum due to a malfunction in varicose (enlarged) veins. To prevent infertility, this condition may require treatment.

required unless the scrotum is so swollen that it is uncomfortable.

Treatment. *Surgery.* Surgery is necessary when a hydrocele needs treatment. Also, the fluid can be drawn off (aspirated) with a needle and syringe. This procedure is simple but, because the fluid usually will accumulate again, it is seldom done. In addition, needle aspiration is potentially hazardous because of possible introduction of infection. Thus, aspiration should be used only in patients for whom surgery has too high a risk.

VARICOCELE

Signs and Symptoms
• Swelling in the scrotum, usually on the left side. The swelling is painless, and the area feels like a bag of worms. This sensation may nearly disappear when you lie down.

A varicocele is a swelling in the scrotum caused by varicose (enlarged) veins. The blood backs up in the veins leading from the testicles because of a problem with valves located inside the veins.

The Diagnosis. Your physician will carefully feel the swollen scrotum and may shine a light at the swollen area. If the problem is a varicocele, the light will not shine through the blood in the veins. A painless ultrasound examination also may be used.

How Serious Is a Varicocele? The varicocele itself is not a serious disorder. The problem is that the backed-up blood in the testicles can cause infertility. If this is the case, surgical tying off (ligation) of the varicocele can restore fertility.

Treatment. *Surgery.* When infertility is caused by a varicocele, surgery is necessary to ligate the varicocele. This surgical procedure often can be done on an outpatient basis. Unless a varicocele causes infertility, however, surgical ligation is rarely necessary.

ORCHITIS

Signs and Symptoms
• Pain in the scrotum;
• Swelling, generally on one side of the scrotum only;
• A feeling of weight in the scrotum.

Orchitis is an inflammation of the testicle. The most common cause of orchitis probably is the disease mumps, most often in adults who have mumps (see page 865). Orchitis also may occur due to infection of the prostate or the epididymis. Many diseases that are much less common may have orchitis among their manifestations.

The Diagnosis. Your physician will carefully feel the swelling in your scrotum. Because the symptoms of orchitis are similar to those of epididymitis (see page 1115) and other conditions affecting the testicles, your physician also may take a urine sample and perform other tests to identify other infections that may be associated with it.

How Serious Is Orchitis?   Orchitis can permanently damage one or both testicles to cause infertility and diminished size of the organ.

Treatment. *Medication.* Orchitis associated with bacterial infections generally is treated with antibiotics. However, orchitis associated with viral infections such as mumps is treated only by conservative means such as rest and medications to relieve pain.

UNDESCENDED TESTICLE

Signs and Symptoms
• Scrotum contains one rather than two testicles.

Before birth, the testicles develop inside the male infant's abdomen. Usually, they move down into their permanent place in the scrotum at about 1 month before birth. A small percentage of male infants are born with one or both testicles undescended.

In most of these babies, the testicles will move into the scrotum on their own during the first few years of life, without any medical intervention. In some cases, however, medication or surgery may be necessary. A testicle that remains undescended by age 5 years may become infertile later in life.

There are less common causes that may require extensive study for diagnosis. Sometimes, both testicles are present but one is smaller than normal.

The Diagnosis. Your physician can confirm the absence or the stunted development of a testicle by feeling the scrotum. Other tests may be required before determining the appropriate action for correcting the condition.

How Serious Is Undescended Testicle? The absence of a testicle is not serious. In the case of infants or young children, the condition often corrects itself or can be corrected with medication or surgery. After age 5, however, the situation can lead to later infertility. Even after it descends or after surgical correction, a testicle that was undescended will be more vulnerable to cancer than a normal testicle.

Treatment. *Medication.*   Hormones often are given to induce an undescended testicle to descend into the scrotum.

Surgery.   For testicles that do not descend early in life or in response to hormones, surgery is required to preserve future fertility and to lessen later vulnerability to testicular cancer. The best age for the treatment is 12 to 18 months.

CANCER OF THE TESTICLE

Signs and Symptoms
• A lump or swelling in a testicle;
• Possible local pain or tenderness;
• A heavy feeling in a testicle (sometimes).

Cancer of the testicle often begins in the cells that produce sperm. The cancer first is noticed as a pea-sized hard lump on the testicle. This lump usually is not painful to the touch. In the early stages, there are no other symptoms. Most men discover the tumor themselves (see Self-Examination of the Testicles, page 1116). The earlier this discovery is made, the better. Usually, the cancer affects only one testicle.

Cancer of testicle

A painless lump in the testicle may indicate cancer. Consult your physician immediately. The earlier it is treated, the greater your chance of cure.

Testicular cancer is more common in younger men, particularly between ages 15 and 35, and it is more common in white men than in black men. If one or both testicles are undescended at birth, the risk of cancer in either testicle later in life is greater. If detected and treated early, testicular cancer often can be cured.

The Diagnosis. A self-examination can detect the presence of a possible growth or tumor within the scrotum. Regardless of whether or not pain is associated with the growth, if you discover such a lump visit your physician without delay. An ultrasound examination may be performed to confirm the diagnosis.

A tumor on the testicle is almost always malignant (cancerous), but examination by a physician is required to determine if in fact a tumor is present. Other conditions affecting the testicles and scrotum can produce a lump that feels quite similar (see Epididymitis, page 1115; Scrotal Masses, page 1115; Hydrocele, page 1116; Varicocele, page 1117; and Orchitis, page 1117), and some of them are harmless.

If you do have a tumor on a testicle, surgical removal is necessary. If the tumor is malignant, blood tests, x-rays, and other tests may be necessary to determine if the cancer has spread to other parts of the body.

How Serious Is Cancer of the Testicle? Overall, about 70 percent of the men who are found to have cancer of the testicle live for 5 years or more after treatment (5-year survival rate). However, this includes cancers discovered at a late stage. The most common type of testicular cancer, seminoma, can be cured in nearly all cases if it is discovered and treated early.

Treatment. *Surgery.* Surgical removal of the affected testicle is necessary. This does not imply any loss of manhood because the remaining healthy testicle can maintain the body's normal sexual and hormone-production functions. If both testicles are lost, infertility will result. However, male hormones given by injection about every 3 weeks will maintain an essentially normal sexual function.

Other Therapies. Radiation therapy and chemotherapy may be used to prevent the spread of cancer to other parts of the body or to combat it if spread has begun.

PENIS, URETHRA, AND BLADDER

The penis functions both as a sexual organ and to transport urine. Each function sometimes can be affected by infections and other problems. The urethra, a tube that runs the length of the penis through the center, transports semen and urine.

Urine originates in the kidneys (see page 882) and is conveyed by the ureters to the bladder, a storage pouch within the abdomen, before it is excreted from the body through the urethra. Although the distance from the bladder to the outside is much longer in men than in women, infecting organisms sometimes can travel the entire length of the urethra into the bladder.

CYSTITIS

Signs and Symptoms
- Painful urination (a burning or itching feeling);
- Frequent or urgent need to urinate;
- Cloudy, malodorous, bloody urine (sometimes);
- Lower abdominal pain (sometimes);
- Slight fever (sometimes).

Cystitis is an inflammation of the bladder, usually the result of an infection. The term comes from the Greek word *cyst* for bladder. Rarely, the inflammation is caused by something other than an infection, such as in interstitial cystitis. Because of the length of the urethra in men, when men develop cystitis it often is caused by some problem, such as an enlarged prostate, that has interfered with the urinary tract.

Cystitis is uncommon in men. Although it is easy to treat, the underlying problem must be treated as well to avoid recurrence.

The Diagnosis. A urologist will diagnose cystitis based on the description of the symptoms and on tests. These tests may include analysis of urine, cystoscopy (visualization of the urethra and bladder with a special viewing device) (see page 904), and a special type of x-ray called an intravenous pyelogram (IVP, see page 885). Cultures of the urine may be needed to identify the bacteria that may be causing the infection.

How Serious Is Cystitis?   Cystitis is not serious if it is treated promptly and properly. If the cystitis and the underlying cause are not treated, however, the cystitis can become chronic and disabling.

Treatment. *Medication.*   Antibiotics are given to combat the infection that causes the cystitis. Additional medications, or surgery, may be required to correct an associated underlying problem.

PENILE WARTS

Signs and Symptoms
• Warts on the shaft or head of the penis.

Warts on the penis are similar to warts found elsewhere on the body. All warts, including penile warts, are caused by a virus. This means that warts are contagious. Warts in the genital area can be transmitted to or received from one's partner during sexual activity. Consequently, if you have penile warts, both you and your sexual partner may require treatment.

The Diagnosis.   Penile warts are diagnosed on the basis of their appearance. Sometimes a growth on the penis may look like a wart but in reality be a symptom of a venereal disease or a malignant tumor. If

your physician suspects one of these other problems, tests will be performed to provide a diagnosis and to permit planning of effective treatment.

How Serious Are Penile Warts?   Penile warts are harmless. However, they should be treated because they can easily spread to a sexual partner and can also proliferate on your penis.

Treatment. *Medication.*   Your physician will prescribe a preparation (such as tincture of podophyllum resin) to apply to the warts in order to remove them. (Do not purchase over-the-counter wart paints yourself and apply them to the penis because they are designed for skin that is less sensitive than the skin of the penis.) Sometimes, more involved treatment is necessary to remove the warts, such as cryosurgery, laser surgery, or electrodesiccation surgery.

URETHRITIS

Signs and Symptoms
• Burning pain when urinating or ejaculating;
• Need to urinate frequently;
• Discharge from the tip of the penis.

Urethritis is an inflammation of the urethra, the duct in the penis through which urine and semen pass. It often is caused by a sexually transmitted disease, particularly gonorrhea or chlamydiosis (see page 875). Sometimes the cause is unknown. The discharge that often is associated with urethritis can vary in color from clear to yellow and can vary in consistency from thin to thick. Urethritis generally is easy to cure. The affected person's sexual partner probably should be treated as well. Urethritis is sometimes associated with a form of arthritis called Reiter's syndrome (see page 1001).

The Diagnosis.   Pain on urination and a discharge from the penis are reasons to visit a physician. He or she will test both the urine and the discharge fluid to identify the infecting organism.

How Serious Is Urethritis?   In most cases of urethritis the infection goes away after treatment. Sometimes, repeated treatments are necessary. In a small number of cases,

---

NONINFECTIOUS URETHRAL DISCHARGE

This rare but disconcerting condition may occur in men who abruptly cease normal sexual activity, perhaps due to the illness of their partner or some other reason not having to do with the man's own health. A man with noninfectious urethral discharge may observe spots on his undershorts or a urethral discharge during bowel movements.

The discharge is merely the passage of normal prostatic fluid. It will cease over time or upon resumption of his usual sexual patterns.

the urethritis resists treatment and urethral stricture, epididymitis, prostatitis, or other complications will occur.

Treatment. *Medication.* Antibiotics are given to treat urethritis. The sexual partner probably also will require treatment.

URETHRAL STRICTURE

Signs and Symptoms
- Difficulty urinating;
- Painful urination.

Urethral stricture is a narrowing of the urethra (the narrow tube through the penis that transports urine and semen) to such a degree that the passage of urine is impeded. This is a rare condition. There are various causes of urethral stricture, including injury to the penis or disease that produces scar tissue which gradually shrinks and narrows the urethral passage. In extreme instances, the passage can even be blocked. Urethral stricture may become evident a number of years after an acute episode of gonorrhea.

The Diagnosis. Visit a urologist if you have difficulty or pain in urinating. A number of infections and conditions other than urethral stricture can be responsible. Your physician will examine your penis and may perform various tests, including examination of the urethra with a thin, flexible instrument called a cystoscope (see page 904).

How Serious Is Urethral Stricture? To restore the ability to urinate normally and painlessly, the urethral stricture must be treated. Usually, the first approach is to stretch the urethra by dilating it with a thin instrument (called a sound) that is inserted into the urethra; local anesthesia is used. This treatment must be repeated a number of times. If the passageway does not remain adequate after repeated dilations, a surgical procedure may be necessary.

The severity of the stricture usually is monitored by using the cystoscope. If a surgical procedure is performed, it is done with special instruments through the cystoscope.

BALANITIS

Signs and Symptoms
- Irritation and redness of the end of the penis.

Balanitis is an inflammation of the glans or tip of the penis. Balanitis is a fairly common genital ailment. It is more frequent in uncircumcised males, particularly if the foreskin is narrowed so that it cannot be retracted easily, than in those who have been circumcised.

There are various types of balanitis. The underlying causes include urinary tract infection, irritation from clothing that rubs against the penis or from chemicals used in cleaning or manufacturing the clothing, and reaction to contraceptive creams. Men with diabetes are especially prone to balanitis as a result of the high sugar content of their urine. Yeast infection also is a common cause.

The Diagnosis. If you have a penis irritation that does not go away in a day or two, visit your physician or a urologist. Your physician will examine your penis and may perform tests to rule out other, more serious, types of infection. If balanitis is diagnosed, your physician probably will analyze your urine to see if you have diabetes.

Treatment. The principal treatment for balanitis is cleanliness (see Hygiene for Men, below). In an uncircumcised man whose foreskin cannot be easily retracted, circumcision may be needed to prevent or relieve balanitis. Use of antibiotics or antifungal

---

HYGIENE FOR MEN

Wash your penis and scrotum the same way you wash other parts of your body: with soap and water every day. If your penis is uncircumcised, don't forget to pull back the foreskin and clean the head of the penis beneath it. These basic hygienic practices will help keep the genitals clean and free from minor infections.

Look for signs of disease as you clean. Possible trouble signs include sores or growths. If you find any, visit a doctor (see Self-Examination of the Testicles, page 1116).

Washing will not prevent acquiring a sexually transmitted disease, however. For suggestions on avoiding venereal disease, see Venereal Disease in Men, page 1122.

VENEREAL DISEASE IN MEN

Venereal (sexually transmitted) diseases can have tragic consequences. Venereal diseases are transmitted by contact with an infected person through sexual intercourse, anal intercourse, or oral sexual activity. In the case of AIDS (acquired immune deficiency syndrome) possible routes of transmission are infected semen, saliva, and blood, particularly blood on hypodermic needles shared by infected drug addicts. The symptoms of a venereal disease do not develop immediately after invasion by the organism, and the course and consequences of the disease vary with the disease itself (see Sexually Transmitted Diseases, page 875, and AIDS, page 848).

Wearing a condom during sexual activity offers much protection against acquiring or passing along a venereal disease. However, use of condoms does not offer foolproof protection from venereal diseases. The only certain way to avoid acquiring a venereal disease is to engage in sexual activity only with a trusted, noninfected partner.

PRIAPISM

This very rare condition occurs as a result of some type of spinal cord disorder, of leukemia, or of inflammation of the urethra. It is a sustained, often painful, erection that occurs without sexual stimulation.

In priapism, the penile shaft is firm but the head of the penis (glans) is soft. The penis becomes filled with blood as during a normal erection, but the blood does not drain out and the erection does not go away as it normally would after sexual activity or stimulation ceases. The name priapism derives from the Latin name for a male fertility god in classical mythology, Priapus.

If you have a painful erection that does not go away, seek medical help. Prompt treatment is necessary to preserve the ability of your penis to have a normal erection. Your physician will examine the penis and perform tests to determine the underlying cause.

agents may be required to cure bacterial or yeast infections.

CURVATURE OF THE PENIS

Signs and Symptoms

- Painful (sometimes) bend in the penis that develops during an erection and makes sexual intercourse difficult or impossible.

Curvature of the penis, also known as Peyronie's disease after the French physician who first described it, mainly affects men ages 40 to 60. Scar tissue (or plaque) forms inside the penis around the cylindrical structures that run the length of the penis and fill with blood during an erection. Why the scar tissue forms is not understood.

The Diagnosis. If you have curvature of the penis, you can feel the plaque that causes it as a ridge running along the penis beneath the skin.

How Serious Is Curvature of the Penis? The symptoms often are mild and do not always grow worse with time. In many cases, the disease goes away on its own, but this may require several years. Various treatments have been tried without any real proof of success. The best approach is to give the condition a chance to improve on its own. If it does not, consult a urologist.

PARAPHIMOSIS

Signs and Symptoms

- Painful swelling in the end of an uncircumcised penis;
- Retracted foreskin that cannot be pulled back over the head of the penis to cover it.

Emergency Symptoms

- Severe swelling in the end of an uncircumcised penis.

Paraphimosis occurs when the foreskin of an uncircumcised penis becomes trapped in the retracted position and cannot be returned over the glans or head of the penis. Consult a urologist or an emergency room physician immediately. Surgical treatment by circumcision or partial circumcision will probably be necessary to release the foreskin. If treatment is prompt, permanent damage to the penis generally can be avoided.

CANCER OF THE PENIS

Signs and Symptoms

- Pimple-like, painless sore on the penis, particularly at the end;
- Other types of painless sores or warts on the penis.

Cancer of the penis is rare. When it occurs, it most often affects uncircumcised males who do not keep the area beneath their foreskin clean. In its early stages, small, painless growths occur on the penis, usually near its end. Without surgical removal and tests, these growths may be indistinguishable from the ordinary penile warts which are harmless. As the malignant growth progresses, there may be pain and bleeding.

The Diagnosis. Any growth on the penis is a good reason to see a urologist promptly. Through examination and possible surgical removal and tests of the growth, your doctor can determine whether or not the growth is malignant. If it is found to be malignant, more tests will be necessary to see whether the cancer has spread to other parts of your body and to plan the best treatment to combat spread.

How Serious Is Cancer of the Penis?
As with any other form of cancer, cancer of the penis can be life-threatening. The earlier it is detected and treated, the better are the chances for curing it.

Treatment. *Surgery.* Removal of the malignant growth, and possibly of adjacent portions of the penis, will be required. If a large portion of the penis must be removed, as with an advanced cancer, often a portion can be left that is sufficient for sexual activity and urination.

Other Therapies. Radiation therapy and chemotherapy may be used to prevent or to combat the spread of the disease to other parts of the body.

URINARY INCONTINENCE

Signs and Symptoms
- Inability to control urination, some or all of the time;
- Involuntary urination upon coughing, sneezing, laughing, running, or other physical activity involving the abdominal muscles (called stress incontinence).

Urinary incontinence—the inability to keep urine in your body until you decide to release it—can have several different causes. The muscular and neural systems that control the retention or release of urine are complex, and they can be affected by illness, medications, urinary tract infections, prostate gland problems, an operation on the urinary tract, and even psychological factors such as depression, anger, or confusion. Fatigue and immobilization also have an effect.

In children, problems of bed-wetting are common (see page 1015). After puberty, however, urinary incontinence is rare until the late decades of life. It is estimated that a third or more of elderly people who are hospitalized or live in long-term-care facilities are incontinent. Among older persons living at home, the percentage is much smaller, around 10 percent. Urinary incontinence is more frequent in women than in men.

In many cases, bladder control can be regained by treating the underlying cause, by use of drugs, or by modifying daily habits. If urinary incontinence persists, special aids are also available to help manage the problem.

The Diagnosis. The symptoms of urinary incontinence are obvious. First, visit a urologist. This physician will ask questions about the medications you take, operations you have undergone, and infections that you may have experienced. Your penis, rectum, and abdominal area will be examined, and a urine specimen will be taken for analysis. Sometimes, a painless ultrasound examination, a special x-ray called an intravenous pyelogram (IVP, see page 885), or cystoscopic examination (see page 904) may be required.

How Serious Is Urinary Incontinence?
People with urinary incontinence often withdraw socially. This is unfortunate. Normal daily hygiene and appropriate use and changing of pads or diapers generally will prevent offensive odors. Treatments are available, and there are ways to live with the problem if it persists.

Other risks include infectious reactions to urine on the skin or to the catheters sometimes used to control incontinence.

Treatment. *Self-Help.* Your physician may advise specific exercises to strengthen the pelvic area or bladder training techniques to regain control of urination. Often, a simple adjustment in daily routine—such as altering the times that you take medication or the hours you sleep—can make the difference. With some people, remembering to go to the bathroom is difficult, and use of an alarm can help. It is also handy to have a urinal nearby if the bathroom is distant or if handicaps make getting there in time a problem.

When incontinence cannot be eliminated, special aids can help. Absorbent undergarments are available that neutralize the odor of urine and keep the skin fairly dry. Devices can be used to catch the urine, such as a type of condom that fits over the penis and drains urine through a tube into a plastic bag. There is also a type of foam rubber clamp that can be worn around the penis, which occasionally is helpful. For more difficult cases, a catheter is placed through the penis to the bladder, to drain the urine to an external plastic bag (the plastic bags are emptied and cleaned or changed as needed).

Medication. Your physician may prescribe medications to combat incontinence.

Surgery. The underlying cause of the incontinence, such as prostate gland problems, sometimes requires surgical correction (see below). In some types of incontinence problems, your urologist may recommend a surgically implanted artificial sphincter which allows the patient to control its open (voiding) and closed (continent) settings.

DISORDERS OF THE PROSTATE GLAND

The prostate gland is located within the pelvis, beneath the bladder. It surrounds the urethra, the duct through which urine passes. This gland plays an important function in reproduction by contributing fluids to the semen that, among other things, appear to improve the survival of ejaculated sperm within the vagina's acidic environment. As men age, it is common for the prostate gland to enlarge and thus interfere with urination. This can be corrected surgically. Other prostate problems covered in this section include infections (prostatitis) and cancer.

ENLARGED PROSTATE

Signs and Symptoms
- Need to urinate frequently;
- Difficulty in starting to urinate;
- Decreased strength and force of urine stream;
- Inability to sleep through the night without getting up to urinate;
- Dribbling after the end of urination.

Emergency Symptoms
- Complete inability to urinate.

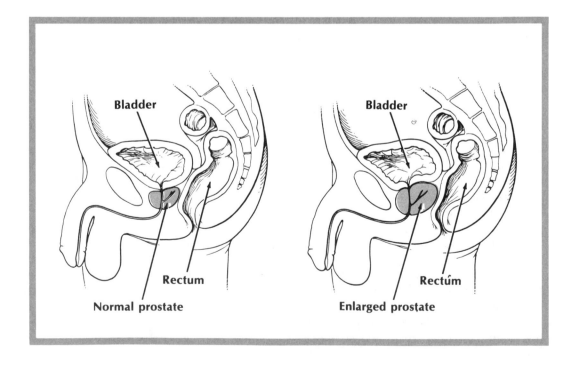

An enlarged prostate can produce difficulty in urination because the flow of urine is restricted.

The prostate gland, present only in males, has an important sexual function: contributing fluids to the semen used to transport sperm. As a normal result of aging, the prostate gland often enlarges, starting in the late 40s. Because it surrounds the urethra, growth of the prostate can restrict the flow of urine through the urethra during urination. If the enlargement is sufficient, the restriction can lead to the symptoms described above.

An enlarged prostate gland is also called benign prostatic hypertrophy. The word "benign" distinguishes this condition from cancerous growth of the prostate, which can also occur (see Cancer of the Prostate, page 1126). The word "hypertrophy" means an increase in size.

The National Institutes of Health reports that more than four of every five men between the ages of 50 and 60 have benign enlargement of the prostate gland. However, only about 1 in 10 of them will require a surgical procedure to relieve the obstruction caused by the enlarged gland, although the probability of an operation being required to remove the prostate at some time during a man's life now is estimated to be between one in four or five.

Many men with an enlarged prostate gland will have occasional pain and disability. The symptoms vary in severity, from slight difficulty in urinating to nearly complete loss of control of urination. Men are usually annoyed by the symptoms, and in some cases they are alarmed by them. As the enlargement continues, the symptoms usually worsen, often insidiously. However, this condition can be readily corrected by an operation, generally without complications.

The Diagnosis. If you have an enlarged prostate gland, in all likelihood you will notice some of the symptoms listed above and will ask your physician about them. Your physician can examine your prostate by inserting a gloved finger well into the rectum and feeling the gland with it. Also, a urine test may be performed, the bladder may be examined with a cystoscope (see page 904), or an ultrasound scan of the prostate gland may be made (see page 1287). An important consideration is determining if the enlargement is benign or malignant (cancerous).

How Serious Is an Enlarged Prostate?
An enlarged, noncancerous prostate gland is not serious unless its growth progresses to the extent that urination is extremely difficult or impossible, the bladder becomes infected (cystitis), or the kidneys are damaged as a result of the backed-up urine.

The condition can be corrected surgically, most often with a transurethral prostate resection (see below). This procedure is successful in most cases. In a small number of instances, however, it can lead to an inability to control urination or the loss of sexual potency.

Treatment. Surgical treatment can decrease the size of the prostate gland, or it can remove it and thus eliminate the condition. Today, the most common surgical procedure is transurethral prostate resection

TRANSURETHRAL PROSTATE RESECTION

The surgical procedure now chosen by most urologists to decrease the size of an enlarged prostate is transurethral prostate resection. The word "transurethral" refers to the fact that the procedure is done via the urethra, the tube that transports the urine from the bladder through the penis. The patient is anesthetized, generally with a spinal anesthetic but sometimes with a general anesthetic. Then, a thin tube called a resectoscope or operating cystoscope is carefully inserted into the urethra and manipulated so that its end, where the electric cutting device is located, enters the prostate.

This device is equipped with a miniature telescope. While viewing the urinary tract through the telescope, the urologist controls the cutting device and carefully removes small pieces of the enlarged part of the prostate gland. In effect, the urologist cores out a channel for an unhindered flow of urine.

After the operation, the resectoscope is removed and a catheter is inserted through the urethra into the bladder, where it remains for a day or two so that the bladder can void while the enlarged channel heals. The hospital stay generally is about a week.

Transurethral prostate resection usually relieves all of the symptoms caused by the enlarged prostate without complications. After prostate surgery, it is common for some or all of the semen to enter the bladder rather than be ejaculated through the penis during sexual activity (known as retrograde ejaculation, described on page 1144). There is no harm in this—the semen is then voided with the urine—but it can impair fertility. In some cases the prostate again becomes enlarged, requiring another operation. In rare cases, prostate surgery can lead to impotence or to complete inability to control urination.

(TUR), which is performed without any incision in the abdomen. Sometimes, however, because of the size of the gland, surgical removal of the prostate through the abdomen is necessary.

Physicians are evaluating a new technique in which a small balloon is introduced through the penis into the prostate and inflated, thus enlarging the opening through the prostate.

In the future, medicines that shrink the prostate gland may become available.

ACUTE PROSTATITIS

Signs and Symptoms
- Sudden moderate to high fever;
- Chills;
- Urination is frequent and difficult;
- Urgent need to urinate;
- Pain in the lower back and in the area between the rectum and the testicles;
- Pain or a burning sensation while urinating;
- Blood in the urine (sometimes).

Acute prostatitis is a sudden infection of the prostate gland (acute means sudden). A portion of the prostate, or all of it, will be inflamed. Acute prostatitis often leads to cystitis as well. It requires prompt treatment. Abscesses can develop in the prostate and, in extreme cases, the flow of urine can be blocked altogether.

The Diagnosis.   If you have symptoms of acute prostatitis, visit a physician without delay. Your physician will examine your prostate gland with a gloved finger inserted into your rectum. In acute prostatitis, the gland will be extremely tender. Also, a urine sample will be obtained for the tests needed to identify the bacteria causing the infection.

How Serious Is Acute Prostatitis?   Untreated acute prostatitis can lead to abscesses of the prostate or complete retention of urine. Acute prostatitis generally can be corrected with antibiotics. In severe cases, hospitalization may be necessary. Although acute prostatitis is generally cured, in some cases chronic prostatitis follows.

Treatment.   *Medication.*   Antibiotics, given by mouth or intravenously, are used to treat acute prostatitis.

CHRONIC PROSTATITIS

Signs and Symptoms
- Urination is frequent and difficult;
- Urgent need to urinate;
- Pain in the pelvis and genital area;
- Fever, chills, painful ejaculation, blood in the urine (occasionally).

Chronic prostatitis (chronic means long-lasting or recurring) is an infection of the prostate gland. In some cases chronic prostatitis follows acute prostatitis. The symptoms generally are milder than those of acute prostatitis. This ailment may or may not be associated with other urinary tract infections.

The Diagnosis.   If you have the symptoms of chronic prostatitis, visit your physician who will examine your prostate gland with a gloved finger inserted into the rectum. A urine sample will be taken for tests to identify the infecting organism. Other tests also may be required.

How Serious Is Chronic Prostatitis?
Chronic prostatitis affects different people to different degrees. The symptoms can range from discomfort to pain. Chronic prostatitis sometimes is due to bacteria that can cause, or have spread from, other urinary tract infections which should be eliminated.

Treatment.   *Self-Help.*   Hot sitz baths sometimes provide relief from the symptoms of chronic prostatitis. Massage of the prostate by a physician formerly was a frequent means of treatment but is less commonly used today.

Medication.   Antibiotics are often given to treat chronic prostatitis. Sometimes, anticholinergic drugs are used to relieve symptoms.

CANCER OF THE PROSTATE

Signs and Symptoms
- Decreased strength of urine stream;
- Dribbling after the end of urination;
- Difficulty starting to urinate;
- Hip or back pain;
- Urination or ejaculation is painful;
- Blood or pus in the urine.

Cancer of the prostate gland is common—it ranks third among the types of cancer that kill American men. Its symptoms also overlap with those of benign (noncancerous) prostate gland enlargement, a very common condition among middle-aged and older men, which means that prostate cancer may be mistaken for benign prostate enlargement, giving the disease time to spread.

Prostate cancer is most frequent in men ages 60 to 80. It is more common in black men than in white men. Its cause is unknown. The prostate enlargement that is common as men get older does not lead to prostate cancer.

If detected early, cancer of the prostate can be cured. It can be detected early, before it causes symptoms, by digital rectal examination, a routine procedure in which the physician inserts a gloved finger into the rectum and feels the prostate gland. This examination should be performed during the regular checkup in men 40 or more years old.

Once the symptoms of prostate cancer begin to appear, cure is less likely. This is why the regular digital examination is so important.

The Diagnosis. Prostate cancer is best found by the digital rectal examination during the regular checkup. If a hard lump is present on the gland, other tests, such as x-rays and blood and urine analyses, are performed. A small portion of the prostate gland will be removed for examination under a microscope to determine if it is malignant. This sample is often taken with a needle inserted through the skin between the scrotum and the rectum or through the surface of the rectum itself; local anesthesia is used for this procedure.

If the sample proves malignant, more tests will be required to determine whether the cancer has spread to other parts of the body and to plan a treatment program.

Sometimes the presence of cancer will not be apparent on digital examination and the diagnosis of cancer will be established only on microscopic examination of the tissue removed during the course of operation. A blood test may indicate an abnormality, but usually only after the cancer has spread beyond the gland itself.

Cancer of the prostate tends to spread to the bones, and occasionally the diagnosis is made in the course of investigating progressive back pain. Bone scans are often used to determine whether the malignancy has spread to the skeleton.

How Serious Is Cancer of the Prostate?
If found early, cancer of the prostate can be cured. When the cancer has had time to spread to other sites in the body, cure is still possible but less likely. Treatment is then directed primarily at slowing the progress of the disease and relieving symptoms.

Treatment. Surgery. Surgical removal of the prostate gland is often called for if the disease has not spread. If the disease is advanced, orchiectomy (surgical removal of the testicles, sometimes referred to as castration) may be recommended to eliminate the male hormones that promote the growth of prostate cancer. Orchiectomy generally causes impotence. An alternative to orchiectomy is administration of female sex hormones.

Other Therapies. Radiation therapy is sometimes used if the cancer remains confined to the prostate. If the cancer has spread, a combination of chemotherapy and radiation therapy may be used.

Promising new drugs for use in treating prostate cancer that has spread are now available. These medications block the production of male hormones. They include leuprolide and flutamide.

SEXUAL PROBLEMS OF MEN

These problems include difficulties in achieving an erection, ejaculating too soon, and other problems associated with erection and ejaculation. Male sexual problems range in seriousness from quite minor to some that may be very damaging to one's self-image or sex life. Fortunately, effective treatment is available.

The cause of and the solution to such sexual problems frequently involve the sexual partner as well (see Health Problems of Partners, page 1129).

CHAPTER 36

HEALTH PROBLEMS OF PARTNERS

CHAPTER CONTENTS

NORMAL REPRODUCTION

In normal reproduction, the sperm (the male reproductive cell) fuses with the egg (the female reproductive cell). Genetic information contained in the two parent cells mixes. From this fused cell, an embryo begins to develop; 9 months later, after the embryo has undergone incredible development within the uterus of the mother, a baby is born. To understand the workings and the problems of the reproductive systems, we must understand the steps that must occur for successful fertilization.

Sperm cells are produced by the male's testicles under the influence of male hor-

During each menstrual cycle, an egg is released by one of the ovaries. This is called ovulation. The egg travels into the fallopian tube. If fertilization is to occur, sperm ejaculated into the vagina must swim up through the uterus and into the fallopian tube, where the sperm penetrates the egg (see insets). The fertilized egg travels into the uterus, where it imbeds itself in the wall of the uterus (endometrium).

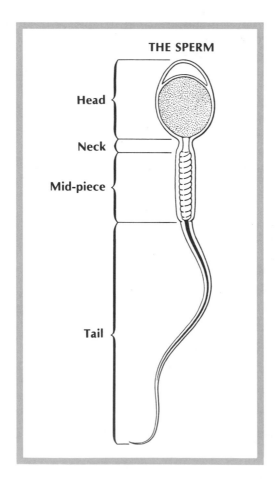

THE SPERM

mones. From the testicles, the sperm travel through several internal organs before they reach the penis. These organs include the prostate gland and the seminal vesicles, which secrete fluids that create a healthy environment in which the sperm can live. The mixture of these fluids and the sperm, known as semen, is stored in the seminal vesicles until ejaculation.

During sexual intercourse, semen is ejaculated from the penis into the vagina. Although sperm comprise only a small portion of semen, a single ejaculation contains as many as a quarter billion of them. Each sperm cell is equipped with a long whip-like tail that provides mobility to enable it to reach the egg. Many sperm are produced because few, if any, survive to reach the egg.

In the female, eggs are produced by the two ovaries. At birth, every female has a supply of egg cells in each ovary that will be released during her sexually mature stage of life. During each menstrual cycle, one of the ovaries releases one, and occasionally more, of these eggs.

Once released, the egg must travel a short distance from the ovary to the entrance of a fallopian tube, which joins an ovary and the uterus (or womb) and is used to transport the egg. The egg travels slowly, requiring several days to travel through the tube. If a sperm cell is able to "swim" successfully from the point in the vagina where it left the penis all the way up through the uterus and into the fallopian tube, fertilization can occur.

Once a single sperm successfully penetrates the egg, a membrane forms around the egg to prevent any other sperm from entering it. The fertilized egg then continues its passage down the fallopian tube for several more days, dividing and growing as it travels. When the fertilized egg reaches the interior of the uterus, it implants itself in the wall of the uterus. This embryo, or fetus, will develop from this point until birth (or miscarriage). (For further discussion of the function and malfunction of the reproductive organs, see pages 167, 1053, and 1111.)

INFERTILITY

Infertility is a common problem in partners. Fortunately, major advances have been made in recent decades, and the problem of infertility can be solved in many cases. This section outlines the methods used in the evaluation of infertility, the major causes of it, and the various options for treating it. The section concludes with ethical considerations of fertility therapy.

Problems of infertility can include problems with the sperm, problems with the egg, or difficulties encountered in their union. Infertility problems also can result from sexual dysfunction, which is discussed later in this chapter. To physicians, the term infertility usually means the inability to become pregnant after 1 year of frequent sexual intercourse without using any contraception. Three out of four fertile couples will become pregnant within this time.

For many couples, "under-fertility" is often a better term—that is, despite the absence of pregnancy, fertility is still possible, but the odds are not as good as they might be (for example, more than a year might be required before pregnancy occurs).

Note that infertility is not the same thing as sterility, which means the inability to conceive a child under any circumstances. With infertility, the possibility of conceiving a child has by no means been ruled out. To many people and their physicians, the diagnosis of infertility may best be regarded as a challenge.

MAGNITUDE OF THE PROBLEM

About 10 to 15 percent of couples are infertile (according to the definition given above). Of these couples, the man is the infertile partner in about 30 percent of cases and contributes to the infertility problem in an additional 20 percent of cases; the woman is infertile 50 to 70 percent of the time. In both men and women, various factors can account for infertility.

EVALUATION

If you and your partner are unable to achieve conception within a reasonable time and would like to do so, seek help. The woman's gynecologist, the man's urologist, or the family physician can determine whether there is a fertility problem that requires a specialist or clinic that treats infertility problems.

Although either partner or both partners can be infertile, physicians usually begin evaluation with the man because it is much easier to perform the tests necessary to evaluate male infertility. The woman's tests not only are more complex but also entail more risk. If tests for the man do not find a source of the infertility, then the woman can be evaluated.

Before embarking on infertility tests, a couple should be aware that a certain amount of commitment is required. The physician or clinic will need to determine exactly what your sexual habits are and, moreover, may make recommendations about how you should change those habits. The tests and periods of trial and error may extend over several months. Evaluation is expensive and in some cases entails operations and uncomfortable procedures, and the expenses may not be reimbursable by many medical plans. Depending on the cause, there is no guarantee, even after all the tests and counseling, that conception will occur.

However, for couples eager to have their own child, such evaluation is the route to take. It may result in a successful pregnancy.

Tests for the Man.

For a man to be fertile, his testicles must produce enough sperm, the sperm must be able to pass unobstructed through his body, and the sperm must be ejaculated effectively into the woman's vagina. Tests for the man attempt to determine whether any of these steps are impeded.

The first step is a general physical examination. This includes examination of the genitals and questions concerning your medical history, illnesses or disabilities, medications, and sexual habits.

Your physician probably will require a specimen of ejaculated semen. This is generally obtained by masturbating, or interrupting intercourse, and ejaculating the semen into a clean container. Your physician will provide instructions. Such a specimen may be required more than once.

The semen is then analyzed by a laboratory, and the quantity, color, and presence of infections or blood are noted. Principally, however, the analysis is of the sperm themselves. The laboratory will determine whether the number of sperm present in the ejaculate is enough for fertility and whether the shape, appearance, and motility (activity) of the sperm indicate that they are healthy enough for fertility. A needle biopsy of the testicle is often the most definitive way to identify the cause of an abnormal result of semen examination. This usually can be performed in a urologist's office.

Other tests also are required sometimes, such as a blood test to determine the level of testosterone or other hormones.

Tests for the Woman.

If tests for the man do not reveal the cause of infertility, testing for the woman is the next step. For a woman to be fertile, her ovaries must release healthy eggs regularly and her reproductive tract must allow the eggs and sperm unobstructed passage for a possible union in the fallopian tubes.

A general physical examination is the first step. This includes an ordinary gynecological examination (see page 1055). Your physician will ask many questions concerning your health history, illnesses, medications, menstrual cycle, and sexual habits.

Specific fertility tests follow. The first thing that your physician must establish is that healthy eggs are released. There are different methods of making this determination. In a common method, temperature charting, you take your temperature each morning before rising and record the temperature on a chart during one complete menstrual cycle. The temperature normally rises slightly when ovulation—the release of an egg—occurs.

Another test you can do is a home LH-monitoring test. LH refers to luteinizing hormone, which affects ovulation and the preparation of the uterus for receiving a fertilized egg. This simple urine test makes it possible for you to monitor the hormone yourself.

Another useful test is the cervical mucus test. This test is performed at about the time when ovulation should occur, and at a time between 2 and 16 hours after intercourse. The physician takes a tiny sample of the mucus lining your cervix, which is the lower portion of the uterus where it meets the vagina. The procedure is painless. The sample is examined under a microscope to determine how well sperm penetrate and survive.

Endometrial biopsy, another test, can help to determine whether and when ovulation is occurring and whether the lining of the uterus is hormonally prepared. In this test, the physician takes a small sample of tissue from the uterine lining shortly before the beginning of the menstrual period.

A blood test is sometimes performed to determine the levels of hormones involved in successful ovulation and, sometimes, to look for infections.

Once one or more of these tests has been performed, your physician will know whether ovulation occurs and whether sperm can survive in the reproductive tract. If no problems have been uncovered, additional information may be needed.

Hysteroscopy is a procedure in which a small instrument is used to examine the interior of the cervix and uterus for irregularities that might lead to infertility.

Hysterosalpingography is a test that also is used to evaluate the condition of the uterus as well as the fallopian tubes. This test sometimes is done under general anesthesia. A fluid is injected into the uterus and an x-ray is obtained to determine whether the fluid progresses out of the uterus and up the fallopian tubes. Blockages or problems often can be located, and these can be corrected with medications or operation.

Another test is laparoscopy; it involves a brief operation, with either local or general anesthesia, to insert a thin viewing device to examine the fallopian tubes, ovaries, and uterus. A small incision is made beneath the navel, and a needle is inserted into the abdominal cavity; a small quantity of gas (usually carbon dioxide) is pumped into the abdomen to create a space for entry of a laparoscope, a thin, illuminated telescope.

Through the telescope, the physician can spot blockages or irregularities of the fallopian tubes and uterus; often, a dye is injected into the cervical canal and through the uterus and fallopian tubes to determine whether they are open. At the end of the procedure, the gas and laparoscope are drawn out and the incision is closed. The test may help to identify blockages or other problems that could be corrected surgically. This can be done either in the hospital or on an outpatient basis.

These are the primary types of tests used to determine the possible causes of female infertility. Not everyone needs to undergo all, or even many, of the tests before the cause is found. Which tests are used and their sequence depend on discussion and agreement between you and the physician or clinic involved.

In up to 20 percent of infertile women, regardless of which tests are used, no cause can be found.

CAUSES

The cause of infertility can involve the man, the woman, or both. The physical examinations and tests discussed above should help your physician or clinic to pinpoint the cause.

Sometimes the problem is not really one of infertility but a more general sexual problem. For example, an impotent man might be fertile if he could obtain an erection to have intercourse. Similarly, premature ejaculation, before the penis is very far into the vagina, greatly lessens the chances of a sperm meeting the egg. These and other general sexual problems are discussed in the section Sexuality and Sexual Dysfunction (see page 1137).

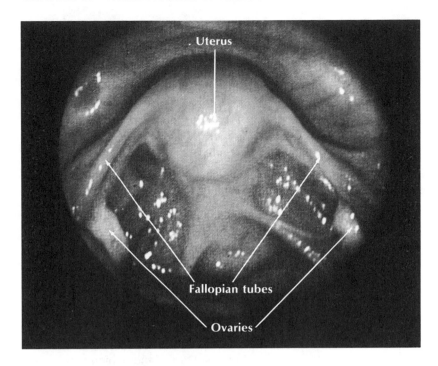

By using a laparoscope, your physician can visualize your uterus and other pelvic organs.

Aside from such basic mechanical problems, the prime cause of infertility in a man is likely to be a problem with the sperm. Azoospermia is the complete absence of sperm in the semen, generally due to a disorder of the testicles or a blockage in the passage leading from the testicles. In oligospermia, sperm are present in the semen but not in enough quantity to fertilize an egg readily. The causes of these and other disorders of the sperm include problems with the testicles, hormone disorders, and infections.

An important cause of male infertility is varicocele (see page 1117), a problem of varicose changes in veins surrounding the testicle, which can sometimes be corrected surgically. The varicosities prevent normal cooling of the blood reaching the testicles and thereby raise the testicular temperature—a factor that impairs sperm production. Several other problems with the testicles also can be responsible for infertility.

Hormone disorders often can be identified by a blood test, and these sometimes can be treated. Sexually transmitted diseases or other infections can block the passageways through which sperm travel, or they can injure sperm (impairing their ability to reach the egg) or kill them. Injuries also can affect sperm production. Mumps (and other infections) sometimes can cause an inflammation of one or both testicles (orchitis) that can permanently impair or prevent sperm production in the affected testicle (see also page 1117).

In some men, sperm production is perfectly normal but the sperm are ejaculated into the bladder rather than out the penis (see Retrograde Ejaculation, page 1144).

In women, the failure to release an egg each menstrual cycle, called anovulation, is responsible for infertility problems in up to 15 percent of cases. It can be caused by various factors. If menstruation does not occur or occurs only occasionally, there may be a problem with the way the uterus or ovaries developed. Even if a woman has normal periods, however, she still can have impaired ovulation.

Hyperprolactinemia, a condition in which the blood contains an excess amount of the hormone prolactin, can cause anovulation. The hypothalamus, a part of the brain, produces hormones that normally stimulate a woman's pituitary gland, which in turn triggers the release of an egg. If the hypothalamus does not secrete the hormones, no egg is released. Additional causes of anovulation include chronic debilitating diseases such as uncontrolled diabetes or thyroid disease.

When ovulation is normal, the problem lies elsewhere. Abnormalities of the fallopian tubes are the problem, or part of the problem, as often as a third of the time. Tumors or irregularities in the formation of the fallopian tubes can block passage of the egg. In a condition called endometriosis, some of the tissue that lines the uterus and is shed each month during the menstrual period remains in the abdomen somewhere outside the uterus. This tissue can interfere with the passage of released eggs to or through the fallopian tubes, causing infertility (see page 1101).

Sometimes, ovulation occurs normally and the egg passes successfully through the fallopian tubes, only to encounter other problems. These include luteal-phase defects, in which something (frequently a hormonal abnormality) interferes with the further development of the egg once it has been released.

Uterine factors are sometimes a cause of infertility. These include an irregular shape of the uterus, an unconventional positioning of the uterus within the abdomen (see page 1098), or tumors (see page 1099). Surgical correction may or may not restore fertility. Similarly, cervical factors can be responsible for infertility; these include cervix irregularities or growths that block the sperm or problems with the cervical mucus that damage the sperm or impede its passage.

Immunological factors also can be responsible. A few women are allergic to sperm, and their bodies produce antibodies that kill the sperm before they have a chance to penetrate an egg. A physician can suggest various ways to avoid this problem.

Similarly, some men produce antibodies that are meant to fight an infection but inadvertently attack sperm instead. Treatment of the infection should eradicate this problem.

In men as well as women, numerous diseases that can affect the genitourinary tract can cause infertility. These include the sexually transmitted diseases (see page 875).

Pelvic inflammatory disease is caused by sexually transmitted diseases such as gonorrhea, chlamydial infection, and vaginitis and, less commonly, by tuberculosis and anaerobic streptococcal infection (see also page 1104). These diseases can cause problems depending on the amount of fallopian tube inflammation and the amount of irritation at the end of the tube and around the ovary. Even with severe pelvic inflammatory disease with known tubal and ovarian involvement, aggressive treatment with antibiotics and conservative operation allow subsequent fertility in 25 to 30 percent of cases.

THERAPY

The numerous treatments for infertility depend on the cause. Recent developments in therapy have increased the number of once-infertile couples who can have their own child.

Some causes of infertility cannot be corrected. However, even then, various means of insemination or embryo transfer may be possible so that the woman can still become pregnant.

This section divides infertility therapy into two categories: 1) restoring or bringing about fertility, and 2) artificial fertilization.

Therapy To Achieve Fertility.   One of the easiest means of treating infertility for many couples is advice on when and how often to have intercourse to improve the chances of achieving fertility. This means is particularly effective in couples with impaired fertility rather than infertility—for example, when the man has oligospermia (see page 1133). In addition to giving suggestions on the frequency of intercourse, and how to time it to best match the ovulatory cycle, your physician can give other advice, such as recommending that the woman remain supine (on her back) and with her knees bent for some minutes after intercourse to keep her organs in the best position for the further movement of the sperm toward the egg.

General sexual problems, such as impotence or premature ejaculation, also can be treated to improve fertility. These problems and their treatment are discussed in the section Sexuality and Sexual Dysfunction (see page 1137).

When the source of infertility lies in the man's sperm (or lack of it), restoring or initiating fertility is sometimes possible. For example, varicocele, a common source of problems with the sperm, can be corrected surgically, and in some instances this also will restore fertility. Problems with the testicles, prostate gland, seminal vesicles, and urethra also can be treated (see Health Problems of Men, page 1111).

When sperm production is impaired because of damage to the sperm-producing areas of the testicle, drug treatment has been of little use. In extremely rare instances when sperm production is impaired because of a pituitary gland problem, the use of human chorionic gonadotropin or human pituitary gonadotropin has been helpful. When infections hamper sperm production, block the transport of sperm, or damage or kill the sperm, treatment of the infection often restores fertility. This is particularly true of sexually transmitted diseases, and both partners must be treated.

In the woman, treatment also depends on the results of the examination and tests. Treating any infection or underlying illness is, as usual, the first step. If the fertility problem is related to anovulation (failure to release an egg), your physician can attempt to bring about ovulation. Generally, clomiphene citrate, human menopausal gonadotropins, or gonadotropin-releasing hormones with or without human chorionic gonadotropin are administered. Occasionally, an ovarian operation is necessary to bring about ovulation.

Blockages, tumors, or other problems in the fallopian tubes usually are repaired surgically. Microsurgical techniques permit delicate operations on the fallopian tubes. Not all fallopian tube damage can be repaired surgically, however.

Endometriosis (see page 1101) can be treated with medications, including oral contraceptives taken in low doses. Sometimes surgical removal of the endometrial tissue is necessary. Correction of endometriosis can improve fertility.

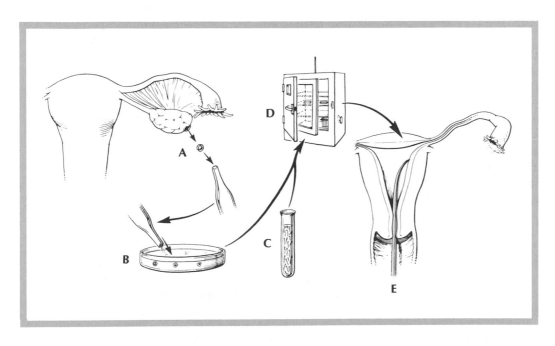

In in vitro fertilization, eggs are removed from the ovary (A). The eggs and sperm from a donor are combined in a Petri dish and placed in an incubator (B, C, and D). If fertilization occurs, the embryo is transferred to the uterus by means of a cannula (E).

Artificial Fertilization. When a couple remains infertile despite treatment of the cause, when the cause is determined but cannot be treated, or when the cause cannot be determined, pregnancy is often still possible. The techniques used involve artificially fertilizing an egg from the woman with sperm from the partner or from another man. The fertilization can take place inside the woman's body or outside the body, in which case the fertilized egg is then transferred to inside the body (embryo transfers).

The term test-tube babies actually is inaccurate because the baby is developed within the mother; only fertilization and the very earliest development of the fertilized egg (embryo) take place in a test tube. The correct term is in vitro fertilization. Once the subject of headlines, it is now routine in specialized clinics. It does, however, require a

surgical procedure, and it is costly and difficult.

With in vitro fertilization, eggs are removed from the woman's ovary—with laparoscopy (see page 1297) or with ultrasonography (see page 1287) to locate the follicle in the ovary so that a needle can be inserted into the follicle for retrieval of the eggs. Semen is obtained from the male partner or from a donor. Attempts are then made to fertilize an egg with a sperm in a laboratory under optimal conditions. If fertilization occurs, the embryo is transferred to the uterus of the woman (embryo transfer). The technique achieves pregnancy in about one of five or six cases.

The partner's semen can be used for artificial insemination if it contains healthy sperm. The semen is collected, and the physician places it directly into the woman's

ETHICAL CONSIDERATIONS IN FERTILITY THERAPY

Determining the cause of infertility and treating it is a demanding task both for the partners and for the physician or clinic. It requires much energy over a protracted period. New techniques are being developed constantly, and physicians are pleased to be able to use them for a couple's benefit.

Measure Your Own Attitudes
It is important for a couple considering fertility therapy to examine their own attitudes toward such therapy. Just because something can be done doesn't mean that it should be done. Attitudes toward conception vary greatly. Some couples believe that if having sexual intercourse does not produce a child, then they should accept the situation; this may be a religious or an ethical position. Conversely, some couples are so eager to have their "own" child that they believe that to achieve that end no tests are too prolonged, no therapy too

complicated, and no expense, procedure, or hardship too great.

Most couples find themselves somewhere between these two positions. Fertility clinics, and physicians who specialize in fertility problems, often are prepared to discuss ethical issues with you. They can help you to define or discover your own attitudes. These discussions should include what can realistically be expected. Even though medical science has provided many new techniques, they all have their limitations and rates of success that are not 100 percent.

Don't Take It Personally
Being infertile does not mean that a man is any less manly or that a woman is any less feminine. Infertility does not make anyone "incomplete" or "defective." It has nothing to do with attractiveness or sexual prowess. Moreover, it is not a negative comment on a couple's relationship.

Medically speaking, infertility is simply the existence of some obstacle in the long and exceedingly complex chain of events that lead

to pregnancy which makes it difficult for you to have children. It need not be viewed as a tragedy.

Consider the Ethical Questions
When fertilization is not possible through sexual intercourse but only through other methods such as artificial insemination, some couples believe that a line has been crossed and ethical considerations are raised.

A significant distinction for many people is donor sperm from someone other than the husband. Using sperm from a stranger raises many ethical issues: Who was he? (Most sperm banks ensure anonymity.) What sort of person was he? Is he the real father, or is the male partner the real father? Does the donor have any rights concerning the child? Might future court decisions award donors visitation rights?

In the end, only you and your partner can answer such questions and address such issues. But the time to consider your ethical positions on fertility therapy is *before* pregnancy occurs as a result of such therapy.

uterus at the time of ovulation. In other words, the more variable transit of the semen after sexual intercourse is not relied on; instead, to reduce the element of chance, it is placed where fertilization is most likely to occur.

Artificial insemination also can be performed with semen from a donor. Fertility clinics and physicians specializing in fertility have access to sperm banks and other sources of healthy sperm. If the partner does not produce sperm or not enough sperm for successful fertilization, a donor's sperm may be used. Sometimes sperm from both the partner and the donor are mixed before being transferred to the woman.

Artificial insemination has a higher success rate with donor sperm than with the partner's sperm. However, the use of someone else's sperm does raise questions in the minds of some couples (see Ethical Considerations in Fertility Therapy, page 1136).

With a slightly different technique, called gamete intrafallopian transfer, a mixture of sperm taken from the partner or a donor and eggs from the woman is placed directly in the fallopian tube. This also is done with laparoscopy. The intent is to encourage fertilization to occur "naturally" within the woman. As with in vitro fertilization, the success of this procedure is by no means ensured.

SEXUALITY AND SEXUAL DYSFUNCTION

Sexual dysfunction simply means problems or obstacles encountered in the course of sexual intercourse. The problems can be experienced by either the man or the woman. It is rare, however, for only one of the partners to be affected; for example, premature ejaculation, a problem in the man, will likely lead to sexual satisfaction problems for the woman.

This section first discusses problems that can occur in the woman: desire disorders, sensation disorders, and orgasm disorders. Because these problems are not always easy to distinguish, read all three sections if you suspect you have one of these dysfunctions.

The second part of this section covers problems in the man: impotence, erection abnormalities, and premature ejaculation. The solution to sexual problems in either partner, as will be seen, often entails the understanding and cooperation of both partners.

DESIRE DISORDERS IN WOMEN

Signs and Symptoms
- Diminished or absent sexual desire;
- Insufficient sexual desire to sustain interest in sexual activity.

Sexual desire is an interest in having sexual activity with a partner. Sometimes sexual activity, including orgasm, may take place even though the desire for it is lessened or nonexistent.

How much desire is "too little" is, of course, a personal judgment that will differ from woman to woman. If you wish you had more sexual desire, then you probably are experiencing too little.

On average, men desire sexual relations more often than women; the fact that your partner desires sex more frequently than you do does not necessarily mean that you have a desire problem. Instead, it suggests a disparity in desire between the two of you. In such cases, counseling is sometimes in order; it generally results in a compromise and better understanding on the part of both partners.

In the female (as in the male), sexual desire can stem from various sources, including the senses of sight, touch, hearing, and smell, and from thoughts and emotions. The attractiveness of a partner and the nature of the relationship with the partner can figure heavily in the presence or absence of sexual desire. Desire lessens somewhat during the later years of life.

It is important to realize that diminished or absent sexual desire during one sexual encounter or another is not a sign of a problem; this happens to any woman, is perfectly normal, and is generally transient. Diminished or absent desire that persists over time, however, can create problems for a woman's self-image and damage the sexual life of both partners.

Causes can be nonphysical, physical, or both. Among nonphysical causes, discord with one's partner is common, as is depression. Physical causes include various illnesses, hormonal imbalances, and side effects of medications. When desire disorders do not cure themselves, treatment is usually possible.

The Diagnosis. Although a physician is not needed to diagnose a desire disorder (you will be able to recognize this yourself), he or she can be helpful in separating it from other possible problems and in suggesting treatment. Your physician will ask questions concerning your relationship with your partner, your physical condition, the medications you are taking, and your history of illnesses.

How Serious Are Desire Disorders? In and of themselves, desire disorders are not harmful. Most, in fact, are merely passing events in a marriage or relationship. A persisting desire disorder, however, can have a negative effect on the sex lives of both partners and can damage a woman's self-image.

Treatment. If a physical illness is present, your physician will treat the illness. Similarly, your physician may replace or eliminate medications that you take to determine whether they have an impact.

Most commonly, however, the cause is nonphysical. Your physician may suggest counseling of one or both partners with a therapist or may offer some guidelines or specific programs to follow to increase desire.

SENSATION DISORDERS IN WOMEN

Signs and Symptoms
- Diminished or nonexistent sexual excitement during sexual activity;
- A dry, rather than lubricated, vagina during sexual intercourse, despite ample opportunity for sexual stimulation during foreplay;
- Sometimes, painful intercourse.

There is a fine distinction between desire disorders (see page 1137) and sensation disorders. With a sensation disorder, the desire for sexual activity is present but pleasurable sensations are not obtained from such activity. In other words, you would like to have

sex, but when you do your body does not seem to cooperate and usually shows this by failing to secrete enough vaginal lubrication. The sexual act does not excite you as it should.

As with other sexual problems, the first thing to realize is that an occurrence or two does not mean that you have a problem. A sensation disorder has to persist for it to be a problem at all.

The causes of a sensation disorder are varied. Nonphysical causes predominate; they include anger or hostility toward the partner, depression, and stress. To appreciate the sensations involved during sexual activity, one has to be able to focus on them, and anything that interferes with this can be at the root of the problem.

Lack of stimulation by the partner also can be a cause. Sufficient foreplay is important; failing to respond to a partner who does not provide as much foreplay as you want is not a sensation disorder at all—it is a normal reaction to inadequate sexual stimulation. The same applies during the sexual act itself: a sensation disorder is present only if ample attention is paid to your sexual needs without resulting in excitation.

A physical sensation disorder is dyspareunia (painful intercourse). Several physical ailments affecting the genital area can be responsible for this condition, including vaginal irritations, infections, growths, and reactions to devices or substances used for contraception.

The absence of sufficient vaginal lubrication due to a lack of ample foreplay or desire also can, of course, cause painful intercourse. After menopause, the mucus lining of the vagina generally becomes somewhat thinner and drier, and previously pleasurable intercourse may become painful.

The Diagnosis. If you suspect that you have a sensation disorder, discuss this with your physician. Your physician will ask questions concerning your physical health, the medications you take, your relationship with your partner, and your experiences during sexual intercourse.

If intercourse is painful, a pelvic examination will be necessary (see page 1055). Your physician also will ask questions to help pinpoint when you experience the pain and where in the vagina; for example, if deep thrusts hurt, your physician may suspect damage to the uterus.

How Serious Are Sensation Disorders?
A persisting sensation disorder can damage your sex life, taking the pleasure out of sex. It also can cause problems for your partner, who knows that he is not satisfying you. Beyond these consequences, however, physical damage does not generally result from a sensation disorder. If an inflammation, growth, or injury is present, however, continued intercourse can aggravate the condition.

Treatment. If you have an illness that causes a sensation disorder as a secondary effect, your physician will treat it. The medications you are taking or the contraceptives you are using may be altered or eliminated to determine whether they affect your sexual responsiveness. In addition, vaginal lubricants can be used during intercourse to alleviate a common source of pain.

In some cases, however, treatment will be directed toward nonphysical causes, and counseling may be necessary. The counseling may include recommending specific measures to help you and your partner regain the pleasurable sensations associated with normal sexual activity.

If an underlying problem in the relationship between you and your partner is the cause of the sensation disorder, marital counseling or other forms of therapy may be advised.

ORGASM DISORDERS IN WOMEN

Signs and Symptoms

- Failure to attain orgasm during sexual activity.

Some women never attain orgasm and yet have pleasurable sexual experiences, some obtain orgasm only part of the time, and others have orgasm every time they have intercourse. It is a change in these patterns leading to dissatisfaction with sexual activity that warrants evaluation.

Orgasm disorders are closely related to sensation disorders (see page 1138). In general, if you do not experience ample pleasurable sensations from sexual activity, you will not experience orgasm either. In some cases of orgasm disorder, a woman does experi-

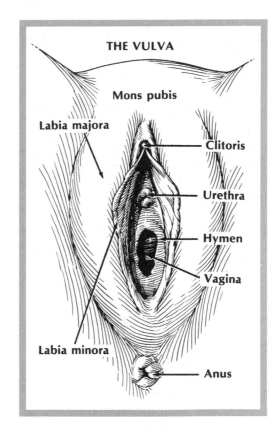

THE VULVA

Mons pubis

Labia majora

Clitoris

Urethra

Hymen

Vagina

Labia minora

Anus

ence orgasm but has to work unreasonably hard or long to attain it.

Orgasm is a complex event, involving sexual desire and sexual stimulation. Foreplay and sexual intercourse itself must reasonably approximate the needs of the particular woman in terms of the way it is done and how long it lasts. Communicating these needs to a responsive partner will relieve many orgasm disorders.

It is also important to realize that a large percentage of women—estimates range from a third to two-thirds of all women—require stimulation of the clitoris to reach an orgasm. Do not assume that you have an orgasm disorder until your partner or you have thoroughly experimented with direct stimulation of the clitoris before, during, or after intercourse and you find you still cannot attain orgasm.

Causes can be nonphysical, physical, or both. A common physical cause is simply that intercourse hurts. Physicians refer to this as dyspareunia. Disorders in the female genitourinary tract, such as minor injuries or abrasions and infections, or reactions to contraceptive creams or devices can cause painful intercourse, as can a lack of ample vaginal lubrication. Sometimes dyspareunia is experienced after menopause, when the vaginal lining becomes somewhat drier and thinner; use of lubricants can overcome this condition. Endometriosis also can be a cause of dyspareunia (see page 1101).

Nonphysical causes can include problems in the relationship with the partner, depression, anger, or other factors that affect the ability to focus on pleasurable sexual sensations. A few women inhibit their orgasm out of fear of "letting go" or losing control, perhaps believing that this implies dependence on the partner.

The Diagnosis. You, rather than your physician, are the one who knows you are not experiencing orgasms. It is helpful to discuss the problem with your physician, how-

ever, so that he or she can determine the cause and suggest the appropriate course of action to take to regain (or initiate) the ability to have orgasms.

Your physician will ask questions concerning your physical health, the medications you take and the contraceptives you use, your relationship with your partner, and your experiences during sexual intercourse. If intercourse is painful, your physician will perform a pelvic examination.

How Serious Are Orgasm Disorders?
A persisting orgasm disorder can render your sex life unsatisfying or less satisfying than it might be. This is its most serious consequence. However, some women who do not experience orgasms often enjoy foreplay and sexual stimulation during intercourse a great deal and do not think that they are missing anything by not having an orgasm. This is a judgment a woman must make on her own.

Physical consequences of orgasm disorders themselves are rare. If an inflammation or injury is present, however, continued intercourse can aggravate the condition, and it should be treated.

Some women find the inability to have orgasms damaging to their self-image, although this need not be the case. The problem usually can be corrected; when it cannot, a woman is not rendered any less feminine, in any way "incomplete," or unable to enjoy sexual activity with her partner.

Also, your partner can be disturbed by your orgasm disorder, feeling that he fails to satisfy you. Reassurance concerning your enjoyment of the act even in the absence of orgasm can be helpful.

Treatment. If you have an illness or injury that causes an orgasm disorder, your physician will treat it. The medications you take or the contraceptives you use may be altered or eliminated to determine whether they affect your responsiveness.

In most cases, treatment will be directed toward nonphysical causes and will involve suggestions or counseling. Experimenting with clitoral stimulation before, during, and after intercourse may solve the problem. Your physician may suggest counseling, which may include specific measures to help you and your partner regain the pleasurable sensations associated with sexual

LOSS OF SEXUAL DESIRE IN WOMEN

It is normal for a woman to experience sexual desire from puberty until well beyond menopause. Diminished sexual desire or a loss of desire altogether is generally due to some specific problem or situation. The most common cause in a woman is day-to-day discord with her partner. This is present, to one degree or another, in about three of four cases that are discussed with physicians.

The second most common cause of desire problems is inadequate stimulation by the partner. A man who focuses merely on satisfying himself can rarely satisfy a woman. A well-intentioned, considerate partner may satisfy a woman and himself simultaneously.

Sometimes a woman fails to discover her potential in sexual relationships because of inadequate knowledge of her anatomy, of the importance of timing during the sex act, or of the need to communicate her needs to her partner. Gradually, as a consequence

of bland or unsatisfying sexual experiences, she can sometimes lose interest. Worse, such an absence of desire is sometimes reinforced by the "common wisdom," from an earlier era, that it is unseemly for a woman to experience desire, to experience very much desire, or to continue experiencing it after childbearing years; such attitudes are as wrong today as they were then.

Physical problems are sometimes the cause of a loss of desire. The presence of some disease or disability can diminish desire, and many medications also suppress feelings of sexual desire as a side effect.

Loss of desire generally can be reversed. A physician can guide you to a therapist who can help resolve problems with your partner. Your therapist also can suggest measures to help you regain sexual desire. In the case of a physical problem, your physician can treat the particular ailment or can suggest substitute medications that do not suppress desire.

activity. The use of vaginal lubricants also may be helpful.

Your physician also may suggest a set of simple exercises (known as Kegel's exercises, see page 1091) that can help you develop the muscles in the outer third of the vagina that are involved in pleasurable sensations. These same muscles also help control the flow of urine.

If an underlying problem in the relationship between you and your partner is a possible cause of your inability to experience orgasm, marital counseling or another form of therapy may be advised.

IMPOTENCE

Signs and Symptoms
• Inability of the penis to become erect or to stay erect.

Impotence is a persistent inability to obtain an erection or to keep it long enough for sexual intercourse. The name comes from the Latin word *impotentia*, which means lack of strength.

It is important to realize that an occasional episode of impotence happens to most men, is perfectly normal, and is nothing to worry about. When it proves to be a pattern or a persistent problem, however, impotence can be a detriment to a man's self-image as well as to his sexual life. Fortunately, impotence often can be cured.

A first step toward curing impotence is to understand how an erection occurs. The penis has two cylindrical, sponge-like structures that run along its length parallel to the urethra (the tube that carries semen and urine). When a man is sexually aroused, nerve impulses cause the blood flow to the cylinders to increase to about 7 times the normal amount. This sudden influx of blood expands the sponge-like structures and thus straightens and stiffens the penis, producing an erection. Continued sexual arousal or excitation maintains the higher rate of blood flow, keeping the erection. After ejaculation, or when the sexual excitation passes, the excess blood drains out of the spongy tissue and the penis returns to its nonerect size and shape.

Note that three important things take place to produce the erection. The first step is sexual arousal, which men obtain from the senses of sight, touch, hearing, and smell and

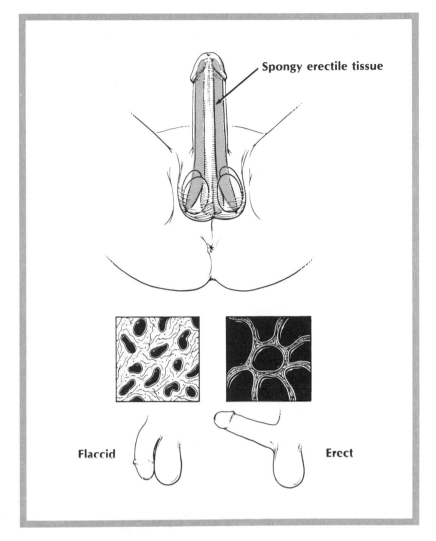

Spongy erectile tissue

Flaccid   Erect

In an erection, two cylindrical, sponge-like erectile structures become engorged with blood. After orgasm, excess blood drains from the spongy tissue, leaving the penis flaccid.

from thoughts. The second step is communication of the sexual excitation by the body's nervous system from the brain to the penis. The third step is a relaxing action of the blood vessels that supply the penis, allowing more blood to flow into the shafts that produce the erection. If something affects any of these three factors—arousal, nervous system response, or vascular system response—or the delicate balance among them, impotence can result.

Diminished sexual desire or even loss of sexual desire is not the same thing as impotence (see Loss of Sexual Desire in Men, page 1145). Impotence refers to the inability to have an erection and to use the penis for sexual activity when desire and opportunity are present.

Impotence affects about 10 million American men. It affects more older men than younger men—nearly 20 percent of men are impotent at age 60 years and more than 70 percent are impotent at age 80 years. However, impotence is by no means an inevitable consequence of aging, and treatment in older men is often as effective as it is in younger men.

Nonphysical causes account for more than half of the cases of impotence. The main nonphysical cause is stress or anxiety. If a man cannot relax and focus on the sexual situation, or if he is overwhelmed or confused by circumstances, it is difficult for the three-stage erection process to take place. This happens to almost everyone at some time.

Impotence is also an occasional side effect of psychological problems such as depression. Negative feelings toward the sexual partner—or expressed by the sexual partner—such as resentment, hostility, or lack of interest also can be a factor in impotence.

The important thing is not to assume that an episode of impotence means that you have a permanent problem and should expect it to happen again during the next sexual encounter. Because thought processes are so important in erection, such a negative assumption can, in some cases, bring the problem about. The best thing to do if you experience an episode of impotence is to forget it and expect a more successful experience at another time. Such an episode is not a lasting comment on a man's virility or masculinity.

It is important too for the man experiencing transient or persisting impotence to remember his sexual partner. To a greater or lesser degree, a woman may consider an erection as a comment on her desirability; lack of an erection may communicate undesirability to the partner, and reassurance is helpful. A woman's self-image can be damaged by her partner's impotence, but this can be avoided if the man makes it clear that she attracts him or if the woman herself realizes that impotence is only rarely caused by lack of interest.

Physical causes account for nearly half of the cases of impotence. These include (from the most to the least frequent) diabetic neuropathy, cardiovascular disorders, prescription medicines, operation for cancer of the prostate, fractures that injure the spinal cord, multiple sclerosis, hormone disorders, and alcoholism and other forms of drug abuse.

The physical and nonphysical causes of impotence interact. For example, a minor physical problem that slows sexual response may cause anxiety about attaining an erection, and the anxiety worsens the impotence.

The Diagnosis.   If episodes of impotence keep occurring, consult your physician. Your physician will ask questions about how the impotence developed, medications that you take, physical ailments, and factors such as stress.

If your physician suspects mainly nonphysical causes, he or she may ask whether you obtain erections during masturbation, with a partner, or while you sleep. Most men experience many erections (without remembering them) during sleep. A simple test—

In men who are incapable of attaining erection, special devices may be implanted surgically. Among the varieties of implants in use today are semirigid implants that maintain a firmness at all times but allow the penis to be tucked close to the body when not in use for intercourse (top drawings), and an inflatable device that uses fluid reservoirs and a hand pump you operate mechanically to produce erection (bottom drawing).

wrapping a special perforated tape around the penis before sleeping—can confirm whether you have nocturnal erections. If the tape is separated in the morning, your penis was erect at some point during the night. Tests of this type confirm nonphysical causes.

If your physician suspects that physical causes are involved, other tests, such as angiography to determine the adequacy of the arterial circulation of the genital organs, neurological evaluation to exclude neuropathy, and measurements of the male hormone level in the blood, may be performed. Prescription drugs may be eliminated or replaced one at a time to see whether they are responsible.

How Serious Is Impotence? Impotence often can be cured. When it cannot, a penile implant may be used to achieve erection, making an active sexual life possible. If left untreated, persisting impotence can damage one's sexual life as well as the self-image of one or both partners.

Treatment. *Psychological Therapy.* If nonphysical causes are predominantly or entirely responsible for impotence, your physician may suggest visiting a psychiatrist, psychologist, or sex therapist, either alone or with your partner.

Medication. Hormones can be given for some cases of impotence. Sometimes you can inject a drug that causes an erection directly into your penis.

Medications that you take for other conditions may be replaced or eliminated if they are thought to cause the impotence as a side effect.

Surgery. Vascular reconstruction may be performed if your impotence is caused by obstructed arteries leading to the penis.

If the impotence is not correctable by any of the other therapies, a permanent penile implant can be put in place. This type of operation has been performed successfully on thousands of men. There are three common types of implants: 1) a malleable (semirigid) implant, 2) a multipart inflatable implant, and 3) a self-contained inflatable implant. The semirigid type remains firm all the time but permits the penis to be tucked close to the body. The inflatable types have fluid reservoirs that you can operate when

you want to have an erection. Also, a newly developed external vacuum device offers a noninvasive alternative to surgically implanted penile prostheses.

ERECTION ABNORMALITIES

Signs and Symptoms
- Inability of the penis to become or stay erect;
- A painful (sometimes) bend in the penis during an erection;
- A prolonged, painful erection.

An erection is a prerequisite for intercourse and most other sexual activity. Problems with erection, of whatever type, can hamper sexual activity. The three main kinds of erectile abnormalities are impotence, Peyronie's disease, and priapism.

The first abnormality, impotence, was discussed on page 1141. The second type of erection abnormality is Peyronie's disease (curvature of the penis). This is less common than impotence. It affects men mainly between the ages of 40 and 60 years, can make sexual intercourse difficult or impossible, and is caused by scar tissue that forms inside the penis for reasons that are unknown. It is not related to any infection, tumor, contagious disease, or sexual practice. Most cases of Peyronie's disease disappear spontaneously within 1 to 3 years after onset. If the degree of curvature precludes intercourse (it usually does not), surgical procedures can correct this deformity (see Curvature of the Penis, page 1122).

Priapism, the third type of erectile abnormality, is a prolonged, painful erection of the penis with no associated sexual excitement. (The name is derived from the Latin name for a male fertility god in classical mythology, Priapus.) In its effect, priapism is the opposite of impotence. This is a rare, potentially dangerous condition that requires prompt medical treatment (see Priapism, page 1122).

BLOOD IN THE SEMEN

Signs and Symptoms
- Blood in the semen.

Blood in the semen (hematospermia) alarms many men but seldom should. Hematospermia is sometimes known as hemospermia. The color of the semen ranges from pink to red. If you or your partner sees blood in your ejaculated semen but you have no other symptoms, you probably do not have any physical disorder.

To make sure, however, visit your physician and have a thorough physical examination of your genital area, including your prostate and testicles. If your physician finds nothing wrong, further tests usually are unnecessary. You may or may not notice bloody semen again; but, in any case, it is not cause for alarm.

The source of the blood in hematospermia is not clear. It probably comes from the vessels lining the seminal vesicles and may be the result of some harmless inflammation.

PREMATURE EJACULATION

Signs and Symptoms
- Ejaculation during foreplay with a sexual partner, or at a point during intercourse too soon to satisfy the partner.

The only thing wrong with premature ejaculation is its timing—too soon, before either partner has had an opportunity to enjoy the sexual act fully. In rare cases, merely touching a woman is enough to bring about ejaculation. More commonly, ejaculation occurs when the penis first enters the vagina or very shortly after it enters the vagina.

Premature ejaculation is a common sexual problem, especially for young men. The cause is rarely physical, and treatment that involves the partner's help is almost always successful.

Premature ejaculation can be recognized without a physician's aid and is not serious. However, it has a detrimental effect on the sex life of both partners—a responsive female partner does not have time to attain orgasm, and the male partner experiences orgasm but after so little sexual activity as to deprive him of much of the pleasure involved. On occasion, men become so frustrated at premature ejaculations that they become impotent. Such anxiety is unnecessary because the solution is simple.

Treatment.   Premature ejaculation can be treated with the "squeeze" technique. The method works as follows.

Begin sexual activity as usual, including penile stimulation, until you feel almost ready to ejaculate. Then have your partner squeeze the end of the penis, at the point where the glans joins the shaft, for a period of several seconds. After the squeeze is released, wait for about half a minute, and then go back to foreplay. You will notice that squeezing the penis causes it to become less erect but that when sexual stimulation is resumed it soon regains full erection.

If you again feel that you are about to ejaculate, have your partner repeat the squeeze process. By repeating this as many times as necessary, you can reach the point of entering your partner without having ejaculated. After a few practice sessions, the feeling of knowing how to delay ejaculation will become a habit without the squeeze technique and you will continue through successful intercourse.

RETROGRADE EJACULATION

Signs and Symptoms
- Little or no semen is ejaculated from the penis during a sexual climax.

Retrograde ejaculation is a fairly unusual, and harmless, phenomenon in which, rather than emerging from the end of the penis, the semen enters the bladder during orgasm. The word retrograde in the name refers to the backward direction of the semen.

Retrograde ejaculation may be distinguished from absence of ejaculation by voiding through a red-colored cloth immediately after intercourse or masturbation. When retrograde ejaculation occurs, the cloth acts as a strainer to trap the seminal discharge which will appear on the red cloth. With absence of ejaculation, no seminal discharge will appear on the cloth.

Absence of ejaculation usually is due to a functional inability to achieve orgasm. Sexual counseling should be considered. In certain instances, absence of ejaculation may be due to injury of the seminal vesicles or some types of genitourinary surgery.

Various conditions can cause retrograde ejaculation, including diabetes, prostate surgery, urethral surgery, and use of mood-altering or antihypertensive drugs. It is most likely to occur among men who have diabetes.

The Diagnosis. You will notice the symptom of retrograde ejaculation. A physician can confirm the diagnosis by tests such as a test of your urine after ejaculation to see if it contains a large quantity of sperm.

How Serious Is Retrograde Ejaculation?
Retrograde ejaculation is harmless. Semen that enters the bladder is simply expelled with the urine during urination. However, retrograde ejaculation does prevent fertility if no semen at all goes out the penis or diminishes fertility if a decreased quantity of semen emerges.

Treatment. *Medication.* If the retrograde ejaculation is caused by drugs that you are taking, the drugs can be stopped or you can switch to others in an effort to restore normal ejaculation.

Retrograde ejaculation may also be corrected by certain prescription drugs such as ephedrine, adrenaline, or Ornade (a combination of chlorpheniramine and phenylpropanolamine). Infertility due to retrograde ejaculation sometimes can be reversed by artificial insemination with sperm obtained by catheterization immediately after intercourse.

LOSS OF SEXUAL DESIRE IN MEN

Men can have various problems with their erections and with ejaculation that complicate sexual activity. But what about when the urge to have sex itself goes away?

A complete absence of sexual desire is unusual, but lessened sexual desire is not. Sometime after about age 60 years, most men experience somewhat diminished sexual desire, although this varies greatly from one man to another. The first cause to suspect is some physical ailment. Illnesses that cause persistent pain, weakness, or fatigue are prone to lessen sexual desire, as are emotional factors such as depression, anger toward your partner, and stress. Apathy or lack of enthusiasm from your partner also can lead to dampened desire.

In addition to the physical and nonphysical causes of loss of desire, the medications taken to combat these disorders can often cause such loss. When this is the case, substitute medications generally can be found.

In many men, loss of desire may occur because of inadequate communication of arousal needs between partners and poor timing of the act of intercourse. It is also important to realize that impotence usually does not imply a lack of desire but is a problem that your physician can treat.

Loss of desire often can be cured. If you experience a persisting loss of sexual desire, do not assume that this is the natural course of events. Seek help from your physician. Changes in medication, counseling, or other forms of therapy may be in order.

SEXUAL CRISES

The problems described thus far in the chapter—although inconvenient or even dismaying—for the most part are not emergencies. The rest of this chapter addresses true crisis situations: rape, physical abuse, and sexual abuse of adolescents.

The section on rape is addressed to the adult or teenager who has been raped and needs to know where to turn or to the concerned friend or parent who wants to help. The section on physical abuse concerns bodily harm inflicted by one partner on another, regardless of whether or not sexual activity is involved. The section on sexual abuse of adolescents offers practical advice on where victims can seek help.

Although females are the prime victims of all three types of crimes, males are also sometimes victims.

RAPE

Signs and Symptoms
• Forced sexual intercourse, oral sexual activity, or anal intercourse.

Lack of consent is the factor that differentiates rape from acceptable sexual activity: rape is forced on you, sometimes by violence or threats of violence and sometimes by deception.

Women of all ages, from infancy through old age, can be rape victims. The rapist can be a stranger, but in about half of cases the rapist is known to the victim. About half of the instances of rape occur in the victim's own home. Rapists are often members of the extended family. In 90 percent of cases, the rapist is of the same race as the victim. In some instances, the rapist is the husband.

Although rape of a man is more rare than rape of a woman, men can be the victims of rape, by other men or by women. They suffer the same types of mental damage and require the same care as women.

Regardless of the identities of the victim and the rapist, rape is psychologically and sometimes physically devastating. Rape is a crime, although it is one of the most difficult crimes to prosecute successfully. The recognition that forced sexual activity by one's own spouse can constitute rape is fairly recent and even more difficult to prosecute successfully. Nevertheless, if you have been raped, once you have sought the help that you need, you should also report the crime to the police.

Most rapes are planned by the rapist and are not the result of impulse—although the victim may be picked on impulse. The rapist is often not after sexual pleasure but needs an outlet to express anger and aggression.

Many techniques can be used to avoid becoming a rape victim (see Rape Prevention, page 1147). If you are attacked by a potential rapist, how to resist—or whether to resist at all—depends on the individual and the circumstances. One technique is to stall for time, in the hope that someone may come along and help. Some women have avoided rape by saying they have a sexually transmitted disease or by disgusting the rapist by urinating or defecating. Resistance possibilities that are more active include the use of any self-defense techniques you are proficient at, such as screaming, breaking a window, or kicking the attacker forcefully in the testicles to disable him long enough to enable you to escape.

However, if you think you will be harmed if you resist, or if resistance does not work, submit. It is preferable to being killed or seriously injured. Note that as far as later prosecution goes, rape is a crime regardless of whether you resist or submit.

If you have been raped, you should seek immediate medical care at a rape treatment center at a major hospital, from your regular physician, or from a hospital emergency room (see also page 290). If you are not certain where to go, look in the telephone book under "Rape" for the number of a local rape hotline, which can provide advice on a physician to see and other help, including personal support and legal advice. If pos-

sible, do not wash before you are examined by a physician.

The physician who examines you has two jobs: first and foremost, treating any injuries and providing psychological support; second, obtaining evidence that can be used to prosecute the rapist. Taking evidence involves asking you to describe the rape. In addition, the physician will examine you for the presence of semen, blood, or other materials from the rapist that could be used as evidence.

How Serious Is Rape?   A rape victim has endured a terrible experience. In most cases, the physical consequences are not long-lasting, and in fact there may not be any at all. Wounds and scratches heal; if there is a possibility of sexually transmitted disease or pregnancy, medications can be given.

The emotional and psychological consequences are often harder to deal with. Women may become unreasonably fearful (as opposed to rationally cautious) as a result of having been raped, may become depressed, or may have trouble with existing or future relationships with men. Sometimes women wrongly assume that they are to blame for the rape or for not resisting effectively.

Even if a woman manages to avoid all of these pitfalls, explaining what happened to the physician, to the police, and to family and friends is an ordeal. If the rapist is caught, recounting the experience in court is another ordeal, and it frequently is made worse by the ignorance and insensitivity with which many rape cases are handled.

However, lasting emotional and psychological consequences of having been raped can be avoided or overcome through counseling with someone who is trained in helping rape victims.

Treatment.   Your physician will treat the physical injuries. He or she can also refer you to a rape crisis center or community organization that will provide counseling and other support.

If there is a possibility of pregnancy as a result of the rape, the physician may give you a drug known as diethylstilbestrol (DES), which may prevent pregnancy. Medications can be prescribed to reduce the risk of acquiring a sexually transmitted disease. A follow-up examination and tests are generally necessary after several weeks to determine whether pregnancy has occurred or if a venereal disease has been acquired.

Sympathetic counseling is a cornerstone of effective rape treatment.

PHYSICAL ABUSE

Signs and Symptoms

- Deliberate abuse of your body by another;
- Deliberate abuse of your body by another during or in connection with sexual activity.

If someone is attacked and beaten on the street, an obvious crime of violence has been committed, and the first places to which most of us would turn are the police and a hospital. If you have been injured by a stranger, seek such help without delay.

Our principal concern here, however, is physical abuse that can be fully as damaging but occurs in a more "seemingly normal" situation—generally the home. The person inflicting the abuse can be a husband, friend, wife, relative, or someone else known to the victim. (Rape, a particular form of physical abuse, is discussed on page 1145; the sexual abuse of adolescents is discussed on page 1148.)

Some cultures, primarily in the past, held that a man had the right to beat his wife if he were so inclined and that she should put up with it. This attitude is no longer acceptable, but remnants of it can still be encountered. It should be clear in your mind that it is wrong if your spouse (husband or wife), friend, or someone else abuses your body. You do not have to put up with it; help is available.

The most common pattern of physical abuse is spouse abuse, typically a husband beating his wife when he is drunk or upset. The wife flees or recovers from the beating and hopes that it will not happen again, but often it does. The person inflicting the abuse has psychological problems that are unlikely to simply go away on their own. In many cases, the beatings will continue for years, as long as what is left of the relationship lasts or until the wife dies.

Husbands are also the victims of physical abuse by wives. Friends, lovers, and relatives are the victims of abuse by other friends, lovers, or relatives. Regardless of the

---

RAPE PREVENTION FOR WOMEN: SOME HELPFUL TIPS

Like most crimes, sexual assault cannot always be prevented, but you can take steps to reduce your risks. Some examples follow.

Sexual Limits

How friendly is too friendly? This is a judgment call—one that you must make whenever you are alone with a man. Always remember that you have the right (but not the obligation) to establish limits and that it is okay to change those limits as required by the circumstances. When it comes to sexual intercourse, you should never feel pressured.

Communication

Make your limitations known to the other person. Avoid sending any messages (verbal or nonverbal) that could be misleading.

Know Yourself

Pay attention to your emotions. Do not let circumstances override your good judgment. If it *seems* as though you are being pressured, then you *are* being

pressured, and it is time to say "Good-by."

Be Observant

Sometimes you can anticipate circumstances that can lead to rape. For example, avoid eye contact with an individual who stares at you. If someone seems to enjoy sitting or standing too close to you, move aside. If an individual is blocking your way, walk in another direction (confidently, avoiding eye contact). Avoid people who speak or act as though they know you intimately when they do not.

Assert Yourself

If someone grabs or pushes you or disregards your negative response to any physical or verbal act, tell the individual, in a firm tone of voice, to "bug off." The language may seem unrefined or rude, but in circumstances such as this you may need to be uncharacteristically direct. Always remember that it is okay to become angry. Also, it is important to react quickly with your negative response. If assertiveness is a problem for you, consider an assertiveness training course. Such courses are available in most communities.

---

combination, abuse is wrong and the victim is entitled to help and protection.

One type of physical abuse is connected with sexual activity. A relatively small number of people, of either sex, experience heightened sexual response when pain or humiliation is associated with the activity. For example, a sexual sadist may obtain sexual pleasure by inflicting harm on his or her partner. A sexual masochist receives sexual pleasure by experiencing such pain. Both sadism and masochism run the gamut from minor or even feigned pain to torture and ritual murder.

Some aggression during sexual activity is perfectly normal and it does not imply that either partner is a sadist, masochist, or potential sex offender. Probably the clearest dividing line between the acceptable and the unacceptable for most people is pain: when something hurts, you avoid it or stop it. If a partner expects your participation in some activity that hurts you and you do not enjoy it, then that activity is physical abuse.

In other words, physical abuse can be connected or not connected with sexual activity. The result for the victim in either case is the same: physical and mental suffering, often prolonged because of repeated episodes.

The Diagnosis.   The deliberate infliction of harm on your body, regardless of whether or not sexual activity is involved, constitutes physical abuse. See a physician or go to a hospital emergency room for treatment of the physical injuries.

Equally important is ensuring that the abuse stops. Your physician or hospital personnel can refer you to persons who can provide sympathetic counseling and intervention. Many communities have organizations that provide safe shelter for battered wives who fear reprisals or greater abuse.

The police also can be helpful, but they are equipped to respond to emergency situations and not to solve long-term problems. For example, a woman may call the police to get her husband to stop beating her, or the neighbors may call. The husband will be reprimanded and possibly jailed, but the situation generally will be repeated in the future. Your physician, social workers, hospital emergency personnel, or counselors on spouse-abuse hotlines are more able to set you on the right track toward solving the problem permanently.

How Serious Is Physical Abuse?   Severe physical injuries, including death, can result. Even minor injuries that accumulate over time can be debilitating. The emotional and psychological damage inflicted by abuse can be just as devastating as the physical damage.

Treatment.   Cuts, broken bones, and other physical injuries will require medical care, including operation for severe injuries. Your physician or a hospital emergency room can provide such care. Counseling is necessary to help you avoid further abuse; a physician,

nurse, social worker, or worker for a spouse-abuse hotline can put you in touch with organizations or individuals who provide such counseling. They can also help you seek safe shelter if you are in imminent danger.

For emotional rehabilitation after abuse, a psychiatrist, psychologist, or social worker can be helpful.

If you decide to help the abusing partner seek care for his or her behavior problems, your physician, a marriage counselor, or a social worker should be able to provide referral for such care.

SEXUAL ABUSE OF ADOLESCENTS

Signs and Symptoms
• Forced sexual activity or sexual contact against your will.

This section is addressed to the adolescent who believes that he or she has been abused sexually. In addition, a parent who suspects that the teenager is being abused by another adult, sibling, or friend can read this to determine how the problem can be handled.

"Abuse" is anything that is done to your body without your consent or approval. Sexual abuse includes sexual intercourse without consent (which is rape), forced oral sexual contact, forced anal intercourse, or any other activity involving unwilling exposure of your body or unwilling contact with someone else's body. (For more about rape, see page 1145.) Sexual abuse can happen to people of either sex, and it is against the law.

The sexual abuser can be a parent, brother or sister, friend, acquaintance, or unknown adult or teenager. Abuse happening within the family also is wrong. For example, a father does not have the right to sexually molest his daughter, even if the mother knows about it and does nothing. Seek help.

There are two ways to deal with sexual abuse. The best way—unfortunately, it is not always possible—is to prevent the abuse from happening. Prevention methods include not associating with persons likely to inflict abuse; taking safety precautions about being out at night, locking doors, and the like; saying "no"; resisting physically; and trying to get away. If someone threatens you with a weapon or overwhelming force, however, physical resistance may only result in worse abuse, injury, or death.

The second method is making sure that physical abuse does not happen again. If you are abused sexually, tell your parents and the police, who will advise you on how to prevent its happening again. If a parent is the one inflicting the abuse, go straight to a physician, a hospital emergency room, the police, your clergy, or a relative you can trust. Physicians are required by law in all states to report cases of child abuse (which includes adolescent sexual abuse) to the proper authorities.

In addition, many communities have groups that offer free emergency counseling to child-abuse victims and rape victims. Experienced, sympathetic counselors can give you anonymous advice on the next step to take.

Sometimes adolescents—particularly younger adolescents—are in doubt about exactly who their body belongs to. It is simple: you need only remember that your body belongs only to you. If someone is abusing it, seek help from relatives, the police, or a physician to see that the abuse stops.

The Diagnosis.   See your physician or go to a hospital emergency room to discuss sexual abuse. If you do not know what physician to go to or if you are not near a hospital, ask a reliable adult for advice or phone a child-abuse hotline. A physician can help

you to recover physically and emotionally from the experience and can help to ensure that it does not happen again. In addition, a physician can note physical evidence of abuse or rape for possible use in legal prosecution of the abuser (see Sexual Assault and Sexual Abuse, page 290).

How Serious Is Sexual Abuse in Adolescents?   Most sexual abuse in adolescents does not leave lasting physical injuries. The body can recover from the wounds and fractures. You also can recover from the emotional effects of abuse. However, if the abuse continues, it can damage your ability to form normal, trusting relationships with people. Continued abuse also increases the possibility of serious physical harm.

For the person inflicting the sexual abuse, it is very serious: he or she is committing a crime.

Treatment.   A physician can treat physical injuries caused by the abuse. He or she also may refer you for counseling with social workers or other professionals so that you can express your feelings about the abuse. Talking about it with someone who understands can help you to work through the emotional problems that the abuse causes.

If the abuse is occurring within the home and if social workers believe that the abuse will continue there, they will find you a new home or foster-care environment where you can live in safety.

CHAPTER 37

THE SKIN

CHAPTER CONTENTS

HEALTHY SKIN, HAIR, AND NAILS

Your skin is a unique and remarkable organ. The 2 square yards of skin that covers the average adult constitutes approximately 15 percent of the total weight of the body.

One square inch of your skin contains millions of cells as well as many specialized nerve endings for sensing heat, cold, and pain. In addition, each square inch contains numerous oil glands, hair follicles, and sweat glands. There also is an intricate network of blood vessels that nourish this complex structure.

Your skin protects your vital organs. It also serves as your heat regulator. Capillaries and blood vessels in the skin dilate or constrict in response to your body temperature. When you are hot you sweat, and the evaporation of the sweat on your skin lowers your body temperature. When your body is chilled, these blood vessels become narrowed and your skin becomes pale and cold. This constriction decreases the flow of blood through your skin and so reduces the heat loss and conserves heat for the main part of your body. Your sweat glands also excrete waste products such as urea, although this is a minor pathway of waste disposal compared to your kidneys, by means of the urine.

By its texture, temperature, color, and clarity, your skin gives information about your general health. Sensory nerves send signals to your brain about hazards. A group of specialized nerve endings in your skin can arouse your nerve and endocrine systems to sexual excitement.

Although the average thickness of your skin is 1/10th of an inch, it ranges from very thin on your eyelids and inner folds of your elbows to very thick on the palms of your hands and soles of your feet. It is composed of three layers—the epidermis, the dermis, and the subcutaneous tissue.

The epidermis is the top layer, the skin you see. The outermost surface of the epidermis is made up of dead skin cells. Squamous cells lie just below the outer surface; basal cells are at the bottom of the epidermis.

It takes approximately 1 month for new skin cells, manufactured in the living epidermis, to move upward to the outer surface. As the cells move away from their source of nourishment, they become smaller and flatter, changing into a lifeless protein called keratin. Once on the surface, they remain briefly as a protective cover and then flake off as a result of washing and friction. Thus, the skin is a dynamic organ, constantly being replenished.

The cells that manufacture skin constitute about 95 percent of your epidermis. The remaining cells produce a black pigment, melanin. Melanin provides the coloring of your skin and helps protect it from ultraviolet light.

People of all races are born with the same number of pigment cells (melanocytes). However, the rate at which melanin granules are formed in these cells and their degree of concentration in the epidermis are inherited characteristics and major factors in differences in skin color.

The dermis, found beneath the epidermis, makes up 90 percent of the bulk of your skin. It is a dense bed of strong, white fibers (collagen) and yellow, elastic fibers (elastin) through which blood vessels, muscle cells, nerve fibers, lymph channels, hair follicles, and glands are interspersed. The dermis gives strength and elasticity to your skin. As you age, the dermis becomes thinner and the skin becomes more transparent, which accounts for the prominence of blood vessels in the skin of the elderly.

Beneath the dermis lies the subcutaneous tissue which is composed largely of fat and

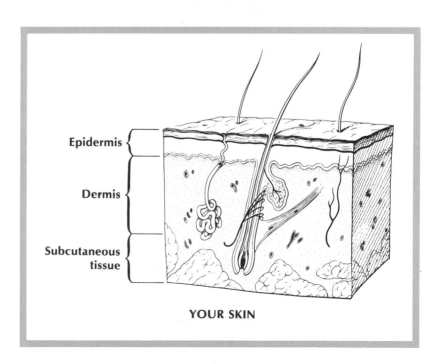

YOUR SKIN

Epidermis

Dermis

Subcutaneous tissue

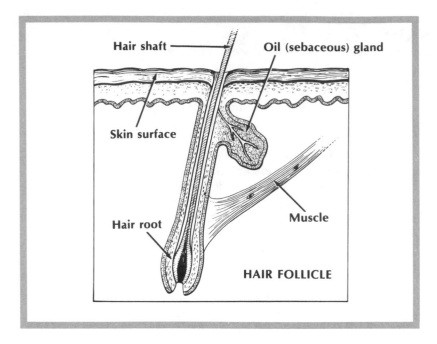

Hair shaft — Oil (sebaceous) gland

Skin surface

Hair root

Muscle

HAIR FOLLICLE

glands that secrete at times of stress or emotion. In the ear they form a portion of the earwax; elsewhere they produce body odor. They are found most abundantly under your arms and around your nipples and genitals.

The human being is a hairy animal; only the lips, palms, and soles are truly hairless. Your scalp hair, like your skin, protects your scalp from excessive sun exposure and your head from trauma. It is a visible indicator of your age and, to some extent, of your general health.

Each hair grows from a single live follicle that has its roots in the subcutaneous tissue of your skin. The oil from the oil gland next to it provides gloss and, to some degree, waterproofing for the hair. The hair follicle is nourished by the minerals, proteins, vitamins, fats, and carbohydrates brought to it by tiny capillaries. Your hair, like the surface of your epidermis, is made up of the dead protein keratin. Hair also contains melanin. Just as the pigment cells determine your skin color, the number of melanin granules in your hair determines its color.

Your fingernails and toenails also are products of your epidermis and are composed of the protein keratin. Each nail grows outward from a nail root that extends back into a groove of skin.

Your fingernails normally grow at the rate of ⅛th inch a month, approximately 2 to 3 times faster than your toenails. Growth slows in old age. Sudden or significant changes in the appearance of your nails can be a first signal of illness.

With severe malnutrition, after an injury, or during a course of some kinds of chemotherapy, hair and nail formation is impaired. During the several weeks of such impaired formation, the shaft of the growing hair thins and even may break off; similarly, an area of thinning of the nails can be seen. The width of this zone of thinning of nails or the length of this portion of the hair shaft that is thinned corresponds to the duration of the injury or the use of chemotherapy. Contrary to common belief, the structure of the nails is not related to the structure of bone, and taking extra calcium will not strengthen brittle nails. Neither will taking gelatin.

Problems such as acne, dermatitis, hair loss, fungal infections of your nails, and many other skin, hair, and nail conditions are usually best treated by a physician called a dermatologist.

through which blood vessels and nerves run. This layer, which specializes in manufacturing fat, is unevenly distributed over your body. The roots of your oil and sweat glands are located here. Subcutaneous tissue thins and disappears with aging.

Oil glands (sebaceous glands) are distributed throughout your skin but are most concentrated in your scalp, face, mid-chest, and genitals. They are attached to the hair follicles and secrete an oily substance (sebum) that rises through the follicle to the surface of the skin. The oily sebum, which is made up of fatty acids, cholesterol, various hydrocarbons, unsaturated alcohols, and waxes, lubricates and protects your skin.

There are two types of sweat glands. The *eccrine* glands are distributed throughout your body, but your palms, soles, forehead, and underarms have the richest supply. The *apocrine* glands are specialized sweat

Skin fold — Nail

Root

YOUR FINGERNAIL

PROPER SKIN CARE

The single most important goal in caring for your skin is to protect it against ultraviolet light. Regardless of your skin color or type or your age, you must monitor your exposure to the sun—and its ultraviolet rays—in order to prevent unnecessary deterioration and, eventually, skin cancer.

Dark skin can tolerate more sun than fair skin can, but any skin can become blotchy, leathery, and wrinkled from continued overexposure. Protective clothing, sunscreen preparations, and daily lubrication or moisturizing are routinely needed (see How To Avoid Sunburn, page 1165).

Proper cleansing is another important strategy in protecting your skin. The best procedures and cleansing ingredients are determined by the type of skin you have—oily, dry, balanced, or a combination of these (see What Is Your Skin Type?, page 1154).

If you use cosmetics, be sure to match them to your skin type: an oil base is suitable for dry skin; a water base is suitable for oily skin.

For women, the first step in facial cleansing is the removal of eye makeup products. Use cotton balls to avoid damaging the delicate tissue around your eyes.

When washing your face, use tepid (never hot) water and a facecloth or sponge to remove dead cells. Use a mild soap for your face and skin; a superfatted variety of soap may be better if your face skin is dry. Oily skin may need to be cleaned two or three times each day.

In general, when washing your body avoid very hot water and strong soaps. Bathing will dry out your skin. If you have dry skin already, limit use of soap to your face, underarms, genital areas, and hands and feet. After bathing, remove the excess water from your skin by brushing rapidly with the palms of your hands. Then, apply a bath oil and rub the oil-water mixture into your skin until it is dry. Legs, arms, and the sides of your body become particularly dry in the winter and are in need of this attention. The oil not only lubricates your skin but also prevents evaporation of water added to it by the bath.

Some men have unusually sensitive skin. Others sometimes injure their faces by the way they shave. Always use a sharp blade when shaving with a blade razor. Soften your beard by applying a warm facecloth for a few seconds; then use plenty of shaving cream. Pass the blade over your beard only once, in the direction of hair growth. Reversing the stroke to obtain a close shave can cause a skin irritation called razor burn. When using an electric razor, too vigorous a shaving method also may irritate your skin. Various preparations are available to lessen the skin irritation that may occur from use of an electric razor.

Women who shave their skin for cosmetic purposes also need to avoid skin irritation. When using hair removers (depilatories) for the first time, the preparation should be applied to a small area as a test to determine whether the product is irritating to your skin.

If you develop a skin problem, do not neglect it. See a dermatologist. The benefits of good skin care will become increasingly apparent to you and to others as you grow older.

WHAT IS YOUR SKIN TYPE?

The skin of your face is generally the best guide in classifying skin type. Examine your skin closely, especially the pores.

Oily Skin
Oily skin is caused by overactivity of the sebaceous glands. Oily skin is thick and has large pores. Oily skin has a greater tendency to develop acne but not wrinkles. Most people with oily skin also have oily hair.

Dry Skin
Dry skin is caused by underactivity of the sebaceous glands, environmental conditions, or normal aging. Dry skin is usually thinner and more easily irritated. It often is associated with dry hair and small pores. There is a greater tendency to develop wrinkles but not acne. Your skin tends to become drier as you age.

Balanced Skin
Balanced skin is neither oily nor dry. It is characterized by fine texture, smoothness, and few problems. However, it has a tendency to become dry as a result of environmental factors and aging.

Combination Skin
Combination skin consists of oily regions—often on the forehead and around the nose—and regions that are balanced or dry.

PHOTOGRAPHIC GUIDE TO COMMON SKIN DISORDERS

The color and texture of your skin can reveal a great deal about the health of your skin and your health in general. Often, the first clue to illness is revealed in the form of a rash or a welt, a growth or a blemish. At other times, the skin disorder is in itself the only abnormality. The photographs that follow provide an overview to a variety of skin disorders. Because skin ailments can vary widely in their manifestations, it is important to consult your physician if you are uncertain as to the cause of any skin blemish.

CHILDHOOD ILLNESSES
All highly contagious

Measles (Rubeola)—Red, blotchy rash first appearing on the face (A) or behind the ears, then spreading to the chest, back, and finally to the arms and legs. In addition, small white spots appear on the inside lining of the cheek (B). (See page 861.)

German Measles (Rubella)—Fine, pink rash that appears on the face, trunk (shown above), and then on the arms and legs. It generally lasts 2 or 3 days. (See page 862.)

Roseola—Begins with a high fever. As the fever subsides, a rash may appear on the trunk and neck. The rash may last a few hours to a few days. (See page 862.)

Scarlet Fever—Rash appearing on the neck and chest (but not the face), then spreading to the entire body. The rash has a sandpaper consistency. Often, the rash is most severe on the armpits and groin. (See page 866.)

Mumps—Characterized by swollen, painful glands just beneath the angle of the jaw, causing cheeks to puff out. (See page 865.)

Chickenpox (Varicella)—Itchy, red rash that breaks out on the face, scalp, chest, back, and, to a lesser extent, arms and legs. The spots quickly fill with a clear fluid, rupture, and then turn crusty. Spots at various stages of development may occur at the same time. (See page 864.)

SKIN DISORDERS AT BIRTH AND INFANCY

Diaper Rash (Diaper Dermatitis)—Most often results from reaction of sensitive skin to contact with urine and stool. Often disappears without treatment. (See pages 16 and 71.)

Candidiasis—Fungal infection may appear on the buttocks and genitals as bright red spots that come together to form a solid red area with a scalloped border. (See pages 16 and 1177.)

Cradle Cap (Seborrheic Eczema)—Common problem that generally occurs in infancy. Dry, scaly patches give scalp a dirty appearance. A yellow crust may form over the scales. In addition, scaly patches may occur around the hairline, eyebrows, eyelids, nose, and ears. (See pages 16 and 72.)

Infantile Eczema (Atopic Dermatitis)—Rough, red, patchy rash usually associated with extremely dry skin. May be a reaction to an irritant such as food, clothing, baby powder, or urine. Itching is associated with the rash. (See pages 16, 459, and 1157.)

Milia—Small white bumps or cysts on a newborn's face or, less often, the trunk. They resemble whiteheads and usually disappear without treatment within a few weeks. (See pages 17 and 72.)

BIRTHMARKS (HEMANGIOMAS)

There are many forms of birthmarks. Hemangiomas are one common type. These are benign tumors made of newly formed blood vessels. They characteristically are bright red or sharply protruding lesions that may appear anywhere on the body.

Port-wine Stain—Maroon or red skin discoloration. Most common site: the face. (See page 18.)

Strawberry Hemangioma—Often appears on the face, scalp, back, or chest, but may occur anywhere on the body. (See page 17.)

Cavernous Hemangioma—Typically a red-blue, spongy mass made up of tissue filled with blood. (See page 18.)

DERMATITIS IN ADULTS

The term dermatitis, which describes irritated, inflamed skin, may be used interchangeably with the term eczema. There are many forms, including those shown below:

CONTACT DERMATITIS

Direct contact with any one of various substances can cause contact dermatitis. (See pages 457 and 1155.)

Poison Ivy—Characterized by an itchy rash consisting of small bumps, blisters, and general swelling. (See page 457.)

Nickel Dermatitis—Contact with chemicals such as the nickel contained in this purse-strap buckle causes this rash. (See page 1155.)

Dishpan Hands—Common reaction to a variety of household chemicals. (See page 1155.)

Neurodermatitis—Characterized by scratch marks (excoriations) and small, flat growths (plaques) of various sizes, with definite margins. The growths become thickened and leatherlike (lichenified). Often called lichen simplex chronicus. (See page 1156.)

Stasis Dermatitis—Thickening and itching of the skin at the ankles, often associated with varicose veins. At times the skin becomes inflamed, or open ulcers slowly develop around the ankles and heels. The skin often becomes irregularly thickened from continued scratching. (See page 1157.)

▲ **Seborrheic Dermatitis**—Greasy-appearing, scaly, itchy areas at the sides of the nose, between the eyebrows, behind the ears, or over the breastbone. Dandruff is mild seborrheic dermatitis of the scalp. (See page 1157.)

◀**Prickly Heat Rash**—Characterized by rash of pinhead-sized bumps surrounded by a zone of red skin. This lesion itches intensely. Typically, it occurs on the neck, upper chest, groin, and armpits. Associated with excessive perspiration. (See page 1156.)

NONCANCEROUS (BENIGN) SKIN DISORDERS

Seborrheic Keratoses—Benign skin tumors that commonly appear after age 40. These oval growths have a waxy, wart-like, scaly, slightly elevated surface. Their color varies from yellow to dark brown or black. They have a pasted-on appearance. Occasionally, they appear singly but most often are seen in large numbers. (See page 1168.)

Cutaneous Tag (Acrochordon)—Tiny, harmless, painless tumor that protrudes on a narrow stalk. It is soft and normally skin-colored but may appear darker. (See page 1168.)

Actinic Keratoses (Solar Keratoses)—Gritty, scaly, gray-to-dark-pink patches on the face, scalp, and back of hands. They have a sandpaper-like surface that is more felt than seen. Probable cause: long-term, excessive exposure to ultraviolet radiation in sunlight. (See page 1169.)

Cherry Angioma—Benign skin tumor of unknown origin that appears most frequently after age 40. Characterized by a small, smooth, cherry-red bump on the skin. Most commonly found on the torso. It ranges in size from that of a pinhead to ¼ inch across. (See page 1169.)

Liver Spots (Senile Lentigines)—Harmless, flat patches of increased pigmentation that range from freckle-size (see arrow) to a few inches across. They are light brown to black in color and may occur on your face or the backs of your hands. (See page 1169.)

Sun-damaged Skin—Characterized by coarse wrinkles, sagging folds, sallowness, roughness, excessive dryness, or leather-toughness. The cause: long-term, excessive exposure of unprotected skin to ultraviolet radiation. (See page 1167.)

Wart (Verruca Vulgaris)—Benign tumor caused by a virus that stimulates rapid multiplication of skin cells. Warts are contagious by contact and most commonly occur on the hands or feet. (See page 1170.)

Keloid—Overproduction of scar tissue. Consists of flesh- or lighter-colored, nodular or rigid growths on the skin. A keloid is harmless but may be tender, itchy, or displeasing in appearance. (See page 1170.)

MOLES (PIGMENTED NEVI)

Moles are benign accumulations of pigment cells. They may contain hairs, stay smooth, or become raised or wrinkled. **Important:** Consult your physician about any change in the color or size of a mole, or if itching, pain, bleeding, or inflammation develops. (See page 1170.)

SKIN CANCERS—MELANOMAS

Melanomas are the most lethal forms of skin cancer. These skin growths require prompt diagnosis and treatment. There are four main types of melanomas:

Superficial Spreading Melanoma—Characterized by variations in color and an irregular border. Most frequent sites for this common type of melanoma are the torso and limbs. (See page 1171.)

Acral Lentiginous Melanoma—Freckle-like melanoma of the extremity. Skin around or under a fingernail or toenail is commonly affected. (See page 1171.)

Nodular Melanoma—From its inception, this growth is raised above the skin surface. There is no most-frequent site. Because invasion into the lower skin occurs early, prompt treatment is especially crucial. (See page 1171.)

Lentigo Maligna Melanoma—Most often afflicts elderly people. Occurs primarily on sunlight-damaged skin of the face or backs of the hands. Always preceded by lentigo maligna, a flat, tan-to-brown area that may exist for many years or decades before the cancerous cells begin to penetrate deeper into the skin. (See page 1171.)

OTHER SKIN CANCERS

Basal Cell Cancer—The most common malignant skin tumor. Characterized by a pearly or waxy bump on the skin of the face, ears, or neck, or may be a flat, flesh-colored or brown, scar-like lesion on the chest or back. (See page 1171.)

Kaposi's Sarcoma—Red-purple nodules anywhere on the skin (as above), or dark-blue or purple-brown nodules on the toe or leg (lower right). Now occurring with greater frequency because of its association with acquired immune deficiency syndrome (AIDS). (See page 1172.)

Squamous Cell Cancer—Normally painless unless it ulcerates. Generally occurs in areas regularly exposed to sunlight. Lesion generally firm, red, nodular, or flat, with a scaly or crusted surface. Occurs on the face, ears, neck, hands, or arms. (See page 1171.)

PIGMENTARY CHANGES, HAIR AND NAILS

◀ ▲ **Vitiligo**—If you have black skin, vitiligo can turn your skin patchy white (left). If you have white skin, you may first become aware of vitiligo during the summer season, when depigmented areas of your skin become more noticeable as the rest of your skin tans. (See page 1163.)

Chloasma—Patches of darker skin, most commonly found on the face. May be associated with pregnancy or use of birth control pills. Chloasma results from excessive melanin in the skin. (See page 1163.)

Alopecia Areata—Sudden hair loss. Usually starts abruptly with one or more circular bald patches that may overlap. The bald areas are smooth and painless. The cause is unknown. (See page 1185.)

Paronychia—Superficial infection of the skin around the nail, most commonly caused by staphylococci or a fungus (*candida*). Skin next to the nail becomes red and swollen. (See page 1186.)

Leukonychia—White nails, either completely or in spots or patches under the nails. (See page 1186.)

Hirsutism—Excess hair. Normally develops over a few months. (See page 1184.)

FUNGAL INFECTIONS

Fungal infections are caused by microscopic plants that become parasites on your skin. Susceptibility to these infections is increased by poor hygiene, continually moist skin, or minor skin or nail injuries. (See page 1177.)

Ringworm (Tinea Corporis)—Itchy, red, scaly, slightly raised, expanding rings on the trunk, face, or groin/thigh fold. The ring grows outward as infection spreads and the central area becomes less actively infected. (See page 1177.)

Tinea Versicolor—Tissue-thin coating of fungus on your skin, characterized by small, slightly scaly, pale patches on the upper body and neck or face. (See page 1177.)

Intertrigo—Red, moist patches rimmed with small red bumps under the breast, in armpits, navel, groin, or buttock/thigh fold, or between fingers or toes. (See page 1177.)

Jock Itch (Tinea Cruris)—Red, moist, well-marked patches in the groin area. (See page 1178.)

Onychomycosis—Fungal infection of the fingernails (above) or toenails. (See page 1186.)

Athlete's Foot (Tinea Pedis)—Itchy, red, soggy, flaking, and cracking skin between toes, or a few fluid-filled bumps on sides or sole of the foot. There also may be extreme dryness with small white scales on the sides or sole of your foot or palms of your hand. (See page 1178.)

Cystic Acne—Most severe form of acne. Results from hair follicles that are plugged by skin oils or dead cells from sebaceous glands. The resulting rupture within your skin may form boil-like infections. (See page 1158.)

Acne Rosacea—Chronic inflammation of the cheeks, nose, chin, forehead, or eyelids, with pimple-like pustules in the reddened area. (See page 1159.)

Hives (Urticaria)—Acute hives (left) are characterized by raised, red, often itchy welts of various sizes that appear and disappear at random on the surface of the skin. If persistent, chronic hives (right) develop. (See page 460.)

Dermographism—Welts that develop where the skin is scratched. (See page 460.)

Angioedema—Large welts that develop below the surface of your skin, particularly on the eyes and lips, but also on the hands and feet and even in the throat. (See page 460.)

ORAL DISORDERS

Cold Sores (Herpes Simplex)—Often called fever blisters. Single or clustered, small, fluid-filled blisters on a raised, red, painful area of the skin. The blisters form, break, and ooze; then a yellow crust forms and finally sluffs off to uncover pinkish, healing skin. (See page 1175.)

Canker Sore (Aphthous Ulcer)—Occurs singly or in clusters on the inside surfaces of the cheeks or lips, on the tongue, at the base of the gums, or on the soft palate. It is a painful ulcer sore with a white or yellow center and a red border. (See pages 577 and 1175.)

Oral Thrush (Candidiasis)—Slightly raised, creamy-white, sore patches in your mouth or on your tongue. If patches are brushed off, bleeding may result. (See pages 18, 578, and 1177.)

Oral Lichen Planus—Small, pale pimples that form a lacy network on the tongue or cheeks, or shiny, slightly raised patches on the tongue or cheeks. (See pages 578 and 1161.)

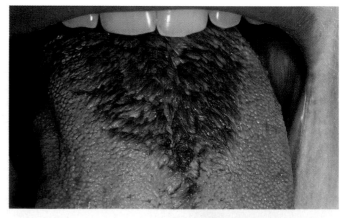

Leukoplakia—Thickened, hardened, white patch on the cheek or tongue. If the patch develops in the mouth of a smoker as the body's natural protection against the heat of tobacco smoke, the condition is referred to as smoker's keratosis or snuff keratosis. This may be a precancerous lesion. (See page 578.)

Black, Hairy Tongue—Hair-like projections that grow profusely on the tongue, giving it a hairy appearance. The tongue usually is not sore, but the appearance can be alarming. Growths can be removed by brushing gently with a toothbrush. (See page 580.)

EYE DISORDERS

Stye (Hordeolum)—Bacterial infection near the root (follicle) of an eyelash. Similar to a boil or pimple. Often painful. (See page 753.)

Chalazion—Painless swelling of the eyelid, resulting from blockage of one of the small glands that produce part of the tear layer. (See page 753.)

Conjunctivitis—Inflammation of the transparent membrane that lines the eyelid. Characterized by redness and a gritty sensation in the eye, along with itching. Often, a discharge forms a crust during the night. If caused by a virus, this disorder is commonly known as pinkeye. (See page 759.)

Orbital Cellulitis—Swelling and redness of the eyelid, followed rapidly by pain and decreased vision. There may be displacement of the eye due to swelling. Requires prompt (emergency) treatment. (See page 761.)

Xanthelasma—Soft, yellowish, fatty, flat lesions that appear on eyelids, near your nose. May suggest elevated concentrations of cholesterol and triglycerides. (See page 1168.)

Iris Melanoma—Development of a brown or black spot in the iris may suggest a melanoma, a type of cancer of the eye. If this occurs, see your ophthalmologist promptly. (See page 762.)

SKIN INFECTIONS

Impetigo—Fairly common superficial infection caused by bacteria (staphylococci, streptococci, or both) that usually invade at the site of a skin abrasion, scratch, or an insect bite. Infection starts with a red sore that blisters briefly and then oozes during the next few days to form a thick crust. (See page 1173.)

Carbuncle—Cluster of boils that form a connected area of infection under the skin. Swelling, redness, and pain may spread. Generally appears on your upper back or the nape of your neck. (See page 1174.)

Cellulitis—Generally caused by bacterial infection. Painful area of hot, red, swollen skin. (See page 1174.)

Folliculitis—Small, white-headed pimples around hair follicles. This is a superficial infection that generally is caused by staphylococci, bacteria, or fungi. (See page 1173.)

Shingles (Herpes Zoster)—Characterized by pain or a tingling sensation in a limited area of one side of your face or torso. Red rash follows, with small, fluid-filled blisters. (See page 1176.)

Genital Herpes (Herpes Simplex 2)—Lesion in the genital area, characterized by water blisters (vesicles) or open sores (ulcers). The ulcers begin as small, tender, red bumps and become water blisters within days. Pain or itching occurs. The blisters rupture, becoming ulcers that ooze or bleed. After 3 to 4 days, scabs form and the ulcers heal. (See page 877.)

Human Bite—Fight bites occur when, in the act of striking another person, the assailant cuts his or her hand or knuckles on the victim's teeth. Bacteria often enter the wound, causing infection. This injury requires prompt treatment. (See pages 257 and 1181.)

Molluscum Contagiosum—A common viral infection of the skin, characterized by tiny, pearl-like projections with a core of white, cheesy matter. Contagious by contact. (See page 1177.)

Portuguese Man-of-War Sting—Red, hive-like lesions in a line, along with stinging pain. Caused by contact with a toxic venom from Portuguese man-of-war. (See pages 260 and 1179.)

INFESTATIONS AND BITES

Lice—These tiny insects most frequently are transmitted by contact from person to person. (See page 872.)

Scabies—Caused by tiny mites that burrow into your skin. Characteristic burrow looks like a thin, irregular pencil mark. Causes severe itching. (See page 872.)

Head Lice—Found on the scalp and easiest to see at the nape of the neck and over the ears. Small nits (eggs) resembling tiny pussy-willow buds can be found on the hair shafts. (See page 872.)

Chigger Bite— Characterized by small red pimples and sometimes by hives. Intense itching is present at the site where the chigger inserts its feeding tube. Chiggers and ticks feed on human and animal blood. (See page 874.)

Lyme Disease— Caused by tick bite; results in red rash that usually occurs at the site of the bite, followed by flu-like symptoms such as headache, chills, fever, body aches, and stiffness. Central portion of the rash clears as the rash spreads outward. (See pages 259 and 854.)

Tick Bite—Small, hard, itchy lumps surrounded by a red halo. (See pages 259 and 874.)

Spider Bite (Brown Recluse)—Fluid-filled bump forms at site of the bite, then sluffs off, sometimes leaving a large, deep, growing ulcer. (See pages 257 and 1179.)

MISCELLANEOUS SKIN DISEASES

Nummular Dermatitis—Inflammation of the skin in which the lesions are shaped like small coins. (See Contact Dermatitis, page 1155.)

Perioral Dermatitis—Inflammation of the skin around the mouth. (See Contact Dermatitis, page 1155.)

Pityriasis Rosea—Common rash characterized by mild itching and red spots on the torso, upper arms, neck, and thighs. Frequently affects young people. A single, scaly, red patch on the torso may be the first sign. After several days, more spots may appear. Probably caused by a virus. Rash disappears in 3 to 12 weeks. (See page 1161.)

Ichthyosis—An inherited skin disorder in which the skin has a fish-scale appearance. (See page 1162.)

Spider-Burst Veins—Collection of bluish veins seen through the skin of the leg. (See page 1167.)

Dry Skin (Asteatosis)—Itchy, scaly skin. This common problem occurs particularly when air is low in humidity. Skin may become cracked. Round patches of irritated skin may develop. Most common sites are lower legs, upper arms, sides, and thighs. (See page 1161.)

Drug Rash—Skin changes may include redness, hives, blisters, and bleeding into the skin. Itching usually is present. Caused by an allergic reaction to a medication. (See page 1163.)

Psoriasis—Common skin disease characterized by flare-ups and partial remissions. Sometimes portions of the skin are covered with dry, red patches with silvery scales. These lesions may itch. Small, scaling dots may also be present. Most common sites are the trunk, knees, elbows, and scalp. Pits or ridges may develop in the nails. (See page 1160.)

Scleroderma—Progressive systemic disorder with skin manifestations of thickening and tightening of the skin, especially on arms, face, and hands, resulting in loss of flexibility. (See page 1007.)

Raynaud's Disease—A condition in which the fingers and toes turn white on exposure to cold, with an accompanying stinging pain. The skin may turn blue or red before it recovers. (See page 840.)

SKIN DISORDERS

Because it is a complex organ constantly exposed to the elements, your skin is susceptible to various problems. Taking care of your skin can prevent many skin disorders.

Your skin protects your body from the environment. It is surprisingly resistant to a wide variety of insults. However, it may become irritated and inflamed, a condition called dermatitis. Its capillaries may become enlarged as a result of sunburn, hives, or rosacea. Any of the production activities within your skin can go awry—for example, too much oil (acne), too many new skin cells (psoriasis), or too much or too little melanin (pigmentary changes).

The skin disorders described below are not life-threatening or contagious. However, they can cause acute discomfort or make you upset about your appearance. Your symptoms may disappear in a week, may require surgery, or may necessitate a long-term treatment program.

The term dermatitis, which is used interchangeably with eczema, simply means an inflammation of the skin. It has many causes and may appear in a number of different guises including contact dermatitis, prickly heat rash, lichen simplex chronicus (neurodermatitis), atopic dermatitis, stasis dermatitis, and seborrheic dermatitis.

CONTACT DERMATITIS

Signs and Symptoms
- Redness and itching;
- Blisters and weeping from the sores in severe cases;
- Skin changes are sharply limited to the area of contact with the causative agent.

Direct contact with one of various substances can cause a skin inflammation physicians call contact dermatitis (see color photograph, page B-3). The rash caused by exposure to poison ivy is a good example of this problem, although the sensitivity of skin varies considerably among individuals (see page 457). If you are sensitive to material in a watchband or ring, skin beneath the object can become inflamed. Another example of contact dermatitis is the red, sore eyelids that can follow use of certain cosmetic products or contact with other materials brought to the eyelids by your fingers.

The Diagnosis.   If your dermatologist suspects that your skin problem is the result of a contact sensitivity, he or she may do skin testing by applying small amounts of different substances to your skin under an adhesive covering and examining the test sites 48 hours later. This is called patch testing. If your skin responds to one or more of these substances (relatively few patients have such a response), the problem is known as allergic contact dermatitis. When virtually everyone who contacts a specific substance reacts with dermatitis, the ailment is known as irritant contact dermatitis. In contact dermatitis, only the areas of skin contacted by the offending substance react. The area with the greatest exposure reacts most severely.

In allergic contact dermatitis, it is not unusual for the allergen to be something that you have used for years with no problem. Mild chemicals such as hexachlorophene in soap, acetone in nail-polish remover, thimerosal in contact lens solutions, and

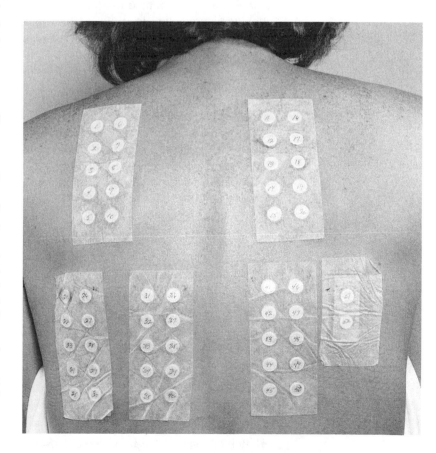

Patch testing can be helpful in determining whether you are allergic to a specific substance.

PRICKLY HEAT RASH

To some of us, hot weather means the arrival of prickly heat. This condition is characterized by a rash of pinhead-sized bumps surrounded by a zone of red skin (see color photograph, page B-3).

Prickly heat itches intensely; often, there is an accompanying prickling, stinging sensation. Typically, it occurs on the neck, upper chest, groin, and armpits. The medical name for the most common variety of prickly heat is miliaria rubra.

Excessive perspiration produces prickly heat because the moisture damages cells on the surface of your skin. These damaged cells form a barrier that blocks the free flow of sweat out to the surface of your skin. Instead, the sweat accumulates beneath your skin.

The best treatment for prickly heat is prevention: avoid situations that lead to excessive perspiration. If you already have a prickly heat rash, keep the affected area cool and dry and the problem probably will clear up spontaneously within a few days.

An air-conditioned environment can be most helpful. Also, avoid antiperspirants, lotions, insect repellents, or powders if you are still perspiring. After your skin is cool and dry, use a calamine-type lotion to help relieve the symptoms.

---

household cleaning products can produce contact dermatitis after repeated use for a long time. Other hard-to-identify causes include ingredients in medicinal lotions (antihistamines, antibiotics, or antiseptics), plants (ranging from trumpet creeper to mangoes), rubber, metals (such as nickel), dyes, cosmetics, and chemicals used in manufacturing (such as those used in making shoes or clothing).

Some substances cause dermatitis only when they contact your skin in the sunlight (see Photosensitivity, page 1165). Typical examples include shaving lotions, sunscreens, ointments containing sulfa drugs, some perfumes, and coal-tar products. Other possible causes of contact dermatitis are airborne, such as ragweed pollen or insecticide spray.

Treatment. Treatment consists primarily of identifying the offending agent and avoiding it. Sometimes, hydrocortisone-containing creams or slightly astringent wet dressings may be beneficial.

NEURODERMATITIS

Signs and Symptoms
- Itching, aggravated by nervous tension;
- Thickening of circumscribed patches of skin;
- Scratch marks (excoriations).

Although the conditions are not precisely the same, the names neurodermatitis and lichen simplex chronicus often are used interchangeably (see color photograph, page B-3). In simple terms, these common skin disorders consist of small flat growths (plaques) of various sizes (1 to 10 inches in diameter) with definite margins that have become thickened and leather-like (lichenified).

Lichen simplex chronicus is usually the result of something—often a tight garment—that rubs or scratches, or causes you to rub or scratch, an area of your skin. This leads to thickening of the skin which, in turn, produces itching and thereby encourages more rubbing or scratching. This problem also may occur in a plaque of psoriasis or in the skin about the anus.

Generalized neurodermatitis is a condition closely related to localized neurodermatitis but tends to involve more of the body. The affected skin tends to be less leathery. Long-standing neurodermatitis may lead to brownish pigmentation. This condition often is associated with nervous tension and anxiety.

Treatment. The primary treatment for these skin problems is to stop the scratching. Perhaps by simply understanding that the disorder is the result of the irritation you are causing, you may be able to stop or to minimize your tendency to irritate the area with your hands or fingernails. If you have trouble ignoring the area, a dressing that is difficult to remove, and that is left on for a week or more, may help.

Your physician may recommend hydrocortisone-containing lotions to decrease the itching and inflammation. These often can be purchased as over-the-counter preparations. If the inflammation is more severe, your physician may prescribe a stronger cortisone preparation. Also, the thickened plaques may be thinned by applying salicylic acid-containing ointments that have a peeling effect.

Sedatives and tranquilizers may help, but your physician will want to monitor your use of these substances because they can be addictive.

ATOPIC DERMATITIS

Signs and Symptoms
- Itchy, thickened, fissured skin, most often in the folds of the elbows or back of the knees.

Atopic dermatitis (infantile eczema, see color photograph, page B-2) is often associated with allergies such as asthma (see page 466), nasal congestion (see page 461), and hives (see page 460). Frequently, it runs in families. It usually begins in infancy as areas of scaling and redness concentrated in the folds of the elbows or knees. This ailment causes severe itching.

Atopic dermatitis may wax and wane in severity during childhood and adolescence. It tends to become less of a problem in adult life (see page 16).

Treatment. Treatment consists of applying hydrocortisone-containing lotions. If your skin cracks open, physicians sometimes prescribe wet dressings with mildly astringent properties. If itching is severe, antihistamines may help. Diphenhydramine has a substantial sedative action in addition to being an effective antihistamine and may be chosen for use at night.

STASIS DERMATITIS

Signs and Symptoms
- Thickening and itching of the skin at your ankles.

Varicose veins, or other chronic conditions involving vessels other than arteries, in the legs can lead to buildup of fluid (edema) in tissues beneath the skin (see also Varicose Veins, page 839). As a result, these areas are poorly nourished by blood and become fragile. Because they have less supporting tissues, the ankles are often the site of involvement. Sometimes, the skin becomes inflamed, or open ulcers develop around your ankles and heal very slowly. This condition is called stasis dermatitis (see color photograph, page B-3). Although initially the skin may become thin, it later becomes irregularly thickened, perhaps in response to itching and continued scratching.

Treatment. Treatment consists of correcting the condition that causes water to ac-cumulate in your ankles for extended periods. This may involve varicose vein surgery.

Another treatment option is elevating your legs well above the level of your heart for a week or more. This is usually done in a hospital, under the direction of a physician specializing in the care of varicose veins. When you are allowed to begin walking again, you may need elastic support stockings for your lower legs.

Wet astringent dressings also may be used to soften the thickened, yet fragile, skin and to control infection.

SEBORRHEIC DERMATITIS

Signs and Symptoms
- Greasy-appearing, scaling, itching areas at the sides of your nose, between your eyebrows, behind your ears, or over your breastbone.
- Stubborn, itchy dandruff.

Seborrheic dermatitis (see color photograph, page B-3) is characterized by greasy scaling and a somewhat reddened appearance of the skin, predominantly in the folds at the sides of the lower portions of the nose, above the bridge of the nose, and over the breastbone. It also occurs beneath the breasts, in the folds of skin in the genital regions, and around the umbilicus in obese persons.

Some people seem to be born with a tendency to have seborrheic dermatitis and will never completely get rid of it, although treatment will help keep it under control. Another manifestation may be scaling and itching of the scalp (see Dandruff, page 1158).

In folds of skin kept moist by contact with other skin (i.e., beneath breasts, about the genitalia), secondary infections with yeast may contribute to the problem. These infections may flare up in persons who are taking antibiotics.

Treatment. Treatment consists of frequent shampooing of the scalp followed by careful rinsing. Application of hydrocortisone-containing creams or solutions may soothe the skin. Your dermatologist may recommend a specific shampoo. You also may need treatment for a secondary infection.

DANDRUFF

Everyone has some degree of scaling of the skin on their scalp because of the normal process of shedding the outer layer of cells. If the flaking becomes obvious on your hair and clothing, it is commonly called dandruff (see color photograph, page B-3).

The cause of dandruff is unknown. It is a mild form of seborrheic dermatitis (see page 1157) and is considered to be caused by overactive oil glands or, perhaps, a yeast infection.

You probably can recognize ordinary dandruff. If your dandruff persists or you have very large flakes together with symptoms around your nose, ears, or chest, you may have a more severe form of dandruff or perhaps even psoriasis of the scalp (see page 1160). If you have questions about its seriousness, consult your dermatologist.

Treating Your Dandruff

Over-the-counter dandruff shampoos usually contain sulfur, salicylic acid, selenium, or tar as their active ingredient.

Shampoo daily, leaving the lather on for a few minutes before rinsing. Sometimes flaking can be caused by a residue of shampoo in your hair, so you need to rinse very thoroughly. Finish up with a conditioner to help smooth out any tangles. A conditioner is an after-shampoo rinse that coats the hair to make it softer and more manageable. Neither your dandruff nor a daily shampoo will cause hair loss.

When your dandruff clears up, shampoo as needed. Occasional use of a dandruff shampoo can help keep a mild condition in check.

If your flaking persists despite home remedies, your dermatologist may prescribe a rub-on steroid lotion to suppress the flaking or a stronger salicylic acid or tar medication to loosen the scales so that you can wash them away more easily.

OVERTREATMENT DERMATITIS

Signs and Symptoms
- Redness and sensitivity of the skin in areas that have been vigorously treated for another skin disorder.

A common skin problem actually is the result of overtreatment. Dermatologists often see people who have inflammation of the skin (dermatitis) that has persisted for several weeks or months and worsened, in spite of frequent application of a number of ointments or other treatments.

Typically, there is no way that the underlying disorder can be identified. The inflammation resulting from the excessive treatment obscures the underlying disease that may or may not still be present.

Treatment. In this situation, all treatment other than the most soothing measures must be discontinued for a week or two. It is often hard to accept this idea. However, only after the withdrawal of all medications is it possible to assess the problem. In the meantime, the problem may have lessened considerably or even disappeared.

ACNE

Signs and Symptoms
- Blackheads or whiteheads on face, neck, shoulders, or back;
- Pimples (zits);
- Cysts.

Acne occurs when the hair follicles of your skin become plugged. Each follicle contains sebaceous glands that secrete a fatty oil (sebum) to lubricate your hair and skin.

When sebum and dead cells are produced faster than they can exit from the pore, they solidify as a white, cheesy plug. This plug may close off the pore, causing the follicle wall to bulge, and thus creates a whitehead. If the pore stays open, the top surface of the plug may become darkened, causing a blackhead. Blackheads are neither caused nor colored by dirt.

Pimples are infections that develop when whiteheads rupture the follicle wall. After the rupture, solidified sebum, dead cells, and bacteria invade your skin. Ruptures deep within your skin form boil-like infections called cystic acne (see color photograph, page B-9).

In some situations, the sebaceous gland continues to secrete material that does not rupture through the skin. Instead, a flattened, pliable lump forms under the skin. This is called a sebaceous cyst or wen. Sometimes the lumps can be an inch or more in diameter. Generally, there is no discoloration or pain unless the cyst becomes infected.

Three out of four teenagers have some acne. It is most prevalent in adolescence because hormonal changes stimulate the sebaceous glands during these years, increasing sebum production and the chances of acne. Aggravation of acne in later life may occur with menstrual periods, the use of birth control pills, and stress. Sudden onset of severe acne in a mature woman can be due to a tumor that affects hormone production. This requires prompt medical attention.

Application of oil or grease to your skin can aggravate acne. This includes use of oil-based makeup, suntan oil, or hairdressing as well as oils from machinery or cooking.

The Diagnosis.   Acne usually is easy to diagnose. Pimple-like pustules alone, with no blackheads or whiteheads, may be another skin disease (see Rosacea, below) or a reaction to medications such as corticosteroids.

How Serious Is Acne?   Acne often is a chronic problem from puberty through early adulthood. It eventually clears up in most cases, but permanent scars may remain. Medical treatment usually provides visible improvement within a few months, but the condition can affect self-esteem, confidence, personality, and social life.

Treatment.   Your acne may require a lengthy, consistent treatment involving four basic steps. The first step is to identify everything that aggravates your acne and to avoid these things. The second step is to follow your physician's advice in regard to removing blackheads and mature pimples or to have this done by a professional. Step three is to use a cleansing agent or soap that dries out your skin enough to cause minor shedding of skin so that the follicular plugs flake. The fourth step is to promote skin peeling within your follicles, either by using one of the medications described below or by using a sunlamp (with proper caution).

Medication.   Two types of medication are used for acne. The first is topical. This consists of a skin lotion that dries up the oil and promotes peeling. Over-the-counter lotions are mild and contain benzoyl peroxide, sulfur, resorcinol, or salicylic acid as the active ingredient. Stronger lotions containing these ingredients or a vitamin A acid (tretinoin or retinoic acid) require a prescription and supervision by your dermatologist.

The second type is taken orally. For severe acne, your dermatologist may prescribe either an antibiotic (tetracycline) or a new form of vitamin A acid (isotretinoin) if your acne is cystic. Both of these can cause side effects and neither should be used during pregnancy. The vitamin A preparation in particular is recognized as causing birth defects. Because such harmful effects are likely to occur during the very early stages of pregnancy, even before you are certain you are pregnant, do not use this drug if you are not using birth control measures.

Surgery.   Cystic acne and sebaceous cysts may require minor surgery under local anesthesia for drainage and removal.

Cosmetic surgery is sometimes used to diminish the scars left by acne. The main procedures are dermabrasion or peeling by freezing or chemicals. If your skin tends to form scar tissue (see Keloids, page 1170), these procedures can make your complexion much worse.

Peeling procedures eliminate superficial scars. Dermabrasion, usually reserved for more severe scarring, consists of abrading the skin with a rapidly rotating wire brush. A local anesthetic or topical freezing of the skin is used during the procedure. General anesthesia ordinarily is not required. Generally, dermabrasion is done as an outpatient procedure.

ROSACEA

Signs and Symptoms
- Red areas on face;
- Inflammation of cheeks, nose, forehead, and chin;
- Red, bulbous nose.

Rosacea (see color photograph, page B-9) is a chronic inflammation of the cheeks, nose, chin, forehead, or eyelids. The cause is unknown. The symptoms are due to enlargement of blood vessels just under the skin. This occurs most frequently in fair-skinned people who blush easily.

It usually begins between ages 30 and 50 years. Although it is more common in women, men are more likely to have the severe form with a bright red, bulbous nose.

Because there may be pimple-like pustules in the reddened areas, the condition used to be called acne rosacea. This name is misleading because the blackheads and whiteheads of acne are not associated with rosacea.

Treatment. Rosacea is not life-threatening, but it seriously affects your appearance. The redness sometimes can be minimized by avoiding hot or spicy foods, hot beverages, and alcohol. Consult your physician if these avoidance measures do not decrease the redness to your satisfaction.

Long-term treatment with an antibiotic (such as tetracycline) almost always is effective in controlling the eruption. The dose of the antibiotic is gradually decreased to maintain control; eventually the drug can be discontinued without recurrence of the rosacea. Later, laser treatment can eliminate persistent blood vessels and improve your complexion.

PSORIASIS

Signs and Symptoms
- Dry, red patches of skin covered with silvery scales;
- Small scaling dots (most commonly seen in children).

Emergency Symptoms
- Reddening and scales affecting entire skin.

Psoriasis (see color photograph, page B-16) is a common skin disease characterized by flare-ups and partial remissions. The attacks can range from a few spots of dandruff-like scaling to large areas with major eruptions. The most common locations are elbows, knees, trunk, and scalp; pits or ridges may develop in the nails.

The eruptions take various forms including pustules, skin cracking, itching, minor bleeding, or aching joints. Psoriasis is not contagious.

Psoriasis apparently develops from a genetic predisposition that affects the life cycle of skin cells. Normally, about a month is required for new cells to move from the lowest skin layer, where they are produced, to the outermost layer, where they die and scale off in tiny flakes. With psoriasis, however, the entire cycle takes only 3 or 4 days. The result of this speed-up in the cycle is that dead cells accumulate rapidly, forming thick scales.

Psoriasis flare-ups are often triggered by skin injuries such as a cut, burn, rash, or insect bite. They also can be precipitated by medications, viral or bacterial infections, excessive alcohol consumption, being overweight, lack of sunlight, a bad sunburn, stress, or by constant friction on the skin.

Approximately 3 million Americans have psoriasis and 100,000 of these people have severe symptoms. It can strike suddenly at any age, but the onset usually is gradual and begins between ages 15 and 35. It is most common in white-skinned people.

The Diagnosis. The diagnosis usually is by physical inspection. Your doctor may need a skin sample (biopsy) for microscopic analysis to rule out other disorders or a fungal infection.

How Serious is Psoriasis? Psoriasis ranges from mild to severe and chronic. Although it cannot be cured, treatment for different levels of severity is generally effective when the disorder flares up.

If almost all of your skin is affected, this is an acute attack requiring emergency treatment. Acute secondary infections also can start during any flare-up. A secondary chronic condition of arthritis develops in nearly 1 out of 10 cases, more frequently in women (see Psoriatic Arthritis, page 1001).

Treatment. *Self-Help.* Self-help for psoriasis includes maintaining good general health and especially avoiding having a sore throat. Maintaining a normal weight lessens aggravation of the psoriasis when it occurs in creases or folds of the skin. Exposure of psoriatic areas to sunlight may help resolve some patches.

Avoid scratching, rubbing, or picking at the patches of psoriasis. These habits cause thickening of the patches.

Medication. In mild cases, over-the-counter coal-tar soaps, shampoos, cleansers, or ointments used together with bath oils will suffice. Your dermatologist can help devise a treatment suited to your needs and, if necessary, may prescribe stronger coal-tar or corticosteroid preparations.

Affected patches in the scalp are more resistant to therapy and may require a phenol and sodium chloride (salt) lotion or a stronger tar preparation in addition to a daily tar shampoo.

In disabling cases, an anticancer drug called methotrexate is taken orally to slow down the rapid production of skin cells. This is used only when no other therapy has worked; it may cause liver damage after long-term use.

Phototherapy.   Severe cases of psoriasis often require phototherapy at a hospital or psoriasis-care facility for about 3 weeks. After your skin is sensitized by application of coal-tar ointment (Goeckerman therapy), your skin will be exposed to ultraviolet light. A new class of oral medications (psoralens) are used with ultraviolet A light irradiation to control the psoriasis in some people. This is called PUVA therapy.

LICHEN PLANUS

Signs and Symptoms
* Itchy spots on wrists, legs, torso, genitals, mouth, and lips.

Lichen planus is a rare, recurrent, itchy rash characterized by shiny reddish purple spots on the skin and gray-white ones in the mouth. (See color photograph, page B-10.) Most commonly it appears in mid-life. The initial attack may persist for weeks or months, and recurrences can continue over many years. Oral symptoms, consisting of a dryness and metallic taste or burning in the mouth, may appear first and be the only evidence of the disease.

The cause of lichen planus is unknown. Flare-ups are thought to be related to stress. The rash may produce ridges in your nails and leave behind dark spots on your skin.

The diagnosis is by inspection or biopsy.

Treatment.   Corticosteroid ointment may relieve itching. Corticosteroid tablets (prednisone) are prescribed for severe cases.

PITYRIASIS ROSEA

Signs and Symptoms
* Mildly itchy red spots on torso, upper arms, neck, and thighs.

Pityriasis (scaling) rosea (rose-colored) is a common benign rash (see color photograph, page B-15). It most frequently affects young people.

A single scaly red patch on the torso may be the first sign. After several days more spots appear. It is thought to be caused by a virus. The rash usually disappears in 3 to 12 weeks.

Your physician may perform blood tests to rule out other diseases.

Treatment.   Treatment of this eruption should be gentle because irritating your skin may cause the eruption to spread to other areas of your body. Mild lubricants and anti-itching (antipruritic) lotions may control the itching. Hydrocortisone cream also may help.

Moderate sunbathing helps, but avoid sunburn. Your physician also may recommend antihistamine tablets.

DRY SKIN

Signs and Symptoms
* Itchy, scaly skin.

Dry skin, also known as asteatosis or winter itch, is a common problem that occurs especially in older people (see color photograph, page B-15). It is particularly annoying in the winter, when the cold air outside and the heated air inside are low in humidity. Asteatosis is a common winter complaint in the Midwest.

The symptoms are the result of loss of natural moisture and oil from the skin. Your skin may become cracked. Round patches of irritated skin may develop, resembling ringworm (see page 1177). The most common sites are the lower legs, upper arms, sides (flanks), and thighs.

Treatment.   To help decrease the dryness that causes asteatosis, adjust your bathing habits in winter. Take shorter baths in tepid water; apply soap only to your face, armpits, genital and anal areas, and hands and feet. Dry off gently. After bathing, apply bath oil immediately to the moist skin to give a protective coating.

Bathe less frequently, and moisturize your skin daily. Bathing does not contribute to dryness of your skin so long as you limit use of soap and lubricate your skin immediately afterward with a bath oil or other lubricant. Also, use a humidifier during the winter.

If your symptoms persist, apply an over-the-counter hydrocortisone (corticosteroid) cream to your skin. For a severe rash with itching, your physician may prescribe a stronger corticosteroid preparation to lubri-

ITCHING

The medical term for itching is "pruritus"—but whatever you call it, it can be a miserable, distressing condition.

Causes

Itching can be a manifestation of a systemic condition such as: liver disease with obstruction of the bile ducts; some blood disorders (polycythemia, see page 492; leukemia, see page 484; Hodgkin's disease, see page 489); and, rarely, cancer. Kidney failure (see page 906) may cause severe itching when there are high levels of urea and other waste products in the blood. It may be caused by penetration of the skin by larvae of the hookworm family of parasites (see page 871). This includes swimmer's itch and creeping eruption caused by the larvae of cat and dog hookworm and ground itch caused by the true hookworm.

Many external skin disorders can have itching as a major problem, including: insect bites, atopic dermatitis, hives (urticaria), lichen planus, and skin parasites (scabies) (see also pages 1178, 1157, 1163, 1161, and 872, respectively). Aging skin often is more likely to itch. Some drugs can cause itching without causing a rash; aspirin and codeine-related pain relievers are examples.

Neurodermatitis (see page 1156) (lichen simplex chronicus) is characterized by itching and is perpetuated by the scratching of the itch. This rubbing produces an area of thickening (lichenification) of the skin. The thickened skin causes you to rub or scratch some more.

Emotional stress can contribute to or aggravate the sensation of itching, no matter what the initiating or underlying cause may be. If emotional factors are the primary cause, the condition may be known as psychogenic itching. Some persons develop the conviction that their itching is due to a parasite. This is often associated with other symptoms such as burning sensations in the tongue and may constitute a major psychiatric problem.

Treating the Itch

We have many medicines that are effective for relieving or moderating pain, but we have no medicine that will specifically lessen itching.

Antihistamines will relieve the itching of hives but not other forms of itching. Most antihistamines do have a mild sedative effect, however, and may help you get to sleep. Tranquilizers also may be helpful in this indirect manner.

If itching is the result of stress or psychogenic causes, your physician may refer you to a psychiatrist for help.

Creams or ointments containing hydrocortisone may help control the itch of insect bites, atopic eczema, or neurodermatitis.

Perhaps the most common cause of itching is the dry skin associated with aging. Here are some self-help measures you can try: keep your bathwater lukewarm and limit the time of immersion; use minimal amounts of soap; lubricate your skin after bathing; avoid alcohol-containing lotions; apply bath oil immediately after bathing and daily to affected areas; keep room temperatures cool; keep humidity up by using a humidifier—just short of the point at which water condenses on your windows.

You can use Aveeno (a form of oatmeal soap available at your drugstore) in your bathwater for severe itching arising from dry skin. Much the same effect can be obtained from an oatmeal bath or a starch-and-soda bath.

For the oatmeal bath, tie a handful of oatmeal into a piece of cotton cloth. Boil it just as you would cook the oatmeal. Then use this "oatmeal sponge" while you bathe in a tub half full of lukewarm water.

To prepare a starch-and-soda bath, add half a 16-oz. box of baking soda and one 16-oz. box of laundry starch to a tub half full of lukewarm water. Mix well, and then bathe but do not use soap.

An Aveeno, oatmeal, or starch-and-soda bath sometimes will help you get through a difficult day or night when no other remedy seems to help.

cate your skin and lessen the itching. If you have a general, persistent itching, consult your physician. This may be a symptom of other disorders.

ICHTHYOSIS

Signs and Symptoms
• Dry, scaly skin starting in early childhood.

Ichthyosis is also called fish-scale disease because of the appearance of its characteristic rash. Ichthyosis is the most common form of inherited skin disease (see color photograph, page B-15).

This disorder usually first occurs in childhood, between ages 1 and 4 years. Sometimes it disappears entirely for most of the adult years, only to return in later years.

The rash is most noticeable on the elbows, knees, and hands. It usually worsens in the winter. Ichthyosis may be associated with atopic dermatitis (see page 1157).

Treatment. Rub white petroleum jelly (Vaseline) on your affected areas and wrap them in plastic overnight. Applications of lactic acid lotion or cold cream can help if done twice a day.

HIVES

Signs and Symptoms
- Red or pink, itchy bumps on the skin;
- Swelling of the skin.

Hives, also called urticaria, is one of the more common skin diseases (see color photograph, page B-9). Typically, the condition appears as a reaction to internal or external allergens.

For a detailed discussion of Hives, see page 460.

PIGMENTARY CHANGES

Signs and Symptoms
- Slowly growing white patches of skin;
- Dark brown patches of skin.

Skin color is the result of the melanin pigment created in the skin cells. Occasionally, something happens to this coloring mechanism and an area of skin starts producing too much melanin and so becomes darker (chloasma) (see color photograph, page B-7). The reverse also occurs—when no melanin is produced in a patch of skin, it becomes white. When a white patch grows periodically, you may have a skin disorder called vitiligo (see color photograph, page B-7).

Chloasma patches are most common on the face and seldom spread very far. They often are associated with pregnancy or use of birth control pills in women, although both men and women get them for no apparent reason.

Vitiligo patches can start at any age, although most often they first appear between ages 20 and 30. They may begin on your face above the eyes or on your neck, armpits, groin, hands, or knees. They are often symmetric and can spread over your entire body. Heredity is often a factor.

The cause may be destruction of melanin-producing cells by the immune system; in some cases, there are associated disorders such as thyroid problems (see page 730) or pernicious anemia (see page 479).

Neither vitiligo nor chloasma is life-threatening. Cosmetics or skin dyes often are used to hide the patches. Vitiligo patches become sunburned easily and use of a sunscreen lotion is necessary.

Treatment. Repigmentation and depigmentation treatments are used to restore uniform skin color. Repigmentation of vitiligo patches is done by exposure to sun or ultraviolet light after sensitizing the area with topical or oral medications (psoralens). This works for 6 out of 10 affected persons if used two to three times weekly for as long as 2 to 3 years. Side effects may occur.

Depigmentation is done by applying lotions (benoquine or hydroquinone) that bleach your chloasma patches or whiten your remaining skin if you have vitiligo.

DRUG RASHES

Signs and Symptoms
- Skin changes, including redness, hives, blisters, and bleeding into the skin;
- Itching.

You may have an allergic reaction to any over-the-counter drug or to one prescribed by your physician (see color photograph, page B-15).

When a rash develops while you are taking any kind of medicine, that medicine must be suspected as a cause of the rash. Your family physician or a dermatologist can help in sorting out the possible causes.

Drug reactions can involve more than an itch or rash—there may be fever, seizures, nausea, vomiting or diarrhea, heartbeat irregularities, difficulty breathing or asthma, or decreased urine flow. In addition, laboratory tests may demonstrate an effect on your hemoglobin value or white blood cell count. Thus, the signs and symptoms of a drug reaction are extremely varied.

Skin rashes take various forms. This increases the difficulty of determining the cause of the rash. Rashes from drugs usually occur soon after you take your first dose of the medication. This time relationship may alert you to further problems.

Fever is the earliest sign of many drug re-actions. Fortunately, rashes usually are seen early during the course of a drug reaction and will warn you that you may be experiencing a drug reaction. If you take multiple medications, a persistent rash is a warning to seek medical help (see Adverse Drug Reactions, page 1230).

Treatment.   If your rash is due to a medication, when you stop taking the drug the signs and symptoms will usually cease. However, if the drug was prescribed, consult your physician before discontinuing its use.

If your rash is itchy, oatmeal baths or wet dressings may sooth it (see Itching, page 1162). Topical hydrocortisone cream also may help. Antihistamines are sometimes of benefit for certain types of drug rashes.

SUNBURN

Signs and Symptoms
* Red, tender, swollen skin;
* Water blisters.

Emergency Symptoms
* Fever, chills, nausea, or delirium.

Sunburn is the result of overexposure to the sun's ultraviolet radiation. Only short-wavelength ultraviolet light causes sunburn unless you become photosensitive (see page 1165).

The ultraviolet content of sunlight varies. It is greater at higher elevations. It is not filtered out by clouds or haze. Cold air does not reduce ultraviolet radiation from the sun. Reflected ultraviolet light from snow, sand, water, and other surfaces can burn as severely as direct sunlight.

The swollen, red skin of a sunburn is due to congestion in the capillaries that supply blood to your skin. Although any ultraviolet radiation can penetrate your skin, only short wavelengths affect the capillaries, under normal conditions. The darker your skin, the less these rays penetrate because they are absorbed by the melanin pigment.

Mild sunburn or exposure to sun may stimulate your skin to produce extra melanin as protection against further ultraviolet penetration. More melanin means a deeper tan,

if the additional pigment is distributed evenly. Otherwise, it forms freckles, liver spots, or discolored splotches. Your melanin production and dispersal are genetic. There is nothing you can do to change your tanning capacity.

Your natural skin color is an important factor in your susceptibility to sunburn, but other factors also contribute. You are most likely to sunburn without tanning if you have light-colored skin, blue or green eyes, and blond or red hair. Resistance to sunburn and easy tanning are most likely if you have dark brown eyes, brown or black hair, and brown or black skin.

The Diagnosis.   Symptoms of sunburn do not appear until a few hours after exposure, but the pain, redness, and occasional blistering of sunburned skin are unmistakable.

If you have complications such as a rash or itching, you may have sun poisoning (an allergy to sunlight after severe sunburn) or photosensitivity (see page 1165).

How Serious Is Sunburn?   The effect of sunburn is like that of any burn, but its development is relatively slow, rather than rapid as from a heat burn. There is damage to your skin. If the sunburn is severe, skin cells die and blisters form. The skin then heals over in a period of a week or two.

Damage to your skin cells from recurrent sunburn is cumulative, and continued overexposure to ultraviolet radiation produces long-term effects. These can include skin discolorations, actinic keratosis (see page 1169), and skin cancer (see page 1170). Ninety percent of all skin cancer is due to this irreversible damage.

Treatment. *Medication.*   Treat your sunburn by application of hydrocortisone cream several times daily (available over-the-counter). Leave the water blisters intact to speed healing. If they break open on their own, remove the skin fragments and apply an antibacterial ointment on the open areas to help prevent infections. Keep the wounds clean. And take aspirin several times daily.

If your sunburn is severe, contact your physician even before the symptoms and signs are fully developed. Your physician may elect to prescribe oral corticosteroid treatment to decrease the reaction and prevent some of the symptoms.

HOW TO AVOID SUNBURN

At one time a deep tan was regarded as fashionable, even glamorous. Physicians encouraged people to sunbathe. It was considered to be healthful.

Today, we recognize that chronic overexposure to the ultraviolet radiation in sunlight causes your skin to age prematurely. Wrinkles form. But most importantly, skin cancer may develop. Now there is evidence that persons who receive blistering sunburns as youths are the ones most likely to have malignant melanoma, the most serious type of skin cancer (see page 1171), in later years.

If you expect to be exposed to sunlight for lengthy periods, get protection. Wear a hat. Select shirts with long sleeves and avoid shorts.

When possible, plan out-of-doors recreational activities for early-morning or late-afternoon hours to avoid ultraviolet radiation which is most intense from 10 a.m. to 2 p.m.

Whenever outdoors for sustained periods, use a premium-quality sunscreen lotion. A sunscreen will not totally prevent tanning but can protect you from burning. Coconut oil, cocoa butter, or baby oil do not make you tan faster, and they provide very little protection from ultraviolet radiation.

Good sunscreens contain either *para*-aminobenzoic acid (PABA) or benzophenone. Some contain both. (PABA can cause a rash.)

Your sunscreen will work best if you apply it at least half an hour before exposure. Alcohol-based sunscreens seem to penetrate deeper and afford the best protection.

Sunscreens are rated by their sun protection factor (SPF) in a range from 2 to 45. Follow your physician's instructions as to the correct rating for your type of skin. (It's probably best to use a sunscreen with an SPF rating of at least 15.) Reapply your sunscreen frequently during exposure. Protection diminishes with evaporation of the product. Bathing and perspiration can wash it away.

Sand, water, and other surfaces reflect light that can burn as severely as direct sunlight.

Sunscreens also should be used for winter exposure. The greatest hazard in winter months is on cloudy days after a fresh snow. Radiation is increased at higher altitudes, and skiers should always use a sunscreen.

The delicate skin around your eyes, nose, and lips needs extra protection. Some people prefer a sun blocker, such as zinc oxide or titanium dioxide, which stops all radiation from reaching the skin. Others use a special lip sunscreen with an SPF rating of 15 or higher.

Forego perfumes or after-shave lotion before sun exposure. Such preparations may produce discolored patches on your skin. If you have had sun-sensitive reactions in the past, read about photosensitivity (see below; for a list of sensitizing substances, see below).

After your sun exposure, bathe or shower away perspiration, salt, pool chemicals, and sunscreen products. Follow this with application of a lubricant to your skin.

PHOTOSENSITIVITY

Signs and Symptoms
- Redness;
- Rash;
- Blistering or swelling.

Photosensitivity is a heightened reaction of skin to light from the sun or artificial sources, usually following consumption of medications or foods.

Certain medications are known to cause photosensitive reactions in some people. These include anticancer drugs, water pills, tranquilizers, antibiotics of the tetracycline family, antidepressants, antihistamines, birth control pills, Retin-A, anticonvulsants, antidiabetic or high blood pressure (antihypertensive) medications, sulfonamides (usually prescribed for urinary tract infections), and topical antiseptic creams.

Some skin products also can cause a reaction. This is called photocontact dermatitis.

Common photocontact sensitizers include plants (such as limes, parsley, celery, carrots, mustard, or figs), artificial sweeteners (cyclamates), antibacterial deodorant soaps, perfumes containing bergamot, sandalwood, lavender, or citron oils, skin-bleaching creams, shampoos or soaps with coal-tar ingredients, sunscreens with *para*-aminobenzoic acid, medicated cosmetics, detergents, and after-shave lotions.

Photosensitive reactions are divided into two categories, photoallergic and phototoxic. A photoallergic reaction is a result of changes in your immune system. When this occurs, your skin will have a bad reaction each time it is exposed to sunlight. Your skin becomes red (although not necessarily sunburned) and develops a bumpy rash similar to poison ivy. Discolored patches, blisters, or swelling also can occur. Symptoms can extend to areas not exposed to the light. Photoallergy can strike again, with suddenness, later in life. Once you are sensitized to a substance, you can react again and again. You also can react to substances that are chemically similar.

A phototoxic reaction, on the other hand, will look and feel like an exaggerated sunburn with inflammation, redness, blisters, and the characteristic discomfort. You may have this reaction any time a sufficient amount of the sensitizing chemical is present in your body and you are exposed to the specific wavelength of light.

Treatment.   Your photosensitive reaction usually will disappear within a week after you begin protecting your skin from light exposure and avoiding the sensitizing substance, although in some cases the symptoms linger.

If you have had a photoallergy reaction, it is especially important to wear protective clothing and sunscreens when outdoors. For a severe reaction, your physician may prescribe a corticosteroid ointment or cream or hydroxchloroquine tablets to help suppress photoallergic reactions.

SOLAR ELASTOSIS

Signs and Symptoms
- Loose, sagging, or wrinkled skin;
- Dry, tough, leathery skin.

Elastosis is a degenerative disease of the connective tissues of your skin. This degeneration happens slowly as a result of normal aging. Repeated exposure to ultraviolet radiation, however, can accelerate the rate dramatically by a process called photoaging. The resulting condition is solar elastosis.

Your skin is comprised of two types of connective tissue. One type is a strong, white fiber (collagen); the other is an elastic, yellow fiber (elastin). Ultraviolet radiation penetrates skin and damages these tissues. The amount of collagen is decreased; the amount of elastin is increased but it loses its elasticity. The orderly structural arrangement deteriorates, and abnormal cell growth begins.

Each exposure to ultraviolet light causes slight but irreversible changes, so the damage within your skin accumulates over the years. The signs and symptoms of solar elastosis appear gradually as the skin loses its resilience, flexibility, and water-holding capacity. If you have had excessive sun exposure, by the time you are 30 years old the overexposed areas of your skin can look 15 to 20 years older.

If you sunburn easily and tan poorly, you are most susceptible to solar elastosis. This condition usually occurs in fair-skinned, blue- or green-eyed people with blond or red hair who are frequently exposed to intense sunlight without protection. The risk is highest for sunbathers, farmers, sailors, and others who are often outdoors. Those who live in regions with intense sunlight are more at risk; such areas include higher elevations and the Western plains.

The Diagnosis.   You can see the effects of solar elastosis by comparing your protected skin to overexposed skin. Your dermatologist can confirm the diagnosis by examination which may reveal other symptoms of sun-damaged skin (see page 1164) including solar keratosis (see page 1166).

TREATMENT FOR DAMAGED SKIN

If your skin is damaged by too much sun, retinoic acid (Retin-A), a form of vitamin A used for years to fight acne, might help.

Your dermatologist can prescribe nightly applications of Retin-A cream for mild wrinkles on your face, neck, upper chest, or hands. This treatment will cause peeling in the surface skin and will stimulate new skin growth. It may reverse some deterioration within the dermal layer.

You may even notice a healthier glow.

There are potential side effects, however. These include increased sensitivity, dryness, redness, and excessive peeling of your skin. Less-frequent applications (perhaps three times per week) would then be appropriate.

Avoid the sun when using this medication, or discontinue its use prior to and during exposure. Skin treated with Retin-A should not come into contact with dyes, hair-removal wax, or perfume. Diligent applications of sunscreens and lubricants are very important.

How Serious Is Solar Elastosis? The photo-aging process causes cumulative effects. There is no medical treatment to reverse the damage or to rejuvenate your skin.

If your skin has been damaged enough to cause solar elastosis, you are at increased risk of acquiring skin cancer. See your physician whenever you have a new growth or a change in an existing growth such as a mole.

Treatment. Your dermatologist may recommend lubricating creams to reduce dryness and soften your skin. Facial massages and masks can make your face feel better for a while by toning muscles and stimulating blood circulation. Collagen injections may smooth out minor wrinkles in the short term, perhaps for a month or so.

Your doctor also may recommend chemical peeling, dermabrasion, or a face-lift as a longer-lasting treatment. Retin-A, a derivative of vitamin A, is an effective peeling medication (see page 1166). Dermabrasion is a surgical procedure that removes the outer layer of your skin with sandpaper or, more commonly, a wire brush. Face-lifting is the surgical removal of some facial skin so that the remaining skin is stretched more tightly.

To prevent further damage, avoid sunlight if you can. If you cannot, seek protection (see page 1165).

SENILE SKIN

Signs and Symptoms
- Skin discolorations including liver spots, freckles, and red, yellow, gray, or brown blotches;
- Skin texture changes including coarse wrinkles, sagging folds, sallowness, roughness, excessive dryness, or leathery toughness;
- Skin growths including scaly patches.

The effects of aging on skin are gradual under normal conditions. However, the signs of age may appear faster if you are susceptible to sun damage and expose your unprotected skin to ultraviolet radiation frequently (see color photograph, page B-4).

Senile or sun-damaged skin is irreversible. The separate symptoms and treatments are described in sections on liver spots (see page 1169), solar elastosis (see page 1166), and actinic keratosis (see page 1169), the three

WRINKLED SKIN

Wrinkling is a natural part of aging. As you grow older, your skin gets thinner, drier, less elastic, and more wrinkled, and it tends to lose its youthful color and glow.

Dryness is a result of decreased oil production within your skin. Sagging, wrinkling, and thinning are caused by deterioration in the connective tissue (elastin and collagen) in your dermal layer. Finally, as your blood supply slows, your rosy glow begins to fade.

Although aging of your skin is inevitable, it can be slowed by maintaining good general health and the consistent use of sunscreens whenever you are outdoors.

There is no cure for wrinkled skin. Overexposure to sun and excessive cigarette smoking accelerate wrinkling dramatically. Avoid them. Your physician may prescribe Retin-A (see Treatment for Damaged Skin, page 1166).

SPIDER-BURST LEG VEINS

These really have nothing to do with spiders. However, the pattern of bluish veins seen through the skin of the leg does look a bit like a spider. (See color photograph, page B-15.)

Both the cause and the prevention are unknown. Unlike more serious varicose veins (see page 839), spider-burst veins generally are painful only to your vanity: for some people, wearing a skirt or shorts is no longer an option because of worries about the appearance of the purple-blue veins on the legs.

The easiest course is to ignore the veins: they are a common, mild, and medically insignificant variety of varicose veins. However, if the unsightly blood vessels do concern you or, more importantly, they prevent you from taking part in activities you otherwise would enjoy, sclerotherapy is a treatment option.

What Is Sclerotherapy?
The procedure is done while you are standing. The physician slowly injects a solution into one or several of the visible veins. Treating each vein requires only a few minutes. Then, a small bandage is wrapped snugly around your leg over the veins and is left on for 24 hours.

The procedure collapses the veins, which prevents blood from flowing into them and eliminates the discoloration. The treatment has no significant effect on circulation in the leg.

Are There Side Effects?
In most people, the color of the spider-burst veins fades within a week or so and is gone in a month. In about one in three of those who undergo the procedure, a yellow-brown discoloration may appear in the area and takes weeks or even months to fade. In rare instances, this discoloration persists longer.

principal problems associated with senile skin.

Sun damage also increases your chances of skin cancer (see page 1170) significantly, so, as you age, watch for early signs of these malignant growths.

Your susceptibility to sun damage is greatest if you are green- or blue-eyed, are fair-skinned, have blond or red hair, and sunburn easily. Sun protection (see page 1165) is critical if you spend time outdoors.

Treatment. For treatment of specific symptoms, see the sections referred to above. In general, however, it is wise to apply adequate lubrication and sunscreen lotions. Also, consult your physician about new growths or changes in existing ones.

XANTHELASMA AND XANTHOMA

Signs and Symptoms
- Soft, fatty bumps beneath the surface of your skin.

Both xanthelasma and xanthoma are yellowish bumps that appear beneath the skin. These bumps have sharply defined margins.

Xanthelasmas (see color photograph, page B-11) are flat and appear in the skin of your eyelids near your nose. They do not hurt and they may be harmless, but you should have your blood tested for increased concentrations of cholesterol and triglycerides.

Xanthomas are a symptom of an underlying metabolic disorder that increases the fat (lipid) concentration in the blood. Xanthomas can appear anywhere on your body but most commonly occur over joints or tendons. With certain disorders they often appear where your skin receives persistent pressure, such as on your knees, elbows, hands, feet, or buttocks. Xanthomas are flat and can vary from less than 1 inch to more than 3 inches across. They are associated with diabetes mellitus (see page 707), primary biliary cirrhosis (see Cirrhosis, page 653), some malignancies, and a number of inherited metabolic disorders such as familial hypercholesterolemia (evelated cholesterol).

Consult your physician if you wish to have a xanthelasma or xanthoma removed. But be aware that they may reappear.

BENIGN SKIN TUMORS

Benign skin tumors are very common and usually are harmless. As you grow older you are likely to have a number of them. With the exception of actinic keratoses (see page 1169) and certain moles (see page 1170), benign tumors do not require removal unless they are irritating or cosmetically displeasing. As a precaution, however, consult your physician about any new growth or change in an old one. Several kinds of benign patches, lumps, and bumps that can occur on your skin are described in the pages that follow.

CUTANEOUS TAGS

Signs and Symptoms
- Small protrusions of skin on your neck, armpits, upper trunk, and body folds.

Cutaneous tags, also called acrochordons or skin tags, are tiny benign tumors of unknown origin that protrude from your skin on a narrow stalk. (See color photograph, page B-4.) They are soft and normally skin-colored but may appear darker.

Skin tags are common, especially after middle life, and usually are painless, but they can become irritated by friction from clothing.

Treatment. Treatment is unnecessary unless the tag is bothersome. Your physician can remove it, without scarring, by freezing it with liquid nitrogen (cryotherapy), cutting it off, or burning it off with electricity.

SEBORRHEIC KERATOSIS

Signs and Symptoms
- Yellow, brown, or black growths on face, chest, shoulders, and back.

Seborrheic keratoses are benign skin tumors of unknown origin that commonly appear on light-skinned people after age 40. (See color photograph, page B-4.) The oval growths have a waxy, wart-like, scaly, slightly elevated surface and range from ⅓ to 1 inch or more across. Their color varies from yellow to dark brown or black. They have a pasted-on appearance. Occasionally, they appear singly but most often are seen in large numbers. They are not caused by exposure to sunlight or by viruses.

Treatment. Seborrheic keratoses are normally painless and require no treatment unless they itch, irritate, or detract from your appearance. The growths are never deeply rooted, so removal is simple and nonscarring. Your physician can freeze them off with liquid nitrogen (cryotherapy) or can use a surgical procedure.

ACTINIC KERATOSIS

Signs and Symptoms
- Gritty, scaly, gray-to-dark-pink patches on face, scalp, and back of hands.

Actinic or solar keratosis occurs mostly in fair-skinned persons with sun-damaged skin. (See color photograph, page B-4.) Initially, the keratoses are flat and scaling; later, they have hard, wart-like surfaces. Their sandpaper-like surface is more easily felt than seen. Actinic keratoses are considered to be benign tumors, but they may be signs of precancerous changes in your skin.

Treatment. Prompt medical attention is needed because 20 percent of untreated keratoses develop into squamous cell skin cancer (see page 1171). Your physician can remove them by freezing with liquid nitrogen (cryotherapy) or by using topical medication, electrical burning, or surgery. A sample of the tissue is studied for signs of cancer.

BIRTHMARKS

Signs and Symptoms
- Skin marking that develops before or shortly after birth.

Several kinds of common birthmarks are termed hemangiomas. They are benign, usually painless, markings of unknown origin caused by a proliferation of blood vessels at the site.

For a detailed discussion of Birthmarks, see page 17.

CHERRY ANGIOMA

Signs and Symptoms
- Small, smooth, cherry-red bump on skin.

Cherry angioma is a benign skin tumor of unknown origin that appears most frequently after age 40. (See color photograph, page B-4.) It can occur almost anywhere on your skin but most commonly is found on the torso. These tumors range from pinhead size to ¼ inch across. Large angiomas can bleed profusely when they are injured.

Treatment. A cherry angioma is painless and harmless, but you may want it removed for cosmetic reasons. It is superficial, so your physician can remove it easily by freezing it with liquid nitrogen (cryotherapy) or destroying it by a minor electrosurgical procedure.

LIVER SPOTS

Signs and Symptoms
- Flat, light-brown to black spots on your face or backs of hands.

Liver spots, also known as senile lentigines, are harmless flat patches of increased pigmentation that range from freckle-size to a few inches across. (See color photograph, page B-4.) They are extremely common after age 55 and occur most commonly on the backs of the hands or the forehead. Although frequently associated with overexposure to sun, they also can occur from unknown causes.

Treatment. Most people seek no treatment. For cosmetic reasons, liver spots can be lightened with skin-bleaching products or can be removed by freezing with liquid nitrogen (cryotherapy). Recurrence or appearance of new spots can be minimized by using high-protection sunscreen lotion.

MOLES

Signs and Symptoms
• Flesh-colored, brown, blue, or black spots on the skin.

Nearly everyone has moles. (See color photograph, page B-5.) These benign tumors are nests of pigment cells. They may contain hairs, stay smooth, become raised or wrinkled, and even fall off in old age.

Moles are usually harmless, but they can become cancerous. Consult your physician about changes in color or size, or if itching, pain, bleeding, or inflammation develops. Certain moles (in particular, those that are irregularly shaped, have a mixed brown and black color, are congenital, or are located around the nails or genitals) should be monitored by a physician (see Malignant Melanoma, page 1171).

Treatment.   Treatment usually is unnecessary. For cosmetic reasons, a mole can be removed surgically. If changes develop in a mole, your physician may remove it for microscopic examination.

KELOIDS

Signs and Symptoms
• Flesh- or lighter-colored nodular or ridged growths on the skin.

A keloid is an overproduction of scar tissue, sometimes called hypertrophic scar-

ring. (See color photograph, page B-5.) It occurs at the site of a skin injury (operation, vaccination, severe acne, burn, or even a minor scratch). It is fairly common on black skin and much less common on white skin.

Your keloid is harmless, but it may be tender, itchy, or displeasing. Some keloids stop growing or even disappear by themselves.

Treatment.   Surgical removal often causes further scarring unless it is followed by x-ray treatment or injection of steroids at the site. Small keloids may be removed by freezing with liquid nitrogen (cryotherapy).

WARTS

Signs and Symptoms
• Small, hard, flesh-colored, white, or pink granulated lumps on the skin.

The common wart, verruca vulgaris, is a benign tumor caused by a virus that stimulates rapid multiplication of skin cells. (See color photograph, page B-5.) Warts are contagious by contact and most commonly occur on the hands or feet (plantar warts).

Warts are harmless and many disappear by themselves within 2 years. Plantar warts, however, are often painful from the pressure of standing on them.

Treatment.   Treatment might be unnecessary. Over-the-counter medications may remove a wart. If this fails, your physician can prescribe stronger preparations or remove it by freezing (cryotherapy), electrical burning, minor surgery, or laser surgery.

SKIN CANCERS

If you observe any changes in an existing growth on your skin or a new growth that ulcerates without healing, seek medical attention. This could be skin cancer. The cure rate for skin cancer is high with early treatment, but neglect can lead to disability or even death.

More than 90 percent of skin cancers occur on areas regularly exposed to ultraviolet radiation, and this exposure is considered to be the chief cause. Other contributing factors include: genetic predisposition (evi-

denced by light-colored skin, blue eyes, blond or red hair); chemical pollution; and x-ray radiation. Inorganic arsenics, which were used in medical treatments before 1970 and are still used in herbicides, may contribute.

Identification of skin cancer in its earliest stage allows for early treatment and a high cure rate. This section will help you become familiar with the various forms of skin cancer and show you how to check your skin periodically for such lesions and how to use sunburn protection routinely to guard against the development of skin cancer (see How To Avoid Sunburn, page 1165).

BASAL CELL CANCER

Signs and Symptoms
- Pearly or waxy bump on the skin of your face, ear, or neck;
- Flat, flesh-colored or brown scar-like lesion on chest or back.

Basal cell cancer is the most common form of malignant skin tumor, accounting for 75 percent of all skin cancers (see color photograph, page B-6). When the basal cells in your epidermis become cancerous, they form a painless bump or flat lesion that may ulcerate after a few months, enlarge slowly, and never heal completely.

Because these cancers usually occur on unprotected areas of skin, repeated overexposure to ultraviolet radiation is thought to be a primary cause. Genetic predisposition also may be a contributing factor. Fair-skinned, blue-eyed, red-haired persons are the most vulnerable. Onset most commonly occurs after age 40.

Basal cell cancer remains a local growth and only very rarely spreads to other parts of the body. Lack of medical attention can allow the growth to invade nearby tissues and underlying structures including your nerves, bones, or brain.

Treatment.   Diagnosis requires a skin biopsy of your bump or lesion. Treatment depends on the cancer's size, depth, and location and may include scraping and cauterization, surgical excision, cryosurgery, x-ray radiation, or a series of microscopically controlled shaved excisions (Mohs' surgery).

With early treatment, the cure rate exceeds 95 percent. However, you will need to use high-protection sunscreens diligently to avoid further growths. Also, have regular medical examinations.

SQUAMOUS CELL CANCER

Signs and Symptoms
- Firm, red nodule or flat lesion with scaly or crusted surface on face, ears, neck, hands, or arms.

Squamous cell cancer is a malignant tumor that arises from the midportion of the epidermal layer of the skin. (See color photograph, page B-6.) It is more aggressive than basal cell cancer; it can spread (metastasize) to other locations including lymph nodes or internal organs.

The tumor initially is painless, although pain may develop if it ulcerates and never completely heals. It begins in normal skin, in a burn or scar, or at a site of chronic inflammation. It may originate from a precancerous skin tumor that occurs in sun-damaged skin (see Actinic Keratosis, page 1169).

This cancer appears most frequently on skin regularly exposed to sunlight, and ultraviolet radiation is considered to be the main cause. Genetic predisposition may be a contributing factor. Fair-skinned, blue-eyed, blond or red-haired persons are most vulnerable. The onset most commonly is after age 50.

Treatment.   Diagnosis requires biopsy of your nodule or lesion. Treatment will depend on the cancer's size, depth, location, and signs of metastasis. Surgical removal of the tumor and the skin around it, together with x ray treatment, may be necessary. A skin graft might be needed to replace excised skin. For cancers that recur after surgical removal, Mohs' surgery (a series of microscopically controlled, shaved excisions) may be necessary.

With early treatment, the cure rate is approximately 95 percent. Persistent use of high-protection sunscreens will tend to minimize further development of such lesions. Regular medical examinations for possible recurrence are important for proper follow-up.

MALIGNANT MELANOMA

Signs and Symptoms
- Superficial spreading melanoma: small lesion with irregular border and red, white, blue, or blue-black spots on trunk or limbs;
- Nodular melanoma: shiny, firm, pearl to black bumps or lesions anywhere on skin;
- Acral lentiginous melanoma: dark lesions on palms, soles, tips of fingers and toes, or mucous membranes;

- Lentigo maligna melanoma: large brownish spot with darker speckles on skin overexposed to sun.

Malignant melanoma is the most deadly but least common skin cancer. It typically arises painlessly from cells that produce the skin's pigment (melanin). Approximately 70 percent of these cancers appear on normal skin; 30 percent arise from an existing mole that has undergone sudden changes (color, size, pain, itching, bleeding, swelling).

The cancer first spreads in the surrounding skin and is highly curable at this phase. If not treated, the tumor then spreads downward into other areas of the skin or to lymph nodes or internal organs.

Superficial spreading melanoma accounts for 70 percent of cases and strikes at any age. Nodular melanoma may ulcerate and fail to heal completely. It can develop anywhere on the skin, usually between ages 20 and 60.

Acral lentiginous melanoma accounts for 10 percent of the cases and is more common in old age. Lentigo maligna melanoma occurs in 5 percent of cases. It frequently afflicts the elderly and is associated with senile skin (see page 1167). A benign brownish spot may appear several years before turning cancerous. (See color photographs, page B-6.)

Sunlight is considered to be the chief cause of melanoma. Fair-skinned, blue-eyed, blond or red-haired persons are most vulnerable, and dark skin is the most resistant. Certain moles that may transform into melanoma can run in families. Other contributing factors are listed in the introduction to this section (see Skin Cancers, page 1170).

The incidence of malignant melanoma has doubled among Americans during the past 20 years. In various forms, it can strike at any age, but men have a higher mortality rate.

The Diagnosis. Your physician may be able to diagnose a melanoma from visual inspection. A skin biopsy must be performed to confirm the diagnosis. If there is a possibility of spread of the melanoma to other locations, further testing, including a complete physical examination with chest x-ray and CT scan (see page 1286), may be needed.

How Serious Is Malignant Melanoma?
Prompt treatment in the early stages provides a cure in 85 percent of the cases. When the tumor has grown downward or spread to the lymph nodes or other organs, the 5-year survival rate is 30 percent.

Treatment. Surgical removal of the tumor, together with a wide margin of normal skin and even nearby lymph nodes in some cases, may be required. This may be followed by a skin graft to the site of operation. Other treatment may include anticancer drugs and immunotherapy. In immunotherapy, a vaccine is injected to stimulate your immune system to destroy cancerous tissue.

Periodic medical examinations for evidence of recurring melanoma is a necessary part of the follow-up process for long-term management of this cancer.

KAPOSI'S SARCOMA

Signs and Symptoms
- Aggressive form: Red-purple nodules anywhere on the skin;
- Indolent form: Dark blue or purple-brown nodules on the toe or leg.

Kaposi's sarcoma is a malignant condition sometimes associated with other cancers, including leukemia or lymphoma. (See color photograph, page B-6.) The early lesions are red to purple and resemble a birthmark (hemangioma). Older lesions become brown to black, are flatter, and occur with scarring of the skin.

The disease appears in two forms: aggressive and indolent. The aggressive form occurs both internally and externally. It is now occurring with greater frequency due to its association with acquired immune deficiency syndrome (AIDS). If linked with the multiple disorders of AIDS (see page 848), this is a dangerous cancer.

The dark tumors of the indolent form, which are caused by blood vessel involvement, can spread to your hands and arms or can produce fungus-like growths, or both. This cancer may penetrate your underlying tissue and invade bone, lymph nodes, and internal organs.

Treatment. After diagnosis by examination and skin biopsy, your treatment may include x-ray therapy or chemotherapy. Elastic support hose to reduce swelling may provide some symptomatic relief.

SKIN INFECTIONS

Because your skin is your first line of defense, it often is called upon to deal with attacks from unwanted bacteria, viruses, fungi, and insect venom. If bacteria become established in a wound, they can cause a number of illnesses; bacteria or other foreign invaders may infect hair follicles or develop in skin, as occurs in erysipelas (see page 1174) or shingles (see page 1176).

Skin infections range from localized, superficial infections (like impetigo) to widespread, life-threatening infections. The symptoms depend on where the infection develops and the organism that is causing it.

IMPETIGO

Signs and Symptoms
• Itchy, red sores with yellow or gray crusts on face, legs, or arms.

Impetigo is a fairly common superficial skin infection caused by bacteria—staphylococci, streptococci, or both. (See color photograph, page B-12.) It may occur on normal skin, but the bacteria usually invade at the site of a skin abrasion, scratch, or insect bite or as a secondary complication to other skin diseases such as dermatitis (see page 1155).

The infection starts as a red sore that blisters briefly and then oozes during the next few days to form a sticky crust. The sore tends to grow and is contagious through bacteria in the blister's fluid. Physical contact—including scratching—can spread the infection to other parts of the body or even to other people.

An ulcerating form of impetigo, ecthyma, appears as itchy, thick, brown-black crusts ringed by red skin. In rare instances, the bacteria may infect the bloodstream and, in children, lead to kidney disease (see Acute Glomerulonephritis, page 893).

The incidence of impetigo is highest among children who live in poor hygienic conditions. In adults it appears mostly as a complication of another skin problem.

Your physician will diagnose impetigo by examination and culture of tissue from your infection.

Treatment. Topical medications are effective in limited and minor infections. For more extensive infections, your physician may prescribe antibiotics (such as penicillin or erythromycin) to be taken orally. Several washings daily with antibacterial soap or cleanser soften crusts so that they can be gently removed. To avoid spreading the infection, towels, clothing, and razors should not be shared, and skin contact should be avoided until the condition clears. The sores heal slowly, but the cure rate is very high.

FOLLICULITIS

Signs and Symptoms
• Small, white-headed pimples around the hair follicles.

Folliculitis is a superficial infection of the hair follicles. (See color photograph, page B-12.) These infections are common and usually are caused by staphylococci or fungi. They can occur anywhere on your skin as a result of clothing friction, hair follicle blockage, or injury. For example, shaving your neck or underarms can produce a rash of them that becomes chronic unless treated.

Barber's itch is a staphylococcal infection of the hair follicles of the bearded area, especially the upper lip near the nose. Itching may occur a day or two before the pinhead-sized pustules erupt. Shaving is a major aggravating factor.

A similar eruption due to a fungal infection is referred to as tinea barbae. Antifungal treatment is required for this.

Pseudofolliculitis barbae occurs primarily in black males when the hair of the beard grows into an adjacent hair follicle and forms a small, curled-up mass within the follicle. Chronic infection is present.

Treatment. Mild folliculitis can be treated by a topical antibiotic alone. More extensive folliculitis, such as that involving the beard, requires hot tap-water compresses and oral antibiotics. If folliculitis of the beard is present, use a new razor blade each day for shaving. Take care to avoid reinfections from contaminated clothing or reuse of razor blades.

Pseudofolliculitis barbae may respond only if the infected person does not shave.

BOILS AND CARBUNCLES

Signs and Symptoms
- Swollen and tender nodule on your skin, usually pink or red;
- Spreading area of swelling, redness, and pain in skin;
- Fever or exhausted feeling.

A boil (furuncle) is a local infection in one or more hair follicles and usually is caused by staphylococci. When there are multiple boils anywhere on the body, the condition is called furunculosis. In contrast, a carbuncle is a cluster of boils that forms a connected area of infection under the skin. (See color photograph, page B-12.) These infections are easily spread by contact with other parts of the body and other people.

Sometimes a boil will go away after the initial stage of itching or mild pain. More often, however, it grows rapidly over a few days; as pus collects within the lesion, pressure and pain increase. It comes to a head with a white or yellow center in the nodule and then bursts, drains, and heals. It may recur later near the same site and go through the same cycle.

Boils are very common, and most persons get one at some time during their lifetime. A boil can occur anywhere on your skin but is most likely to appear on your face, neck, armpits, buttocks, or thighs.

Carbuncles commonly appear on the upper back and on the nape of your neck. They are less common than boils. Men are more prone to have them than women. Carbuncles develop slowly and may not reach your skin's surface to drain on their own.

Boils and carbuncles occur under various circumstances including poor hygiene, rundown physical condition, friction by clothing, and disorders including acne, dermatitis, diabetes mellitus, and pernicious anemia.

The Diagnosis. You may not need a diagnosis unless your infection persists beyond 2 weeks, recurs, or is located on your spine or in the middle of your face. The diagnosis may require culture of the pus to determine the specific bacteria that caused the boil. Further tests of your blood and urine may be necessary if your physician suspects an underlying disorder.

How Serious Are Boils and Carbuncles? A boil usually will burst within 2 weeks. Any carbuncle or boil that persists longer might spread the infection to your bloodstream or internal organs. Internal staphylococcal infections, which are life-threatening, often start from skin infections.

A boil or carbuncle on or near your nose, cheeks, forehead, or spine can spread even more rapidly to become a brain abscess or spinal abscess (see page 532). Prompt medical treatment can help prevent these serious complications.

Permanent scarring can occur from a boil or carbuncle, especially if it is improperly treated. The frequent occurrence of boils may indicate an underlying disorder that needs medical attention.

Treatment. Application of a warm tap-water compress to the boil for about 30 minutes every few hours will either cause it to regress and disappear or, more likely, to burst and drain much sooner. Never squeeze or lance your boil because you might spread the infection. Wash the infected area frequently with antibacterial soap, and prevent the drained matter from contacting other skin areas.

Your physician may prescribe oral antibiotic treatment for a carbuncle or boil that persists or is located on your face or spine. Surgical drainage is used for some boils and carbuncles.

ERYSIPELAS AND CELLULITIS

Signs and Symptoms
- Painful area of hot, red, swollen skin with lines or blisters on your face, arm, or leg.

Cellulitis is an acute inflammation of the connective tissue in your skin that results from a bacterial infection. (See color photograph, page B-12.) It usually occurs with dermatitis, a fungal infection, or after a skin injury and may be accompanied by a fever (see Wound Infections, page 1180).

Erysipelas is a severe streptococcal cellulitis in which the infected area is shiny and sharply defined. It is characterized by high fever and recurrences. Gangrene is possible from these infections.

Treatment. After an examination, your physician may prescribe an antibiotic. This treatment usually stops the infection within a week. Elevating the infected area and applying hot, moist compresses to the site will help.

The pain may be sufficiently severe that your physician also may prescribe a medication for pain relief.

LYMPHADENITIS AND LYMPHANGITIS

Signs and Symptoms
- Swollen areas of skin, sometimes with redness and pain.

Lymphadenitis is an infection of lymph nodes by bacteria, viruses, fungi, or other disease-producing microorganisms; lymphangitis is a similar infection of the lymphatic channels. Pus-filled abscesses and cellulitis (see page 1174) also may occur.

Lymphangitis causes a throbbing pain in the area of the wound, malaise, a fever of 100-104°F, loss of appetite, sweating, and chills. A red streak may be evident running from the site of the infection up the extremity. Immediate treatment is essential. This infection can spread very rapidly—often in just a few hours—and may be fatal.

Diagnostic tests may include blood analyses and a lymph node culture or biopsy.

Treatment. Treatment varies depending on the source of the infection. If antibiotic treatment begins immediately, the disease usually is brought under control in a few days and you should recover completely. Also apply hot, moist compresses or a heating pad, elevating the area (if possible), and take aspirin. Abscesses may require drainage by your physician.

COLD SORES AND CANKER SORES

Signs and Symptoms
- Single or clustered, small, fluid-filled blisters on a raised, red, painful area of skin;
- Painful ulcerous sore inside your mouth, with a white or yellow center and red border.

Cold sores, also called fever blisters, are very common infections. (See color photograph, page B-10.) They can appear anywhere on your body but are most likely to be on your gums, the outside of your mouth and lips, nose, cheeks, or fingers.

This infection is caused by the herpes simplex virus and is transmitted by contact with another person's active infection. Eating utensils, towels, and razors are other common sources. Type 1 herpes is usually responsible for fever blisters. Type 2 is responsible for genital herpes (see page 877).

Symptoms of your initial herpes infection may start as long as 20 days after exposure to the virus and may last for 7 to 10 days. The blisters form, break, and ooze; then a yellow crust forms and finally sloughs off to uncover pinkish, healing skin.

The virus reverts to a latent form within your nerve cells and may emerge again as an active infection on or near the original site. You may experience an itch or heightened sensitivity at the site preceding each attack. Recurrences are generally milder than the initial infection and are triggered by menstruation, sun exposure, or any illness with fever.

A canker sore lasts for 1 to 2 weeks. (See color photograph, page B-10.) In later stages of healing, it develops a gray membrane covering. Minor injuries, such as denture friction or biting the inside of your mouth, often precipitate development of a lesion.

Canker sores also commonly recur; they are thought to be a localized immune system reaction to unknown causes. These sores usually start between age 10 and 40 and may recur for years with one or more ulcers. Recurrences can be unpredictable or may be triggered by stress, fatigue, or food allergies. A tingling or burning sensation may precede an attack. This is followed by a red spot or bump where an ulcer will appear. Severe attacks may have additional symptoms of fever, listlessness, and swollen glands. Women are more prone to develop canker sores than men. Sometimes there is a family history of the disease.

The Diagnosis. Both infections are usually diagnosed by examination. Your physician may require a culture of material from your sore or a blood test to confirm the presence of herpes simplex virus.

How Serious Are Cold Sores and Canker Sores? Treatment is often effective in alleviating cold sores. However, there are potentially serious complications from this infection. The infection can spread to your eye; this is the most frequent cause of corneal blindness in the United States.

If you have a cold sore, avoid contact with infants, anyone who has atopic dermatitis (see page 1157), or those using an immune-system suppression medication (cancer and organ transplant patients). Your virus can cause a life-threatening condition in them.

Treatment. To reduce discomfort from a canker sore, avoid spicy and acidic foods. Apply ice to relieve the pain of a cold sore. In addition, for your cold sore your physician may prescribe an antiviral medication in ointment or tablet form.

Recurring canker sores usually are treated with mouthwashes. For severe attacks, your physician may prescribe a solution containing an antibiotic or an antihistamine or suggest the use of a corticosteroid preparation applied locally or taken by mouth.

SHINGLES

Signs and Symptoms

- Pain or tingling sensation in a limited area of one side of your body or face; a red skin rash follows, characterized by small, fluid-filled blisters.

Shingles (herpes zoster) is a localized infection caused by the same virus that causes chickenpox. (See color photograph, page B-13.) After an occurrence of chickenpox, the virus often becomes dormant within the nerve cells. It can emerge years later as shingles.

The symptoms occur in a sequence as the virus reactivates. The reasons for this reactivation are not known. The initial sensation is pain or tingling as the virus proliferates along one of the peripheral nerves that spread outward from your spine. It affects only the area of your face or body served by that nerve. A rash appears 2 or 3 days later, after the virus gets to the nerve endings in your skin.

Over the next 3 to 5 days, the rash reaches its maximum extent. This can be a rectangular belt on one side of your body from spine to breastbone (zoster is Latin for belt), over an extremity, or on one side of your face or head. The blisters dry up in a few days, forming crusts that fall off 2 or 3 weeks after your initial symptoms.

Each year, about 300,000 Americans have a shingles infection. It can occur at any age but is most common after age 60. Recurrence is possible and is more likely when you are taking a medication that suppresses your immune system. If you did not have chickenpox as a child and are exposed to the virus, you will probably have a serious case of chickenpox rather than shingles.

The Diagnosis. The diagnosis is based on the history of your symptoms and the characteristic appearance of the rash.

How Serious Is Shingles? Shingles normally is not a serious condition, although you may have continuing pain for months or even years along the peripheral nerve involved. This is called post-herpetic neuralgia and occurs in 50 percent of those who have had shingles and are over age 60.

When a major nerve in your face, the trigeminal nerve, is affected, the rash can occur on your face and inside your mouth or eye. If you have shingles, any pain in your eye requires prompt medical attention because an eye infection can lead to permanent damage to your sight.

Shingles can be debilitating if your immune system is weakened or you have certain forms of cancer including leukemia and Hodgkin's disease. Medications taken after transplantation surgery, for example, suppress your immune system and make you vulnerable to shingles.

Treatment. The natural course of a shingles rash cannot be changed by any treatment, but you can obtain some relief by soaking your blistered areas with cool, wet compresses (aluminum acetate solution) and applying a soothing lotion. Analgesics such as aspirin may help alleviate the milder pain of post-herpetic neuralgia. Stronger painkillers occasionally are needed for more serious discomfort.

Your physician might prescribe corticosteroids in the early stages of your infection to minimize the subsequent neuralgia, atropine for eye infections, or an antiviral agent such as acylovir when your immune system is impaired.

MOLLUSCUM CONTAGIOSUM

Signs and Symptoms

• Tiny, pearl-like papules on the skin with a core of white, cheesy matter.

Molluscum contagiosum is a relatively common viral infection of the skin. (See color photograph, page B-13.) Each small, globular papule characteristically has a small black dot on its summit. In children, nodules usually appear on the face, trunk, or limbs. The infection is contagious by contact. In adults, common sites are the genitals, abdomen, and inner thighs. It frequently is spread through sexual contact.

The firm nodules are often painless and disappear within a year. If the nodules and surrounding skin are injured, local spreading can occur.

Treatment. Left untreated, more lesions may occur by the shedding of the virus from lesions to normal skin. Your physician can remove the nodules by freezing, surgical scraping, or squeezing out the core matter.

FUNGAL INFECTIONS

Signs and Symptoms

• Itchy, red, soggy, flaking, and cracking skin between toes;
• Itchy, fluid-filled bumps on sides or sole of your foot;
• Extreme dryness with small, white scales on the sides or sole of your foot or the palm of your hand;
• Itchy, red or grayish, scaling patches on the scalp with partial baldness or broken hairs;
• Itchy, red, scaly, slightly raised, expanding rings on the trunk, face, or groin/thigh fold.
• Red, moist, well-marked patches, rimmed with small, red bumps in armpits,

navel, groin or buttock/thigh fold, under the breasts, or between fingers or toes;
• Reddened areas with white patches inside the mouth or cracks at the mouth corner.
• Small, slightly scaling, pale patches on the upper body, neck, or face.

Fungal infections are caused by microscopic plants that become parasites on your skin. Your body hosts a great variety of microorganisms including mold- and yeast-like fungi. Some serve useful purposes, or cause no problems. Others can proliferate as infectious colonies.

Athlete's foot, jock itch (see page 1178), and ringworm of the skin or scalp (see below) are caused by mold-like fungi called dermatophytes. These fungi live on dead tissues of your hair, nails, and the outer layer of your skin. Your susceptibility to infection by them is increased by poor hygiene, continually moist skin, and minor skin or nail injuries.

Ringworm often affects children. (See color photograph, page B-8.) The characteristic rings may be irregular and can expand beyond the scalp. The ring grows outward as the infection spreads and the central area becomes less actively infected. This type of infection is very contagious and can be passed from shared hats, combs or brushes, and barber tools. It is also possible to be infected with scalp or skin ringworm from pets or domestic animals.

Some fungal infections are referred to as yeast or *Candida* infections. These ailments result from infection with a fungus of the genus *Candida*. Examples include diaper rash and oral infections, called oral thrush, which is common in babies (see color photographs, pages B-2 and B-10). Chafing can occur in folds of skin of overweight people. Genital infections (see page 1087) can be transmitted sexually.

Your susceptibility to a *Candida* infection is increased under certain conditions including pregnancy, obesity, endocrine disorders such as diabetes mellitus, cancers such as leukemia, inherited or AIDS-produced immune system deficiencies, and use of certain medications (antibiotics effective against various organisms or large doses of adrenal corticosteroids).

Another type of yeast infection, tinea versicolor, appears as a tissue-thin coating of fungus on your skin. (See color photograph, page B-8.) The only symptoms are patches of discolored skin that slowly grow. Tinea versicolor is common among teenagers and young adults.

The Diagnosis. Skin changes associated with fungal infections often are quite specific. Thus, your physician may only need to examine your skin to make the diagnosis. At other times it will be necessary to obtain material from the lesion for laboratory analysis.

How Serious Are Fungal Infections? These infections are rarely life-threatening.

They can range from mild to severe attacks and often persist or recur. Treatment is generally successful, but long-term medication and continued use of preventive measures may be required, particularly for infections in your nails.

A skin infection by *Candida* can spread through your bloodstream to internal organs. This is rare, but prompt medical attention is necessary if you have a fever, eye pain, visual disturbances, or symptoms of meningitis (see page 527). *Candida* infections have been blamed for a wide variety of symptoms, including chronic fatigue syndrome (see page 853), but evidence for this is lacking.

JOCK ITCH AND ATHLETE'S FOOT

Jock itch and athlete's foot are skin conditions caused by fungi that thrive in warm, moist areas. (See color photographs, page B-8.) They are common in athletes as well as in people who are obese or who perspire a great deal. In both cases, itching and a rash are the primary symptoms.

Jock itch consists of itching in the groin and anal area; with athlete's foot there is itching, stinging, and burning on the soles of the feet, on the palms, and between the fingers and toes. Cracking of the skin and peeling may occur as well.

These infections are mildy contagious and are transmitted by contact in public showers and swimming areas, by sharing towels, or by using contaminated bath mats. Extreme dryness on your soles or palms is more likely to be associated with fungal infections of your nails (see page 1186).

Good personal hygiene is essential in preventing or treating jock itch and athlete's

foot. To prevent jock itch, keep the area clean and dry, avoid chafing, and launder athletic supporters frequently. To treat it, dust the area with antifungal drying powders two or three times a day (no more or your irritation may become worse). Antifungal creams are available for use at bedtime.

Wearing sandals when bathing or using foot troughs at the local shower or pool entry have not been proven to help prevent athlete's foot. The key to prevention: keep your feet dry. Always dry them thoroughly after bathing. Antifungal powders also can help.

Avoid socks manufactured from synthetic fibers. Synthetic fibers do not absorb moisture very well. Instead, select socks made from cotton, wool, or a combination of these. And change your socks frequently. Wear well-ventilated shoes with leather soles, not shoes with synthetic uppers and hard rubber soles. Also, alternate daily among two or more pairs of shoes. Each pair then can dry completely and will absorb more moisture when worn.

Treatment. For athlete's foot, skin ringworm, and jock itch, apply over-the-counter antifungal agents (miconazole, clotrimazole, Whitfield's ointment, or Castellani paint). Your physician may prescribe an antifungal medication to be taken orally if one of these infections is chronic or severe, or for scalp ringworm. Antibiotics may be prescribed if a bacterial infection develops.

Diaper rash in babies and chafing (intertrigo) infections in adults are treated by applying over-the-counter antifungal agents together with keeping the area clean and dry and dusting it with antifungal powder. The same medications are available in lozenge or mouthwash form for oral thrush infections. For severe or persistent *Candida* infections, your physician may prescribe an antifungal medication to be taken orally. Because there are potentially serious side effects from long-term oral use of antifungal medications, medical supervision is necessary during this treatment.

For tinea versicolor, frequent showering can help. Also apply sulfur medications (such as sodium thiosulfite or sodium hyposulfite) to your skin overnight for a month. An alternative medication is selenium sulfide, which is used as an application over a 5-day period.

INSECT BITES

Signs and Symptoms
- Itchy, red bumps;
- Red, painful, ulcerating sore;
- Local numbness or pins-and-needles sensation.

Emergency Symptoms
- Swollen face, widespread numbness, muscle cramping, breathing difficulty, headache, nausea, or fever;
- Coma.

Symptoms of insect bites are caused by the injection of venom or other agents into your skin. Most often the reaction is local and temporary. However, if you are hypersensitive to the venom or the venom is exceptionally potent, your entire body can be affected.

The bite of a black widow spider feels like a pinprick. Some people are not aware they've been bitten. At first, there may be only slight swelling and faint red marks in the area of the bite. Within a few hours, however, intense pain and stiffness begin. Other symptoms may include chills, fever, nausea, and severe abdominal pain. Generally, the pain lessens after a few hours but may return over the next 2 to 3 days.

Bites by the brown recluse (see color photograph, page B-14) and other spiders cause a mild stinging followed by local redness and intense pain within 8 hours. A fluid-filled bump forms at the site and then sloughs off, sometimes leaving a large, deep, growing ulcer. Your body reactions can vary from a mild fever and rash to nausea and listlessness.

Most ant bites cause only local redness and swelling. Fire ants, however, can produce many small, fluid-filled bumps that ulcerate like spider bites.

Other biting insects usually inject their chemicals as they feed on you. These insects include mosquitoes, fleas, flies, bedbugs, and chiggers.

Stings by bee, wasps, and hornets inject venom that causes immediate pain and rapidly growing red bumps. A flying insect sting will subside and turn itchy in a few hours, unless you have an allergic reaction (see Insect Bite Allergies, page 472).

The Diagnosis. An insect bite or sting sometimes is easy to recognize because you feel the sting when it happens. At other times, bites just seem to appear. If you have a severe reaction, knowing what bit you will help your physician determine the treatment.

How Serious Are Insect Bites? Symptoms from a typical bite or sting generally last a few hours or days. On the other hand, if you are allergic to bee stings, or if you receive multiple stings, this can be life-threatening and requires emergency treatment. About one in one hundred Americans are allergic to bee stings. These stings cause more deaths than snake bites. Poisonous spider bites are rarely fatal, but small children and the elderly are especially vulnerable.

Treatment. Mild insect bites are generally treated by applying ice cubes to decrease pain and over-the-counter hydrocortisone cream or calamine lotion to relieve itching or inflammation. Your physician may prescribe corticosteroid cream for more severe reactions.

Bee stingers must be carefully removed. Immediate injections of antihistamine and an anti-spasm drug may be required for more severe reactions. If faintness, listlessness, or shortness of breath occurs, seek emergency medical care immediately. Your physician can prescribe an emergency medical kit for you to keep handy if you are hypersensitive to bee or hornet stings.

Persons with black widow spider bites may require hospitalization and are treated by hot soaks, intravenous infusion of calcium gluconate to relieve cramps, and injections of antivenin. Brown recluse spider bites are treated with corticosteroid injections and surgical scraping of the ulcer.

PORTUGUESE MAN-OF-WAR STINGS

Signs and Symptoms
- Stinging and pain;
- Red, hive-like lesions in a line;
- Shortness of breath, nausea, stomach cramps, and emotional upset.

The Portuguese man-of-war is a colony of free-floating individual organisms. Like the jellyfish, it is invertebrate (without a backbone). It is easily recognized by the highly characteristic blue or red bell-shaped body that floats at the surface of the water and ranges from less than 1 inch to more than a foot in width. A cluster of tentacles hangs beneath the body of the man-of-war. Most are short and frilly; however, one or more can be many feet long. These long fishing tentacles are responsible for the stings.

If you touch one of these tentacles it will whip around the contact area and inject a toxic venom into your skin. Because the venom (a neurotoxin) remains potent long after the man-of-war is dead, wading in shallow water or walking along the beach can be hazardous. The tentacles discharge their venom for long periods, even after being separated from the main body of the man-of-war. The venom is carried into the victim by tiny barbs on the tentacles.

You may encounter the man-of-war in the waters and on beaches of the Atlantic Ocean, ranging from Canada to the West Indies, and of the Mediterranean Sea. They also are found in the Pacific Ocean near Hawaii and southern Japan.

How Serious Are Man-of-War Stings?

Death from man-of-war stings is unusual, but symptoms can be painful. Common symptoms range from mild prickling to severe burning and numbness. A red line develops on the area of the skin exposed to the tentacles. Sometimes a string of welts or blisters develops. (See color photograph, page B-13.)

Severe stings can lead to muscle cramps, fainting, cough, vomiting, and difficulty with breathing. In rare cases, a potential fatal reaction (see Anaphylaxis, page 474) may occur.

Treatment. Here are practical tips for coping with man-of-war stings.

WOUND INFECTIONS

After an injury that causes a break in the skin or after an operation, various wound infections may occur. Among them is cellulitis (inflammation of the skin, see page 1174). Others, that can result in death or decay of tissues (gangrene), are discussed below.

Necrotizing Subcutaneous Infection

This is a severe infection caused by bacteria that infect the tissue through wounds. The primary symptoms are swelling, discoloration, and death of the surrounding tissue. The skin around the wound becomes hot, inflamed, tender, and red. If the infection worsens, the skin becomes discolored and gangrene may develop.

This infection most often is caused by aerobic bacteria (which require oxygen to live) or anaerobic bacteria (unable to live in the presence of oxygen). In treating it, your physician will select an antibiotic. To determine the correct antibiotic to prescribe, your doctor will take a sample of pus for culture to identify the bacteria present. The wound often must be thoroughly opened so that all infected tissue can be removed.

One operation usually is not sufficient to remove all of the dead tissue. Most often, a second may be required. If the infection involves an arm or leg, amputation eventually may be necessary.

Gas Gangrene

Gangrene is death of the tissue. Gas gangrene results when a wound becomes infected by certain bacteria, usually *Clostridium*. This infection causes sudden pain and swelling around the wound, a moderate increase in temperature, a decrease in blood pressure, and a rapid heartbeat. Skin around the wound becomes pale due to fluid that builds up under it. A watery, foul-smelling, brownish-red fluid is released later. The tissue changes from pale to dusky to highly discolored as the infection worsens. Left untreated, stupor, delirium, coma, and death result.

Treatment consists of penicillin given intravenously. Surgical removal of infected tissue is essential, and removal of surrounding tissue usually is necessary.

Cutaneous Abscess

This is a pus-filled sore on the skin caused by bacteria, usually occurring after a minor wound. Some-times the lymph glands in the area become swollen, and you may have a fever.

Treatment consists of opening the infected area, thoroughly cleaning and irrigating the wound with saline, and packing it with gauze for 24 to 48 hours to absorb the pus and discharge. Application of heat and, if possible, elevating the affected area help to relieve the inflammation. Administration of antibiotics through a needle into a muscle or through a vein often is appropriate treatment for these infections.

Animal Bites

Cats and dogs cause most of the bite wounds seen in hospital emergency rooms. Cat bites are the most likely to cause a bacterial infection. If you are bitten by a cat or dog and have not had a tetanus shot recently, you may need a booster (see page 858).

In all cases, prompt, thorough cleaning of the wound is essential. This often involves opening the wound and removing all areas of infected tissue. Antibiotics are usually given. Also, soak your wound in warm water and, if possible, elevate and immobilize the affected part.

Get out of the water. The pain and cramps can be disabling, and drowning can result.

Inactivate the stinging. Sprinkle the area with meat tenderizer, vinegar, salt, sugar, or even dry sand and gently rub this material into the wounds. This often offers quick relief.

Cleanse the wound. After waiting 15 to 20 minutes, gently wash the area with sea water. Do not use fresh water and do not rub the skin because either action could trigger discharge of more venom.

Remove the stinging tentacles. Apply a paste made of sea water and sand (or baking soda, talcum powder, or flour). Scrape the residue with a knife or other sharp object such as a clam shell. It is best to wear gloves or use a towel in removing the residue.

Apply 0.5 percent hydrocortisone cream (available without a prescription) to relieve redness and swelling. A local anesthetic ointment (such as benzocaine) helps relieve pain, and a calamine-type lotion lessens itching. Mild analgesics such as aspirin and acetaminophen are often used but prescription pain killers may be necessary after severe stings.

Extra clothing is your best protection from the man-of-war, particularly a wet suit or body stocking if you are swimming in waters where they are found. Also, wear sneakers or plastic beach shoes while walking along the beach. And watch where you step.

HUMAN BITES

Animal bites are commonplace: about 1,000 people visit hospital emergency rooms each day for treatment of dog or other animal bites. Human bites are less common but represent an equally serious medical problem.

There are two kinds of human bites. A "true bite," like most animal bites, is the injury that results from flesh being caught between the teeth of the upper and lower jaws. "Fight bites" occur when, in the act of striking another person, an assailant cuts his or her knuckles on the victim's teeth. (See color photograph, page B-13.)

While such bites may seem superficial, the cut (laceration) may extend below the skin, injuring tendons and joints. The human mouth also contains many bacteria, and the saliva that enters at the site of the puncture may cause serious infections. There is little risk of rabies, but there is danger of transmission of the hepatitis B virus.

You may fear embarrassment or even legal action if you go to the emergency room for treatment of a fight bite. However, remember that you risk a prolonged hospital stay, permanent joint stiffness, and even amputation if a serious infection is not promptly treated. Whether yours is a true bite or a fight bite, seek help before the risks become more serious.

HAIR

Hair is composed of keratin, the same protein that makes up nails and the outer layer of skin. The part seen rising out of the skin is the hair shaft or strand. There may be about 100,000 of them on the average head.

Below your skin is the hair root which is enclosed by a sack-like structure called the hair follicle. Tiny blood vessels at the base of the follicle provide nourishment. A nearby oil-producing gland keeps the hair shiny and somewhat waterproof.

Each strand consists of three layers. The outermost layer, or cuticle, is thin and colorless. The middle layer, or cortex, is the thickest. It determines your hair color and whether your hair is straight or curly.

Your hair color is due to melanin from your pigment cells. Blondes have few melanin granules in the cortex layer and brunettes have many. The innermost layer, or medulla, is nearly colorless and does not extend all the way to the tip of the hair shaft. Light reflected from the medulla creates the sheen and the variations in color tone.

Like skin cells, hair grows and is shed regularly. You normally lose 50 to 100 strands a day. The average rate of growth is about ½ inch a month. Each hair grows for 2 to 6 years and then rests. At any time, about 85 percent of your hair is growing and the other 15 percent is resting. After its rest period, the hair falls out and a new one starts to form.

Your hair says a lot about you. Getting it to make the statement you want may not be easy. Americans spend a great deal of time and money to curl, color, spike, slick, restore, or remove their hair. This section describes some of the problems you can have with your hair, as well as how to take proper care of it.

FEMALE-PATTERN BALDNESS

Signs and Symptoms
- General thinning of hair all over the head;
- Moderate loss of hair on the crown or at your hairline.

It is normal for a woman's hair to thin out gradually as she grows older. You might have as much hair at age 80 as you did at 18, but this would be unusual. The other extreme, extensive hair loss, is thought to be the result of inheriting, from both of your parents, genes that tend toward baldness. The hair loss in women is far less prominent than the usual male-pattern baldness.

The distribution of your hair is largely controlled by your endocrine system through a group of hormones known as androgens.

Major changes in your androgen production can have a significant effect on your hair. For example, you may find that during or after the hormonal changes of menopause, the hair on your head is definitely thinned out while your facial hair is coarser.

Hair loss in women also can occur from poor nutrition, pregnancy, internal or scalp disorders, hair damage, and medications. Sometimes there is a temporary hair loss (see page 1185) when some substance or condition is causing a transitory problem.

Treatment. Your physician can diagnose female-pattern baldness by ruling out other causes for your hair loss. A dermatologist can advise you on various methods that might stop the hair loss or restore the hair that is lost. These methods, which are discussed in the section on making hair grow (see this page), include use of surface medications such as hormonal creams, irritants or sensitizers to promote hair growth, minoxidil treatments, and transplants.

You also may want to seek the advice of a hair-care expert in choosing a new hairstyle or perhaps a hairpiece that flatters you.

MALE-PATTERN BALDNESS

Signs and Symptoms
- Receding hairline;
- Moderate to extensive loss of hair, especially on the crown.

The pattern of male baldness is very common. It usually begins at your hairline, which gradually recedes to form an "M" shape. You also may find your hair is finer and does not grow as long as it once did. The hair on the crown of your head begins to thin out and eventually the top points of the "M" meet the thinned spot on your crown. Over time, you are left with a horseshoe pattern of hair around the sides of your head.

The explanation for this pattern is probably your genetic inheritance, which is complex and not well understood. Baldness is also due to aging and is affected by hormones called androgens, controlled by your endocrine system, which are the major determining factor for hair distribution in both sexes.

Your hair grows in a cycle as described in the introduction to this section (see page

---

CAN LOST HAIR GROW AGAIN?

Even after your hair is lost, the roots usually remain alive. This suggests the possibility of new growth.

Cortisone tablets taken orally sometimes promote hair growth. Unfortunately, prolonged use can cause physical or mental side effects, and the new hair usually falls out when you discontinue the tablets. Other forms of cortisone are rubbed or injected into your scalp. Their effect is often temporary, and this treatment is practical and effective only for small areas.

Another method uses chemical irritants which are rubbed onto the scalp to cause chronic skin inflammation. Sometimes this makes hair grow. Allergen sensitizers are also applied to the scalp to stimulate hair growth. These methods require professional supervision and are time-consuming but effective in some people.

Another approach uses minoxidil. This drug was developed to treat high blood pressure and had the unanticipated side effect of stimulating hair growth, sometimes in unwanted areas. For treating baldness, it is used as a topical lotion. The hair produced is usually fuzzy, the treatment is expensive, and so far the results are varied.

The most successful method for treating male- and female-pattern baldness is hair transplantation. The dermatologist implants tiny plugs of skin, each containing about 10 hairs, into your scalp. These plugs are taken from a donor site, usually on the back or side of your head. Scars at the site are covered by the remaining hair. The transplanted hairs fall out in about 3 weeks, but new hairs are soon produced. Up to four transplantation sessions, at 4-month intervals, may be needed. This treatment also is expensive.

PROPER HAIR CARE

Each year, Americans spend millions of dollars on hair-care products and treatments. Unfortunately, some of these efforts are too rough or done too frequently. The result is hair damage rather than hair care. Damaged hair stays damaged until it grows out and is cut off. This can take many months, because your hair grows only about ½ inch each month.

Your hair requires gentle handling. Wet hair is especially fragile because it might become stretched. A natural bristle brush is preferred over a synthetic one because the synthetic material may cut the hair. Brush the hair gently from the scalp to disperse scalp oil over the hair. If you prefer a comb, use a wide-toothed comb to avoid injury to your hair.

Certain hairstyles and treatments can cause breakage or root damage. Avoid excessively tight braiding, buns, or ponytails, and do not roll your hair too tightly in curlers. Teasing and back combing should be done gently or not at all. Too much exposure to sun, wind, or swimming-pool chemicals will dry out your hair and cause it to knot.

The quality of your hair reflects in part the adequacy of your diet: regular, well-rounded meals are best for you and your hair. Consuming extra protein or amino acid preparations will not promote hair growth. Crash diets and eating disorders such as anorexia nervosa can damage hair dramatically. Various claims are made for the value of analysis of hair samples, but the process has no validity and

can be considered one of the many scams aimed at appealing to people concerned about their health.

If done gently, daily shampooing will not damage your hair. The amount of washing will depend on the type of your hair, the weather, your physical activity, and perhaps even your occupation.

For proper washing, wet your hair completely with warm water. Put the shampoo on with your hand and massage gently, using your fingertips instead of your nails as you work the lather outward from your scalp. Rinse thoroughly.

Buy shampoos tailored to your hair type—oily, dry, or normal. Protein shampoos do not penetrate your hair, but they do coat it, giving your hair more bulk. A protein shampoo acts as a shampoo and conditioner in one. Permanent-waved, straightened, or dyed hair needs low pH shampoos. Excessive flaking may require dandruff shampoos (see Dandruff, page 1158). Follow your shampoo with a cream rinse or conditioner. These products lubricate your hair between washings and help minimize damage from brushing or combing. Those containing protein ingredients may also thicken your hair temporarily.

Towel dry by patting gently. Whenever possible, let your hair dry naturally in the air. If a blower is necessary, use it on a low setting and leave your hair slightly damp. If you brush or comb your hair while it is wet, you pull out much more hair than you would by gently untangling it with your fingers and waiting until it is damp or dry before you carefully brush or comb it.

A styling gel or mousse can give your hair more body or thickness. They do not necessarily damage

your hair, but you may experience extra dryness, especially at the hair ends.

Hair bleaches chemically alter the melanin granule in the middle layer of each hair strand. Despite careful treatment, persistent bleaching eventually damages even healthy, strong hair shafts, but it does not injure the roots from which future hair growth takes place.

Hair dyes work more like paint by covering hair strands with color or by mixing with the melanin granules without altering them. Dyes come in temporary form, which eventually wash out, and semi-permanent and permanent forms, which penetrate your hair. Before using one of the permanent forms, conduct a patch test to check for possible irritation. Permanent dyes require prior bleaching. Thus, the dying process does damage hair.

Curling is safest if you twist your hair into pin curls overnight. Use of hot rollers or curling irons gives the best results for coarse hair, but they may damage strands or roots when used to excess. For safe curling of fine hair, let it air dry and wind it loosely around sponge rollers.

Permanent waving is safe for healthy hair, but you may find it results in increased dryness and splitting. Straightening and permanent waving use the same chemical methods to change the properties of hair strands. The initial (waving) solution dissolves a chemical linkage in the hair. After the hair is arranged in its new, curly configuration, application of the second solution, the neutralizer, restores the linkage. Like other aggressive cosmetic treatments, permanent waving can be damaging when done to excess.

HIRSUTISM

There is a paradox about hair. An ample and healthy head of it generally is regarded as beautiful. But the presence of hair in inappropriate locations is not. Among women, for example, hair on the cheeks, upper lip, underarms, or legs is considered, by many women and men, to be unattractive.

The amounts of normal facial and body hair vary greatly from one person to another. Our society regards the norm to be almost no hair on the face, body, arms, or legs of women and only moderate body and extremity hair for men.

Many women develop considerable amounts of body and facial hair during puberty; in some cases, even faint mustaches appear. The normal secretion of androgen hormones produces many changes in a young girl's body, including hair growth in the pubic and armpit regions. Some women—mainly those of southern European or Middle-Eastern ancestry—develop noteworthy amounts of facial and body hair; others, typically of northern European extraction, do not.

In women, the amount of hair usually increases slowly with age, even past menopause. Men similarly may develop considerable body hair as they age.

The presence of too much hair is called hirsutism. How much is too much is largely a matter of personal perception. Part of the solution to a cosmetic problem of excessive hair is the simple acceptance that the amount you have is right for you. On the other hand, if you have a sudden increase in hair (for example, over a period of a few months), consult your physician. There may be a medical cause. Your doctor will consider the possibility of an adrenal or ovarian tumor (see pages 722 and 1107, respectively). Some drugs, such as the antiseizure medication Dilantin, may also cause growth of body hair; certain vitamin preparations contain testosterone and cause increased growth of facial and body hair. The eating disorder anorexia nervosa (see page 1019) often is associated with an increase in fine body hair. Sometimes hirsutism occurs for no known reason (see Idiopathic Hirsutism, page 722.)

If excessive facial or body hair is a cosmetic worry to you, several treatment approaches are available. Here are some cosmetic treatment options:

Plucking

This is the most common cosmetic method. It is safe and works well if your problem is a few scattered hairs. Wash the area first and dab on a little alcohol with a cotton ball. Use good tweezers to remove the hair by pulling it out in the direction it is growing. Plucking is a temporary solution. It does not make hair grow back darker or coarser. Check with your physician before plucking hair from a mole. Plucking causes rupture of the hair bulb and associated bleeding. The possibility of an infection in the follicle is always present.

Shaving

Shaving is another popular, but temporary, method. This can be very irritating to your skin if you do it haphazardly (see Proper Skin Care, page 1154). Women commonly shave their underarms and lower legs, but shaving is also safe for facial hair. Shaving does not make your hair grow faster, darker, or coarser (more bristly).

Pumice and Other Abrasives

The use of abrasive agents, such as a pumice stone, is the oldest method of hair removal. This is slow and tedious, and the vigorous rubbing can irritate your skin. You may find it useful for scattered hairs, but it is not practical for large areas.

Bleaching

Bleaching is commonly used for large areas, such as forearms or thighs, to make unwanted hair less conspicuous. Use a product especially designed for this purpose, and follow the directions. Be sure to do the patch test on a small area to check for possible irritation.

Waxing

Wax removal is popular among American women for removing hair on the upper lip, chin, and legs. Wax is melted and applied to the area. After it cools and sets, it is quickly stripped off in the direction of the hair growth. The results last longer than other temporary methods because the hair is pulled out below your skin's surface. New hairs generally appear after a month. Waxing can be painful and may irritate your skin. It should be done by a trained cosmetician. As with plucking, infection of the hair follicles may occur.

Hair Removers

Depilatories are chemical agents that dissolve hair protein. You can buy them in foam, cream, or lotion form. Follow the directions, and test the product on a small area of your skin for possible irritation. Some women find depilatories inconvenient because they must stay on for 10 to 15 minutes. Do not use these products on injured or inflamed skin.

Electrolysis

The most permanent method of

hair removal is electrolysis. A very fine needle is inserted into each hair follicle and a burst of electric current is delivered through the needle to destroy the hair root. The hair grows back about 30 percent of the time. Infections, scar- ring, or discoloration around the follicle may occur, so this proce- dure is best done by a trained electrologist. It is wise to have the electrologist do a few hairs (per- haps six) and observe the results before embarking on an extensive program of hair removal. You may need several sessions because the maximum removal rate is about 100 hairs per visit. Electrolysis can be long, tedious, and expensive, but it might be a permanent solu- tion to unwanted hair.

1181). At the end of its cycle, each resting hair falls out and a new hair normally forms in the root. In male-pattern baldness, the rate of growth and the intervals in between periods of growth shorten. Thus, the periods of growth occur more often but more and more roots fail to produce new hair at the end of each cycle.

You may want to check with your physi- cian to be sure that your hair loss is not the result of some medical problem (see Tempo- rary Hair Loss, below).

Treatment. A dermatologist can advise you on various methods that might restore lost hair (see Can Lost Hair Grow Again?, page 1182).

You may want to check with hair-care experts about hairpieces, weaving tech- niques, or changing your hairstyle. For some men, shorter hair minimizes the contrast produced by male-pattern baldness and cre- ates a distinguished image. Schemes for growing hair are among the more common health-oriented scams. Evaluate any such proposal carefully.

TEMPORARY HAIR LOSS

Signs and Symptoms
- Small bald patch(es) on the scalp;
- General thinning of scalp hair;
- Loss of scalp, eyebrow, and eyelash hair;
- Complete loss of hair over the body.

Gradual hair loss can occur for a wide variety of reasons including excessive hair styling treatments, tight hairstyles, compul- sive abuse (twisting, rubbing, or pulling), skin diseases or infections, internal disorders, high fever, stress, poor nutrition (a crash diet or anorexia), use of birth control pills, and medical treatments such as with anticancer drugs.

Sudden hair loss most commonly is due to alopecia areata, a condition that occurs in 2 percent of the population. Alopecia areata starts abruptly with one or more circular bald patches, up to 3 inches across, that may overlap. These bald areas are smooth and painless. (See color photograph, page B-7.)

The cause of alopecia areata is unknown. Suspected factors include stress, family pre- disposition, and autoimmune reactions to your own hair follicles.

In 90 percent of the cases, the hair grows back within 6 to 24 months. The outcome is worse if the episode occurs early in life or if you lose all scalp hair in a single episode.

To diagnose alopecia areata, your physi- cian will perform a complete medical history and examination. Testing may be needed if an underlying disorder might be the cause.

Treatment. Treatment will depend on curing or controlling any underlying condi- tion, if one exists. Your physician may sug- gest various techniques to make your hair grow (see page 1182).

FINGERNAILS AND TOENAILS

Your nails are produced from cells in the tips of your fingers and toes and are composed of laminated layers of a protein called "kera- tin." Each nail grows toward the end of your finger or toe from a nail root that extends back into a groove of skin. Just in front of your nail root is your cuticle skin which is attached to the nail surface and helps protect the new keratin cells that slowly emerge from below.

Your nails can give the first signal of an illness. They occasionally provide clues for diagnosis as well as information about your age and diet. They also assist you with the tasks of daily living, although you may not be conscious of how much you use them until an injury, infection, or other disorder limits your use of them. The following section describes the disorders that may develop in your nails and how to take proper care of your nails.

PARONYCHIA

Signs and Symptoms
- Red, swollen area on the skin next to a nail.

Paronychia is a superficial infection of the skin around the nail, most commonly caused by either staphylococci or yeast. (See color photograph, page B-7.) It is usu-ally the result of an injury such as biting off a hangnail, or is caused by manipulating or pushing back the cuticle. *Para* means along-side and *onyx* means nail in Greek.

Bacterial paronychia usually is a sudden and painful infection. Superficial pus blisters may appear. Pressing the affected area can produce oozing pus.

Another form of paronychia is caused by fungal infections and is common among per-sons with diabetes mellitus and persons who have their hands in water for long periods. Fungal infections develop slowly but tend to persist. Sometimes both bacteria and fungi are present, causing greater swelling and pus.

An acute infection can extend around your nail and cuticle to invade beneath them in a painful abscess. Your cuticle becomes raised. The nail may become detached. Nail distortion or discoloration might occur. Al-though rare, the infection can penetrate into your finger and attack tendon tissue. Red lines along your skin are a signal that bacte-ria have entered your bloodstream. If this occurs, see your physician. The diagnosis may require a pus culture to determine which type of microorganism is causing your paronychia.

Treatment.   Hot soaks will help decrease inflammation of the tissues. These should be followed by topical application of an anti-bacterial agent (for bacterial infections) or 1 percent gentian violet solution if a fungal in-fection is present.

FUNGAL INFECTIONS OF THE NAILS

Signs and Symptoms
- Thickened, lusterless fingernails or toe-nails with discoloration or crumbling edges.

Fungus spores may attach themselves to the dense bed of keratin cells that make up your nails. These microscopic plants can di-gest the keratin and live within it. The result-ing infection, known as onychomycosis (tinea of the nails), can persist indefinitely. (See color photograph, page B-8.)

You can contract such infections in sev-eral ways including walking barefoot in pub-lic places or as a complication of athlete's foot (see page 1178) or paronychia (above).

DISCOLORATION OR DEFORMATION OF NAILS

Nails can be discolored or de-formed in many ways. Minor injury is the most common cause. The black spot under your thumbnail after a ham-mer blow is blood. White, cloud-like marks on the tips are the result of minor trauma. Splitting, peeling, or brittle-ness usually are signs of over-exposure to strong soaps or chemicals. Tight or ill-fitting shoes can cause ingrown or thickened toenails. Proper care is important to prevent bacteria and other infectious organisms from gaining entry into tissues and possibly your bloodstream (see Proper Care of Nails, page 1187).

Discoloration occurs with a number of ailments includ-ing fungal infections that can turn your nails yellow, gray, brown, or black. Injury, chem-ical exposure, or a reaction to medication also can cause an array of colors.

Internal disorders can de-form your nails. Clubbing of your nails, a condition in which your fingers or toes thicken and the nails wrap around them, may indicate a problem in your lungs.

It is not unusual for your nails to be affected during an illness and to recover after-ward. However, your nails grow slowly: about ⅛ inch a month for fingernails and about 1/24 inch for toenails. Damage can be repaired only by the slow process of new growth. After your underlying disorder is under control or cured, your nails will gradu-ally return to normal. But re-port any new changes in color or markings to your physician.

PROPER CARE OF NAILS

Perhaps the single most important element in taking care of your nails is to avoid biting, picking, or injuring them. Even a minor cut alongside your nail can allow bacteria or fungi to enter and cause an infection. Because your nails grow slowly, an injured nail retains signs of its injury for several months.

Exposure to detergents and chemicals can weaken, split, and discolor your nails. To protect them, wear rubber or disposable plastic gloves with cotton liners. Between uses, turn rubber gloves inside-out to dry. This prevents microorganisms from growing in them.

Trim Fingernails Weekly

Weekly trimming is important because nails that are smooth and cared-for are less likely to be damaged.

To trim your fingernails, use an emery board and sharp manicure scissors or clippers. If your nails are brittle or thick, trim them after bathing, when they are softer. Bevel the edges with the fine side of the emery board. If you prefer long nails, be careful to avoid accidental injury and accumulations of dirt under the edge.

Never Trim Cuticles

Although fashion encourages trimmed cuticles, avoid this practice. It can result in a point of entry for bacteria and fungi and thus promote infection.

Use Polish-Remover Sparingly

Despite advertising claims, most polishes are identical chemically. They make your nails stronger only in the sense that the polish itself coats and thus protects the nail. If you polish your nails, apply several thin coats instead of one heavy one. Minimize use of nail-polish remover. It can weaken and dry your nails. Touch up chips with polish and apply new polish over old to avoid use of remover for as long as possible.

Avoid Nail-Care Products

Nail strengtheners can discolor or break your nails. Artificial nails may produce reactions beneath your nails. Cuticle removers are corrosive alkali-based products that destroy the naturally protective bands around your nails. There is no scientific evidence that gelatin capsules, calcium tablets, or other vitamin or protein products improve and strengthen your nails.

Cut Toenails Straight

Trim your toenails straight across and not too short. This needs to be done only about once a month because toenail grow more slowly

To avoid ingrown toenails, cut your nails straight across and not too short.

than fingernails. They also tend to be thicker, especially on your great toe, so the best time for a trim is after bathing.

Take Care of Ingrown Toenails

Ingrown toenails usually occur on the big toe. They form when the edge of your nail curls and grows into the soft underlying tissue. They are caused by improper cutting of nails, by the way your nails grow (faster at the edge than at the center), and by pressure from ill-fitting shoes. Women who routinely wear pointed-toe, high-heeled shoes are especially likely to have this problem. If you have a slightly ingrown nail, pare off the excess nail and put tiny bits of sterile cotton under the affected edge to lift it up. Change the cotton daily until the pain and redness subside. If an infection develops (evidenced by severe pain and a discharge of pus), see your physician.

If you have a hangnail, do not attempt to pull it off. Pulling almost always rips into living tissue. Instead, clip it off neatly, leaving a slight angle outward. This may help prevent recurrence. Lubrication with hand lotion also can help prevent hangnails.

Healthy nails are smooth, without ridges or grooves. They are uniform in color and consistency and free of spots or discoloration. Remember this: no nail-care product can give you healthy nails. The only way you can help your nails to look their best is to protect them from damage and irritants (chemicals and detergents), then clean and trim them regularly.

The associated fungal infection of the foot or hand can be mild and produce no inflammation or it can be acute with blisters and painful swelling. Once the nails are involved, they may become thickened, detached, and shed, or the nail even may be destroyed. An accumulation of keratinous debris is usually found beneath the free edge of the infected nail.

Your physician's diagnostic tests may include scraping up some of the debris beneath the nail edge for microscopic examination to identify the fungus. The presence of a fungus will rule out other diseases of the nails.

Treatment. There are no good treatments for fungal infection of the nails. Solutions, creams, or ointments do not penetrate the nail, although they may help to control fungal infection of the surrounding skin. If you have a fungal infection that is disabling, or if the infection is excessively disfiguring, your physician may prescribe a systemic antifungal preparation. Sometimes it is difficult to tell whether these medications are effective. In addition, the nails grow so slowly that it takes 6 to 12 months to grow new nails free of infection. Once the drug is stopped, the fungus may return or the nails may remain permanently free of infection.

PART V

MODERN MEDICAL CARE

The following chapters are intended to help you make your way through the sometimes confusing world of modern medical care. Among other key concerns addressed are finding a suitable doctor, dealing with your medical bills, and numerous other issues, including cancer and the complex world of medicinal drugs.

CONTENTS

CHAPTER 38

THE HEALTH-CARE SYSTEM

CHAPTER CONTENTS

THE HEALTH-CARE SYSTEM TODAY

The American health-care system is perhaps the finest in the world. Our medical schools and teaching hospitals, the level of training offered to physicians and nurses, and the use of highly advanced medical technology attract some of the finest students from not only the United States but also many foreign countries. American medical institutions, both public and private, are at the forefront of research.

In the following pages we will consider the system as it functions today in order to provide an understanding of the training medical professionals receive, the economics of the health-care business, and the range of facilities available to suit the varied needs of you and your family.

THE ADVANCE OF TECHNOLOGY

Consider the long-established tradition of the visit to the physician's office. At first glance this may seem unchanged from the way it was 50 years ago: the physician takes your blood pressure, listens to your chest with a stethoscope, and thumps your knees with a little rubber hammer. Yet, thanks to technological advances, much has changed.

Now, your physician may have an electrocardiograph machine or other test equipment on the premises. When your physician suspects certain health problems, he or she can choose from among various diagnostic tests. Your physician can prescribe from an immense range of new as well as older medications. Some of the newest medications are the products of genetic engineering techniques—techniques unheard of only a few years ago.

Now, many operations, such as reattaching the nerves and blood vessels of severed limbs, are performed with the aid of microscopes for more precise work. Microsurgery was unavailable a few years ago. Heart surgery using various newly developed methods saves the lives of people who formerly would have died. Some types of organ transplantations, such as kidney, have become routine. Large numbers of Americans have undergone successful cataract surgery performed with new technology on an outpatient basis.

Technology has also helped us to avoid operations. Now, kidney stones can be broken up by directing sound waves at the body (see Kidney Stone Lithotripsy, page 900). Arthroscopic surgery has avoided major surgery and lengthy rehabilitation for knee injuries (see Arthroscopy, page 968). Recently developed drugs have helped to lower the risk of further heart attacks among patients who have already had a heart attack, without the need for cardiovascular surgery.

Even with problems for which scientists have not yet found a cure, such as many forms of cancer and AIDS, strides are being made in prolonging life as well as in prevention. Progress has been made in cancer treatment with chemotherapy and irradiation. Genetic engineering has made available new forms of medications. Research continues at an intense pace, resulting in greater understanding of the human immune system.

The advance of technology in medicine, with the associated progress in surgical techniques, instrumentation, and materials, has had positive results. The chances are you know someone who is alive today thanks to a pacemaker, a CT scan that revealed a suspected problem early enough for it to be corrected, or a medication that keeps a serious condition under control.

There also is a negative side to these advances in technology. When a new machine, technique, or medication becomes available, often the full range of benefits along with the most effective means of using it are still being determined. As a result, the tendency may be to use it not only when it is clearly needed but also in marginal situations in which the benefits may or may not ultimately be found to outweigh the risks and discomfort. These new techniques or medications often are very expensive as well.

Overuse of technology is relatively unusual. The efforts to cut the sometimes staggering costs of medical care have emphasized the need to find the most appropriate use of new technology. Many of today's physicians emphasize the importance of patient education, counseling patients on lifestyle changes and offering support and understanding as well as a willingness to undertake heroic technological measures when appropriate.

To the researcher in medicine, the closing decade of the 20th century is an exciting time. Many barriers seem about to tumble as new discoveries seem to be occurring at a breathtaking pace. Almost daily, our understanding of cancer, Alzheimer's disease, AIDS, and other serious human afflictions grows. The potential of biotechnology and genetic engineering has barely been tapped. The further development of these and other areas in medical technology holds promise for us all.

HEALTH CARE IN EVOLUTION

The American health-care system has many parts (most of which will be described in this chapter). It may be hard to think of the one-physician rural clinic and the skyscraper hospital staffed with specialists as belonging to the same system, but they do. And all parts of the system have felt the impact of some recent trends.

One trend is toward specialization. Before World War II, most people had a family physician who was a general practitioner. Today, general practitioners are rare, and the physician who provides your basic care is more likely to be a specialist in internal medicine or in family medicine. Most American medical school graduates go on to train in one of the 23 approved medical specialties (see Medical Specialties, page 1195).

Most graduates will go into private practice, either alone (solo practice) or with a group of physicians (group practice). In private practice, the physician cares for patients in his or her office or in a hospital setting. Payment comes directly from the patient or from insurance or government-furnished funds. Nonprivate practice may take the form of salaried employment in government public health posts, in medical schools, in research and teaching positions (although many physicians on medical school faculties are permitted to practice part time), or in hospitals in the fields of anesthesiology, pathology, radiology, or emergency room care.

Another trend is the changing nature of medical practices. Before World War II, in all likelihood your family physician was a solo practitioner. He or she often made house calls. Although some of us still receive our medical care this way, physicians today are likely to be part of a group practice, a health maintenance organization (HMO), or a clinic rather than in a solo practice. The costs, to physicians, of practicing medicine have increased, and the new clinical and group arrangements are one way to meet these costs. Such arrangements also offer physicians an opportunity to work in a more medically stimulating environment, benefiting from the experience of other physicians and sharing facilities, equipment, and expertise.

Another change from the recent past is that health care now is much more complex. There used to be just the physician and the hospital. Although these remain the cornerstones of the health-care system, the traditional idea of the physician has been changed to include many different specialized physicians and even nurse-practitioners. In addition to that at hospitals, care is delivered in clinics, HMOs, neighborhood health centers, freestanding emergency centers, nursing homes, and hospices, all of which are discussed in this chapter.

A key reason for the continual evolution of health-care delivery systems is financial; another is the spread of specialization. All of the advances in medicine have made it a much more complicated field of knowledge than it used to be. It was once possible for a physician to have some familiarity with the whole range of medicine and to keep up with the new developments published in technical journals. Now there is too much to learn. With the explosion of new technology, medications, and other options for cures, it is a formidable challenge for your physician to be current, even in his or her own specialty.

It is important to find one physician—a general practitioner, internist, pediatrician, or family medicine specialist—to take on the overall responsibility for your care and the care of your family. Sometimes, this "primary-care physician" actually is a team of physicians. Thus, one physician (or team) will be familiar with your medical history and problems. It is to this person (or team) that you go with your health concerns and for routine checkups. When necessary, your primary-care physician or team will refer you to a specialist and will keep track of what that specialist recommends.

You can find such a physician or team in private practice, in a group practice, in a

HMO, or in one of various types of clinics (these facilities are described later in the chapter). It is well worth the trouble to seek out such a physician or team to handle your general care. Your health will benefit.

Another area of change in the health-care system is the matter of how the costs of medical services are paid for. Medical care was once paid for by those able to pay, and physicians and hospitals could afford to charge little or nothing for those unable to pay. This has changed to a significant extent, due both to greater costs produced by scientific technological advances and to increased regulation by Medicare and insurance companies of fees that can be charged. The introduction of the federally funded Medicare program for the aged and of the state-funded Medicaid program for people with low incomes has lessened but not solved the problems of lower-income groups. In addition, conventional group insurance programs, paid for jointly by employers and employees, have become much more common.

The result of having more sources of funding for medical care is a greater number of patients seeking the help of physicians and health-care facilities. This has led to more medical care reaching those who need it, whether or not they can afford it. To those of us who can afford to pay insurance premiums, it has led to options such as whether to join an HMO for prepaid care or to remain under the care of physicians that we arrange for individually.

Despite expanded coverage of funding for medical care, many people today do not receive adequate medical care. Medicare does not pay all expenses for the elderly, nor does Medicaid pay them for the poor. The result is that many forgo care. A century ago, many Americans never visited a physician except in an emergency; this is still true, as can be seen in many a hospital emergency room. Perhaps the greatest tragedy are the children born in poverty to mothers who did not receive proper prenatal care and who also will not benefit from appropriate medical attention during their childhood.

There are two major problems to be solved: 1) providing access to medical care for everyone, and 2) controlling cost. Although health insurance, federal funds, and community welfare services cover payment for most of our population, there are some who fall through the cracks and, because they cannot pay, do not seek medical care until seriously ill.

Striking a balance between giving good medical care and lowering costs or at least restraining further increases is a difficult challenge. It raises fundamental questions.

Should further development of health-care techniques be discouraged because of potential costs? True, some useful techniques have proven to be extremely expensive. Equally true, other advances, such as polio immunization, have proven to be inexpensive to apply, especially in comparison with the alternative of providing treatment to those who without immunization would have been stricken with polio.

How much can use of tests and treatments be restricted without significantly impairing the quality of medical care? Ethical considerations in life-and-death decisions, which have become of greater magnitude with advances in technology, may be further complicated by the need for cost containment. There is no easy solution to the cost-versus-care paradox.

The challenges remain formidable, as they have been throughout the evolution of the American health-care system. The remainder of this chapter describes the contemporary health-care system—who the professionals are, how to pay the bills, and the facilities where health care is given. The more you know about who the players are and how the system works, the better your chances of seeking and finding appropriate, affordable, and quality care for you and your family.

THE PROFESSIONALS

When you seek health care, you must interact with physicians, nurses, and other health-care professionals. This section describes the diverse kinds of physicians, beginning with the various training regimens and including an explanation of when and why specialization takes place. Then we look at nurses, including some of the newer roles that they have taken on. Also included are brief descriptions of doctors of osteopathy, allied-health-care professionals, and sources of nutritional advice.

TRAINING THE M.D.

The physician, or medical doctor (M.D.), is the person ultimately responsible for delivering health care. Although the health-care system could not function without the nurses or other professionals, it is the physician on whom final responsibility falls for your care.

To become a physician requires, first, an undergraduate college degree. Medical school follows, with its 4-year curriculum. The first 2 years of medical school traditionally focus on the scientific foundations of medicine, including courses in human anatomy, physiology, genetics, biochemistry, microbiology, pharmacology, and behavior, along with an introduction to patient care. In the third and fourth years the focus of medical school is patient care. While continuing to take classes, the medical student also works with physicians in treating patients. The main areas of medicine covered during these third and fourth years are internal medicine, surgery, pediatrics, obstetrics and gynecology, family medicine, and psychiatry.

After successfully completing a 4-year medical school program, the student receives the M.D. (Doctor of Medicine) degree. To obtain a state license to practice medicine, however, the M.D. must pursue graduate training in a hospital or other health-care facility. Formerly, the first year after the M.D. degree was spent in an internship that provided experience in the common areas of medicine.

In more recent years, the first year is usually the beginning of a residency program in family medicine, internal medicine, or some other specialty. At the end of 1 year of such training and experience, the physician may take an examination to obtain a state license to practice medicine as a general practitioner.

At present, it is uncommon for physicians to actually start their practice at this point in their training.

The state license to practice must be renewed annually. A state licensing board not only examines the credentials of and gives

MEDICAL SPECIALTIES

The primary specialties are organized under the general direction of the American Board of Medical Specialties. In addition to the specialties, there are many subspecialties with their boards which operate within the authority of one or another of the primary boards. Thus, if your physician is a gastroenterologist, he or she initially received board certification in internal medicine, followed by subspecialty certification in gastroenterology. The specialty and subspecialty boards include:

Specialties

Allergy/Immunology
Anesthesiology
Colon/Rectal Surgery
Dermatology
Emergency Medicine
Family Practice
Internal Medicine
Neurological Surgery
Nuclear Medicine
Obstetrics/Gynecology
Ophthalmology
Orthopedic Surgery
Otolaryngology
Pathology
Pediatrics
Physical Medicine and
    Rehabilitation
Plastic Surgery
Preventive Medicine
Psychiatry and Neurology
Radiology
Surgery
Thoracic Surgery
Urology

Subspecialties

Diagnostic Laboratory
    Immunology
Critical Care Medicine
Dermatopathology
Dermatological Immunology
    /Diagnostic Laboratory
    Immunology
Geriatric Medicine
Cardiovascular Disease
Critical Care Medicine
Diagnostic Laboratory
    Immunology
Endocrinology and
    Metabolism
Gastroenterology
Geriatric Medicine
Hematology
Infectious Disease
Medical Oncology
Nephrology
Pulmonary Disease
Rheumatology
Critical Care Medicine
Nuclear Medicine
Radioisotopic Pathology
Critical Care
Gynecologic Oncology
Maternal and Fetal Medicine
Reproductive Endocrinology
Hand Surgery
Blood Banking
Chemical Pathology
Cytopathology
Dermatopathology
Forensic Pathology
Hematology
Immunopathology
Medical Microbiology
Neuropathology
Radioisotopic Pathology
Diagnostic Laboratory
    Immunology
Pediatric Cardiology
Pediatric Critical Care
    Medicine
Pediatric Endocrinology
Pediatric Hematology-
    Oncology
Pediatric Nephrology
Pediatric Pulmonology
Neonatal-Perinatal
    Medicine
Child and Adolescent
    Psychiatry
Nuclear Radiology
Pediatric Surgery
Surgical Critical Care
General Vascular Surgery

examinations to physicians wishing to practice in that state but also hears reports of inappropriate or unprofessional behavior by physicians. When necessary, the board may revoke the license of a physician. A physician who moves from one state to another must obtain a license in the state to which he or she is moving. Often this can be done by reciprocity—that is, the second state recognizes the credentials from the first state. However, some states insist on the physician taking all of the qualifying examinations.

The majority of physicians now continue their graduate education (residency) beyond the first year. They work as residents at a hospital or health-care facility for another 2 to 6 years or longer, gaining knowledge and experience in their medical specialty. Then they have the option of being examined and certified by the board in charge of their particular specialty (there are 23 of these). Many specialties are broadly based. For example, the fields of family medicine, internal medicine, general surgery, and pediatrics encompass a wide range of problems. Some physicians choose to go into medical research or teaching, in addition to or in place of a clinical practice of medicine.

Why do physicians put in those many years of specialty training—in addition to their 4 years of college and 4 years of medical school—in order to specialize? Perhaps one reason is the human desire to master a discipline. Medicine is such a broad and complex field that any one physician reasonably can expect to grasp only a small portion of it, a specialty, and to be able to apply it in any depth.

Once the physician starts to practice, his or her education is by no means over. Physicians continue their postgraduate education, by means of brief intensive courses, to keep up with developments in their fields. Some states require physicians to obtain a specified amount of continuing education to keep their licenses. The medical boards that govern particular specialties also have continuing education requirements which may be more stringent than those of the states. In addition to formalized postgraduate courses, the main ways that physicians attempt to keep abreast of the medical information explosion is through reading medical journals and attending conferences.

NURSES

In using the health-care system, you sometimes encounter nurses more frequently than you encounter physicians. This is especially true in hospitals where much of the care is provided by nurses.

Like the physician, the nurse has the goal of helping you to get well. The nurse observes symptoms and listens to your description of them. He or she helps to carry out the treatment plan and to evaluate the results. Included in the care provided by the nurse often is information for you and your family on how to manage health-care problems at home.

When both physician and nurse are involved in treating a health problem, the nurse plays a supporting and assisting role. Frequently, there also is a slight difference in the nurse's focus, with the physician concentrating on the medical problem and the nurse focusing more on how the person reacts to and deals with the problem and its accompanying symptoms and discomforts.

The initials R.N. after a person's name mean Registered Nurse. To be an R.N., a man or woman must first complete a course of study. There are several options: nursing

DOCTORS OF OSTEOPATHY

Osteopathy was founded by Andrew Taylor Still (1828–1917). His original premise was that, under most circumstances, the body has the ability to heal itself. Consequently, treatment offered by a doctor of osteopathy (D.O.) is intended to enable the body to restore itself by removing internal or external roadblocks to normal function. D.O.s emphasize the treatment of the musculoskeletal system, often with manipulation.

Today, D.O.s have a training regimen, scope, and licensing procedure similar to those of the traditional medical profession. However, there is a different division of responsibilities in that osteopathy has only 16 primary specialties (compared to 23 for traditional M.D.s).

In the past, D.O.s did not recommend the use of medications or surgery to cure disease. Today, however, the gap between M.D.s and D.O.s is narrowing. The majority of doctors of osteopathy now use much the same approach to the care of patients as medical doctors do.

OTHER PROFESSIONALS

In addition to physicians and nurses, many other individuals are vital to delivering effective health care. Other types of health-care professionals are listed here, together with a brief description of what they do.

Attendants and *orderlies* provide a variety of basic services such as transporting patients and helping nurses in health-care facilities.

Dental hygienists clean teeth, take dental x-rays, and perform other preventive dental services.

Emergency medical technicians (EMTs) offer emergency care, including life support, and transport the sick and injured to medical facilities.

Home health aides help the homebound with dressing, grooming, and eating and perform simple nursing tasks such as changing bandages (see Home Care, page 1267).

Laboratory technicians perform tests and analyses on blood, urine, and other materials to help in diagnosis and in monitoring the progress of a patient.

Medical records personnel keep patient files up to date and accessible.

Midwives attend women in labor and assist in the delivery of babies as well as in prenatal care.

Nurses' aides carry out nonspecialized basic tasks in health-care facilities, such as feeding and bathing patients and making beds.

Occupational therapists help the injured or disabled to regain the ability to carry out everyday tasks, including suggesting possible physical modifications around the home.

Optometrists test vision and prescribe eyeglasses.

Opticians grind and fit eyeglass lenses and contact lenses.

Pharmacists formulate and dispense medicines according to physicians' prescriptions.

Physical therapists help the injured or disabled to regain lost physical functions, using techniques such as exercise, massage, and ultrasound.

Physicians' assistants examine patients, diagnose some health problems, and suggest a course of treatment, under a physician's supervision.

Podiatrists treat injuries and other problems of the feet.

Psychologists diagnose and treat mental health problems through techniques such as counseling and therapy.

Radiology technicians help in taking and developing x-rays, CT scans, and other types of tests based on radiation.

Recreational therapists use group activities including music and games to help improve the communication or behavior patterns of withdrawn, depressed, and other patients.

Registered dieticians help to specify and to modify the types of foods eaten in order to address specific health conditions.

Respiratory therapists use respirators and other devices to improve breathing ability and capacity.

Social workers provide counseling about health-related and other problems and offer aid in obtaining financing, care after hospital dismissal, and other needed services.

Speech therapists treat disorders and injuries that affect the ability to speak, such as helping a child to overcome a lisp or an adult to regain speaking skills after a stroke.

---

credentials may be earned at a 2- or a 4-year college or university or in a 3-year diploma program in a hospital. Having earned a degree or diploma, a nurse must then pass a licensing examination in the state where he or she intends to practice. Some nurses also have postgraduate degrees.

The initials L.P.N. mean Licensed Practical Nurse. The L.P.N. course of study is shorter and less academically oriented than that of the R.N. The L.P.N. generally provides services under the guidance of an R.N.

Although most nurses are generalists, some specialize. In hospitals or clinics, some nurses work in a particular area of care such as cardiology, pediatrics, or psychiatry.

Other specialized types of nurses include the nurse-anesthetist, nurse-clinician, nurse-educator, nurse-midwife, and nurse-practitioner. The nurse-practitioner performs the same basic tasks as a physician, examining and treating patients, frequently in a setting where physicians are scarce or unavailable. However, they cannot write prescriptions.

Most nurses work in hospitals. Some nurses work in clinics, in physicians' offices, for home-care agencies, or in private practice (especially the nurse-practitioner and nurse-midwife). Nurses' aides are persons who have little or no formal instruction but have learned their skills by working under the supervision of R.N.s and L.P.N.s. They provide many valuable services in the hospital setting.

From the origin of the nursing profession in the 1800s, educating others about sound health practices has always been a focus. Education is accomplished in the form of lectures and demonstrations given by nurses to groups as well as the practical advice traditionally given to individuals. Nurses also conduct research and publish their results in respected journals, in addition to keeping abreast of new developments in nursing and medicine and attending professional conferences.

CHIROPRACTIC

After graduation from a junior college, a person who wishes to be a chiropractor attends a chiropractic college for several years. Upon graduation, he or she must pass a state examination in order to practice.

In most states, chiropractors are not permitted to prescribe medications for health problems, nor do they recommend or perform surgery. Instead, they manipulate the vertebrae of the spine and the body's joints and muscles. One of the basic premises of chiropractic is that the manipulation improves the flow of nerve impulses to the brain, thus increasing the body's own ability to solve its health problems. This theory was originated by David Palmer (1845–1913).

Other theories have since been incorporated into the training of chiropractors, although the focus on manipulating the spine remains, even for treating respiratory ailments and high blood pressure. A drawback of single-focus approaches to health care is that serious, correctable conditions and diseases can go untreated although the patient believes that meaningful treatment is being received. The American Medical Association does not recognize the chiropractic specialty as a legitimate medical field. Some insurance companies do cover chiropractic treatment.

Whom should you believe about the usefulness of chiropractors? Ask your physician. He or she knows you and your medical problems best. Some of the techniques of massage and physical therapy used by modern chiropractors are similar to those used by physical therapists and can help to restore and improve physical functioning.

On the other hand, a chiropractor is not an appropriate choice for a primary-care physician. Chiropractic's narrow approach and the limited medical training given the chiropractor leave this type of practitioner unskilled in the essential diagnostic role a physician must perform. In most cases, the chiropractor is ill-equipped to diagnose or effectively treat most serious medical problems.

NUTRITIONAL ADVICE

Nutrition is now a much-discussed topic. Almost daily, news sources offer stories regarding the health value of this or that nutrient or additive. In the supermarket you are bombarded with competing claims on packages. Where can you turn for sound advice on nutrition?

First, to your physician. Contemporary medical training places more emphasis on the importance of nutrition in preventing and treating disease than previously was the case. Many physicians also have special training and interest in nutrition and are affiliated with leading nutrition organizations such as the American Board of Nutrition, American College of Nutrition, American Institute of Nutrition, and American Society for Clinical Nutrition.

Your physician also can recommend a registered dietician (R.D.). Registered dieticians are registered with the American Dietetic Association (ADA). These professionals have college training and formal clinical experience in nutrition and have to pass an examination. Some states formally license dieticians, who are then known as licensed dieticians (L.D.s). After passing the examinations, dieticians can legitimately use the R.D. or L.D. title.

The term "nutritionist" is less clearly defined. Anyone can proclaim himself or herself a nutritionist. Legitimate nutritionists have a minimum of a 4-year college degree in nutrition. Many work with government and public health food programs. Conversely, dieticians focus on giving advice to individuals and work in private practice as well as in hospitals and clinics.

Some call themselves "nutritionists" merely to sell services or products. Ask about their training. The best nutritionists come from well-recognized universities and have a degree in nutrition, dietetics, or food science. Be wary of products such as weight-loss preparations or dietary supplements recommended by "nutritionists"—they may have manufactured the title as well as the product.

Seek nutritional advice from someone who has the R.D. or L.D. title or from an M.D. Your physician, local hospital, or health department can suggest qualified dieticians.

HOW TO PAY YOUR MEDICAL BILLS

Medical costs never seem to go down but continue to soar. Proposals and legislation aimed at lowering costs or at limiting the benefits of directly paid government programs or at spreading care more equitably are virtually always pending.

In the United States, physicians and hospitals usually bill for individual services rendered—so much per office visit, a certain amount per day of stay in a hospital, a certain fee for a particular laboratory test. This fee-for-service arrangement can become expensive, especially if a lot of services are involved, such as with an operation. Most of us are not in a position to be able to pay extensive medical expenses on short notice.

The medical expenses will be less of a burden for the person who has extensive health problems if they are added together for everyone and then averaged out. This is the philosophy behind health maintenance organizations (HMOs; see page 1200), conventional group insurance policies (both of which are described below), and government-aided insurance supported by tax dollars. In a large group, many people may need a few hundred dollars of medical care each year, some may not see a physician in 10 years, and an occasional person may incur hospital and surgical fees of a quarter million dollars. Care offered as a group plan would charge each of these people the same or nearly the same fee.

This type of averaged coverage for costs of medical care is offered to Americans in four main ways: conventional insurance, Medicare, Medicaid, and prepaid health plans. With Medicare and Medicaid, the government assumes a major share of the costs.

Medicare is available to all Americans age 65 or above, to some handicapped persons, and to certain persons with kidney disease who qualify under the end-stage renal disease program (see Chronic Renal Failure, page 909). It is supported by the federal government and covers some, but by no means all, medical care. A deductible amount, which varies each time the government modifies Medicare provisions, must first be paid by the patient before Medicare payment begins. For those expenses that are covered, reimbursement is for a large percentage but not the total. The remainder is then paid for by the patient through privately purchased major medical plans or by Medicaid.

Medicaid is also a government-supported program administered by the state with funds coming from both the state and federal governments. The coverage is for those whose incomes fall below a particular level, regardless of their age. Persons with Medicaid coverage have little or no out-of-pocket expenses. The specific coverage of Medicaid varies a good deal from state to state, however, and both Medicare and Medicaid are subject to constant revision.

Your local Social Security Administration office can supply details on current Medicare coverage. For Medicaid information, contact your local welfare agency, social services agency, or Social Security Administration office.

CONVENTIONAL HEALTH INSURANCE

Most large employers offer some type of health coverage plan for their employees. The choice is typically between conventional group insurance and joining a health maintenance organization (see page 1200). Depending on the employer and the coverage offered, the employee may pay for a portion of the insurance coverage as a payroll deduction, and the employer pays for the remainder as a "benefit." Some policies offer coverage for spouses and dependents at rates that are higher than coverage for a single person.

If you leave your job and want to continue that policy's coverage on your own, you can do that through your old employer if new coverage is unavailable elsewhere, although at greatly increased rates. It may be cheaper to obtain new coverage as a member of another group. Group insurance policies are available to the self-employed or unemployed through various organizations to which they may belong.

The tendency in conventional insurance is for the insurance company to reimburse you for those medical expenses arising from illness or injury, including costs of surgery, hospital stays, some prescriptions, and some types of rehabilitation therapy. Maternity expenses are usually covered as well. There is generally a waiting period between the date when your coverage under the policy starts and when maternity benefits or coverage for treatment of long-term illnesses takes effect.

Visits to a physician for regular checkups are not always reimbursed. However, if you have some particular problem to discuss with your physician during the visit, your insurance company may cover it.

Before expenses are reimbursed, there generally is a deductible amount that must be paid by you first ($200 or $500 per year are typical deductibles). Expenses beyond that often will be reimbursed in large part (such as 80 percent) rather than fully.

Major expenses, such as for surgery and hospital stays, are reimbursed up to a point that the insurer determines is usual, customary, and reasonable. For example, if your surgeon charges $3,000 for an operation, and the insurer determines that the maximal reasonable charge for that particular operation is $2,000, the insurer will pay the lesser amount or a percentage of it. The remaining amount you can pay privately or through additional insurance coverage such as major medical insurance. Employers and group plans frequently offer major medical insurance in addition to their basic policy. You also can purchase it privately.

The thing to understand about conventional insurance is that there is no "standard" insurance. Even insurance plans that have paid the hospital bills of generations of Americans, such as Blue Cross/Blue Shield, offer different levels or degrees of coverage according to the specific policy that the employer or other group asked the company to write. The coverage varies greatly.

What your particular policy covers will be explained by the policy. Many companies summarize the coverage in a pamphlet, but looking at the actual policy or contacting a knowledgeable representative of the insurance company or the insurance plan's administrator at your job will give you more precise details.

All insurance policies have caps (limits) on what they will pay. For example, a policy might pay for up to 3 months of hospitalization (but no more), 100 home visits a year from a registered nurse, or $1,000,000 in total benefits over a lifetime. It is a good idea to determine what these caps are before disaster strikes. Insurance agents can advise you on additional insurance that you can purchase to cover costs above the specified caps.

Medical expenses are sometimes covered by private insurance policies that people may not be aware of. Worker's compensation applies to injuries sustained on the job, and automobile insurance may cover medical expenses arising from car accidents. Homeowners' policies often contain some liability coverage for visitors who are injured. Athletic associations frequently cover injuries sustained by athletes during sporting events.

HEALTH MAINTENANCE ORGANIZATIONS

The health maintenance organization (HMO) offers medical coverage in a way that is fundamentally different from private insurance. An HMO is a group of providers including physicians, nurses, and other health-care specialists. You become a member of an HMO for a fixed monthly fee.

The system works this way. When you or a family member want a regular medical checkup, you visit a physician who is associated with the HMO. If you become ill, sustain an injury, or need surgery, the HMO will provide and pay for the medical services you need, either at its own facilities or at an affiliated hospital. Emergency services are covered wherever they are provided.

The idea behind HMOs is that they attempt to offer more complete medical coverage, ranging from the preventive physical examinations that conventional insurance usually does not cover to the serious problems that conventional insurance usually does cover.

Many employers will pay some or all of the cost of belonging to an HMO, as an alternative to paying for some or all of an employee's coverage under a group insurance policy. It is also possible to join an HMO as an individual or as a member of an interest group (a union, professional association, or the like) that you belong to.

There are drawbacks to HMOs. At most HMOs, you can only visit the HMO's own physicians or those to whom the HMO refers you. This means that you are not free to choose your own physician. You must choose from among those who are members of the HMO. If you need treatment or hospitalization for a serious illness such as cancer, the HMO may not send you to the specialists or hospital that you would have chosen yourself.

Keep in mind that, as with any health insurance program, the coverage is never truly total. HMO policies frequently contain exclusions (particular types of medical care that are not covered, such as vision and hearing problems) and caps (maximums on the amount that will be spent). Read descriptions of HMO coverage carefully or ask a knowledgeable HMO administrator.

On the other hand, there are advantages to HMO care. These include coverage that is usually more complete than with conventional insurance, ready access to a physician as well as other health-care professionals at a location that has your medical history file on hand, and no financial penalty for visiting a physician for a minor problem or a checkup.

PREFERRED PROVIDER ORGANIZATIONS

Preferred provider organizations (PPOs) represent an attempt to deliver medical care at a lower cost. A PPO is a network of physicians designated by a particular insurance company to provide medical services. The physicians agree, in negotiations with the insurance company, to offer medical services at fees that are lower than the going rate in exchange for a steady supply of patients.

A PPO is not a health-care organization like a HMO. It is merely a modification of the stipulations of some conventional insurance policies to favor certain physicians. The physicians submit bills for each service rendered, in the same way as any physician in private practice.

Some insurance companies offer inducements to the insured person to use a PPO

UTILIZATION REVIEW BOARDS

Just as an auditor goes over a firm's financial ledgers to look for irregularities, a utilization review board is charged with the task of determining whether hospital care is justified. Since the introduction of Medicare in 1966, utilization review boards have sprung into existence across the country. Currently, the government, private insurance companies, and HMOs all make extensive use of utilization review boards.

Utilization review boards focus on the care offered to individual patients as well as on overall patterns of care over time. Case by case, the boards check to see that the services rendered were medically necessary, and that they could be provided only in the hospital setting. Utilization review boards are alert to any evidence of abuse of hospital services.

Utilization review can take place at various times, such as before admission to the hospital, upon admission, during dismissal planning, or before settling insurance claims. The second opinion program that insurance policies commonly require before an operation is approved is a form of utilization review.

Sometimes utilization review boards monitor the quality as well as the costs of care. Quality and cost are not necessarily in conflict: poor-quality care may make additional, subsequent care necessary, subjecting the patient to repeated procedures and incurring added costs.

The operation of the utilization review boards lowers costs by shortening hospital stays but adds to the administrative costs of health care.

physician. For example, the insurance company may pay the full cost of care rather than a percentage of this cost or may waive the deductible.

The intent is to lower costs—for the insurance company, the employer paying part of the bill for insurance coverage, and the insured person who pays the remainder. The use of PPOs is growing, but the concept is still relatively new, and a consensus has not yet been reached on whether the quality of care is compromised. The utilization review board (see above) is a control mechanism incorporated into all PPOs.

HEALTH-CARE FACILITIES

The American health-care system offers health care to its medical consumers in many settings. The majority of health care takes place in the outpatient or office setting or in the hospital.

Most hospitals can be considered to be

general or comprehensive, although many will lack some services such as neurological surgery or emergency room care. In addition, there are specialized hospitals that cover only a limited category of services. Examples of these are hospitals that restrict care and operations to diseases of the eye, orthopedics, obstetrics, or other specialties.

In recent years, there has been an increase in the types of facilities that serve the health consumer. These facilities have been developed in response to experimentation with new means of delivering health care and of cutting costs.

This section describes various types of health-care facilities other than hospitals. Specialized facilities such as mental health centers, nursing homes, and hospices are described, as are the hospital outpatient department, office practice, freestanding emergency centers, neighborhood health centers, and rehabilitation centers.

OFFICE-BASED PRACTICES

The three main types of office-based practice are solo practice, group practice, and HMO. In solo practice, a physician works alone rather than with partners or in a clinic. General practitioners, internists, and other specialists can be found in private practice. A nurse or assistant may help the physician with the workload. When you are under the care of a physician in solo practice, he or she is on call for emergency advice 24 hours a day. When your physician is on vacation or ill, he or she will advise you of who to consult if necessary during the interim.

A group practice can include two or more physicians. The rationale is to share the 24-hour-a-day care burden as well as the office and personnel expenses. In addition, it is helpful for a physician to be able to talk over some cases with a colleague. For the patient, group practice differs from single-physician practice mainly in that you may already know the replacement physician when yours is on vacation or sick. Some groups include various specialists, another advantage if you need them. Larger groups also may have clinical support facilities such as on-site laboratories.

The bill for care in solo or group practice is paid for by conventional medical insurance, Medicare or Medicaid, and the patients themselves.

The HMO is another type of group practice (see Health Maintenance Organizations, page 1200).

If you need hospital care, a solo, group-practice, or HMO physician will send you to the hospital with which he or she is affiliated.

HOSPITAL OUTPATIENT DEPARTMENTS

A hospital outpatient department may offer health services by appointment or on a walk-in basis. The full range of facilities of the hospital are used to provide the services—physicians, nurses, laboratories, operating rooms, recovery rooms—but you leave the same day that you come in, without occupying a hospital bed overnight.

In recent years, the proportion of hospital services offered on an outpatient basis has greatly increased. Many operations—such as hernia repair, breast biopsy, cataract removal, and operations on children—are now routinely performed on an outpatient basis, whereas not so long ago they often involved a stay in the hospital.

Not all hospitals have an outpatient department. Virtually all that do not, however, provide outpatient care in their emergency department or emergency room.

A main advantage (to you, your insurer, or both) of outpatient care is lower cost. Another is that you can spend any recovery period necessary (as from an operation) at home, where the environment probably is more cheerful than in a hospital.

For surgical procedures or involved tests, have someone accompany you to the hospital, to stay with you while you wait, and to take you home after the procedure. One of the drawbacks of outpatient surgery is that you really do not feel like going anywhere when the anesthesia first wears off, yet you have to go home. Another drawback is that, if unforeseen complications arise that cannot be managed by telephone, you will have to return to the hospital.

FREESTANDING EMERGENCY CENTERS

The freestanding emergency center (sometimes called an "urgicenter" because urgent cases are treated there) is like a hospital's emergency room without the hospital attached. The freestanding emergency center does not have the extensive resources of a hospital emergency room to draw on. The freestanding emergency center generally is a private, profit-making facility and may not provide the level of follow-up attention that a hospital or your physician would provide.

Freestanding emergency centers provide treatment on a drop-in basis, like hospital emergency rooms, but typically with shorter waits. The care offered is usually confined to minor emergencies, such as closing and suturing wounds or treating a high fever, that do not require hospitalization.

Many of the medical procedures performed in a freestanding emergency center could be done just as well in a physician's office or clinic, but these centers are open for more hours (some never close) and do not require an appointment. The care at freestanding emergency centers generally costs more than in a physician's office or clinic but is less than the charges in a hospital emergency room.

Freestanding emergency centers vary in the quality of care they provide. Therefore, before using one (and, if possible, before the emergency), ask your physician for an opinion concerning its competence and to find out if the center has arrangements for transferring severely ill or injured patients to a hospital when necessary.

NEIGHBORHOOD AND PRIMARY HEALTH-CARE CENTERS

A neighborhood health-care center or primary health-care center offers clinical care by appointment or on a drop-in basis. The purpose of these government-supported centers, which originated in the 1960s, is to provide medical care in either rural or urban areas that do not have enough (or any) physicians and hospitals. Payment is by Medicaid, Medicare, conventional insurance, or directly by the person needing care (sometimes on a sliding-fee scale based on ability to pay). Some centers offer care to migrant farm workers as well as to residents of the area.

The services offered by neighborhood or primary health-care centers vary depending on the size of the facility and what other types of health-care arrangements the area

has. In general, they offer the kinds of medical care and procedures that would be available in a clinic or hospital outpatient department. Unfortunately, many of the centers closed in recent years for lack of funding.

NURSING HOMES

Nursing homes offer care and supervision to those requiring help with such daily activities as eating, dressing, bathing, or going to the toilet. Ongoing skilled nursing and medical attention is also available in some homes. Most nursing home residents are elderly; about 5 percent of those over age 65 and about 20 percent of those over 85 live in nursing homes.

Admission to a nursing home is no longer considered to be the "last stop." Now, physicians may recommend a stay in a nursing home during recovery from a stroke, hip fracture, or illness. People often leave nursing homes to return to independent living arrangements.

There are two main types of nursing homes: skilled-care homes and intermediate-care homes. A skilled-care home offers 24-hour nursing services as well as restorative, physical, occupational, and other therapies. An intermediate-care home offers fewer of these intensive nursing and rehabilitative services. Both types of homes provide supervision and help with daily activities. Most nursing homes are or are becoming skilled-care homes.

Most nursing homes are for-profit businesses. These homes should provide as pleasant an atmosphere as possible for their occupants. (For advice on selecting a nursing home, see Selecting a Good Home, page 246.)

A hospital dismissal planner, private care manager, or hospital-based social worker may be able to suggest nursing homes that do not have prohibitively long waiting lists and can advise on financing nursing home care. Although the cost of nursing home care is high, financial assistance is sometimes available from Medicare, Medicaid, private health insurance, the Veterans Administration, trade unions, or fraternal organizations.

For someone who does not require constant or extensive care and help, a nursing home may not be the place to go. A number of alternative forms of care are available for those who just need a little help or nursing attention, including home care (see page 1267), adult day-care, day hospitals, and medical day-care. Retirement communities and special housing designed for the elderly are other options. Before you decide on a nursing home, see When Is a Nursing Home Appropriate? (page 247).

HOSPICES

A hospice provides care for those who are dying and for their families. Some hospices are small, independent institutions, and others are part of a hospital. The hospice movement began in Europe and has recently taken hold in this country.

The philosophy behind a hospice is that the person who has no medical hope of recovery—the dying person—should be made as comfortable as possible. If someone is terminally ill, a hospital's normal routine, with its busy atmosphere, numerous interruptions, and focus on getting better, is probably irrelevant and disturbing.

A hospice addresses the two biggest fears that dying people have—the fear of pain and the fear of being alone. The staff of a hospice administers appropriate pain relief, provides nursing care, and offers plenty of reassurance. The staff and family see to it that the individual is not alone during this last and important phase of his or her life.

Admission to a hospice program must be requested by the terminally ill person together with a physician. Sometimes, hospice care begins in the home until the person becomes too ill; care then continues in an institution. Ideally, the same care-givers are involved in both settings.

After the death, many hospices also help the family to manage their bereavement.

Medicare and other types of insurance provide coverage for some hospice care (see also page 1251).

MENTAL HEALTH FACILITIES

Mental health services are available in various settings. For the sudden crisis situation, there is the hospital emergency room. For problems that require less-immediate atten-

tion, access to psychiatrists and psychologists is to be found in three main settings.

The first is in a private, office-based practice. The cost of visiting a psychiatrist or psychologist in private practice can be high but is sometimes covered in part by insurance.

The second setting is the community-based mental health clinic which has a staff of mental health professionals. Community-based centers generally receive some type of government support. The cost to you will be lower than that for visiting a professional in private practice. Sometimes costs are determined on a sliding-fee scale based on the ability to pay.

Community-based centers, ideally, will devote a portion of their efforts to the care and supervision of mentally ill persons living in group homes. With the introduction of antipsychotic medications in the last few decades, it has been possible to dismiss many persons from state mental hospitals. In addition, many such hospitals have been abandoned in the interest of economy. Unfortunately, group homes have not been able to care for some of the more severely disabled. When an affected person fails to take the prescribed antipsychotic medication, his or her condition may deteriorate. This person may become another member of the homeless group.

The third main setting where psychiatrists and psychologists are accessible is in a hospital-run mental health clinic or outpatient department. Not all hospitals provide outpatient mental health services.

Some mental and emotional problems require the long-term care that is possible only with institutionalization. Every state and many larger cities and counties have some type of residential mental health facility. Admission to a residential facility is usually through the recommendation of a physician and the consent of the family of the person being admitted.

The quality of care in residential institutions varies greatly. Some are overwhelmed with more patients than the staff and facilities can reasonably care for. Take a look at the facility before trying to get someone admitted, and if anything about it disturbs you, discuss alternatives with your physician.

Private residential mental health facilities are also available. These tend to offer a better staff-to-patient ratio. They may have a waiting list, and they tend to be substantially more expensive.

Group homes are also available for the mentally retarded and mentally ill. These are usually foster homes that provide a safe living environment, personal care, and some activities and social contact. The focus is on custodial care, however, rather than on therapy to enhance recovery.

Many adult day-care centers and nursing homes also admit patients with mental problems. Again, in such facilities treatment of mental disabilities tends more to the custodial than to the restorative.

For people with long-term but minor mental health problems, home care may be a viable alternative to residence in an institution (see Home Care, page 1267).

MATERNAL AND CHILD CARE

Many community health centers have maternal and child care programs which can provide care both before and after the baby is born. Funding for these programs comes from federal and other governmental sources, which means that care is often free if your income is below a specified level.

Child care should begin early, during the second month of pregnancy. Care of the mother and child should continue at regular intervals through the remainder of the pregnancy. We cannot overemphasize the importance of sound nutrition and of good health habits during the prenatal period. Prenatal medical care and good nutrition greatly decrease the infant mortality rate as well as problems associated with pregnancy and childbirth. The result is a healthier baby and mother. (See also Concerns During Pregnancy, page 181.)

The newborn infant, and later the child, should continue to receive regular medical attention, including counseling on nutrition and help with health problems that arise.

REHABILITATION CENTERS

The focus of rehabilitation care is on helping someone to regain some or all of the physical abilities that have been lost or impaired through injury, illness, or disease.

For example, if a runner injures an Achilles tendon, physical therapy using ultrasound may help speed the tendon's natural healing process and the runner's ability to return to running. The physical therapist also can recommend specific exercises to help avoid recurrence of the problem.

In the case of someone who has suffered a stroke, physical and occupational therapy helps restore use of the muscles affected by the stroke, and speech therapy can assist in restoring lost speech capacity if the stroke affected the brain's speech center.

The Services. Rehabilitation care is provided by various specialized types of therapists. Generally, someone in need of rehabilitation is referred to a therapist by a physician who may also monitor the course of recovery.

Physical therapists help to restore use of muscles and parts of the body by using heat, cold, massage, whirlpool baths, ultrasound, and other techniques as well as restorative exercises. Occupational therapists help to restore the ability to carry out daily functions, including adaptation to handicaps, use of devices such as wheelchairs, and advice on modifying the home environment. Speech therapists use special techniques to help correct speech disorders or restore speech lost through stroke or other injury. Inhalation therapists use respirators and other breathing aids to help restore normal breathing capacity. Hearing therapists help with damaged hearing function and hearing aids. Dieticians or nutritionists provide advice on diet adaptations to recover from, or avoid, particular types of problems. Physiatrists and other physicians coordinate the efforts of other members of the team. Usually, conferences among the team members will be held periodically (often once a week) to discuss the program and make decisions regarding the care of an individual patient.

The Settings. Rehabilitation services can be obtained in various settings. Many hospitals offer rehabilitation services on an outpatient basis. Rehabilitation services may or may not be separated within the hospital into a specific department, but most hospitals are good sources for the therapists who help with rehabilitation.

Sports medicine clinics, freestanding or as departments of hospitals, can be found across the country. The physicians and therapists at such clinics help not only injured athletes but also nonathletes who need to regain or improve their use of limbs and muscles.

Skilled-care nursing homes frequently provide physical and occupational therapy and sometimes other forms of therapy such as speech therapy. Physicians often suggest a stay in a nursing home, for recovery from a stroke or serious illness, before returning home. During such a stay, rehabilitation can be the focus of both the patient and the medical team, provided the nursing home is set up to offer skilled medical care rather than merely custodial care. Evaluate nursing homes (see Nursing Homes, page 246) and their ability to provide rehabilitation services before selecting one.

Physical therapists, occupational therapists, speech therapists, and other types of therapists also can be found in clinical practice, private office-based practice, and some health maintenance organizations.

Therapists can make home visits to persons unable to leave home conveniently. Many community-based as well as profit-making home health service agencies can provide needed therapists for rehabilitation (see Home Care, page 1267).

How do you find a therapist if you need one? If you were hospitalized, the medical team in the hospital—in particular, the dismissal planner—would advise on follow-up therapy needs for rehabilitation. If you have not been hospitalized but believe you need rehabilitation therapy, ask for your physician's opinion on this and for recommendations on where you can obtain the needed care.

There are many organizations that will provide advice and help to people in need of rehabilitation. These include Rehabilitation International, the National Rehabilitation Association, the Easter Seal Society, the National Amputation Foundation, the Disabled American Veterans Association, and numerous organizations concerned with specific types of disabilities and illnesses (blindness, hearing impairment, cancer, arthritis, and so on).

Within limits, many types of insurance cover some therapy for rehabilitation purposes.

CHAPTER 39

USING THE SYSTEM

CHAPTER CONTENTS

YOUR PERSONAL PHYSICIAN

Our knowledge of illness and our ability to treat it are growing rapidly. In fact, the time has long passed when a single physician can be expected to know everything about the thousands of ailments, common and uncommon, that have been identified. As a result, specialties and subspecialties have developed as medicine seeks to manage this explosion of knowledge.

One result of the increasing specialization is that some people believe they can get the best care by seeing a specialist for whatever part of their body is bothering them. Perhaps a visit to a gastroenterologist is necessary for an intestinal problem, or to an orthopedist for joint problems, and so on. Also, today people are much more mobile than they were in the past—it's the exception for an individual to spend his or her entire life in the same town (and under the long-term care of the same physician). One result of these two trends is that many people no longer have an individual they would describe as their personal physician.

Yet the personal physician can still be found. He or she is someone you trust, have confidence in, and are comfortable with. In some situations, more than one physician will serve as your personal physician. This may occur in a group or HMO setting (see Health Maintenance Organizations, page 1200) in which you may see different physicians but all of your medical records are together for easy access and review.

It is important that your physician be able to advise you candidly when your personal life and habits affect your health. Your personal physician is better able to care for you if he or she is knowledgeable about the health of other family members and is aware of diseases that occur with high frequency in your family. Your physician should also know about sources of tension in the workplace or at home that may affect your health.

A good personal physician will serve as a "gatekeeper," helping you obtain specialty consultations when needed and making sure that one treatment is not in conflict with another. This role is particularly important when you have long-term or multiple health problems that require consultation with specialists. Your personal (primary-care) physician is generally responsible for coordinating and overseeing your preventive care, treatment when a problem arises, and rehabilitation after treatment.

In medicine today, this physician is usually a specialist in family practice, internal medicine (for adults), or pediatrics (see Medical Specialties, page 1195). Family practice has been in existence as a specialty of its own, with board certification, since 1970. To be certified in family practice, a physician must complete 3 years of advanced training in family medicine. He or she will have had some training in almost every aspect of medicine, including obstetrics and pediatrics. An internist is a physician who diagnoses and treats medical diseases of adults. He or she also can deal with nearly every health problem you might have. Pediatricians diagnose and treat medical diseases of children.

Earning the M.D. degree requires 4 years of medical school. Following that academic training, the personal (primary-care) physician enters a training program in his or her chosen specialty, which generally lasts 3 years. After finishing a specialty training program, a physician may choose to obtain further training in a subspecialty. For example, someone trained in the specialty of internal medicine may obtain further training in the subspecialty of cardiology (study of heart disorders). Occasionally, a physician with subspecialty training may still serve as your personal physician (see Understanding the Specialties, page 1214).

In addition to such educational and training experiences, your physician should also offer you the ability to care for you as a person.

FINDING A PERSONAL PHYSICIAN

The first step in finding a personal physician is to assemble a list of names. Don't worry about how long your list is at this stage—you can narrow it down later.

Before you move into a new community, ask your current physician for recommendations. You can also obtain names from various sources. One good place to start is your local or county medical society, which should be able to provide you with a list of physicians in your area. Consumer affairs groups may have information or may even have a guidebook on local physicians.

Your local hospital is another possible source of names, as are the yellow pages of your telephone book (look for internists, pediatricians, and general or family practitioners). Your local library has several directories, including the American Medical Directory, that list physicians. This directory has information about every physician who belongs to the AMA. Included are their addresses, ages, education (undergraduate and medical), certifications as specialists, and the specialty associations they belong to.

Ask your friends and colleagues for recommendations. Inquire about availability and promptness for returning telephone calls if you have a medical question. In the same way, no matter where you obtain names, take into account accessibility. Include only those physicians whose offices are located within or near your community and are easily accessible from your home or office.

Call the office of each of the physicians on your list. You will most likely speak to a receptionist or medical assistant. Introduce yourself and tell him or her you are looking for a physician.

Take note of the receptionist's tone. Is it warm, friendly, concerned? Are your questions answered directly?

Ask what hospital the physician is affiliated with, what the fee schedules are for checkups and office visits, and what the physician's office hours are. Does the receptionist give you directions to the office? How accessible is it?

Inquire about the kind of coverage the physician has for emergency situations that occur outside normal office hours. Find out how much time the physician allots for appointments. Your physician should allow at least a half hour for a routine initial examination; subsequent appointments should last at least 10 minutes. If you have particular religious or other strong feelings that may affect the kind of care you seek, inquire about the physician's willingness to accommodate these concerns.

Using what you have learned and your own instincts, narrow your list to two or three physicians. Now call back the physicians on your list and inform the receptionists again that you are looking for a physician and would like to make an appointment for a brief consultation. Be prepared to pay for the time—remember, you will be building a long-term relationship with this person, one that implies responsibilities (one of them financial) on your part too.

When you actually go to meet each physician, take note of the office. Is it clean, cheerful, and comfortable? How crowded is it? Are you greeted pleasantly? Are there magazines—including health publications? Take note of how long you have to wait in the reception area.

When you meet the physician, remember that the primary questions you need answers to are: Is this person well qualified by both education and experience? Does the individual care about you as a person? Are you comfortable talking to him or her? Do you feel relaxed in his or her presence; do you get the feeling the physician is in a hurry and you feel rushed? Are you encouraged to ask questions, and do you understand the answers? Does the physician use a lot of medical jargon? Are the fees reasonable?

One question you might want to ask is how the physician would treat a terminally ill patient. This may surprise the physician, but it is one way to find out about his or her philosophy. All in all, the physician should be well trained, experienced, warm, friendly, concerned, professional, and well respected in the community. Choose one who closely fits these criteria, one in whom you would be comfortable entrusting your health.

SECOND OPINIONS

Given the various treatments and the technology available today and the high cost of many of them, getting a second opinion has become almost standard practice before proceeding with many treatments. In fact, some health insurance agencies insist that a second opinion be obtained before certain surgical procedures are performed.

The decision to get a second opinion can be initiated by either you or your physician. A good physician who is uncertain about a diagnosis will have no reservations about referring you to a specialist. In fact, the physician may be glad to have the diagnosis confirmed by another trained professional. Second opinions are sometimes useful when the diagnosis is clear but the choice of treatments is less so; often, several significantly different treatments are available for a particular disease. Therefore, if a diagnosis is very serious, if the treatment advised by your physician is risky, experimental, or controversial, or if major surgery appears necessary, a second opinion may be in your best interest.

If you are the one requesting a second opinion, don't feel you have to be secretive about it. Let your physician know you would like a second opinion just to confirm the diagnosis or the appropriateness of the procedure. Remember, your physician's principal concern is to try to ensure your continued good health.

COMMUNICATION BETWEEN PATIENT AND PHYSICIAN

Traditionally, the advice of physicians has been accepted without question. Today, however, there is a growing recognition that this system of one-way communication is not healthy for either physician or patient. Better care may result when you are an active participant in your medical care.

The highest-quality medical care results from a partnership between you and your physician. To make an accurate diagnosis, your physician needs information only you can provide. In the same way, many treatments require that you help your physician—and yourself—by following his or her instructions precisely. (A frequent cause of the failure of a treatment is the failure of the patient to follow instructions precisely.)

For the best health care, work with your physician to determine which treatment is best for you. Ask questions. Understand what your health-care providers are doing and why. Have a clear understanding of what to expect from your disorder and its treatment.

Feel free to contact your physician to discuss unexpected events, discomforts, or other problems. Essential to proper physician-patient communication is your confidence both in your physician's abilities *and* in his or her openness in listening to your concerns and observations. Your side of the bargain is your willingness to listen and be guided by the advice you are given.

YOUR EXPECTATIONS AND RESPONSIBILITIES

Becoming a partner with your physician in maintaining your health is not always easy. The time when this partnership becomes most important is when you or a loved one is sick—yet it is at times of illness that feelings of fear and helplessness can make communication more difficult.

As a patient, you have certain expectations and responsibilities. For example, expect the following:

1. Information: as much information as you want about your illness;
2. Time: a reasonable amount of time to ask questions and discuss concerns;
3. Cost estimates: information on how much your care will cost;
4. Consultations: reasonable access to your physician. Don't expect to see your physician at any time day or night; but you should be able to consult your physician as your medical condition dictates and as your physician's schedule permits;
5. Emergency contacts: to know where care is available in an emergency if your own physician cannot be reached;
6. Timely appointments: to be seen within a reasonable time of your scheduled appointment except in extenuating circumstances;
7. Changes in physicians: to be able to change physicians at any time and expect that your medical information will be promptly forwarded to your new physician;
8. Confidentiality: that your condition and your medical records are your business and your physician's. If you need to consult a specialist, however, keep in mind that he or she may also need to review your records. For some conditions (such as certain infectious diseases), your physician is required by law to notify government authorities. However, your records generally are not to be released to insurance companies, employers, or other individuals unless you approve their release;
9. Decision-making ability: to participate in decisions made about your care based on your knowledge of your illness.

To fulfill your responsibilities, inform your physician of all information that might relate to your illness. Information that may seem completely unrelated—concerning your medical history, family, home and work situation—may have a direct and sometimes crucial impact on your current problem.

Be on time for office appointments; if you are unable to be there as scheduled, cancel at least 24 hours in advance. As a courtesy to your physician (whose schedule may be busy indeed) and to ensure that you get what you need from your appointment, plan what you want to ask ahead of time. Stop your physician and ask for an explanation if you don't understand something.

Once a treatment is prescribed, follow it accurately—but if you can't, let your physician know. There may be an alternative treatment you can try. Be patient—often a treatment takes time to have an effect, but inform your physician promptly of any adverse effects, worsening symptoms, or complications.

WHEN TO CHANGE PHYSICIANS

A good physician will welcome your taking an active role in your health care. If your physician puts you off and seems to resent your reasonable questions, consider getting another physician.

Even though physicians provide services like other professionals, services physicians provide are unique, involving an intimacy not found in relationships with other service providers. It takes time to build these relationships. Confidence and trust between you and your physician are essential. Take time to select one carefully. Invest time in getting to know him or her. Avoid jumping from physician to physician. If something annoys you, or if a misunderstanding arises, discuss it.

Some circumstances may amount to a basic incompatibility between you and your physician. Do you feel you can't trust your physician? Are you uncomfortable talking about personal aspects of your life or illness? Is your physician condescending or brusque? Do you think he or she isn't always straightforward and honest with you? Do you often believe that you aren't getting your physician's complete attention? Are you rushed during appointments? Is your physician unavailable, or is after-hours coverage inadequate? Are your philosophies and lifestyles incompatible? Does your physician fail to follow through on problems when they arise?

If the answer to all or many of these questions is "yes," it may be an indication to change physicians.

If you decide to change, let your former physician know and know why. Although it is easier simply to leave, give your physician an opportunity to hear why the physician-patient relationship failed. Also, you will need to have your medical records forwarded to your new physician.

THE MEDICAL EXAMINATION

Most adults need a thorough medical examination at least every few years—more frequently if there is a specific health problem that requires continuing care (see Periodic Medical Examinations: How Often Should I Consult My Physician?, page 1212). A physician is less likely to be able to provide you with appropriate preventive care and accurate diagnoses if he or she sees you only when you are sick.

Before heading to your physician for a checkup, think about what you want to discuss. This step may save you from forgetting a question you wanted to ask. Prepare a written list summarizing symptoms that concern you, medications you are taking, and questions you want to ask. Such a list should not be extensive; just jot down five or six items that you want to be sure not to forget.

It is especially helpful to think about your symptoms before you see your physician. For example, if you have a specific medical complaint such as abdominal discomfort, tell your physician what the discomfort feels like, how intense it is, how long it lasts, where it occurs, how far the pain spreads from its beginning point, what precipitates the pain, what makes it better, what makes it worse, whether it is associated with any other symptoms, and how often it occurs.

If this is your first visit to a new physician, he or she should obtain your complete med-

PERIODIC MEDICAL EXAMINATIONS: HOW OFTEN SHOULD I CONSULT MY PHYSICIAN?

The answer to this question varies, depending on whom you ask. Consult your physician if you have pain or other symptoms. On the other hand, the absence of disagreeable symptoms does not necessarily guarantee that you are in good health.

In the early stages, many diseases, including diabetes, high blood pressure, and some forms of cancer, are asymptomatic (without symptoms) but are detectable and treatable. Many conditions can be cured or at least controlled if they are found early. The main goals of a periodic medical examination are to diagnose treatable, asymptomatic diseases and to correct modifiable disease risk factors. These goals imply a comprehensive physical examination and laboratory evaluation (see The Medical Examination, page 1211).

How often should you have a medical examination? This is a difficult question to answer because all of us have different needs. Nevertheless, there are guidelines that may be useful to you in discussing this issue with your physician. The following guidelines are for people who have no symptoms of disease.

Regular Physical Examinations

The interval between examinations depends on your age. If you are between 18 and 30 years, every 5 or 6 years is appropriate, perhaps at ages 18 and 24 years. After age 30 years, every 3 years is probably a better frequency. Between 40 and 60 years an every-other-year schedule is sensible; after age 60 years, have a checkup annually.

Self-Examination

Self-examinations are also important. Men should begin regular self-examination of the testicles during the teenage years (see Self-Examination of the Testicles, page 1116). Women of childbearing age or older should examine their breasts monthly (see Breast Self-Examination, page 1076).

In addition to periodic health checkups and self-examinations, specific studies can help keep you healthy. Here are guidelines to aid you in discussing this with your physician.

Annual Pelvic Examination and Pap Smear

Women should schedule these tests annually from the time they become sexually active (see The Pelvic Examination, page 1055, and The Pap Smear, page 1096).

Mammography

If you are younger than 40 years you probably do not need mammography unless you develop a problem or are in a high-risk category (for instance, if you have a family history of breast cancer). If you are between 40 and 49 years of age, have no symptoms or lumps, and have no family history of breast cancer, have mammography done to determine a "baseline" (a test to determine what is normal for you) and then a repeat test every 2 years. After the age of 50 years, have mammography annually. If you have a family history of breast cancer, have mammography once a year regardless of age (see also page 1080).

Screening for Colon Cancer

You should first have this test (involving examination of a stool sample for microscopic blood) at approximately age 40 years and then at each subsequent general health examination. At age 50 years, request this test annually.

Digital Rectal Examination

This should be done at the time of each general comprehensive physical examination.

Proctosigmoidoscopy

In the absence of any family history of colon cancer, this examination (which involves insertion of a device into the rectum) should be done initially at age 45 years and every other year thereafter (see also page 641).

Blood Lipid Measurements

Your blood cholesterol, HDL-cholesterol, and triglyceride values should be determined as early as possible (preteen years, for example), particularly if there is a family history of atherosclerosis. If test results are within normal limits, further testing should then be performed at least every 5 years.

Chest X-Ray

When to obtain a chest x-ray is somewhat controversial. In the absence of any heart or lung disease, it may not be necessary before age 40 years. It is reasonable to have a baseline chest x-ray at approximately age 40 years and to repeat the test as recommended by your physician.

Glaucoma Screening

This brief, painless eye examination should be done at age 40 years and repeated as recommended by your physician.

Resting Electrocardiography

Before age 40 years, have a baseline test; repeat as recommended by your physician.

Blood Pressure Measurement

Have your blood pressure determined at every physical examination or more often if so advised by your physician.

ical history. If you are seeing a physician for a specific ailment, going through a complete medical history and describing past illnesses may seem irrelevant to the problem at hand. However, a current illness often has roots in or may be affected by past medical conditions. Be prepared to give a description of illnesses experienced by your parents, siblings, and grandparents (see How To Gather a Family History, this page). Inform your physician of prior illnesses, hospitalizations, accidents, operations, or allergies. You will be asked a long list of questions reviewing each of your body's systems. Your physician should take detailed notes of any past problems.

THE PHYSICAL EXAMINATION

Your physician will supply you with a dressing gown and ask you to undress so that he or she can perform a physical examination. To provide you with complete, quality care, your physician must be informed of all the details of your health history and be able to examine all parts of your body. However, this examination will be performed with professionalism, humanity, and respect for you as an individual.

Physical examinations may vary slightly, but the basic elements of a thorough examination are the same. Your height and weight will be checked. Your physician will check your blood pressure. He or she will record your heart rate and will listen to your heart closely with a stethoscope, ideally while you are lying down and while you are sitting up. Your physician will also use the stethoscope to listen for any abnormal sounds in your lungs and abdomen. Your eyes, ears, nose, and throat, as well as the skin on your face, will be examined. Your physician will check the extent of your visual field (that is, your side vision).

Your abdomen will be carefully palpated to check for enlargement of the liver, spleen, or aorta or any other abnormalities. You may be asked to walk a few steps so that any abnormalities of gait or balance can be observed. Your physician will feel for pulsations of arteries in your neck, groin, knees, and feet. Your neck, armpits, and groin will be examined for the presence of swollen lymph nodes. Your reflexes will be checked by tapping your knees and ankles with a small rubber hammer.

HOW TO GATHER A FAMILY HISTORY

In preparation for your medical examination, gather information about any childhood illnesses, accidents, or operations. You will also be asked to offer additional information about other members of your family and their illnesses.

Obviously, it is important for your physician to know about any genetic diseases that are clearly inherited (Huntington's disease and sickle cell anemia are two examples). Such ailments are passed from parents to children, although not every child in each generation will be affected.

At the same time, many common diseases have apparent familial links. For example, if your father has heart disease, it does not necessarily mean you will have heart disease also. But it is important for your physician to know about the history of this illness in your family so that any symptoms can be caught early and preventive steps can be taken to reduce other controllable risk factors (see page 787).

To assemble a family history, make a list of any chronic diseases affecting your parents, grandparents, brothers, sisters, children, and sometimes aunts and uncles. Keep track of whether they are on the maternal or paternal side of your family. Such diseases include high blood pressure; cancers of the breast, uterus, and colon; diabetes; arthritis; Alzheimer's disease; allergies; emphysema; heart disease; and kidney disease. Also record any unusual diseases, even those that you have no reason to believe have an inherited tendency.

Take note of any twins born in your family or any miscarriages. Finally, note whether any immediate relatives died at a young age from an illness. Pass this information on to your primary physician to be included in your medical record.

For women, the examination will often include a breast and pelvic examination, which usually includes a Papanicolaou smear (see The Pelvic Examination, page 1055, and The Pap Smear, page 1096). These can be performed as part of the regular physical examination, unless you prefer—or your physician recommends—a gynecologist. Both men and women should have a rectal examination, and men should have their prostate gland palpated. Samples of your urine or blood may be taken for testing.

The examination will proceed smoothly, without interruption, and will be thorough and methodical. The steps in the examination probably will not be limited to those mentioned above, especially if your physician suspects a problem, past, present, or future, that requires further examination, questioning, or testing.

You will be encouraged to ask your physician questions and to amplify any points on which you have information, such as any scars, sensitive areas, or family traits.

At the end of the examination, your physician will forthrightly discuss the findings. Review the important points with your physician to make sure you understand them.

LABORATORY TESTS

Routine laboratory tests are likely to be done in conjunction with the physical examination. These include a urinalysis, an x-ray of the chest, and blood tests. Electrocardiography may also be done, particularly if you are older than 40 years.

The blood tests are of two categories or groups. The hematology group tests measure the number of white and red blood cells and also the number of platelets. The hemoglobin concentration is measured, and the varieties of white cells are enumerated. All this is done in an automated procedure. Figures are given for the average size and hemoglobin content of the red blood cells.

The purpose of hematology group testing is to identify any evidence of the different kinds of anemia, leukemia, and other disorders of the blood-forming system.

The second category of blood tests consists of several chemistry measurements—blood sugar and other substances, enzymes that reflect liver and kidney function, electrolytes, and blood fat concentrations, such as cholesterol and triglycerides. Your physician will obtain measurements of other substances in your blood if the physical examination or your symptoms suggest the possibility of particular diseases or disorders. A blood test for syphilis will be done in some circumstances.

Such routine tests done on a person who has no symptoms of illness and no abnormal findings on physical examination only occasionally will reveal a previously unsuspected illness—and thus it is argued that in the interest of cost-containment they should not be performed. Most people, however, want the reassurance of normal laboratory tests and place value on these. Furthermore, having an electrocardiogram and a good-quality chest x-ray on file may be very useful in the future for comparison purposes, particularly if you should develop new symptoms and have equivocal findings on an electrocardiogram or chest x-ray at a later time.

When the test results are complete, your physician will discuss them with you. If the initial tests suggest some type of abnormality, your physician may recommend further testing.

UNDERSTANDING THE SPECIALTIES

Your primary-care physician should be responsible for providing you with general health care on a regular basis. However, there may be times when your personal physician is not completely certain about a diagnosis or what is the best treatment for your symptoms. In such circumstances, you, your physician, or both of you may think a second opinion is appropriate, a situation that does not necessarily reflect on your physician's confidence or competence.

Consulting another physician, one with special training, is appropriate in several circumstances, as in the following:

1. If you have a rare disease or an unusual manifestation of a common disease;
2. If you need a special procedure or operation;

3. If you are not responding to therapy;
4. If your disease is progressing especially rapidly or new complications are developing.

Getting a second opinion may be initiated by your physician, by you, or by your insurance company, many of which now insist on second opinions before they will pay for a procedure.

A wide variety of specialists are experts in particular organ systems and diseases. Often, areas of expertise overlap. For instance, if you have been diagnosed as having lung cancer, you may see a lung (pulmonary) specialist, a cancer specialist (oncologist), a radiotherapist (who will supervise radiation therapy), and a thoracic surgeon. All are medical doctors.

Do not be surprised if different physicians recommend slightly different treatments. Keep in mind that medicine is not an exact science. Different physicians—each of whom may be highly qualified and experienced practitioners—may favor different choices from among the therapies available for the same disease. All treatments may be effective, but each will have advantages and disadvantages. So keep in mind that a specialist's opinion is just an opinion. Look to your primary-care physician to help you determine which treatment is best for you.

Finding a specialist for your disease can be as simple as obtaining the names of several physicians from your personal physician and making an appointment with one of them; often your physician or the nurse will contact the specialist, brief the second physician about your case, and even schedule an appointment for you. Or you can locate a specialist on your own, much the same as you would look for a primary-care physician (see Your Personal Physician, page 1208). If you live in a rural area or have an especially rare or complex medical problem, you may have to go to a major teaching hospital to find an appropriate specialist.

Before you see the specialist, put together a short list of questions that you want answered. When you visit a specialist, he or she is likely to ask you about your medical history again and may repeat some of the tests you have already undergone. Nevertheless, make sure that a copy of your medical records reaches the specialist. And feel free to ask how much the consultation will cost. For a review of all the specialties, see page 1195.

REASONABLE EXPECTATIONS FROM MEDICAL CARE

What can we reasonably expect from medical care? The answer to that question is complicated and subjective. A range of factors, including our health at any given moment and our experience with medicine in the past, all have an impact on our hopes, worries, and health concerns. To make matters more complicated, the rapidly escalating cost of health care raises questions such as how much are we willing—or able—to pay for health care.

Let's start with statistics. On average, the life expectancy is now almost 75 years, as opposed to that in the year 1900, when the average person could reasonably expect to die before reaching age 50 years. People are living longer, mainly because many of the acute and infectious diseases that once struck people down at a relatively early age have been largely conquered. In recent years, mortality rates for most cancers have not changed a great deal, but death rates have declined for the most frequent causes of death, including heart disease, stroke, diabetes, and peptic ulcer. Also, the infant death rate, on average, has also declined—although there remains a significant difference in death rates in infants of mothers with little or no prenatal care and poor access to the health-care system.

Developments in medical research have resulted in a steadily increasing ability to predict, detect, diagnose, and treat countless diseases. As people live longer, chronic diseases occupy more of your physician's time. An increased emphasis on preventive medicine is spurring life-style changes by Americans that also may result in lower disease and death rates.

Remember that, despite remarkable advances, modern medicine does not have all the answers. However, in partnership with your physician, many medical concerns and discomforts can be relieved. Diseases that in years past caused early death can be prevented or treated more effectively. Many serious disorders can be diagnosed earlier, when treatments are much more effective. And for disorders that cannot be cured, effective means of relieving pain and of prolonging or ensuring a better quality of life are increasingly available.

THE HOSPITAL STAY

Suppose your physician has decided that you should be admitted to the hospital. Going to a hospital 150 years ago was strictly a last-resort measure. Today, however, hospitals offer the highest-quality medical care possible—and rarely is a hospital stay to be regarded as anything like a final event.

In a hospital, skilled teams of physicians, nurses, technicians, therapists, dieticians, and support staff work together to provide care. High-technology medical equipment is available to perform a vast array of medical tests and procedures. Still, staying at a hospital can be a frightening prospect—it means that you are sick enough, or require a procedure that is serious enough, to require a stay in the highly sophisticated environment of a hospital.

ENTERING THE HOSPITAL

What should you bring with you? You do not need to bring much—a change of clothing for the trip home, slippers, reading or other material to pass the time, a minimal amount of cash, and basic toiletries. Also, bring a form of identification, insurance information, any medical records, any medications you take, and whatever else your physician suggests you may need. The hospital will supply you with a hospital gown (you may want your own pajamas), meals, and most of the other services you require.

Once you get to the hospital, your first stop will probably be the admitting office. You will meet with an admitting officer to review your medical history, financial information, insurance forms, and the hospital's fees and to obtain a room assignment.

Many hospitals provide you with a plastic card used for billing purposes. An identification bracelet will be placed on your wrist. The bracelet lists your name, age, hospital identification number, any allergies you

---

THE HOSPITAL VISIT

Of the 30 million Americans admitted to hospitals annually, probably one or more of them will be a friend or relative of yours.

Visits from you may help advance the person on the road to recovery. This is not an area in which clinical analyses reveal statistical findings; however, many physicians can tell you stories about how visits from friends and relatives proved to be strong medicine for some of their patients.

Unfortunately, many people feel ill at ease in a hospital setting and are reluctant to call on a recuperating patient. However, as is so often the case, knowing a bit of the basic etiquette of the circumstances may well make the situation seem easier and more natural.

These basic guidelines may help make visiting a sick friend less uncomfortable.

Phone Ahead
Let the person know you are coming. Hospitals have routines—tests or rounds in the morning, per-

haps—that should not be interrupted. Perhaps your friend or relative relishes a nap at 3:00 P.M. or simply is not ready for visitors. Set up a convenient time for both of you.

Do not interrupt at mealtime—it's difficult to eat comfortably and talk too.

Keep the Visit Brief
The person you are visiting is ill or recuperating, and resting is part of recovering. Talking and visiting may be draining, so 10 or 20 minutes is probably the ideal duration.

Obey Hospital Regulations
Stop and check in at the nurses' station on the way to the person's room. Visit during scheduled visiting hours. If you are bringing plants or foods, check with the nurses first; the person may be on a special diet and certain hospital units do not allow plants. Do not interfere with care—if a nurse or physician arrives, ask whether you should leave.

Sit Down, Listen
Pull up a chair (do not sit on the

bed) and try to be at eye level with the person. Never probe about what is wrong or what is going to happen: let the patient tell you whatever he or she is comfortable in sharing. Keep your personal hospital experiences to yourself. Let the patient talk at his or her own pace and steer the conversation.

Express Your Feelings
Do not hesitate to express affection. A sincere hug, kiss, pat on the arm, or squeeze of the hand can express more than you can say.

Commonsense Rules
Even if it is not forbidden (it usually is), do not smoke. Do not offer medications; that is the job of the physician and the hospital personnel.

Check first before you bring children—they can often lift spirits, but they may not be welcome. If youngsters do accompany you, keep the visit short.

If you are ill, stay home: the person in the hospital does not need to be exposed to another ailment.

have, and perhaps other information. It is important that you wear this bracelet throughout your stay.

If you enter the hospital as an emergency patient, the entry procedure may be somewhat different. An admitting officer probably will obtain the necessary information from a family member or, if you are well enough, will visit you in your room.

DURING YOUR STAY

After being admitted, you will be escorted to your room. You will meet members of the nursing staff who will be responsible for your daily care. If you have questions during your hospital stay, contact your nurse or physician. If you are unhappy with some aspect of your care, discuss the situation with your nurse or physician. If your complaint is not resolved, check to see if the hospital has a patient representative or ombudsman. These people work to clear up such problems.

Every hospital has specific routines and policies regarding visiting hours, patient meals, services, and other practical aspects of day-to-day life in the hospital. Usually, policies, procedures, and services of hospitals are described in printed literature that patients receive on admission. These policies generally vary, depending on which unit of the hospital you are in. For instance, visiting hours will be different for an intensive-care unit than for a general-care unit.

Reasons for being admitted to the hospital are constantly monitored by utilization review boards. If a case can be made that your care could be given in a nonhospital setting, the board may refuse to authorize admission and you may be responsible for all or a portion of your hospital bill. Hospitals maintain a system of surveillance that helps avoid these situations. Your physician will discuss this with you if the nurses and physicians responsible for surveillance think that hospitalization has not been justified or that you have remained in the hospital longer than necessary.

LEAVING THE HOSPITAL

Once your physician determines you are well enough to leave, you will be dismissed from the hospital. Before you leave, dismissal planning can be arranged. Dismissal planning involves making arrangements for any home medical care you will need, determining what follow-up appointments you should have, and teaching you how and when to take your medications and do other procedures relating to your illness.

SURGERY

You and your physician have discussed your illness. You have reviewed all the alternative treatments and their risks and benefits and have decided that the best course of action involves surgery.

For most people, entering the hospital for an operation is a frightening prospect. However, taking an active role in your care and making sure you understand the process may go far toward relieving your anxieties. An understanding of what is going on helps reduce the fear factor in most situations.

Be particular about whom you choose to perform your operation. Usually your primary physician will recommend a surgeon, but you want to be sure to pick a surgeon with extensive experience and a good track record for the operation you are to undergo. Also, choose a good facility, one that is well equipped, is adequately staffed, and has a blood bank. During the operation, a team of professionals is responsible for bringing you through it safely. This team consists of your surgeon, an anesthesiologist, nurses, and, sometimes, physicians-in-training who assist with the operation. Your personal physician may also be in attendance. You need to feel confident that each member of the team is highly skilled.

PRESURGICAL EVALUATION

Before you undergo an operation, your physician is responsible for going over your medical history in detail and uncovering any medical conditions, reactions, or allergies that may affect the outcome. As much as possible, existing medical problems will be corrected before an operation. At most hospitals, the anesthesiologist will conduct his or her own evaluation and has the responsibility of refusing to administer anesthetics if the risk is judged to be too great.

Be sure to inform your physician of any medications you are taking, including diuretics, aspirin, and even seemingly insignificant over-the-counter medications. These are easy medications to overlook because they are used so commonly, but they can have a significant effect on your recovery. For example, aspirin can interfere with the ability of blood to clot. This could increase the risk of excessive bleeding during or after your operation.

As part of your presurgical evaluation, you may undergo several laboratory tests, particularly if you are older than 40 years or have other medical problems. These tests may include electrocardiography to evaluate your heart and a chest x-ray. Often, blood tests are done.

If you have a history of a diseased valve in your heart, you will receive antibiotics as a preventive measure before such operations as dental extractions, hemorrhoid operations, or other procedures that may involve tissue contact with bacteria (see Infective Endocarditis: Protection and Prevention, page 824).

ANESTHESIA

The practice of modern surgery has been made possible by the development of anesthesia, which enables your physician to perform an operation without you experiencing much or any pain. Various anesthetic techniques are available.

In most instances, the anesthesiologist will visit you before your operation. He or she will review any pertinent medical problems with you and ask some additional questions. The anesthesiologist may ask you whether any family members have had adverse reactions to anesthetics because there are several inherited disorders that can cause severe reactions to certain anesthetics.

The anesthesiologist will recommend a type of anesthetic on the basis of your physical and emotional status and what operation is being done. For most operations it is imperative that you not eat anything within at least 8 to 10 hours before you receive an anesthetic. This precaution helps to prevent you from vomiting during or after the sur-

gery. Children younger than 3 years may drink clear liquids (water, apple juice, grape juice, or soft drinks—but no milk) up to 4 hours before the operation.

The three main categories of anesthesia are local, regional, and general.

Local Anesthesia. Local anesthesia is considered the safest form. An anesthetic is administered into the skin at or near the site of the operation. The injection numbs the area to pain and any other sensation, usually for a relatively short time.

You remain conscious during the operation. Local anesthesia is used for localized operations or for certain other more extensive operations in patients for whom general or regional anesthesia is too risky.

For some operations done with the patient under local anesthesia, a catheter is placed in one of your veins (usually in an arm) so fluids can be infused intravenously. This will also serve as an access to give sedatives and other medications. A solution containing sugar and salt may be infused to help prevent dehydration. For the other types of anesthesia, an intravenous line always will be used.

Regional Anesthesia. Regional anesthesia is similar to local anesthesia in that you remain conscious. However, in most instances you are also sedated. There are four main types of regional anesthesia: spinal, epidural, caudal, and major nerve block.

The major advantages of regional anesthesia are that it can be used for more extensive procedures than local anesthesia and that only the region of the body that is anesthetized is affected. Therefore, other regions of your body, such as your heart, lungs, and brain, are relatively unaffected. Regional anesthesia also can be used to provide excellent relief of pain after the operation. Depending on your health and the operation you are having, it may be the safest form of anesthesia for you.

Spinal anesthesia can be used for most operations below the navel, such as hernia repair, rectal, bladder, prostate, and pelvic operations, and operations on the legs and hips. The anesthetic is injected through a small needle into the fluid-filled space surrounding the spinal cord. The injection, which generally is painless, is made while you are lying on your side or sitting. Side effects, such as nausea and vomiting, difficulty breathing, light-headedness, or pain, occur infrequently during the operation and usually can be managed easily. After the operation, you may have some minor discomfort at the site of the injection. Headaches, which may last for several days, occur only rarely.

Epidural and caudal anesthesia can be used for many of the same procedures for which spinal anesthesia is used. The injection is made just outside the sac that contains the spinal fluid. The advantage of these techniques is that a small catheter can be placed to allow easy reinjection during longer operations and for treatment of pain for several days after the operation. Injections of narcotics (such as morphine) through these catheters provide excellent pain relief with very few side effects and help you recover from your operation faster.

Regional nerve blocks are most commonly used in the arms, but they can be used in almost any area of the body. A small needle is placed into the area through which a major nerve passes. Often you will feel a sensation of a mild electric shock in the region of this nerve, such as in a finger. This tells the anesthesiologist that the needle is in the correct place. A local anesthetic drug is then injected through this needle and the intended area of your body will become numb and immobile. Side effects, such as minor pain during the operation, are rare, and persistent numb areas or tingling, which may last several days or longer, is extremely rare.

General Anesthesia.   General anesthetics are administered either by inhalation or by intravenous injection. These drugs circulate in your bloodstream to all areas of your body, including your brain, and cause loss of consciousness.

Because general anesthetics affect all areas of your body, such as the heart and lungs, side effects are more common. However, most of these side effects are temporary and easily managed by the anesthesiologist or a nurse anesthetist who is with you throughout your operation.

All general anesthetics depress your breathing and alter the function of your heart, and they may affect your blood pressure. To prevent problems, an anesthesiologist or nurse anesthetist continually monitors your blood pressure, heart rate and rhythm, breathing, and temperature. In most in-

stances a breathing tube is placed to ensure adequate breathing.

Other side effects that may occur after general anesthesia, such as nausea and vomiting, sore throat, muscle pain, and other aches and pains, usually are of short duration or are easily treated. More serious complications, such as heart attack, kidney damage, and stroke, are extremely rare. They almost never occur in the absence of preexisting conditions. Proper screening and treatment of any serious medical illnesses in advance of the procedure, as well as careful monitoring of your vital signs during the operation, greatly reduce all of these risks.

THE OPERATION

In most cases you will be brought to the operating room on a rolling table and then transferred and positioned comfortably on the operating table. During the operation, the table may be rotated and tilted to allow complete access to the site of the operation.

Your medical team will take great care to avoid an infection. The area to be operated on is shaved and disinfected. An initial shaving is often done before you come to the operating room. All instruments and supplies are carefully sterilized, and the team wears gowns and masks. Your blood pressure, heart rate, and breathing are monitored carefully throughout the operation and after the procedure. Solutions of salt or glucose (sugar) are given slowly into a vein to maintain normal levels of water in your body and to serve as an avenue for giving drugs, if necessary, during the operation. If a general anesthetic is given, either intravenously or by inhalation, a device is used to help you breathe.

POSTOPERATIVE RECOVERY

After the operation, you are moved to the recovery room until you wake up. It is important that close monitoring be maintained throughout the recovery period because occasionally complications develop. If possible, you will be placed on your side with your head down so that secretions and any vomit from your mouth will drain instead of being breathed in (aspirated).

After some major operations, such as complicated neurological or cardiac procedures, you will be moved to an intensive-care unit (ICU). The intensive-care unit is equipped with complex monitoring equipment, mechanical devices to assist breathing, and resuscitation equipment, all of which are maintained by a highly trained staff of physicians and nurses. Fluids and blood are administered through an intravenous tube in your arm. If your intestines have been operated on, you probably will have a tube exiting from your nose to drain intestinal secretions and swallowed air. As soon as your intestines resume normal functions, the tube will be removed.

Once you have recovered sufficiently and no longer require the close monitoring and sophisticated life-support systems of the ICU, you are moved to a general unit. You will be encouraged to do deep-breathing exercises and to walk, both of which assist in your recovery. Besides providing for your care, your nurse also will educate you on any special care you must have after you leave the hospital. Finally, when your physician decides you are well enough to go home, you will be dismissed.

After dismissal you probably will come back to the hospital or your physician's office for follow-up examinations. Your physician will advise you as to when and how quickly you can resume normal activities.

AMBULATORY SURGERY

Ambulatory surgery, same-day surgery, and outpatient surgery are all terms for the same concept. Given the high cost of staying overnight at a hospital and government pressures to keep costs lower, same-day surgery has become increasingly popular.

A number of surgical procedures can be performed on an outpatient basis. Generally this means you come to the facility, have the operation, and leave on the same day. A family member or friend should come with you.

You can have same-day surgery at either an outpatient (or ambulatory) clinic within a hospital or at a freestanding "surgicenter." The advantage of an ambulatory center at a hospital is that complications can be dealt with more easily if they arise, whereas a surgicenter may be some distance from a hospital.

Some of the surgical procedures that can be done on an outpatient basis include simple hernia repairs, tissue biopsies, abortions, D & Cs (dilation and curettage), vasectomies, and some cosmetic procedures.

The initial steps are not much different from those for inpatient procedures (see above). A physician or nurse will take your medical history and tell you what to expect. Tell your physician or nurse if you are diabetic. An identification band may be placed on your wrist.

If you are going to receive an anesthetic, you must not eat or drink anything for 8 to 10 hours before the operation, unless instructed otherwise by your physician. Children younger than 3 years may drink clear liquids (water, apple juice, grape juice, or soft drinks—but no milk) up to 4 hours before the operation.

In addition, if you receive an anesthetic, do not drive yourself home afterward. Have a family member or friend drive for you.

Leave your jewelry and valuables home or give them to the person accompanying you. Wear comfortable clothing that is easy to remove, and do not wear makeup or nail polish. If you wear contact lenses, glasses, false teeth, or a removable bridge, make sure you bring along a case to put them in. The center will provide you with a hospital gown and slippers.

After the operation, a nurse will give you instructions on how to care for yourself at home.

MALPRACTICE AND LAWSUITS

Malpractice occurs when a physician's care of a patient is somehow negligent. The physician does something that a reasonable physician in the same or similar circumstances would not do, causing injury to the person.

The number of malpractice cases brought to court in the United States has increased in recent years. One result is that rates of malpractice insurance for physicians have spiraled upward. An expensive malpractice suit, settlement, or judgment increases the cost of malpractice insurance for all physicians, not just the one being sued. This is an important factor in the high cost of medical care today.

BRINGING A MALPRACTICE SUIT

If you suffer long-term injury due to negligence on the part of your physician, you have the right to bring a malpractice suit. If you die, a survivor can file a suit.

The first step in bringing a malpractice suit is consultation with an attorney, who will gather the medical records and history and then submit them to an expert physician to determine whether there is a valid case. Because the opinions of physicians may differ, the lawyer may get a second or even a third opinion. The physician's lawyer will usually obtain a statement from the patient describing the events that led to the damages.

Even after you have a lawyer and the suit is filed, the outcome is by no means ensured. Many cases are settled out of court before a judge and jury ever hear one word of the evidence. Yet, despite headlines about enormous malpractice judgments, most cases that go to trial are resolved in favor of the physician.

If the defending physician feels strongly that he or she followed standard medical practices, the case may go to trial. In most cases, the court will require the plaintiff to call an expert witness (that is, another physician who is qualified to testify about the case).

A responsible lawyer will consider a case seriously and in detail before deciding whether to bring a claim. And a patient or surviving family of a patient should consider seriously whether they want to go through the trauma and expense of a court trial.

Many malpractice suits could be prevented if better communication existed between patients and physicians. All too often, it is miscommunication between physician and patient or the patient's incomplete understanding of the proceedings that results in the pain, expense, and other hardships associated with a malpractice suit.

INFORMED CONSENT

Few procedures or treatments in medicine are entirely risk-free. To make sure patients are informed of these risks beforehand, the medical profession adopted a rule called informed consent. This requires physicians to explain to you certain significant risks that are involved in a particular treatment. Depending on the situation, the physician may be required to explain the diagnosis, the nature of the treatment, any risks or side effects involved, the consequences of not receiving the particular treatment, and any alternative treatments that are available. Sometimes you will be asked to sign a form stating that this information has been explained. You and your physician may both benefit from having a member of your family included in the discussion.

You have the ultimate control of your body and the right to refuse a particular treatment. However, if you have a psychiatric illness, if you are a minor, or if you are under the influence of medication, illegal drugs, or alcohol, you may not be able to give your consent.

QUACKERY

The ancestor of today's medical quack sold "life-saving elixirs" from the back of a horse-drawn wagon. The so-called magical potions of yesteryear may have faded into history, but medical quackery—defined as the promotion of medical schemes or remedies that are known to be useless or are unproven, for a profit—still is alive and well.

Each year, one out of every four Americans will use quack medical treatments. They will spend a total of at least $25 billion for these treatments. At best, the drugs, devices, and lifestyles are worthless; at worst, they lead to physical harm and even death.

So why is quackery so successful? Its success lies in the fact that it takes advantage of a basic human vulnerability—the yearning for a quick cure, whether it be for cancer, AIDS, arthritis, obesity, male baldness, or other human complaints, simple or serious.

Oddly, medical quackery knows no educational boundaries; in fact, recent studies show that people with a college education are actually more likely to use unproven treatments than those with less-formal education.

Often those who use fraudulent medical cures are isolated and lack the support of family and friends. Some people have absolute faith in the written word, believing that if something is published, it must be true. Disease, or the fear of one, may result in a frantic willingness to try anything. Because medicine has no cure for many problems, some people turn to quack remedies as a last hope.

THE DANGERS OF QUACK MEDICINES

Instead of offering hope, fraudulent medical treatments can provide a threat. Besides being useless, sometimes they are actually dangerous. They may consist of medications that are harmless when taken in moderation but harmful when taken in doses prescribed by the quack. Another potential risk is that manufacturers of quack drugs often do not produce their products under the strict quality control measures required of legitimate drug companies. These drugs also may contain substances that, although safe by themselves, become harmful when mixed or taken in combination with certain foods, drink, or other drugs that you may be taking.

Quack medicines also can be dangerous to your financial well-being. The American Medical Association estimates that most victims of fraudulent medical treatments spend $500 to $1,000 annually. Of the $25 billion estimated to be spent on quack medicine each year, some $5 billion is spent on ineffective treatments for cancer. It is estimated that people older than 65 years, many of whom are on fixed incomes, spend a total of at least $10 billion annually. Often those who spend the most on quack medicines are the least able to afford them.

Another risk of quack remedies is that if you trust the miraculous promises of the quack you may be losing precious time while you are pursuing a nonexistent cure instead of an actual one. Some cancers and other diseases respond well to medical therapy, especially if detected and treated early.

Quack medicine promoters may play on your emotions, making you feel at fault for having a disease or failing to recover. This feeling of guilt may affect your loved ones also, causing them to pursue quack remedies as a cure. Finally, fraudulent promoters may try to generate anxiety to sell solutions to medical problems you do not really have.

One classic ploy used by purveyors of quackery is the testimonial. In fact, someone you know may even have tried a quack medicine and found it to work. However, this does not mean the medicine produced the "cure."

Many chronic or incurable diseases wax and wane. Symptoms sometimes will disappear, only to recur later. If you happen to be taking a quack medicine at a time when symptoms disappear, you may be led to believe that the quack remedy was the cause. Also, the placebo effect is a well-documented medical phenomenon. Placebos have no active ingredients, but if a person believes they do, scientists hypothesize that certain chemicals in the brain may be activated that actually cause symptoms to diminish. However, quack medical treatments can make for expensive placebos.

IDENTIFYING FRAUDULENT MEDICAL "CURES"

Identifying quack medicine is not always easy. Although most fraudulent promoters are simply looking for a quick buck or personal fame, some are sincere people who are misled. Some have fake degrees from mail-order "diploma mills." Others have actual degrees but are no longer following the high standards of their field or proclaim themselves to be "doctors"— even though their degrees are not in medicine but are in some other, often unrelated, field. Promoters often cloak their advertising in official-sounding, scientific language.

Some things to watch out for are promotions of medical treatments described with adjectives such as "secret," "proven," "miracle," "foreign," "breakthrough," and "overnight." Also beware of glowing testimonials from happy patients. Quacks tend to claim they are fighting against a conspiracy of established physicians who are unwilling to acknowledge new treatments. They claim their product provides a complete cure for various problems without any side effects.

Quacks also may promote a "holistic" approach that provides total health and emotional well-being, but they are vague as to what that means. Quacks often make the offer sound safe, with money-back guarantees. Finally, they often exert pressure, claiming that this is a "limited offer," available for only a short time. Medical quackery can range from black-and-white mail-order advertisements for "quick-loss" diets to sophisticated promotions seen on television.

THWARTING QUACKERY

Three federal institutions—the Food and Drug Administration, the Federal Trade Commission, and the US Postal Service (which can take action against anyone who uses the mail to promote fraud)—work to prevent quackery. However, the large volume of fraudulent promotions overwhelms the small enforcement staffs and limited budgets designated for fighting quackery. And it often takes a long time to stop a determined quack. In a classic case, it took the FDA 16 years of litigation to get the word "liver" removed from a product named Carter's Little Liver Pills.

The best ally you have in avoiding quackery, therefore, is yourself. If you are being pressured to spend money for a "quick cure," resist it. Beware of vague, dramatic claims. Find out exactly what the treatment is supposed to do and what evidence exists to prove it is effective. Ask your physician, pharmacist, or registered dietician for advice, and ask if your medical insurance will help pay for the treatment. Get other, independent opinions from local health organizations or consumer groups.

Finally, remember that if it sounds too good to be true, it probably is.

CHAPTER 40

THE MODERN PHARMACY

CHAPTER CONTENTS

MEDICATIONS AND YOU

The modern pharmacy does not offer magical cures for all or even most diseases and disorders. However, today's medicine chest does contain an ever-increasing variety of tablets, capsules, lozenges, syrups, suppositories, powders, topical solutions, creams, gels, and other preparations. Many of these medicaments do serve to relieve, calm, soothe, relax, and, yes, even help cure us of some of our aches, pains, and other complaints.

On average, seven prescriptions are filled annually for every man, woman, and child in the United States. Also, more than a half million over-the-counter products are now on the market. In fact, Americans annually spend more than *30 billion dollars* for medications and pharmaceutical products.

That is not to say, however, that all of these drugs are without risks. In fact, thousands of Americans are hospitalized each year because of inappropriate use of medicines. In some cases, the problem is the result of a drug sensitivity or allergy; in others, especially the elderly, the interaction of multiple drugs can lead to uncomfortable or dangerous side effects. In still other instances, the problem results from known and predictable side effects of certain drugs, but such side effects occur infrequently enough that the efficacy of the drug outweighs such potential dangers (see Adverse Drug Reactions, page 1230).

No matter what your age or condition, there are fundamental rules to follow when taking medications. Here are the rules.

Communicate with your physician about all aspects of your health. Whether your physician is treating you for a cold or for cancer, he or she needs to know your medical history. In particular, inform your physician about any chronic disease you have (especially heart disease, hypertension, or glaucoma), whether you are taking prescription medications, and whether you are allergic to certain drugs. In such instances, a prescription that for most people is entirely safe could be life-threatening.

Advise your physician of any over-the-counter (OTC) drugs you are taking, including laxatives or antacids; aspirin or acetaminophen; cough, cold, or hay fever medicines; or mineral or vitamin supplements. Nonprescription drugs can be potent, and some can cause serious reactions when mixed with prescription drugs. A proper dose of OTC drugs may be less than the amount recommended on the label, especially in elderly and very young people.

Tell your physician if you are or are planning to become pregnant. Numerous drugs can cross the placenta to your unborn fetus; some can result in birth defects. Your physician may change your medications if you are pregnant or breast-feeding to avoid affecting your fetus or child.

Tell your physician how much alcohol you consume. Be accurate: do not underestimate your consumption.

Follow the instructions you are given. If your prescription says "Take three times a day after meals," do not take it twice or four times a day.

Anyone who uses more than the recommended dosage is in danger of an overdose. The "more is better" theory does not apply to drugs. Avoid doubling the amount you take if you miss a dose.

Read the label carefully; follow the instructions there or those given by your physician. Make sure the instructions are clear. For example, if your prescription label directs you to take your medicine "four times a day," it could mean that you should take the medication with every meal and at bedtime. Or, it could mean that you should take it at precise 6-hour intervals around the clock. Ask your physician or pharmacist to clarify exactly when you are to take your medicine.

If the bottle says a liquid preparation is to be shaken before you take it, shake it. If you are to take a drug before, with, or after a meal, do as instructed. Failure to follow such instructions can result in unwanted side effects or inadequate concentrations of the drug in your body. Follow all instructions, not just those you find convenient.

Never increase the number of tablets or capsules you are taking without first consulting your physician; in the same way, do not stop taking a drug just because your symptoms seem to lessen. Take your medication for the entire length of time prescribed, even if symptoms for which you are using the drug have disappeared. Talk to your physician before discontinuing use of the drug.

If you are taking numerous medications on a daily basis, keep a record of what you take (see Keep a Medicine Calendar, page 1232).

Never take medications in the dark. This is a potentially dangerous practice. It can lead you to take the wrong medication or the wrong quantity. A missed dose of one drug or too much of another can be hazardous to your health.

Inform your physician of side effects. Discuss any side effects with your physician immediately. If the drug makes you feel ill, feverish, or nauseous or if you vomit after taking the drug, if you develop hives, if you experience headache or dizziness or have blurred vision or a ringing in your ears, if you become short of breath, or if you experience other symptoms after taking a drug, consult your physician immediately. It may be the wrong drug for you (see also Recognizing Side Effects, page 432).

Be familiar with the drugs you take. Remember names of medications you are taking. Read labels carefully. Ask your physician how the drug works. Make a special effort to understand your physician's explanation.

Ask your physician about potential side effects, about any dietary restrictions you should follow, whether you should avoid alcohol while taking the drug, or if there are other concerns of which you should be aware. If you get a renewal prescription and it is different from what you had been taking, ask why.

Have all prescriptions filled at one pharmacy. This can help you avoid problems of interactions. Your pharmacist is trained to know how drugs work and interact. In preparing, packaging, and recording each of the prescription drugs you purchase, your pharmacist can help monitor the mix of medications. He or she also can advise you when to take your medicines and how to take or use them properly. Your pharmacist also may alert you to possible side effects and tell you what to do in case of an adverse reaction.

Store and dispose of medications properly. Keep medicines out of the reach of children; do not save old medications past their point of usefulness (see Your Home Medicine Chest, page 1229).

Do not share prescription medications with others: the purpose of controlling the availability of prescription drugs is to ensure that appropriate medications are given to people who can tolerate, need, and will be helped by them. A well-intentioned friend or relative with leftover pills is a poor substitute for a physician who is familiar with your medical history and general health.

Avoid mixing drugs and alcohol. Use of many drugs along with alcohol can cause harmful interactions. In particular, sedatives and tranquilizers pose a danger. Discuss your consumption of alcohol with your physician. Ask whether there are risks of interactions with medicines prescribed for your use. (See also Dependence on Tranquilizers, page 436, and Dependence on Analgesics, page 436.)

Keep medicines in their original containers. Keep all medications in their original, labeled prescription containers. Never mix medications in the same container. Prescription vials are designed to protect medications from light and moisture. If you have a problem with the size of a container, ask your pharmacist to split the supply into multiple containers. If you have trouble opening a container with a safety cap, ask your pharmacist for a nonsafety cap for your medication.

Keep phone numbers handy. Keep the names of telephone numbers of your physician, pharmacist, nearest poison control center, and rescue squad on or near your phone.

DRUG CLASSIFICATIONS

Mastering the complexities of the modern pharmacy is not necessary or even plausible for the average consumer. However, a working familiarity with certain basic distinctions among and facts about the range of drugs you take can help you use today's medicines as safely and efficiently as possible.

Over-the Counter Versus Prescription Drugs. Over-the-counter (OTC) drugs are those you can purchase *without* a prescription. Examples are aspirin, many cough medicines and cold remedies, and innumerable other drugs offered to help you deal with ailments ranging from rashes to constipation to menstrual discomfort.

Prescription drugs are those that appear on government listings of controlled substances. They may be purchased only from a licensed pharmacy and require a prescription. They include a wide range of medications, from powerful painkillers to anticancer medications to familiar antibiotics such as penicillin.

Is It a Generic or a Brand Name Drug?
When a drug is discovered or produced in a laboratory, the name it is first given is its *generic* name, a name designated by a committee of drug experts and approved by governmental agencies. This name identifies the drug as unique and distinguishes it from all others. The generic name is not proprietary (that is, it is not owned by one company or individual).

When the drug is first allowed to be sold to the public, it is usually given another name, a *brand* name, by the original manufacturer. In general, the Food and Drug Administration (FDA) licenses a manufacturer to sell a given drug for a fixed period. During that time, the manufacturer owns the exclusive (proprietary) right to sell that medication and attempts to establish the drug in the marketplace under its own brand name.

Typically, the brand name of a drug is shorter and easier to pronounce and remember than the generic name. Examples are brand name drugs such as Librium (chlordiazepoxide), Tylenol (acetaminophen), Valium (diazepam), and Dilantin (phenytoin).

After the patent expires, the drug becomes public property. The initial manufacturer continues to own exclusive rights to the brand name it established, but other drug companies can manufacture and market the drug under its generic or their own brand name. Some drugs (for example tetracycline and prednisone) are sold primarily under generic names. More often, drugs are sold under both generic and various brand names.

One example is the pain reliever and anti-inflammatory agent acetaminophen: it is sold as a generic drug (acetaminophen) and under the brand names Tylenol, Anacin-3, Datril, and Panadol, among others. To complicate matters further, both generic and brand name drugs may be sold as combination drugs, in which two or more medications are blended and sold under brand or generic names.

The expiration of the proprietary license to manufacture a drug means that other makers can enter the marketplace, and, in many cases, the resulting competition lowers the price of the drug.

Price is usually the principal advantage of purchasing a generic rather than a brand name drug. However, critics of the pharmaceutical industry suggest that manufacturing standards for generic drugs are less than those of the brand name drugs originally produced.

Your physician, working with your pharmacist, is your best guide in selecting the right drug—and the right form (brand name or generic)—for your disorders. If cost is a concern and generic versions of a drug you are taking on a maintenance basis are available, discuss the matter with both your physician and your pharmacist.

In certain instances pharmacists may fill prescriptions with generic medicine instead of the brand name drug specified by the physician. If you or your physician wants to be sure the drug prescribed is a brand name product, be sure your physician includes the words "dispense as written" on the prescription form (or similar words depending on your state's regulations).

ADMINISTERING MEDICATION

Pills.   When you swallow a pill (whether it is a capsule, tablet, caplet, or some other form), it travels down your esophagus to your stomach and, eventually, to your intestines, where the medication is absorbed by your bloodstream and distributed throughout your body. That is the route it is supposed to take.

Studies have found, however, that pills often stick to the inner lining of the esophagus (the muscular tube that carries liquids and foods from your throat to your stomach). If the medication dissolves there, it can cause irritation, sometimes leading to vomiting or chest pains.

Here are ways to help ensure that your pills make it to their destination.

• Drink at least half a glass of water when taking a pill. Sip a little water first to lubricate your esophagus. Swallow the pill with a mouthful of water; then drink the rest to wash the medication down.

- Stand up or sit up straight when taking a pill. Remain upright for at least a minute and a half after you swallow it.
- Consider an alternative form of your medicine. If you have problems swallowing medications, consult your physician or pharmacist. Your medication may be available in a form that is easier to swallow, such as a liquid.
- If a pill sticks in your esophagus, eat a bulky food such as a banana. The bulk of the banana passing down your esophagus may carry the pill with it.

Other Medications. Other forms of delivery also can be difficult. Use the following techniques to simplify self-administration of ointments, drops, suppositories, and douches.

Eye Ointment. Wash your hands first—always. Then lie down or sit with your head tilted back. Draw the lower eyelid down, look upward, and place approximately a half-inch bead of the ointment along the inside margin of your eyelid. Do not touch your eye or eyelid with the tube. Close your eye, then gently remove any excess ointment from your eyelashes with a tissue.

YOUR HOME MEDICINE CHEST

Having a designated area—whether it is over the bathroom sink, beside your bed, or a corner of a kitchen cupboard—can help you keep medications you need to take organized and easy to find. A medicine chest also can help keep your medicines safely out of the reach of children.

Where Should It Be?
Most bathrooms have built-in medicine cabinets; yet bathing and showering areas, because of humidity produced by hot water, are less-than-perfect locations for storing drugs. Your refrigerator is also an inappropriate storage area for most drugs. The best place is a locked cabinet in your bedroom.

Be Concerned for Children
Regardless of location, your medicine cabinet should keep prescription and nonprescription drugs safely away from the reach of children. Even if visits from youngsters are rare, take care to keep drugs out of their reach. Also, buy childproof packages, especially if

you have young children, grandchildren, or very young guests.

Be especially careful to properly store medications you take daily. Never take storage for granted. Remember that it is easy to absentmindedly leave medications on a kitchen counter or bedside table where a toddler may find their bright colors irresistible. If you have drugs that must be refrigerated, put them on a high shelf that is well out of the reach of children.

Discard Outdated Drugs
Flush unused, outdated prescription drugs down the toilet. Medicine deteriorates over time. If you develop the same health problem you had several years ago, do not resume taking leftover medicine. Instead, consult your physician and get a new prescription.

Keep medicines in their original containers, otherwise you or members of your family may get confused. Taking the wrong medicines or inappropriate combinations of medicines can be dangerous. If the label gets separated from a medicine container and there is any doubt as to its contents, discard the medicine immediately.

What Should It Contain?
In addition to whatever prescription or over-the-counter drugs your physician recommends for your use, there are other key items a well-equipped household should have on hand, such as the following.

Pain relievers: aspirin or, for children, aspirin substitutes such as acetaminophen.

Ipecac: a liquid used to promote vomiting and used in certain kinds of poisoning emergencies (see Handling Poisoning Emergencies, page 299).

Bandages: adhesive strip bandages, adhesive tape and sterile gauze pads, elastic bandages, and surgical bandages (Steri-Strips).

Tools, including scissors to cut bandages and tweezers to remove splinters.

A thermometer (include a rectal-type thermometer if you have an infant).

Absorbent cotton and rubbing alcohol.

Over-the-counter pharmaceuticals, including antidiarrheal medication, insect repellant, antacids, cough syrup, calamine or other mild lotion for itching, a sunscreen to prevent sunburn, and skin creams or lotions to treat sunburn.

Eye Drops.   Position yourself in the same way as for administering eye ointment. Have clean hands, tilt your head back, draw the lower eyelid down, and look upward. Place the drops behind your lower eyelid. Avoid putting drops directly on the cornea, and do not touch the dropper itself to your eye. Close your eye, then gently remove any excess solution from the eyelashes or lid with a tissue.

Nose Drops.   Lie down or sit with your head tilted back. Check the tip of the dropper to be sure it is not chipped or cracked. Breathing through your mouth, place the prescribed number of drops in your nose. Do not touch the sides of your nasal openings with the dropper. Remain reclined or seated with your head tilted for several minutes so the medication can spread through your nasal cavity.

Ear Drops.   Check the tip of the dropper to be sure it is not chipped or cracked. Tilt your head so that the affected ear is angled upward. Straighten the ear canal to receive the medicine by drawing your earlobe down and back. Then deliver the prescribed number of drops into your ear, avoiding touching your ear canal with the dropper.

Suppositories.   For a rectal suppository, wear rubber gloves. If you have hemorrhoids, coat the suppository well with petroleum jelly. Lie on your side and insert the suppository, pointed end first, high into the rectum. Push the bottom of the suppository sideways to be sure that some portion of it touches the bowel wall. If you have trouble retaining the suppository, you may not have inserted it high enough. You also may find it helpful to hold your buttocks together for a short while after inserting the suppository.

Douches.   Use a thoroughly cleaned and rinsed syringe (unless the douche is of the disposable type, in which case use each fresh syringe and bag only once). Using slightly warm or tepid water, fill the bag with the solution. Administer the douche while lying or sitting. If lying, draw your knees up and raise your hips. Insert the syringe into the vagina. After douching, cleanse or dispose of the douching equipment.

ADVERSE DRUG REACTIONS

Pharmacokinetics is the study of how drugs work in the body. This relatively new medical discipline examines, among other things, the time required for drugs to be absorbed, how they are distributed in the body, how long they remain effective, and how they are eliminated from your body.

Through the study of pharmacokinetics, we are coming to understand more about the interactions that determine specific drug effects and the individual diversity of different drug responses. We also are learning that virtually no drug is entirely without side effects in all individuals.

Some adverse drug reactions are the result of overdose: intentionally or accidentally, people take too much of a drug and their systems react. Some are the result of kidney or liver disease, which makes individuals more susceptible to certain kinds of drug toxicity.

Depending on several factors, including your body weight, health, and age, most drugs on the market are safe and are associated with only minor or rare potential complications. When prescribing a drug for your use, your physician may alert you to possible side effects. Your pharmacist, too, may brief you on how to take the drug and also about its risks. In the case of over-the-counter drugs, the packaging in which the medications are sold frequently offers warnings regarding side effects.

In the case of many prescription drugs, a complete list of potential side effects can be frightening. However, few drugs on the market today produce significant side effects in more than a small fraction of persons who take them. Elderly people are more likely to experience side effects (see Drugs in the Elderly, page 434).

Among the serious potential side effects are drug allergies, anaphylactic reactions, and the complications of multiple drug use.

Drug Allergy.   Allergic reactions to most drugs are uncommon, but they do occur occasionally. Sometimes the potentially toxic effects of an uncharacteristic reaction are mistaken for a drug allergy.

Follow your physician's directions carefully when taking a medication. If unusual symptoms develop, consult your physician immediately.

Some of us process (metabolize) drugs in an unusual manner. Again, if unusual symptoms occur after you take a drug, consult your physician.

Rash is the most common allergic drug reaction. More serious reactions may include wheezing and difficulty in breathing, an itching sensation over your entire body, and even shock (see Shock, page 303).

Penicillin and related drugs are responsible for many allergic reactions to drugs. The reactions range from mild rashes to hives to immediate anaphylaxis (see below). Most people who develop reactions have minor rashes, and only those who are extremely sensitive have the strong reaction of anaphylaxis.

Among the other drugs that can cause allergic reactions are antibiotics such as sulfas, barbiturates, anticonvulsants, insulin, and local anesthetics. In addition, contrast dyes injected into blood vessels to help outline major organs in x-ray studies contain iodine, which in some people is an allergen (the substance that stimulates an allergic reaction). Aspirin produces hives in many sensitive people.

If you know you are allergic to certain drugs—avoid them. This means alerting your physician or dentist to your sensitivity before treatment. People sensitive to aspirin should avoid all aspirin-containing drugs.

Wear a medical alert necklace or bracelet indicating your allergy, or carry a card that provides this information (see also Drug Allergies, page 471).

Anaphylaxis. Anaphylaxis is the most dangerous of allergic responses; it is also the least common.

The anaphylactic reaction is not limited to the site of the irritation. A mild reaction may cause only generalized hives and intense itching, but a severe reaction is life-threatening. The most characteristic symptom is a constriction of the passageways in the bronchial tract or throat or both and an accompanying difficulty in breathing.

Shock—a sudden drop of blood pressure that causes rapid pulse, weakness, paleness, mental confusion, nausea and vomiting, unconsciousness, and cardiovascular collapse—also may occur. Shock can cause death if not treated immediately.

In sensitive people, drugs such as penicillin, aspirin, insulin, and the contrast injection agents used in some x-ray studies can result in anaphylaxis in a matter of minutes or even seconds.

The standard treatment for anaphylaxis is an injection of epinephrine (adrenaline), which opens the airways and blood vessels. Cardiopulmonary resuscitation (CPR) and emergency tracheostomy (making an opening in the windpipe) sometimes have to be performed as lifesaving measures (see Anaphylaxis, page 307, and Cardiopulmonary Resuscitation, page 270.)

The Hazards of Multiple-Drug Use. A drug that is entirely safe when taken on its own can become a health hazard if taken in combination with another drug or several other drugs. Such pharmaceutical interactions are sometimes also called problems of polypharmacy.

As you age, changes occur in your body that put you at greater risk for problems with medication. For example, the proportion of your body that is made up of water and lean muscle tissue decreases while the percentage of fat increases. Therefore, drugs that your body stores in fat tissue (called fat-soluble drugs) can accumulate to higher levels as you grow older. Also, as you age your liver and kidneys become less efficient at breaking down and eliminating drugs, so medications remain in your body longer. Buildups of drugs can result, with potentially dangerous side effects.

If you have several illnesses, each new symptom may result in a visit to your physician—and a new prescription. Too often, physicians give prescriptions without regard to medicines already being consumed. Beware of this.

Do not expect a medicine for every new symptom. Sometimes a symptom can be eliminated simply by reducing the dosage of another drug or by reorganizing the sequence in which you take medications.

With multiple drug use, it is hardly surprising that people often become confused and take too little or too much of one or more drugs, or experience unwanted side effects from drug interactions.

You may need assistance in following drug therapies, especially if you have multiple diseases that require the correct use of several medicines each day.

Review the schedule of all of your medicines with your physician on every visit, particularly if a new medicine is added, to determine whether the schedule can be simplified (see Keep a Medicine Calendar, below).

FOOD AND DRUG INTERACTIONS

The drugs you take and the foods you eat are both processed and absorbed by your stomach and intestines. Thus, it should come as no surprise that certain foods and certain drugs, when taken in combination, can have results that differ from results you might experience if you were to consume the same substances on separate occasions.

Sometimes a combination can be beneficial. At other times, the interactions can be dangerous. In any case, your physician and pharmacist should anticipate such potential problems and give you specific instructions on how and when to take your drugs.

A few general guidelines and explanations also may help.

- Follow all instructions. Listen to your physician or pharmacist. Read the label too. If the instructions are to take your medication with a meal, do so.
- Drink at least half a glass of water when taking a medication. This helps ensure that the pill goes down. It also can aid absorption and may eliminate or decrease potential stomach irritation.
- Instructions to take a drug on an empty stomach mean you should take it at least 1 hour before or 2 to 3 hours after eating.
- In the absence of other instructions, take the drug at a time when you are most likely to remember to take it.
- Take the drug at the same time each day. If you vary your routine from one day to the next, the effects of the medication can change.
- Do not drink tea, coffee, or other hot beverages with your medications. Hot temperatures destroy the effectiveness of many drugs.
- Beware of alcohol interactions: if the medication is labeled (or your physician warns you) "Do not take with alcohol"— then do not. Alcohol has potentially lethal interactions when taken with certain prescription medications, but even some over-the-counter medications can make you especially drowsy when combined with alcoholic beverages.
- Never play pharmacist. Do not open, crush, or dissolve tablets or capsules without checking first with your physician or pharmacist. If you find a particular drug difficult to take because of a disagreeable taste, mix it with juice or applesauce—but do not mix more than one dose at a time—and take all of it immediately. If the drug/food mixture is left around, someone else might take it.

KEEP A MEDICINE CALENDAR

Ask your primary-care physician to help you work out a medicine calendar. This is a master schedule of drugs you take and when they are to be taken.

When you visit your physician, take along all medicines you currently are using. This might include medicines prescribed by other physicians and over-the-counter medications you take for minor ailments (such as antacids; constipation remedies; cough syrups, hay fever, cold, and cough remedies; and even mineral and vitamin supplements).

Together with your physician, work out your medicine calendar by identifying each drug and assigning regular consumption times and dosages for each.

The effort required in preparing your calendar will help make your physician more aware of the drugs you take and may eliminate unnecessary drugs or reduce the frequency or dosage of others. As a result, you are less likely to experience unwanted drug interactions.

Your physician also may be able to simplify the drug-taking process: certain medicines can be taken together, perhaps just before or after meals. By consolidating and organizing the ritual of taking your medicines, your physician may help you avoid missing dosages and taking the drugs at times of the day when they are less likely to be effective.

THE DRUG INDEX

Here are some of the categories into which most of the commonly prescribed medications are divided. Use this index in conjunction with the Drug Directory (see page 1299) to identify the nature and function of drugs you are taking.

Amphetamine-like drugs: drugs that act like amphetamines. These mood-elevating drugs work on chemical messengers (neurotransmitters) in the brain. Most often they are used as antidepressants or appetite suppressants.

Anabolic steroids: drugs closely related to natural hormones of the male and that mimic their effects. These drugs are used in treating various skeletal and growth disorders and certain types of anemia. Athletes sometimes use anabolic steroids to build up body tissue—a practice that is unhealthy, unwise, and illegal.

Analgesics: pain-relieving drugs. These drugs are generally divided into two categories: narcotic and nonnarcotic pain-relieving drugs.

Narcotic analgesics, most of which are derived from opium, are used for relief of severe pain. Nonnarcotic analgesics are used to relieve mild pain. Some also reduce inflammation. See Anti-inflammatory agents.

Androgens: hormones that stimulate the production of male sexual characteristics.

Angiotensin-converting enzyme inhibitors: drugs that block the formation of a natural body chemical and dilate small arteries, thereby reducing blood pressure.

Antacids: drugs used for relief of symptoms of indigestion or disorders caused by excess acid. These medications work by neutralizing stomach acids.

Antiacne agents: drugs used in the treatment of acne.

Antialcoholic drugs: drugs used in the treatment of alcoholism. When alcohol is consumed in conjunction with antialcoholic drugs such as disulfiram, the result is flushing, headache, chest pain, nausea, weakness, and repeated vomiting.

Antianxiety agents: also called anxiolytics, sedatives, or tranquilizers, these drugs relax muscles, reduce tension, and may be used to treat insomnia. Two families of antianxiety drugs are some of the barbiturates and the benzodiazepines.

Antiarrhythmics: medications used to control unwanted variations in heart rhythms. Digitalis is one antiarrhythmic drug; certain recent varieties are classified as beta-adrenergic blockers or calcium channel blocking drugs. See Calcium channel blockers.

Antiasthmatics: drugs used in the treatment of asthma. These medications work by dilating (expanding) airways in the lungs.

Antibacterials: see Antibiotics.

Antibiotics: drugs used to fight bacterial infection. Penicillin is a naturally occurring variety, but synthetic antibiotics include cephalosporins.

Anticancer drugs: see Cytotoxic drugs.

Anticoagulants: drugs prescribed to prevent blood from clotting. One variety, the thrombolytics, often is used in emergency cases to dissolve clots that are producing heart attack. They commonly are called blood thinners.

Anticonvulsants: drugs used to prevent seizures.

Antidepressants: mood-lifting drugs. This category of drugs is generally divided into two kinds: tricyclics and monoamine oxidase inhibitors (MAOIs).

Antidiabetic agents: drugs used in the treatment of diabetes. Antidiabetic drugs are used to restore the body's ability to use sugar normally. Insulin is one variety; it usually is used in people whose bodies produce little or no natural insulin. Insulin is administered by subcutaneous injections. Other antidiabetic drugs, called hypoglycemic drugs, are given orally.

Antidiarrheals: drugs used to relieve diarrhea.

Antiemetics: medications used to treat nausea and vomiting.

Antiepileptics: see Anticonvulsants.

Antifungals: drugs used to treat infections caused by fungi.

Antiglaucoma agents: medications used to treat glaucoma. These drugs act to reduce pressure in the eye.

Antihistamines: drugs used to treat allergies, asthma, nausea, motion sickness, nasal congestion, coughing, and itching. Antihistamines work to prevent the secretion of histamine, which contributes to these symptoms.

Antihypertensives: medications prescribed to reduce high blood pressure (hypertension). Antihypertensives also are classified as belonging to one of several drug families according to the way they work. The subdivisions include drugs that increase the rate at which your body eliminates urine and salt (see Diuretics), drugs that block many of the effects of epinephrine (adrenaline) in your body (see Beta-adrenergic blockers), drugs that block the entry of calcium into the walls of your small arteries (see Calcium channel blockers), and drugs that block formation of a natural body chemical and dilate small arteries (see Angiotensin-converting enzyme inhibitors). The calcium channel blockers and the angiotensin-converting enzyme inhibitors both cause the walls of your small arteries to dilate.

Anti-infectives: drugs used to fight infection. These drugs are used to combat bacterial, yeast, or other infections of the urinary tract, vagina, and gastrointestinal tract.

Anti-inflammatory agents: drugs used to reduce inflammation. Inflammation results in an increased blood flow, which in turn produces swelling, redness, pain, and heat. One of the body's defense mechanisms, inflammation occurs in response to infection and certain chronic diseases such as rheumatoid arthritis. Aspirin and corticosteroids are anti-inflammatory drugs.

Anti-itching drugs: drugs used to reduce itching.

Antimicrobials: non-antibiotic drugs used to treat infections of the body, especially of the gastrointestinal tract, by microbes (germs).

Antiparkinsonians: drugs used to treat the trembling, rigidity, or other symptoms of Parkinson's disease.

Antipruritics: see Anti-itching drugs.

Antipsychotic agents: drugs used to treat a type of psychiatric disorder.

Antipyretics: fever-reducing drugs. These drugs, including aspirin and acetaminophen, directly affect the temperature-regulating center in the brain, the hypothalamus.

Antispasmodics: drugs used to relieve involuntary muscle spasms such as may occur in the gastrointestinal tract or urinary bladder.

Antivirals: drugs used to treat viral infections.

Anxiolytics: see Antianxiety agents.

Appetite suppressants: diet medications, used for short periods to help treat obesity.

Barbiturates: see Antianxiety agents.

Benzodiazepines: see Antianxiety agents.

Beta-adrenergic blockers: also known as beta blockers, these are heart drugs. They work by blocking the stimulating effect of epinephrine (adrenaline) on your heart, thereby reducing heartbeat and decreasing oxygen requirements. They also are effective for reducing blood pressure.

Bronchodilators: drugs that open (dilate) main airways (bronchi) in your lungs. They are used to treat asthma and certain allergies.

Calcium channel blockers: also known as calcium blockers, these are heart drugs. They function by blocking entry of the mineral calcium into your cells, reducing the tendency of your small arteries to narrow (vasoconstriction). They also are effective for reducing blood pressure.

Carbonic anhydrase inhibitors: see Antiglaucoma agents.

Chelating drugs: drugs that bind to unwanted metals in your body and carry them out through the urine. They commonly are used to treat lead poisoning.

Cholesterol-reducing agents: drugs used to lower blood cholesterol concentrations in people with atherosclerosis.

Corticosteroids: used principally as anti-inflammatory drugs (see Anti-inflammatory agents). Various corticosteroid drugs are used to treat arthritis, bursitis, certain skin diseases, adrenal gland insufficiency, thyroiditis, some cancers, and other disorders.

Cough suppressants: often called antitussives. They are used to suppress coughs.

Cytotoxic drugs: anticancer drugs. They are a broad category of drugs used to treat various cancers by different means.

Decongestants: drugs used to relieve nasal congestion. They work by constricting blood vessels in your nose, which serves to reduce swelling. They are used to treat sinusitis, allergies, and acute upper respiratory infections.

Digitalis preparations: heart drugs. They are used to treat heart failure by stimulating the heart to increase the force of its contractions. They also are effective for treating atrial fibrillation, a heart rhythm abnormality.

Diuretics: also called water pills, these drugs increase the volume of urine and salt released by the kidneys. Most often, diuretics are used to treat hypertension and congestive heart failure.

Estrogen hormones: female sex hormones that stimulate and maintain female sex characteristics. They are either natural or synthetic. Estrogens are used to treat menstrual and menopausal disorders and also are used as oral contraceptives.

Expectorants: drugs that stimulate the expulsion of mucus or phlegm from the lungs or throat. They often are one of several ingredients in cough medications.

Fever-reducing drugs: see Antipyretics.

Gout medications: drugs used to treat gouty arthritis. Varying types of gout drugs work to decrease the amount of uric acid in the body, either by limiting its production or by promoting its excretion.

H₂ blockers: see Histamine blockers.

Heart rhythm regulators: see Antiarrhythmics.

Histamine blockers: drugs used to treat ulcers and related disorders in which there is excess stomach acid. These medications work to inhibit the secretion of gastric acid.

Hypnotics: sleeping medications. Barbiturates and benzodiazepines are the two most common types of hypnotic drugs.

Hypoglycemics: see Antidiabetic agents.

Immunosuppressants: drugs that impair the workings of the body's immune system. They are used to treat disorders such as rheumatoid arthritis, ulcerative colitis, and some cancers and to prevent the body's rejection of transplanted organs.

Laxatives: constipation drugs. A range of laxatives are available that work to increase the action (motility) of the intestines or to stimulate the addition of water to the stool to increase its bulk and ease of passage.

Male sex hormones: see Androgens.

Monoamine oxidase inhibitors (MAOIs): see Antidepressants.

Muscle relaxants: drugs used to relax muscles. They are used to treat muscle spasms associated with injury of muscles, bones, and joints.

Nitrates: heart drugs. They often are used in patients with angina.

Nonsteroidal anti-inflammatory drugs (NSAIDs): see Analgesics and Anti-inflammatory agents.

Penicillin: see Antibiotics.

Phenothiazines: drugs used for their antipsychotic effect. Occasionally they are used to control vomiting.

Salicylates: see Analgesics and Anti-inflammatory agents.

Sedatives: see Antianxiety agents and Hypnotics.

Sulfa drugs: see Antibiotics.

Tetracyclines: see Antibiotics.

Thrombolytics: see Anticoagulants.

Tranquilizers: see Antianxiety agents and Antipsychotics.

Vasodilators: heart drugs. These medications stimulate the arteries of the heart to enlarge (dilate). They often are used to treat angina pectoris.

Xanthines: drugs used to dilate bronchial passageways.

CHAPTER 41
CANCER

UNDERSTANDING CANCER

We often refer to cancer with universal dread—yet, more than 3 million Americans who were found to have cancer 5 or more years ago are alive today. Most of these 3 million can be considered cured; others still may have evidence of cancer. Clearly, a diagnosis of cancer is not a certain death sentence.

Another common misunderstanding is that cancer is a single deadly disease. In fact, there are more than 100 different types of cancer. Some cancers can affect just one organ, and others are more generalized. In each of its types, however, cancer always consists of an uncontrollable growth and spread of abnormal cells.

Many people have a morbid fear of cancer, perhaps because to them it is an incurable, wasting disease. The facts do not support this idea. About 4 of every 10 people who are found to have cancer this year will be cured (cured is defined as being free of any evidence of the disease for 5 years or more). These cured individuals will have the same life expectancy as others of the same age and sex who have never had cancer.

Despite such impressive statistics, cancer remains a serious disease. Annually, more than 1 million persons are given a diagnosis of cancer (this excludes non-melanoma skin cancer). Cancer causes about 500,000 deaths each year, and nearly one of every three persons alive in this country today will have cancer at some time in the future.

Why cancer develops in some people who are exposed to potentially cancer-causing agents but not in others is not fully known. But we do know that most cancers develop slowly. It may be 5 to 40 years after exposure to a cancer-causing agent before there is any evidence of the disease. Cancer of the lung, for example, may not appear until 25 years or more after sustained exposure to tobacco smoke. This long delay between exposure and development of the disease may partly explain why so many people ignore the warnings associated with smoking (see Tobacco, page 407).

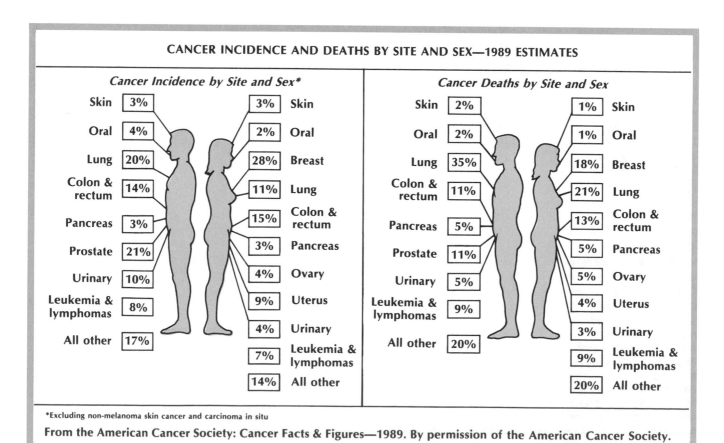

CANCER INCIDENCE AND DEATHS BY SITE AND SEX—1989 ESTIMATES

Cancer Incidence by Site and Sex*

Male			Female	
Skin	3%		3%	Skin
Oral	4%		2%	Oral
Lung	20%		28%	Breast
Colon & rectum	14%		11%	Lung
Pancreas	3%		15%	Colon & rectum
Prostate	21%		3%	Pancreas
Urinary	10%		4%	Ovary
Leukemia & lymphomas	8%		9%	Uterus
All other	17%		4%	Urinary
			7%	Leukemia & lymphomas
			14%	All other

Cancer Deaths by Site and Sex

Male			Female	
Skin	2%		1%	Skin
Oral	2%		1%	Oral
Lung	35%		18%	Breast
Colon & rectum	11%		21%	Lung
Pancreas	5%		13%	Colon & rectum
Prostate	11%		5%	Pancreas
Urinary	5%		5%	Ovary
Leukemia & lymphomas	9%		4%	Uterus
All other	20%		3%	Urinary
			9%	Leukemia & lymphomas
			20%	All other

*Excluding non-melanoma skin cancer and carcinoma in situ

From the American Cancer Society: Cancer Facts & Figures—1989. By permission of the American Cancer Society.

THE BIOLOGY OF CANCER

Your body is a living, growing system that contains billions of cells. These cells carry out all of your body's functions, such as metabolism, transportation, excretion, reproduction, and locomotion.

Growth and development are the result of increases in numbers of new cells and their changes into different types of tissue. New cells are created through the process of cell division (mitosis). Different types of cells are created by an accompanying process called cell differentiation (differentiation is the process by which cells acquire a specialized function). Cell division results in the normal pattern of human growth; cell differentiation makes possible the normal pattern of development.

The biology of cancer and cancer cells is different, however, and the distinctions are important to understanding cancer.

Basically, there are three types of cells in our bodies: static cells (differentiated cells), expanding cells (undifferentiated cells), and renewing cells (also called stem cells, they give rise to other kinds of cells). For example, the cells of muscle and nerve tissue are static (differentiated) because after they reach a specific size they lose their ability to divide and produce new cells. These cells are said to be highly differentiated and cannot be replaced if damaged or lost because they can no longer reproduce.

The expanding cells (undifferentiated cells) of the body also stop growing when the organ or tissue reaches its normal adult size. But the key difference between static and expanding cells is that, if the tissue is damaged or a portion of it is removed, the expanding cell can "switch on" and grow again. The liver, kidney, and hormone-secreting glands are examples of organs that contain these types of cells. If any part of these organs is damaged through illness or is removed surgically, the remaining cells can divide and grow until the organ is restored to normal or nearly normal function.

The renewing (stem) cells die and are replaced at regular intervals. For example, the cells that make up your skin, hair, the lining of your intestinal tract, and your blood all are constantly being replaced as they become old and die, either through normal processes or through injury or disease.

These renewing cells are controlled by an internal mechanism that maintains a balance between cells that are dying and new cells that are developing to replace them.

The ability of renewing cells to obey signals to stop growing distinguishes their rapid growth from the uncontrolled growth of cancer cells. Unlike other cell types, cancer cells lack the control mechanism that switches off growth in normal cells.

Cancer cells are similar in a way to uncontrolled stem cells. They can be differentiated or undifferentiated—but they continue to divide without restraint. They displace their neighbor cells by crowding them out. The growth of cancer cells also affects the function and growth of normal cells by competing with them for available nutrients.

Contrary to popular belief, cancer cells do not grow faster than normal cells. However, they live longer and divide more times, thus creating a greater proportion of cancer cells in the growth process.

Not all cells that are unable to regulate their growth and maturation are cancer cells. Some cells may divide rapidly and grow into masses called tumors but they are benign because they lack other characteristics of malignancy.

What produces cancer cells? Studies suggest that many cancers are associated with a rearrangement in the chromosomes in the cell. Current research in the fundamental biological steps that cause cancers is now beginning to explain how a normal cell can be transformed into a cancer cell.

Genes are segments of large molecules known as deoxyribonucleic acid (DNA) which are essentially chemical "blueprints" that are the basis of heredity. Genes are located in the nucleus of every cell. The sequence of chemical components in your genes is the blueprint—the genetic information—for the manufacture of the proteins that control how your body cells work. These genes make each of us unique.

Oncogenes (*oncos* from the Greek for mass or tumor) are special kinds of genes that may cause cells to divide abnormally. The normal form of an oncogene (called a proto-oncogene) is part of our normal complement of genes. The proto-oncogenes are present in all of our cells. In normal cells, the

CANCER WARNING SIGNS

According to the American Cancer Society, if you have any of these seven warning signs, *consult your physician immediately.*

Change in bowel or bladder habits

Sore that does not heal

Unusual bleeding or discharge

Thickening or lump in a breast or elsewhere in your body

Indigestion or swallowing difficulty

Obvious change in a wart or mole

Nagging cough or hoarseness

---

proto-oncogene can be changed to a cancer-causing gene (oncogene) by a process genetic specialists call point mutation. By this, we mean that some cancers develop at the point where one of the components of the gene is changed or mutated. This change occurs to a component that regulates the effects of the oncogene. In other cancer cells, proto-oncogenes may be moved from their normal place in the DNA to another site and are thus changed to cancer-causing (oncogenic) genes. In addition, some infectious cancer-inducing viruses can inject their own oncogenes into normal cells. The new oncogenes inserted by viruses seem not to be regulated (controlled) by normal cell processes. The cells thus lose their ability to control their activity and they divide abnormally.

proto-oncogenes appear to be under strict control as they regulate cell division and cell differentiation. They also seem to control the growth of cells required to repair injured body tissue, such as after surgery. In addition, they play a role in organ development.

The strict control of proto-oncogene function in normal cells can be impaired by agents that induce cancer. For example, a

In all instances, the proteins made under direction by the oncogenes are produced in vastly larger amounts. Ultimately, these proteins cause the cell to grow abnormally and cause cancer.

CANCER PREVENTION

There are no guarantees—yet taking some precautions to avoid cancer risk factors makes good sense. Try to follow these guidelines.

Tobacco Use
In a word, *don't.* Smoking is responsible for more than four of every five deaths from lung cancer and for about 30 percent of all cancer deaths (see Tobacco, page 407). Use of smokeless tobacco puts you at increased risk of cancer of the mouth, larynx, throat, or esophagus (see the Risks of Chewing Tobacco, page 410).

Sun Exposure
Recent research points to the sun as the chief villain in almost all of the half-million annual cases of non-melanoma skin cancer. Limit your exposure to the sun, especially if you are light-skinned. Use a sun blocker, too (see How To Avoid Sunburn, page 1165).

Alcohol
Be reasonable in your consumption of alcohol. Heavy drinkers are at increased risk of oral cancer and cancers of the larynx, throat, esophagus, or liver (see Alcohol Abuse, page 417).

Menopause Treatments
The use of estrogen by mature women for treating the symptoms of menopause poses certain risks for endometrial cancer. Weigh carefully the benefits and risks of estrogen replacement therapy in discussing its use with your physician (see Menopause, page 1067).

Radiation Exposure
Excessive exposure to ionizing (x-ray) radiation poses an increased risk of cancer (see Radiation and Your Health, page 333). There may be a potential risk with radon in the home (see The Radon Risk, page 335). Most medical x-rays are adjusted to deliver the lowest dose possible without sacrificing the quality of the image and without subjecting you to excess radiation.

Industrial Exposure
Exposure to nickel, chromate, asbestos, vinyl chloride, and certain other industrial agents increases the risk of certain cancers.

Nutrition
What you eat may have an effect on your cancer risk. Diets high in fats or salt-cured, smoked, or nitrite-cured foods may be potentially hazardous; on the other hand, foods rich in vitamins A and C or high in fiber may help lower your risk for certain cancers (see Diet and Cancer Protection, page 369).

Oncogenes and their protein products comprise, however, only one of a series of abnormalities that must occur for a cell to become malignant. Our understanding of the workings of most cancer cells and our ability to interrupt their reproduction are, at best, primitive. However, research is advancing our knowledge of cancer and its workings—at the same time that a wide range of both proven and experimental approaches to treating cancer in its many guises are saving innumerable lives.

CANCER DIAGNOSIS

The best diagnosis of cancer is an early diagnosis. The earlier the cancer is detected, the greater the chances it can be treated before it spreads to other tissue or organs in the body. With the cancer screening procedures available today, many cancers can now be detected early enough to be cured.

Every diagnosis of cancer attempts to identify the type and location of the cancer. Each type of cancer has its own characteristic rate of growth, tendency to spread, and particular set of target tissues or organs to which it is likely to spread. Identifying the kind of cancer enables your physician to anticipate how it is likely to behave and to plan appropriate treatment procedures. The diagnosis also involves determining the extent to which the cancer has already spread (staging). Finally, your physician needs to assess how the malignancy may have affected or will affect your health.

Among others things, these determinations will guide your physician as to the type of treatment suited to your cancer. You should not be alarmed if the diagnosis and staging of the disease require several days or weeks. An accurate diagnosis, on which your entire therapy program will be based, usually requires laboratory study of a tissue sample (biopsy), x-rays, and other laboratory procedures.

CANCER SCREENING

Screening tests vary in complexity and cost. Most of the widely used tests are designed to discover common forms of cancer in persons at highest risk.

Cancer screening tests must be practical. This means that the test should detect the cancer early enough that the chances for a full recovery are still high.

Safety is also important. The test itself should not pose a dangerous health hazard. Twenty years ago, the mammography procedure used to detect breast cancer had a relatively high radiation exposure and itself may have been a factor in cancer development. Today, however, mammography exposes women to only small amounts of radiation so the examination is much safer.

Periodic screening tests for cancer do not have the same preventive value in all cases and all types of cancer. With lung cancer, for example, frequent x-rays of the chest or analysis of sputum will not significantly improve your chances of surviving a bout with lung cancer, especially if you smoke. Although early detection is important, the survival rate with lung cancer is still less than 15 percent. Consequently, if you smoke or are exposed to chemicals in your home or work environment, see your physician about the advisability of screening for lung cancer. But even more crucial than watching for indications of the disease is exercising all options available to you that will reduce your exposure to the potential carcinogens. Quitting smoking is one such strategy.

Other cancers can be detected early enough that survival rates significantly improve. The following cancer screening tests are part of a cancer prevention program recommended by the American Cancer Society.

Breast Cancer

Warning signs: Any lump or thickening in the breast or bleeding or discharge from the nipple.

Cancer risk factors: Breast cancer most often occurs in women over age 50; in women who have never had children, had their first child after age 30, have never breast-fed, are more than 40 percent over their ideal weight, or who reached sexual maturity late or had a late menopause; and in women from families in which there is a history of premenopausal breast cancer in mother or sisters.

Checkup guidelines: Every woman should examine her breasts carefully and expertly once a month (see Breast Self-Examination, page 1076).

In addition, women between the ages of 20 and 40 should have their breasts examined by a physician every 3 years; women over the age of 40 should have this examination every year. If you are less than 40 years old, you probably do not need a mammogram unless you are in a high-risk group such as having a family history of breast cancer. If you are between 40 and 49 years of age, have no symptoms or lumps, and have no family history of breast cancer, have a baseline mammogram (see page 1080). After age 50, have a mammogram annually. If you have a family history of breast cancer, have a mammogram annually regardless of your age.

Testicular Cancer

Warning signs: Any lump on the testicle or change in its size.

Cancer risk factors: Strikes younger men more often than older men (uncommon after age 40); undescended testes (see page 1118).

Checkup guidelines: Men of all ages, starting in late teenage years, should examine their testes monthly (see Self-Examination of the Testicles, page 1116).

Colorectal Cancer

Warning signs: Any rectal bleeding or long-term change in your bowel habits.

Cancer risk factors: History of colorectal polyps (see page 635) or of colorectal cancer in a family member or chronic ulcerative colitis (see page 639).

Checkup guidelines: Men and women over age 40 should have a digital rectal examination annually. Moreover, men and women over age 50 should have a sigmoidoscopic examination at least every other year (see page 641) and a stool test for blood each year (see page 641).

Lung Cancer

Warning signs: Nagging cough, coughing up blood, and persistent attacks of pneumonia or bronchitis; chest pain.

Cancer risk factors: Heavy smoking and exposure to environmental pollutants, particularly asbestos (see Asbestosis, page 942).

Checkup guidelines: Every person over age 40 should have a baseline chest x-ray. Subsequent chest x-rays should be done at the discretion of your physician.

Cervical Cancer

Warning signs: Abnormal vaginal bleeding.

Cancer risk factors: Having had genital herpes or genital wart infections; sexual intercourse shortly after reaching puberty or having many sexual partners.

Checkup guidelines: Women who have reached age 18 or who are sexually active should have a Pap test (see page 1096) and pelvic examination annually. Your physician may decide that, after three or more consecutive satisfactory normal annual examinations, the Pap test can be performed less frequently.

Endometrial Cancer

Warning signs: Abnormal vaginal bleeding.

Cancer risk factors: History of infertility or failure to ovulate; late onset of menopause or prolonged estrogen therapy after menopause; obesity; heavy smoking.

Checkup guidelines: Upon reaching menopause, women who have had a history of infertility, obesity, failure to ovulate, abnormal uterine bleeding, or estrogen therapy should have an endometrial biopsy (see page 1099).

Urinary Tract and Bladder Cancer

Warning signs: Blood in the urine; back pain; loss of weight and appetite; persistent fever; anemia.

Cancer risk factors: Most common in men over age 50; heavy smokers; history of chronic urinary tract infections.

Checkup guidelines: The routine urine analysis performed during your complete physical examination will reveal if there is any blood in your urine (hematuria). If hematuria is found, your physician may do a cystoscopic examination with biopsy if abnormal tissue is found (see page 904). Your physician also may obtain an x-ray of your kidney (see The Kidney X-Ray, page 885).

Oral Cancer

Warning signs: Any change of color in your mouth or sore that fails to heal in your mouth.

Cancer risk factors: Most common in men over age 45, heavy smokers, and users of smokeless (chewing) tobacco, especially when coupled with heavy use of alcohol (see page 702).

Checkup guidelines: If you have a sore that fails to heal, see your physician or dentist.

Throat Cancer

Warning signs: Hoarseness.

Cancer risk factors: Heavy smoking, particularly if coupled with substantial use of alcohol.

Checkup guidelines: Examination by a throat specialist in the event of a change in the character of your speech lasting more than a few weeks, or annually if you are a heavy smoker.

Prostate Cancer

Warning signs: Difficulty in urination; incessant pain in the lower back, pelvis, or upper thighs; blood in the urine.

Cancer risk factors: Most common among men over age 70.

Checkup guidelines: If you are over age 40 you should have a digital rectal examination at the time of your periodic medical examination (see page 1127).

Skin Cancer

Warning signs: A small lesion with irregular border and red, white, blue, or blue-black spots on trunk or limbs; shiny, firm bump or lesions from pearl to black anywhere on the skin; dark lesions on palms, soles, tips of fingers and toes; large brownish spot with darker speckles on skin exposed to sun; red-purple spots anywhere on the skin; purple-brown or dark blue nodules on toes or leg; pearly or waxy bump on face, ear, or neck; flat, flesh-colored or brown scar-like lesion on chest or back; firm, red nodule or flat lesion with scaly or crusted surface on face, ears, neck, hands, or arms; change in a mole or any sore that fails to heal.

Cancer risk factors: Fair skin, blue eyes, or red hair in men and women; severe sunburn in childhood; family history of birthmarks or moles (dysplastic nevus syndrome).

Checkup guidelines: If you have any skin lesion that has the warning signs listed here, see your physician.

See also Periodic Medical Examinations, page 1212.

CANCER CLUSTERS IN POPULATIONS

At times, cancer seems to occur more frequently in certain groups or in certain geographic locations. Such clusters of cancer suggest that some factor in the environment may be responsible.

A well-demonstrated example is the occurrence of a particular lung tumor (mesothelioma) among industrial workers exposed to asbestos. This tumor occurs at a much greater frequency in asbestos-exposed persons who also smoke (see also Asbestosis, page 942). Another example is the high frequency of cancer of the stomach in Japan, although no single environmental factor has been identified with certainty to explain the Japanese susceptibility to this tumor.

Occasionally, data collected by public health facilities will show an increased frequency of a disease in a certain community. A search then begins for an explanation. Most often, such clusters are explained by the laws of chance.

The mathematical expression of the laws of chance tells us not only that most communities or groups of people of similar age and background will have about the same frequency of various diseases but also that, from time to time, there will be a concentration of one disease or another in certain groups of people. This statistical phenomenon might be compared to dealing a hand of cards. Usually the cards in a hand will be fairly evenly distributed among the four suits, but you also can expect that now and then you will be dealt a hand composed almost entirely of one suit. Mathematicians can calculate the exact odds that such an event will occur.

It is important to separate the clusters of cancer that are merely statistical from those that are caused by environmental factors. Quite properly, much attention and concern are being expressed these days about exposure to substances that have been shown to produce cancers in laboratory animals. However, it is also important to remember that scientific *proof* that a cluster of cancers is in fact a consequence of exposure to potentially toxic substances known to be present in a given community depends on careful statistical comparison of the exposed group of persons with people known to have little or no exposure.

LIVING WITH CANCER

More frequently than ever before, cancer can be cured. The probability of a complete cure and extended survival is continually improving because of our growing knowledge and understanding of the biology of cancer. As a result, new therapies that selectively kill cancer cells are steadily being developed. These therapies are not only more effective but also safer.

The management of pain also has been greatly improved over the years to the point that most pain, even that of terminally ill cancer patients, can be decreased. In the following pages, we describe the treatments now available, how to go about getting appropriate care, and other key issues in living and dealing with cancer and its treatment.

CANCER TREATMENT

No two cancer treatment regimens are the same; each person with cancer is unique. But the basic therapeutic options available to most persons with cancer are similar: surgery, radiation therapy, and chemotherapy.

Why one form of treatment is more appropriate than another in a given person depends on the individual diagnosis, the stage to which the disease has developed, and other factors such as the person's age, sex, general health, and, in women, menopausal status.

A critical part of the diagnosis is determination of whether the cancer has spread. A diagnostic process called staging determines what other tissues or organs may have been invaded by the tumor. Staging not only helps your physician plan the treatment but also evaluates the likelihood of its success or failure. For example, your physician may learn whether a localized treatment such as surgery or radiation therapy would be sufficient or whether a systemic form of treatment such as chemotherapy will be needed to kill cancer cells that have spread to other parts of your body.

Surgery.   Surgery has long been the foundation of cancer treatment. The goals of surgery can vary. It can be done to determine whether or not the growth is malignant, to remove a cancerous growth from the body, or to learn if malignant cells have spread to other parts of the body.

Sometimes surgery is directed primarily toward relief of obstruction of bile ducts or of the intestine. At other times, when it is not possible to remove all of the cancerous growth, the surgeon will remove as much as possible (a debulking procedure) in order to make chemotherapy or radiation more effective.

Surgery is most successful if the cancer has not spread. Sometimes, however, cancer cells that break off from the site where the cancer first appeared (the primary tumor) may travel through blood or lymph vessels to other sites within the body to form secondary tumors. In these instances, the cancer is said to have metastasized. If cells spread before the primary growth is removed, cancer may recur at other locations, even after the primary tumor has been excised.

If the cancer is widespread, surgery is unlikely to cure it. Occasionally, a single secondary tumor appears after removal of the primary cancer and, in some cases, the surgical removal of this single lesion makes a cure possible. This situation may occur in cancer of the colon or testes, among others.

Radiation Therapy.   By careful aiming and regulation of dose, high-energy radiation can be used to destroy cancer cells. Radiation therapy (also referred to as radiotherapy, x-ray therapy, cobalt treatment, or irradiation) is either part of the treatment or the only treatment for about half of all cancer patients. This form of treatment is effective only for those cancer cells within the area receiving the radiation (the field).

Radiation may be used before surgery to shrink a cancerous tumor, after surgery to stop growth of any remaining cancer cells, or alone or with anticancer drugs to destroy a malignant tumor. It is particularly effective when used to treat certain types of localized cancers such as malignant tumors of the lymph nodes or vocal cords.

Like surgery, however, radiation usually is not curative if the cancer cells have spread throughout the body or outside the area of radiation. It can be used even if a cure is not probable because it can shrink tumors, which decreases the pressure and pain they cause, or it can stop their bleeding.

Generally, radiation produces less physical disfigurement than radical surgery does, but it may produce troublesome side effects. These side effects are related to the damage x-rays do to normal tissue. You may have to cope with irritated skin, swallowing difficulties, dry mouth, nausea, diarrhea, hair loss, and a loss of energy. How serious and extensive these side effects become depend on where and how much radiation is used.

Chemotherapy. If cure by surgery or radiation is not possible, treatment with anticancer drugs may be appropriate, an approach termed chemotherapy. For some types of malignancy, such as Hodgkin's disease (see Lymphomas, page 489), leukemia in children (see Leukemias, page 484), or cancer of the testes (see page 1118), chemotherapy may produce a cure even when the cancer is widespread. In other cases in which the cancer is not curable, chemotherapy can relieve symptoms and enhance the quality of life for a patient.

Cancer chemotherapy does not always mean the use of only a single drug. Combination chemotherapy consists of giving a group of drugs that work together to kill cancer cells. If anti-cancer drugs are used in an attempt to destroy any cancer cells that may remain after surgery or radiation therapy, it is referred to as adjuvant chemotherapy. Adjuvant chemotherapy (the Latin *adjuvans* means aiding) is a preventive measure commonly used for cancer, such as breast cancer that has spread into the lymph nodes of the armpit and was discovered at the time of initial surgery.

Anti-cancer drugs can affect normal tissue cells as well. The normal cells most likely to be affected are those that divide rapidly, such as in the bone marrow, gastrointestinal tract, reproductive system, and hair follicles. These cells usually recover shortly after the treatment.

Depending on the specific drugs used, chemotherapy can produce various side effects similar to those of radiation therapy. These toxic reactions include loss of hair, sores in the mouth, difficulty swallowing (esophagitis), dry mouth, nausea, vomiting, diarrhea, bleeding, and infection. Less common problems include damage to the heart, liver, lungs, or kidneys.

In general, these effects of chemotherapy

and radiation are reversible and can be minimized when experienced cancer specialists supervise the treatments.

Immunotherapy. The body's immune system (see The Workings of the Immune System, page 844) acts as a surveillance system to guard against the presence of what it interprets to be foreign substances. For example, the immune response to the presence of an organ that was transplanted from an unrelated donor might be rejection of the organ.

Cancer cells also are seen as foreign. For years, researchers have been trying to enhance the natural immune reaction toward cancer cells. When used as a method of treatment, this technique is called immunotherapy.

Immunotherapy involves the use of biologic agents, known as lymphokines, that normally are produced by white blood cells. The best-documented immunotherapy agent is interferon which is produced by the body in response to a viral infection.

Until recently, the results of immunotherapy against cancer were disappointing, but researchers recently have had success controlling a few types of cancer with one type of interferon, interferon alpha. Specifically, interferon often produces remarkable improvement in people with a rare cancer known as hairy cell leukemia. It also provides limited benefit against certain types of lymph tissue cancer. Unfortunately, inter-

Radiation therapy can be used to effectively destroy cancer cells. During treatment, the device slowly rotates to deliver radiation more effectively.

feron therapy produces little or no improvement against the major cancer killers that arise in the lung, breast, and digestive tract.

We are learning more about how the immune system recognizes and attacks malignant cells. This major field of cancer research eventually may lead to effective immunotherapy techniques against many types of cancer.

CHOOSING A PHYSICIAN AND A PLACE FOR CANCER TREATMENT

The choice of physician and hospital, as well as all decisions about your diagnosis, treatment, and rehabilitation, should be shared. With the complexity involved in all these decisions, they are too important to be left to any one person, including you.

If you suspect that you have cancer or cancer has been diagnosed, the best policy is to share your fears and concerns with family members and loved ones. People who know and care about you can be helpful in sharing the pain and responsibility of making critical decisions.

Never relinquish your responsibility for your health out of a feeling of helplessness. No situation need ever be beyond your control. You always have the option and obligation to ask questions, change your mind, and express your fears to everyone involved. You may not be able to change the diagnosis—but you can and should be the decision-maker regarding your care and treatment.

The Physician. The American Cancer Society (ACS) recommends that a team be formed to help you during this period. This team includes not only yourself, your family, and loved ones but also a variety of medical professionals, primarily physicians and other health professionals trained to deal with one or another aspect of your illness: radiotherapists, surgeons, and medical oncologists (cancer specialists) as well as dieticians, physical therapists, and others. To coordinate the diagnostic and therapeutic efforts that may be considered, it is recommended that you appoint what the ACS calls a physician advisor or primary-care physician.

The physician advisor may be your personal family physician or a specialist who is directing the overall treatment of the cancer. What is important to understand is that the physician you select should be qualified to advise you on the entire process—diagnosis, treatment, and rehabilitation. Moreover, he or she should be available to provide long-term, continuing care.

If for any reason you are not comfortable in your relationship with your physician, tell him or her what bothers you. If you remain dissatisfied with any aspect of your care, get a second opinion from another physician (see Second Opinions, page 1209). Do this as soon as possible because most people find it difficult to start over once a physician begins the treatment.

This is also the time to talk about your physician's willingness to involve other physicians in your treatment. Questions like these need not be difficult to ask or answer. Your physician should be happy to answer intelligent and thoughtful questions because this suggests the prospect of an open and frank relationship. If, on the other hand, this does not occur, look elsewhere.

Cancer Centers. Your physician advisor will conduct some of the initial diagnostic tests, such as a Pap smear or biopsy. If the diagnosis requires tests for which this physician's office is not equipped, you may be referred to a specialist at a medical center.

Depending on the type of cancer and the treatment you require, you may find yourself spending a substantial amount of time at a medical center specializing in the treatment of cancer. Your physician advisor will help you locate and evaluate an appropriate center. Another source of information is the American College of Surgeons. A rule of thumb is the greater the number of beds in the hospital (perhaps 500 or more), the more likely it will have experience in treating cancer patients.

Usually, a hospital directly connected to or controlled by a medical school offers a broader range and higher quality of care because these institutions draw prominent clinicians, researchers, and educators for their medical facilities and teaching staff. Teaching hospitals (those in which residents are trained, although there may be no medical school directly affiliated with the hospital) also often are good facilities, although their services are usually not as extensive as those found in a hospital/medical school tandem.

Your illness may require you to go to more than one medical center. One center may provide the diagnosis, another may conduct the treatment based on the diagnosis, and a third may provide the rehabilitation.

Most large local or community medical centers are equipped to treat cancer cases that do not require a high degree of specialization. However, if you need a complicated or experimental treatment or if physicians at your local hospital are inexperienced in treating your specific type of cancer, you might be referred to a specialized cancer center.

In teaching hospitals (hospitals with residents), there often are carefully organized trials of treatments in progress. Some of these trials compare new modes of therapy with the best currently available treatment. Other trials are to study new agents or approaches in a non-comparative manner. If you are offered a chance to enter one of these trials, you will be given a frank and comprehensive description of the risks and possible benefits. While such clinical trials are clearly experimental, the careful application of these therapies, whether new or old, generally will provide some of the best treatments currently available.

CANCER FACILITIES

The National Cancer Institute (NCI) has designated 20 medical centers throughout the United States as Comprehensive Cancer Centers. These centers provide leadership in cancer research. They develop comprehensive programs involving scientists and physicians from many fields.

In addition to providing state-of-the-art diagnosis and treatment of cancer, comprehensive cancer centers conduct interdisciplinary programs in basic laboratory and clinical research, cancer control, and education.

There also are clinical centers that are supported by the National Cancer Institute. These offer many of the same services that are available at the Comprehensive Cancer Centers.

Comprehensive Cancer Centers offer the most extensive range of cancer treatment found in the United States, including therapies that are still considered investigational. If the medical center at which you are to be treated is not a Comprehensive Cancer Cen-

ter, you may want to ask whether it has a clinical cancer center. If not, learn if it has an approved cancer program sponsored by the American College of Surgeons. These are programs that have met specific requirements and standards for the treatment of malignant diseases.

COMPREHENSIVE AND CLINICAL CANCER CENTERS SUPPORTED BY THE NATIONAL CANCER INSTITUTE

The National Cancer Institute supports a number of cancer centers throughout the country that develop and investigate new methods of cancer diagnosis and treatment. Information about referral procedures, treatment costs, and services available to patients can be obtained from the individual cancer centers listed below.

Alabama   **The University of Alabama at Birmingham Comprehensive Cancer Center**
1918 University Boulevard
Basic Health Sciences Building, Room 108
Birmingham, AL 35294

California   **The Kenneth Norris Jr. Comprehensive Cancer Center and The Kenneth Norris Jr. Hospital and Research Institute**
University of Southern California
1441 Eastlake Avenue
Los Angeles, CA 90033-0804
Jonsson Comprehensive Cancer Center (UCLA)
10-247 Factor Building
10833 Le Conte Avenue
Los Angeles, CA 90024-1781

Connecticut   **Yale University Comprehensive Cancer Center**
333 Cedar Street
New Haven, CT 06510

District of Columbia	**Georgetown University/ Howard University Cancer Research Center** (comprehensive) 2041 Georgia Avenue, NW Washington, DC 20060 **Vincent T. Lombardi Cancer Research Center** (comprehensive) Georgetown University Medical Center 3800 Reservoir Road, NW Washington, DC 20007	**New York**	**Memorial Sloan-Kettering Cancer Center** (comprehensive) 1275 York Avenue New York, NY 10021 **Columbia University Cancer Center** (comprehensive) College of Physicians and Surgeons 630 West 168th Street New York, NY 10032 **Roswell Park Memorial Institute** (comprehensive) Elm and Carlton Streets Buffalo, NY 14263
Florida	**Sylvester Comprehensive Cancer Center** University of Miami Medical School 1475 Northwest 12th Avenue Miami, FL 33136	**North Carolina**	**Duke University Comprehensive Cancer Center** P.O. Box 3843 Durham, NC 27710
Illinois	**Illinois Cancer Council** (a consortium that includes two clinical centers) **Illinois Cancer Council** 36 South Wabash Avenue Chicago, IL 60603 **University of Chicago Cancer Research Center** 5841 South Maryland Avenue Chicago, IL 60637	**Ohio**	**Ohio State University Comprehensive Cancer Center** 410 West 12th Avenue Columbus, OH 43210
		Pennsylvania	**Fox Chase Cancer Center/University of Pennsylvania** (comprehensive) 7701 Burholme Avenue Philadelphia, PA 19111 **University of Pennsylvania Cancer Center** (comprehensive) 3400 Spruce Street Philadelphia, PA 19104
Maryland	**The Johns Hopkins Oncology Center** (comprehensive) 600 North Wolfe Street Baltimore, MD 21205		
Massachusetts	**Dana-Farber Cancer Institute** (comprehensive) 44 Binney Street Boston, MA 02115	**Texas**	**The University of Texas M.D. Anderson Cancer Center** (comprehensive) 1515 Holcombe Boulevard Houston, TX 77030
Michigan	**Meyer L. Prentis Comprehensive Cancer Center of Metropolitan Detroit** 110 East Warren Avenue Detroit, MI 48201	**Washington**	**Fred Hutchinson Cancer Research Center** (comprehensive) 1124 Columbia Street Seattle, WA 98104
Minnesota	**Mayo Comprehensive Cancer Center** 200 First Street Southwest Rochester, MN 55905	**Wisconsin**	**Wisconsin Clinical Cancer Center** University of Wisconsin 600 Highland Avenue Madison, WI 53792

For additional information about cancer, write to the Office of Cancer Communications, National Cancer Institute, Bethesda, MD 20892, or call the toll-free telephone number of the Cancer Information Service at 1-800-4-CANCER.

Spanish-speaking staff members are available to callers from the following areas (daytime hours only): California, Florida, Georgia, Illinois, New Jersey (area code 201), New York, and Texas.

In Hawaii, on Oahu call 524-1234 (from neighboring islands call collect).

NUTRITION AND CANCER

A person who has cancer and is in sound nutritional shape is better able to tolerate the side effects of chemotherapy, radiation, and surgery. Furthermore, good nutrition improves the sense of well-being, enhances tissue function and repair, and improves the immune function of the person with cancer. However, a common and difficult problem often associated with cancer has been weight loss and malnutrition. This is sometimes called cancer cachexia.

Many factors can contribute to weight loss. The disease or its treatment can decrease appetite and food intake (anorexia) or interfere with the consumption, digestion, absorption, or utilization of food by your body.

Many cancers affect the nutritional status adversely even before the diagnosis or treatment. Depending on the type of cancer, malnutrition may result from anorexia, obstruction (blockage) by a tumor that impairs food intake or digestion, malabsorption of nutrients in the gastrointestinal tract, or disturbances in fluid balance due to vomiting and diarrhea.

Often, a person with cancer who experiences severe anorexia simply cannot eat in spite of his or her understanding that nourishment is required. For various reasons, many people with cancer are either unable to taste their food or experience changes in taste. It is not uncommon for them to find that they often feel full after eating only a few bites of food.

The radiation, surgery, and chemotherapy used as treatment for cancer may predispose to nutritional problems such as nausea, alterations in taste and smell, sore mouth, diarrhea, anorexia, or difficulty in swallowing.

The treatment also may increase the body's need for calories and protein to rebuild damaged tissues.

Recent advances in the subject of nutrition have been very helpful in the management of cancer cachexia. Today, in most cases, weight loss is not considered an unavoidable consequence of cancer. There are many simple constructive steps that you can take to improve intake and ensure maintenance of your body weight. In addition, new feeding techniques such as tube feedings, intravenous feedings, and improved oral supplements have been developed that enable almost everyone, even those with complicated nutritional problems, to improve their nutritional status.

Your physician, often in consultation with a dietician who is especially knowledgeable about cancer and nutrition, can offer you further advice concerning nutrition.

Clinical studies have shown that a sound nutritional state can improve a person's chance of undergoing successful treatment and withstanding the rigors of cancer, but no conclusive evidence exists to indicate that decreased or excessive amounts of any nutrient have a beneficial role in the treatment of cancer. (See Nutrition and the Cancer Patient, page 368. See also Diet and Cancer Protection, page 369.)

CANCER PAIN

Cancer does not always cause pain. More than half of all cancer patients do not experience exceptional pain; often the pain is moderate and far less intense than that experienced in some forms of arthritis or nerve disorders. In general, pain relief can be achieved by tumor control with surgery, radiation therapy, or chemotherapy.

Some persons with cancer do have episodes of more severe pain; in general, the more advanced the cancer, the greater likelihood of some periods of severe pain.

When cancer pain that is not relieved initially by cancer treatment does occur, there are many other ways of obtaining relief. Through a combination of pain-relieving drugs and non-drug methods, most people with cancer can function as well as the other symptoms of the disease will permit. As a result, one of the primary goals of cancer treatment is to decrease pain with as few side effects as possible.

Causes of Pain. Cancer pain depends on the type of cancer, the stage of the disease, and your tolerance for pain. Cancer pain can be dull, aching, sharp, constant, intermittent, mild, moderate, or severe. It may be caused by pressure of the tumor on a nerve, poor circulation because of blocked blood vessels, blocked organ in the body, bone fractures, infection, or side effects from surgery. Nonphysical responses to the cancer, such as anxiety or depression, can make the pain seem worse.

Pharmacological Relief of Pain. The principal treatment for cancer pain is pain-relieving drugs (analgesics). These drugs fall into two categories: nonsteroidal anti-inflammatory drugs (NSAIDs), including aspirin, ibuprofen, and acetaminophen, and narcotics such as codeine and morphine.

Many patients fear that aspirin is not strong enough to treat their pain. Yet, aspirin can be highly effective and provide the same amount of pain relief as many of the more powerful painkillers. In combination with codeine or meperidine (Demerol), aspirin can provide effective control of mild to moderate pain.

Most NSAIDs are prescription drugs. The benefit of these agents is that they are slightly more potent and more convenient to take than aspirin and they require fewer pills per day.

The more powerful painkillers used to treat moderate to severe pain are narcotics. Many cancer patients fear an addiction if they take narcotics as a part of their cancer treatment. This fear is largely unfounded.

Drug addiction can occur in patients with cancer pain but, when the narcotic is used under proper medical control, the chance is very small. Besides, if a narcotic is needed to relieve severe pain for a long period of time, the comfort it provides is often more important than any possibility of an addiction.

Sometimes tranquilizers are used in combination with analgesics. The tranquilizers offer no relief of the pain, but they may help you tolerate the discomfort and can be an integral part of treatment.

In some cases, larger doses of narcotics or tranquilizers can cause confusion or delirium. This may limit their usefulness.

Radiation therapy delivered to a selected site, such as a bone involved with cancer, can shrink the tumor and lessen or eliminate the pain.

Nerve pathways that carry pain impulses to the brain can be blocked either by the injection of certain substances into or around the nerve or by surgery. These procedures have risks and some are considered experimental. However, for those who cannot tolerate the side effects of other pain medications, these methods can be helpful. For some cancers, such as pancreatic cancers, these procedures have become almost routine.

Your physician may suggest some behavioral modification methods, in combination with other pain-relief methods, to increase pain control; these methods include relaxation techniques, hypnosis, and biofeedback and often help people to decrease their anxiety and to build their confidence in coping with pain.

CANCER REHABILITATION

Rehabilitation, a significant part of the treatment of cancer, is often planned before the treatment begins. The choice of your treatment may dictate the scope and nature of your rehabilitation.

Whatever form the rehabilitation takes, the goal is always the same: to restore you to as normal a lifestyle as possible. This might mean job retraining, homemaker services, an exercise program, or learning to use a prosthesis. Such wide-ranging skills and services usually call for a team approach. Depending on need, you may see a

number of health-care professionals besides your primary physician. These include physiatrists, social workers, physical therapists, and occupational therapists.

Some of the more common rehabilitation efforts involve: a speech therapist or speech pathologist who can help with retraining for speech after a surgical procedure on the larynx or mouth (see page 703); an enterostomal therapist who instructs in the use of the artificial opening, made as a result of either colon or bladder surgery, for eliminating body wastes (see Ileostomy and Colostomy, page 638; Bladder Cancer, page 902); or a physical or occupational therapist to help in learning how to use an artificial limb. The initial stage of the rehabilitation can be started in the hospital, or all of the rehabilitation may be offered in the home or in an outpatient center.

Do not be discouraged if you find your initial efforts difficult and the results disappointing. Progress may come slowly and the work may be hard. But do not give up and withdraw from the rehabilitation program that has been designed for you. Follow your therapist's instructions. If you have problems, do not hesitate to discuss them with your therapist, physiatrist, or physician advisor.

To help during this transition in your life, there are many volunteer support groups made up primarily of patients who have recovered from cancer. Their desire is to help the person with cancer through the usually difficult period of adjustment during and after treatment. One of the best known is the Reach to Recovery program of the American Cancer Society for women recovering from breast cancer. If you inform your physician that you would like to talk with someone from this group, a volunteer will pay a visit while you are still in the hospital. Two other volunteer cancer support groups are the Ostomy Rehabilitation Program for people with abdominal stomas and the Laryngectomee Club for those who lose their natural voice because of cancer surgery.

Older people may find returning to normal life especially difficult; many youngsters do too. These behaviors, which may involve depression or a refusal to try to adjust, can place added stress on the other members of the family. CanSurmount is an organization devoted to the support and care of those recovering and their families during this period. I CAN COPE is another volunteer group that advises the patient and family on cancer therapy, treatment side effects, nutrition issues, and other topics of interest.

You can learn the whereabouts of the nearest chapter of these or other such support groups by calling the American Cancer Society (ACS) in your area. The ACS also can help you with problems of transportation and home-care items and with contacting community groups such as Community Mental Health and Family Services.

It is important to understand that this is a time in your life when you must learn to accept help. Going it alone is probably unwise and may be impossible. You can benefit greatly from allowing people who have themselves recovered from cancer to advise and support you.

HOSPICES

The word hospice comes from the Latin word for guest; it is the root that forms the words hospital, hospitality, and hostel. Hospice conveys a sense of caring and shelter.

In the Middle Ages, the hospice was a way station for travelers. Today, hospice has another meaning: a hospice is a program—sometimes within the confines of a medical center—that offers a coordinated, interdisciplinary program of care and services for terminally ill people and their families.

The Team Approach. At the heart of the hospice approach is the team. Hospice workers, who include physicians, nurses, social workers, and clergy, provide an integration of various skills to help both the dying person and the family. Physicians and nurses provide medical services; social workers can assist with psychosocial support for the person and family and help with financial planning, insurance, and funeral arrangements; clergy offer spiritual counseling for both the dying person and his or her family; and volunteers help the hospice staff with clerical assistance and the person and family with their daily needs (for example, transportation, meal preparation, looking after the one who is ill).

In this setting, the entire staff concerned with delivery of care meets frequently. Everyone's opinion counts, especially that of the patient. The goal is to allow the person to live his or her last days in comfort and to adequately prepare for death. The care offered to the family does not suddenly stop at the person's death—the hospice team continues to provide care for the family in the form of bereavement services.

Palliative Care. The hospice concept is not a resignation to death, as many people believe. Hospice care neither hastens nor postpones death. Rather, the emphasis at a hospice is on quality of life with the focus on symptom control and psychosocial counseling rather than reversal of the disease process.

Planning the care involves education of the terminally ill patient and his or her family. In some cases, the individual with the terminal ailment can decide what medications to take and when. Careful consideration is given to all options, and a decision is made in conjunction with the hospice team.

Patient and Family. In the hospice system, patients are not passive recipients of medical care nor are the families mere bystanders. The person receiving hospice care is encouraged to make decisions about his or her treatment, relationships with other people, personal business, and preferences about burial and memorial services.

One goal of hospice care is to treat the entire unit of care—that is, the terminally ill person *and* the family. Efforts of the team are directed to supporting the family and its needs, as well as those of the terminally ill person. Family members may assume an active role as care-givers. They may learn to administer drugs. They also come to understand what to expect when a loved one is at the point of death.

Types of Hospices. There now are many hospices across the United States. The services are offered in a range of formats. In some instances, hospice care is offered at home but in coordination with a program at a local hospital; in some communities, there are independent hospices with no formal ties to any medical institution. Some hospitals also have rooms designated for hospice care.

Whatever the details of a particular hospice's organization, the emphasis in most programs is on home care, with short-term in-hospital care when necessary. What distinguishes the hospice is the nature of the care: the goal is to affirm life yet to accept death as a normal process. Through personalized service and a caring community of people, hospice care-givers aim to help the dying person and his or her family to prepare for a death that is satisfactory to them.

To find what hospice services are available in your region, contact: National Hospice Organization, 1901 N. Ft. Myer Dr., Arlington, VA 22209.

CANCER IN CHILDREN

Cancer is rare in children. In addition, the most progress has been made—and the chances of cure are highest—in those cancers that affect children. Only 25 years ago, almost all children with cancer died from it, usually within a year. Modern treatment now makes prolonged survival and cures not only possible but likely with most kinds of childhood cancer. At least half of all American children with cancer now survive it.

Still, many types of cancer are life-threatening, especially if they are not detected early and treated properly. Cancer remains responsible for more deaths than any other type of disease in school-age and preschool children (only accidents claim more lives in these age groups).

The most common childhood cancer is leukemia (see Leukemias, page 484). With new treatments, the outlook for children with this disease has brightened considerably in recent years. The other major class of childhood cancers are brain tumors (see page 537). Other cancers common in children are kidney cancer (see Cancer of the Kidney or Ureter, page 901), bone cancer (see Bone Tumors, page 988), soft tissue sarcomas (see page 978), and lymphomas (see page 489).

The causes of these cancers remain unknown. However, some agents such as certain chemicals and viruses are thought to trigger some cancers by altering the genetic material of normal cells. Cancer is not contagious. We all have oncogenes (see The Biology of Cancer, page 1239), the genes that can activate cells to become cancerous. It is not yet clear what turns them on or off.

It is important to choose carefully where to have your child treated for cancer. With the help of your child's physician, seek out a center where the staff is experienced at providing the latest advances in treatment for children with cancer. The center and its staff also should offer the emotional support that the entire family needs (see Cancer Facilities, page 1247).

A team of specialists in childhood cancer is necessary to deliver the best treatment. This therapy is complex and often requires a combination of surgery, chemotherapy, and radiation. People with the needed expertise are usually gathered only in cancer centers, children's hospitals, or large medical centers.

Such centers are often affiliated with major medical schools located in big cities. Perhaps you live far from the nearest center. If so, it is usually sufficient for your child's care to be planned, started, and directed from there. In close cooperation with a cancer center staff, a local physician can provide some of the treatment and interim tests. This kind of arrangement minimizes the cost and the change in location for the child and family.

Both you and your child's health-care team should prepare your child thoroughly for all the new experiences involved in these treatments. Be truthful with your child. Be supportive. Reassure your child that everybody is trying to make him or her better. Make sure that your physicians and nurses help answer all of your child's health-related questions.

HOW TO DEAL WITH CANCER IN YOUR CHILD

Especially when it involves your child, a diagnosis of cancer can conjure up feelings of dread and devastation. However, because of technological advances and drug treatments, the outlook is much improved. With the increasing survival rates there has come a better understanding of the emotional needs of children who have cancer and of their families.

Pediatric oncology (cancer) teams generally consist of physicians, nurses, social workers, and clergy who are trained to deal with these kinds of emotions. They are able to provide comprehensive care that supports the entire family through the course of the disease and are able to anticipate adjustments of families and to plan needed interventions. Social workers help families to deal with the diagnosis of cancer in a psychologically healthy manner. The ability to

cope as a parent is essential because your sick child may have years of precious life ahead.

Of equal importance is retaining a healthy relationship within the family. This is not always easy because of the additional stress created by your sick child. Sisters, brothers, and spouses all have needs, but these sometimes are forgotten. Parents who listen to their other children and their needs and who leave openings for them to voice their thoughts and concerns are establishing a trusting, open, caring, and honest relationship that will last a lifetime.

Very few families undergo treatment for cancer without considerable economic stress involving medical bills, lodging, meals, transportation, needs of other family members at home, and so forth. Financial burdens begin at the time of diagnosis and can extend well beyond the time of illness. Early assessment, by social workers, of financial plights and job-related issues is crucial and can uncover possible supports for the family. The assessment also serves as a warning to families regarding the magnitude of expenses at the initial diagnosis and for the future.

Another pertinent issue to your child is school reentry. School personnel need to be educated regarding your child's cancer and the specific implications it will have for both your child and the school. Appropriate behavior and academic expectations must be discussed. An opportunity for discussion with school administrators and personnel gives much-needed reassurance and helps to dispel misconceptions.

It is important for the entire family to return to normalcy. Children are very resilient and wish to be treated the same as they were before the cancer diagnosis and to have a life that is not totally focused on their illness.

It is painful to think about a child with cancer. Some parents want to run; some wish to avoid the diagnosis. But, overall, parents who accept the pain and take a look at the realities of the specific illness are much better equipped to cope with future concerns and problems. There are bewildering emotions to confront: confusion, denial, fear, anger, guilt, grief, and hope. You may have experienced any or all of these feelings at different times with different degrees of intensity, but the ultimate message you must receive from the cancer team is that you are not alone in this experience.

Social workers are aware of the multiple implications of childhood cancer. Early assessment and ongoing evaluation of stresses are provided throughout the disease to help with changing needs and to provide continued psychological and emotional support to your child and the family.

It is easy to become cynical and bitter. The optimism of the meaning and value of life becomes threatened with the injustice of cancer in a child. Along with many emotions (grief, anger, guilt, fear), most parents discover riches they never before appreciated: closeness and support of family, friends, church, and community and availability of a good medical team that provides the care.

CHAPTER 42

DEATH AND DYING

CHAPTER CONTENTS

DEALING WITH DEATH

Whether death is embraced as a part of life or feared as a tragic loss, dealing with it rarely is easy.

The circumstances in which a death occurs have a great deal to do with how we react: for most of us, the sudden and shocking death of a child is quite different from the final end to the pain of a long-suffered illness an elderly person may experience. Yet, what makes death difficult for most of us is that we tend to deny that it can occur.

We whisper about death as if it were something to be ashamed of. In part this may account for why so many of us feel confused or guilty about the prospect of our own death or that of someone else. Because death challenges our understanding of the mystery of life, it always will be held in awe. Perhaps, if we can come to understand the medical and legal facts of death we will have less fear and be able to deal more immediately with the reality of death.

It is important to realize that death is quite different from dying. Death is an end point, the event in which life ceases. But dying is an essential part of the life process. For many dying persons, life's experiences still have significant meaning and importance.

In our society, death has come to be expected at the end of a long and fruitful life; yet, no matter when it comes it always seems too soon. New discoveries in science raise expectations for cures and medical miracles. As a consequence of these and other factors, when death occurs we often are more surprised than understanding and accepting of the event.

TERMINAL ILLNESS

Death is inevitable. But it appears in many different guises. Sometimes it is sudden and comes without warning; at other times, it marches relentlessly into a person's life.

A terminal illness is one example of a circumstance in which the dying person, his or her physician, and perhaps a circle of family and friends are given time in which to prepare for death. We can discuss with family members issues such as nutritional support, continuation of medical treatments, and resuscitation. We can make clear whether or not an autopsy is to be performed, organs are to be donated, or the body is to be given to science. We can review the details of funeral or burial arrangements if we wish or any business that affects our legal will.

As fearful as it may be, the reality of death usually moves the dying to some level of acceptance. However, for the families, prolonged terminal illness brings out complicated and painful emotional reactions. In some instances, the bereaved may be so pained by the issue of someone's death that they will choose to ignore it or to avoid any talk of it, even with the dying person. Such silence from friends and families may add to the ordeal of the terminally ill person.

Although the time of dying may be traumatic for everyone involved, it is also a time to come to terms with the passing of a life. Dying well can be filled with moments of grateful remembrance.

SHOULD THE DYING PERSON BE TOLD?

Most dying people can and should be told of their impending death. In general, dying persons want to be informed of the reality of their situations. In most cases, a properly informed person is fortified, not undermined.

Dying people often dread abandonment, humiliation, and loneliness at the end of their lives. They believe that their personal relationships will suffer during this time and that they will not be treated as normal human beings while they die.

These concerns are reinforced if the dying person is denied the right to dignity and an opportunity to talk about the natural fears of, and wonderment about, death.

The person who is terminally ill may find it easier to talk to someone who is not a relative. Most hospitals have a supportive care program with trained staff members who can make it easier for the dying person and his or her family to negotiate this difficult time. In some instances, the psychiatric social worker or hospital chaplain can be present to tell the person or to make it easier for the person and family members to talk about their fears of death. Once the terrible silence is broken, both the person and his or her family have the opportunity to talk about the future of family members.

THE ACT OF DYING

Pain, both physical and emotional, is usually the principal fear of a dying person. The good news is that today the available methods of pain control make it possible to provide relief, with a minimum of side effects to compromise the comfort or dignity of the dying person.

Many large hospitals operate pain clinics or hospice programs (see Hospices, page 1251) that are staffed by teams of specialists available to your physician. Today, most physical pain can be successfully treated with effective painkilling drugs. Biofeedback and relaxation therapy are often used to alleviate the sensation of pain. These approaches alone, however, cannot always relieve pain, particularly the profound psychological pain in someone who is dying (see Cancer Pain, page 1249).

Dying has been characterized as a five-stage process. The initial stage is denial and isolation; anger and resentment follow. The third stage involves an attempt to "bargain" and perhaps postpone the inevitable. A period of depression and an accompanying sense of loss follow. Finally, at the fifth stage the dying person is able to accept the reality of death.

Most terminally ill people are shocked when told that they are dying. First they express disbelief. When they reach the point at which they no longer can deny the fact of their approaching death, their bafflement is replaced by anger. At this stage, anger and resentment may be directed toward anyone and everyone, including those helping and loving them. They often feel as if they have been cruelly robbed of the rest of their lives.

Frequently, the third stage prompts a profound question: "Why me?" At this point, the person attempts to negotiate or postpone what is inevitable. Often the person tries to bargain with God or fate; usually the desired "deal" involves a period of time without pain and discomfort. If eventually the person can surmount the denial, anger, and futile bargaining, depression may set in.

Once the depression lifts, the final stage of this process of dying often is acceptance. The acceptance does not necessarily bring happiness or even understanding. Rather, the acceptance on the part of the dying person involves an understanding that he or she can die in the manner he or she wishes.

Not everyone goes through these stages in the same manner. Some may skip a stage; others may experience two or three at the same time; and some may experience them out of order. But ultimate acceptance of one's pending death often involves these steps.

APPROACHING DEATH

The experience of dying can be strongly influenced by the behavior and attitudes of those who care for the dying person, especially loved ones. For example, dying people frequently demand that they not be left alone. They fear not only the moment of death with its uncertainties but also that they might be abandoned.

Offering consolation and reassurance at these moments is difficult but necessary. Many dying people are made less fearful when comforted in the values of their faith traditions. There is comfort in being assured that most people near death do not feel pain but rather grow relaxed and fall asleep.

There are various signs that the moment of death may be near. The dying person may become fidgety or restless and have difficulty breathing. A physician may provide medications to make the person more comfortable in such circumstances. In some cases, especially if the dying person is willing and alert, breathing can be eased if he or she can be placed in a sitting position or allowed to lie on one side with a pillow under his or her head.

Even though the dying person may not be able to communicate, he or she often can hear much of what is being said. Despite any sense of powerlessness you may feel, your very presence can be the comfort the dying person seeks. Remember, it is feeling that they are abandoned by loved ones that dying persons fear most when they approach the moment of death.

If talking to the person makes you uncomfortable but you want to be present and of some comfort, simply hold the person's hand. Physical contact at this time can be comforting. Sometimes, silence is the best approach.

ROLE OF THE CLERGY OR CONFIDANT

A dying person often needs someone to talk to, a person to whom he or she can look for honesty and acceptance in searching for the meaning of life and death.

The dying do not need pity. They do need understanding and empathy. Feelings of helplessness may make the dying and their loved ones uncomfortable. A member of the clergy who is experienced in dealing with death and dying can help the dying person and his or her family explore thoughts and feelings they may need to share.

The dying are often reluctant to reveal their feelings of guilt and anxiety. If they see the confusion and fear that their dying is causing, they may not want to subject their families to any more pain. The dying rightly feel that most others, even friends and family, may not be able to understand what they are going through. Even though, or perhaps because, he or she is a virtual stranger, a hospital chaplain may be someone who can enable the dying person to talk more freely.

A member of the clergy or a confidant often can help a dying person work through the transition from life to death. Sometimes this includes a strengthening and healing of family relationships. A growing closeness may be experienced through faith traditions and practices.

The confidant should be helpful but not too helpful. He or she should be perceptive enough to recognize that a dying person does *not* always need or desire comfort or assistance.

Finally, the confidant can help the dying person say what needs to be said and do what needs to be done. For example, saying goodbye at this time may be painful but necessary.

MAKING DECISIONS

With the advent of drugs, surgical techniques, and life-sustaining technologies, modern medicine can prolong the lives and ease the pain of seriously ill people. In this age of extraordinary life-support capabilities, physical death due to the natural failure of the heart or lungs sometimes can be postponed until life-prolonging measures are withdrawn.

Recent legal decisions support the rights of people, and in particular those who have had a prolonged illness, to live their final days as they choose. These court decisions reflect society's evolving perspective that dying involves the whole person—not only physical but also emotional and spiritual aspects.

The criteria on which a decision is made that a person is to die are an issue that is hotly debated in hospital wards and courts of law. The arguments are complex and often contradictory, but one key theme recurs. Whenever possible, the choice of whether or not to proceed with extraordinary measures should be a matter for the dying person to decide.

Living Will. Today, many people want a voice in determining the treatment they are to receive if they become terminally ill and are unable to communicate their wishes. A living will offers this capability. It becomes active only if you lose your mental competence or suffer an injury or disease that impairs your ability to communicate.

Living wills are written in general language because no one can anticipate all possible circumstances. They can follow a general guideline or be quite specific. For example, your living will might prohibit heroic procedures, but that leaves it to your physician to make certain distinctions: is the use of a respirator a heroic measure? What about a blood transfusion? As new technologies are developed and yesterday's heroic treatments become routine, the problem becomes increasingly complicated.

To draft a living will, it is useful but not essential to get help from an attorney. It is also important to realize that all living wills have limitations because few of us can predict our way of death. You might consider stating in your living will your wish that extraordinary technological procedures not be used when your condition is terminal. But at what point is a condition to be considered terminal? This remains a subject of considerable debate.

A living will may seem to you to be an appropriate step, but by itself it carries only moral force in stating your preferences. To give legal authority to living wills, most states have passed statutes often called natural death acts. In these states, the statutes interpret the extent of the authority and the legal force of the living will.

The statutes are not uniform among states. Each state's law has unique characteristics. To ensure that your living will conforms to your state's requirements and will have the intended effect, be familiar with the appropriate laws in your state. Some states have laws that include forms you can use for this purpose.

In addition to a living will, you may want to consider a document invoking a durable power of attorney. This document gives the person you select the authority to act as your proxy should you become incapacitated.

Under the law of some states the proxy may make more than financial decisions for you. He or she also may make medical decisions. Usually this person is a trusted friend or relative but not one of your direct heirs. By naming one person to speak on your behalf, you lessen the danger that your wishes will be misinterpreted or ignored. Also, your proxy can respond specifically to the unique questions that your condition creates. The combination of a durable power of attorney and a living will provides maximum personal participation in the face of many medical situations that require difficult decisions. Discuss these decisions with your family so that your wishes are well understood.

Discontinuing, Withholding, or Limiting Treatment.　If you become terminally ill, you should, if possible, participate in decisions made about the treatment you are to receive. And your wishes should be communicated to all care-givers and respected by them.

A serious illness may reach a point at which further treatment may just prolong the process of dying. At this point, you and your family, with help from your physician and perhaps a clergy member, may agree to stop further treatment except to ease pain and provide comfort. You and your family also may decide not to carry out cardiopulmonary resuscitation if it only prolongs the dying process.

Decisions that involve highly sensitive ethical matters may bring out differences of opinion among family members. Intentionally removing life-support systems may not present a dilemma for someone who sees the choice only in terms of death with dignity, whereas another relative could be quite unable to consider this because it would violate deep beliefs about the preservation of life.

The correct course of action is not always obvious. Discussions in the family may grow heated and give rise to yet more questions. This is why it is best to communicate your feelings early and clearly to those whom you entrust with your life.

Laws regarding living wills often include a disclaimer specifying that the law's intent is not to authorize euthanasia or assisted suicide. The Council on Ethical and Judicial Affairs of the American Medical Association has made it very clear that "active euthanasia" is a euphemism for the intentional killing of a person and that this is not part of the practice of medicine, whether or not there is consent from the patient. The Council statement further notes that the intentional termination of the life of one human being by another (so-called mercy killing) is contrary to public policy, medical tradition, and the most fundamental measures of human value and worth.

The American College of Physicians draws a firm line between not using life-sustaining interventions and active euthanasia or assisted suicide. Medical killing would involve the administration of a lethal agent (such as a deliberate overdose of morphine) to a person with the clear intention of causing immediate death. Although a person may refuse some medical therapies and the physician may comply with this refusal, the physician should never intentionally and directly cause death or assist a patient to commit suicide. This type of euthanasia remains illegal in the United States. Even if legalized, according to the American College of Physicians, such an action would violate the ethical standards of medical practice.

The practical boundary between euthanasia (an act of willfully ending a life) and death with dignity will always be obscure. Some treatments have a double effect. On one hand, the primary effect of a narcotic such as morphine is to relieve pain, but an inescapable secondary effect is depression of the drive to breathe, which can lead to death.

Life-supporting medical technology, much like nuclear power, is a double-edged sword. Its use has permitted physicians to resuscitate patients who might not have

"DO NOT RESUSCITATE" ORDERS

The directive "do not resuscitate" (DNR) means that cardiopulmonary resuscitation (CPR) is not to be done in the event of stoppage of heart action or breathing.

CPR is intended to be used when the threat of death occurs suddenly and unexpectedly in an apparently healthy person. It is ordinarily not appropriate in a patient with a terminal, irreversible illness when death is to be expected at any time. Furthermore, CPR is rarely effective for elderly persons who experience stoppage of breathing or heart action that occurs outside the hospital or is not observed when the episode occurs so that the duration of the stoppage is unknown.

The initials DNR are ordinarily prominently displayed on the charts of patients in hospitals or nursing homes when it has been decided that CPR is not to be used. The decision to place DNR on the chart is made by the patient and the physician; if the patient is not competent, it is made by the relatives and the physician. Sometimes the decision is part of a living will (see page 1258).

The decision as to whether or not to use CPR should not have to be made in an emergency situation. This is the reason for making the decision early and making everyone who might be involved aware of it. Placing "DNR" on the patient's chart does not imply that any lesser quality of care will be given.

In addition to deciding about the use of CPR, questions regarding use of other life-sustaining measures such as antibiotics, kidney dialysis, blood transfusions, and respirators (aids to breathing) will arise in the care of the person with a terminal illness. It is best that discussions of such measures be carried out before the patient has lost his or her decision-making capacity and before a medical crisis has occurred.

Another issue is whether to use artificial feeding, usually by means of a tube through the nose into the stomach, to treat an otherwise healthy person who becomes permanently unconscious. There are several difficult questions: Is an unconscious person completely unaware of his or her surroundings? If feedings are discontinued, will the person experience thirst and hunger? Is withdrawal of such feeding for an otherwise nonterminally ill person a form of euthanasia?

Active euthanasia, or mercy killing, is the intentional killing of a person, such as by the injection of a large dose of morphine. Active euthanasia includes a practice sometimes referred to as assisted suicide in which one person furnishes the means for another person to end his or her life. This can imply a tacit encouragement on the part of the patient to proceed with the suicide. Active euthanasia is illegal in all jurisdictions of the United States and, even if it were legalized, it would be contrary to ethical standards for a physician to participate in such an action.

Passive euthanasia is a term sometimes applied to the withholding of treatment that might be life-saving. An example might be the decision not to use antibiotics when pneumonia develops in a terminally ill person. Under some circumstances, this may be an appropriate action.

Many difficult decisions are made in the care of a terminally ill person. In making such decisions, unique factors must be weighed. Although there are no rules, general principles of ethical behavior for physicians are formulated and revised from time to time by authoritative sources such as the American Medical Association and the American College of Physicians.

survived several decades ago. But this new ability brings with it complicated moral problems never encountered before.

For physicians, one of the biggest challenges is to continue to keep the dying person and members of the family informed of potential "heroic measures." For most people, the challenge is to discover, often by discussion with their physician, the personal impact of life-sustaining treatments. It is the well-informed patient who is most likely to exercise the right to participate in medical decision-making wisely.

DEATH

Of late we have developed the capacity to keep people alive in circumstances in which it was not possible in years past. Consequently, these new life-sustaining technologies have virtually transformed our definitions of death.

Only a few years ago, anyone who had lost consciousness, was unable to breathe, and had no heartbeat was considered to be dead. Today, however, in some instances life-support systems can revive such a person and, in part, continue to support or to replace some of these necessary functions. This remarkable ability to sustain life has brought with it certain ethical, legal, and medical problems.

With the advent of new technologies, physicians now are often able to maintain heart or lung function even when the entire brain ceases to function. However, most states recognize that a person is legally dead when either there is irreversible cessation of circulation and respiration or irreversible cessation and function of the entire brain including the brainstem (which controls breathing).

THE BUSINESS OF DEATH

Death is a legal event that calls for several formalities. Before a funeral can take place, you must secure a medical death certificate that shows the cause of death and formally registers the death. In some instances, the death may have to be investigated by the medical examiner or the coroner, and an autopsy may be required if the death resulted from an accident, is unexpected and unexplained, or is a suspected homicide or suicide (see Autopsies, page 1262). After these matters have been taken care of, the family usually arranges with a funeral home for any final arrangements.

The death certificate is a document that legally certifies the cause of death. It is completed by a licensed physician who usually has been in attendance at the time of death. If the physician has examined or treated the patient regularly or shortly prior to death, he or she generally is not obliged to examine the body before signing the certificate.

Sometimes, deaths must be investigated by the medical examiner or coroner. He or she will establish the cause of death and sign the certificate rather than the family physician or the physician in attendance.

The funeral director can be helpful in making virtually all of your other decisions concerning the funeral and burial arrangements. You may even want to make these arrangements before or during the time of the terminal illness.

ORGAN DONATION

As a result of technological advances, livers, corneas, hearts, kidneys, and a wide variety of other organs and tissues now can be transplanted. However, these operations are possible only when the needed organs are donated.

If you are willing to donate organs for use after your death, register as a designated organ donor. Arrangements can be made either by executing a living will or, in some states, by having a notation added to your driver's license. In some cases, the pain of an impending death may be eased by arranging for an organ donation that saves the life of another person—or even, in some cases, several persons.

Organ transplantation is less common at hospitals outside major medical centers. However, all hospitals are now required by law to inform relatives of potential donors about the United Network for Organ Sharing (UNOS), established in 1984 by the National Organ Transplantation Act. UNOS maintains an extensive computer network to ensure equitable distribution of donated organs.

If you would like to become an organ donor, discuss the procedure for UNOS registration with your physician or a local hospital administrator.

First, the funeral director will come to the home or hospital to collect the body and bring it to the funeral home. Later, members of the family will meet with the funeral director (usually at the funeral home) to discuss arrangements. Family members should make it quite clear how elaborate or simple the funeral will be and how the details are to be handled. Because these are emotionally difficult times and funeral arrangements can be expensive, you may want to seek help in making these decisions from someone who is not personally involved, such as a member of the clergy, a close friend, or an attorney.

Funeral and burial decisions include the type and location of the funeral service and the final disposition of remains (that is, burial or cremation). If the body is to be donated to research, the funeral director will deliver the body to the designated institution.

Funeral ceremonies can be held at the funeral home or a place of worship or both. If the family has no church affiliation, the funeral director can recommend a member of the clergy. In addition to the funeral service, there is often a brief committal or interment ceremony at the grave site.

Fees and terms of payment are made with the funeral director at the time funeral arrangements are agreed to. Usually, payment is not required in advance, but these expenses become the first legal obligation of the estate of the deceased.

After the funeral, a probate judge will designate the executor or personal representative of the estate. This is often a member of the family, the family attorney, or a close friend. The executor is responsible for the financial affairs of the deceased, which may include the funeral expenses.

After all payments are made, any remaining assets are distributed according to the deceased's will or the laws of the state in which the person lived. Specific procedures may vary from state to state.

AUTOPSIES

"Autopsy" comes from Greek words meaning to see with one's own eyes. It is a detailed examination of the body to determine the cause of death. It is performed by a medical specialist, a pathologist, who reports findings to the attending physician. Upon request, the attending physician will discuss findings with the family.

In the 1940s, an autopsy was performed after about half of all hospital deaths; but for several reasons it now occurs only 10 to 15 percent of the time. Some physicians believe that modern diagnostic measures performed during the life of the patient establish the cause of death so well that autopsy is superfluous. Others think that today's sophisticated technology has replaced autopsy as a way to help educate young physicians on understanding how a disease affects the human body. In many cases, families are reluctant to permit an autopsy. They believe the procedure to be degrading or that the deceased has "suffered enough."

All of these factors add up to a marked decline in autopsies. This is unfortunate because they still play an important role.

Benefits to the Surviving Family Members. *Hereditary Disorders.* Autopsy can reveal conditions that may affect offspring and siblings. If polycystic kidney disease (see page 886) is found, close relatives of childbearing age may want genetic counseling before they have children.

Emotional Security. Members of the family may feel guilty that they did not do more to prevent the death of a loved one. In the case of a fatal heart attack, family members might berate themselves for not insisting that the deceased take it easier. An autopsy may uncover that the person had a preexisting heart condition that could have taken his or her life at any time.

Insurance Settlements. Knowing the cause of death can help resolve disputes that affect the benefits survivors receive. In the case of a person with heart problems who dies in a fall, the insurance benefits may vary depending on whether death was accidental or the result of a long-term heart ailment.

Benefits to Medical Science. Much of what we know about diseases, including statistical information, was discovered and confirmed through autopsies.

Medical Research. Advances in medical knowledge depend in part on study of human tissue removed at autopsy. Pathological observations truly have taught us a great deal about human disease. For example, such data helped to confirm the association between cigarette smoking and lung cancer. Autopsies discovered the nature and character of hyperparathyroidism (see page 732), viral hepatitis (see page 650), and the effects of toxic chemicals and other industrial hazards on the lungs.

Quality Assurance. Physicians use autopsy data to assess their skills in diagnosis and treatment. Autopsy findings also help measure the overall quality of care in a hospital and community.

Vital Statistics. The way people die keeps changing. Deaths from infectious diseases are less common today, but degenerative illness takes a greater toll. Public health officials use information from autopsies to monitor these trends. Death statistics influence government spending for health care, the enactment of safety standards, and the design of medical equipment.

Emerging Illness. Early identification of AIDS, legionnaires' disease, toxic shock syndrome, and deaths from poisoned medicine all came from autopsy studies. So did knowledge of environmental hazards such as the link between asbestos exposure and cancer.

Arranging for an Autopsy. Autopsies usually are required by state or local law when death results from an accident, is unexpected or unexplained, or is a suspected homicide or suicide. Otherwise, autopsies cannot be performed unless the next of kin grants permission.

Read the consent form carefully. When you sign the consent form, you can order a limited autopsy that restricts the procedure to specific parts of the body. However, this may limit the amount of useful information and leave some questions unanswered. The procedure is usually handled discretely and in a confidential setting. Consent forms generally permit removal of internal organs and tissue.

There are many misconceptions about autopsy (and tissue removal). For example, a properly done autopsy will not disfigure the body, and at an open-casket funeral service observers will not be able to tell that an autopsy was performed. Autopsy does not prevent embalming of the body, nor need it delay the funeral. Also, the majority of religious faiths do not prohibit autopsy.

In most instances, when you grant permission for an elective autopsy, the bill will be paid by the hospital. Medicare will not pay for the procedure. When death occurs outside a hospital and family members request an autopsy, they usually must pay for it.

If you want an autopsy performed after your death, make a provision in your will that refers to this elective procedure. Then be sure to notify your loved ones of the provision, because the reading of your will may come days or weeks after burial. If you have prepared a letter of last instructions, your wishes concerning the autopsy should be addressed. Knowing your preference will spare your loved ones the burden of decision-making during a time of grief.

We believe that physicians should recommend this procedure more often and survivors should request it more frequently. Without the data gained from autopsies, family members may have to cope with unanswered questions. Furthermore, valuable information is lost on the possible cause and effectiveness of treatment of many diseases, especially cancer and heart disease. Through autopsy findings, the dead can help the living.

BEREAVEMENT

Bereavement is your response to a loss. It usually refers to subjective feelings after the loss of a loved one, usually through death, but also after the dissolution of a relationship. We experience many losses throughout our lives, and the longer we live, the more losses we suffer. Our ability to adapt to the stress of these losses in our lives often influences our health.

Grief and the effect it has on our daily routine of living can have an adverse effect on our health. Grief and the loneliness of bereavement can contribute to depression, excessive use of alcohol, and even suicide.

A death of a loved one is never easy to accept, and a sudden loss can be especially distressing. On the other hand, a long, terminal illness prior to the death of a loved one can be emotionally, physically, and financially draining. To protect yourself from a grief-related illness, you must take care of your health during your bereavement. Monitor any medical problems you had before the loss and seek professional help if new symptoms develop.

Although there are cultural norms for mourning, there is no single right way to grieve, nor is there a fixed timetable for coping with grief. Some people may recover from their grief in a month, but bereavement more often is measured in years rather than weeks or months.

During your bereavement, seek help from clergy, friends, and counselors. And remember, it is entirely appropriate—and essential for both your mental and your physical health—to express your emotions. Healthy mourning is the process by which we come to accept our losses, so we can go on with our lives. Covering your feelings either emotionally or with tranquilizers may prolong the mourning process.

People cope with their grief in different ways. This can be explained partly by differences in cultural heritage. Some people grieve openly, others privately. And it is not always evident that someone is grieving.

Nevertheless, grief needs to be expressed or processed one way or another so it can be healed. If it is not, symptoms such as erratic behavior or failing health may appear (see Grief Responses, page 1027).

CHILDREN AND DEATH

Death is a crisis which should be shared by everyone in the family. Children, however, are often overlooked in a time of grief and even denied the opportunity to grieve with other family members. Instead, they are offered a silence and secrecy that isolates them from the changing reality of the rest of the family.

Informing children that one of their parents is going to die, or that they themselves are dying, is difficult for everyone, including physicians and nurses. At the same time, children have a right to know about anything that affects them or their family. Not telling them is a breach of trust and, in truth, most children, like adults, have a sort of sixth-sense that alerts them when something is wrong either in themselves or in the family.

Why They Need To Know. Children are quite capable of sensing when a parent is seriously ill, but young children in particular usually cannot interpret their suspicions. They require help in integrating their observations into their day-to-day reality. If left alone with his or her suspicions, the small child may somehow feel responsible for the illness or death of a loved parent.

When informed of the facts in a manner they can grasp, most children have a remarkable capacity for dealing with truth. Even the weight of very sad truths is preferable to the anxiety of too much uncertainty. If you inform them, they will no longer feel cut off from that part of the family that "knows," you won't need be so secretive, and, finally, you may find that your young children can be a comfort to you and others. Instead of burdening them with the darkness of unspoken fears, discussing the issue of death and loss with them permits them to live more freely.

When and From Whom. Unless the dying parent feels that the child or children will become unduly upset were they to hear the news from him or her, it is generally best for the mother and father to together tell the child or children. This makes it more real for everyone. And your tears are not to be disguised. On the contrary, they give permission for the child to cry and to grieve with you. If you are not available or are unable to tell the child, ask a close relative who is loved by the child. Finally, the task can be left to a nurse or physician. However, they may be viewed by a young child as strangers and, thus, their word is subject to disbelief.

When should children be told? The simple answer is, as soon as possible. Children should be told about your health status immediately after the initial diagnosis. Also keep them informed as your treatment progresses and tell them how it is affecting your health. Any change they see in your appearance or disposition should not go unexplained. Children of different ages should probably be told individually; but after the initial disclosure, efforts should be made to make it a shared experience among all the children.

How Much. Children need to be told as much as they can understand. There is no single "right" way to tell children about death. They should be told what has happened and what will happen. Parents should be guided by their own styles and what they feel comfortable in discussing. At all times they should be told that no matter what the outcome the children will always be loved. They should be encouraged to ask questions, and these questions should be answered simply. Ask them how they feel because they may not ask about that which they fear. At no time should you lie, make promises you may not be able to keep, or be afraid to say, "I don't know."

Different Ages. The youngest children fear being separated from their parents. Being left in the care of strangers may suggest to them that they have been abandoned. During this period, discipline can be difficult because they may need to seek attention. If you suspend the normal rules of conduct, it may be alarming to them. It is more appropriate that you be reassuring of your love while expecting the same cooperation and good behavior from them. As the children come to learn what is happening, they should be assured that nothing they said or did, including any possible bad behavior, caused the illness or death.

Very young children (under age 3 years) believe that everything is possible; there are no limits to the powers of their parents. To preschoolers, death is still reversible; nothing is final. School-age children less than age 9 usually are able to understand that death is a biological event rather than someone appearing or disappearing in a supernatural form. But it is only at about age 9 that they are able to grasp that death is the final, universal end of human life.

Because school-age children can become overly concerned about details and misjudge their significance, guard against overcommunicating with specific data. Teachers and school counselors can be helpful in weighing the gravity and meaning of the information the children have learned from you.

After the Death of a Parent.   The death of a parent is a powerful event in the life of a child. Many children are able to resume a normal lifestyle in a matter of weeks and fully recover from the trauma. Others suffer the effects of an unhealed wound throughout their childhood and adult lives. Why one child is able to recover from the death of a parent and another is not depends in part on how the child is told and how the rest of the family accepts the loss.

Children initially may deny the reality of the death, express anger, or act out in rebellion. They also may repress any feelings associated with the loss. Children should be encouraged to share their emotional experience to whatever degree they can. Allow their friends to come into the home during the time of mourning. Their friends can be a comfort, and the friends' knowing about the death can deepen the reality of the loss for the child.

Keep in mind that children have a remarkable capacity for adjustment. The changes they see in themselves, in the world around them, and in those who surround them constitute an endless string of events to be absorbed. Whether the news is bad or good, children usually succeed in working their way through life's events—even those that seem quite unfair and unreasonable, like the death of a beloved parent. Rarely are there lasting scars.

CHAPTER 43

HOME CARE

For many people, the best place to get well is at home. During illness or recuperation from an injury, the sophisticated medical facilities and specialized professional staff of a hospital often are unnecessary. Similarly, services provided by a nursing home are not needed. As you recover from most illnesses or injuries, your own home is the most comfortable place to be.

Another major advantage of care at home is that it is less costly. Benefits can be paid for longer periods and be adjusted as needs vary and your condition stabilizes or improves.

When given their choice, people tend to feel better, eat better, and get well quicker at home. These reasons in large measure explain today's trend toward home care. In the following pages, the whys and wherefores of home care are introduced; matters such as planning a sickroom, caring for a child who is ill, and dealing with convalescence are addressed. The types of home health services that are available to assist with home care are described. Also covered are adult day-care, vocational rehabilitation programs, home health-care kits, and independent living centers.

HOME HEALTH SERVICES

Skilled medical, nursing, and rehabilitation services can be provided right in your home by outside organizations. These kinds of assistance are known collectively as home health services. Many organizations in the United States provide home health services, including several private companies such as the Visiting Nurse Association (which began in the 19th century), hospitals, nursing homes, community social service agencies, and city and county health departments.

Services available to you depend on your needs and the particular program or programs that exist in your area. Agencies that offer skilled nursing care can provide a nurse to monitor your health status, give injections, change bandages, and perform other nursing tasks. Sometimes various forms of therapy are also available in the home, including physical, occupational, speech, hearing, and respiratory therapies. Most agencies provide social workers and some even have dental care, laboratory testing, and pharmacists. Meals and housekeeping services are available.

Home-care agencies that offer such skilled nursing, therapeutic, and supplemental services will do so under the direction of your physician. A medically trained case worker or case manager may be responsible for coordinating the care given to you or the individual in need of the help.

Many organizations offer supportive rather than skilled services. With these, a home aide regularly spends time in the home, perhaps every day, although in some cases alternate days or even once a week is sufficient. The aide may help with basic tasks such as bathing, dressing, shopping, cooking, eating, and doing housekeeping chores. A home aide also can handle certain simple nursing tasks, such as taking a temperature. For many people, help with some everyday activities can make it possible to continue to live independently at home rather than in a nursing home.

Since the 1960s, a home service that has improved the lives of countless elderly people is Meals-on-Wheels. Local Meals-on-Wheels services often are administered through senior citizens' centers. In many communities, this service delivers one hot, nutritional meal a day at a low cost, either 5 or 7 days a week. Meals-on-Wheels is a great help to people who find it difficult to prepare a balanced meal. Some communities also have other nutrition services such as group dining for the elderly.

SOURCES OF HELP FOR HOME CARE

To find out which services are available where you live, ask a hospital dismissal planner, hospital-based social worker, local or county health department, senior citizens' center, or your physician. In addition, churches, synagogues, welfare departments, and charitable organizations such as the United Way often can provide information on services available. You can also look in the Yellow Pages under "Nurses" or "Home Health Agencies."

If you live in an area that has multiple home care alternatives, compare the services offered. Important points to determine are whether your insurer approves the agency, whether the services match your present and future needs, the amount of medical or skilled supervision that the agency offers, which hours a day or week are covered, and whether replacement aides are available to fill in when regularly assigned individuals cannot come. Speak with people who have actually used the service to get their opinion.

Medicare, Medicaid, private insurance, and other programs often pay for home health services, although usually with limitations (see Reimbursement for Home Health Services, below). A prescreening evaluation may be required.

REIMBURSEMENT FOR HOME HEALTH SERVICES

Home health services are paid for in five main ways: by Medicare; Medicaid; insurance carriers; health maintenance organizations; or the person being cared for (or the family), sometimes on a sliding-fee scale.

Medicare. Medicare covers people age 65 years or older as well as some disabled people. Medicare pays for some home health services, but not all. Visits by nurses or by physical, speech, or other therapists may be covered. The services of someone to help with chores around the house and with bathing and dressing generally are not covered. However, personal care services such as bathing and dressing can be covered by Medicare if skilled services such as nursing, speech, or other therapy are being provided. For more information, contact your local Social Security Administration office or senior citizens' center.

Medicaid. Medicaid covers people of all ages with low incomes, but coverage varies drastically from state to state. Some home health services may be covered in your state but, again, inquire at your local social services, welfare, or Social Security Administration office.

Private Insurance Carriers. Private insurance policies may pay for some home health services. Find out from the person who handles benefits at your place of employment, from your insurance agent, or directly from the insurance company.

Other Sources. In addition to the medical insurance your company provides or that you buy for yourself, do not overlook two other possible sources of reimbursement: automobile insurance policies (if you were injured in an automobile accident) and workmen's compensation insurance (if you were injured on the job).

Health Maintenance Organizations. Health maintenance organizations (HMOs) generally offer some home care on a limited basis. Coverage will vary depending on the rules of the particular organization. Ask an administrator at your HMO (see also page 1200).

Direct Payment. Of course, home health services also can be paid for directly. Most nonprofit and government-aided home health care organizations, when their costs are not completely covered by the sources mentioned above, bill for their services on a sliding-fee scale based on ability to pay. For-profit private agencies generally do not use a sliding-fee scale.

Understand Your Coverage. The above-listed sources may provide partial or total reimbursement for home health services. However, determining exactly what coverage a particular source offers may not be as easy as it should be.

Begin by reading the insurance policy yourself (not merely a brochure summarizing the benefits). Then speak to a knowledgeable person in the organization. Persist until you are able to determine exactly what the benefits are. Home health services may be referred to under a different name or under a broader category, so even if it appears at first that home care services are not covered, be sure you read the fine print or have it explained to you.

Regardless of the type of coverage, there will be limits, as with any insurance policy. In the case of home health services, limits usually are placed on the types of services (for example, skilled nursing), the length of visits (the number of hours), and the number of visits (for example, per week, per year, or for the life of the policy).

EQUIPMENT NEEDS

If you are cared for at home, you may require or benefit from special equipment, such as a wheelchair, walker, or even a hospital bed. Drugstores and medical supply houses rent, sell, and service such items.

For expensive equipment, renting is a money-saving alternative because the need for the equipment may be temporary. Drugstores and medical supply houses also stock a range of other sickroom supplies useful in home care.

Alternatively, the American Cancer Society, the Arthritis Foundation, the Easter Seal Society, the American Diabetes Association, and other comparable organizations sometimes are able to lend medical and nursing equipment.

Talk to your physical therapist, hospital discharge planner, or physician; they may be aware of wholesale distributors or other sources of these goods at reasonable prices. Do not hesitate to shop around. Even if you are buying only medication, the monthly costs can be high, and the markup may vary greatly.

HOME HEALTH CARE

At some point, everyone needs home care. For most of us, a childhood illness meant staying home and being nursed back to health. As adults, when sick with the flu or a cold, we recover at home, ideally with bed rest. Home care for a more serious or prolonged illness or during a period of recovery from an injury or stroke is essentially a variation on the same, familiar theme.

In the case of the elderly, home care may be one alternative to a nursing home; other possibilities include adult day-care, medical day-care, and day hospitals. Certain developments and retirement communities may provide assisted living, transitional care, and respite care. (These topics are discussed later in this chapter; see also Community Services, page 245.)

The requirements of the person being cared for at home vary with his or her daily activities, the available services, and the other care-givers in the household. Most often, total responsibility falls on the shoulders of one person; sometimes the burden is simply too much for the health and well-being of that individual. Care-givers also need a break, and many agencies can provide temporary, around-the-clock assistance if there is a mechanism for payment. Home care should lie within the limits of a family's physical, emotional, and financial resources.

THE ROOM

Locate the room used for home health care on the ground floor and near a bathroom. The reasons are safety and to save the person requiring home care the risk (and energy drain) of having to negotiate stairs. In addition, the care-giver is also saved the time and trouble of trips up and down the stairs many times a day.

If possible, have the person being cared for sleep in the same bed used before the illness: recovery implies a return to normality. Sometimes a small thing such as sleeping in one's own bed offers a psychological lift. If falling out of bed is a possibility, a guardrail can be added.

If a special bed is required, hospital beds can be rented or purchased from a medical supply house or drugstore. They have the advantages of being adjustable and sufficiently high to make care somewhat easier. However, a hospital bed has the marked disadvantage of giving a familiar room a "hospital look," which may have a negative impact on the person being cared for.

Unless the person being cared for has very serious disabilities, not only the bedroom but also other rooms may need some changes. A recliner or a suitable ordinary chair will be used when the person is out of bed. It may be necessary to try out more than one chair or type of recliner to find one that suits the energy level and physical abilities of the individual.

Arrange the bedroom or the parts of the house where the person will spend the most time for maximal comfort and convenience. A bedside table or the type of table that fits over the bed is a must.

Because a person's quality of life and recovery are linked to one's sense of well-being, a feeling of independence should be provided. If the person values familiar objects, place them in his or her room, ideally in their usual places. Items of convenience—remote control for the television, a telephone, books and magazines, tissues, wastebasket—should be within reach of the person whose mobility is limited. Some items might be kept in a bedside caddy that fastens onto the side of the bed.

At the same time, make sure that the bed, table, and other areas are easily accessible to care-givers. Remove objects that can be readily tripped over, such as throw rugs or superfluous furniture.

Alternatively, encouraging mobility may be a part of the recovery process. Do not make life too easy for the person who should be gaining strength and independence. One way to encourage someone to get out of a bed that has been rendered perhaps too comfortable is to locate some items of interest—such as magazines, the television, or the recliner—across the room or in a different room.

MEDICATIONS

One of the main functions of a nurse in a hospital is to give the correct medications at the proper times. At home, this becomes the responsibility of the care-giver.

Make sure that medicines are given exactly as your physician prescribes, both in dose and frequency. Know medications by their dosage (usually in milligrams) as well as by their color and shape. Always be alert to the possibility of side effects. The physician may tell you which side effects might be expected. Sometimes multiple medications interact in ways the physician did not anticipate. If the person cared for develops unexpected, new, or worsening symptoms, inform the physician.

MAKING THE BED

Because the bed will be a place where a great deal of time is spent, change the sheets, covers, and pillowcases frequently. Some commonsense rules are as follows.

If the person is in bed all the time, the bed needs to be made every morning and evening.

Tuck in the sheets. Cotton sheets are preferable to synthetic sheets because they absorb moisture.

An old mattress that slopes to the side can present a hazard for falling while getting in and out of bed. Replace it with a firmer new one or put a bed board beneath it.

The person in bed probably will prefer more than one pillow, arranged so that the head and shoulders are supported. Occasionally turning the pillows over provides a thoughtful touch of comfort.

Use props and wedges to help someone sit up in bed. Place a cushion between the feet and the board at the foot of the bed to prevent discomfort from pressure in the raised or sitting position.

FEEDING

Meals are a social activity and key source of pleasure for someone who must spend a great deal of time in bed. Follow diet instructions given by your physician, nutritional therapist, or nurse. Vary the diet as much as possible, and include foods the person especially enjoys. Enhance the pleasure of mealtime with appropriate treats, careful food preparation, and attractive presentation.

Many people confined to their beds can still feed themselves from a tray beside the bed or from an over-the-bed table. Use bendable straws for the beverages. If the person cannot eat alone and spoon-feeding is necessary, you may find that pureed and finely cut foods are the easiest for you or another care-giver to feed and for the sick person to eat. Test foods to be sure that they are not too hot. To keep them warm, insulated dishes or single-serving vacuum containers are available.

If you encounter difficulties with feeding or if the person being cared for does not eat the food or loses weight, report these problems to the physician or visiting nurse.

BATHING

Bathing presents a special challenge in home care. Bathing is a personal activity that people generally prefer doing alone. To help retain as much privacy as possible, helpful bathing products may be rented or purchased.

Often all that is required is a tub bench (a special seat that runs across the bathtub) or a grabrail mounted on the wall near the tub. With such aids, the person with impaired balance or limited mobility may be able to get safely in and out of the tub or shower alone. Place a nonslip rubber mat or adhesive strips on the tub bottom; make sure that there is no towel or mat on the floor that the person can slip on.

In considering bathroom safety, remember that another bathroom danger is burns. Disabled people may find themselves trapped in a running bath or shower, unable to move away from water that has suddenly turned scalding hot (or, for that matter, icy cold). Faucets are available (and are required by law in new construction in some states) that automatically turn off when a preset temperature is exceeded. The temperature of the hot water can be adjusted at the hot water tank. Set the temperature no higher than is necessary for washing dishes or clothes.

A bell or cordless intercom in the bathroom is a good idea so a person can summon help if it is needed.

For the person who is unable to leave the bed to bathe, a sponge bath can be given in the bed. When administering a sponge bath to a bed-bound person, the following suggestions may make the task easier.

1. Place a disposable or rubber pad under the person.
2. Uncover and wash a small part of the body at a time, to avoid chilling.
3. Use comfortably warm water. Place a towel between the part of the body being washed and the bed.
4. Use soap sparingly, mainly on the face, under the arms, and for the genital area. Remember, soap is an irritant if it is not rinsed off.
5. When drying, pat with the towel rather than rubbing. (Rubbing can encourage bedsores.)

BEDPANS AND BED URINALS

The person unable to leave the bed requires a bedpan or (for men) bed urinal. A few simple considerations can make their use a little easier.

Keep the pan or urinal in a warm place; a cold container can be a disagreeable shock.

When positioning the pan for use, maneuver it under the buttocks. If the person cannot sit in bed, roll the person to the side, slide the pan under (pressing it down into the mattress as far as possible), and roll the person back.

Privacy is as important—perhaps more so—to the bed-bound person as to the rest of us, so provide as much as possible. Leave the room or draw a curtain while the person is actually using the bedpan. Be patient, making sure to allow the person enough time.

Many people are able to get up out of bed but are unable to make the trip to the bathroom, particularly if the bathroom is a long walk or a flight of stairs away. In such cases, a commode may be the solution. A commode is simply a chair with a toilet-like attachment under the bottom, which can be removed for easy cleaning. An apparatus designed to assist in lifting a person to reach the commode is available.

If the person can reach the bathroom, the toilet may require some modification for safe use. A grabrail on the wall near the toilet, or freestanding rails on either side of the toilet, can be installed to enable many people to raise and lower themselves safely. If the toilet is too low, special seats that raise the height are available.

BEDSORES

Bedsores, also known as pressure sores or decubitus ulcers, sometimes develop on weight-bearing parts of the body, especially where the bones are near the skin (in particular, the hips, shoulder blades, elbows, base of the spine, knees, ankles, and heels). In some individuals, just a few hours of constant pressure can be enough to initiate a bedsore.

A bedsore begins as a reddened, sensitive patch of skin and progresses to become a sore or ulcer. It may or may not be painful. Treatment of a bedsore requires the attention of a nurse or physician, and healing may take a long time. Prevention is therefore the best approach.

Bedsores are prevented by frequent positioning: be sure the bedridden person moves himself or herself regularly to keep pressure from building on one spot. If the person cannot move alone, help him or her to move.

Change position at least every 2 hours. Use of pillows or foam wedges is the easiest way to shift the load of a heavy or paralyzed individual.

Splints placed at pressure points are also helpful. Special anatomically shaped cushions, such as those used in wheelchairs, can be placed in the bed to distribute weight more evenly and so help keep pressure from building in one spot. Also helpful are synthetic sheepskin bed pads, air mattresses, and "egg-crate" pads (foam padding resembling the cardboard packaging in which eggs are traditionally sold). Specially designed pads for heels and elbows are also available. You can rent bed cradles from medical supply houses; these can raise the weight of covers off the body and create a tent-like structure.

Changes in bedding, a balanced diet, and exercise are important for avoiding bedsores. Even the bed-bound person can exercise; if the person cannot do it alone, then movement of the joints by others will help prevent bedsores.

VOMITING

If the person is liable to vomit, keep a bowl within easy reach. Some people can handle vomiting on their own and prefer to be left alone until they are done. Others feel comforted with someone nearby. In either case, offer water to rinse out the person's mouth afterward, and sponge off his or her face.

Avoid solid food after a vomiting episode. Encourage liquids to replace lost body fluids. The nurse or physician can advise on which liquids are best. Tea, diluted fruit juice, water, chicken broth, and gelatin are among the liquids most easily tolerated. If the vomiting is a new symptom, inform your physician.

CARING FOR SICK CHILDREN

Although the symptoms of a child's illness can be dramatic—high fevers, for example—recovery is usually easier and quicker than for adults. However, children need a great deal more reassurance and companionship during illness than adults, so although the nursing experience is likely to be shorter, it can be more demanding.

Giving Medicine. Many children resist taking medication. To sidestep such resistance, approach this task in a natural, matter-of-fact way. Apprehension on your part or the expectation of resistance can often become a self-fulfilling prophecy.

Most medications can be mixed with food or liquids. Check with your physician or your pharmacist about whether the medication is to be taken on an empty stomach; even then it may be acceptable to take it with a small amount of food. Juices and pop, applesauce, and ice cream with chocolate sauce work well to disguise the taste of many medications.

Do not try to get your child to take medication by promising a treat or, worse, telling him or her that the medication is candy. It is essential that all children make a clear distinction between medicine and candy and learn to take all medications while supervised by an adult.

Medications are generally available in a liquid suspension for younger children. Most are quite palatable. A graduated syringe is available from your pharmacist. This pump device allows the proper amount of medication to be placed in the back corner of your child's mouth.

It is important to give medications exactly as prescribed, in both the correct dose and at the correct interval. Give medications at evenly spaced intervals throughout the day rather than giving the dosages in a shorter period of time. Do not stop giving your child medication when he or she begins to show signs of improvement unless specifically instructed to do so. Moreover, do not attempt to prescribe for yourself or your child different doses or remnants of old prescriptions.

Fevers. Sudden occurrence of fever usually means that an infection has developed. Viral infections, strep throat (see page 1295), and ear infections (see Acute Ear Infection, page 680) are the most common causes of fever in children. The more serious illnesses can, of course, cause fever also, but fortunately they are not common.

A temperature greater than 99.5°F (37.5°C) by mouth or more than 100.5°F (38°C) by rectum is considered a fever. The only difference in thermometers is the tip; always use a round-bulb thermometer for taking a rectal temperature. Your physician or nurse can help you learn how to read a thermometer (see How To Take a Temperature and How To Read A Thermometer, page 859).

Children tolerate most fevers quite well. Fevers often provoke far more anxiety than they deserve. Among parents, a common concern is that there is some critical level of fever that can cause convulsions (see Febrile Seizures, page 73) or brain damage. This is not the case.

Less than 5 percent of all children are prone to febrile seizures. These seizures are more closely related to how rapidly the fever rises than to any critical level. Although frightening, children with febrile seizures rarely have long-term ill effects. Moreover, high fever by itself does not cause brain damage.

Contact your physician if your child's fever is accompanied by 1) considerable listlessness, irritability, or severe headache, 2) persistent vomiting or stomachache, or 3) a bulging of the soft spot (fontanelle) on the scalp of an infant. Also call your physician if the fever occurs during the first few weeks of life or if there is high fever that is not responding to acetaminophen. Be guided more by how your child is acting rather than by any particular temperature.

Lowering fevers unnecessarily may prolong the course of a child's illness. If your child is very uncomfortable, however, you can do the following.

1. Let heat escape. Do not bundle your child up.
2. Provide plenty of liquids to drink.
3. Give acetaminophen in the recommended dosage. This is available in liquid, chewable, and suppository forms. Physicians no longer recommend routine use of aspirin for treating fever in children because of the risk of Reye's syndrome (see Reye's Syndrome, page 531).
4. If necessary, you can sponge your child with warm (tepid) water. Do not allow your child to become chilled.

A high fever is not necessarily a cause for alarm. If in doubt, check with your physician. Alternatively, the absence of a high fever does not mean an ailing child does not require medical care. If your child shows symptoms that alarm you at any time, contact your physician.

Feeding.　Follow your physician's instructions on what to feed your child. These instructions will vary depending on the illness. If the child's symptoms include fever, vomiting, or diarrhea, provide plenty of liquids. Relax household rules such as a restriction on soda pop if making it available helps get sufficient liquid into your child. When vomiting or diarrhea is present, restrict the diet as instructed by your child's physician. In these circumstances, sugar-containing sodas often may be preferable to the sugar-free varieties.

If your child's physician has not specified a particular diet, relaxing usual dietary restrictions also may help encourage your child to eat.

Getting Up.　When your child feels well enough, allow him or her to get out of bed. Only in rare cases will physicians instruct otherwise. During a convalescent period, your child may be out of bed part of the time and back in bed when tired. Children are often better than adults at letting their physical condition guide them in how much they can manage.

Long-Term Convalescence.　Long-term care of a child with a disease or injury follows the same procedures as used for an adult (described earlier in the chapter). The principal difference with children is that keeping them busy and occupied (with toys, reading, and suitable television programs) requires more effort on the part of the caregiver.

Unless your child has a contagious disease, you may want to arrange for occasional visits from other children for prescribed periods that suit the convalescent child's energy level, interests, and attention span. Encourage your child to participate in the normal activities of the home as much as possible.

RETURNING TO INDEPENDENCE

Home care is not static. Whether the care at home follows dismissal from a hospital or the occurrence of an illness or disability that is treated at home from the start, the ultimate aim of convalescence is a return to one's former status.

Convalescence presents special challenges for the care-giver. There are common pitfalls to avoid. For example, avoid becoming so bound up in the job of delivering care or coordinating home health services that you forget the ultimate goal: a return to independence.

Sometimes the person being cared for becomes needlessly accustomed to being waited on. This pattern can prolong care beyond what the condition warrants. Like a spoiled child, the ill or injured person—whether child or adult, male or female—can consciously or unconsciously perpetuate the period of care. A return to normal activities can be retarded or even put off altogether.

If you are the patient, do not confine yourself to bed. Getting out of bed and moving about is an important aspect of home care unless your physician recommends otherwise. As you remain confined to bed, your unused muscles weaken and bone loss accelerates (see Osteoporosis, page 982). The longer the time spent in bed, the more difficult the regaining of mobility becomes.

Moreover, some potentially fatal infections and conditions, such as pneumonia (see page 917), thrombophlebitis (see page 838), and pulmonary embolisms (see Pulmonary Embolism, page 947), are more likely to develop in persons who are confined to bed.

Approach getting up for the first few times carefully and gradually. Your blood pressure and balance need to adjust. Sit on the edge of the bed a few minutes before trying to stand up. Standing or even sitting up the first few times may make you feel dizzy and weak. Next, take a short, slow trip from your bed to a recliner or chair. Have someone assist you if you are unsteady. As your strength increases and you regain the ability to move about, the trips can become longer, with less assistance required.

A physical or occupational therapist (or both) can be useful during convalescence. Physical therapists recommend exercises

ADULT DAY-CARE

An important consideration of home care is the person providing the care. Caring for an injured or disabled person over a long period can be extremely taxing. In a large family in which some family members spend significant amounts of time at home and can share the care-giving responsibility, the burden will be felt the least. But if care is being provided by one person, who may very well have to work, be in poor health, or in any case have his or her own life to lead, home care can be an unacceptable burden.

Adult day-care can offer an alternative. It is a service whereby someone who cannot be left alone is looked after in a supervised setting during the day. Adult day-care is suitable for the person who is disabled, is recuperating, or requires help performing everyday activities and who is able to leave the home. Depending on the program, people can attend for part

of the day for one, two, or more days a week. Transportation to and from the day-care center often can be arranged.

At the day-care center, the person has an opportunity to socialize with others and to read or watch television. A midday meal is served. Some centers arrange formal activities.

A variant of the adult day-care center is the medical day-care center. Here, medical and nursing attention are provided in addition to the supervision, social activities, and food. The person can visit the facility on an as-needed basis for some particular medical procedure, nursing care, or a type of therapy that is required. Such a visit might be necessary once or twice a week or every day.

Medical day-care is often located in a hospital or a skilled nursing home, but you return home every night.

Similarly, some communities offer day-care specifically aimed at individuals with mental illnesses or disabilities. At such a center, psychological services as well as

supervision and activities are offered.

The advantage of adult or medical day-care is an easing of the burden for the care-giver. It provides a chance to work, run errands, pursue interests, or simply relax. In addition, skilled medical, nursing, or mental health services may be available that cannot be so readily obtained at home.

The person requiring care may also benefit from a change of scene and care-givers. Alternatively, however, the person may find the day-care center a dreary and unpleasant place to spend time. Check the facility yourself for your impression of the quality of care and the atmosphere.

Your hospital dismissal planner, physician, visiting nurse, or social worker should be able to tell you whether your community has facilities for adult day-care. Adult day-care also may be offered by community health centers, psychiatric facilities, the Salvation Army, and other service organizations. (For further discussions of other alternatives, see page 245.)

aimed at specific disabilities as well as at general recovery. Physical therapists also can offer massage, ultrasound therapy, and other healing treatments. Occupational therapists help you to relearn particular skills useful in daily living, how to use prostheses or mechanical devices, and how to make modifications in your home environment to promote independence.

Other types of therapists can help you recover from a specific illness. If you have suffered a stroke (see Stroke, page 508), a speech therapist may help you regain impaired language skills. Arrangements can be made for a home program. Talk to the coordinating home health service organization or individual. Therapists are also available in clinics, hospital outpatient departments, and private practice.

Some organizations also offer vocational rehabilitation and job placement. (See Rehabilitation Centers, page 1205.)

The recovery period is a dynamic time. As people come a few steps nearer to independence, they may become harder to handle. Some are eager to resume normal activities all at once, thinking they are completely recovered when in fact they are only on the way to recovery. Others are disappointed at their rate of recovery or at the discovery that they are not well "all at once." These attitudes can lead to relapses, setbacks, and depression.

The physician, therapist, or visiting nurse can help guide both care-giver and patient as to what degree of recovery might be reasonably expected within a particular time. You must remember that as a care-giver your responsibilities involve not only helping the person's body or mind to recover its health. You also need to take an active role in helping the patient recover self-confidence and good spirits, an equally important but less quantifiable task.

REHABILITATION PROGRAMS

Specialized programs exist for rehabilitation after certain acute illnesses. Depending on the type and severity of the illness or injury, rehabilitation may involve more than one step. If you have had a stroke, for example, rehabilitation will begin with physical and speech therapy soon after the stroke. If you have lost a limb through injury or cancer, physical therapists will help you learn how to use an artificial limb.

A second step may involve the services of another type of specialist, the occupational therapist. The word "occupation" in the title is misleading because occupational therapy is not aimed at helping carry out a particular job but at regaining the ability to handle everyday tasks. The occupational therapist visits your home and takes careful stock of what you can and cannot do and of barriers and obstacles to everyday tasks in your home. The therapist might suggest rearranging furniture, adding a wheelchair ramp, and the like. Aids to bathing and grooming may

be recommended. The occupational therapist promotes a return to one's previous lifestyle.

In addition, an occupational therapist tries to identify, and if necessary reawaken, an interest in hobbies or going places or whatever might help rekindle optimism and an active interest in life—which is vital to regaining or maintaining health. Educating care-givers about when to help and when to let someone do things alone is another function.

A specialized step beyond physical and occupational therapy is vocational rehabilitation. Various organizations promote a return to the work force for people with a disability or illness that does not affect their ability to work but might make them appear to others as less than able (or, initially, to themselves). Vocational rehabilitation programs offer specific job training to overcome a handicap. Many such programs will help with job placements.

HOME MEDICAL TESTING KITS

Your pharmacy or drugstore has a selection of kits that can be used to perform medical

tests at home, without the involvement of a physician or health-care professional. The types of kits available at present include the following:

1. Pregnancy tests to determine whether you are pregnant;
2. Ovulation prediction tests to help determine the best time for intercourse that may lead to conception;
3. Sugar tests, of either urine or blood, to determine whether diabetes is present;
4. Other urine tests, such as for excess protein (which may signal a kidney problem);
5. Tests to detect hidden blood in the stool, which may indicate a tumor in the colon.

Like most tests in a medical laboratory, home tests use urine, blood, or stool. The kits are relatively inexpensive. The containers, test strips, and other paraphernalia contained in the kit are thrown away after use. Some kits contain enough supplies to perform the test more than once.

The advantage of doing a test with a kit is convenience and a reduced cost over having a medical laboratory perform the test. However, there are several disadvantages.

First, there is the risk of simply doing the test wrong—and therefore getting a misleading result. The instructions contained in the kit have to be followed exactly or the test will not work properly. A physician or health-care professional in a medical laboratory is less likely to make a mistake because he or she has more expertise and experience and better equipment.

Second, medical tests do not always work right. This is true for tests done at home and for tests performed in a medical laboratory. A certain percentage of tests have results that suggest that something is true when it is not (false positive). For example, a false-positive test result would indicate that you do have hidden blood in the stool when in fact you do not, or that you are pregnant when you are not.

Alternatively, a certain percentage of test results indicate that something is not true when it is (false negative). For example, a false-negative test result would indicate that your blood glucose concentration is normal when it is not, or that you are not pregnant when you are. A physician is in a better position to judge false-negative and false-positive test results based on other medical evidence, training, and experience.

Third, you may interpret the result incorrectly. Changes in the appearance of the test, such as the color, may be confusing.

Finally, after performing the test, it is often very difficult to decide what to do next. For example, if you are certain there is blood in your stool but the test indicates otherwise, should you still see your physician?

In fact, it is often necessary to see your physician or have the test repeated by a medical laboratory no matter what the result, so you end up duplicating the expense. Use these home testing kits with caution: they are not a substitute for appropriate medical care, especially when you think you may be at risk of a serious medical condition.

INDEPENDENT LIVING CENTERS

There are alternatives to home care that the care recipient may find less restrictive and more conducive to an independent, healthy life. Independent living centers are one such alternative. These are specially designed for people who can function basically on their own but may need a little help.

An independent living center contains separate living quarters for each person, couple, or family. The center offers some services that are shared by all—usually meal preparation and monitoring. Meals are typically served in a common area that doubles as, or is near to, a central room for socializa-

tion and meetings. If residents want to, they can prepare their own meals in their own kitchens.

Monitoring is handled in various ways, such as an alarm in each apartment that is connected to a control desk or nursing station that may be able to offer paramedical assistance. The living center also may incorporate elements of assistance into its architectural design, such as guardrails in bathrooms and in common hallways, wheelchair ramps, conveniently located kitchen cupboards, and easy-to-use appliance controls.

GROUP HOMES FOR THE MENTALLY RETARDED AND MENTALLY ILL

People with mental or emotional handicaps present a special challenge in home care. For example, a young mentally retarded man who is a rational, cheerful, capable person may need a little help with some daily activities.

Ideally, these individuals would be cared for at home in a family setting in which one or more family members were at home rather than out to work and were physically and mentally alert themselves. "Cared for" may even be a misnomer: for example, an elderly woman may only need someone to tell her when to take her pills, or the young man described above may need someone to tell him when it is time to wash his hair and to suggest activities when he is bored. This is not necessarily intensive or continuous care, nor is it always burdensome.

Group homes for the mentally retarded and mentally ill offer such care when there is no family to provide it. In the best of these homes, the environment is like a "home." Residents have some independence in their living arrangements, such as their own rooms with their personal belongings, but they receive care by aides to help carry out grooming and daily activities and by mental health professionals to help in the treatment of, or rehabilitation from, their mental problems. Such group homes are a type of foster care in which all the residents have mental rather than physical problems. This is different from the typical nursing home or foster home, which has a population of people with both physical and mental difficulties.

Although an independent living center does not offer nursing care, residents can individually arrange for such care from the various home health service agencies that are available through the center or from other community sources.

Retirement communities are the most familiar type of independent living center. These are common in areas with large populations of retired people, such as Florida and Arizona, but they can be found throughout the country. The living standards offered, and the costs, vary greatly. Some centers receive government funding and charge rent to residents on a sliding-fee scale based on the ability to pay. As a rule, this type of center has a lengthy waiting list and demands a significant amount of independence. Senior high-rise centers usually do not provide meals.

Another type of living alternative is offered by nonmedical residential institutions. Accommodations range from independent apartments at one extreme to shared rooms at the other. In addition to providing meals and monitoring, such institutions offer help with personal care, housekeeping, and shopping. Some offer continuous personal and nursing care, and there is little if any distinction between these institutions and nursing homes.

Foster homes also offer what amounts to home care in a group setting. Often these are called "board-and-care" homes. Residents may, for example, have their own rooms but share common areas for meals and socializing. Nursing care, continuous or intermittent, may be offered in a foster home.

APPENDICES

CONTENTS

APPENDIX I

MEDICAL TESTS

APPENDIX CONTENTS

THE KINDS OF DIAGNOSTIC TESTS

To reach a diagnosis, your physician requires information. Your medical history, the symptoms you report, and the physical examination he or she conducts are ways your physician obtains this information.

In addition, your physician will order diagnostic tests to obtain more information about you. In the pages that follow, we describe various medical tests—blood tests, tissue sample tests (biopsies), imaging tests (in which x-ray or other technologies are used to create an image of an area within your body)—and other tests as well.

The diverse kinds of diagnostic tests can be divided into two broad categories: invasive and noninvasive.

Invasive tests require direct "invasion" of the interior of your body; noninvasive tests are done outside your body. Invasive tests are performed to get a better view of your internal organs or to remove tissue (biopsy) for study. Noninvasive tests measure function or produce an indirect view of the inside of your body, as in many x-ray procedures.

The value of diagnostic testing depends on factors such as need, what can be reasonably discovered, and risks posed, if any. Before undergoing any test that is not routine, understand the procedure, risks, possible alternatives to the tests, and anticipated benefits.

BLOOD TESTS

Blood tests are used to rule out or to help diagnose disease. Routine blood tests can detect the possible presence of a wide variety of conditions including various types of anemia, infections, and leukemia, to name only a few.

The drawing of a small amount of blood into a vial usually takes only a few seconds and can be done in a laboratory, in your physician's office, or in a hospital. Special preparations are not necessary. (Some tests require overnight fasting; others require no fasting at all. Follow your physician's instructions.)

Blood can be drawn from many sites. If only a drop or two is necessary, the blood usually is drawn from a fingertip and is placed in a small container called a capillary pipette.

If more than a drop of blood is required, the person drawing it will select a vein, cleanse the skin over it with alcohol, and then gently insert a thin needle. Blood will pass through the needle into an attached sterile syringe. Then the needle is withdrawn and the puncture wound can be wiped again with an antiseptic.

In most routine examinations, blood testing includes a complete blood cell count (CBC), a chemistry group, and blood lipids. Literally hundreds of other blood tests can be obtained. Common ones include thyroid

studies (to determine the output of the thyroid gland) and coagulation studies (to determine the rate at which the blood thickens or clots). Your physician will choose the most appropriate tests for you.

Below we describe in more detail some of the principal types of blood tests.

COMPLETE BLOOD CELL COUNT (CBC)

The CBC is the most common blood test of all. It usually is part of a complete health checkup. The term "count" refers to the counting of each type of blood cell in a given volume of your blood.

The CBC measures the amount of hemoglobin, the percentage of the sample that is composed of red blood cells (hematocrit), the number and kinds of white blood cells, and the number of platelets. Like routine urinalysis, this test can signal the possible presence of a wide variety of conditions including various types of anemia, infections, and leukemia.

BLOOD CHEMISTRY GROUP

Often automated, the blood chemistry group tests may include an analysis of electrolytes (sodium, potassium, chloride, and phosphorus) and glucose (blood sugar), a series of liver function tests (including studies for bilirubin), and tests for uric acid, creatinine (a kidney function test), and albumin (a major protein in the blood). Sometimes, different combinations of tests are used.

LIPIDS

Another common blood test is for lipids. This test measures the blood level of fats including total cholesterol, high density lipoprotein (HDL) cholesterol, and triglycerides, all of which may be indicators of risk for coronary artery disease (see What Do Measurements of Blood Fats Mean?, page 789).

ERYTHROCYTE SEDIMENTATION RATE

This blood test, also called sed rate or ESR, determines the rate at which red blood cells settle to the bottom of a container. If the cells settle faster than normal, this can suggest an infection, anemia, inflammation, rheumatoid arthritis, rheumatic fever, or one of several types of cancer.

COAGULATION TESTS

Coagulation tests detect abnormal levels of substances in your blood that control the speed at which your blood clots. For example, tests of the partial thromboplastin time (PTT) and prothrombin time (PT) can help identify blood clotting diseases and liver diseases and are commonly used in monitoring patients taking blood thinning medications (anticoagulants).

DRUG TESTS

It often is helpful to know the amount of a drug in the blood (in general or at a specific time), such as the heart drug digoxin (Lanoxin). Drug tests (there are many) can reveal this information precisely.

ENZYME TESTS

Your blood can be tested for levels of enzymes that may indicate damage to certain organs such as the liver, pancreas, or heart. For example, certain enzymes are normally found in large amounts within liver cells but in small amounts in the blood. When large amounts are found in the blood, the possibility of liver disease has to be considered.

Other enzymes ordinarily found in the heart may leak into the blood from damaged heart cells after a heart attack (myocardial infarction). If you experience chest pain, a test for these enzymes may be done.

THYROID STUDIES

These tests measure blood levels of certain hormones including thyroxine, thyroid-stimulating hormone, and others. Such stud-

A NOTE ON TEST RESULTS

To be of value, test results must be accurate. How can accuracy be checked?

To help ensure dependability of blood tests, for example, solutions with known amounts of the substance being sought are interspersed with blood samples being analyzed. Another check on accuracy is the periodic testing of unknown samples prepared by other laboratories. In both cases, the results provide a way to judge accuracy (or inaccuracy) of testing procedures. Even with these precautions, however, errors can occur.

All variations in test results are not to be blamed on laboratory error. For instance, the amounts of the substances in your blood can vary from day to day or even from hour to hour. Also, some substances in your blood can interfere with test procedures and lead to false results.

There may be only a small difference between normal and abnormal results. Normal values for a substance in the blood usually are established by analyzing blood from a group of people who are in good health. The range of normal is commonly set by selecting values that will include 95 percent of the results of tests done on these normal people. The line between normal and abnormal is set in an arbitrary manner—thus there usually is overlap between test results that suggest disease and those that do not.

If a laboratory measures 15 or 20 different substances in your blood, there is a good chance that one or more of these results will fall outside the normal range. If the apparently abnormal tests are repeated, they are likely to give results within the normal range. But a deviation from the normal range due to early or minimal disease will continue to be found on repeated testing. Sometimes, repeated testing is necessary to determine whether a marginal test result is the result of disease.

ies are useful in distinguishing among the possible causes of thyroid disorders.

ARTERIAL BLOOD GAS ANALYSIS

This test measures the acidity (pH) of your blood and the amount of oxygen and carbon dioxide dissolved in it. The procedure differs somewhat from a standard blood test. Still, it takes only a few seconds and can be performed in a laboratory, a physician's office, or a hospital.

The skin over the artery to be punctured is cleaned with an antiseptic and a local an-esthetic is injected. (An artery is chosen, rather than a vein, because the blood sample must be freshly oxygenated from the heart and lungs.) The selected artery, usually in the wrist, is punctured with a sterile needle attached to a disposable syringe. The interior of the syringe is oil-coated to prevent room air from contaminating the blood sample. The physician or technician draws a sample of blood and then removes the needle from the artery. The blood sample is transferred from the syringe into sterile tubes that are placed in a blood gas analyzer.

After the blood sample has been drawn, you will be asked to apply pressure to the puncture site and rest quietly for 15 minutes before resuming normal activities.

BIOPSIES

A biopsy is the removal of a sample of tissue for study, usually under a microscope. The sample can be removed with a needle, with a knife (sometimes through a surgical incision), or by a special device inserted through an endoscope (an instrument gently inserted into a natural opening in the body. Most samples are treated chemically and sliced into very thin sections. These sections are placed on glass slides, stained (to enhance contrast), and studied under a microscope by a pathologist (a person who specializes in changes in body tissue) or a hematologist (a specialist in blood and blood-forming tissues) or both. Some samples do not require staining and can be interpreted almost immediately by a pathologist. This procedure (which was developed at the Mayo Clinic) is called frozen section and can be useful in diagnosing cancer within minutes after the sample is obtained. Biopsies are necessary to rule out disease or to confirm diagnoses such as cancer.

Virtually all of the fiberoptic instruments used in examining the trachea (windpipe), lungs, and upper and lower gastrointestinal tract also can be used to obtain tissue from the body. These instruments include bron-choscopes, colonoscopes, proctosigmoido-scopes, and esophagogastroduodenoscopes. Rigid instruments (such as cytoscopes) are also used to perform biopsies.

BONE MARROW ASPIRATION AND BIOPSY

A needle can be used to obtain material from your bone marrow for study. This needle rests in a slender sleeve of metal (stylet) that cuts a tiny channel for the needle to pass through. The needle is sharp enough and strong enough to penetrate the thin bone of the breast (sternum) or the back of the pelvic bone for aspiration (sucking up, like a vacuum cleaner) of the bone marrow into a syringe.

Bone marrow aspiration is used in the diagnosis of a wide variety of disorders of the blood or blood-forming organs, including anemia, leukemia, and lymphoma. Bone marrow aspiration also is used to evaluate the effectiveness of chemotherapy on malignancies involving the bone marrow. The test takes a few minutes and usually can be performed in a physician's office, a laboratory, or a hospital.

You will receive a local anesthetic at the site from which the bone marrow sample is to be taken. After the skin is sterilized with an antiseptic, your physician will insert the aspirating needle into the spongy marrow-filled bone of your pelvic bone or breast bone. Less than a teaspoon of marrow will be withdrawn.

You may feel some pressure as the biopsy needle is inserted, and there will be a dull, deep pain when the marrow is removed. But the pain will be only momentary. The needle then is removed, a bandage is placed on the wound, and the specimen is immediately prepared for microscopic examination.

Bone marrow aspiration differs from a bone marrow biopsy in that for biopsy a small solid core of marrow tissue is removed intact. Aside from that, the procedures are essentially the same and often are performed at the same time (see page 1284).

After the procedure, the puncture site may be tender and bruised for several days. The principal risk is bleeding from the puncture site, but this is rare.

LIVER BIOPSY

This safe and relatively simple procedure is used in the diagnosis of liver diseases such as cirrhosis, hepatitis, and cancer. It also may be used to determine the effects of drugs on the liver. The test usually is performed on an outpatient basis or in a hospital.

You may be asked to refrain from eating or drinking for several hours before the test. Before the test starts, you will disrobe and put on an examination gown.

During the procedure you will be asked to lie absolutely still on an examining table. The area where the biopsy needle is to be inserted (between or under the right ribs) will be cleansed and anesthetized. Then you will be asked to inhale deeply and to hold your breath as the needle is gently inserted through the skin and into the liver.

When the needle has reached the liver, it is rotated and then removed. This takes only a few seconds. The tissue specimen captured by the needle is placed in a sterile container and sent to a pathology laboratory for study.

After the procedure, a dressing will be placed on the tiny wound. For the next 3 to 4 hours, bed rest is recommended. Your pulse and blood pressure will be taken periodically. If light-headedness occurs, particularly when you stand up after the initial observation period of 3 to 4 hours, consult your physician. He or she will want to rule out bleeding after the biopsy. Occasionally, a mild, non-aspirin-containing analgesic is given.

ENDOSCOPIC TESTS

An endoscope is an instrument used to examine the interior of a hollow organ or cavity. It consists of either a flexible or a rigid hollow tube connected to an optical system that allows the person who looks through the tube to see tissues at the far end of the tube.

The endoscope has become indispensable for diagnosing a wide range of ailments in many different specialties. To the pulmonary (lung) specialist, the endoscope (known as a bronchoscope) is the key piece of equipment for examining the trachea and bronchial tree. It is used to help locate tumors, constrictions or secretions, and bleeding sites in the bronchial tubes and to diagnose lung cancer, tuberculosis, and other pulmonary diseases (see Bronchoscopy, page 940).

The gastroenterologist, who is concerned with the stomach, intestines, and other digestive organs, also uses an endoscope. The gastrointestinal procedures include gastroscopy (which provides a direct view of your esophagus, stomach, and duodenum), sigmoidoscopy (for examining your rectum and sigmoid portion of your large intestine), and colonoscopy (for examining the lining of your colon from the anus to the junction of your small and large intestines) (see Upper Gastrointestinal Endoscopy, page 611; Colonoscopy, page 637; and Screening for Colon Cancer, page 641).

Other specialties use endoscopes to look at joints (see Arthroscopy, page 968), bladder (see Cystoscopy, page 904), and other organs.

LARYNGOSCOPY

This procedure gives your physician a direct view into your larynx (voice box). Problems such as a tumor or a foreign object or nerve injury are often diagnosed in this fashion. This procedure usually is performed in a hospital.

You will be asked to refrain from eating for several hours before the procedure; then you will disrobe and put on an examination gown.

A local anesthetic may be sprayed into your nose and throat to decrease discomfort. Then a fiberoptic endoscope is inserted into your nose and carefully threaded down your throat into your larynx. The light and the lens system of the endoscope make it possible for your physician to view your larynx and, usually, to diagnose or rule out a health problem. A rigid laryngoscope also is commonly used. This is inserted through the mouth.

There are no serious risks with this procedure, although you may experience some temporary soreness in your nose and throat and you may cough up a small quantity of blood.

BODY SCANS

The x-ray examination is not new—it has been used for viewing such structures as bones, heart, and lungs for nearly a century.

PELVIC ULTRASONOGRAPHY IN PREGNANCY

This painless procedure allows your physician to see the fetus inside your uterus without exposing you or your fetus to x-rays. The image, known as a sonogram, is used to evaluate many important aspects including: the position, size, gestational age, and growth rate of the fetus; unexplained vaginal bleeding or lack of menstrual flow; and painful cramps. It also can be used to distinguish between tumors and cysts and to detect multiple pregnancy.

Early in pregnancy, ultrasonography is used to distinguish between normal intrauterine pregnancy and pregnancies that occur elsewhere such as in the fallopian tubes (tubal pregnancy).

The procedure takes about 15 minutes and can be performed in a laboratory, a physician's office, or a hospital on an outpatient basis. If you are at an early stage in your pregnancy, you will be asked to drink several glasses of water about an hour before this examination (for best results your bladder must be full). Also, a plain water enema may be recommended because this can produce a better outline of the intestine. In later stages of pregnancy, when the goal is to determine the age of the fetus, ingestion of water is not needed.

You will be asked to disrobe and wear a special gown. A jelly-like material or mineral oil will be applied to your abdomen, and then the transducer, a device that looks somewhat like a wand, will be passed over this lubricated area. The transducer sends high-frequency sound waves into the tissue. An oscilloscope translates the reflected sound waves into electrical impulses and displays the result as an image. These pictures can be photographed for later analysis.

Breast x-rays (see Mammograms, page 1080), dental x-rays (see page 397), barium x-rays of the esophagus, stomach, and intestine (see page 613), and other such examinations utilize traditional technology. Examination of many internal organs has improved dramatically in the last decade with the advent of computerized scanning equipment. The three new types of scanning most commonly available are computerized tomography (CT), magnetic resonance imaging (MRI), and ultrasonography.

The MRI and CT techniques are similar in that they both provide an image of the inside of the body, but they use different methods for producing their pictures: CT uses a very thin x-ray beam, and MRI uses a magnetic field. Both CT and MRI are safe, painless procedures that are often done on an outpatient basis.

CT SCANNING

A CT scan is many times as sensitive as an ordinary x-ray. It is produced by an x-ray beam that goes through your body. The CT equipment receives and analyzes the x-ray beam that emerges on the other side. The resulting picture can reveal soft tissue structures not identifiable on a standard x-ray.

You will be asked to lie flat on a movable table; then the table is guided into the center of the CT scanner. This instrument resembles an enormous doughnut. While you remain still, x-rays in a complete circle are beamed through segments of your body and are picked up by detectors. This information is fed into a computer which gathers the data and converts it into a video or photographic image which your radiologist can then interpret. A "dye" (contrast medium) is sometimes injected through a vein to enhance the contrast of the image. (This liquid contains iodine, so before the test begins you will be asked if you are allergic to iodine.) (See page 539.)

MAGNETIC RESONANCE IMAGING

An MRI device also can produce a picture of the inside of your body. But MRI uses magnetism and radio waves rather than x-rays or contrast dyes to produce its image. This picture is clearer than ordinary x-rays. Also, it does not use ionizing radiation as do conventional x-rays and CT scans.

MRI is based on magnetic properties in the interior (nucleus) of all atoms, including those in living tissue. When radio waves are directed to a specific part of your body, they cause the nuclei of atoms there to give off energy. This energy is detected, and a computer translates the emerging pattern of magnetic energy into an image that your radiologist can interpret (see page 539).

ULTRASONOGRAPHY

Images of the inside of your body also can be produced with sound waves. Called ultrasonography, this technique uses a wand-like device (transducer) that can produce and receive high-frequency sound waves (ultrasound); these sound waves are inaudible to the human ear. After they pass into the tissue, the reflected sound waves are transformed into an image that can be displayed on a video screen and photographed for study.

In recent years, the use of ultrasonography has expanded substantially. Now, this safe procedure is used to examine a wide range of tissues including organs in the abdomen, the thyroid and parathyroid glands, and the prostate. The test can observe and measure the flow of blood in your veins and arteries. Ultrasonography has also proved to be valuable during pregnancy for viewing the unborn fetus in the womb.

RADIONUCLIDE (NUCLEAR) SCANS

This imaging process uses small amounts of radioactive material (radioisotopes) that are attached to various substances (radiopharmaceuticals). The preparations are introduced into the body by injection, inhalation, or swallowing. Then, special detectors produce pictures of the radioisotopes in internal organs, permitting your physician to examine the size, shape, and function of the organs. The images also can help to distinguish between normal and abnormal tissue. This scanning procedure is somewhat the reverse of a traditional x-ray; instead of the x-rays coming from *outside* the body, the radiation source is *inside* the body.

To some extent, the radioactive material will be distributed throughout your body. Therefore, this type of scanning will not be used if you are pregnant or if you are breast-feeding an infant—unless the information needed is of vital importance and cannot be obtained in another way. If you are breast-feeding or think you may be pregnant, inform your physician of this before any radioisotope study begins.

BONE SCAN

This procedure is useful in diagnosing cancer, infection, or the cause of unexplained bone pain, such as a subtle or hidden bone fracture. Bone scanning can be performed in an outpatient or a hospital setting.

You receive an injection of a special radiopharmaceutical preparation (a technetium-99m diphosphonate compound). Then, you wait several hours while the material is absorbed by your bones and eliminated by your kidneys. During that time you will drink several glasses of water and you will need to urinate frequently to help remove most of the material from your system (some of the material remains). Then you can leave the laboratory if you wish until the scans (pictures) are to be taken, approximately 3 hours after the injection.

For the scanning, you will be asked to lie still on a table. A special (gamma) camera will record pictures of the pattern of radiation from the radiopharmaceutical that has localized in your bones. An uneven distribution of the radiopharmaceutical suggests a problem. Areas of increased accumulation of radiopharmaceutical are called "hot spots." A bone fracture will show up as such a hot spot.

After the procedure, special care is not required.

LUNG SCAN

Lung scanning most commonly is used to determine if there is a blood clot in a lung (pulmonary embolism). The entire procedure takes about 45 minutes and can be performed in a hospital or an outpatient laboratory.

You inhale a small amount of radioactive material and hold your breath while images are recorded. Following this, a small amount of radioactive material will be injected into a vein and images again are recorded, this time while you are in several different positions.

After the procedure, special care is not required.

LIVER SCAN

This radioisotope study helps to determine the size, shape, and function of the liver. It can detect the presence of cysts, abscesses, or tumors in the liver as well as evidence of cancer that may have spread into or from the liver. The procedure also can reveal the damage done to the liver by hepatitis, cirrhosis, or abdominal injury. Sometimes it is used to determine a suitable site for a needle biopsy (see Biopsies, page 1284, and Liver Biopsy, page 1285). A liver scan takes about 30 minutes. It can be performed in a hospital or in an outpatient laboratory.

You may be asked to disrobe before the procedure. Then, a radioactive material will be gently injected into a vein in your arm. (This may cause mild discomfort.) During the procedure, you will be asked to lie down and to move into different positions while a special (gamma) camera records images of radioactive material that has gathered (localized) in your liver.

After the procedure, special care is not required.

RADIOACTIVE IODINE UPTAKE TEST AND THYROID SCAN

The radioactive iodine uptake (RAIU) test and the thyroid scan are two methods for measuring the size, structure, and function of the thyroid gland. They are valuable in the diagnosis of an overfunctioning thyroid gland (hyperthyroidism) and also are used to evaluate thyroid nodules. Both tests can be done on an outpatient basis or in a hospital.

Depending on the purpose of the test, you may be asked to temporarily discontinue any thyroid medication you may be taking. Also, depending on the type of RAIU test used, you may be asked to swallow radioactive iodine in a capsule or in liquid form. Then you can leave. You return for the measurement 6 or 24 hours later, or at both times.

For the RAIU test, you will be asked to lie on your back on a table with your head stretched backward. An instrument will be held over your neck to measure radioactivity. The procedure, which measures the ability of your thyroid gland to concentrate the radioactive iodine, may require measurements at several intervals.

The thyroid scan is slightly different in that it produces an actual image of your thyroid gland. This study requires an injection (or swallowing) of the radiopharmaceutical preparation. The gamma camera detects radiation from the radioisotope that has collected in your thyroid gland and then produces an image on the screen. The image can be interpreted on the screen or photographed for further study by your physician.

After the procedure, special care is not required.

SCANNING FOR INFECTIONS

There are two types of studies with radioactive preparations (labeled with radioisotopes) that look for infections: the gallium scan, and the indium-labeled white blood cell scan. The procedures are similar, but different isotopes are used.

A special (gamma) camera records the radiation given off by the radiopharmaceutical, and images of abnormal tissues are quite different from those of normal tissues, allowing your physician to detect possible sites of infection (see Radionuclide [Nuclear] Scans, page 1287).

Gallium Scanning. This procedure uses a radiopharmaceutical (gallium-67) that is given intravenously and then collects (localizes) in abnormal tissues such as sites of infection or inflammation and in some tumors.

After you receive an injection of the radiopharmaceutical, you can leave. You will be asked to return for imaging at various times. Imaging may begin as soon as 6 hours later but more often you will be asked to return to the hospital or outpatient laboratory 24 or 48 hours later. In the meantime, you may be directed to take a laxative to help remove the unnecessary radioactivity from your bowel.

A special (gamma) camera will record several images over your abdomen, chest, or some other area where an infection may be suspected. The scanning procedure takes about 1 to 1½ hours.

You may be asked to return on several consecutive days so that changes in the radioisotope location can be recorded. This procedure may suggest to your physician other areas requiring examination by means of other techniques such as ultrasonography, CT, or some other x-ray procedure (see Body Scans, page 1286).

After the procedure, special care is not necessary.

Indium-Labeled White Blood Cell Scanning. This relatively new procedure uses a sample of your own white blood cells which is removed and labeled with a radioisotope and then returned to your bloodstream. These specially marked cells will collect at sites of active infection or inflammation.

Your physician might ask you to discontinue any antibiotics you may be taking before this test (but do so only on the specific advice of your physician).

First, one or two syringes containing your blood are taken. In a laboratory, the white blood cells in the sample are separated from the red cells and plasma. Then, a radioisotope (indium-111) is added to the white blood cells, thus labeling them. Two or 3 hours later, these labeled white blood cells are returned to your body by injection.

Images are made approximately 6 or 24 hours after the injection of your labeled white blood cells. The pictures show where the labeled white cells have collected. The painless procedure takes 1 or 2 hours and usually is performed in a hospital or outpatient laboratory.

Once the procedure is finished, special care is unnecessary.

HEART SCANS

Two key radionuclide procedures are available for scanning the heart—thallium imaging, and radionuclide angiography. The procedures are the same, but different preparations (radioisotopes) are used to reveal different aspects of heart function.

In both tests, a radiopharmaceutical is given. Then, a special (gamma) camera detects the radiation given off by the radiopharmaceutical and records an image of the heart. The image of an abnormal heart may be quite different from that of a normal one, which aids in evaluating the health of the heart and in diagnosing heart ailments.

Thallium Imaging. Thallium is a radiopharmaceutical preparation that collects in the heart muscle. The study may be performed at rest or after you exercise. A thallium scan can show areas of actual heart damage (myocardial infarction) or areas that are not getting enough blood (ischemic myocardium) and are thus candidates for damage.

You may be asked to stop taking any heart medicines for a day or two before the test, but do not do so unless your physician specifically tells you to. Before the test, eat only a light meal. Usually electrocardiogram (ECG) leads are placed on your chest (see Electrocardiography, page 1293).

If the test is to be done after you exercise, electrocardiogram and blood pressure readings will be made while you are exercising on a treadmill. Just before the end of your workout, the thallium preparation will be injected into a vein in your arm.

Immediately after exercising you will lie down while a special (gamma) camera records many images of your heart. (Some cameras rotate around your body.) A few hours after the first images are made, you will return and another set will be made. Completion of each set of images requires 45 minutes to 1 hour. The procedures are performed in a hospital or outpatient laboratory.

You will be told not to drink clear liquids and not to exercise between the first and second sets of pictures. Special care or precautions are unnecessary after the procedure is complete.

Radionuclide Angiography. This procedure can reveal how effectively your heart is functioning. It can be done while you rest or during exercise or in both circumstances.

You will receive an injection of a chemical (stannous pyrophosphate). About a half hour later, a small amount of your blood will be drawn into a syringe that contains a radioisotope (technetium-99m). The blood and radioisotope are mixed and allowed to remain together for 10 minutes, during which time your red blood cells absorb the radioisotope. Then, these labeled cells are injected back into your blood.

Your physician may ask you to discontinue any heart medicines for a day or two before the test, but do not do this unless it is specifically requested. Do not eat a major meal within the 3 hours before the test.

The scanning procedure itself will require 1 to 2 hours and is performed in a hospital or an outpatient laboratory. During the scanning your electrocardiogram will be recorded from leads attached to your chest. A special (gamma) camera will be placed over your heart in several positions to produce the images of your heart created by gamma rays given off by the labeled blood cells. These images can be made while you are at rest and while you exercise on a bicycle, either upright or lying down. Changes in the radioactivity within your heart during exercise show how well your heart muscle contracts. The findings from this test, which includes an electrocardiogram, can reveal useful information on the general health of your heart.

Once the procedure is finished, special care or precautions are unnecessary.

HEART CATHETERIZATION

The heart catheterization procedure enables physicians to view and evaluate the shape and function of your heart's chambers and valves. The examination can detect inherited heart defects, the presence of aneurysms or blood clots in the heart, and narrowed or closed (occluded) coronary arteries (see Scans and Coronary Angiogram, page 805).

By measuring blood pressure and blood flow above and below the aortic valve, this procedure also can help determine the size of the opening of the aortic valve. This information is important in determining whether surgery may be needed to replace a malfunctioning aortic valve. This test should almost always be performed in a hospital.

You will be instructed not to eat any food or drink any liquids for at least 8 hours before the procedure. You will disrobe and wear a gown during the test.

Before the catheterization begins, you will receive a mild sedative, but you will remain conscious during the procedure. At certain times you will be asked to take deep breaths, which improves the quality of the x-ray pictures that are made during the examination.

Leads (wires) of an electrocardiograph machine will be placed on your chest so that your physician can monitor the action of your heart throughout the test. A needle attached to a tube and bottle of 5 percent dextrose in water will be placed in your vein.

An artery in your arm, leg, or groin will be selected for insertion of the tube (catheter) that is to be gently guided into your heart or other area. The insertion site is cleansed with an antiseptic and draped in a sterile fashion. A local anesthetic is injected into the skin and deeper tissues; there should be no further pain after this.

When the catheter is in place, a contrast medium (dye) will be delivered through the catheter to your heart or coronary arteries to provide a clearer x-ray picture. If your physician also wants to widen your blood vessels, you may be asked to hold a nitroglycerin tablet under your tongue. Results of the catheterization are monitored on a television screen during the test. (These video images also can be photographed for further study.) Then the catheter is removed and the examination is complete.

For the first 20 to 30 minutes after removal of the catheter, direct pressure is placed on the insertion site. You will be kept in bed for at least 8 hours. Your vital signs will be checked periodically. If needed, you will also be given pain medication, and the insertion site will be checked for soreness, swelling, or blood loss.

Although this is a common procedure, serious risks are associated with it. For example, if the catheter loosens an existing blood clot or cholesterol deposit within an artery, the result can be a stroke or heart attack. In rare instances, the heart or kidneys can be damaged. Anyone with a blood-clotting disorder or poor kidney function is at increased risk. Still, the risk of a serious complication (such as stroke, heart attack, or even death) is approximately 1 in 1,000. The risks are lowest in young, healthy persons and highest in older persons with serious medical problems.

Because of risks associated with this test, a surgical team usually is available during the catheterization procedure and can be called upon in the event surgery is required.

RIGHT HEART OR PULMONARY ARTERY ANGIOGRAPHY

To study the right atrium and ventricle and its valves (tricuspid and pulmonic) or the pulmonary arteries, a catheter can be placed in a large vein in your leg or arm and advanced into your heart or into the main artery of your lungs (pulmonary artery). Contrast medium (dye) is then injected through the catheter and an x-ray picture of your pulmonary arteries is produced. If a blood clot is discovered during the procedure, it is usually treated with a powerful anticoagulant drug. Rarely is surgery required to remove a blood clot in the pulmonary arteries.

SPECIAL X-RAY PROCEDURES

ARTHROGRAPHY

An arthrogram is an x-ray of a joint, especially a knee, ankle, or shoulder. It is used to detect suspected tears in cartilage and other joint abnormalities. It takes less than an hour and is performed with x-ray guidance. It can be done in an outpatient setting or a hospital.

You will be given a local anesthetic, and then a liquid contrast medium (dye) will be injected into the joint to enhance clarity of the pictures that are to be made. (If your physician chooses to draw fluid from the joint for other studies, this will be done before the contrast medium is administered.) You may be asked to move the joint to help distribute the dye throughout the area. The joint then will be examined with a fluoroscope, and x-rays will be made.

After the procedure, rest the joint for at least a day, or as long as your physician recommends, before resuming normal activity. You may experience some swelling or discomfort in the joint. This should pass in a day or two. If it does not, see your physician (see Arthroscopy, page 968.)

CEREBRAL ARTERIOGRAPHY

Cerebral arteriography is performed by injecting a contrast medium (dye) into a major artery leading to the brain. The dye spreads to other areas of the brain.

For a detailed discussion, see Cerebral Arteriography, page 513.

KIDNEY X-RAY

This procedure, which also is called intravenous pyelography (IVP) or excretory urography, provides images of the kidneys and lower urinary tract.

For a detailed discussion, see The Kidney X-Ray, page 885.

BILE AND PANCREATIC DUCT X-RAYS

X-ray examination of the bile and pancreatic ducts can identify gallstones, narrowings (strictures), cancer of the pancreas or bile duct, or other abnormalities. Contrast medium (dye) is injected into the bile ducts and pancreatic duct through an endoscope.

For a detailed discussion, see X-Raying the Bile and Pancreatic Ducts, page 664.

MYELOGRAPHY

Myelography is an x-ray examination of the space around the spinal cord. A lumbar puncture (also called a spinal tap) is done and a radiopaque dye (contrast medium) is injected into the space around the spinal cord. Once the dye is injected, x-rays are made to show the configuration of the space around the spinal cord and whether it is distorted by the presence of a slipped disc (herniated intervertebral disc), spinal cord tumor, an abnormal collection of blood vessels, or other disorders.

For a detailed discussion, see Myelography, page 555.

OTHER EXAMINATIONS

FLUORESCEIN ANGIOGRAPHY

Fluorescein angiography (or eye angiography) produces photographs of blood vessels in the eye to help in evaluating eye disorders including retinopathy, tumors, and circulatory or inflammatory disorders of the eye. The test takes about 30 minutes and can be performed in a physician's office or in an ophthalmological photography laboratory.

A technician or physician will place drops in your eyes to dilate your pupils. After the pupils have dilated, you may be asked to loosen any constricting clothing around your neck before being positioned at the camera.

Fluorescein dye will then be injected into a vein in your hand or arm. After the dye has moved to your eyes, several photographs will be made in rapid sequence. Another series of photographs will be taken several minutes later.

After the procedure, some discoloration, soreness, or swelling may appear at the site of the puncture, although this is unusual. Your vision may be blurred from the eyedrops for the rest of the day. In addition, your skin and urine may appear slightly discolored for a day or two after the procedure.

ECHOCARDIOGRAPHY

This procedure uses a device that detects sound reflected from the beating heart and creates an image from which the size, shape, and motion of the heart can be determined. *For a detailed discussion, see The Echocardiogram: Images Made With Sound, page 827.*

OPHTHALMOSCOPY

This examination permits your physician to see the back of your eye (the fundus) to examine your retina, optic disc, and the network of tiny vessels that supply your eye with blood. This is an important part of every complete physical examination because the fundus can reveal useful information about your general health. The fundus is the only place in your body where veins and arteries can be observed directly, without an invasive procedure.

If you have high blood pressure, changes in these vessels can indicate the severity of your problem (see High Blood Pressure, page 796). Early clues to circulatory disturbances in your brain may appear in the vessels at the back of your eye. Specifically, particles of cholesterol-containing material or crystalline plaques may be a clue to atherosclerosis (see Atherosclerosis, page 786). Changes in these blood vessels also can suggest complications of diabetes.

Your optic nerve also will be examined. This nerve, which looks like a cream-colored disc, gathers together all the nerve fibers from the retina to transmit visual images to your brain. This disc is actually an extension of your brain. When a person has a disease that causes increased pressure in the skull, such as a brain tumor or meningitis, the optic disc may appear blurred or swollen.

Although eye specialists include this procedure as part of a complete eye evaluation, the more limited test (often called a funduscopic examination) frequently is performed by family physicians, internists, and neurologists. The examination takes only a few minutes.

Your physician may place one or two drops of medicine into your eyes to dilate your pupils. This may cause blurring of your close vision for a short time. Then, the room light may be dimmed and the examination is begun.

As you pick a point to stare at, your physician will shine a light from the ophthalmoscope into each eye and look through the pupil to the fundus.

This is a painless procedure. However, if you receive eye drops, your eyes may be sensitive to light for several hours afterward because your pupils are dilated. Do not drive until your pupils have readjusted to bright light and your vision is no longer blurred.

IMPEDANCE PLETHYSMOGRAPHY AND VENOGRAPHY

These procedures are used to detect blood clots in deep veins of your body, particularly in your legs. Detection of blood clots is important because clots can lead to a pulmonary embolism (see page 947).

Impedance Plethysmography. This procedure generally takes between 30 and 45 minutes and can be performed in a laboratory, a physician's office, or a hospital.

No special preparation is necessary. You probably will be asked to undress and wear a special gown. Electrodes are attached above the calf of your leg and a blood pressure cuff is wrapped around your thigh and inflated as if your blood pressure is to be taken on your thigh. A machine records the electrodes' readings both when the cuff is inflated and when it is deflated. If the size of your leg does not change normally during and after inflation of the cuff, a blood clot may be present within your leg.

Venography. Venography often is performed after impedance plethysmography suggests that a blood clot may be present. Sometimes it is the only procedure performed to diagnose blood clots. This is an x-ray procedure that produces images of the veins in the legs and feet. It takes between 45 minutes and 1 hour and can be performed in a laboratory, a physician's office, or a hospital.

You may have to fast for 4 hours prior to the procedure, and you probably will be asked to undress and wear a special gown. A local anesthetic will be injected into the area where a liquid contrast medium (dye) will be injected to enhance the clarity of the x-ray pictures to be made. The site for this injection is a large vein in your foot or ankle. As the contrast medium is injected, you may feel a warming or mild burning sensation in your leg. Your veins can then be observed by means of an x-ray procedure called fluoroscopy—and x-rays can be recorded for further study.

At some point during the test you may be asked to flex your calf muscles or push your foot against the physician's or technician's hand to help direct more blood into the veins of your leg. A tourniquet is often placed around the leg to force the contrast medium into the deeper veins.

After the procedure, your pulse, blood pressure, and temperature will be checked. You will be observed for swelling, soreness, redness, bleeding, or infection due to the puncture. You may experience a sensation of nausea or mild light-headedness or have a mild headache for a few hours. If these symptoms persist, inform your physician.

ELECTRICAL TESTS

Your body generates electrical currents as you go about your normal activities. Scientists have detected electrical activity in the brain, muscles, heart, and other organs and tissue and have devised unique ways of recording this activity. Studying these recordings can reveal abnormalities that can be used to diagnose disorders.

ELECTROCARDIOGRAPHY (ECG)

This test measures the pattern of electrical impulses generated in your heart. It can help identify damage to the heart muscle, irregular rhythms, enlargement (hypertrophy) of a chamber of your heart, or damage caused by a heart attack, and it can measure the effectiveness of a pacemaker. Electrocardiography, which records the electrical forces produced during each heartbeat, has become one of the most common cardiac diagnostic tests. The procedure takes only a few minutes, is painless, and can be performed routinely in a physician's office.

Generally, no special preparations are necessary. Your physician may ask you not to eat or drink foods containing caffeine for 24 hours before this test. After you have undressed from the waist up, you will be asked to lie on a comfortable bed or examining table and relax. After a jelly-like substance is applied, electrodes will be attached to your wrists, ankles, and chest. During the procedure breathe normally but do not move or talk, because any disturbance may distort test results.

After the procedure, the electrodes and jelly are removed and you can resume normal activities (see Twenty-Four-Hour Cardiac Monitoring, page 818).

EXERCISE TOLERANCE TEST

This test reveals the efficiency and function of the heart under stress.

For a detailed discussion, see The Exercise Tolerance Test, page 804.

ELECTROENCEPHALOGRAPHY (EEG)

Electroencephalography measures the waves of electrical activity produced by the brain. Often, it is used in diagnosing and managing seizure disorders. If you are awake when the recording is made, the test will take about 30 minutes. (Some EEG tests are done while you sleep.) Most often, the test is performed in a hospital but can be done in a laboratory or physician's office.

If you are taking antiseizure medications, continue taking them unless otherwise instructed by your physician. Tell the person performing the test about any medicines you are taking. Because electrodes will be attached to your scalp, shampoo your hair before the test to help remove any hair spray, tonic, or oil.

As many as 16 to 30 small electrodes will be attached to your scalp with paste or an elastic cap as you relax on your back in a bed or reclining chair. The test is painless, but you must remain motionless. Periodically you may be asked to breathe deeply and steadily for 3 minutes or to stare at a patterned board; or a light may be flashed in your eyes. These actions stimulate the brain. The electrical impulses from your brain are detected by the electrodes and sent on to the electroencephalography machine which records the impulses (brain waves) on a continuously moving paper sheet.

If the test is to be a sleep electroencephalogram, you will be asked to stay awake the night before or to get very little sleep. To help you fall asleep, you may be given a sedative before this test begins.

After the test, paste used to attach the electrodes to your scalp may be washed off with ordinary shampoo.

ELECTROMYOGRAPHY (EMG)

Electromyography measures the tiny electrical discharges produced in muscles. A variation of this test, the nerve conduction study, can measure the speed at which nerves carry electrical signals.

Electromyography is used to help diagnose muscle or nerve disorders such as muscular dystrophy (see page 978) and amyotrophic lateral sclerosis (see page 523) and some problems involving the spinal cord. Nerve conduction tests, also referred to as electroneurography, are often used to diagnose peripheral nerve disorders including carpal tunnel syndrome.

Electromyography usually is performed on an outpatient basis. It takes about an hour to complete. If many muscles are studied, however, the test will take longer.

Tell your physician or the technician conducting the test the names of any medicines you have taken in the previous 2 days. You will be asked to disrobe and wear a gown.

In electromyography, a thin needle electrode is gently inserted into each muscle to be studied. You may feel a brief, sharp pain each time this needle is inserted but, because nothing is injected through it, this pain usually is less than that from a typical hypodermic injection. A fine wire leads from the needle to an electronic instrument that detects electrical currents in your muscle. The patterns of electrical activity are recorded when the muscle is at rest and as you voluntarily tighten it. These patterns can be viewed on a screen and may be recorded on film for further analysis.

Nerve conduction tests are performed in somewhat the same manner except that needles are not used. Two small, disc-like recording electrodes are taped to your skin directly above the nerve to be studied or above a muscle connected to that nerve.

Then, a small instrument with metal prongs applies a mild shock over the nerve. This electrical signal moves down the nerve, passing under the disc-like electrodes. By comparing the recording of the signal at each electrode site and calculating the time it took to travel between them, the speed of conduction along the nerve is easily determined. The nature of the signal from the nerve or muscle also helps to determine whether nerve or muscle fibers have been damaged by disease.

MICROBIOLOGICAL TESTS

Any body fluid or tissue can be cultured if the presence of a microorganism is suspected. (A culture is the growing of a microorganism in a laboratory for study.) All cultures require enough time for the organism to grow to sufficient numbers to be identified; some cultures, such as those for tuberculosis or fungi, sometimes require months. Once there are sufficient organisms in the culture, the infecting agent can be identified and its susceptibility to various antibodies can be evaluated.

Most cultures are obtained to identify a bacterium that may be causing an infection. Cultures also are obtained for the diagnosis of tuberculosis or a fungal infection. It also is possible to culture some viruses.

THROAT CULTURE

This is a common microbiological test in cases of pharyngitis, an inflammation or infection of the throat caused by various bacteria, viruses, or fungi.

If you have a sore throat, especially if accompanied by fever, swollen glands, or pus (exudate) in your throat, your sore throat may be caused by *Streptococcus* bacteria. This infection is commonly called strep throat. Because inadequate treatment of this type of sore throat can lead to rheumatic fever or acute glomerulonephritis (see page 893) be sure to have a throat culture.

Obtaining a specimen for a throat culture takes only a few seconds and is most often done in a laboratory or a physician's office.

Using a tongue depressor to permit a clear view through your mouth, your nurse or physician will look for redness and pus on your tonsils or on the back of your throat. If a throat culture is needed, a sterile swab will be rubbed over the back of your throat to obtain a sample of the secretions there. The swab is sent to a laboratory for analysis.

Some physicians use a rapid streptococcal test which gives a fast diagnosis when it is positive. Because these rapid tests detect only one-half to two-thirds of sore throats caused by *Streptococcus,* a negative rapid test needs to be confirmed by throat culture.

SYNOVIAL FLUID ANALYSIS

This test examines the lubricating (synovial) fluid secreted by synovial membranes, the membranes that line joints in your body. The test is useful in the diagnosis of some types of arthritis (primarily those caused by infection, gout, or pseudogout). Obtaining the sample for the test takes about half an hour and usually is done in a physician's office or hospital.

No special preparations are necessary. The skin over the joint is cleaned with an antiseptic. Usually, a local anesthetic is injected. Using a thin needle, your physician will withdraw a sample of fluid for analysis, including culture of the fluid if infection is a possible diagnosis and examination for crystals to diagnose gout or pseudogout. If needed, medication (usually a corticosteroid preparation) can be injected into the joint space through this needle after the specimen is taken.

After the test there often is slight pain at the puncture site, but this is brief. Discomfort also may occur when the needle penetrates the joint lining, but this also is relatively mild and brief. After the procedure is complete, the antiseptic is washed off and a small bandage is applied. If cortisone was injected, the joint space may be slightly uncomfortable for several hours but then will feel better.

Avoid excessive use of the joint for a few days even though the pain and swelling may diminish. If pain worsens or if the joint becomes red and warm, contact your physician immediately. He or she may want to examine the area to make sure there is no infection.

CEREBROSPINAL FLUID ANALYSIS

For this test, a small amount of cerebrospinal fluid is removed from your spinal column by lumbar puncture (spinal tap) for analysis. Analysis of this fluid can help in the diagnosis of meningitis, hemorrhage around the brain and spinal cord, tumors, syphilis, infections of the central nervous system, or non-inflammatory conditions of the central nervous system. The procedure can be conducted on an outpatient basis in a hospital, in a laboratory, or in a physician's office and requires only a few minutes (see Lumbar Puncture, page 530).

REPRODUCTIVE AND UROLOGICAL TESTS

The functions of the reproductive and urological organs require diverse, specialized tests that aid in examination of these organs and in the diagnosis of their disorders.

HYSTEROSALPINGOGRAPHY

In this test, x-ray pictures of the interior of the uterus and fallopian tubes are obtained. The pictures are used to evaluate infertility in women by detecting abnormalities in the fallopian tubes such as adhesions, obstructions, injuries, or the presence of foreign objects. The test takes about 30 minutes and can be performed in a laboratory, in a physician's office, or in a hospital.

You will disrobe and wear a gown. Once you lie down on the examining table and place your feet in the stirrups, an instrument called a speculum will be carefully inserted into your vagina. A hook-like instrument (tenaculum) will be used to hold your cervix in place.

A liquid contrast medium (dye) is then gently injected through a small tube into the uterus and fallopian tubes. There may be slight discomfort when the contrast medium reaches your uterus. If the tubes are blocked, the point of obstruction will be visible on the viewing screen of an x-ray device (fluoroscope). You may be asked to change positions occasionally so that better x-ray pictures can be obtained.

After the test, you may feel cramps, nausea, or dizziness but these symptoms will pass. You also may have a bloody vaginal discharge.

COLPOSCOPY

This procedure often is the first test done after a Pap smear gives abnormal results (see The Pap Smear, page 1096). The test provides a magnified view of the vagina and cervix and is used to confirm cervical cancer, evaluate any lesions on the vagina, or monitor daughters of mothers who took the female hormone diethylstilbestrol (DES) during their pregnancy, who may be at increased risk for vaginal and cervical cancer (see page 1091). The test takes about 15 minutes and is done in a physician's office.

Advise your physician of any medications you are taking. You will disrobe and wear a gown. On the examining table, you place your feet in the stirrups and then a colposcope will be inserted into your vagina. This instrument can give your physician a clear view of your vagina and cervix. If a biopsy is required, the specimen will be taken at this time. Any minor bleeding that may occur will be stopped before the colposcope is removed.

LAPAROSCOPY IN WOMEN

This procedure provides direct visual examination of your reproductive organs. It is used to detect endometriosis, ectopic pregnancy, pelvic inflammatory disease, cancer, or other causes of pelvic pain. The procedure usually is done in a hospital and takes more than 2 hours to complete.

Do not eat or drink for 12 hours before the test. You will disrobe and wear a gown. Once you receive an anesthetic (either a general or a local), a small incision will be made in your abdomen and a needle will be inserted to inflate your abdomen with a gas (carbon dioxide). Then, a laparoscope, a long metal tube with a lens and tiny light source on one end, will be inserted to examine the interior of your abdomen.

The anesthetic makes this procedure virtually painless. A special dye may be injected through the cervix into the uterine cavity to check for obstructions in the fallopian tubes. Minor surgery, such as a tubal ligation (female sterilization), may be performed at this time. Once the laparoscope is removed, stitches are used to close the small incision.

If you received a general anesthetic, your vital signs will be checked for the next 4 hours. Any pain in your abdomen should disappear within 2 days.

CYSTOSCOPY

Cystoscopy provides the opportunity to view your bladder and urethra. It is used to diagnose urinary tract disorders that produce symptoms such as painful urination, slowness of urinary stream, incomplete emptying, dribbling and leakage of urine, and blood in the urine.

For a detailed discussion, see Cystoscopy, page 904.

URINE TESTS

A routine urinalysis is a part of most comprehensive health examinations. Urinalysis includes tests for glucose (sugar), protein, bilirubin, and ketones in the urine. None of these substances are present normally, and their presence usually is an indication of a disease process.

The urine sediment also is examined under the microscope for the presence of white and red blood cells and debris. Detection of these substances may indicate the presence of an infection, tumor, or a disorder of the kidneys, ureter, or bladder, and further testing may be required.

Besides the routine urinalysis, there are many other specific tests that can be done on the urine. Most of these involve the detection of abnormal substances produced by your body or cultures if an infection is suspected. Urine can be analyzed for the presence of many drugs, including illicit drugs. Some of these tests can be done on a routine sample of urine; others require careful timing or even collection of the sample under sterile conditions.

In some instances, you will be asked to obtain a clean-catch urine collection. In this situation, you will be asked to void several ounces of urine into a toilet before collecting the sample of urine for analysis.

APPENDIX II

THE DRUG DIRECTORY

APPENDIX CONTENTS

UNDERSTANDING YOUR MEDICINES

UNDERSTANDING YOUR MEDICINES

Thousands of drugs are available in pharmacies from coast to coast. We discuss many of these preparations elsewhere in this book, generally in conjunction with specific diseases.

This appendix is devoted to a brief and simple listing of some common prescription and over-the-counter medications that you may use.

Scientists are continually at work developing new drugs. Pharmaceutical manufacturers constantly compete to be first in marketing effective new preparations. As a result, new products are released almost daily.

Because of this continuous advance in knowledge and the changing nature of the marketplace, a Drug Directory such as this would require many hundreds of pages to be complete. Our purpose is more modest.

In these pages, you will find entries for drugs we know to be commonly prescribed or recommended by physicians nationwide. We include generic and brand names. (This list is not comprehensive and does not represent an endorsement of any product or company.)

A generic name is the name given to a drug when it is first developed. This name identifies the drug as being unique from all others. In this directory, generic names are shown in **boldface type**. In *italic type,* we list some of the brand names under which certain generic medications are sold. The brand name is the proprietary name assigned to the drug by each manufacturer (see Drug Classifications, page 1227). Unless the drug listed is identified as a nonprescription (over-the-counter) drug by the letters OTC, it is available only by prescription.

In the Drug Index (see page 1232), we list principal categories into which most of the commonly prescribed medications are divided. For example, in the Drug Index you will find ANALGESIC, the drug category (painkiller) in which acetaminophen belongs. Acetaminophen is the generic name. Many brands are available.

In taking any drug, it is important to follow the instructions you are given and to take precautions regarding proper dosage, storage, and administration of the drug (see The Modern Pharmacy, page 1225, for specific advice). Be alert for side effects of the drug. Side effects usually are minor but sometimes can be serious. Should such symptoms as dizziness, nausea, abdominal discomfort, or other untoward reactions occur, consult your physician or pharmacist immediately (see Adverse Drug Reactions, page 1230).

Accutane: Brand name of the anti-acne drug isotretinoin.

Acetaminophen: Analgesic drug. OTC.

Acetaminophen with Codeine: A combination analgesic drug.

Acetylsalicylic Acid: The formal name for aspirin.

Achromycin: Brand name of the antibiotic tetracycline.

Actifed: Brand name of the combination drug containing triprolidine and pseudoephedrine, for treatment of allergy or colds. OTC.

Actinomycin D: A cytotoxic drug.

Acyclovir: An antiviral drug.

Adapin: Brand name of the antidepressant drug doxepin.

Advil: Brand name of the analgesic drug ibuprofen. OTC.

Afrin: Brand name of the decongestant drug oxymetazoline. OTC.

Albuterol: A bronchodilator drug.

Aldactone: Brand name of the diuretic drug spironolactone.

Aldomet: Brand name of the antihypertensive drug methyldopa.

Aldoril: Brand name of the combination diuretic drug methyldopa and hydrochlorothiazide.

Allopurinol: A drug for gout (uric acid inhibitor).

Alprazolam: An anti-anxiety drug.

Aluminum Hydroxide: An antacid. OTC.

Alupent: Brand name of the bronchodilator drug metoproterenol.

Amiloride: An antihypertensive and diuretic drug.

Amitriptyline: An antidepressant drug.

Amoxicillin: An antibiotic drug.

Amoxicillin/Clavulenic Acid: An antibiotic drug.

Amoxil: Brand name of the antibiotic amoxicillin.

Ampicillin: An antibiotic drug.

Anaprox: Brand name of the analgesic drug naproxen.

Antivert: Brand name of the antinausea and motion sickness drug meclizine.

Anusol-HC: Brand name of the suppository or cream used to treat anal itching and discomfort; contains bismuth, zinc oxide, and hydrocortisone.

Armour Thyroid: Brand name of thyroid hormone.

Aspirin: An analgesic, antipyretic, and anti-inflammatory drug. Also known by its chemical name, acetylsalicylic acid or ASA. OTC.

Atenolol: An antihypertensive and heart drug.

Atenolol/Chlorthalidone: An antihypertensive combination drug.

Ativan: Brand name of the anti-anxiety drug lorazepam.

Attapulgite: An antidiarrheal drug. OTC.

Augmentin: Brand name of the antibiotic amoxicillin/clavulenic acid.

Azatadine: A decongestant and antihistamine drug.

Bactrim: Brand name of the combination antibiotic trimethoprim/sulfamethoxazole.

Beepen VK: Brand name of the antibiotic penicillin VK.

Benadryl: Brand name of the antihistamine diphenhydramine. OTC.

Benzoyl Peroxide: An anti-acne drug. OTC.

Bisacodyl: A laxative. OTC.

Bismuth Subgallate: A topical preparation for anal discomfort and itching.

Bismuth Subsalicylate: A liquid or tablet preparation for heartburn, upset stomach, and indigestion. OTC.

Brethaire: Brand name of the bronchodilator drug terbutaline.

Brethine: Brand name of the bronchodilator drug terbutaline.

Bricanyl: Brand name of the bronchodilator drug terbutaline.

Brompheniramine: An antihistamine and decongestant drug. OTC.

Bumetadine: A diuretic drug.

Bumex: Brand name of the diuretic drug bumetadine.

Busiprone: An anti-anxiety drug.

BuSpar: Brand name of the anti-anxiety drug busiprone.

Butalbital/Acetaminophen: A migraine analgesic.

Butalbital/Aspirin: A migraine analgesic.

Butalbital/Codeine: A migraine analgesic.

Calan SR: Brand name of the antihypertensive drug verapamil.

Capoten: Brand name of the antihypertensive and heart drug captopril.

Captopril: An antihypertensive and heart drug.

Carafate: Brand name of the drug sulcrafate that protects the lining of the stomach.

Carbamazepine: An anticonvulsant drug.

Cardizem: Brand name of the heart drug diltiazem.

Catapres: Brand name of the antihypertensive drug clonidine.

Ceclor: Brand name of the antibiotic cefaclor.

Cefaclor: An antibiotic drug.

Cefadroxil: An antibiotic drug.

Cemastine/Phenylpropanolamine: An allergy or cold treatment.

Cephalexin: An antibiotic drug.

Chlorothiazide: An antihypertensive and diuretic drug.

Chlorpheniramine: An antihistamine drug. OTC.

Chlorpropamide: A hypoglycemic (antidiabetic) drug.

Chlor-Trimeton: Brand name of the antihistamine drug chlorpheniramine. OTC.

Cholestyramine: A cholesterol-reducing drug.

Cimetidine: A histamine-blocker ulcer drug.

Cipro: Brand name of the antibiotic ciprofloxacin.

Ciprofloxacin: An antibiotic drug.

Clearasil: Brand name of the anti-acne drug benzoyl peroxide. OTC.

Clinoril: Brand name of the analgesic and anti-arthritic drug sulindac.

Clonidine: An antihypertensive drug.

Clorazepate: An anti-anxiety drug.

Clotrimazole: A topical antifungal drug.

Codeine/Iodated Glycerol/Chlorpheniramine: A cough suppressant and expectorant combination drug.

Colace: Brand name of the stool softener docusate. OTC.

Colchicine: A gout drug.

Compazine: Brand name of the antinausea drug prochlorperazine.

Corgard: Brand name of the antihypertensive and heart drug nadolol.

Cortisporin: Brand name of the anti-inflammatory and antibacterial mixture polymyxin B/bacitracin/neomycin/hydrocortisone.

Coumadin: Brand name of the anticoagulant drug warfarin.

Cromolyn Sodium: An anti-allergy drug.

Cyclobenzaprine: An antispasmodic drug.

Cyclopar: Brand name of the antibiotic tetracycline.

Dalmane: Brand name of the hypnotic and sedative drug flurazepam.

Darvocet: Brand name of the combination analgesic drug propoxyphene and acetaminophen.

Delsym: Brand name of the drug dextromethorphan, used in treating the cough associated with the common cold. OTC.

Deltasone: Brand name of the corticosteroid drug prednisone.

Desipramine: An antidepressant drug.

Desyrel: Brand name of the antidepressant drug trazodone.

Dexbrompheniramine/Pseudoephedrine: A drug used in treating allergies and colds. OTC.

Dextromethorphan: A cough suppressant drug. OTC.

Dextromethorphan/Guaifenesin: An expectorant and cough suppressant combination drug. OTC.

Dextromethorphan/Iodated Glycerol/Chlorpheniramine: A cough suppressant and expectorant combination drug.

Diaβeta: Brand name of the hypoglycemic (antidiabetic) drug glyburide.

Diabinese: Brand name of the hypoglycemic (antidiabetic) drug chlorpropamide.

Diazepam: An anti-anxiety drug.

Diclofenac: An anti-inflammatory drug.

Diflunisal: An anti-inflammatory drug.

Digoxin: A heart drug.

Dilantin: Brand name of the anticonvulsant drug phenytoin.

Diltiazem: A heart drug.

Dimetane: Brand name of the antihistamine and decongestant combination drug brompheniramine and phenylpropanolamine. OTC. This medication becomes a prescription drug for cough suppression if codeine is added.

Dimetapp: Brand name of the antihistamine and decongestant combination drug brompheniramine and phenylpropanolamine. OTC.

Diphenhydramine: An antihistamine and cough suppressant drug. OTC (in some preparations).

Dipivefrin: A glaucoma drug.

Dipyridamole: An anticoagulant drug.

Diuril: Brand name of the antihypertensive and diuretic drug chlorothiazide.

Docusate: A stool softener. OTC.

Dolobid: Brand name of the anti-inflammatory drug diflunisal.

Donnagel: Brand name of the antidiarrheal combination drug hyoscyamine/atropine/hyoscine. OTC.

Donnatal: Brand name of the antispasmodic combination drug hyoscyamine/atropine/hyoscine/phenobarbital.

Doryx: Brand name of the antibiotic doxycycline.

Doxepin: An antidepressant drug.

Doxycycline: An antibiotic.

Drixoral: Brand name of the decongestant combination drug pseudoephedrine and dexbrompheniramine. OTC.

Dulcolax: Brand name of the laxative bisacodyl. OTC.

Duraquin: Brand name of the anti-arrhythmia heart drug quinidine.

Duricef: Brand name of the antibiotic cefadroxil.

Dyazide: Brand name of the antihypertensive and diuretic combination drug triamterene/hydrochlorothiazide.

EES: Brand name of the antibiotic erythromycin.

Elavil: Brand name of the antidepressant drug amitriptyline.

E-Mycin: Brand name of the antibiotic erythromycin.

Enalapril: An antihypertensive drug.

Entex LA: Brand name of the decongestant and expectorant combination drug phenylpropanolamine/guaifenesin.

Epinephrine: An anti-asthmatic, anti-glaucoma, and decongestant drug. OTC (in some preparations).

ERYC: Brand name of the antibiotic erythromycin.

Erythromycin: An antibiotic drug.

Erythromycin/Sulfisoxazole: A combination antibiotic.

Esidrix: Brand name of the diuretic drug hydrochlorothiazide.

Estraderm: Brand name of the topical preparation of estrogen (applied as a patch).

Estrogen: Generic name for female sex hormones.

Famotidine: A histamine-blocker ulcer drug.

Feldene: Brand name of the anti-arthritic drug piroxicam.

Fenoprofen: An analgesic and anti-arthritic drug.

Fioricet: Brand name of the migraine analgesic combination butalbital, acetaminophen, and caffeine.

Fiorinal: Brand name of the migraine analgesic combination butalbital, aspirin, and caffeine.

Fiorinal/Codeine: Brand name of the migraine analgesic combination butalbital, codeine, caffeine, and aspirin.

Flagyl: Brand name of the antimicrobial drug metronidazole.

Flexeril: Brand name of the antispasmodic drug cyclobenzaprine.

Flunisolide: A nasal decongestant drug.

Fluocinonide: A topical anti-inflammatory drug.

Fluoxetine: An antidepressant drug.

Flurazepam: A hypnotic and sedative drug.

Folex: Brand name of the cytotoxic drug methotrexate; also used in treating rheumatoid arthritis and psoriasis.

Furosemide: A diuretic drug.

Gemfibrozil: An antilipidemic (cholesterol-reducing) drug.

Glipizide: A hypoglycemic (antidiabetic) drug.

Glucotrol: Brand name of the hypoglycemic (antidiabetic) drug glipizide.

Glyburide: A hypoglycemic (antidiabetic) drug.

Guaifenesin: An expectorant drug. OTC.

Halcion: Brand name of the sedative and hypnotic drug triazolam.

Hydrochlorothiazide: An antihypertensive and diuretic drug.

Hydrocodone/Acetaminophen: An analgesic combination drug.

Hydrocortisone cream: A corticosteroid drug used topically. OTC up to 0.5 percent; greater than 0.5 percent, by prescription only.

Hydrodiuril: Brand name of the antihypertensive and diuretic drug hydrochlorothiazide.

Hyoscyamine/Atropine/Hyoscine: An antidiarrheal combination drug. OTC.

Hyoscyamine/Atropine/Hyoscine/Phenobarbital: An antispasmodic drug.

Ibuprofen: An analgesic drug. OTC up to 200 milligrams; by prescription only for over 200 milligrams.

Iletin: Brand name of the diabetic drug insulin.

Imodium: Brand name of the antidiarrheal drug loperamide. OTC for liquid preparations; by prescription only for tablets.

Indapamide: An antihypertensive and diuretic drug.

Inderal: Brand name of the anti-arrhythmia heart drug propranolol.

Indocin: Brand name of the analgesic and anti-inflammatory drug indomethacin.

Indomethacin: An analgesic and anti-inflammatory drug.

Insulin: An antidiabetic agent.

Intal: Brand name of the anti-allergy drug cromolyn.

Isoptin: Brand name of the antihypertensive drug verapamil.

Isosorbide Dinitrate: A heart (anti-anginal) drug.

Isotretinoin: An anti-acne drug.

Kaopectate: Brand name of the antidiarrheal drug attapulgite. OTC.

Keflex: Brand name of the antibiotic cephalexin.

Keftab: Brand name of the antibiotic cephalexin.

Ketoprofen: An analgesic and anti-arthritic drug.

Klotrix: A potassium supplement.

K-Tab: A potassium supplement.

Labetalol: An antihypertensive and heart drug.

Lanoxin: Brand name of the heart drug digoxin.

Lasix: Brand name of the diuretic drug furosemide.

Levodopa/Carbidopa: A combination antiparkinsonism drug.

Levonorgestrel: A component of oral contraceptives.

Levothroid: Brand name of the synthetic thyroid hormone thyroxine.

Levothyroxine Sodium: Thyroid hormone.

Lidex: Brand name of the topical anti-inflammatory drug fluocinonide.

Loniten: Brand name of the antihypertensive drug and hair growth stimulant minoxidil.

Lo/Ovral: Brand name of the combination oral contraceptive drug norgestrol/ethinyl estradiol.

Loperamide: An antidiarrheal drug. OTC.

Lopid: Brand name of the antilipidemic (cholesterol-reducing) drug gemfibrozil.

Lopressor: Brand name of the antihypertensive and heart drug metoprolol.

Lorazepam: An anti-anxiety drug.

Lotrimin: Brand name of the topical antifungal drug clotrimazole.

Lortrisone: Brand name of the topical antifungal combination drug clotrimazole and betamethasone.

Lovastatin: An antilipidemic (cholesterol-reducing) drug.

Lozol: Brand name of the antihypertensive and diuretic drug indapamide.

Macrodantin: Brand name of the antibiotic nitrofurantoin macrocrystals.

Magnesium Carbonate: An antacid. OTC.

Magnesium Hydroxide: An antacid. OTC.

Magnesium Trisilicate: An antacid. OTC.

Maxzide: Brand name of the antihypertensive and diuretic combination drug triamterene/hydrochlorothiazide.

Meclizine: An antinausea and motion sickness drug. OTC (in some preparations).

Meclofenamate: An analgesic and anti-inflammatory drug.

Meclomen: Brand name of the analgesic and non-steroidal anti-inflammatory drug meclofenamate.

Medrol: Brand name of the anti-inflammatory (corticosteroid) drug methylprednisolone.

Medroxyprogesterone: Progesterone hormone drug.

Metamucil: Brand name of the bulk-forming laxative psyllium. OTC.

Methotrexate: A cytotoxic drug; also used in treating rheumatoid arthritis and psoriasis.

Methyldopa: An antihypertensive drug.

Methyldopa/Hydrochlorothiazide: An antihypertensive and diuretic combination drug.

Methylphenidate: An amphetamine-like drug.

Methylprednisolone: An anti-inflammatory (corticosteroid) drug.

Meticorten: Brand name of the corticosteroid drug prednisone.

Metoclopramide: An antinausea drug.

Metoprolol: An antihypertensive and heart drug.

Metoproterenol: A bronchodilator and anti-asthmatic drug.

Metronidazole: An antimicrobial drug.

Mevacor: Brand name of the antilipidemic (cholesterol-reducing) drug lovastatin.

Mexate: Brand name of the cytotoxic drug methotrexate; also used in treating rheumatoid arthritis and psoriasis.

Miconazole: An antifungal drug.

Micro-K: A potassium supplement.

Micronase: Brand name of the hypoglycemic (antidiabetic) drug glyburide.

Milk of Magnesia: Brand name of the antacid magnesium hydroxide. OTC.

Minipress: Brand name of the antihypertensive drug prazosin.

Minocin: Brand name of the antibiotic minocycline.

Minocycline: An antibiotic drug.

Minoxidil: An antihypertensive drug and hair-growth stimulant.

Moduretic: Brand name of the diuretic combination drug amiloride/hydrochlorothiazide.

Monistat: Brand name of the antifungal drug miconazole.

Motrin: Brand name of the analgesic drug ibuprofen. OTC for 200 milligrams; by prescription only for over 200 milligrams.

Nadolol: An antihypertensive and heart drug.

Naldecon: Brand name of the allergy and cold combination drug phenylephedrine/phenylpropanolamine/phenyltoloxamine/chlorpheniramine.

Nalfon: Brand name of the analgesic and anti-arthritic drug fenoprofen.

Naprosyn: Brand name of the analgesic and anti-inflammatory drug naproxen.

Naproxen: An analgesic and anti-inflammatory drug.

Nasalcrom: Brand name of the anti-allergy drug cromolyn.

Nasalide: Brand name of the nasal decongestant drug flunisolide.

Neo-Synephrine: Brand name of the decongestant drug phenylephrine.

Nicorette: Brand name of a nicotine tobacco substitute.

Nicotine: A tobacco substitute.

Nifedipine: A heart drug.

Nitro-Dur: Brand name of the heart drug nitroglycerin.

Nitrofurantoin Macrocrystals: An antibiotic drug.

Nitroglycerin: A heart drug.

Nitrostat: Brand name of the heart drug nitroglycerin.

Nordette-28: Brand name of the oral contraceptive combination ethinyl estradiol/levonorgestrel.

Norethindrone/Ethinyl Estradiol: A combination oral contraceptive drug.

Norfloxacin: An antibiotic drug.

Norgestrol/Ethinyl Estradiol: A combination oral contraceptive drug.

Normodyne: Brand name of the antihypertensive and heart drug labetalol.

Noroxin: Brand name of the antibiotic norfloxacin.

Norpramin: Brand name of the antidepressant drug desipramine.

Nortriptyline: An antidepressant drug.

Novafed: Brand name of the decongestant drug pseudoephedrine.

Nuprin: Brand name of the analgesic drug ibuprofen. OTC.

Omnipen: Brand name of the antibiotic ampicillin.

Orasone: Brand name of the corticosteroid drug prednisone.

Ortho-Novum: Brand name of the oral contraceptive combination drug norethindrone/ethinyl estradiol.

Orudis: Brand name of the analgesic and anti-arthritic drug ketoprofen.

Oxycodone/Acetaminophen: An analgesic combination drug.

Oxycodone/Aspirin: An analgesic combination drug.

Oxymetazoline: A decongestant drug. OTC.

Pamelor: Brand name of the antidepressant drug nortriptyline.

Panadol: Brand name of the analgesic drug acetaminophen. OTC.

PCE: Brand name of the antibiotic erythromycin.

Pediazole: Brand name of the antibiotics erythromycin and sulfisoxazole, used as a combination drug.

Penicillin V: An antibiotic drug.

Pentoxifylline: A drug used to improve blood flow.

Pen-Vee K: Brand name of the antibiotic penicillin V.

Pepcid: Brand name of the histamine-blocker ulcer drug famotidine.

Percocet: Brand name of the analgesic combination drug oxycodone and acetaminophen.

Percodan: Brand name of the analgesic combination drug oxycodone/aspirin.

Persantine: Brand name of the anticoagulant drug dipyridamole.

Phenergan: Brand name of the antihistamine drug promethazine.

Phenobarbital: An anticonvulsant and sedative drug.

Phenylephedrine/Chlorpheniramine/

Pyrilamine: A decongestant and antihistamine combination drug.

Phenylephedrine/Phenylpropanolamine/Phenyltoloxamine/Chlorpheniramine: A combination allergy and cold drug.

Phenylephrine: A decongestant drug.

Phenylpropanolamine/Guaifenesin: A decongestant and expectorant combination drug.

Phenytoin: An anticonvulsant drug.

Piroxicam: An anti-arthritic drug.

Polymox: Brand name of the antibiotic amoxicillin.

Polymyxin B/Bacitracin/Neomycin/ Hydrocortisone: An anti-inflammatory and antimicrobial combination drug.

Potassium Chloride: A potassium supplement.

Prazosin: An antihypertensive drug.

Prednisolone: A corticosteroid drug.

Prednisone: A corticosteroid drug.

Premarin: Brand name of the oral or vaginal female hormone estrogen.

Probenecid: A gout drug.

Procardia: Brand name of the heart drug nifedipine.

Prochlorperazine: An antinausea drug.

Proloid: Brand name of natural thyroid hormone preparation.

Promethazine: An antihistamine drug.

Propine: Brand name of the glaucoma drug dipivefrin.

Propoxyphene/Acetaminophen: An analgesic drug.

Propranolol: An anti-arrhythmia heart drug.

Proventil: Brand name of the bronchodilator drug albuterol.

Provera: Brand name of the progesterone hormone drug medroxyprogesterone.

Prozac: Brand name of the antidepressant drug fluoxetine.

Pseudoephedrine: A decongestant drug. OTC.

Psyllium: A bulk-forming laxative. OTC.

Questran: Brand name of the cholesterol-reducing drug cholestyramine.

Quinidine: An anti-arrhythmia drug.

Quinora: Brand name of the anti-arrhythmia heart drug quinidine.

Ranitidine: A histamine-blocker ulcer drug.

Reglan: Brand name of the drug metoclopramide. Used to stimulate muscular action (contractions) of the stomach.

Reserpine: An antihypertensive drug.

Restoril: Brand name of the sedative and hypnotic drug temazepam.

Retin-A: Brand name of the anti-acne drug tretinoin.

Rifadin: Brand name of the antibiotic rifampin.

Rifampin: An antibiotic drug.

Rimactane: Brand name of the antibiotic rifampin.

Ritalin: Brand name of the amphetamine-like drug methylphenidate.

Robitussin: Brand name of the expectorant drug guaifenesin. OTC.

Robitussin-DM: Brand name of the expectorant and cough suppressant combination drug dextromethorphan/guaifenesin. OTC.

Rogaine: Brand name of the antihypertensive drug and hair-growth stimulant minoxidil.

Rynatan: Brand name of the decongestant and antihistamine combination drug phenylephedrine/chlorpheniramine/pyrilamine.

Seldane: Brand name of the antihistamine drug terfenadine.

Selenium: A dandruff treatment. OTC.

Selsun Blue: Brand name of the dandruff treatment selenium. OTC.

Septra: Brand name of the antibiotic combination trimethoprim-sulfamethoxazole.

Sinemet: Brand name of the antiparkinsonism combination drug levodopa/carbidopa.

Sinequan: Brand name of the antidepressant drug doxepin.

Sinex: Brand name of the decongestant drug phenylephrine.

Slo-Bid: Brand name of the bronchodilator drug theophylline.

Slow-K: A potassium supplement.

Sodium bicarbonate: An antacid. OTC.

Spironolactone: A diuretic drug.

Stuartnatal 1+1: Brand name of a multivitamin supplement for pregnant and lactating women.

Sucralfate: A drug that has protective properties for the lining of the stomach.

Sudafed: Brand name of the decongestant drug pseudoephedrine. OTC.

Sulindac: An analgesic and anti-arthritic drug.

Sumycin: Brand name of the antibiotic tetracycline.

Synthroid: Brand name of the thyroid hormone levothyroxine sodium.

Tagamet: Brand name of the histamine-blocker ulcer drug cimetidine.

Tavist-D: Brand name of the allergy and cold combination treatment cemastine/phenylpropanolamine.

Tegretol: Brand name of the anticonvulsant drug carbamazepine.

Temazepam: A sedative and hypnotic drug.

Tenoretic: Brand name of the antihypertensive combination drug atenolol/chlorthalidone.

Tenormin: Brand name of the antihypertensive and heart drug atenolol.

Terbutaline: A bronchodilator drug.

Terfenadine: An antihistamine drug.

Tetracycline: An antibiotic drug.

Theo-Dur: Brand name of the bronchodilator drug theophylline.

Theophylline: A bronchodilator drug.

Thyrolar: Brand name of synthetic thyroid hormones.

Thyroxine: A synthetic thyroid hormone.

Timolide: Brand name of the antihypertensive and antiglaucoma drug timolol.

Timolol: An antihypertensive and antiglaucoma drug.

Timoptic: Brand name of the antihypertensive and antiglaucoma drug timolol.

Tinactin: Brand name of the topical antifungal agent tolnaftate. OTC.

Tolectin: Brand name of anti-inflammatory drug tolmetin.

Tolmetin: An anti-inflammatory drug.

Tolnaftate: A topical antifungal agent. OTC.

Transderm-Nitro: Brand name of the heart drug nitroglycerin. Applied as a patch.

Tranxene: Brand name of the anti-anxiety drug clorazepate.

Trazodone: An antidepressant drug.

Trental: Brand name of the drug pentoxifylline, used to improve blood flow.

Tretinoin: An anti-acne drug.

Triamterene/Hydrochlorothiazide: An antihypertensive and diuretic combination drug.

Triazolam: A sedative and hypnotic drug.

Trimethoprim/Sulfamethoxazole: An antibiotic combination drug.

Trimox: Brand name of the antibiotic amoxicillin.

Trinalin: Brand name of the decongestant and antihistamine combination drug azatidine and pseudoephedrine.

Tri-Norinyl: Brand name of the oral contraceptive combination drug norethindrone/ethinyl estradiol.

Triphasil-28: Brand name of the oral contraceptive combination drug ethinyl estradiol/levonorgestrel.

Triprolidine/Pseudoephedrine: An allergy and cold treatment. OTC.

Tussi-Organidin: Brand name of the cough suppressant and expectorant combination drug codeine and iodinated glycerol.

Tussi-Organidin DM: Brand name of the cough suppressant and expectorant combination drug dextromethorphan/iodinated glycerol.

Tylenol: Brand name of the analgesic drug acetaminophen. OTC.

Tylenol with Codeine: Brand name of the analgesic combination drug acetaminophen/codeine.

Tylox: Brand name of the analgesic combination drug oxycodone/acetaminophen.

Valium: Brand name of the anti-anxiety drug diazepam.

Valrelease: Brand name of the anti-anxiety drug diazepam.

Vasotec: Brand name of the antihypertensive drug enalapril.

Veetids: Brand name of the antibiotic penicillin V.

Ventolin: Brand name of the bronchodilator drug albuterol.

Verapamil: An antihypertensive drug.

Vibramycin: Brand name of the antibiotic doxycycline.

Vicodin: Brand name of the analgesic combination drug hydrocodone/acetaminophen.

Voltaren: Brand name of the anti-inflammatory drug diclofenac.

Warfarin: An anticoagulant drug.

Wymox: Brand name of the antibiotic drug amoxicillin.

Xanax: Brand name of the anti-anxiety drug alprazolam.

Zantac: Brand name of the histamine-blocker ulcer drug ranitidine.

Zovirax: Brand name of the antiviral drug acyclovir.

Zyloprim: Brand name of the gout (uric acid inhibitor) drug allopurinol.

APPENDIX III

CONVERSION TABLES
WEIGHTS AND MEASURES

APPENDIX CONTENTS

LINEAR MEASUREMENTS

Millimeters, Centimeters, Meters, and Kilometers		Inches, Feet, Yards, and Miles
1.0 millimeter (mm)	=	0.04 inch (in.)
1.0 centimeter (cm) = 10 mm	=	0.39 in.
2.54 cm	=	1.0 in.
30.48 cm	=	1.0 foot (ft) = 12 in.
0.9144 meter (m)	=	1.0 yard (yd) = 3 ft
1.0 m = 100 cm	=	39.37 in.
1.0 kilometer (km) = 1,000 m	=	0.622 mile (mi)
1.609 km	=	1.0 mi = 5,280 ft

SAMPLE CONVERSIONS FOR METRIC HEIGHTS AND WEIGHTS

Height				Weight	
cm	Feet	Inches (approx.)		Kilo-grams	Pounds
15	0	6		1	2.2
30	1	0		5	11
45	1	6		10	22
60	1	11½		15	33
75	2	5½		20	44
105	3	5		25	55
115	3	9		30	66
120	3	11		35	77
125	4	1		40	88
130	4	3		45	99
135	4	5		50	110
140	4	7		55	121
145	4	9		60	132
150	4	11		65	143
155	5	1		70	154
160	5	3		75	165
165	5	5		80	176
170	5	7		85	187
175	5	9		90	198
180	5	11		95	209
185	6	1		100	220
190	6	3		105	231
195	6	5		110	242
200	6	7		115	253
205	6	9		120	264
210	6	11		125	275
215	7	1		130	286

VOLUME

Milliliters and Liters		Ounces, Quarts, and Cubic Inches
1.0 milliliter (mL)	=	0.034 fluid ounce (fl oz)
16.3866 mL	=	1.0 cubic inch (in.^{3})
16.3866 mL	=	0.558 fl oz
29.57 mL	=	1.0 ounce (fl oz) = 1.8047 in.^{3}
0.9463 liter (L)	=	1.0 quart (qt) = 32.0 fl oz
1.0 L = 1,000 mL	=	1.057 qt

WEIGHT

Milligrams, Grams, and Kilograms		Grains, Ounces, and Pounds
1.0 milligram (mg)	=	0.015 grain (gr)
64.8 mg	=	1.0 gr
1.0 gram (g)	=	15.0 gr
1.0 g	=	0.035 ounce (oz)
31.1 g	=	1.0 oz
453.59 g	=	1.0 pound (lb) = 16 oz
1.0 kilogram (kg) = 1,000 g	=	2.2 lb

SAMPLE CONVERSION FROM METRIC WEIGHT

Symbol	When You Know	Multiply by	To Find
g	grams	0.035	ounces (oz)
kg	kilograms	2.2	pounds (lb)

TEMPERATURE

CENTIGRADE TO FAHRENHEIT

Multiply centigrade degrees by $9/5$ and add 32 to the result.
(Example: 25°C $\times$ $9/5$ = 45 + 32 = 77°F)

FAHRENHEIT TO CENTIGRADE

Subtract 32 from Fahrenheit degrees and multiply the result by $5/9$.
(Example: 77°F − 32 = 45 $\times$ $5/9$ = 25°C)

°F	96	97	98	98.6 / 99	100	101	102	103	104	105
°C	35.6	36.1	36.7	37 / 37.2	37.8	38.3	38.9	39.4	40	40.6

HOUSEHOLD MEASURES

1 teaspoon	=	1/8 fluid ounce
3 teaspoons	=	1 tablespoon
1 tablespoon	=	1/2 fluid ounce
16 tablespoons (wet)	=	1 cup
12 tablespoons (dry)	=	1 cup
1 cup	=	8 fluid ounces
1 pint	=	2 cups or 16 fl oz

Note: Household measures are imprecise. For example, a household teaspoon is defined as containing between 3 and 5 milliliters. Thus, *never* substitute household equivalents for more precise dosages prescribed by your physician.

APPENDIX IV

GLOSSARY

APPENDIX CONTENTS

UNDERSTANDING MEDICAL TERMS

UNDERSTANDING MEDICAL TERMS

The language of medicine is rich with specialized, polysyllabic words. This wealth of vocabulary is a mixed blessing. Your physician can use precise terminology to describe conditions and symptoms to his or her colleagues. Yet in some cases, that same terminology can be confusing, worrisome, or irritating to the uninitiated listener.

In the text of this book, we have tried to use language familiar to the layperson whenever possible to enhance the readability and utility of the book. In most cases, when a medical term is introduced, we define it first and then put the term in parentheses.

However, for those instances in which terms prove confusing or unclear, we have assembled the glossary that follows. In it you will find a wide range of commonly used medical terms.

Given limitations of space, we have not incorporated the names of all or even most ailments discussed in the book; those are defined in entries devoted to them in the text and can be found by using the index at the back of this volume. Similarly, drug terms are found in The Modern Pharmacy (see page 1225) and terms that describe testing procedures are in Appendix I: Medical Tests (see page 1281).

Abortion: The ending of a pregnancy by expulsion or extraction of the fetus from the womb before it is viable, usually before the 20th week of gestation.

Abrasion: A spot rubbed bare of skin or mucous membrane; or, the normal wearing of tooth enamel by chewing.

Abscess: A localized formation of pus in a cavity caused by the disintegration or displacement of tissue due to bacterial infection.

Acute: Term used to describe disorders or symptoms that occur abruptly or disorders or symptoms that run a short course; opposite of chronic.

Addiction: Physical or emotional (or both) dependence on a substance (most often alcohol or another drug), usually requiring increasing amounts.

Adhesion: A union of two surfaces, as in a wound healing.

Adrenal glands: Endocrine glands that produce a range of hormones, including epi-nephrine, norepinephrine, and the corticosteroid hormones.

Adrenaline: See *Epinephrine.*

Aerobic: Requiring the presence of oxygen. Aerobic exercise, for example, is vigorous, requiring increased oxygen consumption. See also *Anaerobic.*

Afterbirth: The placenta and membranes discharged from the uterus after childbirth.

Albumin: A protein found widely in animal and plant tissues; its presence in the urine is one sign of kidney disease.

Aldosterone: Adrenal hormone that affects the body's use of sodium, chloride, and potassium.

Allergen: Any substance that produces an allergic reaction. Common allergens include animal fur, house dust mites, pollen, and certain foods.

Allergy: An exaggerated reaction to a substance or condition produced by the release of histamine or histamine-like substances in affected cells. Symptoms may include rashes, nasal congestion, asthma, and occasionally shock. See also *Histamine.*

Alveoli: Microscopic air sacs in the lungs where gases are exchanged; or, tooth socket.

Amanita mushrooms: Group of mushrooms, most of which are highly poisonous when eaten.

Ambulatory: Able to walk.

Amino acid: A component of protein, containing nitrogen. The body produces many amino acids; those it needs but cannot synthesize are known as essential amino acids and must be obtained through the diet.

Amnesia: Loss of memory.

Amniotic fluid: The protective liquid surrounding the fetus in the womb.

Amputation: The act of cutting off or removing a limb or other body part.

Anaerobic: Able to live without oxygen, as certain bacteria; or, a type of exercise in which short, vigorous bursts of activity requiring little additional oxygen are performed. See also *Aerobic.*

Anaphylaxis: An immediate and sometimes life-threatening allergic hypersensitivity reaction. Symptoms can include shock, breathing difficulty, itching and hives, convulsions, and coma. See *Shock.*

Androgen: A hormone such as testosterone and andosterone responsible for the development of male characteristics. Produced in the testes in the male; also found in small amounts in females.

Anemia: Condition characterized by a reduced number of red blood cells, amount of hemoglobin, or amount of blood.

Anesthesia: Partial or complete loss of feeling or sensation sometimes accompanied by loss of consciousness. Local anesthesia is accomplished by the injection or topical application of drugs. General anesthesia, which includes loss of consciousness, is accomplished by the inhalation or injection of drugs into the muscles or bloodstream.

Aneurysm: The local swelling or bulging of a blood vessel, usually an artery, to form a sac.

Angina pectoris: Episodic pain in the chest due to a temporary inadequacy of the blood supply to the heart.

Angioedema: Allergic swelling of the mucous membranes, tissues beneath the skin, or an internal organ.

Anorexia: Loss of appetite, often due to depression, fever and illness, widespread cancer, or addiction to alcohol or drugs.

Anorexia nervosa: Loss of appetite caused by an emotional disturbance; it most often affects young women between 12 and 21 years old and can result in severe loss of weight and even death.

Antibody: Protein of the immune system that counteracts or eliminates foreign substances known as antigens.

Antidote: Substance that neutralizes the effects of a poison.

Antigen: Substance foreign to the body that causes antibodies to form.

Anus: Outlet of the rectum, through which fecal waste passes.

Aorta: Largest artery in the body; it carries blood from the heart's left ventricle and distributes it throughout the body.

Aphasia: Loss of the ability to speak or to understand speech because of brain injury.

Aplastic: Arrested development of a tissue or an organ.

Apnea: Temporary cessation of breathing.

Aqueous humor: Transparent fluid that flows between the anterior and posterior chambers of the eye.

Areola: Circular, pigmented area around the nipple of the breast.

Arrhythmia: Irregular heartbeat.

Arteriole: Tiny artery that joins a large artery to a capillary.

Arteriosclerosis: Condition in which the walls of arteries become hard and thick, sometimes interfering with blood circulation.

Artery: Blood vessel that carries blood from the heart to other tissues of the body.

Arthroplasty: Surgical replacement or repair of a joint.

Asphyxia: Suffocation due to insufficient oxygen intake.

Aspiration: Removal of fluids by suction from cavities such as the nose, throat, or lungs; or, the inhalation into the lungs of fluids, such as water in drowning or stomach contents in vomiting.

Asthma: Condition characterized by congestion of the bronchial tubes, causing wheezing, coughing, and difficult breathing.

Asymptomatic: Without symptoms.

Ataxia: Incoordination of voluntary muscle movements.

Atherosclerosis: Condition in which fatty deposits accumulate in the lining of the arteries, resulting in smaller, less flexible pathways for the blood.

Atresia: Congenital absence of an opening in the body.

Atria: Cavities or chambers such as the upper chambers of the heart, which receive blood from veins and pass the blood to the ventricles. (Singular form is **atrium.**)

Atrophy: Wasting of tissue or organ due to disease or lack of use.

Aura: Sensation felt before the onset of a convulsion or migraine headache.

Autoimmune response: Reaction of the body against one or some of its own tissues that are perceived as foreign substances, resulting in production of antibodies against that tissue.

Autonomic nervous system: Portion of the nervous system that regulates involuntary body functions.

Autopsy: Examination of tissues and organs of the body after death.

Avulsion: Forced tearing away of a body part or structure such as a limb or tooth.

Bacteria: Single-celled microorganisms, some of which cause disease and some of which are beneficial to biological processes.

B cell: Lymphocyte of the bone marrow that works as part of the immune system by producing antibodies to fight infection.

Benign: Essentially harmless; not progressive or recurrent.

Bicuspid: One of four teeth in the adult mouth having two points, located between the canine and molar.

Bile: Bitter-tasting fluid produced by the liver and temporarily stored in the gallbladder before discharge into the small intestine. In the small bowel the bile facilitates the digestion of fats.

Bilirubin: Orange or yellowish pigment in bile that is the result of breakdown of hemoglobin. An excess of bilirubin produces jaundice.

Biofeedback: Behavior training program that teaches a person how to control autonomic reactions such as heart rate, blood pressure, skin temperature, and muscular tension.

Bladder: Membranous sac that holds secretions, most commonly the sac that collects urine before its elimination.

Blood pressure: Constant force placed on the walls of the arteries. See also *Diastole* and *Systole.*

Bone marrow: Soft material found inside bone cavities that is the site of formation of blood cells.

Bowel: Lower or large intestine. The small intestine is sometimes called the small bowel.

Brainstem: Portion of the brain that connects the hemispheres with the spinal cord. Consists of medulla oblongata, pons, and midbrain.

Brand name drug: A drug carrying a trademark name designated by its manufacturer.

Bronchi: The two main breathing tubes leading from the trachea to the lungs.

Bronchiole: One of the subdivisions of a bronchus or bronchial tube.

Bruise: Injury in which blood vessels beneath the skin are broken and blood escapes to produce a discolored area.

Bursa: Fluid-filled sac near or involving a joint or bony prominence that helps to reduce friction between a tendon or bone or between bone and skin during movement.

Cachexia: Malnutrition and wasting due to illness.

Calcitonin: A hormone produced by the thyroid gland that affects the amount of calcium in the blood.

Calculus: Accumulation of mineral salts in various parts of the body or on the teeth, which resemble stone.

Callus: Area of thickened skin.

Calorie: The amount of heat needed to raise the temperature of 1 gram of water by 1° centigrade.

Cancer: General term for various illnesses characterized by abnormal growth of cells, forming malignant tumors that can develop in various parts of the body. See also *Malignant* and *Benign.*

Canine: One of four teeth found between the molars and incisors; also known as eye teeth.

Capillaries: Minute blood vessels connecting the smallest arteries to the smallest veins.

Carbohydrate: A group of compounds composed of starches or sugars and found primarily in breads and cereals and in fruits and vegetables.

Carcinogen: Potential cancer-causing agent.

Cardiac: Pertaining to the heart.

Cardiac arrest: Sudden stopping of circulation by cessation of the heartbeat.

Cardiopulmonary: Pertaining to the heart and lung.

Cardiopulmonary resuscitation (CPR): Technique for reviving a person whose heart and breathing have stopped and who is unconscious.

Cardiovascular: Pertaining to the heart and blood vessels.

Caries: Decay of tooth or bone due to bacteria; also known as cavities.

Carotid artery: Principal artery of neck; carries blood to head and brain.

Cartilage: Dense, white connective tissue located in the joints, nose, and ear.

Cataract: Opacity of the eye lens that obstructs vision.

Catheter: Small, flexible tube that may be inserted into various parts of the body to inject or remove liquid.

Cerebellum: Portion of the brain responsible for coordinating movements.

Cerebrovascular: Pertaining to the blood vessels of the brain.

Cerebrum: Largest portion of the brain, containing the two hemispheres; responsible for thinking, feelings, and voluntary movement.

Cervix: The neck of an organ, such as the neck of the uterus.

Cesarean section: Surgical removal of a baby from the womb through an incision in the abdomen.

Chemotherapy: Treatment of disease by

using chemicals that have a direct effect on the disease-causing organism or disease cells; widely used in the treatment of cancer.

Cholesterol: Fat-like substance synthesized in the liver and found in the blood, brain, liver, and bile and as deposits in the walls of blood vessels. Essential to the production of sex hormones. Found in foods of animal sources and thought to contribute to heart disease when eaten in large quantities over a long period of time.

Choroid: Membrane of the eye between the sclera (white) and the retina; together with the iris and ciliary body it makes up the uvea.

Chromosome: One of 46 rod-shaped structures in the nucleus of each cell that carry information regarding heredity.

Chronic: Term used to describe long-lasting diseases or conditions.

Chyme: Mixture of partly digested food and digestive secretions found in the stomach.

Cilia: Eyelashes; or, other small hair-like projections lining the nose and bronchi.

Claudication: A cramping of the calf muscles with exercise, produced by inadequate blood flow.

Clinical: Pertaining to information gathered from working with patients, as distinct from laboratory findings.

Clitoris: Small, erectile organ of the external female genitalia.

Coagulate: To solidify or change from a liquid to a semisolid, as when blood clots.

Cochlea: Snail-shaped tube of the inner ear that is the receptor for hearing.

Cognitive: Pertaining to the mental process of thought, including perception, reasoning, intuition, and memory.

Coitus: Sexual intercourse between a man and woman in which the man inserts his penis into the woman's vagina.

Colic: Pain in abdomen produced by intermittent spasm of the intestines. In infants, it may be manifested by episodes of crying, with a distended abdomen and the legs drawn up to the chest.

Collagen: Fibrous protein found in connective tissues such as skin, bone ligaments, and cartilage.

Colon: The large intestine running from the small intestine to the anus. It is responsible for extracting water from undigested food and storing the waste, which is eliminated in bowel movements.

Colorectal: Pertaining to the colon and rectum.

Colostrum: The thin, lemon-colored liquid produced by a mother's breasts in the first day or so after giving birth. Its antibodies are beneficial to the infant.

Coma: An abnormal state of deep unconsciousness due to illness or accident.

Conception: Fertilization of an egg by sperm.

Concussion: Temporary disturbances of brain function due to a blow or fall.

Congenital: Term used to describe something present at birth, especially an abnormality.

Congestion: The presence of excessive blood or fluid, such as mucus, in an organ or tissue.

Conjunctiva: Transparent membrane that lines the eyelid and covers the front of the eyeball (except for the cornea).

Constipation: The difficult passage of hard, dry stools.

Contracture: Permanent tightness or shortening of a muscle due to disease.

Contrast agent: A liquid substance ("dye") opaque to x-rays that is taken into the gastrointestinal tract or injected into a blood vessel or into the fluid-filled space around the spinal cord to permit x-ray visualization of structures of the body that could not otherwise be seen by x-ray.

Contusion: Bruise.

Convulsion: A sudden attack usually characterized by loss of consciousness and severe, sustained, rhythmic contractions of some or all voluntary muscles. Convulsions are most often a manifestation of a seizure disorder (epilepsy).

Cornea: Transparent part of the eye through which the iris and pupil may be seen.

Coronary: Related to arteries that supply blood to the heart.

Corticosteroids: Hormones produced by the cortex of the adrenal glands; also, artificial hormones used as medications.

Cranium: Portion of the skull that houses the brain.

Creatinine: One of the non-protein constituents of blood and urine. It is found in high amounts in the blood of persons with renal failure.

Curettage: Scraping of a cavity, such as the uterus.

Cuspid: Tooth with one point, located

between the incisors and bicuspids toward the front of the mouth, sometimes called the canine tooth.

Cyanosis: Bluish discoloration of the skin due to lack of oxygen.

Cyst: A closed sac or cavity filled with a fluid, gas, or semisolid substance.

Debility: A state of physical weakness.

Dehydration: Excessive loss of body fluids.

Delirium: A state, usually temporary, of mental confusion, sometimes characterized by disordered speech and often accompanied by hallucinations.

Delusion: Belief held despite evidence as to its falsehood.

Dementia: Mental deterioration due to organic causes.

Dentin: The tissue of a tooth beneath the enamel and enclosing the pulp cavity.

Deoxyribonucleic acid (DNA): A substance found in the nucleus of cells that carries genetic and hereditary information.

Depression: A feeling of extreme sadness and discouragement. Symptoms also may include disruption of sleeping and eating patterns and lack of energy.

Dermatitis: Inflammation of the skin, often characterized by itching and redness.

Dermis: The layer of skin beneath the epidermis.

Detoxification: Process of cleansing the body of a drug such as alcohol.

Dextrose (glucose): A simple sugar that is found in the blood and is a main component of honey and corn syrup.

Diabetes mellitus: Disorder characterized by high levels of glucose in the blood. Diabetes mellitus may be caused by a failure of the pancreas to produce sufficient insulin or by resistance of the body to the action of insulin.

Diagnosis: Identification of a disease or disorder by a physician.

Dialysis: Technique of removing waste and toxins from the blood, used primarily when the kidneys malfunction or in cases of overdose of a drug.

Diaphragm: Muscle that separates the abdomen from the chest; or, a rubber or plastic cup that fits over the cervix to help prevent conception.

Diastole: Period during the heart cycle in which the muscle relaxes, followed by contraction (systole). In a blood pressure reading, the lower number is the diastolic measurement.

Digit: A finger or toe.

Dilate: To expand or open an organ such as the pupil of the eye or a passageway such as an artery.

Disc: A plate-like structure such as the cartilage cushion found between each vertebra.

Dislocation: Displacement of a bone from its normal position in a joint.

Dominant: A mode of inheritance in which only a gene from one parent is required for a trait to appear in an offspring. See also *Recessive.*

Duodenum: The part of the small intestine closest to the stomach.

Dura mater: The tough outer membrane covering the spinal cord and brain.

Dysplasia: Abnormal development of tissue.

Ect-, Ecto-: Prefixes meaning outside.

Ectopic: Abnormal placement, such as of a fertilized egg in a fallopian tube.

Eczema: Acute or chronic inflammatory condition of the skin characterized by itching and scaling.

Edema: Swelling of body tissues due to excessive fluid.

Effusion: Accumulation of fluid in body cavities or between tissues.

Ejaculation: Ejection of semen during male orgasm.

Embolism: Obstruction of a blood vessel by a blood clot, air bubble, fat deposit, or other foreign substance.

Embryo: The human organism from the time of implantation in the uterus to the end of the second month.

Emetic: Substance that induces vomiting.

Emission: Discharge of fluid.

En-, Endo-: Prefixes meaning inside or within.

Endocardium: The thin, inner membrane that lines the heart muscle. See also *Epicardium* and *Myocardium.*

Endoscope: An illuminated optical instrument used to study the inside of a hollow organ or cavity.

Enema: Injection of fluid into the rectum and colon to induce a bowel movement to empty those structures.

Enzyme: A complex protein present in digestive juices or within cells that acts as a catalyst for chemical reactions.

Epicardium: The thin, exterior membrane that protects the heart muscle. See also *Endocardium* and *Myocardium.*

Epidermis: Outer layer of skin.

Epiglottis: Flap of cartilage that covers the larynx.

Epilepsy: See *Seizure.*

Epinephrine and Norepinephrine: Naturally occurring hormones that increase heart rate and blood pressure and affect other body functions.

Erection: Swelling and stiffening of the penis, characteristic of sexual arousal.

Erythema: Area of reddened skin due to dilatation of capillaries beneath the skin.

Erythrocytes: Red blood cells.

Esophagus: Tube that connects the throat with the stomach.

Estrogen: Hormone produced primarily in women that contributes to the development of secondary sex characteristics and cyclic changes such as menstruation and pregnancy. Oral replacement doses of estrogen are often used to lessen the effects of menopause. The hormone is also produced in small quantities in men.

Ethanol: Grain alcohol.

Eustachian tube: Tube connecting the middle ear to the pharynx.

Faint: To lose consciousness briefly as a result of insufficient blood to the brain.

Fallopian tube: One of two tubes, located on each side of a woman's uterus, that convey the egg from the ovary to the uterus.

False labor: Irregular pains and contractions that give a pregnant woman the illusion that labor has begun.

Fats: A group of organic compounds that are composed of fatty acids. Fats are either saturated or unsaturated. Unsaturated fats are classified as either monounsaturated or polyunsaturated.

Febrile: Feverish.

Feces: Body waste such as food residue discharged from the bowels.

Femur: Thighbone.

Fertility: The ability to conceive a child.

Fertilization: Process of conception in which the sperm and ovum meet, usually in the fallopian tube.

Fetus: A child in the uterus from the second month of pregnancy to delivery.

Fiber: Food substance that resists chemical digestion and passes through the system essentially unchanged. Fiber adds bulk to the diet and aids in the removal of feces.

Fibrillation: Quivering or uncontrollable contraction of heart muscles, causing irregular heartbeat.

Fibroid: Common term for fibroma, a benign tumor of connective and muscular tissue, usually of the uterus.

Fibula: The smaller of two bones that run from the knee to the ankle.

Flatulence: Excessive gas in the stomach and intestine.

Fluoride: Element found in nature. Adequate consumption of fluoride helps prevent tooth decay and possibly strengthens bone.

Follicle: Small tubular gland or sac in the skin or ovary; or, an aggregation of cells in a lymph node.

Fontanelle: The soft spot atop an infant's head where the four bones of the skull have yet to join.

Forceps: Surgical instrument, resembling pincers, that is used for grasping or compressing tissue.

Fracture: To break or crack a bone; or, a break or a crack in a bone.

Fructose: A sugar found in fruit, corn syrup, and honey.

Fungus: Organism of plant origin that lacks chlorophyll; some fungi can cause irritation or disease.

Gallbladder: Sac located under the liver. It stores bile secreted from the liver and then releases it into the small intestine.

Gamma globulin: A protein found in the blood that helps fight infection.

Ganglion: Mass of nerve tissue made up mostly of nerve cell bodies. Also, a cystic tumor in a tendon sheath.

Gangrene: Death of body tissue, usually due to a lack of blood supply; the tissue shrinks and turns black.

Gastric: Pertaining to the stomach.

Gastrointestinal tract: The stomach and intestines.

Gene: Structure within a chromosome that is responsible for inheritance of a particular characteristic.

Generalized: Overall, not limited to one area of the body.

Generic drug: A drug with a non-trademark name.

Genetic engineering: Manufacture, alteration, or repair of genetic material by synthetic means.

Genitals: Reproductive organs.

Geriatrics: The branch of medicine that specializes in the care of problems related to aging.

Germ: A microorganism that often causes disease.

Gestation: Period of time from conception to birth.

Gigantism: Disorder caused by an over-production of growth hormone by the pituitary gland. It results in excessive height. Also known as giantism.

Gland: Any organ or tissue that releases a substance to be used elsewhere in the body; endocrine glands release hormones directly into the bloodstream.

Globulin: A category of blood proteins of which antibodies are formed.

Glomeruli: Small masses of blood vessels in the kidney, responsible for filtering waste from the blood.

Glucagon: Pancreatic hormone that releases the body's stored sugar (glycogen) from the liver into the blood.

Glucose: Blood sugar, also known as dextrose.

Gluten: Plant proteins found in grains such as wheat, rye, oats, and barley.

Glycogen: Stored form of sugar (glucose) in the liver.

Goiter: Enlargement of the thyroid gland.

Gonadal glands: See *Ovaries* and *Testes.*

Grand mal: Generalized convulsion accompanied by loss of consciousness.

Granulocytes: White blood cells (leukocytes), manufactured in the bone marrow, that contain granules. They digest and destroy bacteria.

Groin: Lower abdominal area where the trunk and thigh meet.

Halitosis: Bad breath.

Hallucination: A false perception with no basis in reality; may be seen, heard, or smelled.

Hamstrings: Muscles at the back of the thigh. The tendons of the hamstring muscles can be felt at the back of the knee.

Handicapped: Impaired physically or mentally so that normal activities are interfered with.

Heart attack: Descriptive term for a myocardial infarction: a painful, and sometimes fatal, incident caused by the blockage of one or more of the coronary arteries resulting in interruption of blood to a part of the heart.

Heartburn: Regurgitation of gastric juices (reflux) from the stomach into the esophagus, causing a burning sensation beneath the breastbone (sternum).

Heart murmur: A sound heard in addition to the normal heartbeat. The condition can be benign or a sign of a diseased heart valve or other heart abnormality.

Hemangioma: Benign tumor of dilated blood vessels.

Hematemesis: Vomiting of blood.

Hematoma: Blood-filled swelling beneath the skin or in an organ, due to injury to a blood vessel.

Hematuria: Blood in the urine.

Hemiplegia: Paralysis of one side of the body.

Hemodialysis: Mechanical removal of chemical waste from the blood.

Hemoglobin: A red, pigmented protein that contains iron and is found in the red blood cells. Hemoglobin serves to carry oxygen to and remove carbon dioxide from body tissues.

Hemoptysis: Coughing or spitting up of blood that comes from bleeding in the larynx, trachea, or lungs.

Hemorrhage: Profuse bleeding (internal or external) caused by damage to a blood vessel.

Hemorrhoid: Swollen vein in and around the anus that may bleed.

Hepatic: Pertaining to the liver.

Heredity: Transmission of genetic traits from parent to child.

Hernia: Protrusion or rupture of an organ or part of an organ into surrounding tissues.

Hiccup: Involuntary spasm of the diaphragm, followed quickly by shutting of the glottis, resulting in a sharp, sudden intake of breath.

High blood pressure: See *Hypertension.*

Hirsutism: Excessive growth of body or facial hair.

Histamine: Body chemical present in tissue that, when released, stimulates production of gastric juices for digestion; or, the active agent of allergic reactions that result when excessive amounts of histamine are released to combat a perceived invader. The site affected becomes swollen and congested, resulting in hives (skin), asthma (lining of the bronchial passages), or hay fever (lining of the nose).

Hives: Eruption of itchy red and white wheals on the skin as a result of excessive histamine release within the skin.

Hormone: A substance (secreted by an endocrine gland) that is carried through the bloodstream to various organs of the body, where it serves to regulate various body functions.

Humoral: Pertaining to body fluids.

Hydrogenation: Process of changing an unsaturated fat to a solid saturated one.

Hymen: Membrane partially covering opening to the vagina.

Hymenoptera: Order of insects that includes bees, wasps, and ants.

Hyper-: Prefix meaning excessive or increased.

Hyperactivity: Condition of disturbed behavior among children, characterized by constant overactivity, distractibility, impulsiveness, inability to concentrate, and aggressiveness.

Hyperglycemia: Condition in which an excess of sugar (glucose) is present in the bloodstream.

Hyperplasia: Excessive growth of tissues in an organ, causing increased size.

Hypertension: Condition in which the blood is pumped through the body under abnormally high pressure; also known as high blood pressure.

Hypo-: Prefix meaning inadequate or insufficient.

Hypochondria: Excessive concern about health.

Hypoglycemia: Condition in which the sugar (glucose) in the bloodstream falls below normal amounts.

Hypotension: Low blood pressure.

Hypothalamus: A portion of the brain; partly responsible for basic functions such as appetite, sleep, body temperature, and procreation.

Hypoxia: Decreased concentration of oxygen in the blood.

Iatrogenic disease: Disorder or disease resulting as a side effect of a prescribed treatment.

Idiopathic: Pertaining to a condition or disease with an unexplained cause.

Ileum: Lower portion of the small intestine.

Ilium: The upper portion of the hipbone.

Immobilize: To make a limb or part immovable in order to aid healing.

Immunity: State of being resistant to a disease, particularly an infectious one.

Immunization: Introduction of antigens into the body in very small quantities in order to stimulate the development of immunity.

Immunoglobulin: A protein that can act as an antibody.

Impacted: Pressed firmly together so as to be immovable.

Impotence: Inability of a man to achieve or keep an erection and engage in sexual intercourse.

Incision: A cut made with a knife.

Incisors: The eight front teeth of the mouth, four in the upper jaw and four in the lower jaw.

Incontinence: Inability to control release of urine or feces.

Indigestion: Incomplete or abnormal digestion.

Infarct: An area of tissue that dies because of blockage of its blood supply.

Infection: Condition in which the body or a part of it is invaded by a microorganism such as a bacterium or virus.

Infectious: Ability to transmit a disease.

Infertility: Inability to reproduce.

Inflammation: Body tissue's reaction to injury from infection, physical blow, or irritation, resulting in swelling, pain, heat, and redness.

Inguinal: Pertaining to the groin area where the trunk and legs meet.

Inoperable: Unsuitable for treatment by surgery.

Insemination: Insertion of semen into the vagina; may result in fertilization of an egg.

Insomnia: Inability to sleep.

Insulin: Pancreatic hormone that enables the body to regulate the amount of sugar (glucose) in the bloodstream.

Intestines: Portion of the digestive tract extending from stomach to anus and responsible for much of the absorption of nutrients. See also *Colon, Duodenum, Ileum,* and *Jejunum.*

Intolerance: Inability to endure, as with pain or a drug therapy.

Intracranial: Within the skull.

Intravenous: Within or into a vein.

Intrinsic factor: A substance found in the gastric juices that allows for the absorption of vitamin B_{12}.

Involuntary: Cannot be controlled through will.

Iris: The round, colored membrane of the eye surrounding the pupil, which serves to control the amount of light reaching the retina.

Ischemia: Local, temporary deficiency of blood within an organ or part of an organ. Often refers to the situation in which an artery is narrowed or blocked by spasm or atherosclerosis and cannot deliver sufficient blood to the organ it supplies.

Isotope: One of a number of chemical elements that have similar structures but not identical weights. Some isotopes are radioactive.

-itis: Suffix meaning inflammation.

Jaundice: A yellowing of the skin produced by blockage of the bile passages or by the liver's inability to metabolize bilirubin.

Jejunum: The portion of the small intestine located between the duodenum and ileum.

Joint: The point of juncture between two or more bones where movement occurs.

Jugular veins: The two veins on the sides of the neck that carry blood from the brain to the heart.

Keloid: Abnormally large scar that forms after surgery or injury.

Keratin: Protein found in hair, nails, and the outer layers of skin.

Ketoacidosis: Sometimes fatal complication of insulin-dependent diabetes that results from too little insulin and that can cause loss of consciousness.

Kidneys: The two bean-shaped organs located in the back portion of the upper abdomen, one on each side of the spine. Responsible for excreting urine and regulating the water, electrolyte, and acid-base content of the blood.

Kyphosis: Excessive curvature of the spine, resulting in humpback, hunchback, or rounding of the shoulders. May result from diseases such as osteoarthritis or rheumatoid arthritis, osteoporosis, or rickets, from conditions such as compression fracture, or from a congenital abnormality.

Labia: Two sets of lip-like genital organs in women. The labia majora are two folds of skin and fatty tissue that protect the vulva; the labia minora are smaller folds inside the labia majora that protect the clitoris.

Labor: Process of muscle contraction by which a baby is born.

Labyrinth: Portion of the inner ear responsible for balance.

Laceration: Flesh wound caused by tearing.

Lacrimal gland: Gland of the eye that secretes tears.

Lactation: Process of production and secretion of milk from the breasts.

Lactose: Sugar found naturally in milk.

Larynx: Structure of the voice box, composed of cartilage housing the vocal cords and the muscles and ligaments used to produce sound.

Lens: Transparent structure in the eye that focuses light to form an image on the back of the retina.

Lesion: Area of tissue either injured as in a wound, abscess, or sore or altered as in a tumor, mole, or cyst.

Leukocytes: White blood cells, used to fight infection.

Libido: Sexual drive.

Ligament: Strong fibrous connective tissue resembling a band or sheet that connects a bone to another bone.

Ligature: Filament (synthetic or natural) for tying off blood vessels during surgery to keep them from bleeding. The procedure itself is called ligation.

Lipid: Descriptive term for a fat or fat-like substance found in the blood, such as cholesterol.

Liposuction: Process of removing fat deposits from beneath the skin by using a suction device.

Lithiasis: Formation of calculi deposits such as gallstones and kidney stones.

Liver: Largest internal organ in the body. It is the site of many metabolic functions, including the secreting of bile, neutralizing poisons, synthesizing proteins, and storing glycogen and certain minerals and vitamins.

Localized: Limited to a discrete area, as in an infection or disease. See also *Generalized* and *Systemic*.

Lordosis: Exaggerated curvature of the lower portion of the spine, causing swayback.

Lumbar: Pertaining to the lower back.

Lungs: The two cone-shaped spongy organs of respiration located around the bronchial tree. The lungs bring air and blood into close contact so that oxygen can be added to the blood and carbon dioxide can be removed.

Lymph: Clear fluid present in lymphatic vessels.

Lymph node: Small round organs (from pinhead-size to olive-size) found throughout the body that produce lymphocytes and monocytes, which help protect the body from invasion by bacteria or other organisms.

Lymphocytes: Disease-fighting white blood cells made in the lymph nodes and distributed throughout the body by way of the lymphatic fluid and blood.

Maceration: Softening of tissue by soaking in liquid.

Macrophage: Cells found throughout the body, particularly in the spleen, that have the ability to ingest other substances such as "old" red blood cells; also important in the immune response.

Malabsorption: Inadequate absorption of nutrients from the small intestine. Symptoms of malabsorption syndrome include loose fatty stools, diarrhea, weight loss, weakness, and anemia.

Malaise: General feeling of illness, discomfort, and uneasiness, often a sign of infection.

Malignant: Virulent, harmful; the term is used to describe cancerous tumors that can grow uncontrollably and spread (metastasize).

Malnutrition: Deficiency of nourishment in the body due to lack of healthful food or improper digestion and distribution of nutrients.

Malpresentation: Abnormal position of the fetus during labor, making normal delivery difficult or impossible.

Mammary gland: Compound gland of the breast that secretes milk.

Mandible: Lower jaw.

Mania: Mental disorder characterized by an intense feeling of elation and excitability, often accompanied by increased activity.

Masticate: Chew.

Mastoid process: Round, honeycombed bone mass located behind the ear.

Maxilla: Upper jaw.

Meconium stool: The newborn's first bowel movement, composed of intestinal secretions and amniotic fluid, usually dark green.

Medulla: Center of an organ, gland, or bone.

Melanin: Pigment that provides color to hair, skin, and choroid of the eye.

Membrane: Thin, soft layer of tissue that lines, separates, or covers organs or structures.

Meninges: The three membranes that cover the spinal cord and brain.

Menopause: The gradual cessation of menstruation, at the end of which a woman is no longer able to reproduce.

Menstruation: Monthly shedding of blood and tissue from the lining of the uterus.

Mesentery: Fold in the abdominal lining that connects the intestine to the back of the abdominal wall and contains the arteries and veins that supply the intestines.

Metabolism: The process by which food is transformed, energy is derived, and tissues are broken down into waste products.

Metastasis: Spreading of a disease from one part of the body to another, usually by movement of cells (as in cancer) or bacteria through the lymph or blood system.

Microbes: One-celled organisms such as bacteria, many of which cause disease.

Micturition: Urination.

Miosis: Abnormal pupil contraction, often a sign of disease or disorder.

Miscarriage: Premature, spontaneous termination of a pregnancy.

Mitosis: Type of cell division in which the new cells have the same number of chromosomes as the parent cell.

Mitral valve: Heart valve that allows oxygenated blood to move into the left ventricle from the left atrium and prevents the reverse flow.

Molars: The grinding or chewing teeth, located at the back of both jaws.

Mono-: Prefix meaning one.

Motility: Ability to move.

Mucous membrane: Thin membrane that lines passages and cavities that are in contact with air, such as nose, mouth, and eyes.

Muscle: Tissue that produces movement by its ability to contract.

Musculoskeletal: Pertaining to the muscles and the skeleton.

Myalgia: Muscle tenderness or pain.

Myelin: White, fat-like substance that forms a sheath around some nerves.

Myocardium: The heart muscle. See also *Endocardium* and *Epicardium.*

Myopathy: Any disease of the muscle.

Narcosis: A state of stupor often induced by drugs or other agents.

Nares: Nostrils.

Natal: Pertaining to birth.

Nausea: Sensation of stomach sickness, often followed by vomiting.

Necrosis: Death of areas of tissue surrounded by healthy tissue.

Neonatal: Pertaining to a newborn up to 6 weeks old.

Neoplasm: New and abnormal growth.

Nephritis: Inflammation of the kidney.

Nephron: A structure of the kidney in which blood is filtered to remove waste and form urine.

Nerve: Bundle of fibers that connect the brain and spinal cord with various parts of the body and through which impulses pass.

Neuralgia: Sharp pain along the course of a nerve.

Neuron: A nerve cell.

Neuropathy: Any nerve disease.

Neurotransmitter: Nerve cell chemicals that act as messengers in the brain and nervous system.

Node: Small round tissue or structure.

Nonsteroidal anti-inflammatory drugs (NSAIDs): Medications used to reduce inflammation that are not cortisone-based.

Norepinephrine (sometimes called Noradrenaline): See *Epinephrine*.

Nucleus: Center portion of all cells, except red blood cells, essential for cell growth, nourishment, and reproduction.

Obesity: Abnormal body weight, usually defined as more than 20 percent above average for age, height, and bone structure.

Occipital: Pertaining to the back of the head.

Occlusion: Closure of a passage such as ducts or blood vessels. In dentistry, the alignment of upper and lower teeth when the jaws are closed.

Occult: Undetectable without magnification.

Ocular: Pertaining to the eye.

Olfactory: Pertaining to smell.

-oma: Suffix meaning tumor.

Oncogenes: Genes present in normal cells that, upon exposure to cancer-inducing viruses, lead to development of tumors.

Optic nerve: Nerve that carries light impulses from the retina to the brain, where they are interpreted.

Orbit: Eye socket.

Orgasm: Climax of sexual intercourse or stimulation of sexual organs. In the man, it occurs when semen is ejaculated, and in the woman it occurs when contractions of the vagina occur.

-osis: Suffix meaning diseased state.

Osseous: Pertaining to bones.

Osteopathy: Any bone disease; or, a school of medicine that specializes in treatment that allows the body to heal itself by removing internal and external roadblocks to normal function.

Ovaries: Gonadal glands in the female that produce eggs (ova) for reproduction and the two female sex hormones, estrogen and progesterone.

Over-the-counter: Sold without a prescription.

Ovulation: Monthly ripening and discharging of an egg (ovum) from an ovary. It occurs approximately 14 days before the onset of the next menstrual period.

Ovum: The female reproductive cell (egg) that is capable of developing into a baby after fertilization by sperm.

Oxytocin: Pituitary hormone that acts in women to stimulate the breasts to release milk.

Pacemaker: A group of cells, known as the sinoatrial node, that are located in the atrium of the heart and serve to regulate the rate and rhythm of the heart. An artificial cardiac pacemaker is an electrical device used to simulate the natural process by generating electrical impulses. An artificial pacemaker can be placed outside or inside the chest.

Palate: The hard roof of the mouth.

Palpate: To feel or examine by touch.

Palpitation: Rapid, violent, or throbbing sensation felt as a result of a fluttering or throbbing of the heart.

Palsy: Paralysis; loss of sensation or ability to move or control movement.

Pancreas: Gland that produces enzymes essential to the digestion of food. The islets of Langerhans within the pancreas secrete insulin into the blood.

Papilla: A nipple-like protuberance.

Paralysis: Complete or partial impairment of the ability to move a part of the body.

Paranoia: Mental disorder characterized by suspicion, delusions of persecution, and jealousy.

Paraplegia: Loss of movement and sensation below the waist, including the legs.

Parasite: An organism that lives on or within another organism at the expense of the host.

Parathyroid glands: Endocrine glands located in contact with the thyroid gland that maintain the level of calcium in the blood.

Parenteral: Methods of administering medication or nutrition other than swallowing, including intravenous, subcutaneous, or intramuscular.

Paroxysm: A sudden attack, such as a spasm or convulsion, or recurrence of symptoms of a disease.

Patella: Kneecap.

Pathogen: Disease-producing microorganism.

Pathology: Study of the cause and nature of a disease.

Pectoral: Pertaining to the chest.

Pelvis: Basin-shaped bone structure connecting the spine with the legs.

Penis: Male organ for urination and copulation.

Pepsin: The main enzyme of the digestive juices of the stomach.

Peptic: Pertaining to digestion or the enzyme pepsin.

Percussion: A method of examination by tapping the fingertips at various points on the body to determine position, size, and consistency of a structure beneath the skin.

Perforation: Process of making a hole, or the hole itself.

Pericardium: Membranous sac enclosing the heart.

Perineum: External area between the vulva and anus in a woman or between the scrotum and anus in a man.

Periodontal: Pertaining to the area immediately around a tooth.

Periosteum: Leather-like tissue that encases bone.

Peristalsis: Wave-like contraction of muscles, particularly in the digestive system.

Peritoneum: Membrane lining the abdominal cavity.

Peritonitis: Inflammation or infection of the peritoneum.

Pernicious: Destructive, sometimes fatal. Pernicious anemia is a particular form of anemia caused by inability to absorb vitamin B_{12} in the intestinal tract.

Perspiration: Sweat, the salty fluid excreted from the sweat glands of the skin.

Pessary: Device inserted in the vagina to support the uterus or, as in the case of a diaphragm, to prevent contraception.

Petechiae: Small subcutaneous hemorrhages that appear during severe fevers. Also, the red spots caused by flea bites.

Petit mal: Mild form of epileptic attack, characterized by a blank stare and cessation of activity.

Pharmacology: Study of drugs and their effects on living beings.

Pharynx: Upper portion of the throat; the passageway for air from the nose to the larynx and for food from the mouth to the esophagus.

Phlegm: Thick mucus, especially from the sinuses or respiratory tract.

Phobia: Persistent, irrational fear.

Pigment: Coloring matter.

Pineal body: Cone-shaped gland at the back of the brain, the function of which is not clearly understood.

Pinna: Exterior part of the ear, the portion that is easily visible.

Pituitary gland: An endocrine gland that produces a range of hormones to help control the body's long-term growth, day-to-day functioning, and reproductive capabilities.

Placebo: Nonmedicinal substance given for psychological benefit or as part of a clinical research study.

Placenta: Spongy uterine structure developed during pregnancy through which the fetus takes nourishment and discards waste. The placenta is shed after delivery, when it is known as the afterbirth.

Plague: Term previously used to describe any deadly contagious epidemic disease. Now used primarily to describe infection by *Yersinia pestis* (bubonic plague).

Plaque: A film or deposit of bacteria and other material on the surface of a tooth that may lead to tooth decay or periodontal disease.

Plasma: Fluid part of the blood and lymph.

Platelet: Colorless round or oval disc found in the blood. Also known as thrombocytes, platelets are necessary for the clotting of blood.

Pleura: The membrane that covers both lungs and the chest cavity.

Poly-: Prefix meaning multiple, more than normal.

Polyp: A usually benign tumor, often with a stem, found commonly in the nose, uterus, and colon.

Postpartum: Pertaining to the time after childbirth.

Prepuce: The fold or foreskin over the glans of the penis.

Primary care physician: Physician responsible for a person's general health care.

Progesterone: Female sex hormone responsible for, among other things, the thickening of the uterine lining before conception.

Prognosis: Prediction of the course and outcome of a disease.

Prolactin: Pituitary hormone that stimulates the breasts to produce milk.

Prolapse: Displacement of an organ or a structure, such as the uterus or bladder, by falling or dropping down.

Prophylaxis: Prevention of disease or its spread by following certain rules or taking specific precautions.

Prostaglandins: A group of extremely active substances found in many parts of the body that affect many organs. Certain prostaglandins have a role in stimulating the uterine contractions of labor and birth.

Prostate gland: Gland located at the base of the bladder in men.

Prosthesis: An artificial organ or part, such as a limb.

Protein: One of many complex nitrogen compounds, composed of amino acids; essential for the growth and repair of tissue.

Prothrombin: A chemical substance found in circulating blood that interacts with calcium salts to form thrombin, a step in the process of blood clotting.

Pruritus: Severe itching.

Psychogenic: Originating in the mind; also pertaining to the development of the mind.

Psychomotor: Pertaining to voluntary physical movement.

Psychosis: Mental disturbance of serious magnitude that is characterized by loss of contact with reality. Delusions and hallucinations are often present.

Psychosomatic: Pertaining to the relationship of the mind and body. Psychosomatic illnesses are those in which a physical disorder is caused or aggravated by emotional factors.

Ptosis: Drooping, as of an eyelid.

Ptyalin: An enzyme found in saliva that helps to break down starch into sugars.

Puberty: Period of rapid change in boys and girls during which secondary sex characteristics mature. In girls (usually between 9 and 16 years) it is marked by menarche (the beginning of menstruation), and in boys (between 13 and 15 years) it is marked by discharge of semen and deepening of the voice.

Pulmonary: Pertaining to the lungs.

Pulse: Expansion and contraction of an artery, evidenced by rhythmical throbbing in response to the expansion and contraction of the heart.

Pupil: The circular opening in the center of the iris through which light passes to the retina. The size of the opening diminishes in bright light and enlarges in dim light.

Purpura: A condition characterized by hemorrhages of tiny blood vessels causing patches on the skin or on mucous membranes. The patches begin as red and then change to purple and then brownish yellow before disappearing.

Purulent: Forming or containing pus.

Pus: Thick, whitish yellow fluid containing leukocytes (white blood cells) and bacteria, formed at the site of certain kinds of infections.

Pylorus: Lower opening of the stomach into the duodenum.

Pyrexia: Fever.

Quadriplegia: Paralysis and loss of function in both arms and the trunk.

Radiation therapy: Treatment of disease by using radiation such as x-rays, radium radiation, ultraviolet rays, and others.

Radius: Smaller of the two bones in lower arm; it connects to the base of the thumb.

Radon: A radioactive gas found in nature that is the byproduct of disintegrating radium.

Rash: Eruption on the skin, usually temporary.

Recessive: A mode of inheritance in which a gene that causes a trait must be present from both parents for the trait to become manifest in an offspring. See also *Dominant.*

Rectum: The section of the large intestine closest to the anus.

Reflex: An involuntary response to a stimulus.

Reflux: Backflow or regurgitation.

Refractory: Stubborn, as in a condition that resists treatment or a nerve or muscle that resists stimulation.

Rejection: Refusal to accept, as with a transplanted organ.

Relapse: Recurrence of disease or symptoms after apparent recovery.

Remission: Abatement of symptoms.

REM sleep: The period of sleep known as rapid eye movement sleep, when dreaming seems to occur and the eyes move cyclically even though closed.

Renal: Pertaining to the kidneys.

Resection: Partial surgical removal of an organ or tissue.

Respiration: Breathing.

Resuscitation: Revival of breathing or heartbeat after apparent death.

Retina: Light-sensitive layer of tissue located at the back of the eye that is composed of rods and cones, and transmits nerve impulses to the brain.

Retinopathy: Abnormality of the retina that may cause deterioration of eyesight.

Rhinovirus: A large subgroup of viruses (probably more than 100) that cause the common cold.

Risk factors: Elements such as chemical, physiological, behavioral, psychological, genetic, or environmental that increase chances of a disease developing.

Rods: Long, slender bodies within the retina that perceive faint light. Also, rod-shaped bacteria.

Root canal: Cavity in the root of the tooth that contains nerves.

Roughage: Indigestible fiber of fruits, vegetables, and cereals that aids in the evacuation of waste.

Rupture: Tearing of tissue (as in a hernia) or breaking of an organ.

Sacroiliac joint: The juncture between the sacrum and the ilium. Not a true joint because there is no movement at this point.

Sacrum: Triangular bone at the base of the spine just above the coccyx. Composed of five fused vertebrae, it is a part of the bony pelvis.

Saline: Salt solution.

Saliva: Fluid, secreted by the salivary and mucous glands of the mouth, that moistens food and begins the process of digestion.

Scapula: Shoulder blade.

Sciatic nerve: Largest nerve in the body, it is formed by the sensory and motor nerves of the legs and feet. It emerges from the base of the spinal cord as a number of roots and then passes through the pelvis and down the back of the thigh.

Sclera: The fibrous outer membrane of the eye, extending from the optic nerve to the cornea.

Sclerosis: Hardening or thickening of an organ or tissue, usually due to abnormal growth of fibrous tissue.

Scrotum: Double pouch that holds the testicles.

Sebaceous glands: Oil glands of the skin.

Sebum: Fatty substance secreted by sebaceous glands to lubricate the skin.

Secretion: The process of producing materials by glands; also, the substance produced.

Seizure: A sudden attack often including convulsions; this symptom, if recurrent, often is referred to as a seizure disorder or as epilepsy.

Semen: Thick, whitish fluid containing reproductive cells (spermatozoa) and other fluids, discharged through the male urethra.

Seminal vesicles: Sac-like structures in the male, located behind the bladder, which secrete fluid that is part of the composition of semen.

Senescence: Process of aging.

Sepsis: State of being infected with disease-causing microorganisms in the bloodstream, usually with an accompanying fever.

Septicemia: Presence of disease-causing bacteria in the blood; also known as blood poisoning.

Septum: A wall dividing two cavities or compartments.

Serum: Watery fluid left after coagulation of the blood to form a clot. Serum containing antibodies to a specific disease may be injected into a person to give temporary resistance to that disease; this is called passive immunity. See also *Vaccine.*

Shock: Clinical condition in which the body reacts to injury or severe pain by dilation or relaxation of blood vessels, producing what can be called circulatory failure. Symptoms include rapid pulse, very low blood pressure, pallor, cold, clammy skin, and sometimes unconsciousness.

Shunt: A passage that diverts blood flow from one main route to another. Often constructed artificially.

Side effects: Unwanted changes produced by medication or other treatment, ranging from trivial and transient (minor headache or dry mouth) to more serious (asthma, gastrointestinal bleeding).

Sinuses: Empty spaces or cavities within bone structure; most commonly, the several sets of cavities adjacent to and connected to the nose by small openings.

Somatostatin: Pancreatic hormone that helps regulate the body's production and release of the pancreatic hormones insulin and glucagon. It is also found in other tissues of the body, where it may have other functions.

Spasm: Involuntary movement produced by a muscular contraction.

Speculum: Device used to examine body canals, including the ear or vagina.

Spermatozoa: Male cells that, upon combining with a female egg, result in fertilization. Produced by the testes and contained within semen. Also referred to as sperm.

Spermicide: Birth control agent used to kill sperm cells.

Sphincter: Circular muscles at an orifice that, upon contraction, close the opening. The body has several sphincter muscles, including those at the anus, bladder, and opening to the stomach from the esophagus.

Sphygmomanometer: Device used to measure blood pressure.

Spinal canal: The cavity that contains the spinal cord and is protected by vertebrae of the backbone.

Spinal column: The bony assemblage of vertebrae that enclose the spinal cord.

Spinal cord: Lengthy, cord-like bundle of nerves that link nerves of the trunk and extremities to the brain.

Spleen: Organ located to the left and just in front of the stomach that stores and at times manufactures blood cells.

Sprain: Joint injury in which ligament damage is sustained.

Sputum: The fluid produced upon coughing or clearing the throat. If certain disorders or infections are suspected, the sputum may be examined in a laboratory.

Staging: The process of categorizing the extent and spread of a cancer for the purpose of planning treatment.

Stenosis: The narrowing or closure of an opening or passageway in the body.

Sterilization: The process by which all microorganisms (bacteria) are removed from a substance, as in the sterilization of surgical instruments to prevent infection. Or, the process, usually surgical, of rendering a man or woman incapable of reproduction.

Sternum: The breastbone, in the upper central portion of the chest and abutted by the ends of the clavicle and the ribs.

Steroids: See *Corticosteroids.*

Stillborn: A fetus dead at birth.

Stomach: A sac-like organ to which food is delivered by the esophagus. After the food is processed mechanically by a churning action and chemically with gastric acids, it passes from the stomach to the small intestine.

Stool: Body waste, such as food residue, excreted from the bowels.

Strain: Muscular injury produced by abuse or overuse of a muscle.

Striae: Streaks or stripes.

Stroke: Medical emergency produced by a blood clot that lodges in an artery and blocks the flow of blood to a portion of the brain, producing symptoms ranging from paralysis of limbs and loss of speech to unconsciousness and death. Less commonly, a stroke may be the result of bleeding into the substance of the brain.

Stupor: A state of reduced consciousness in which responsiveness and feeling are lessened.

Subacute: Term used to distinguish the course of a disease that is not chronic (long-lasting) yet not characteristically of limited duration (acute).

Subcutaneous: Beneath the skin.

Sucrose: The simple sugar processed from sugar cane and sugar beets.

Sunblock: Over-the-counter preparation applied to the skin to limit exposure to the rays of the sun.

Suppository: Pharmaceutical preparation in a solid form, intended to be inserted into an organ such as the rectum or vagina.

Suppuration: The formation and discharge of pus from an injury or infection.

Suture: The process of joining two surfaces by stitching; or, the surgical stitch itself.

Synapse: The junction point between two nerve cells (neurons).

Syncope: Fainting.

Syndrome: A collection of symptoms that characterize an ailment.

Synovial fluid: The clear, fluid lubricant found in a joint.

Systemic: Affecting or pertaining to the entire body rather than one of its parts.

Systole: The portion of the heart cycle during which the heart muscle is contracting.

Tachycardia: Abnormally rapid heart rate (more than 100 beats per minute).

Tartar: Plaque deposits on the teeth that lead to tooth decay.

T cell: A type of white blood cell (lymphocyte) that acts as a part of the body's immune system.

Tendon: Cord-like tissue that connects muscles to bones.

Testes: Gonadal glands in the male that produce male cells (spermatozoa) for reproduction and male sex hormone testosterone.

Testosterone: Male sex hormone produced by the testes.

Thoracic: Having to do with the chest (thorax).

Thorax: The portion of the anatomy below the neck and above the diaphragm; the chest.

Thrombin: An enzyme that is part of the process of blood coagulation.

Thrombocyte: Blood platelet, essential to the clotting process.

Thrombus: A blood clot that blocks (occludes) a blood vessel or heart cavity.

Thymus: A gland located in the upper chest that produces T cells, essential to developing the body's immune response.

Thyroid gland: Endocrine gland that helps control the body's rate of function and contributes to maintaining a balance between the calcium in the blood and in the bones through production of the hormones thyroxine and calcitonin.

Thyroxine: Thyroid hormone that controls the pace of chemical activity in the body.

Tibia: The larger of the two bones in the lower leg; the shin bone.

Tic: An involuntary muscular spasm, usually of the face, head, neck, or shoulder; a twitch.

Tincture: A medication that is a mixture of alcohol and an extract of a vegetable or animal substance.

Tissue: A collection of similar cells that, taken together, form a body structure.

Tonsils: Two masses of lymph tissues, located on either side of the back of the throat, that help filter out unwanted bacteria.

Topical: Pertaining to a certain surface area of the body.

Tourniquet: A bandage or other device that is tightened over an extremity to stop bleeding.

Toxemia: A condition in which toxins circulate throughout the body via the blood.

Toxic: Poisonous.

Toxin: A poisonous compound.

Toxoid: A toxin treated so that it is no longer poisonous but, upon injection into the body, will induce antibodies to form. An example is tetanus toxoid.

Trachea: Anatomical term for the windpipe, the tube that connects the throat (pharynx) to the bronchial tubes in the lungs.

Traction: Mechanical pulling on a body part, used in treating certain fractures and dislocations.

Transfusion: Delivery of blood or a blood component into the bloodstream via injection.

Transplantation: The surgical movement of an organ or tissue from one position (or person) to another.

Trauma: An injury such as a burn, wound, or broken bone.

Tremor: An involuntary quaking; tremor can result from disease, a nervous disorder, the side effect of a medication, or some other cause.

Triceps: Muscle in the forearm that, upon contraction, extends the arm.

Tricuspid valve: Heart valve between the right atrium and the right ventricle.

Trigeminal nerve: The nerve that delivers sensory stimuli to the brain from the face, teeth, and tongue.

Triglyceride: Most common type of fat; most animal and vegetable fats.

Truss: A device used to hold a hernia or organ in position.

Tubule: A small tube or canal, especially in the kidneys.

Tumor: Abnormal growth or tissue that resembles normal tissue but has no function. The tumor may be malignant (cancerous) or benign.

Tympanic membrane: The eardrum.

Ulcer: An open sore on the skin or a mucous membrane.

Ulna: Larger of the two bones in the lower arm.

Ultrasound: Sound waves of a frequency beyond human hearing that, upon penetrating most solid matter, change in velocity depending on the density of the body part or other object being studied. A device that can collect echoes and form an image for diagnostic purposes.

Umbilicus: The scar formed by the removal of the umbilical cord from the fetus at the time of birth; the navel.

Urea: Principal waste product in the urine; a nitrogen-containing by-product of protein metabolism.

Ureter: The tube that delivers urine from the kidney to the bladder.

Urethra: Tube draining the bladder to outside the body; in the male, this canal is also the passage for semen.

Uric acid: A waste by-product of metabolism. When too little is excreted, the buildup can lead to the development of gout.

Urination: Act of voiding fluid wastes (urine).

Urine: Fluid waste produced in the kidneys, stored in the bladder, and released through the urethra.

Urticaria: See *Hives.*

Uterus: Female organ that contains the embryo and fetus. Located in the lower abdomen, the uterus is a pear-shaped, muscular organ sometimes known as the womb.

Uvea: Layer of the eye beneath the sclera, consisting of the iris, ciliary body, and choroid. The visible pigments in the eye are seen in the uvea.

Uvula: Pendulous tissue at the back of the throat.

Vaccination: Injection of a vaccine to create immunity to a specific disease.

Vaccine: Weakened or killed microorganisms or viruses of a specific disease that are introduced into the body in order to stimulate immunity; this is called active immunity.

Vagina: Tube of muscle and membrane connecting the external female genitalia with the uterus.

Vagus nerve: Nerve that serves the esophagus, larynx, stomach, intestines, lungs, and heart.

Varicose veins: Weakened, swollen, or twisted veins.

Vascular: Pertaining to blood vessels; includes veins and arteries.

Vas deferens: Duct that transports sperm from the testes to the urethra.

Vein: Blood vessel that carries blood back to the heart.

Venous: Pertaining to the veins.

Ventricle: One of two lower chambers of the heart; or, any small cavity.

Venule: Small vein.

Verruca: A wart.

Vertebra: One of the 33 bony sections that make up the spine.

Vertigo: Dizziness.

Vesicle: A small sac containing fluid.

Viral: Pertaining to or caused by a virus.

Virulent: Highly poisonous or infectious.

Virus: Tiny organism that causes disease; viruses range from minor (the common cold) to deadly (AIDS).

Viscera: The internal organs, in particular those located within the abdominal cavity.

Vital signs: Breathing, heartbeat, and body temperature.

Vitamins: Organic substances that are found in small amounts in food and are essential for most chemical processes in the body.

Vitreous humor: Gelatinous substance found within the interior of the eye.

Vocal cords: Small folds in the cavity of the larynx (voice box) that are involved in the production of sound.

Vomit: The ejection of partially digested matter from the stomach through the mouth; or, the material itself.

Vulva: External female genitalia, including the clitoris and labia.

Wart: Harmless growth on the skin, produced by a virus.

Wen: Cyst that develops in a sebaceous gland.

Withdrawal: The state experienced when addicting medications, illegal drugs, or alcohol are withdrawn. Symptoms may be physiological or psychological or both.

Womb: The female organ in which the fetus develops. See also *Uterus.*

X-ray: Electromagnetic wave that penetrates most solid matter and will produce an image on film upon emerging from the body part or other object being studied. Also called roentgen ray.

Zygote: The egg after it is fertilized by a sperm.

INDEX